The GALE
ENCYCLOPEDIA of
ALTERNATIVE
MEDICINE

The GALE
ENCYCLOPEDIA *of*
ALTERNATIVE
MEDICINE

THIRD EDITION

VOLUME

3

L–R

LAURIE J. FUNDUKIAN, EDITOR

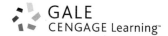

GALE
CENGAGE Learning™

Detroit • New York • San Francisco • New Haven, Conn • Waterville, Maine • London

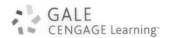

Gale Encyclopedia of Alternative Medicine, Third Edition

Project Editor: Laurie J. Fundukian

Editorial: Donna Batten, Amy Kwolek, Brigham Narins, Jeffrey Wilson

Product Manager: Kate Hanley

Editorial Support Services: Andrea Lopeman

Indexing Services: Factiva, a Dow Jones Company

Rights Acquisition and Management: Robyn V. Young

Composition: Evi Abou-El-Seoud, Mary Beth Trimper

Manufacturing: Wendy Blurton, Dorothy Maki

Imaging: Lezlie Light

Product Design: Pam Galbreath

For product information and technology assistance, contact us at **Gale Customer Support, 1-800-877-4253.**
For permission to use material from this text or product, submit all requests online at **www.cengage.com/permissions.**
Further permissions questions can be emailed to **permissionrequest@cengage.com**

Library of Congress Cataloging-in-Publication Data

The Gale encyclopedia of alternative medicine, 3rd ed. / edited by Laurie J. Fundukian, editor.
     p. cm. --
     Includes bibliographical references and index.
     ISBN 978-1-4144-4872-5 (set) -- ISBN 978-1-4144-4873-2 (vol. 1) --
ISBN 978-1-4144-4874-9 (vol. 2) -- ISBN 978-1-4144-4875-6 (vol. 3) --
ISBN 978-1-4144-4876-3 (vol. 4)
     1. Alternative medicine--Encyclopedias. I. Fundukian, Laurie J. II. Title: Encyclopedia of alternative medicine.
     [DNLM: 1. Complementary Therapies--Encyclopedias--English. 2. Internal Medicine--Encyclopedias--English. WB 13 G1508 2009]

R733.G34 2009
615.5'03--dc22   2008016097

Gale
27500 Drake Rd.
Farmington Hills, MI, 48331-3535

ISBN-13: 978-1-4144-4872-5 (set)   ISBN-10: 1-4144-4872-4 (set)
ISBN-13: 978-1-4144-4873-2 (vol. 1)   ISBN-10: 1-4144-4873-2 (vol. 1)
ISBN-13: 978-1-4144-4874-9 (vol. 2)   ISBN-10: 1-4144-4874-0 (vol. 2)
ISBN-13: 978-1-4144-4875-6 (vol. 3)   ISBN-10: 1-4144-4875-9 (vol. 3)
ISBN-13: 978-1-4144-4876-3 (vol. 4)   ISBN-10: 1-4144-4876-7 (vol. 4)

This title is also available as an e-book.
ISBN-13: 978-1-4144-4877-0   ISBN-10: 1-4144-4877-5
Contact your Gale, a part of Cengage Learning sales representative for ordering information.

Printed in China
1 2 3 4 5 6 7 12 11 10 09 08

CONTENTS

LIST OF ENTRIES

A

Abscess
Acidophilus
Acne
Aconite
Acupressure
Acupuncture
Ademetionine
Adie's pupil
African pygeum
Agastache
Aging
AIDS
Alcoholism
Alexander technique
Alfalfa
Alisma
Allergies
Allium cepa
Aloe
Alpha-hydroxy
Alzheimer's disease
Amenorrhea
Amino acids
Andrographis
Androstenedione
Anemarrhena
Anemia
Angelica root
Angina
Anise
Ankylosing spondylitis
Anorexia nervosa

Anthroposophical medicine
Anti-inflammatory diet
Antioxidants
Anxiety
Apis
Apitherapy
Apple cider vinegar
Applied kinesiology
Apricot seed
Arginine
Arka
Arnica
Aromatherapy
Arrowroot
Arsenicum album
Artichoke
Art therapy
Ashwaganda
Asthma
Astigmatism
Aston-Patterning
Astragalus
Atherosclerosis
Athlete's foot
Atkins diet
Atractylodes (white)
Attention-deficit hyperactivity
  disorder
Aucklandia
Auditory integration training
Aura therapy
Auriculotherapy
Autism
Ayurvedic medicine

B

Bach flower essences
Bad breath
Balm of Gilead
Barberry
Barley grass
Bates method
Bayberry
Bedsores
Bedwetting
Bee pollen
Behavioral therapy
Behavioral optometry
Belladonna
Beta-hydroxy
Beta-methylbutyric acid
Beta carotene
Betaine hydrochloride
Bhakti yoga
Bilberry
Binge eating disorder
Biofeedback
Bioflavonoids
Bioidentical hormone
  therapy
Biota
Biotherapeutic drainage
Biotin
Bipolar disorder
Bird flu
Bites and stings
Bitter melon
Bitters
Black cohosh

Leukemia
Lice infestation
Licorice
Light therapy
Linoleic acid
Lipase
Livingston-Wheeler therapy
Lobelia
Lomatium
Lomilomi
Lou Gehrig's disease
Low back pain
Lung cancer
Lutein
Lycium fruit
Lycopene
Lycopodium
Lycopus
Lyme disease
Lymphatic drainage
Lysimachia
Lysine

M

Macrobiotic diet
Macular degeneration
Magnesium
Magnetic therapy
Magnolia
Maitake
Malaria
Malignant lymphoma
Manganese
Mangosteen
Manuka honey
Marijuana
Marsh mallow
Martial arts
Massage therapy
McDougall diet
Measles
Meditation
Mediterranean diet
Medium-chain triglycerides
Melatonin
Memory loss

Ménière's disease
Meningitis
Menopause
Menstruation
Mercurius vivus
Mesoglycan
Metabolic therapies
Methionine
Mexican yam
Migraine headache
Milk thistle
Mind/Body medicine
Mistletoe
Mononucleosis
Morning sickness
Motherwort
Motion sickness
Movement therapy
Moxibustion
MSM
Mugwort leaf
Mullein
Multiple chemical sensitivity
Multiple sclerosis
Mumps
Muscle spasms and cramps
Music therapy
Myopia
Myotherapy
Myrrh

N

Narcolepsy
Native American medicine
Natrum muriaticum
Natural hygiene diet
Natural hormone replacement
  therapy
Naturopathic medicine
Nausea
Neck pain
Neem
Nettle
Neural therapy
Neuralgia
Neurolinguistic programming

Niacin
Night blindness
Noni
Nosebleeds
Notoginseng root
Nutmeg
Nutrition
Nux vomica

O

Oak
Obesity
Obsessive-compulsive disorder
Omega-3 fatty acids
Omega-6 fatty acids
Ophiopogon
Oregano essential oil
Ornish diet
Ortho-bionomy
Orthomolecular medicine
Osha
Osteoarthritis
Osteopathy
Osteoporosis
Ovarian cancer
Ovarian cysts
Oxygen/Ozone therapy

P

Pain
Paleolithic diet
Panchakarma
Pancreatitis
Panic disorder
Pantothenic acid
Parasitic infections
Parkinson's disease
Parsley
Passionflower
Past-life therapy
Pau d'arco
Pelvic inflammatory disease

PLEASE READ—IMPORTANT INFORMATION

The Gale Encyclopedia of Alternative Medicine is a medical reference product designed to inform and educate readers about a wide variety of complementary therapies and herbal remedies and treatments for prevalent conditions and diseases. Gale believes the product to be comprehensive, but not necessarily definitive. It is intended to supplement, not replace, consultation with a physician or other healthcare practitioner. While Gale has made substantial efforts to provide information that is accurate, comprehensive, and up-to-date, Gale makes no representations or warranties of any kind, including without limitation, warranties of merchantability or fitness for a particular purpose, nor does it guarantee the accuracy, comprehensiveness, or timeliness of the information contained in this product. Readers should be aware that the universe of complementary medical knowledge is constantly growing and changing, and that differences of medical opinion exist among authorities. They are also advised to seek professional diagnosis and treatment for any medical condition, and to discuss information obtained from this book with their healthcare provider.

INTRODUCTION

The Gale Encyclopedia of Alternative Medicine (GEAM) is a one-stop source for alternative medical information that covers complementary therapies, herbs and remedies, and common medical diseases and conditions. It avoids medical jargon when possible, making it easier for the layperson to use. *The Gale Encyclopedia of Alternative Medicine* presents authoritative, balanced information and is more comprehensive than single-volume family medical guides.

Scope

More than 800 full-length articles are included in *The Gale Encyclopedia of Alternative Medicine.* Many prominent figures are highlighted as sidebar biographies that accompany the therapy entries. Articles follow a standardized format that provides information at a glance. Rubrics include:

Therapies

- Origins
- Benefits
- Description
- Preparations
- Precautions
- Side effects
- Research and general acceptance
- Resources
- Key terms

Herbs/remedies

- General use
- Preparations
- Precautions
- Side effects

- Interactions
- Resources
- Key terms

Diseases/conditions

- Definition
- Description
- Causes and symptoms
- Diagnosis
- Treatment
- Allopathic treatment
- Expected results
- Prevention
- Resources
- Key terms

Inclusion criteria

A preliminary list of therapies, herbs, remedies, diseases, and conditions was compiled from a wide variety of sources, including professional medical guides and textbooks, as well as consumer guides and encyclopedias. The advisory board, made up of three medical and alternative healthcare experts, evaluated the topics and made suggestions for inclusion. Final selection of topics to include was made by the medical advisors in conjunction with Gale editors.

About the Contributors

The essays were compiled by experienced medical writers, including alternative healthcare practitioners and educators, pharmacists, nurses, and other complementary healthcare professionals. *GEAM* medical advisors reviewed more than 95% of the completed essays to insure that they are appropriate, up-to-date, and medically accurate.

How to Use this Book

The Gale Encyclopedia of Alternative Medicine has been designed with ready reference in mind:

- Straight **alphabetical arrangement** allows users to locate information quickly.

- Bold faced terms function as *print hyperlinks* that point the reader to related entries in the encyclopedia.

- A list of **key terms** is provided where appropriate to define unfamiliar words or concepts used within the context of the essay. Additional terms may be found in the **glossary**.

- **Cross-references** placed throughout the encyclopedia direct readers to where information on subjects without their own entries can be found. Synonyms are also cross-referenced.

- A **Resources section** directs users to sources of further complementary medical information.

- An appendix of alternative medical organizations is arranged by type of therapy and includes valuable **contact information**.

- A comprehensive **general index** allows users to easily target detailed aspects of any topic, including Latin names.

Graphics

The Gale Encyclopedia of Alternative Medicine is enhanced with more than 400 images, including photos, tables, and customized line drawings.

ADVISORS

An advisory board made up of prominent individuals from complementary medical communities provided invaluable assistance in the formulation of this encyclopedia. They defined the scope of coverage and reviewed individual entries for accuracy and accessibility. We would therefore like to express our appreciation to them:

Mirka Knaster, PhD
author, editor, consultant in
Eastern and Western body-mind
disciplines and spiritual traditions
Oakland, CA

Diana Quinn, ND
Naturopathic Women's
Healthcare, Ann Arbor, MI
Ann Arbor, MI

Suzanna M. Zick, ND, MPH
University of Michigan
Department of Family Medicine
Ann Arbor, MI

CONTRIBUTORS

Margaret Alic, PhD
Medical Writer
Eastsound, WA

Greg Annussek
Medical Writer
American Society of Journalists
and Authors
New York, NY

Barbara Boughton
Health and Medical Writer
El Cerrito, CA

Ruth Ann Prag Carter
Freelance Writer
Farmington Hills, MI

Linda Chrisman
*Massage Therapist and
Educator*
Medical Writer
Oakland, CA

Rhonda Cloos, RN
Medical writer and Nurse
Austin, TX

Gloria Cooksey, CNE
Medical Writer
Sacramento, CA

Amy Cooper, MA, MSI
Medical Writer
Vermillion, SD

Angela Costello
Medical Writer
Northfield, OH

Sharon Crawford
Writer, Editor, Researcher
American Medical Writers
Association

Periodical Writers Association of
Canada and the
Editors' Association of Canada
Toronto, ONT Canada

Sandra Bain Cushman
Massage Therapist
*Alexander Technique Practitioner
and Educator*
Charlottesville, VA

Helen Davidson
Medical Writer
Portland, OR

Tish Davidson, MA
Medical Writer
Fremont, CA

Lori DeMilto, MJ
Medical Writer
Sicklerville, NJ

Doug Dupler, MA
Medical Writer
Boulder, CO

Paula Ford-Martin, PhD
Medical Writer
Warwick, RI

Rebecca J. Frey, PhD
Medical Writer
New Haven, CT

Lisa Frick
Medical Writer
Columbia, MO

Kathleen Goss
Medical Writer
Darwin, CA

Elliot Greene, MA
*Former President, American
Massage Therapy Association*

Massage Therapist
Silver Spring, MD

Peter Gregutt
Medical Writer
Asheville, NC

Clare Hanrahan
Medical Writer
Asheville, NC

David Helwig
Medical Writer
London, ONT Canada

Beth A. Kapes
Medical Writer, Editor
Bay Village, OH

Katherine Kim
Medical Writer
Oakland, CA

Erika Lenz
Medical Writer
Lafayette, CO

Lorraine Lica, PhD
Medical Writer
San Diego, CA

Whitney Lowe, LMT
Massage Therapy Educator
Orthopedic Massage
Education & Research
Institute
Bend, OR

Mary McNulty
Freelance Writer
St.Charles, IL

Leslie Mertz
Medical Writer, Biologist
Kalkaska, MI

Katherine E. Nelson, ND
Naturopathic Physician
Naples, FL

David E. Newton, Ed.D.
Medical Writer
Ashland, OR

Teresa Odle
Medical Writer
Ute Park, NM

Jodi Ohlsen Read
Medical Writer
Carver, MN

Carole Osborne-Sheets
Massage Therapist and Educator
Medical Writer
Poway, CA

Lee Ann Paradise
Medical Writer
Lubbock, TX

Patience Paradox
Medical Writer
Bainbridge Island, WA

Belinda Rowland, PhD
Medical Writer
Voorheesville, NY

Joan M. Schonbeck, RN
Medical Writer
Marlborough, MA

Gabriele Schubert, MS
Medical Writer
San Diego, CA

Kim Sharp, M Ln
Medical Writer
Houston, TX

Kathy Shepard Stolley, PhD
Medical Writer
Virginia Beach, VA

Judith Sims, MS
Science Writer
Logan, UT

Patricia Skinner
Medical Writer
Amman, Jordan

Genevieve Slomski, PhD
Medical Writer
New Britain, CT

Jane E. Spear
Medical Writer
Canton, OH

Liz Swain
Medical Writer
San Diego, CA

Judith Turner, DVM
Medical Writer
Sandy, UT

Samuel Uretsky, PharmD
Medical Writer
Wantagh, NY

Ken R. Wells
Science Writer
Laguna Hills, CA

Angela Woodward
Science Writer
Madison, WI

Kathleen Wright, RN
Medical Writer
Delmar, DE

Jennifer L. Wurges
Medical Writer
Rochester Hills, MI

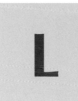

Labyrinth walking

Definition

A labyrinth is a patterned path, often circular in form, used as a walking **meditation** or spiritual practice. A labyrinth's walkway is arranged in such a way that the participant moves back and forth across the circular form through a series of curves, ending at the labyrinths's heart or center. It is unicursal, which means that it has only one entrance and leads in only one direction. Although the word "maze" is often used as a synonym for labyrinthmazes are multicursal in design; the user has to make choices at many points along the path. Mazes often have more than one entrance, and usually contain many wrong turns and dead ends.

The English word labyrinth is derived from the Greek word *labyrinthos*, which in turn may come from *labrys*, the word for the double-headed axe associated with the Minoan culture on the island of Crete that was at its height around 1650 B.C.. According to the Greek historian Herodotus (c. 450 B.C.), King Minos of Crete asked an Athenian architect and inventor named Daedalus to build a house with winding passages for the Minotaur, a monster that his queen had borne after having intercourse with a bull. This mythical Cretan labyrinth was actually a maze rather than a true labyrinth, as it was intended to prevent those who entered it as human sacrifices to the Minotaur from escaping.

Origins

The unicursal designs associated with labyrinths are thought to predate constructed labyrinths. Pottery estimated to be 15,000 years old painted with labyrinthine patterns has been discovered in the Ukraine. The oldest known constructed labyrinths were built in ancient Egypt and Etruria (central Italy) around 4500 B.C., perhaps to prevent evil spirits from entering tombs. It was thought that the evil spirits were repelled by the planned order of the labyrinth's design. Other labyrinths were made by the Romans as mosaic patterns on the floors of large houses or public buildings. These mosaic labyrinths were usually square or rectangular in shape. The Romans also constructed turf labyrinths in fields or other open areas as a test of skill for horseback riders. Traces of Roman turf labyrinths have been found all over Europe.

Labyrinths have been found in many cultures around the world, including ancient India, Spain, Peru, and China. Members of the Tohono O'odham and Pima tribes in southern Arizona have made baskets for centuries decorated with the so-called "man in the maze" design. The labyrinth pattern woven into the basket represents the path to the top of a local sacred mountain known as Baboquivari. More than five hundred ancient stone labyrinths have been identified in Scandinavia. Most are located near the coast, and are thought to have been used for rituals intended to guarantee good fishing or protection from storms.

The best-known labyrinths in the West, however, are those dating from the Middle Ages. They were built as substitutes for going on a pilgrimage to Jerusalem, a journey that was physically or economically impossible for most Christians in Western Europe during this period. Cathedrals were designated as pilgrimage shrines, and labyrinths were embedded in the stone floors of the cathedrals as part of the shrine's design. The labyrinth on the floor of Chartres Cathedral in France was installed around A.D. 1200, and a similar labyrinth in Amiens Cathedral was made around the same time. Tracing the path through the labyrinth, often on the knees, was for many pilgrims the final act of devotion on the pilgrimage. The circuitous journey to the center of the labyrinth represented the many turnings in the journey of life, a journey that required the Church's guidance and support. Medieval labyrinths were circular in shape, the circle being a universal symbol of wholeness, completion, and unity.

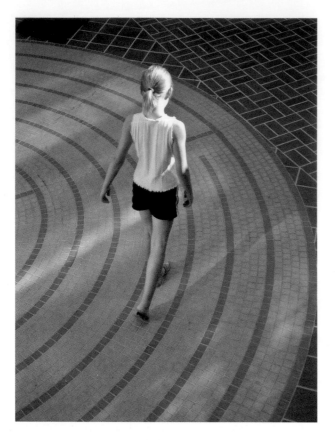

This girl walks on a labyrinth, or a patterned path used for walking meditation or spiritual practice. *(Ginna Fleming / Alamy)*

By the seventeenth century, however, many cathedral labyrinths were removed or destroyed. There is some disagreement among scholars regarding the reasons for their removal. Some experts think that the labyrinths were removed because the cathedral clergy had forgotten their history and original purpose, while others speculate that they were destroyed to prevent children from playing on them during Mass and disturbing worship. Another factor was the growth of rationalism in the seventeenth century and the hostility toward religion that emerged during the French Revolution at the end of the eighteenth century. The labyrinths were regarded as remnants of "superstition" and therefore offensive to "enlightened" people.

The contemporary revival of interest in labyrinth walking began in the early 1990s, when Dr. Lauren Artress, a psychotherapist who was on the Special Ministries staff of Grace Cathedral (Episcopal) in San Francisco, attended a Mystery Seminar led by Jean Houston, who describes herself as "a scholar and researcher in human capacities," and directs the Foundation for Mind Research in Pomona, New York. Dr. Houston presented the labyrinth as a tool for spiritual growth that would lead the seminar participants to their spiritual center. She had taped the forty-foot-wide pattern of the Chartres Cathedral labyrinth on the floor of the meeting room. Dr. Artress felt drawn to return to the labyrinth later that night and found walking through it a powerful experience. She then made a pilgrimage to Chartres itself in 1991, followed by further research into the history and significance of labyrinths. After returning to the United States, Dr. Artress made a canvas version of the Chartres labyrinth for use in the San Francisco cathedral. It was introduced to the public on December 30, 1991, and was used twice a month until 1995, when a permanent outdoor labyrinth made of terrazzo stone was laid down in the cathedral's outdoor garden.

Benefits

In general, labyrinth walking is said to benefit participants by allowing a temporary suspension of so-called left-brain activity—logical thought, analysis, and fact-based planning—and encourage the emergence of the intuition and imaginative creativity associated with the right brain. Lauren Artress has said,

"The labyrinth does not engage our thinking minds. It invites our intuitive, pattern-seeking, symbolic mind to come forth. It presents us with only one, but profound, choice. To enter a labyrinth is to choose to walk a spiritual path."

In addition to helping people open themselves to the nonrational parts of the psyche, labyrinth walking puts them in touch with simple body rhythms. Because labyrinth walking involves physical movement, participants may find themselves becoming more mindful of their breathing patterns, the repetition of their footfalls, and the reorientation of the entire body that occurs as they move through the circular turns within the labyrinth. More particularly, the overall pattern of movement in labyrinth walking—first inward toward the center of the labyrinth and then outward on the return path—holds deep symbolic meaning for many people.

Specific benefits that some people have experienced as a result of labyrinth walking include:

• answers to, or insights, personal problems or circumstances
• a general sense of inner peace or calm
• emotional healing from past abuse or other traumas
• a sense of connection to, or unity with, past generations of pilgrims or family ancestors
• reawakened interest in their specific religious tradition
• greater awareness of their own feminine nature or the feminine principle in nature, often associated with circular shapes and patterns
• stimulation of their imagination and creative powers
• improved ability to manage chronic pain
• faster healing following an injury or surgical procedure

Description

Labyrinth construction and design

Contemporary labyrinths are constructed from a wide variety of materials in outdoor as well as indoor settings. In addition to being made from canvas, mosaic flooring, or paving stones, labyrinths have been woven into patterned carpets, outlined with stones, bricks, or hedgerows, or carved into firmly packed earth. Most modern labyrinths range between 40 and 80 feet in diameter, although larger ones have also been made.

One classification scheme categorizes labyrinths as either left- or right-handed, according to the direction of the first turn to be made after entering the labyrinth. The entrance to the labyrinth is known as the mouth, and the walkway itself is called the path. Classical labyrinths are defined as having a simple path with an equal number of turns and counter-turns. Labyrinths are also classified by the number of circuits in their design, a circuit being one of the circles or rings surrounding the center of the labyrinth. The labyrinth in Chartres Cathedral, for example, is a classical eleven-circuit labyrinth. Three- and seven-circuit classical labyrinths have been constructed in many parts of the United States, while one labyrinth in Denmark has 15 circuits.

Walking the labyrinth

The actual procedure of labyrinth walking is divided into three phases or stages: the journey inward, a pause for **prayer** or meditation at the center, and the return journey. There are no rules or guidelines for the pace or speed of labyrinth walking, although participants are asked to be respectful of others who may prefer a slower pace, and to move around them as gently as possible. Some people choose to dance, run, crawl on their hands and knees, or walk backwards in the labyrinth. With regard to pausing in the center of the labyrinth, people's behavior varies depending on the size of the labyrinth. Labyrinths based on the Chartres model have six "petals" or semicircular spaces surrounding the center, which allows several people to remain for a few minutes to pray, contemplate, or meditate. Smaller labyrinths may have room for only one person at a time in the center, and it is considered courteous to remain there only briefly.

Labyrinth walking can be incorporated into such ritual events as weddings, funerals, and anniversary celebrations, or such personal events as completing one's schooling, taking a new job, or moving to a new area. Some published guides to labyrinth walking include meditations to be used for labyrinth walking during **pregnancy**, or for blessing ceremonies at different seasons of the year.

Preparations

Although one need not be a member of any specific faith or religious tradition to participate in labyrinth walking, spiritual preparation is considered an important part of the activity. Although the walk itself is informal and relatively unstructured, most participants find that a period of quietness to focus their attention on their journey is essential. Some also recommend clarifying one's intention for the walk beforehand; that is, participants should ask themselves whether they are seeking spiritual guidance, healing, closer fellowship with God, discernment, blessing, or the fulfillment of some other purpose. The use of prayers or mantras is suggested as a way to calm and "center" one's spirit at the beginning of and during the walk.

Participants are advised to wear comfortable shoes and clothing for labyrinth walking so that they will not be distracted by physical discomfort or concerns about their appearance. They will be asked to remove their shoes, however, if the labyrinth is made of canvas or woven into a rug; thus it is a good idea to bring along a pair of clean cotton socks or soft-soled slippers.

Precautions

There are no special precautions needed for labyrinth walking other than allowing sufficient time for the experience. Most people find that the walk takes about 45 minutes or an hour, but some take two to three hours to complete their journey. It is best to plan a labyrinth walk for a day or evening without a tight time schedule.

Side effects

No physical or psychological side effects have been reported from labyrinth walking.

Research and general acceptance

Little research has been done within the mainstream or alternative medical communities on labyrinth walking in comparison to other forms of treatment. As of 2004, however, it appeared to be generally accepted as a form of mind-body therapy or spiritual practice that has few if any associated risks and offers spiritual benefits to many people.

Since the mid-1990s, growing numbers of churches and retreat centers in the United States and Canada have built or installed labyrinths. Some communities have also built outdoor labyrinths for the general public. In the early 2000s, health spas and tourist resorts have added labyrinths to their facilities in order to attract visitors interested in wellness programs. A labyrinth locator is available on the web site of The Labyrinth Society.

Training and certification

The Labyrinth Society (TLS), which was founded in 1999, hosts an annual meeting that includes workshops and speakers on labyrinth construction as well as the spiritual aspects of labyrinth walking. TLS does not, however, offer licensing or training programs as of 2004; its membership code of ethics states, "Membership or leadership in this Society does not serve as qualifying evidence of any level of proficiency or ability relating to labyrinths and their uses and shall not be so represented." Membership in TLS is open to anyone interested in "inspir[ing] possibilities and creat[ing]connections through the labyrinth."

Resources

BOOKS

Artress, Lauren. *Walking A Sacred Path: Rediscovering the Labyrinth as a Spiritual Tool.* New York: Riverhead Books, 1995.

Curry, Helen. *The Way of the Labyrinth: A Powerful Meditation for Everyday Life.* New York: Penguin Compass Books, 2000.

Schaper, Donna, and Carole Ann Camp. *Labyrinths from the Outside: Walking to Spiritual Insight—A Beginner's Guide.*

PERIODICALS

Oakley, Doug. "Tourism Officials Push Wellness as Niche Market." *Travel Weekly,* 20 May 2002.

Stone, Victoria. "Discovering the Labyrinth as a Tool for Health and Healing." *Journal of Healthcare Design* 10 (1998): 73–76.

Unsworth, Tim. "The Ancient Labyrinth Makes a Comeback: Walk Through Maze Recalls Our Wandering Journey Through Life." *National Catholic Reporter* 3 October 2003, 10.

ORGANIZATIONS

Labyrinth Enterprises. 128 Slocum Avenue, St. Louis, MO 63119. (800) 873-9873 or (314) 968-5557. Fax: (314) 968-5539. http://www.labyrinth-enterprises.com.

StoneCircle Services. E-mail: info@stonecircledesign.com. http://www.stonecircledesign.com.

The Labyrinth Society (TLS). P. O. Box 144, New Canaan, CT 06840. (877) 446-4520. http://www.labyrinthsociety.org.

Rebecca Frey

Lachesis

Description

Not all products used in alternative healing come from plants. Lachesis is the venom of the bushmaster snake, *Lachesis mutus*. It is used in homeopathic medicine.

L. mutus is a tropical snake that lives in the jungles of Central and South America, growing to a length of 12 feet (3.6 m). It is the largest poisonous pit viper in the Western hemisphere, and second in size in the world only to the king cobra. *L. mutus* is related to the familiar North American rattlesnake.

A large bushmaster can have fangs more than 1 in (2.5 cm) long. Its venom is deadly and kills rapidly by inhibiting nervous impulses or slowly by interfering

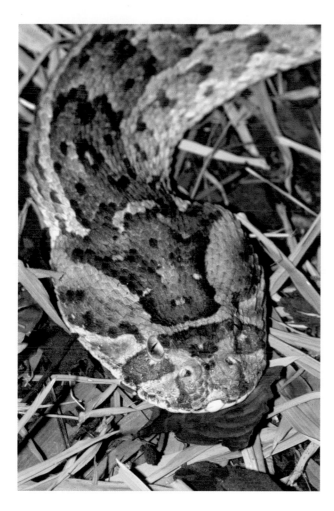

Lachesis is the venom of the bushmaster snake, Lachesis mutus. *(© blickwinkel / Alamy)*

with blood clotting and accelerating the destruction of red blood cells. The bushmaster is also called the surucucu (sometimes spelled surukuku).

General use

Homeopathic medicine operates on the principle that "like heals like." This means that a disease can be cured by treating it with substances that produce the same symptoms as the disease, while also working in conjunction with the homeopathic law of infinitesimals. In opposition to traditional medicine, the law of infinitesimals states that the *lower* a dose of curative, the more effective it is. To achieve a low dose, the curative is diluted many, many times until only a tiny amount remains in a huge amount of the diluting liquid.

In homeopathic terms, fresh *L. mutus* venom was "proved" as a remedy by Constantine Hering around 1830. Although born in what is now Germany, Hering is considered to be the founder of American **homeopathy**. In 1827 he went to Surinam, South America, to conduct biological research for his government. In experimenting with lachesis venom in an attempt to find a homeopathic inoculation for smallpox, he accidentally poisoned himself with a small amount of venom. This led him to his "proof" that lachesis was a homeopathic remedy. Ever the curious scientist, Hering later accidentally paralyzed his right side by continuing to test higher and higher doses of lachesis on himself.

Lachesis is used in homeopathy to treat a wide range of symptoms. These fall into the following general categories of:

- menstrual and menopausal complaints
- throat and mouth complaints
- fear, paranoia, and associated mental complaints
- nervous system complaints
- circulatory complaints

All these complaints exhibit certain patterns or modalities that indicate they should be treated with lachesis. These symptoms may:

- worsen after sleep and upon awakening
- worsen in the spring
- worsen after drinking hot beverages, taking hot baths, or direct exposure to the sun
- worsen if touched or if the body is constricted by tight clothes
- worsen with alcohol consumption
- produce surging waves of pain
- move from the left side to the right side of the body
- result in a mottled, engorged, congested face
- result in a very sensitive neck
- improve from eating
- improve from the onset of bodily discharge
- improve from exposure to cold and fresh air

In homeopathy, certain remedies are thought to be especially effective in people with specific personality and physical traits. The "lachesis personality" tends to be egocentric, self-important, unstable, and jealous. They may be possessive. This personality type often talks about doing great things, but rarely follows through. Physically, lachesis types tend to be overweight and bloated. They often have red hair and freckles.

Lachesis is a major homeopathic remedy for **hot flashes** associated with **menopause**. It is also used to treat premenstrual and menstrual symptoms such as **premenstrual syndrome** (PMS), menstrual **pain**, and short menses.

Throat and mouth complaints are also treated with lachesis. A **sore throat** that worsens when hot liquids are swallowed is a good example of the type of throat complaint for which lachesis is considered appropriate. Similarly, so is a sore throat with left-sided pain or pain in the left ear, and a purplish, engorged throat, swollen gums, tongue, and foul-tasting saliva. The throat, neck, and larynx are extremely sensitive to touch.

Lachesis is used to alleviate certain mental or emotional symptoms. These include suspicion and distrust that can border on paranoia, extreme talkativeness that reflects nervousness and restless, **depression**, petty jealousy, and unsociability.

Circulatory complaints treated with lachesis include:

- swollen and engorged veins that give the skin a bluish cast
- varicose veins
- nose bleeds
- slow-to-heal, bluish wounds
- a throbbing sensation in various parts of the body
- weak, irregular rapid pulse
- palpitations
- fainting

The main nervous system complaint treated by lachesis is cluster headaches. These are headaches that produce pulsating waves of pain, often on the left side, or beginning on the left side then moving to the right. They often precede **menstruation** and improve once menses begins. Petit mal seizures and **angina** are also treated with lachesis.

Other complaints that lachesis is said to alleviate include stomach pains, appendicitis, **vomiting**, and gastrointestinal complaints, anal spasms, bleeding **hemorrhoids**, and cravings for alcohol, coffee, and shellfish.

Preparations

Fresh venom is commercially prepared in a very highly diluted form. It is available in tablets or liquid and is known as lachesis 12X. It can be taken with other complementary homeopathic remedies.

Precautions

No particular precautions have been reported when using lachesis, however, caution must be taken when using this—and any homeopathic treatment. Individuals should consult a licensed homeopath or physician.

KEY TERMS

Angina—Any painful spasm that leaves one feeling choked or suffocated. In common usage, angina usually refers to chest pain associated with a heart spasm.

Petit mal seizures—A less severe form of epileptic seizure.

Side effects

When taken in the recommended dilute form, no side effects have been reported. However, concentrated quantities of the venom cause paralysis and hemorrhaging, and can be fatal.

Interactions

Studies on interactions between lachesis given in homeopathic doses and conventional pharmaceuticals are nonexistent.

Resources

BOOKS

Hammond, Christopher. *The Complete Family Guide to Homeopathy*. London: Penguin Studio, 1995.

Lockie, Andrew. *The Family Guide to Homeopathy: Symptoms and Natural Solutions*. New York: Prentice Hall, 1989.

Lockie, Andrew and Nicola Geddes. *The Complete Guide to Homeopathy*. London: Dorling Kindersley, 1995.

OTHER

Homeopathic Internet Resources. http://www.holisticmed. com./www/homeopathy.html.

ORGANIZATIONS

National Center for Homeopathy, 801 N. Fairfax Street, Suite 306, Alexandria, VA, 22314, (703)548-7790, (703)548-7792 , http://nationalcenterforhomeopathy.org.

Tish Davidson

Lacto-ovo vegetarianism

Definition

Lacto-ovo vegetarians do not eat meat but do include dairy products (lacto) and eggs (ovo) in their **diets**.

Origins

The term "vegetarian" was coined in 1847 by the founders of the Vegetarian Society of Great Britain, although **vegetarianism** as a way of life had existed for thousands of years. The founders of the Vegetarian Society were lacto-ovo vegetarians.

One of the central values that motivated vegetarians is that food choices should not require the death or suffering of animals. Thus, many vegetarians avoid meat but eat dairy products and eggs (on the grounds that store-bought eggs are unfertilized). Some people argue, however, that eating eggs may prevent the life of an animal, so some vegetarians are lacto-vegetarians. **Veganism**, another type of vegetarianism, follows a diet that uses no animal products at all.

Some of the world's oldest religious traditions have advocated vegetarianism as a means to both physical and spiritual health. In the Christian tradition, Trappist monks of the Roman Catholic Church are vegetarian, as are Seventh Day Adventists, who form a group large enough that many studies have been performed on them to determine the health benefits of lacto-ovo vegetarianism. Some vegetarians maintain that there is evidence that Jesus and the early Christians were vegetarians as well. In ancient India, the idea of *ahimsa* developed, which means "not doing harm." Followers of this creed believe that living in a manner that reduces the suffering of other living beings, including animals, is necessary to reach higher levels of spiritual wellness. According to Hinduismm, there is an endless cycle of rebirth and lives until souls reach nirvana. The presence of souls on all levels of animal life precludes meat eating.

The **yoga** system of living and health recommends vegetarianism because its dietary practices are based on the belief that healthy food contains prana. Prana is the universal life energy, which yoga experts believe is abundant in fresh fruits, grains, nuts, and vegetables, but absent in meat because it comes from an animal that has been killed. Some Buddhists are vegetarian because of their spiritual belief in the oneness of all life. Other traditional cultures, such as those in the Middle East and the Mediterranean regions, have evolved diets that consist mainly of lacto-ovo vegetarian foods. The **Mediterranean diet**, which a Harvard study declared to be one of the world's healthiest, is primarily although not strictly lacto-ovo vegetarian.

The list of famous vegetarians forms an illustrious group. The ancient Greek philosophers, including Socrates, Plato, and Pythagoras, advocated vegetarianism. Other famous vegetarians include Leonardo da Vinci, Sir Isaac Newton, the physician Albert Schweitzer, writer George Bernard Shaw, musician Paul McCartney, and champion triathlete Dave Scott. Albert Einstein, although not a strict vegetarian himself, stated that a vegetarian diet would be an evolutionary step forward for the human race.

Vegetarianism in the United States has generally consisted of a small but vocal number of adherents. It has its roots in the mid-1800s, when some people began to question accepted health and dietary practices. In 1839, Sylvester Graham, who invented the graham cracker from whole wheat flour, wrote *Lectures on the Science of Human Life.* A few decades later, Ralph Waldo Emerson and Henry David Thoreau both advocated vegetarianism. In 1883, Howard Williams published *The Ethics of Diet,* which promoted vegetarianism. Williams's book influenced many people around the world, including Russian author Leo Tolstoy and Indian political leader the Hindu Mahatma Gandhi. But vegetarianism remained largely unpopular in the United States during the nineteenth century.

In the twentieth century, vegetarianism steadily gained followers in the United States, although it met considerable resistance from the meat industry and general public. By the 1960s, the consumption of meat in the United States had increased significantly from consumption levels at the turn of the century. Meat and dairy foods made up two of the four recommended food groups designed by the United States government. Some researchers claimed that meat was fundamental to health, while a growing minority of nutritionists began to correlate the meat-heavy U.S. diet with rising rates of **heart disease**, **cancer**, and diabetes.

In 1971, Frances Moore Lappe published her landmark book, *Diet for a Small Planet,* which proposed that vegetarians could obtain a complete source of dietary protein by combining particular foods such as rice and beans. Until that time it was believed by U.S. nutritionists that only meat could supply adequate protein. The book sold millions of copies. Lappe's book argued that meat-centered diets are unhealthy for both people and the environment, and it stressed that meat-eating perpetuated hunger worldwide because animals raised for food consume so much grain. Millions were converted to vegetarianism by this book.

Vegetarianism steadily gained acceptance as an alternative to the meat-and-potatoes regimen of the traditional American diet. Several factors contributed to the U.S. trend toward vegetarianism. Outbreaks of **food poisoning** from meat products, as well as increased concern over such additives in meat as hormones and antibiotics, led many people and professionals to question the safety of meat products. People also became aware of unethical treatment of animals in the meat industry. Then too the environmental impact of an agricultural system based on meat production was examined more closely. Some argued that raising of livestock causes soil erosion, water contamination and shortages, pollution, deforestation, and an inefficient use of natural resources.

The growing health consciousness of Americans is probably the most important reason for the surge of interest in vegetarianism. **Nutrition** experts argue that the high rates of heart disease, cancer, and diabetes are directly related to poor dietary habits, particularly a diet high in **cholesterol** and saturated fat and low in fiber. Nutritionists have repeatedly shown in studies that a healthy diet consists of plenty of fresh vegetables and fruits, complex carbohydrates such as whole grains, and foods that are high in fiber and low in cholesterol and saturated fat. The vegetarian diet fulfills all these criteria.

In alternative medicine, vegetarianism is a cornerstone dietary therapy, used in Ayurvedic treatment, **detoxification** therapies, the Ornish and Wigmore diets, and in treatments for many chronic conditions, including heart disease, diabetes, and cancer.

Benefits

Lacto-ovo vegetarianism is sometimes recommended as a dietary therapy for a variety of conditions, including heart disease, cancer, diabetes, **stroke**, high cholesterol, **obesity**, **osteoporosis**, **hypertension**, **gout**, **gallstones**, **kidney stones**, ulcers, **colitis**, **hemorrhoids**, **premenstrual syndrome**, **anxiety**, and **depression**. Lacto-ovo vegetarianism is an economical and easily implemented preventive practice. It does, however, require self-education regarding how to fashion an adequate diet for those who adopt it.

Preparations

It is generally recommended that a vegetarian diet be adopted gradually, to allow people's bodies and lifestyles time to adjust to new eating habits and food intake. Some nutritionists have designed transition diets to help people become vegetarian in stages. Many Americans eat meat products at nearly every meal, and the first stage of a transition diet is to replace meat in just a few meals a week with wholly vegetarian dishes. Then, particular meat products can be slowly reduced and eliminated from the diet and replaced with vegetarian foods. Red meat can be reduced and then eliminated, followed by pork, poultry, and fish. Individuals should be willing to experiment with

transition diets and need patience when learning how to combine vegetarianism with such social activities as dining out. Many vegetarian cookbooks are available to help vegetarians prepare meals at home.

The transition to vegetarianism can be smoother for those who make informed choices regarding dietary practices. Nutritional guidelines include decreasing fat intake, increasing fiber, and emphasizing fresh fruits, vegetables, legumes, and whole grains while avoiding processed foods and sugar. Other helpful health practices include reading food labels and understanding such basic nutritional concepts as daily requirements for protein, fats, and nutrients. Would-be vegetarians can experiment with meat substitutes, foods that are high in protein and essential nutrients. Many meat substitutes are readily available, such as tofu and tempeh, which are soybean products that are high in protein, **calcium**, and other nutrients. Veggie-burgers can be grilled like hamburgers, and vegetarian substitutes for turkey and sausage have surprisingly realistic textures and tastes.

Precautions

Adopting a lacto-ovo vegetarian diet does not automatically mean an improvement in health. One of the advantages of lacto-ovo vegetarianism is that eggs and dairy products are good sources of the protein, vitamins, and minerals for which vegetarians may have special requirements. Both eggs and dairy products, however, are generally high in calories and contain cholesterol and saturated fat. Studies have shown that some vegetarians consume higher than recommended quantities of fat, and some vegetarians have high cholesterol levels. The lacto-ovo vegetarian diet is most healthful when it uses eggs and low-fat dairy products sparingly to supplement a diet rich in whole grains, fruits, vegetables, and legumes. Another option for lacto-vegetarians is to use only egg whites (which contain no fat) and nonfat dairy products when high cholesterol and fat consumption are problems. Vegetable sources of saturated fat include avocados, nuts, and some cooking oils.

In general, a well-planned lacto-ovo vegetarian diet is healthful and safe and contains all the nutrients needed by the body. Vegetarians who eat few animal products, however, should be aware of particular nutrients that may be lacking in non-animal diets. These are protein, **vitamin A**, **vitamin B$_{12}$**, **vitamin D**, calcium, **iron**, **zinc**, and **essential fatty acids**. Furthermore, pregnant women, growing children, and people with certain health conditions have higher requirements for these nutrients.

Vegetarians should be aware of getting complete proteins in their diets. A complete protein contains all of the essential **amino acids**, which are proteins that are essential to the diet because the body cannot make them. Meat and dairy products generally contain complete proteins, but many vegetarian foods such as grains and legumes contain incomplete proteins, lacking one or more of the essential amino acids. Vegetarians can overcome this difficulty by combining particular foods in order to create complete proteins. In general, combining legumes such as soy, lentils, beans, and peas with grains such as rice, wheat, or oats forms complete proteins. Eating dairy products or nuts with grains also makes complete proteins. Oatmeal with milk combines to make a complete protein, as does peanut butter on whole wheat bread. Proteins do not necessarily need to be combined in the same meal, but generally they should be combined over a period of a few days.

Getting enough vitamin B$_{12}$ may be an issue for some vegetarians, although this vitamin is present in both eggs and dairy products. Vitamin supplements that contain vitamin B$_{12}$ are recommended, as are fortified soy products and nutritional yeast. Research has indicated that vitamin B$_{12}$ deficiency is a risk for vegetarians, especially vegans. Those choosing a vegetarian diet should watch carefully to ensure they get enough active vitamin B$_{12}$ from diet and supplements. Deficiency of this vitamin poses particular risk to pregnant women and nursing mothers.

Vitamin D can be obtained in dairy products, egg yolks, fortified foods, and sunshine. Calcium can be obtained in dairy products, enriched tofu, seeds, nuts, legumes, dairy products, and dark green vegetables, including broccoli, kale, spinach, and collard greens. Iron is found in raisins, figs, legumes, tofu, whole grains (particularly whole wheat), potatoes, and dark green leafy vegetables. Iron is absorbed more efficiently by the body when iron-containing foods are eaten with foods that contain **vitamin C**, such as fruits, tomatoes, and green vegetables. Zinc is abundant in eggs, nuts, pumpkin seeds, legumes, whole grains, and tofu. For vegetarians who eat no fish, getting enough omega-3 essential fatty acids may be an issue, and such supplements as **flaxseed** oil should be considered as well as eating walnuts and canola oil. Vegetarians may also consider buying organic foods, which are grown without the use of synthetic chemicals, as another health precaution.

Research and general acceptance

Walter Willett, chair of the Department of Nutrition at Harvard University and professor of epidemiology and nutrition, has extensively studied the effects of diet on health. His research has shown that about 82 percent of heart attacks, about 70 percent of strokes, more than 90 percent of type 2 diabetes, and more than 70 percent of colon cancer can be prevented with proper nutrition as part of a healthy lifestyle. In addition, he and his colleagues have found that greater meat consumption is associated with a higher prevalence of degenerative arthritis and soft tissue disorders. In addition, a healthy lifestyle that includes low meat intake has been shown to increase longevity.

One major epidemiological study of vegetarianism was done at Loma Linda University in California. Epidemiology is the study of how diseases affect populations as a whole. Researchers analyzed data from over 25,000 people in the Seventh Day Adventist Church, who are lacto-ovo vegetarians. These vegetarians had 14% of the chance of dying from heart disease that meat-eating Americans faced. The Adventists also had significantly longer life expectancy. From this study, researchers estimated that eating meat just once a day triples the risk of dying from heart disease by age 64. It should be noted, however, that Seventh Day Adventists typically do not smoke or drink alcohol, and may have healthier lifestyles in general, affecting rates of heart disease. A study in England analyzed more than 10,000 vegetarians and meat eaters, and researchers concluded there was a direct relationship between the amount of meat consumed and the chances of getting heart disease. Other studies have been performed on population data from World War II. In Norway during the war, the death rate from heart disease and strokes dropped significantly concurrent with the drop in consumption of meat.

Many studies have concentrated on the benefits of eating fruits and vegetables and have shown that eating more fruits and vegetables helps decrease the risk of cancer. Other studies have shown that diets high in fiber, which vegetarian diets tend to be, reduce the risk for heart disease, cancer, and other conditions, including digestive disorders, appendicitis, and osteoporosis (bone loss).

A lacto-ovo vegetarian diet, as prescribed by Dean Ornish, has been shown to improve heart disease and reverse the effects of **atherosclerosis**, or hardening of the arteries. Ornish's diet was used in conjunction with **exercise**, **stress** reduction, and other holistic methods. Ornish allowed only the use of egg whites and nonfat dairy products in his low-fat vegetarian diet. Ornish's groundbreaking clinical research demonstrated that coronary heart disease can be reversed with comprehensive lifestyle changes.

Resources

BOOKS

Bender, D. A. *A Dictionary of Food and Nutrition.* New York: Oxford University Press, 2005.

Berdanier, C., and J. T. Dywer, eds. *Handbook of Nutrition and Food,* 2nd ed. Boca Raton, FL: CRC Press, 2006.

Willett, Walter C., and P. J. Skerrett. *Eat, Drink, and Be Healthy: The Harvard Medical School Guide to Healthy Eating.* New York: Free Press, 2005.

PERIODICALS

Leitzmann C. "Vegetarian Diets: What Are the Advantages?" *Forum of Nutrition* 57 (2005): 147–156.

ORGANIZATIONS

Food and Agricultural Organization of the United Nations, http://www.fao.org.

Food and Nutrition Information Center, National Agricultural Library, United States Department of Agriculture. 10301 Baltimore Ave., Room 105, Beltsville, MD, 20705, (301) 504-5414, http://fnic.nal.usda.gov.

International Food Information Council, 1100 Connecticut Ave. NW, Suite 430, Washington, DC, 20036, (202) 296-6540, http://www.ific.org.

North American Vegetarian Society, PO Box 72, Dolgeville, NY, 13329, (518) 568-7970, http://www.navs-online.org/.

Vegetarian Nutrition Dietetic Practice Group, American Dietetic Association, 120 S. Riverside Plaza, Suite 2000, Chicago, IL, 60606-6995, (800) 877-1600, http://www.vegetariannutrition.net/.

Douglas Dupler
Teresa Norris
Angela M. Costello

Lactobacillus species

Definition

Lactobacillus is a genus of Gram–positive anaerobic bacteria that get their name from the fact that they convert lactose to lactic acid by the process of fermentation. Lactose is a disaccharide sugar, similar

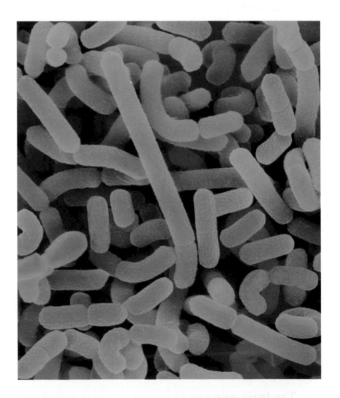

Scanning electron microscope image of lactobacillus acidophilus bacteria. *(Dennis Kunkel / Phototake, Reproduced by permission.)*

to sucrose (ordinary table sugar), that consists of one molecule of glucose and one molecule of galactose bonded to each other. The genus consists of more than 100 species, many of which consist of two or more **strains**. Probably the best known member of the genus is "L. acidophilus"

Description

Lactobacillus is a member of a larger group of bacteria known as lactic acid bacteria (LAB), so named because they convert carbohydrates to lactic acid. Lactobacillus differs from other members of the LAB group in that they are homofermentive, that is, they produce lactic acid only as their primary (>85%) metabolic product. Other LAB produce other fermentative products, such as ethanol (ethyl alcohol), acetic acid, and carbon dioxide in addition to lactic acid. Lactobacillus bacteria are an important component of the gut flora in humans; they are also found in the female genital system. The term gut flora refers to all the bacteria and other microorganisms that live in the human intestinal system and that, for the most part, are benign and play useful roles in the digestive process. Their beneficial function is to some extent a result of their production of lactic acid, which provides an acidic environment in which disease–causing microorganisms are less able to survive. Lactobacillus also occur in many environments other than the human digestive and genital systems, specifically, in any condition in which dead or decaying plant material is available as a food source.

The lactobacilli are of special interest to researchers, at least partly because of their relatively simple genetic and biochemical structure. As of 2008, the genomes of three species, "L. plantarum", "L. johnsonii", and "L. acidophilus" had been completely sequenced, while the genomes of at least four other members of the genus were at least partially determined.

Uses

Historically, lactobacillus bacteria have played a very important role in many kinds of food production. They are used in the manufacture of cheese and yogurt; sauerkraut, pickles, and kimchi; beer, wine, and cider; and silage, fermented plant matter used as feed for domestic animals. Two common species used in food production are "L. casei" and "L. brevis".

The basic principle behind the use of lactobacilli as dietary supplements is that the human digestive system consists of a finely balanced mixture of beneficial ("good") and harmful ("bad") bacteria. Beneficial bacteria contribute to and support many biochemical reactions that promote growth and development, while harmful bacteria attack systems, leading to disease. In healthy individuals, the body maintains a proper balance between "good" and "bad" bacteria. Any number of conditions may cause a disruption in this balance that can result in disease. For example, the use of antibiotics to treat an infectious disease may result in the destruction of beneficial as well as harmful bacteria. Without the benefit of "good" bacteria to keep "bad" bacteria under control, other diseases may develop. For this reason, health care workers routinely recommend that patients on antibiotics supplement the bacteria in their digestive system by eating yogurt containing a lactobacillus to maintain a proper bacterial balance in their digestive systems.

The most common use of lactobacilli in medicine is as **probiotics**. A probiotic is a dietary supplement consisting of microorganisms thought to have potentially beneficial effects in the digestive system of humans and other animals, with the potential for preventing the growth of pathogenic (disease–causing) organisms. The lactobacillus most widely used for this purpose is "L. acidophilus". A number of diseases and disorders for which "L. acidophilus" has been recommended, with greater or lesser scientific support, include:

- acne
- cancer
- cardiovascular disease
- constipation
- Crohn's disease
- diverticulitis
- heartburn
- indigestion
- stomach ulcers
- ulcerative colitis
- urinary tract infections
- vaginal yeast infections
- weakened immune system

The scientific validity of claims such as these is the subject of considerable research. In November 2005, the National Center for Complementary and Alternative Medicine (NCCAM) held a conference of researchers to determine the current state of knowledge about the use of probiotics in general. The conference reported that there is "encouraging evidence" for claims that support the use of probiotics in the treatment of a number of conditions, including treatment for:

- diarrhea, for which the evidence is strongest of any condition
- urinary tract and genital tract infections
- irritable bowel syndrome
- bladder cancer (reduction in the risk of recurrence)
- pouchitis (a condition that develops after surgery for removal of the colon)
- atopic dermatitis (eczema) in children

The conference report also concluded that "in studies of probiotics as cures, any beneficial effect was usually low; a strong **placebo effect** often occurs; and more research . . . is needed in order to draw firmer conclusions."

Side effects

Probiotics have been used extensively for many years, with few or no generally recognized side effects. However, well–controlled scientific studies on the subject are largely absent and need to be undertaken to gain a better understanding for the potential of such effects. Some moderate side effects of using probiotics like lactobacilli are already well known and include bloating, **gas**, and **indigestion**. Theoretically, the introduction of bacteria into the digestive system could result in infectious disease, but virtually nothing is known as to the practical likelihood of such an event.

Interactions

Scientists have hypothesized a number of possible interactions between lactobacillus and various herbs and drugs. Alcohol and antibiotics, for example, may be toxic to lactobacillus and should, therefore, not be taken at or near the same time that a probiotic is ingested. Another hypothesis suggests that lactobacillus thrives in a digestive environment that is only moderately acidic, so that taking a antacid prior to using a probiotic will increase the efficacy of the lactobacillus. Some evidence suggests also that lactobacillus may extend the period over which some drugs remain in the body. As an example, a probiotic may magnify the effects of a drug such as lorazepam, one of whose side effects is drowsiness. Herbal practitioners sometimes recommend that certain foods be taken in conjunction with lactobacillus because they are especially efficient at promoting the growth of the bacteria. These foods include asparagus, bananas, **garlic**, Jerusalem artichokes, and onions. At this point, scientific evidence to support any of the side effects is almost completely lacking.

KEY TERMS

Disaccharide—A type of sugar that consists of two simpler (monosaccharide) sugars.

Gram–positive bacteria—Bacteria that turn purple in the Gram staining process. They lack a secondary outer membrane that allows dye to enter and stain the bacterial cell.

Gut flora—A term used to describe all of the microorganisms living in the digestive system.

Lactic acid bacteria (LAB)—Bacteria that convert carbohydrates to lactic acid as a major metabolic product.

Probiotic—A dietary supplement consisting of microorganisms with potential beneficial effects in the digestive system of humans and other animals and potential blocking effects on pathogenic organisms.

Resources

BOOKS

Dash, S. K.. *The Consumer's Guide To Probiotics: The Complete Source Book*. Topanga, Calif.: Freedom Press, 2005.

Elmer, Gary W., Lynne V. McFarland, and Marc McFarland. *The Power of Probiotics: Improving Your Health With Beneficial Microbes*. Binghamton, NY: Haworth Press, 2007.

Huffnagle, Gary B., and Sarah Wernick. *The Probiotics Revolution: The Definitive Guide to Safe, Natural Health Solutions Using Probiotic and Prebiotic Foods and Supplements*. New York: Bantam Books, 2007.

Lactobacillus acidophilus – A Medical Dictionary, Bibliography, and Annotated Research Guide to Internet References. San Diego: ICON Health Publications, 2004.

Tannock, Gerald W., ed. *Probiotics and Prebiotics: Scientific Aspects*. Wymondham, Norfolk, U.K.: Caister Academic Press, 2005.

PERIODICALS

Alvarez–Olmost, M. I., and R. A. Oberhelman. "Probiotic Agents and Infectious Diseases: A Modern Perspective on a Traditional Therapy." *Clinical Infectious Diseases* (June 2001): 1567–1576.

Cabana, M. D., et al. "Probiotics in Primary Care Pediatrics." *Clinical Pediatrics* (June 2006): 405–410.

Doron, S., and S. L. Gorbach. "Probiotics: Their Role in the Treatment and Prevention of Disease." *Expert Review of Anti–Infective Therapy* (April 2006): 261–275.

Huebner, E. S., and C. M. Surawicz. "Probiotics in the Prevention and Treatment of Gastrointestinal Infections." *Gastroenterology Clinics of North America* (June 2006): 355–365.

Reid, G., and J. A. Hammond. "Probiotics: Some Evidence of Their Effectiveness." *Canadian Family Physician* (November 2005): 1487–1493.

Vanderhoof, J. A., and R. J. Young. "Current and Potential Uses of Probiotics." *Annals of Allergy, Asthma, & Immunology* (November 2004): S33–S37.

OTHER

Aetna InteliHealth. "Lactobacillus acidophilus." http://www.intelihealth.com/IH/ihtIH/WSIHW000/8513/31402/347266.html?d=dmtContent#uses (February 17, 2008).

MedicineNet.com. "Probiotics." http://www.medicinenet.com/probiotics/article.htm (February 17, 2008).

Sahelian, Ray. "Lactobacillus." http://www.raysahelian.com/lactobacillus.html (February 17, 2008).

David Edward Newton, Ed.D.

Laetrile *see* **Apricot seed**

Lapacho *see* **Pau d'arco**

Laryngitis

Definition

Laryngitis is caused by inflammation of the larynx, often resulting in a temporary loss of voice.

Description

When air is breathed in, it passes through the nose and the nasopharynx or through the mouth and the oropharynx. These are both connected to the larynx, a tube made of cartilage. The vocal cords, responsible for setting up the vibrations necessary for speech, are located within the larynx.

The air continues down the larynx to the trachea. The trachea then splits into two branches, the left and right bronchi (bronchial tubes). These bronchi branch into smaller air tubes that run within the lungs, leading to the small air sacs of the lungs (alveoli).

Either food, liquid, or air may be taken in through the mouth. While air goes into the larynx and the respiratory system, food and liquid are directed into the tube leading to the stomach, the esophagus. Because food or liquid in the bronchial tubes or lungs could cause a blockage or lead to an infection, the airway must be protected. The epiglottis is a leaf-like piece of cartilage extending upwards from the larynx. The epiglottis can close down over the larynx when someone is eating or drinking, preventing these substances from entering the airway.

In laryngitis, the tissues below the level of the epiglottis are swollen and inflamed. This causes swelling around the area of the vocal cords and they can't vibrate normally. Hoarse sounds or loss of voice are characteristic of laryngitis. Laryngitis is a very common problem, and often occurs during an upper respiratory tract infection (cold).

Causes and symptoms

Laryngitis is primarily caused by overuse of the voice, a condition faced by people ranging from teachers to performers. Other causes of laryngitis include:

- strain on the larynx from talking or singing for long periods
- shouting or cheering for an extended time
- allergies
- colds or cough
- smoking
- alcohol consumption
- atmospheric conditions like dust in the air
- anxiety
- underactive thyroid
- growths on the larynx

However, the primary medical cause of laryngitis is a viral infection. The same viruses that cause the majority of simple colds are responsible for laryngitis. In extremely rare cases, more harmful bacteria or the bacteria that causes **tuberculosis** (TB) may cause laryngitis. In people with faulty immune systems (like AIDS patients), **infections** with fungi may be responsible for laryngitis.

Symptoms usually begin with a cold. The person may have a sore, scratchy throat, as well as a **fever**, runny nose, aches, and **fatigue**. Difficulty swallowing sometimes occurs, and the patient may have a ticklish **cough** or wheeze. Most characteristically, the patient suffers voice loss or the voice will sound strained, hoarse, and raspy.

In extremely rare cases, the swelling of the larynx may cause symptoms of airway obstruction. This is more common in infants because the diameter of their airways is so small. In that case, the baby may have a greatly increased respiratory rate and exhibit loud, high-pitched sounds with breathing (called stridor).

Diagnosis

Laryngitis is easily recognizable. People realize they can't speak or that their voices are hoarse. In most cases, they know the cause. Laryngitis could be the next phase of the flu or the result of cheering too energetically during a football game. In addition to being an easily recognizable condition, laryngitis is a self-limiting condition that goes away on its own. In most cases, laryngitis can be treated at home.

However, a doctor should be consulted if the laryngitis occurs for no apparent reason or if hoarseness lasts for more than two weeks. A doctor may diagnose another condition such as an underactive thyroid. Symptoms of underactive thyroid include tiredness, **constipation**, aches, and dry skin.

Diagnosis is usually made by learning the history of a cold that is followed by hoarseness. The throat usually appears red and somewhat swollen. Listening to the chest, neck, and back with a stethoscope (an instrument used to hear heart and lungs sounds) may reveal some harsh wheezing sounds when the person breathes.

With chronic laryngitis, TB may be suspected. Using an instrument called a laryngoscope, a doctor can examine the airway for redness, swelling, small bumps of tissue called nodules, and irritated pits in the tissue called ulcerations. Special skin testing (TB testing) will reveal if the person has been exposed to TB.

Treatment

Alternative treatments for laryngitis include various herbal therapies, as well as **reflexology**, homeopathy, **relaxation**, and exercise . Resting the voice is especially important, as is consulting a doctor or practitioner if symptoms last for more than two weeks.

Practitioners who treat laryngitis include naturopathic doctors and ayurvedic doctors. **Naturopathic medicine** focuses on whole body health care; the ayurvedic practitioner concentrates on maintaining balance between the body and the world.

Acupuncture or accupressure, elements of **traditional Chinese medicine** (TCM), may provide some relief. A TCM practitioner may prescribe Throat Inflammation Pills, which are also known as Laryngitis Pills. The pill is an over-the-counter Chinese formula. The usual dosage for adults is 10 pills taken three times daily. This is a short-term treatment and should be stopped after three days.

An ayurvedic practitioner could prescribe an infusion of mint, **ginger**, or cloves, as well as a milk decoction or **licorice** root powder.

Herbal remedies

Numerous herbals can be used to treat laryngitis. Herbal lozenges and throat sprays can provide immediate relief to a raw throat. Herbs that are effective for laryngitis include **thyme**, **horehound**, cardamom, plantain, cinnamon, and **eucalyptus**. Commercial cough medicines that are effective include herbs such as **anise**, **fennel**, and **peppermint**. A person can gargle with warm salt water and slippery elm bark, wild cherry, and mallow.

Echinacea tincture taken in water is recommended to boost the immune system. The tincture consists of 10 drops (1/8 teaspoon or 5/8 ml) of the herb in a glass of water. This mixture is taken frequently, or 5 ml three to four times a day. Antiviral herbs such as usnea, **lomatium**, and ligusticum may help speed recovery.

Poke should be taken as a last resort. It's a strong herb that should be taken only in small amounts and under the direction of a healthcare professional. However, there are many other herbs that can be purchased as packaged cold and throat remedies or used to prepare home treatments.

HYDROTHERAPY. A person can use a vaporizer for relief by inhaling steam. A natural version of the vaporizer is a boiling pot of water with herbs or **essential oils** added. The amount of these ingredients varies. A small handful of **sage** or eucalyptus leaves may be added to the water. When using essential oils, 1-2 teaspoons (4.5-10 g) of an oil such as sage, eucalyptus, **lavender**, benzoin, frankincense, thyme, or sandalwood are added. The pot is removed from the stove and the ingredients are allowed to steep. The person places a towel over the head for a tent-like effect, leans over the pot, and breathes in steam through the mouth.

HERBAL TEAS. Commercial products like horehound tea will provide relief. For brewing tea at home, 1 cup (250 ml) of boiling water is poured over 1-2 teaspoons (4.5-10 g) of an herb. The tea is steeped for about 10 minutes and then strained. Generally, up to 3 cups of tea may be drunk daily.

Helpful herbs for teas include capsicum (cayenne), which is used to treat conditions caused by a cold or flu. Capsicum tea might be a painful treatment if inflammation is severe. Ginger root helps with chest congestion. Other useful herbs include cardamom, eucalyptus, spearmint, **rosemary**, sweet Annie, **nutmeg**, lavender, bee balm, peppermint, tansy, mallows, and **mullein**.

GARGLES. A home gargle is prepared like herbal tea. One cup (250 ml) of boiling water is poured over 1-2 teaspoons (4.5-10 g) of an herb. This mixture is steeped for about 10 minutes and then strained. The solution is gargled for about 10 seconds, and repeated every three to four hours. Herbs recommended for gargling include **coltsfoot**, garden **raspberry**, golden seal, mullein, **plantain**, red sage, **yarrow**, licorice, and **slippery elm**.

Other home remedies

A range of other home remedies will bring relief to laryngitis and its symptoms. These include:

- Drinking more liquids and eating raw fruit and vegetables.
- Eating certain foods. Candied ginger, honey, lemon, and pineapple juice are soothing. Spicy foods with ingredients like garlic, cayenne pepper, horseradish, mustard, or ginger are helpful.
- Using vitamins. They can also help the immune system. The recommended dosages are 1,000-3,000 mg of vitamin C and 10,000-20,000 I.U. of vitamin A (beta carotene).
- Using a compress. A compress is a form of hydrotherapy that starts by placing a warm washcloth on the neck. Next, a long cotton cloth is soaked in cold water. After the cloth is wrung out, it is wrapped around the neck. Then a long piece of wool flannel such as a scarf is wrapped around the wet cloth. The flannel is secured with a safety pin and remains in place for at least 30 minutes. The compress can be worn overnight.
- Relaxing and exercising. Since anxiety can cause laryngitis, both relaxation techniques and physical exercise can reduce stress.
- Breathing deeply. Deep breaths and breathing exercises can make the respiratory system stronger.

Reflexology

Reflexology is a healing method that involves the manipulation of certain parts of the body to bring about balance. For laryngitis, the reflexology focus is on the throat, lung, chest, lymphatic system, and diaphragm points on both feet. Also recommended is manipulation of all points on the sides and bottoms of the toes.

Homeopathy

Homeopathy is a healing method that is based on the theory that "like cures like." The potency of a homeopathic remedy is indicated by an "x." This indicates the number of times that one part of a remedy was diluted in nine parts of a dilutant. Distilled water is the preferred dilutant. The potency of a remedy can also be expressed as "c," the number of times one part of the remedy was diluted in 99 parts of a dilutant.

Homeopathic remedies for laryngitis include:

- Aconite (6x or 12x). It's taken every two hours at the very start of a cold or when the voice is lost and the person has a dry cough. If there is no improvement after four or five hours, another remedy such as spongia tosta is taken.
- Spongia tosta (12x). It's taken four times daily for laryngitis combined with a dry throat.
- Arnica (6x or 12x). It's taken hourly when loss of voice is caused by overuse or trauma.

Allopathic treatment

Treatment of a simple, viral laryngitis relieves the symptoms. Gargling with warm salt water, using **pain** relievers such as acetaminophen, using a vaporizer to create moist air, and resting will help the illness resolve within a week. Over-the-counter remedies such as throat sprays and lozenges may provide relief.

For an infant who is clearly struggling for air, a doctor may put in an artificial airway for a short period of time. This is very rarely needed.

When a doctor is consulted, antibiotics may be prescribed. The person with an underactive thyroid could be prescribed a thyroid hormone supplement. An individual with tubercular laryngitis is treated with a combination of medications used to treat classic TB. For people with fungal laryngitis, a variety of antifungal medications are available.

Expected results

The prognosis for people with laryngitis is excellent because it is a self-limiting condition. Recovery is complete, usually within a week. In the meantime, alternative remedies can provide relief.

Prevention

Prevention of laryngitis is the same as for any upper respiratory infection. People should wash their hands frequently and thoroughly, and should avoid contact with people who might be sick. However, even with relatively good hygiene practices, most people will get about five to six colds per year. It is unpredictable which of these may lead to laryngitis.

Resting the voice is important, particularly for people like teachers, politicians, or actors who talk for long periods. Not speaking for a time is one way to rest the voice. Before giving a lengthy speech or attending an exciting championship game, herbal remedies can be used preventively to soothe the larynx. If **anxiety** provokes laryngitis, a person should practice a relaxation technique or **exercise** to reduce **stress**.

In all cases, **smoking** should be avoided. Since alcohol can irritate the throat, consumption may need to be limited.

Resources

BOOKS

Albright, Peter. *The Complete Book of Complementary Therapies*. Allentown, PA: People's Medical Society, 1997.

Duke, James A. *The Green Pharmacy*. Emmaus, PA: Rodale Press, Inc.,1997.

Fauci, Anthony S., et al., eds. *Harrison's Principles of Internal Medicine*. New York: McGraw-Hill, 1998.

Gottlieb, Bill. *New Choices in Natural Healing*. Emmaus, PA: Rodale Press, Inc., 1995.

Keville, Kathi. *Herbs for Health and Healing*. Emmaus, PA: Rodale Press, Inc., 1996.

Medical Economics Company. *PDR for Herbal Medicines*. Montvale, N.J: 1998.

Stoffman, Phyllis. *The Family Guide to Preventing and Treating 100 Infectious Diseases*. New York: John Wiley and Sons, Inc., 1995.

Time-Life Books Editors. *The Alternative Advisor*. Alexandria, VA: Time-Life Books, 1997.

Tyler, Varro, and Steven Foster. *Tyler's Honest Herbal*. Binghamton, NY: The Haworth Herbal Press, 1999.

ORGANIZATIONS

American Botanical Council. P.O. Box 201660, Austin, TX, 78720. (512) 331-8868. http://www.herbalgram.org

Herb Research Foundation. 1007 Pearl St., Suite 200, Boulder, CO 80302. (303) 449-2265. http://www.herbs.org

OTHER

Holistic OnLine. http://www.holisticonline.com.

MotherNature.com Health Encyclopedia. http://www.mothernature.com/ency.

Liz Swain

Laughter therapy *see* **Humor therapy**

Lavender

Description

Lavender is a hardy perennial in the Lamiaciae, or mint, family. The herb is a Mediterranean native. There are many species of lavendula which vary somewhat in appearance and aromatic quality. English lavender, *L. augustifolia*, also known as true lavender, is commercially valuable in the perfume industry and is a mainstay of English country gardens. French lavender, *L.stoechas*, is the species most probably used in Roman times as a scenting agent in washing water. The species *L. officinalis* is the official species used in medicinal preparations, though all lavenders have medicinal properties in varying degrees.

This fragrant, bushy shrub has been widely cultivated for its essential oil. The tiny, tubular, mauve-blue blossoms grow in whorls of six to ten flowers along square, angular stems and form a terminal spike. These flower spikes stretch upward beyond the

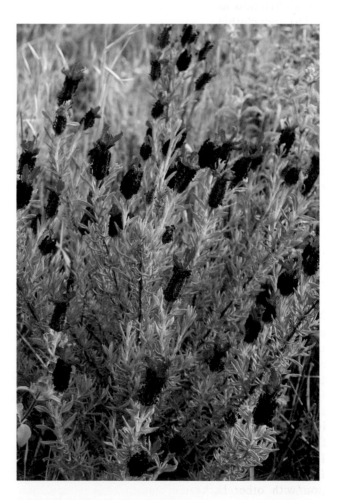

French lavender. (© *blickwinkel / Alamy*)

12-18 inch (3.6-5.4 m) height of the shrub, blooming from June to August. The blossoms are well liked by bees and a good source of honey. The needle-like, evergreen, downy leaves are a light, silver-gray. They are lanceolate, opposite, and sessile, and grow from a branched stem. The bark is gray and flaky. The herb thrives in full sun and poor soil. Ancient Greeks and Romans used lavender blossoms to scent bath water, a common use that gave the herb its name, derived from the Latin *lavare*, meaning to wash.

General use

Lavender is best known and loved for its fragrance. The herb has been used since ancient times in perfumery. As an aromatic plant, lavender lifts the spirits and chases melancholy. Taking just a few whiffs of this sweet-smelling herb is said to dispel **dizziness**. Traditionally, women in labor clutched sprigs of lavender to bring added courage and strength to the task of childbearing. A decoction of the flower may be used as a feminine douche for leucorrhoea. The dried blossoms, sewn into sachets, may be used to repel moths and to scent clothing, or may be lit like incense to scent a room. Because of its fumigant properties, the herb was hung in the home to repel flies and mosquitoes, and strewn about to sanitize the floors. Lavender essential oil was a component of smelling salts in Victorian times.

The essential oil of certain lavender species has a sedative, antispasmodic, and tranquilizing effect. Lavender has been long valued as a **headache** remedy. It can be taken in a mild infusion, or can be rubbed on the temples, or sniffed like smelling salts to provide relief from headaches caused by **stress**. Lavender oil is antiseptic, and has been used as a topical disinfectant for **wounds**. In high doses, it can kill many common bacteria such as typhoid, diphtheria, streptococcus, and pneumococcus, according to some research. The essential oil has also been used as a folk treatment for the bite of some venomous snakes. When used in **hydrotherapy** as part of an aromatic, Epsom salt bath, the **essential oils** of some species will soothe tired nerves and relieve the **pain** of **neuralgia**. They are also used topically on **burns** and have been shown to speed healing. It is also a fine addition to a foot bath for sore feet. Lavender essence makes a pleasant massage oil for kneading sore muscles and joints. Acting internally, lavender's chemical properties increase the flow of bile into the intestines, relieving **indigestion**. Its carminative properties help expel intestinal **gas**. Lavender is an adjuvant and may be used in combination with other herbs to make a tonic cordial to strengthen the nervous system.

KEY TERMS

Adjuvant—A characteristic of an herb that enhances the benefits of other ingredients when added to a mixture.

Carminative—A property of an herb that assists in relieving intestinal gas.

Coumarins—These blood-thinning plant chemicals break down red blood cells. Coumarins are responsible for the fresh- mown lawn aroma that some herbs exude.

Flavonoids—There are numerous phytochemicals known as flavones. Most exert a pharmacological effect, depending on their type. Flavonoids are one type of flavone.

Sessile— A botanical term to describe a leaf that emerges from the plant stem without a stalk.

Tannins—These astringent plant chemicals are the medicinal constituent of an herb that enables it to facilitate healing of wounds.

Volatile or essential oils—Simple molecules that give the plant its scent. When applied to the skin, volatile oil extracts are absorbed into the bloodstream through the fatty layer of the skin.

A 2002 report from Korea showed that **aromatherapy** massage with lavender oil and **tea tree oil** on patients undergoing hemodialysis for kidney failure received relief from the **itching** the treatment often causes.

Preparations

The medicinal properties of lavender are extracted primarily from the oil glands in the leaf and blossom. The plant contains volatile oil, tannins, coumarins, flavonoids, and triterpenoids as active chemical components. These phytochemicals are the plant constituents responsible for the medicinal properties. Lavender's volatile oil is best when extracted from flowers picked before they reach maximum bloom and following a long period of hot and dry temperatures. The flower spikes dry quickly when spread on a mat in an airy place away from direct sun.

Distilled oil: The essential oil of lavender is extracted by steam distillation. Just a few drops of this essential oil are effective for topical applications. Commercial distillations of this essential oil are readily available.

Lavender tea: An infusion of the fresh or dried flowers and leaf can be made by pouring a pint of boiling water over one ounce of the dry leaf and flower, or two ounces fresh herb, in a non-metallic pot. It can be steeped (covered) for about ten minutes, strained and sweetened to taste. It should be drunk while still warm. Lavender tea may be taken throughout the day, a mouthful at a time, or warm, by the cup, up to three cups per day. Lavender works well in combination with other medicinal herbs in infusion.

Lavender oil extract: In a glass container, one ounce of freshly harvested lavender flowers can be combined with 1-1/2 pints of olive oil, sufficient to cover the herb. It should be placed in a sunny window-sill for about three days and shaken daily. After three days, the mixture should be strained through muslin or cheesecloth. More fresh flowers should be added and the process repeated until the oil has the desired aromatic strength. Lavender extract can be safely used internally to treat migraines, and nervous indigestion. A few drops on a sugar cube can speed headache relief. Externally, a small amount of lavender oil, rubbed on sore joints, can relieve rheumatism. The essential oil has also been used to minimize scar tissue when applied to burned skin.

Lavender sachet: Dried lavender blossoms and leaves can be sewn into a small cloth bag to scent linens and deter insects. The bag may be placed beneath the pillow as an aromatherapy.

Lavender vinegar: Fresh leaves and blossoms may be steeped in white vinegar for seven days, then strained and stored in a tightly capped bottle.

Precautions

Lavender has a long history of use as an essential oil and as a mildly sedative tea. When taken in moderation the tea is safe. It is important to note that, as with all essential oils, high or chronic doses of lavender essential oil are toxic to the kidney and liver. Infants are even more easily overdosed than adults.

Interestingly, lavender's relaxant effects were put to the test in a 2002 study on aromatherapy's effects on improved mental or physical performance. It seems that study subjects who smelled lavender actually did worse on mental tests than those who smelled nothing at all. So those choosing to use lavender's soothing effects should perhaps choose the timing carefully.

Side effects

No known side effects.

Interactions

As an adjuvant, lavender can enhance the helpful properties of other herbs when used in combination. **Lemon balm** (*Melissa officinalis*) leaves can be combined with lavender as a headache infusion. For cramping, an infusion of lavender and **valerian** (*Valeriana officinalis*) makes a soothing tea. Lavender's pleasant scent works well to cover disagreeable odors of other herbs in medicinal combinations. A tonic cordial can be made by combining fresh **rosemary** (*Rosmarinus officinalis*) leaves, cinnamon, **nutmeg**, and sandlewood with the lavender blossoms and steeping the mixture in brandy for about a week.

Resources

BOOKS

Blumenthal, Mark. *The Complete German Commission E Monographs, Therapeutic Guide to Herbal Medicines* Massachusetts: Integrative Medicine Communications, 1998.

Bown, Deni. *The Herb Society of America, Encyclopedia of Herbs & Their Uses*. New York: D.K. Publications, Inc., 1995

Kowalchik, Claire and Hylton, William H., Editors. *Rodale's Illustrated Encyclopedia of Herbs*. Pennsylvania: Rodale Press, 1987

Lust, John B. *The Herb Book*. New York: Bantam Books, 1974.

Mabey, Richard. *The New Age Herbalist*. New York: Simon & Schuster, Inc.,1998.

McIntyre, Anne. *The Medicinal Garden*. New York: Henry Holt and Company, 1997.

McVicar, Jekka. *Herbs For The Home*. New York: Penguin Books, 1994.

Peterson, Nocola. *Culpeper Guides, Herbs And Health*. New York: Seafarer Books, Penguin Books, 1994.

Forsell, Mary. *Heirloom Herbs*. New York: Villard Books, 1990.

Phillips, Roger and Foy, Nicky. *The Random House Book of Herbs*. New York: Random House, 1990.

PERIODICALS

Carlson, Mike, et al. "Rosemary on my Mind (Memory Booster)." *Men's Fitness* (August 2002): 28.

Ro, You-Ja, et al. "The Effects of Aromatherapy on Pruritis in Patients Undergoing Hemodialysis." *Dermatology Nursing* (August 2002):231- 238.

Clare Hanrahan
Teresa G. Odle

Lazy eye

Definition

Lazy eye, or amblyopia, is an eye condition in which disuse causes reduced vision in an otherwise healthy eye. The affected eye is called the *lazy* eye.

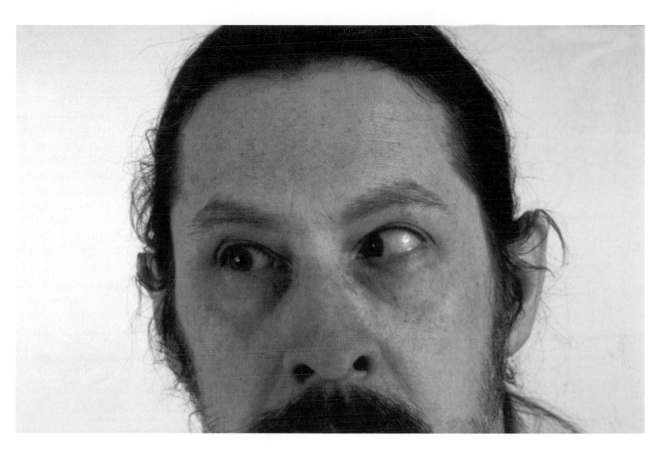

Man with a lazy eye. *(Custom Medical Stock Photo. Reproduced by permission.)*

This vision defect occurs in 2–3% of American children. If not corrected before age eight, amblyopia will cause significant loss of stereoscopic vision, the ability to perceive three-dimensional depth.

Description

In some children, one eye functions better than the other. When a child begins to depend on the stronger eye, the weaker eye can become progressively weaker. Eventually, the weaker eye grows "lazy" from disuse. If left untreated beyond the early child-development years (from birth to seven years old), vision in the affected eye will be underdeveloped due to lack of use.

The impairment of vision in the lazy eye occurs in three phases. In the first (suspension) phase, the brain turns the weaker eye on and off. In the second (suppression) phase, the brain turns off the lazy eye indefinitely. At this point, the eye still has usable vision and can function well if the other eye is covered. In the last (amblyopia) phase, which occurs after age seven, the eye loses all the sensitivity that is essential for good vision because it has not been used for so long.

Lazy eye is a visual problem with potentially serious consequences. If left untreated, the affected child may have permanent loss of vision in the lazy eye. Because of loss of vision in one eye, these children cannot see three-dimensional images very well—all images appear flat. They also have problems with depth perception. This has serious consequences in their future ability to work in professions that require good vision in both eyes. Affected children also have increased risk of blindness should something happen to the good eye.

Causes and symptoms

The following are probable causes of lazy eye:

- Strabismus, or misalignment of a child's eyes (crossed eyes). This is the most frequent cause of lazy eye. Approximately half of all children with crossed eyes will develop a lazy eye. In children with crossed eyes, the images do not coordinate, thus confusing the brain. Therefore, the brain will suppress the image that comes from one eye and predominantly use the image from the stronger eye.

- Anisometropia (unequal refractive power). In this case, there is difference in image quality between the two eyes because one eye is severely nearsighted or farsighted. In other words, one eye focuses better than the other. The brain will mostly use the clearer image from the good eye. The other eye will become underdeveloped due to neglect.
- Congenital cataract. The lazy eye can not see well because its lens is already cloudy at birth.
- Ptosis (drooping eyelid). Vision in the lazy eye is blocked or impaired by the drooping eyelid.
- Corneal scarring. The image quality of the affected eye is poor due to scarring in the cornea.

The following are risk factors for amblyopia:

- Rubella (German measles) or other infections in the mother during pregnancy
- premature birth
- other family members with vision problems in childhood

Lazy eye may not present obvious symptoms. For this reason, it is important for small children to have regular eye examinations.

Diagnosis

Diagnosis of amblyopia is often made during visual screening during routine infant check-ups and in the preschool years (aged three to five). Premature babies need to have more frequent eye exams during early childhood to prevent this and other vision problems. A new photoscreening instrument that has been recently introduced appears to significantly increase the accuracy of diagnosis of these eye problems.

Treatment

The following alternative methods may complement conventional treatment of lazy eye. However, they are not replacements for conventional treatments. Because their effectiveness is not proven, parents should consult their child's ophthalmologist about the appropriate use of these methods (if any) in their child's overall eye treatment program.

Orthoptics (eye exercises)

Eye exercises can be helpful. Orthoptic exercises are designed to help the eyes move together and assist the fusing of the two images seen by the eyes. It can help correct faulty vision habit due to misalignment of the eyes and can teach the child to use both eyes effectively and comfortably. This form of therapy can be used before or after eye-realignment surgery to improve results.

Vision therapy

Vision training is a form of physical therapy for the brain and the eyes. It is a more extensive form of eye exercise and requires more frequent visits.

Acupuncture

One study shows that **acupuncture** treatment may be effective in treating anisometropia, a condition in which one eye focuses much better than the other. Acupuncture can reduce the differences in refractive powers between the eyes so that both eyes can have similar image quality. This helps reduce the amblyopia problem. However, its long-term effectiveness remains unknown.

Allopathic treatment

In order to treat lazy eye, the doctor has to identify and treat underlying causes. Depending on these underlying causes, the doctor may recommend surgical or nonsurgical treatments, as discussed below.

Refractive error correction

If both eyes need vision correction, children are given prescription glasses for better focus and to prevent misalignment of the eyes.

Forcing the use of the lazy eye

In many children with amblyopia, only one eye has a focusing problem or weak muscles. In order to force the affected eye to work, the doctor will cover the strong eye with a patch for most of the day for at least several weeks. Sometimes, this treatment requires as long as a year. The eye patch forces the lazy eye to work and thus, strengthens its vision and its muscles. This is the most common method used to treat lazy eye. To prevent the strong eye from becoming weaken due to disuse, the child is allowed to remove the patch so that he can see with the good eye for at least a few hours each day.

Another way to force the lazy eye to work harder is to use eye drops or ointment to blur the vision in the strong eye so that the child has to use the lazy eye to see. This method is not often used because it is associated with more adverse effects.

Surgical treatments

If the problem is caused by imbalances of the eye muscles and is not treatable with nonsurgical methods, the eye muscles can be realigned surgically to help the eyes coordinate better. Sometimes more than one surgery is required for the correction. Eye patch, glasses, or orthoptic exercises may be necessary following surgery to help the child use both eyes effectively. Long-term follow-up of surgical treatment indicates that it is highly effective in correcting the problem.

In patients whose amblyopia is caused by a congenital cataract in one eye, the cloudy lens is surgically removed and replaced by an intraocular lens. However, after surgery—even with eye glasses or contact lenses—this eye will still have poorer image quality than the good eye. Thus, the risk for amblyopia remains high. Therefore, nonsurgical treatment for lazy eye is often started after cataract surgery.

For a child whose vision is affected by a drooping eyelid, ptosis surgery is needed.

Expected results

With early diagnosis and treatment, children with amblyopia are expected to restore the sight in the lazy eye. However, if left untreated, the weak eye never develops adequate vision and the person may become functionally blind in that eye.

Prevention

Most cases of lazy eye are congenital, occurring since birth. However, if diagnosed early, vision loss in the affected eye can be prevented.

Resources

BOOKS

"Crossed Eyes." In Reader's Digest Guide to Medical Cures and Treatments. New York: Reader's Digest Association, 1996.

PERIODICALS

Broderick, Peter. "Pediatric Vision Screening for the Family Physician." American Family Physician 58, no. 3 (September 1, 1998): 691–700 + . http://www.aafp.org/afp/980901ap/broderic.html.

Mills, Monte D. "The Eye in Childhood." American Family Physician 60, no. 3 (September 1, 1999): 907–18. http://www.aafp.org/afp/990901ap/907.html.

Paysse, Evelyn A., et al. "Detection of Red Reflex Asymmetry by Pediatric Residents Using the Bruckner Reflex Versus the MTI Photoscreener." Pediatrics 108 (October 2001): 997.

ORGANIZATIONS

American Academy of Ophthalmology. P.O. Box 7424, San Francisco, CA 94120-7424. (415) 561-8500. http://www.eyenet.org.

American Association For Pediatric Ophthalmology and Strabismus. c/o Denise De Losada Wilson. P.O. Box 193832, San Francisco, CA 94119-3832. (415) 561-8505. aapos@aao.org. http://med-aapos.bu.edu.

National Association for Parents of the Visually Impaired, Inc. P.O. Box 317, Watertown, MA 02471. (800) 562-6265. Fax: (617) 972-7444. http://www.spedex.com/napvi.

OTHER

"Congenital Eye Defects." The Merck Manual Online. http://www.merck.com/pubs/mmanual/section19/chapter261/261i.htm.

Mai Tran
Rebecca J. Frey, PhD

Lead poisoning

Definition

Lead poisoning occurs when a person swallows, absorbs, or inhales lead in any form. The result can be damaging to the brain, nerves, and many other parts of the body. Acute lead poisoning, which is somewhat rare, occurs when a person ingests a relatively large amount of lead over a short period of time. Chronic lead poisoning—a common problem in children—occurs when small amounts of lead are taken in over a longer period. The Centers for Disease Control and Prevention (CDC) defines childhood lead poisoning as a whole-blood lead concentration equal to or greater than 10 mcg/dL.

Description

Lead can damage almost every system in the human body, and it can also cause high blood pressure (**hypertension**). It is particularly harmful to the

Sources of lead poisoning

Source	Description
Paint	Lead-based paint can be a hazard in older homes. Children eat peeling paint, or come in contact with it during remodeling projects.
Dust and soil	Contamination of soil is usually caused by paint, leaded gasoline, pollution from industrial sites, and smelters.
Foods	Lead can be found in imported canned foods, leaded crystal, and some ceramic dishware.
Activities	Activities such as pottery, stained glassmaking, and furniture refinishing can heighten exposure to lead.
Drinking water	Homes built before 1930 may contain lead water pipes. Newer homes may also contain copper pipes with lead solder.
Traditional remedies & cosmetics	Certain ayurvedic medications, traditionally from India and other Southern Asian countries, may contain lead. Also litargirio (a peach-colored powder used mainly in the Dominican Republic) contains high levels of lead, and the FDA warns against its usage. Kohl is another traditional cosmetic frequently containing high levels of lead.

(Illustration by Corey Light. Cengage Learning, Gale)

developing brain of fetuses and young children. The higher the level of lead in a child's blood, and the longer this elevated level lasts, the greater the chance of ill effects. Over the long term, lead poisoning in a child can lead to learning disabilities, behavioral problems, and mental retardation. At very high levels, lead poisoning can cause seizures, coma, and even death. In one of the rare studies of its kind, the National Center for Environmental Health reported in 2003 that there were about 200 deaths from lead poisoning in the United States between 1979 and 1998. Most of the deaths were among males (74%), African Americans (67%), adults over the age of 45 (76%), and southerners (70%).

Of much greater concern than mortality due to lead poisoning is the number of children who have elevated levels of lead in their blood. Many children are exposed to lead through peeling paint in older homes. Others are exposed through dust or soil that has been contaminated by old paint or past emissions of leaded gasoline. Since children between the ages of 12 and 36 months are apt to put objects in their mouths, they are more likely than older children to take in lead. Pregnant women who come into contact with lead can pass it along to their fetuses.

More than 80% of American homes built before 1978 have lead-based paint in them, according to the Centers for Disease Control and Prevention (CDC). The older the home, the more likely it is to contain lead paint, and the higher the concentration of lead in the paint is apt to be. Some homes also have lead in the water pipes or plumbing. People may have lead in the paint, dust, or soil around their homes or in their drinking water without knowing it, since lead cannot be seen, smelled, or tasted. Because lead does not break down naturally, it can continue to cause problems until it is removed.

Efforts to promote public awareness of lead poisoning problems have had marked success in the United States. The percentage of children under the age of six with unacceptably high concentrations of lead in their blood dropped from 7.6% in 1997 to 1.2% in 2006. In 2008, the CDC expressed confidence that it was approaching the federal government's goal of eliminating childhood lead poisoning by the year 2010.

Causes and symptoms

Before scientists knew how harmful it could be, lead was widely used in paint, gasoline, water pipes, and many other products. In the 2000s, house paint is almost lead-free, gasoline is unleaded, and household plumbing is no longer made with lead materials. Still, remnants of the old hazards remain. Following are some sources of lead exposure:

- Lead-based paint. The most common source of exposure to large amounts of lead among preschoolers, paint chips from older homes that have fallen into disrepair are eaten by children. They may also chew on painted surfaces, such as windowsills. In addition, paint may be disturbed during remodeling.
- Dust and soil. These can be contaminated with lead from old paint or past emissions of leaded gasoline. In addition, pollution from operating or abandoned industrial sites and smelters can find its way into the soil, resulting in soil contamination.
- Drinking water. Exposure may come from lead water pipes, found in many homes built before 1930. Even newer copper pipes may have lead solder. Also, some new homes have brass faucets and fittings that can leach lead.
- Jobs and hobbies. A number of activities can expose participants to lead. These include making pottery or stained glass, refinishing furniture, doing home repairs, and using indoor firing ranges. When adults take part in such activities, they may inadvertently expose children to lead residue that is on their clothing or on scrap materials.
- Food. Imported food cans often have lead solder. Lead may also be found in leaded crystal glassware and some imported ceramic or old ceramic dishes (e.g., ceramic dishes from Mexico). A 2003 study of cases of lead poisoning in pregnant women found that 70% of the patients were Hispanics, most of whom had absorbed the lead from their pottery. In addition, food may be contaminated by lead in the water or soil.
- Folk medicines. Certain folk medicines (for example, alarcon, alkohl, azarcon, bali goli, coral, ghasard, greta, liga, pay-loo-ah, and rueda) and traditional cosmetics (kohl, for example) contain large amounts of lead. Also, certain Chinese and Tibetan herbal remedies and techniques are contaminated with lead and other heavy metals, such as mercury.
- Moonshine whiskey. Lead poisoning from drinking illegally distilled liquor is still a cause of death among adults in the southern United States.
- Gunshot wounds. Toxic amounts of lead can be absorbed from bullets or bullet fragments that remain in the body after emergency surgery. The use of lead in some kinds of ammunition has been banned in the United States, and substitutes for lead in other types of ammunition were being developed as of 2008.
- Imported toys. In 2006, the U.S. Consumer Products Safety Commission announced that a number of toy products imported from China were contaminated with lead paint. One of the worst such episodes occurred in 2007 when more than 1.5 million "Thomas & Friends" wooden railway toys painted with lead were recalled. As of 2008, the scope of this problem had not yet been fully determined, nor had adequate methods for controlling the importation of contaminated toys been established.

Chronic lead poisoning

Some evidence suggests that lead may be harmful to children even at low levels that were once thought to be safe, and the risk of damage rises as blood levels of lead increase. The symptoms of chronic lead poisoning take time to develop, however. Children can appear healthy despite having high levels of lead in their blood. Over time, though, problems such as the following may arise:

- learning disabilities
- hyperactivity
- mental retardation
- slowed growth
- hearing loss
- headaches

Scientists also know that certain genetic factors increase the harmful effects of lead poisoning in susceptible children; however, these factors were not completely understood as of 2008.

Lead poisoning is also harmful to adults, who may develop high blood pressure, digestive problems, nerve disorders, **memory loss**, and muscle and joint **pain**. In addition, it can lead to difficulties during **pregnancy**, as well as cause reproductive problems in both men and women.

In the 2000s, chronic exposure to lead in the environment was found to speed up the progression of kidney disorders in patients without diabetes.

Acute lead poisoning

Acute lead poisoning, while less common, shows up more quickly and can be fatal. In such cases, children are almost always affected. Symptoms such as the following may occur:

- severe abdominal pain
- diarrhea
- nausea and vomiting
- weakness of the limbs
- seizures
- coma

Diagnosis

A high level of lead in the blood can be detected with a simple blood test. In fact, testing is the only way to know for sure if children without symptoms have been exposed to lead, since they can appear healthy even as long-term damage occurs. The CDC recommends testing all children at 12 months of age and, if possible, again at 24 months. Testing should start at six months for children at risk for lead poisoning. Based on these test results and a child's risk factors, the doctor decides whether further testing is needed and how often. In some states, more frequent testing is required by law.

Evidence is emerging to indicate that even lower doses of lead than previously thought can cause neurological damage in children. It may be that virtually no level of lead is safe and that measures need to be taken to remove lead from the environment. As of 2008 in the United States, the CDC recommended that lead blood levels in children not exceed 10 mcg/dL.

Children at risk

Children with an increased risk of lead poisoning include those who have the following features:

- live in or regularly visit a house built before 1978 in which chipped or peeling paint is present, particularly poor children in sub-standard housing
- live in or regularly visit a house that was built before 1978 where remodeling is planned or underway
- have a brother or sister, housemate, or playmate who has been diagnosed with lead poisoning
- have the habit of eating dirt or have been diagnosed with pica
- live with an adult whose job or hobby involves exposure to lead
- live near an active lead smelter, battery-recycling plant, or other industry that can create lead pollution

Adults at risk

Testing is also important for adults whose job or hobby puts them at risk for lead poisoning, including the following:

- glazed pottery or stained glass making
- furniture refinishing
- home renovation
- target shooting at indoor firing ranges
- battery reclamation
- precious metal refining
- radiator repair
- art restoration

Treatment

In the event of emergency poisoning, patients or parents should call 911 or the poison hotline at (800) 222-1222. The first step in treating lead poisoning is to avoid further contact with lead. For adults, this usually means making changes at work or in hobbies. For children, it means finding and removing sources of lead in the home. In most states, the public health department can help assess the home and identify lead sources.

If the problem is lead paint, a professional with special training should remove it. Removal of lead-based paint is not a do-it-yourself project. Scraping or sanding lead paint creates large amounts of dust that can poison people in the home. This dust can stay around long after the work is completed. In addition, heating lead paint can release lead into the air. For these reasons, lead paint should be removed only by a professional who knows how to do the job safely and has the equipment to clean up thoroughly. Occupants, especially children and pregnant women, should leave the home until the cleanup is finished.

Medical professionals should take all necessary steps to remove bullets or bullet fragments from patients with gunshot injuries.

Nutritional therapy

While changes in diet are no substitute for medical treatment, they can complement the **detoxification** process. The following nutritional changes are recommended:

- Increased consumption of fresh vegetables, fruits, beans, nuts, whole grains, and seeds.
- Increased consumption of soluble fibers, such as pears, apples, oatmeal, oat bran, rye flour, dried beans, guar gum, pectin, and psyllium.
- Increased consumption of sulfur-containing foods, such as eggs, garlic, and onions. Garlic has been used successfully to reduce lead poisoning in animals.
- Taking high-potency multivitamin/mineral supplements (1 tablet a day).
- Taking additional supplements of vitamin C, B-complex vitamins, iron, calcium, zinc, L-lysine, L-cysteine, and

L-cysteine supplements. These vitamins, minerals, and amino acids help reduce the amount of lead that the body absorbs. Iron is especially important, since people who are deficient in this nutrient absorb more lead. Thiamine, a B-complex vitamin, has been used to treat lead poisoning in animals.

- A 2002 report stated that eating tofu may lower lead levels in the blood since it is rich in calcium.
- Using a filter to prevent lead contamination in the water. Drinking lots of water (at least eight glasses per day) to help the body excrete the toxin.
- Committing to a three-day fast at the end of every season. Fasting is the oldest method of detoxification. During fasting, patients should take supplements and drink four glasses of juice a day to assist the cleansing process and to prevent exhaustion.

Herbal therapy

Milk thistle (*Silybum mariannum*) protects the liver and assists in the detoxification process by increasing **glutathione** supply in the liver. Glutathione is the enzyme involved primarily in the detoxification of toxic heavy metals including lead.

Homeopathy

Homeopathic medicines can be administered once the source is removed, to help correct any imbalances brought on by lead toxicity.

Allopathic treatment

The American Association of Poison Control Centers maintains a nationwide toll-free hotline for prevention and treatment of poisonings. The number is (800) 222-1222. In the case of any suspected poisoning emergency, they can be contacted 24 hours a day.

Chelation therapy

If blood levels of lead are high enough, the doctor may also prescribe **chelation therapy**. This process involves the use of chemicals that bind to lead and help the body pass it in urine at a faster rate. The four most popular chemical agents used for this purpose, either alone or in combination, are edetate **calcium** disodium (EDTA calcium), dimercaprol (BAL), succimer (Chemet; DMSA), and penicillamine (Cuprimine, Depen). EDTA calcium and BAL are given through an intravenous line or in shots, whereas succimer and penicillamine are given orally. (Although many doctors prescribe penicillamine for lead poisoning, this use of the drug has not been approved by the Food and Drug Administration.)

Expected results

If acute lead poisoning reaches the stage of seizures and coma, there is a high risk of death. Even if the person survives, there is a good chance of permanent brain damage. The long-term effects of lower levels of lead can also be permanent and severe. However, if chronic lead poisoning is detected early, these negative effects can be limited by reducing future exposure to lead and getting proper medical treatment.

Prevention

Many cases of lead poisoning can be prevented. These steps can help:

- Keep the areas where children play as clean and dust-free as possible.
- Wash pacifiers and bottles when they fall to the floor, and wash stuffed animals and toys often.
- Make sure children wash their hands before meals and at bedtime.
- Mop floors and wipe windowsills and other chewable surfaces, such as cribs, twice a week with a solution of powdered dishwasher detergent in warm water.
- Plant bushes next to an older home with painted exterior walls to keep children at a distance.
- Plant grass or another ground cover in soil that is likely to be contaminated, such as soil around a home built before 1960 or located near a major highway.
- Have household tap water tested to find out if it contains lead.
- Use only water from the cold-water tap for drinking, cooking, and making baby formula, since hot water is likely to contain higher levels of lead.
- If the cold water has not been used for six hours or more, run it for several seconds, until it becomes as cold as it will get, before using it for drinking or cooking. The more time water has been sitting in the pipes, the more lead it may contain.
- Individuals who work with lead in their jobs or hobbies ought to change their clothes before they go home.
- Do not store food in open cans, especially imported cans.
- Do not store or serve food in pottery meant only for decorative use.
- Arrange for the house to be inspected for lead. Many state health departments will do this.
- Be aware of the status of imported toys that may have unacceptably high levels of lead.

KEY TERMS

Chelation therapy—Treatment with chemicals that bind to a poisonous metal and help the body pass it in urine at a faster rate.

Dimercaprol (BAL)—A chemical agent used to remove excess lead from the body.

Edetate calcium disodium (EDTA calcium)—A chemical agent used to remove excess lead from the body.

Penicillamine (Cuprimine, Depen)—A drug used to treat medical problems (such as excess copper in the body and rheumatoid arthritis) and to prevent kidney stones. It is also sometimes prescribed to remove excess lead from the body.

Pica—An abnormal appetite or craving for non-food items, often such substances as chalk, clay, dirt, laundry starch, or charcoal.

Succimer (Chemet) or DMSA—A drug used to remove excess lead from the body.

Resources

BOOKS

Greim, Helmut, and Robert Snyder, eds.. *Toxicology and Risk Assessment: A Comprehensive Introduction*. New York: Wiley Interscience, 2008.

IARC Working Group on the Evaluation of Carcinogenic Risks to Humans. *Inorganic and Organic Lead Compounds*. Lyon, France: International Agency for Research on Cancer, 2006.

Toxicological Profile for Lead. Atlanta, GA: Agency for Toxic Substances and Disease Registry, 2007.

PERIODICALS

Erickson, Lori, and Teri Thompson. "A Review of a Preventable Poison: Pediatric Lead Poisoning." *Journal for Specialists in Pediatric Nursing* (October 2005): 171–182.

"Herbal Medicines: Lead Poisoning Associated with Ayurvedic Medicines: 8 Case Reports Title." *Reactions* (July 1, 2006): 11–12.

Nevin, Rick. "Understanding International Crime Trends: The Legacy of Preschool Lead Exposure." *Environmental Research* (July 2007): 315–336.

Rajaram, Shireen S. "An Action-research Project: Community Lead Poisoning Prevention." *Teaching Sociology* (April 2007): 138–150.

Ronchetti, Roberto, et al. "Lead Neurotoxicity in Children: Is Prenatal Exposure More Important than Postnatal Exposure?" *Acta Paediatrica* (October 2006): 45–49.

OTHER

"Lead Poisoning." MayoClinic.com, March 15, 2007. http://www.mayoclinic.com/health/lead-poisoning/FL00068. (February 14, 2008).

Marcus, Steven. "Toxicity, Lead." emedicine.com, December 12, 2007. http://www.emedicine.com/EMERG/topic293.htm. (February 14, 2008).

ORGANIZATIONS

National Center for Environmental Health, Centers for Disease Control and Prevention, 1600 Clifton Rd, Atlanta, GA, 30333, (800) 311-3435, http://www.cdc.gov/nceh/.

National Lead Information Center, National Safety Council, 1121 Spring Lake Dr, Itasca, IL, 60143-3201, (630) 285-1121, http://www.nsc.org/issues/lead/.

Mai Tran
Teresa G. Odle
Rebecca J. Frey, PhD
David Edward Newton, Ed.D.

Learning disorders

Definition

Learning disorders are academic difficulties experienced by children and adults of average to above-average intelligence. People with learning disorders have difficulty with reading, writing, mathematics, or a combination of the three. These difficulties significantly interfere with academic achievement or daily living.

Description

Learning disorders, or disabilities, affect approximately 2 million children between the ages of six and 17 (5% of public school children), although some experts think the figure may be as high as 15%. These children have specific impairments in acquiring, retaining, and processing information. Standardized tests place them well below their IQ range in their area of difficulty. The three main types of learning disorders are reading disorders, mathematics disorders, and disorders of written expression. The male: female ratio for learning disorders is about 5: 1.

Reading disorders

Reading disorders are the most common type of learning disorder. Children with reading disorders have difficulty recognizing and interpreting letters and words (**dyslexia**). They are not able to recognize and decode the sounds and syllables (phonetic structure) behind

KEY TERMS

Dyslexia—An inability to read, write, or spell words in spite of the ability to see and recognize letters. Dyslexia is an autosomal dominant disorder thst occurs more frequently in males.

IQ—Intelligence quotient; a measure of intellectual functioning determined by performance on standardized intelligence tests.

Phonics—A system to teach reading by teaching the speech sounds associated with single letters, letter combinations, and syllables.

written words and language in general. This condition lowers accuracy and comprehension in reading.

Mathematic disorders

Children with mathematics disorders (dyscalculia) have problems recognizing and counting numbers correctly. They have difficulty using numbers in everyday settings. Mathematics disorders are typically diagnosed in the first few years of elementary school when formal teaching of numbers and basic math concepts begins. Children with mathematics disorders usually have a co-existing reading disorder, a disorder of written expression, or both.

Disorders of written expression

Disorders of written expression typically occur in combination with reading disorders or mathematics disorders or both. The condition is characterized by difficulty with written compositions (dysgraphia). Children with this type of learning disorder have problems with spelling, punctuation, grammar, and organizing their thoughts in writing.

Causes and symptoms

Learning disorders are thought to be caused by neurological abnormalities that trigger impairments in the regions of the brain that control visual and language processing and attention and planning. These traits may be genetically linked. Children from families with a history of learning disorders are more likely to develop disorders themselves. In 2003 a team of Finnish researchers reported finding a candidate gene for developmental dyslexia on human chromosome 15q21.

Learning difficulties may also be caused by such medical conditions as a traumatic brain injury or brain **infections** such as encephalitis or **meningitis**.

The defining symptom of a learning disorder is academic performance that is markedly below a child's age, grade capabilities, and measured IQ. Children with a reading disorder may confuse or transpose words or letters and omit or add syllables to words. The written homework of children with disorders of written expression is filled with grammatical, spelling, punctuation, and organizational errors. The child's handwriting is often extremely poor. Children with mathematical disorders are often unable to count in the correct sequence, to name numbers, and to understand numerical concepts.

Diagnosis

Problems with vision or hearing, mental disorders (**depression**, attention-deficit/hyperactivity disorder), mental retardation, cultural and language differences, and inadequate teaching may be mistaken for learning disorders or complicate a diagnosis. A comprehensive medical, psychological, and educational assessment is critical to making a clear and correct diagnosis.

A child thought to have a learning disorder should undergo a complete medical examination to rule out an organic cause. If one is not found, a psychoeducational assessment should be performed by a psychologist, psychiatrist, neurologist, neuropsychologist, or learning specialist. A complete medical, family, social, and educational history is compiled from existing medical and school records and from interviews with the child and the child's parents and teachers. A series of written and verbal tests are then given to the child to evaluate his or her cognitive and intellectual functioning. Commonly used tests include the Wechsler Intelligence Scale for Children (WISC-III), the Woodcock-Johnson Psychoeducational Battery, the Peabody Individual Achievement Test-Revised (PIAT-R), and the California Verbal Learning Test (CVLT). Federal legislation mandates that this testing is free of charge within the public school system.

Treatment

Once a learning disorder has been diagnosed, an individual education plan (IEP) is developed for the child in question. IEPs are based on psychoeducational test findings. They provide for annual testing to measure a child's progress. Students with learning disorders may receive special instruction within a regular general education class or they may be taught in a special education or learning center for a portion of the day.

Common strategies for the treatment of reading disorders focus first on improving a child's recognition of the sounds of letters and language through phonics training. Later strategies focus on comprehension, retention, and study skills. Students with disorders of written expression are often encouraged to keep journals and to write with a computer keyboard instead of a pencil. Instruction for students with mathematical disorders emphasizes real-world uses of math, such as balancing a checkbook or comparing prices.

Ensuring that the child has proper **nutrition** can help in the treatment of learning disorders. Those who do not receive the proper doses that they need may require changes in their **diets**, or supplements are taken. Supplements that may help with learning disorders are **fish oil**, flax oil, primrose oil, and **omega-3 fatty acids**. Eliminating food additives, like colors and preservatives, as well decreasing the child's consumption of refined sugars, can also be helpful.

Meditation is also beneficial. It helps to slow the mind down and take in the surroundings while focusing on the task at hand.

Herbal remedies may also help to focus the mind. **St. John's wort** and *Ginkgo biloba* are used to treat **attention-deficit hyperactivity disorder** (ADHD). Ginkgo is a blood thinner and those considering taking it should consult a doctor beforehand.

Expected results

The high school dropout rate for children with learning disabilities is almost 40%. Children with learning disabilities that go undiagnosed or are improperly treated may never achieve functional literacy. They often develop serious behavior problems as a result of their frustration with school; in addition, their learning problems are often stressful for other family members and may strain family relationships. The key to helping these students reach their fullest potential is early detection and the implementation of an appropriate individualized education plan. The prognosis is good for a large percentage of children with reading disorders that are identified and treated early. Learning disorders continue into adulthood, but with proper educational and vocational training, an individual can complete college and pursue a challenging career. Studies of the occupational choices of adults with dyslexia indicate that they do particularly well in people-oriented professions and occupations, such as nursing or sales.

Resources

BOOKS

American Psychiatric Association. *Diagnostic and Statistical Manual of Mental Disorders*, 4th edition, text revision. Washington, DC: American Psychiatric Association, 2000.

Church, Robin P., M.E.B. Lewis, and Mark L. Batshaw. "Learning Disabilities." *Children with Disabilities*. edited by Mark L. Batshaw. 4th ed. Baltimore: Paul H. Brookes, 1997.

"Learning Disorders. " Section 19, Chapter 262 in *The Merck Manual of Diagnosis and Therapy*, edited by Mark H. Beers, MD, and Robert Berkow, MD. Whitehouse Station, NJ: Merck Research Laboratories, 2002.

Mars, Laura. *The Complete Learning Disabilities Directory, 1999/2000*. Grey House Publishing, 1999.

Osman, Betty B. *Learning Disabilities and ADHD: A Family Guide to Living and Learning Together*. New York: John Wiley & Sons, 1997.

PERIODICALS

Baringa, Marcia. "Learning Defect Identified in Brain." *Science*. 273 (August 1996): 867–868.

Galaburda, D. M., and B. C. Duchaine. "Developmental Disorders of Vision." *Neurologic Clinics* 21 (August 2003): 687–707.

Gillberg, C., and H. Soderstrom. "Learning Disability." *Lancet* 362 (September 6, 2003): 811–821.

Stage, Frances K. and Nancy V. Milne. "Invisible Scholars: Students With Learning Disabilities." *Journal of Higher Education*. 67 (July–August 1996): 426–45.

Taipale, M., N. Kaminen, J. Nopola-Hemmi, et al. "A Candidate Gene for Developmental Dyslexia Encodes a Nuclear Tetratricopeptide Repeat Domain Protein Dynamically Regulated in Brain." *Proceedings of the National Academy of Sciences in the USA* 100 (September 30, 2003): 11553–11558.

Taylor, K. E., and J. Walter. "Occupation Choices of Adults With and Without Symptoms of Dyslexia." *Dyslexia* 9 (August 2003): 177–185.

Witt, W. P., A. W. Riley, and M. J. Coiro. "Childhood Functional Status, Family Stressors, and Psychosocial Adjustment Among School-Aged Children with Disabilities in the United States." *Archives of Pediatric and Adolescent Medicine* 157 (July 2003): 687–695.

ORGANIZATIONS

The Interactive Guide to Learning Disabilities for Parents, Teachers, and Children. http://www.ldonline.org.

The Learning Disabilities Association of America (LDA). 4156 Library Road, Pittsburgh, PA 15234–1349. (412) 341–1515. http://www.ldanatl.org.

National Center for Learning Disabilities (NCLD). 381 Park Avenue South, Suite 1401, New York, NY 10016. (410) 296–0232. http://www.ncld.org.

Paula Ford-Martin
Rebecca J. Frey, PhD

Lecithin

Definition

Lecithin was discovered in 1850 by Maurice Gobley, who isolated it in egg yolks and identified it as the substance that allows oil and water to mix. The name is derived from the Greek word *lekithos*, which means "yolk of egg." Lecithin is a naturally occurring fatty substance found in several foods, including soybeans, whole grains, and egg yolks. It is often used as an emulsification agent in processed foods. It can be taken in various forms as a nutritional supplement, often derived from soybeans. The body breaks lecithin down into its component parts: **choline**, phosphate, glycerol, and fatty acids. The body's highest concentration of lecithin is found in the vital organs, where it makes up about 30% of the dry weight of the brain and nearly two-thirds of the fat in the liver.

General use

Lecithin acts as an emulsifier and helps the body in the absorption of fats. Some studies suggest that soy lecithin improves the metabolism of **cholesterol** in the digestive system. Therefore, lecithin has been touted as a treatment for high cholesterol. It has also been said to be a treatment for neurologic and liver disorders. Promoters claim that supplemental lecithin can be used to help lower cholesterol and deter **memory loss**. Some proponents of lecithin warn that the low fat and low cholesterol **diets** that many Americans follow may lower the amount of lecithin that they consume, creating a deficit and necessitating supplemental lecithin. As Americans eat fewer eggs, meats, and dairy products, the amount of choline that they consume may be less than required. Choline is the key element in lecithin that researchers believe may have a beneficial effect on cholesterol and memory.

Lecithin has been identified as a possible resource for lowering blood cholesterol because of its reputation as a source of polyunsaturated fats. In addition, choline helps the liver metabolize fat and form lipoproteins. However, as of 2008, there was scant evidence to support the use of lecithin in lowering cholesterol. Researchers in some studies have found a drop in cholesterol levels, while others have found no drop in cholesterol levels at all. A group of researchers from the Netherlands who summarized findings in the *American Journal of Clinical Nutrition* concluded that many studies of the effects of lecithin had faulty methods, and the few good studies proved that lecithin was not effective in lowering cholesterol. Subsequently, a group of American researchers solved part of the mystery concerning the fact that eggs, which are packed with cholesterol, do not impact people's cholesterol much if eaten in moderation. The reason seemed to be the lecithin found in eggs that reduces cholesterol's absorption in the bloodstream. Generally speaking, the role of lecithin in reducing blood cholesterol appears to be minimal.

Lecithin is also considered to be of possible benefit to brain function, and supporters claim that it may help prevent **Alzheimer's disease**. Promoters indicate that the choline in lecithin may have the ability to penetrate the blood-brain barrier and impact the production of acetylcholine, a neurotransmitter that facilitates brain function. They claim that long-term use of lecithin as a dietary supplement could help minimize memory loss. However, studies on the use of lecithin for the treatment of Alzheimer's disease have found that it has no marked benefit.

Preparations

Lecithin is derived from soy and is available in capsule, liquid, and granule form. Consumers should not use a synthetic form of the supplement (choline chloride) but should seek one that contains natural phosphatidyl choline. Lecithin from soybeans generally contains about 76% phosphatidycholine. Studies of supplements sold in health food stores show that most contain minimal levels of pure lecithin. In fact, a person might get the same benefit from eating a handful of peanuts. The American Heart Association and the College of Physicians and Surgeons of Columbia University have described lecithin supplements as an expensive and probably unnecessary way of increasing unsaturated fatty acids in one's diet.

Precautions

Consumers should be aware that most nutritional supplements are not regulated by the Food and Drug Administration (FDA) for product safety or effectiveness. Because lecithin is not considered an essential nutrient, as of 2008, no Recommended Daily Allowance (RDA) has been established for this nutrient.

Side effects

There are no major side effects for lecithin as a supplement. In high doses (more than 25 g per day), lecithin can cause sweating, upset stomach, **diarrhea**, **nausea**, and **vomiting**. Pregnant or nursing women and children should avoid the supplement because it has not been adequately tested for safety.

Resources

BOOKS

Daniel, Kaayla T. *The Whole Soy Story: The Dark Side of America's Favorite Health Food.* Washington, DC: New Trends Publishing, 2005.

OTHER

"Lecithin." Drugs.com, 2006. http://www.drugs.com/npc/lecithin.html. (February 14, 2008).

Amy Cooper
Teresa G. Odle
David Edward Newton, Ed.D.

Ledum

Description

Ledum is an evergreen shrub, *Ledum palustre*. This plant grows wild in Canada, northern Europe, and the cooler regions of North America as far south as Wisconsin and Pennsylvania, reaching a height of 1–6 ft (0.3–2 m). It has narrow, dark, aromatic leaves with hairy or wooly undersides. The leaves, either dried or fresh, are used primarily in homeopathic healing, but have also been used in Native American and Russian folk medicine.

During the American Revolution when the British imposed a tax on imported tea, the American colonists used ledum as a tea substitute. Other names for ledum include marsh tea, Labrador tea, wild **rosemary**, James's tea, and *ledum latifolium*.

General use

Homeopathic medicine operates on the principle that "like heals like." This saying means that a disease can be cured by treating it with products that produce the same symptoms as the disease. These products

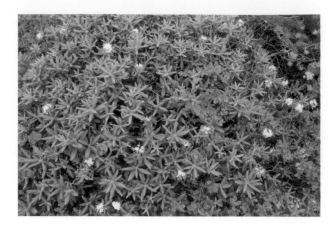

Ledum groenlandicum. *(Erin Paul Donovan / Alamy)*

follow another homeopathic law, the Law of Infinitesimals. In opposition to traditional medicine, the Law of Infinitesimals states that the lower a dose of curative, the more effective it is. To achieve a low dose, the curative is diluted many, many times until only a tiny amount, if any, remains in a huge amount of the diluting liquid.

In homeopathic terminology, the effectiveness of remedies is proved by experimentation and reporting done by famous homeopathic practitioners. Ledum was proved as a remedy by the German founder of **homeopathy**, Dr. Samuel Hahnemann (1775–1843).

In homeopathic medicine, ledum is used first and foremost as a first-aid remedy to prevent infection. It is taken internally for:

- bruises, especially bruises that are improved by the application of cold
- insect stings and animal bites
- puncture wounds, cuts, grazes, and scrapes
- black eyes and other eye injuries

Other homeopathic uses for ledum include the treatment of stiff and painful joints, especially when the **pain** begins in the feet and ankles and moves upward. Ledum is also used for sprained ankles. According to some homeopathic practitioners, ledum is said to take away the craving for alcohol.

Since 1995, ledum has been touted as a homeopathic remedy for **Lyme disease**. Originally prescribed by a holistic veterinarian in Connecticut to treat the symptoms of Lyme disease in horses, dogs, and cats, ledum in the 1M potency is now recommended by some alternative practitioners as a treatment for Lyme disease in humans. There are several anecdotal reports of its success in treating this painful disease.

KEY TERMS

Antioxidants—Enzymes that bind with free radicals to neutralize their harmful effects on living tissue. Ledum appears to be a rich source of antioxidants.

Decoction—Decoctions are made by simmering an herb, then straining the solid material out.

Lyme disease—A chronic, recurrent inflammatory disease carried by deer ticks and caused by a spirochete.

In homeopathic medicine the fact that certain symptoms get better or worse under different conditions is used as a diagnostic tool to indicate what remedy will be most effective. Symptoms that benefit from treatment with ledum get worse with warmth and are also worse at night. Symptoms improve with the application of cold.

Homeopathy also ascribes certain personality types to certain remedies. The ledum personality is said to be discontented and self-pitying. People with the ledum personality may be irritable, angry, impatient, worried, and want to be left alone. People in need of ledum often have restless, disturbed sleep marked by bad dreams.

Ledum is also used in Native American and Russian folk healing. In Russian, ledum is called *bogulnik*. Both these cultures use decoctions or infusions of ledum to treat coughs, **bronchitis**, and bronchial **asthma**. According to historical records, the famous Swedish botanist Karl Linneaus (1707–1778) was the first to record using ledum for sore throats and coughs.

In addition, Russian folk medicine uses ledum mixed with butter to make an ointment that is applied externally to treat scabby **dandruff**, skin **infections**, **bruises**, **wounds**, and bleeding. Used externally, it is believed to act as an antibiotic and an anti-fungal to reduce infection.

Mainstream medical researchers have studied ledum within the field of environmental medicine. Some Russian animal studies from the mid-1990s indicated that ledum offers some protection against radiation damage to the digestive system and the formation of red blood cells. A Canadian study completed in the summer of 2002 reported that ledum is a highly accurate indicator of high environmental concentrations of lead.

Ledum is also being studied for its beneficial effects when eaten as a vegetable. A 2002 report from the School of Pharmacy at the University of London states that ledum has a high level of antioxidant activity, and shows promise as a treatment for **gout**, diseases related to **aging**, and central nervous system disorders.

Preparations

Ledum is prepared by picking the leaves, small twigs, and flowers in the late summer. These can be used fresh or dried to make an infusion (tea) or a decoction. For homeopathic remedies, the dried plant material is ground finely then prepared by extensive dilutions. There are two homeopathic dilution scales, the decimal (x) scale with a dilution of 1:10 and the centesimal (c) scale where the dilution factor is 1:100. Once the mixture is diluted, shaken, strained, then re-diluted many times to reach the desired degree of potency, the final mixture is added to lactose (a type of sugar) tablets or pellets. These are then stored away from light. Ledum is available commercially in tablets in many different strengths. Dosage depends on the symptoms being treated.

Homeopathic and orthodox medical practitioners agree that by the time the initial remedy solution is diluted to strengths used in homeopathic healing, it is likely that very few if any molecules of the original remedy remain. Homeopaths, however, believe that these remedies continue to work through an effect called potentization that has not yet been explained by mainstream scientists.

As an infusion for treating respiratory distress and coughs, 1 oz (30 g) of dried leaves is added to 1 qt (1 L) of boiling water.

Precautions

Puncture wounds from rusty nails, needles, animal **bites**, and similar implements can be serious and may result in **tetanus**. When treating puncture wounds with ledum, patients should make sure their tetanus immunizations are current, monitor their healing, and seek traditional medical help at the first sign of infection.

People who bruise very easily should consult a physician, as this condition is sometimes caused by blood disorders and other serious conditions.

Side effects

Ledum taken in the standard homeopathic dilutions has not been reported to cause side effects. A tea made from ledum has been safely taken for centuries.

Interactions

Studies of interactions between ledum and conventional pharmaceuticals are nonexistent.

Resources

BOOKS

Cummings, Stephen, MD, and Dana Ullman, MPH. *Everybody's Guide to Homeopathic Medicines*, revised and expanded. New York: G. P. Putnam's Sons, 1991.

Hammond, Christopher. *The Complete Family Guide to Homeopathy*. London, UK: Penguin Studio, 1995.

Lockie, Andrew and Nicola Geddes. *The Complete Guide to Homeopathy*. London, UK: Dorling Kindersley, 1995.

Pelletier, Kenneth R., MD. *The Best Alternative Medicine*, Part I: Homeopathy. New York: Simon & Schuster, 2002.

PERIODICALS

Narimanov, A. A. "The Antiradiation Effectiveness of a Mixture of *Archangelica officinalis* and *Ledum palustre* Extracts in the Fractionated Gamma Irradiation of Mice." [in Russian] *Radiobiologiia* 33 (March-April 1993): 280-284.

Pieroni, A., V. Janiak, C. M. Durr, et al. "In Vitro Antioxidant Activity of Non-Cultivated Vegetables of Ethnic Albanians in Southern Italy." *Phytotherapy Research* 16 (August 2002): 467-473.

Pugh, R. E., D. G. Dick, and A. L. Fredeen. "Heavy Metal (Pb, Zn, Cd, Fe, and Cu) Contents of Plant Foliage Near the Anvil Range Lead/Zinc Mine, Faro, Yukon Territory." *Ecotoxicology and Environmental Safety* 52 (July 2002): 273-279.

ORGANIZATIONS

Foundation for Homeopathic Education and Research. 21 Kittredge Street, Berkeley, CA 94704. (510) 649–8930.

International Foundation for Homeopathy. P. O. Box 7, Edmonds, WA 98020. (206)776–4147.

Lyme Disease Foundation, Inc. 1 Financial Plaza, Hartford, CT 06103. (800) 886-LYME. www.lyme.org.

National Center for Homeopathy. 801 N. Fairfax Street, Suite 306, Alexandria, VA 22314. (703) 548–7790.

Tish Davidson
Rebecca J. Frey, PhD

Lemon balm

Description

Lemon balm is a citrus-scented, aromatic herb. It is a perennial member of the Lamiaceae (formerly Labiatae), or mint, family and has proven benefit to the nervous system. This lovely Mediterranean native,

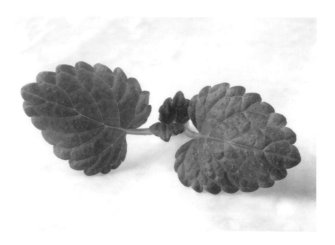

Lemon balm. *(© foodfolio / Alamy)*

dedicated to the goddess Diana, is bushy and bright. Greeks used lemon balm medicinally over 2,000 years ago. Honey bees swarm to the plant. This attraction inspired the generic name, melissa, the Greek word for honeybee. Romans introduced lemon balm (*Melissa officinalis*) to Great Britain where it became a favorite cottage garden herb. The plant has been naturalized in North America.

Lemon balm grows in bushy clumps to 2 ft (0.6 m) tall and branches to 18 in (45.7 cm). It thrives in full sun or partial shade in moist, fertile soil from the mountains to the sea. The heart-shaped, deeply-veined leaves exude a pleasant lemon scent when brushed against or crushed. They have scalloped edges and square stems. The tiny white or golden blossoms grow in the leaf axils, and bloom from June through October. The plant is hardy, self-seeding, and spreads easily in the right soil conditions. The plant has a short rhizome, producing the erect, downy stems. The essential oil content appears to be highest in the uppermost third of the plant.

General use

Lemon balm is a soothing, sedative herb that can relieve tension and lift **depression**. An infusion of this citrus-scented herb will improve digestion, reduce **fever**, ease spasms, and enhance **relaxation**. The plant has antihistaminic properties and helps with **allergies**. Lemon balm infusions, taken hot, will induce sweating. Lemon balm has been used for centuries to calm the mind, improve memory, and sharpen the wit. A daily infusion of lemon balm is said to promote longevity. It is a helpful herb in cases of hyperthyroid activity, palpitations of the heart, and tension **headache**. It can relieve pre-menstrual tension and menstrual

KEY TERMS

Antioxidant—An enzyme or other organic substance that is able to counteract the damaging effects of oxidation in living tissue. The flavonoids in lemon balm appear to have some antioxidative efficacy.

Essential oil—Another term for volatile oil; the aromatic oil that can be obtained by steam distillation from plant parts. Most essential oils are composed of terpenes and their oxygenated derivatives.

Flavonoids—A class of water-soluble plant pigments that have antiviral and other healing qualities. The flavonoids in lemon balm are the source of its antihistaminic effectiveness.

Sedative—A medication or preparation given to calm or soothe nervousness or irritability. Lemon balm has sedative properties.

Volatile oil—The fragrant oil that can be obtained from a plant by distillation. The word "volatile" means that the oil evaporates in the open air.

cramping. It helps promote good digestion, relieve flatulence, and **colic**, and can ease one into a restful sleep. Lemon balm has antiviral and antibacterial properties. Used externally as a skin wash, this gentle herb can ease the sting of insect **bites**, soothe **cold sore** eruptions (herpes simplex), and treat sores and **wounds**. Lemon balm's highly aromatic qualities make it a good insect repellent. It is also valued in **aromatherapy** to relax and soothe a troubled mind. Fresh leaves are often added to salads, or used with fish, mushroom, and cheese dishes. In France, the herb is used in making cordials, and is called *Tea de France*.

Apart from its traditional medicinal uses, lemon balm is used to flavor vermouth and other alcoholic beverages as well as some soft drinks.

Lemon balm contains volatile oils, including citral, citronella, eugenol, and other components as well as flavonoids, triterpenoids, rosmarinic acid, polyphenols, and tannin. Several new flavonoids were discovered in lemon balm in 2002. Flavonoids are a group of water-soluble plant pigments that have antiviral and antioxidative qualities.

Preparations

Lemon balm leaves and flowers are used in medicinal remedies. The herb is at its best when used fresh from the harvest. The leaves may be picked throughout the summer, but the flavor is at its prime just before flowering. When the plant is dried for storage, the volatile oils diminish, reducing the medicinal potency of the herb. Freezing the fresh harvest is a good way to preserve the leaves for later use.

To create a tea, place two ounces of fresh lemon balm leaves in a warmed glass container; bring 2.5 cups of fresh, nonchlorinated water to the boiling point; add it to the herbs; cover; and infuse the tea for about 10 minutes. Once strained, the tea can be consumed warm. The prepared tea will store for about two days in the refrigerator. Lemon balm infusion is a gentle and relaxing tea. It may be enjoyed by the cupful three times a day.

Lemon balm combines well with the leaves of **peppermint** (*Mentha piperita*), and **nettle** (*Urtica dioica*), and the flowers of **chamomile** (*Matricaria chamomilla*).

Precautions

Lemon balm has been used safely for thousands of years. However, pregnant women and individuals with **hypothyroidism** should avoid use unless under consultation with a physician. Use caution when harvesting because of the likely presence of bees.

Side effects

The sedative effect of lemon balm means that it can depress the central nervous system when given in high doses. In addition, it has been reported that persons with **glaucoma** should avoid using essential oil of lemon balm, as it can raise the pressure inside the eye.

Interactions

Lemon balm should be used in lower dosages when combined with other herbs, particularly such other sedative herbs as **valerian**. In addition, lemon balm should not be taken together with prescription sedatives or alcohol, as it can intensify their effects.

Lemon balm has been reported to interfere with the action of thyroid hormones. Persons taking any medication containing thyroid hormones should not take lemon balm.

A physician should be consulted before taking lemon balm in conjunction with any other prescribed pharmaceuticals.

Resources

BOOKS

Blumenthal, Mark. *The Complete German Commission E Monographs, Therapeutic Guide to Herbal Medicines.* Massachusetts: Integrative Medicine Communications, 1998.

Bown, Deni. *The Herb Society of America, Encyclopedia of Herbs & Their Uses*. New York: D.K. Publishing, Inc., 1995.

Gladstar, Rosemary. *Herbal Healing for Women*. New York, Simon & Schuster, 1993.

Lust, John. *The Herb Book*. New York: Bantam Books, 1994.

McVicar, Jekka. *Herbs for the Home*. New York: Viking Studio Books, 1995.

PERIODICALS

Mrlianova, M., D. Tekel'ova, M. Felklova, et al. "The Influence of the Harvest Cut Height on the Quality of the Herbal Drugs *Melissae folium* and *Melissae herba*." *Planta Medica* 68 (February 2002): 178-180.

Patora, J., and B. Klimek. "Flavonoids from Lemon Balm (*Melissa officinalis L.*, Lamiaceae)." *Acta Poloniae Pharmaceutica* 59 (March-April 2002): 139-143.

ORGANIZATIONS

Herb Research Foundation. 1007 Pearl St., Suite 200, Boulder, CO 80302. (303) 449-2265. www.herbs.org.

Southwest School of Botanical Medicine. P. O. Box 4565, Bisbee, AZ 85603. (520) 432-5855. www.swsbm.com.

Clare Hanrahan
Rebecca J. Frey, PhD

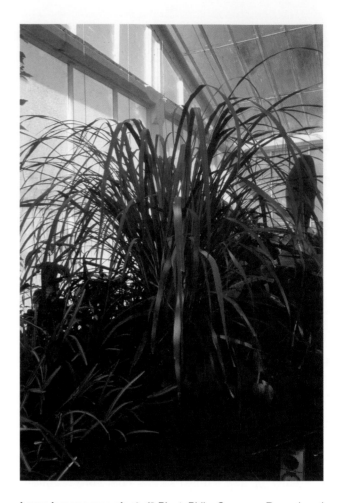

Large lemongrass plant. *(©PlantaPhile, Germany. Reproduced by permission.)*

Lemongrass

Description

Resembling a gigantic weed, lemongrass is an aromatic tropical plant with long, slender blades that can grow to a height of 5 ft (1.5 m). Believed to have a wide range of therapeutic effects, the herb has been used for centuries in South America and India and has also become popular in the United States. Aside from folk medicine, lemongrass is a favorite ingredient in Thai cuisine and dishes that boast a tangy, Asian flavor. While there are several species of lemongrass, *Cymbopogon citratus* is the variety most often recommended for medicinal purposes. Native to Southeast Asia, lemongrass can also be found growing in India, South America, Africa, Australia, and the United States. Only the fresh or dried leaves of lemongrass, and the essential oil derived from them, are used as a drug. *Cymbopogon citratus*, which belongs to the Poaceae family of plants, is also referred to as West Indian lemongrass.

Not to be confused with **lemon balm**, which is an entirely different herb, lemongrass is considered by herbalists to have several useful properties, including antibacterial, antifungal, and fever-reducing effects.

Some of these claims have been supported by animal and laboratory studies. In one test-tube investigation, published in the medical journal *Microbios* in 1996, researchers demonstrated that lemongrass was effective against 22 strains of bacteria and 12 types of fungi. Scientific research has also bolstered the herb's reputation as an analgesic and sedative. A study conducted in rodents suggests that myrcene, a chemical found in the essential oil of *Cymbopogon citratus*, may act as a site-specific **pain** reliever. Unlike aspirin and similar analgesics, which tend to alleviate pain throughout the body, myrcene seems to work only on particular areas. A study involving people indicates that lemongrass may also affect the way the body processes cholesterol.

More recently, lemongrass has been shown to have antimutagenic properties; that is, researchers have found that it is able to reverse chemically induced mutations in certain strains of bacteria.

While they may not be aware of it, most Americans have already tried lemongrass in one form or

KEY TERMS

Analgesic—Any substance that functions as a pain reliever.

Aromatherapy—The use of fragrances, often derived from essential oils, to improve emotional and physical well-being.

Astringent—An agent that helps to contract tissue and prevent the secretion of internal body fluids such as blood or mucus. Astringents are typically used to treat external wounds or to prevent bleeding from the nose or throat.

Citral—A pale yellow liquid drived from lemongrass used in making perfumes and to flavor food.

Essential oil—A general term describing a wide variety of plant-derived oils. They are often used to make soaps and perfumes; candies, soft drinks, processed foods, and other foods and beverages; and certain drugs and dental products.

Lemon balm—A herb with antiviral properties that is also used to alleviate anxiety or insomnia. The botanical name for lemon balm is *Melissa officinalis*.

Myrcene—A compound found in the essential oil of lemongrass that has pain-relieving properties.

Neuralgia—Nerve pain.

Placebo—A sugar pill or inactive agent often used in the control group of a medical study.

another. Citral, a key chemical found in *Cymbopogon citratus*, is an ingredient in a variety of foods and beverages (including alcohol). It can be found in candies, puddings, baked goods, meat products, and even in certain fats and oils. Citral is a pale yellow liquid that evaporates rapidly at room temperature. Like other **essential oils**, lemongrass is also used as a fragrance enhancer in many perfumes, soaps, and detergents.

General use

While not approved by the Food and Drug Administration (FDA), lemongrass reportedly has a wide variety of therapeutic effects. Because the herb has not been studied extensively in people, its effectiveness is based mainly on the results of animal and laboratory studies as well as its centuries-old reputation as a folk remedy. Lemongrass is one of the most popular plant medicines in Brazil, where it is used to treat nervous disorders and stomach problems. In the Amazon, lemongrass is highly regarded as a sedative tea.

When taken internally, lemongrass has been recommended for **stomachaches**, **diarrhea**, **gas**, bowel spasms, **vomiting**, **fever**, the flu, and headaches and other types of pain. The herb (or its essential oil) may be applied externally to help treat **acne**, **athlete's foot**, lower back pain, **sciatica**, **sprains**, tendinitis, **neuralgia**, and rheumatism. To treat circulatory disorders, some authorities recommend rubbing a few drops of lemongrass oil on the skin of affected areas; it is believed to work by improving blood flow. Like many essential oils, lemongrass is also used in aromatherapy.

The link between lemongrass and **cholesterol** was investigated by researchers from the Department of Nutritional Sciences, University of Wisconsin, who published their findings in the medical journal *Lipids* in 1989. They conducted a clinical trial involving 22 people with high cholesterol who took 140-mg capsules of lemongrass oil daily. While cholesterol levels were only slightly affected in some of the participants—cholesterol was lowered from 310 to 294 on average—other people in the study experienced a significant decrease in blood fats. The latter group, characterized as responders, experienced a 25-point drop in cholesterol after one month, and this positive trend continued over the course of the short study. After three months, cholesterol levels among the responders had decreased by a significant 38 points. Once the responders stopped taking lemongrass, their cholesterol returned to previous levels. It should be noted that this study did not involve a placebo group, which is usually used to help measure the effects of the agent being studied (in this case, lemongrass oil).

Considered an antiseptic and astringent, essential oil of lemongrass is also used by some people to cleanse oily skin and help close pores. Some herbalists recommend mixing a few drops of lemongrass with a normal portion of mild shampoo to combat greasy hair. Lemongrass essential oil can also be used as a deodorant to curb perspiration.

Last but not least, the herb has a strong reputation as an insect repellent. It is an important ingredient in several products designed to keep bugs at bay. Some authorities recommend rubbing the crushed herb directly on exposed areas of skin to avoid insect **bites** when enjoying the great outdoors.

The relative safety and stability of lemongrass oil has recommended it to pharmaceutical researchers who are testing new methods of quantitative analysis. Lemongrass oil has been used to demonstrate the superiority of near-infrared spectroscopy to older methods of determining the chemical content of plant oils.

Preparations

The optimum daily dosage of lemongrass, which is available as fresh or dried herb or as lemongrass oil, has not been established with any certainty. Because lemongrass has been recommended for so many different purposes, and can be used internally and externally, consumers are advised to consult a doctor experienced in the use of alternative remedies to determine proper dosage. There is a significant difference between the external use of a few drops of essential oil, and the use of larger amounts of the herb in a tincture or tea.

Lemongrass tea can be prepared by steeping 1–2 tsp of the herb (fresh or dried) in a cup of boiling water. The mixture should be strained after 10–15 minutes. The tea is generally taken several times a day. In *Heinerman's Encyclopedia of Healing Herbs & Spices*, John Heinerman recommends using one cup of lemongrass tea every four hours to reduce fever. In the *Green Pharmacy*, prominent herbalist James Duke recommends drinking one to four cups of lemongrass tea a day to benefit from its anti-fungal properties. The used tea bags can also be applied externally as fungi-fighting compresses, according to the author.

To alleviate gas or persistent vomiting, Heinerman recommends a dose of 3–6 drops of lemongrass oil (the *Cymbopogon citratus* variety). It may be placed on a sugar cube or mixed with 1 tsp of real vanilla flavor before swallowing. For sciatica, lower back pain, sprains, tendinitis, and rheumatism, the author suggests rubbing 10 drops of the essential oil onto the skin of the affected areas.

Precautions

Lemongrass is not known to be harmful when taken in recommended dosages, though it is important to remember that the long-term effects of taking the herb (in any amount) have not been investigated. The essential oil should not be used internally by children, women who are pregnant or breast-feeding, or people with liver or kidney disease.

In rare cases, lemongrass essential oil has caused allergic reactions when applied to the skin. To minimize skin irritation, dilute the oil in a carrier oil such as safflower or sunflower seed oil before application. As with all essential oils, small amounts should be used, and only for a limited time.

Avoid getting lemongrass (herb or oil) in the eyes. Citral has been reported to irritate the respiratory tract in sensitive people as well as the eyes and skin.

Side effects

When taken internally in recommended dosages, lemongrass is not associated with any bothersome or significant side effects. Cases have been reported, however, in which people have developed skin **rashes** after drinking lemongrass tea.

Interactions

Lemongrass is not known to interact adversely with any drug or dietary supplement.

Resources

BOOKS

Gruenwald, Joerg. *PDR for Herbal Medicines*. Montvale, NJ: Medical Economics, 1998.

Price, Shirley. *Practical Aromatherapy*. London, UK: Thorsons/HarperCollins, 1994.

PERIODICALS

Bleasel, N., B. Tate, and M. Rademaker. "Allergic Contact Dermatitis Following Exposure to Essential Oils." *Australasian Journal of Dermatology* 43 (August 2002): 211-213.

Melo, S. F., S. F. Soares, R. F. da Costa, et al. "Effect of the *Cymbopogon citratus*, *Maytenus ilicifolia*, and *Baccharis genistelloides* Extracts Against the Stannous Chloride Oxidative Damage in *Escherichia coli*." *Mutation Research* 496 (September 20, 2001): 33-38.

Wilson, N. D., M. S. Ivanova, R. A. Watt, and A. C. Moffat. "The Quantification of Citral in Lemongrass and Lemon Oils by Near-Infrared Spectroscopy." *Journal of Pharmacy and Pharmacology* 54 (September 2002): 1257-1263.

ORGANIZATIONS

American Botanical Council. PO Box 144345. Austin, TX 78714-4345. www.herbalgram.org.

Herb Research Foundation. 1007 Pearl St., Suite 200, Boulder, CO 80302. (303) 449-2265. www.herbs.org.

International Aromatherapy and Herb Association. 3541 West Acapulco Lane. Phoenix, AZ 85053-4625. (602) 938-4439. www.aztec.asu.edu./iaha/

OTHER

Medline. igm.nlm.nih.gov.

Greg Annussek
Rebecca J. Frey, PhD

Leopard's bane *see* **Arnica**

Leukemia

Definition

Leukemia is a **cancer** that starts in the organs that make blood, namely the bone marrow and the lymph system. Depending on specific characteristics, leukemia can be divided into two broad types: acute and chronic. Acute leukemias are the rapidly progressing leukemias, while the chronic leukemias progress more slowly. The vast majority of childhood leukemias are of the acute form.

Description

The cells that make up blood are produced in the bone marrow and the lymph system. The bone marrow is the spongy tissue found in the large bones of the body. The lymph system includes the spleen (an organ in the upper abdomen), the thymus (a small organ beneath the breastbone), and the tonsils (an organ in the throat). In addition, the lymph vessels (tiny tubes that branch like blood vessels into all parts of the body) and lymph nodes (pea-shaped organs that are found along the network of lymph vessels) are also parts of the lymph system. The lymph is a milky fluid that contains cells. Clusters of lymph nodes are found in the neck, underarm, pelvis, abdomen, and chest.

The cells found in the blood are the red blood cells (RBCs), which carry oxygen and other materials to all tissues of the body; white blood cells (WBCs) that fight infection; and platelets, which play a part in the clotting of the blood. The white blood cells can be further subdivided into three main types: granulocytes, monocytes, and lymphocytes.

The granulocytes, as their name suggests, have particles (granules) inside them. These granules contain special proteins (enzymes) and several other substances that can break down chemicals and destroy microorganisms, such as bacteria. Monocytes are the second type of white blood cell. They are also important in defending the body against pathogens.

The lymphocytes form the third type of white blood cell. There are two main types of lymphocytes: T lymphocytes and B lymphocytes. They have different functions within the immune system. The B cells protect the body by making "antibodies." Antibodies are proteins that can attach to the surfaces of bacteria and viruses. This "attachment" sends signals to many other cell types to come and destroy the antibody-coated organism. The T cells protect the body against viruses. When a virus

enters a cell, it produces certain proteins that are projected onto the surface of the infected cell. The T cells recognize these proteins and make certain chemicals that are capable of destroying the virus-infected cells. In addition, the T cells can destroy some types of cancer cells.

The bone marrow makes stem cells, which are the precursors of the different blood cells. These stem cells mature through stages into either RBCs, WBCs, or platelets.

Chronic leukemias

In chronic leukemias, the cancer starts in the blood cells made in the bone marrow. The cells mature and only a few remain as immature cells. However, even though the cells mature and appear normal, they do not function as normal cells. Depending on the type of white blood cell that is involved, chronic leukemia can be classified as chronic lymphocytic leukemia or chronic myelogenous leukemia.

Chronic leukemias develop very gradually. The abnormal lymphocytes multiply slowly, but in a poorly regulated manner. They live much longer and thus their numbers build up in the body. The two types of chronic leukemias can be easily distinguished under the microscope. Chronic lymphocytic leukemia (CLL) involves the T or B lymphocytes. B cell abnormalities are more common than T cell abnormalities. T cells are affected in only 5% of the patients. The T and B lymphocytes can be differentiated from the other types of white blood cells based on their size and by the absence of granules inside them. In chronic myelogenous leukemia (CML), the cells that are affected are the granulocytes.

Chronic lymphocytic leukemia (CLL) often shows no early symptoms and may remain undetected for a long time. Chronic myelogenous leukemia (CML), on the other hand, may progress to a more acute form.

Acute leukemias

In acute leukemia, the maturation process of the white blood cells is interrupted. The immature cells (or "blasts") proliferate rapidly and begin to accumulate in various organs and tissues, thereby affecting their normal function. This uncontrolled proliferation of the immature cells in the bone marrow affects the production of the normal red blood cells and platelets as well.

Acute leukemias are of two types: acute lymphocytic leukemia and acute myelogenous leukemia. Different types of white blood cells are involved in the two leukemias. In acute lymphocytic leukemia (ALL), the T or B lymphocytes become cancerous. The B cell leukemias are more common than T cell leukemias. Acute myelogenous leukemia, also known as acute nonlymphocytic leukemia (ANLL), is a cancer of the monocytes and/or granulocytes.

Leukemias account for 2% of all cancers. Because leukemia is the most common form of childhood cancer, it is often regarded as a disease of childhood. However, leukemias affect nine times as many adults as children. Half of the cases occur in people who are 60 years of age or older. The incidence of acute and chronic leukemias is about the same. According to the estimates of the American Cancer Society (ACS), approximately 29,000 new cases of leukemia were diagnosed in 1998. Internationally, leukemia is the fourth most common cancer among people age 15 to 19 years old.

Causes and symptoms

Leukemia strikes both sexes and all ages and its cause is mostly unknown. However, chronic leukemia has been linked to genetic abnormalities and environmental factors. For example, exposure to ionizing radiation and to certain organic chemicals, such as benzene, is believed to increase the risk for getting leukemia. A 2003 study from the Electric Power Research Institute showed possible links between metallic drainpipes and childhood baths. Chronic leukemia occurs in some people who are infected with two human retroviruses (HTLV-I and HTLV-II). An abnormal chromosome known as the Philadelphia chromosome is seen in 90% of those with CML. The incidence of chronic leukemia is slightly higher among men than women.

Acute lymphoid leukemia (ALL) is more common among Caucasians than among African-Americans, while acute myeloid leukemia (AML) affects both races equally. The incidence of acute leukemia is slightly higher among men than women. People of Jewish ancestry have a higher likelihood of getting leukemia. A higher incidence of leukemia has also been observed among persons with Down syndrome and some other genetic abnormalities.

A history of diseases that damage the bone marrow, such as aplastic **anemia**, or a history of cancers of the lymphatic system puts people at a high risk for developing acute leukemias. Similarly, the use of anticancer medications, immunosuppressants, and the antibiotic chloramphenicol also are considered risk factors for developing acute leukemias.

The symptoms of leukemia are generally vague and non-specific. A patient may experience all or some of the following symptoms:

- weakness or chronic fatigue
- fever of unknown origin
- weight loss that is not due to dieting or exercise
- frequent bacterial or viral infections
- headaches
- skin rash
- non-specific bone pain
- easy bruising
- bleeding from gums or nose

- blood in urine or stools
- enlarged lymph nodes and/or spleen
- abdominal fullness

Diagnosis

Like all cancers, leukemias are best treated when found early. There are no screening tests available. If the doctor has reason to suspect leukemia, he or she will conduct a thorough physical examination to look for enlarged lymph nodes in the neck, underarm, and pelvic region. Swollen gums, enlarged liver or spleen, **bruises**, or pinpoint red **rashes** all over the body are some of the signs of leukemia. Urine and blood tests may be ordered to check for microscopic amounts of blood in the urine and to obtain a complete differential blood count. This count will give the numbers and percentages of the different cells found in the blood. An abnormal blood test might suggest leukemia, however, the diagnosis has to be confirmed by more specific tests.

A doctor may perform a bone marrow biopsy to confirm the diagnosis of leukemia. During the biopsy, a cylindrical piece of bone and marrow is removed, generally from the hip bone. These samples are sent to the laboratory for examination. In addition to diagnosis, the biopsy is also repeated during the treatment phase of the disease to see if the leukemia is responding to therapy.

A spinal tap (lumbar puncture) is another procedure that the doctor may order to diagnose leukemia. In this procedure, a small needle is inserted into the spinal cavity in the lower back to withdraw some cerebrospinal fluid and to look for leukemic cells.

Standard imaging tests, such as x rays, computed tomography scans (CT scans), and magnetic resonance imaging (MRI) may be used to check whether the leukemic cells have invaded other areas of the body, such as the bones, chest, kidneys, abdomen, or brain. A gallium scan or bone scan is a test in which a radioactive chemical is injected into the body. This chemical accumulates in the areas of cancer or infection, allowing them to be viewed with a special camera.

Treatment

Alternative therapies should be used only as complementary to conventional treatment, not to replace it. Before participating in any alternative treatment programs, patients should consult their doctors concerning the appropriateness and the role of such programs in the overall cancer treatment plan. Appropriate alternative treatments can help prolong a patient's life or at least improve quality of life, prevent recurrence of tumors or prolong the remission period, and reduce adverse reactions to chemotherapy and radiation.

The effectiveness of most anti-cancer drugs used to treat leukemia can be reduced when patients take mega doses of antioxidants. These **antioxidants**, in patients not undergoing chemotherapy, can be very helpful in protecting the body against cancer. However, taken during chemotherapy, these antioxidants protect the cancer cells from being killed by treatment. Because high-dose supplementation of antioxidants can interfere with conventional chemotherapy treatment, patients should only take them at dosages much above the recommended daily allowance (RDA).

Dietary guidelines

The following dietary changes may be helpful:

- Avoiding fatty and spicy foods, which may be harder to digest.
- Eating new and exciting foods. Tasty foods stimulate appetite so that patients can eat more and have the energy to fight cancer.
- Increasing consumption of fresh fruits and vegetables. They are nature's best sources of antioxidants, as well as vitamins and minerals.
- Eating multiple (five or six) meals per day. Small meals are easier to digest.
- Establishing regular eating times and not eating around bedtime.
- Avoiding foods that contain preservatives or artificial coloring.
- Monitoring weight and eating adequate calories and protein.

Nutritional supplements

A naturopath or nutritional physician may recommend some of the following nutritional supplements to boost a patient's immune function and help fight cancer:

- Vitamins and minerals. Vitamins that are of particular benefit to cancer patients include beta-carotene, B-complex vitamins, (especially vitamin B_6, vitamins A, C, D, E and K. The most important minerals are calcium, chromium, copper, iodine, molybdenum, germanium, selenium, tellurium, and zinc. Many of these vitamins and minerals are strong antioxidants. However, patients should not take mega doses of these supplements without first consulting their doctor. Significant adverse or toxic effects may occur at high dosage, which is especially true for minerals. It is prudent to avoid use of antioxidants when undergoing chemotherapy or radiation therapy since these treatments kill the cancer by producing oxidants. Antioxidants can undermine the effectiveness of treatment.

- Other nutritional supplements that may help fight cancer and support the body include essential fatty acids (fish or flaxseed oil), flavonoids, pancreatic enzymes (to help digest foods), hormones such as DHEA, melatonin or phytoestrogens, rice bran, and mushroom extracts. It is best to check with a nutritional physician or other licensed provider when adding these supplements.

Traditional Chinese medicine

Conventional treatment for leukemia is associated with significant side effects. These adverse effects can be reduced with Chinese herbal preparations. Patients should consult an experienced herbalist who will prescribe remedies to treat specific symptoms that are caused by conventional cancer treatments.

Juice therapy

Juice therapy may be helpful in patients with cancer. Patients should mix one part of pure juice with one part of water before drinking. Daily consumption of the following juice may be helpful by reducing toxic burden to the liver:

- carrot and beet juice with a touch of radish or dandelion root
- grapes, pear, and lemon
- carrot, celery, and parsley
- carrot, beet, and cucumber juices

Homeopathy

There is conflicting evidence regarding the effectiveness of **homeopathy** in cancer treatment. Because cancer chemotherapy may suppress the body's response to homeopathic treatment, homeopathy may not be effective during chemotherapy. Therefore, patients should wait until after chemotherapy to try this relatively safe alternative treatment.

Acupuncture

Acupuncture is the use of needles on the body to stimulate or direct the meridians (channels) of energy flow in the body. Acupuncture has not been shown to have any anticancer effects. However, it is an effective treatment for **nausea**, a common side effect of chemotherapy and radiation.

Other treatments

Other therapies that may help the leukemia patient include **meditation**, **qigong**, **yoga**, and **t'ai chi**, all of which can aid in **stress** reduction. Guided imagery can increase immune function and decrease **pain** and nausea.

Allopathic treatment

There are two phases of treatment for leukemia. The first phase is called induction therapy. The main aim of the treatment is to reduce the number of leukemic cells as far as possible and induce a remission in the patient. Once the patient shows no obvious signs of leukemia (no leukemic cells are detected in blood tests and bone marrow biopsies), the patient is said to be in remission. The second phase of treatment is then initiated. This is called continuation or maintenance therapy; the aim in this case is to kill any remaining cells and to maintain remission for as long as possible.

Chemotherapy is the use of drugs to kill cancer cells. It is usually the treatment of choice and is used to relieve symptoms and achieve long-term remission of the disease. Generally, combination chemotherapy, in which multiple drugs are used, is more efficient than using a single drug for treatment.

In 2002, scientists announced the discovery of a gene that triggers the death of leukemia cells. Identification of this gene can lead to better targeting of chemotherapy drugs (that involve a **vitamin A** derivative) for acute promyelocytic leukemia (APL). Another advancement in leukemia treatment occurred in the same year. A new drug was found to cancel the effects of mutations of a gene known as the main culprit in AML, an aggressive, treatment-resistant form of leukemia. Further study was needed on both new discoveries, but they were thought important to improving treatment of two forms of leukemia. Later in 2002, Gleevec, a new antileukemia drug that even proved successful at treating chronic myeloid leukemia, was heralded in clinical trials.

Because leukemia cells can spread to all the organs via the blood stream and lymph vessels, surgery is not considered an option for treating leukemias.

Radiation therapy, which involves the use of x rays or other high-energy rays to kill cancer cells and shrink tumors, may be used in some cases. For acute leukemias, the source of radiation is usually outside the body (external radiation therapy). If the leukemic cells have spread to the brain, radiation therapy can be given to the brain.

Bone marrow transplantation (BMT) is a process in which the patient's diseased bone marrow is replaced with healthy marrow. There are two methods of bone marrow transplant. In an allogeneic bone marrow transplant, healthy marrow is taken from a donor whose tissue is either the same as or very closely resembles the patient's tissue. First, the patient's bone marrow is destroyed with very high doses of chemotherapy and radiation therapy. Healthy marrow from the donor is then given to the patient through a needle in a vein to replace the destroyed marrow.

In the second type of bone marrow transplant, called an autologous bone marrow transplant, some of the patient's own marrow is taken out and treated with a combination of anticancer drugs to kill all abnormal cells. This marrow is then frozen and saved. The marrow remaining in the patient's body is destroyed with high-dose chemotherapy and radiation therapy. The marrow that was frozen is then thawed and given back to the patient through a needle in a vein. This mode of bone marrow transplant is currently being investigated in clinical trials.

Biological therapy or immunotherapy is a mode of treatment in which the body's own immune system is harnessed to fight the cancer. Substances that are routinely made by the immune system (such as growth factors, hormones, and disease-fighting proteins) are either synthetically made in a laboratory or their effectiveness is boosted and they are then put back into the patient's body. This treatment mode is also being investigated in clinical trials all over the country at major cancer centers.

Expected results

Like all cancers, the prognosis for leukemia depends on the patient's age and general health. According to statistics, more than 60% of leukemia patients survive for at least one year after diagnosis.

Acute myelocytic leukemia (AML) has a poorer prognosis rate than acute lymphocytic leukemias (ALL) and the chronic leukemias. In the last 15 to 20 years, the five-year survival rate for patients with ALL has increased from 38% to 57%.

Interestingly enough, since most childhood leukemias are of the ALL type, chemotherapy has been highly successful in their treatment. This is because chemotherapeutic drugs are most effective against actively growing cells. Due to the new combinations of anticancer drugs being used, the survival rates among children with ALL have improved dramatically. Eighty percent of the children diagnosed with

ALL now survive five years or more, as compared to 50% in the late 1970s.

According to statistics, in chronic lymphoid leukemia, the overall survival for all stages of the disease is nine years. Most of the deaths in people with CLL are due to **infections** or other illnesses that occur as a result of the leukemia.

In CML, if bone marrow transplantation is performed within one to three years of diagnosis, 50-60% of the patients survive three years or more. If the disease progresses to the acute phase, the prognosis is poor. Less than 20% of these patients go into remission.

Prevention

Most cancers can be prevented by changes in lifestyle or diet, which will reduce risk factors. However, in leukemias, there are no such known risk factors. Therefore, at the present time, there are no real prevention recommendations for leukemia. People who are at an increased risk for developing leukemia because of proven exposure to ionizing radiation or exposure to the toxic liquid benzene, and people with Down syndrome, should undergo periodic medical checkups. Some experts recommend limiting toxic exposures, eating a whole foods diet, refraining from **smoking**, exercise, and fluids, and even intermittent **fasting** as possible prevention measures. In 2003, new research found that adult women who took aspirin two or more times a week had a 50% lower risk of developing adult leukemia. Scientists continue to work on a possible vaccine for leukemia. They made some progress in 2002, discovering a gene transfer model that might trigger immunity against leukemia cells.

Resources

BOOKS

Berkow, Robert, et al., eds. *Merck Manual of Diagnosis and Therapy*, 16th ed. Merck Research Laboratories, 1992.

Dollinger, Malin. *Everyone's Guide to Cancer Therapy*. Somerville House Books Limited, 1994.

Labriola, Dan. *Complementary Cancer Therapies: Combining Traditional and Alternative Approaches for the Best Possible Outcome*. Roseville, CA: Prima Health, 2000.

Morra, Marion E. *Choices*. Avon Books, 1994.

Murphy, Gerald P. *Informed Decisions: The Complete Book of Cancer Diagnosis, Treatment and Recovery*. American Cancer Society, 1997.

PERIODICALS

"Cancer Killing Gene Found by Dartmouth Researchers." *Cancer Weekly* (April 9, 2002):17.

"Contact Voltage and Magnetic Fields as Possible Factors in Leukemia — Pilot Study." *Journal of Environmental Health* (December 2002):47–51.

"Cytokine and CD154 Gene Transfer Generate Immunity Against Leukemia." *Immunotherapy Weekly* (October 23, 2002):16.

"Drug Blocks Gene Mutation Effect in Lethal Leukemia." *Genomics & Genetics Weekly* (June 21, 2002):13.

"Leukemia Incidence Lowest in Patients 15-30 Years of Age (Incidence Drops at Age 20)." *Internal Medicine News* (May 1, 2002):37.

"New Drug Significantly Improves Survival Even for Patients with Late-Stage Disease." *Cancer Weekly* (December 31, 2002):6.

"Study: Regular Use of Aspirin May Lower Risk of Adult Leukemia." *Women's Health Weekly* (July 10, 2003):36.

ORGANIZATIONS

American Cancer Society. 1599 Clifton Road, N.E., Atlanta, Georgia 30329. (800) 227-2345. http://www.cancer.org.

Cancer Research Institute. 681 Fifth Avenue, New York, N.Y. 10022. (800) 992-2623. http://www.cancerresearch.org.

The Leukemia and Lymphoma Society. 600 Third Avenue, New York, NY 10016. (800) 955-4572. http://www.leukemia.org.

National Cancer Institute. 9000 Rockville Pike, Building 31, Room 10A16, Bethesda, Maryland, 20892. (800) 422-6237. http://wwwicic.nci.nih.gov.

Oncolink. University of Pennsylvania Cancer Center. http://cancer.med.upenn.edu.

OTHER

Rosenberg, Z'ev. "Treating the Undesirable Effect of Radiation and Chemotherapy with Chinese Medicine." *Oriental Chinese Journal*. http://www.healthypeople.com.

Mai Tran
Teresa G. Odle

Lice infestation

Definition

A lice infestation, or pediculosis, is caused by parasites living on human skin. Lice are tiny, wingless insects with sucking mouthparts that feed on human blood and lay eggs on body hair or in clothing. Lice **bites** can cause intense **itching**.

Description

There are three related species of human lice that live on different parts of the body:

- Head lice, *Pediculus humanus capitis*
- Body lice, *Pediculosis humanus corpus*
- Pubic lice, *Phthirus pubis*, commonly called "crab") lice

KEY TERMS

Crabs—An informal term for pubic lice.

Endemic—A condition that is always present in a given population, such as human lice infestation.

Insecticide—A pesticide that kills insects.

Lindane—An organic chloride, neurotoxic insecticide that kills lice.

Malathion—An organic phosphate, neurotoxic insecticide that kills lice.

Neurotoxin—A chemical compound that is toxic to the central nervous system.

Nit—The egg sac laid by adult female lice.

Pediculicide—Any substance that kills lice.

Pediculosis (plural, pediculoses)—A lice infestation.

Permethrin—A synthetic pyrethroid for killing lice.

Petroleum jelly or ointment—Petrolatum, a gelatinous substance obtained from oil that is used as a protective dressing.

Piperonyl butoxide—A liquid organic compound that enhances the activity of insecticides.

Pyrethrin, pyrethroid—Naturally-occurring insecticide extracted from chrysanthemum flowers. It paralyzes lice so that they cannot feed.

Pediculosis capitis is an infestation of head lice. A body lice infestation is called pediculosis corporis. Pediculosis palpebrarum or Phthiriasis palpebrarum, caused by crab lice, is an infestation of the eyebrows and eyelashes.

Lice infestations are not usually dangerous. However, head lice infestations present a serious public health problem because they spread easily among schoolchildren. In general, lice infestations occur in crowded, unsanitary facilities, including prison, military, and refugee camps. Lice infestations also occur frequently among the homeless.

Lice are transmitted through personal contact or infected clothing, bedding, or towels. Pubic lice are sexually transmitted. Lice do not jump, hop, or fly and they do not live on pets.

Head lice infestations are extremely common among children in schools, childcare facilities, camps, and playgrounds. They are the second most common communicable health problem in children, after the **common cold**, and appear to be on the increase. Six to 12 million American children get head lice every year. In developing countries, more than 50% of the general population may be infested. Head lice can affect anyone, regardless of race, sex, socio-economic class, or personal hygiene. However children aged three to ten and their families are most affected. Girls and women are more susceptible than boys and men. Although African American children are much less likely to have head lice than white or Hispanic children, the incidence is increasing, particularly in black children with thick, kinky hair or hair extensions or wraps. In Africa, head lice have adapted their claws to the curly, elliptical hair shafts of blacks. In developing countries, head lice infestations are a significant cause of contagious bacterial **infections**. Neither frequent brushing nor shampooing nor hair length affects the likelihood of head lice infestation.

Head lice live and crawl on the scalp, sucking blood every three to six hours. Their claws are adapted for clinging to hair or clothing. Adult head lice can be silvery-white to reddish-brown. They are about the size of a sesame seed, about 0.6 inches (1–4 mm.) long. Female lice lay their eggs in sacs called nits that are about 0.04 inches (1 mm.) long and are glued to shafts of hair close to the scalp. During her one-month lifespan, a female louse may lay more than 100 eggs. The nymphs hatch in three to 14 days and must feed on blood within one day. Nymphs are smaller and lighter in color than adults and become sexually mature after 9 to 12 days. Head lice cannot survive without a human host for more than a few days at most.

Body lice lay their nits in clothing or bedding. Occasionally the nits are attached to body hair. Body lice nits are oval and yellow to white in color. They may not hatch for up to 30 days. Nymphs mature in about 7 days. Body lice can live without human contact for up to 10 days.

Body lice infestations are usually associated with poor personal hygiene, as may occur during war or natural disasters or in cold climates. Body lice can carry and transmit disease-causing organisms, including those for epidemic typhus, relapsing **fever**, and trench fever. Trench fever is self-limiting. However, typhus and relapsing fever have mortality rates of five to 10 percent. The elderly are most vulnerable to these diseases.

Pubic lice can survive for one to two weeks without human contact and occasionally are transmitted through infected bedding, towels, or clothing. Pubic lice have large front legs and look like tiny crabs. Females are larger than males. Nits hatch in about one week and the nymphs mature in about seven days. Although pubic lice do not carry diseases, they often are found in association with other sexually transmitted diseases.

Causes and symptoms

Lice are endemic in human populations, spreading by personal contact or contact with infested clothing or other personal items. Lice also can be transmitted when unaffected clothing is stored with infested items. Among children, head lice are commonly transmitted by the sharing of hats, combs, brushes, hair accessories, headphones, pillows, and stuffed toys.

Lice infestations are characterized by intense itching caused by an allergic reaction to a toxin in the lice saliva. The itching can interfere with sleep and concentration. Repeated bites can lead to generalized skin eruptions or inflammation. Scratching or scraping at the bites can cause **hives** or abrasions that may lead to bacterial skin infections. Swelling or inflammation of the neck glands are common complications of head lice.

Body lice bites first appear as small red pimples or puncture marks and may cause a generalized skin rash. Intense itching can result in deep **scratches** around the shoulders, flanks, or neck. If the infestation is not treated, complications may develop, including **headache**, fever, and skin infection with scarring. Crab lice in children may be an indication of sexual activity or abuse.

Diagnosis

Lice usually are diagnosed by the itching. However, itching may not occur until several weeks after infestation, if at all. The tickling caused by moving lice may be noticeable. Definite diagnosis requires identification of lice or their nits.

Head lice may cause irritability in children. Scalp irritations or sores may be present. Although head lice in children are usually limited to the scalp, in adults, head lice can spread to eyebrows, eyelashes, mustaches, and beards. An adult louse may be visible as movement on the scalp, especially around the ears, nape of the neck, and center line of the crown—the warmest parts of the head. Since less than 20 mature lice may be present at a given time during infestation, the nits often are easier to spot. Nits vary in color from grayish-white to yellow, brown, or black. They are visible at the base or on the shaft of individual hairs. Applying about 10 ounces (280 grams) of isopropyl (rubbing) alcohol to the hair and rubbing with a white towel for about 30 seconds releases lice onto the towel for identification.

Body lice appear similar to head lice, however they burrow into the skin and are rarely seen except on clothing, where they lay their nits in seams. Over time, body lice infestations can lead to a thickening and discoloring of the skin around the waist, groin, and upper thighs. Scratching may cause sores that become infected with bacteria or fungi.

Pubic lice usually appear first on genital hair, although they may spread to other body hair. In young children, pubic lice are usually seen on the eyebrows or eyelashes. Pubic lice appear as brown or gray moving dots on the skin. There are usually only a few live lice present and they move very quickly away from light. Their white nits can be seen on hair shafts close to the skin. Although pubic lice sometimes produce small, bluish spots called maculae ceruleae on the trunk or thighs, usually it is easier to spot scratching marks. Small, dark-brown specks of lice excretion may be visible on underwear.

Since pediculicides (medications for treating lice) are usually strong insecticides with potential side effects, it is important to rule out other causes of scratching and skin inflammation. The oval-shaped head lice nits can be distinguished from **dandruff** because they are glued at an angle to the hair shaft. In contrast, flat, irregularly shaped flakes of dandruff shake off easily. A healthcare professional needs to distinguish between body lice and scabies—a disease caused by skin mites—and between pubic lice and **eczema**, a skin condition.

Treatment

Most treatments apply to all types of lice infestation and, particularly with head lice, treatments are an area of great controversy. The questionable safety and effectiveness of allopathic (fighting disease with remedies that produce effects different from those produced by the disease) treatments has spurred the search for alternative therapies. With any type of treatment, itching may not subside for several days.

Head lice

Most authorities believe that head lice should be treated immediately upon discovery.Before beginning any treatment:

- Test a small scalp section for allergic reactions to the medication
- A vinegar rinse helps loosen nits
- Wash hair with regular shampoo

Treatments for applying to the scalp and hair include:

- Olive oil or petroleum ointment to smother the lice. Cover the head with a shower cap, four to six hours per day for three to four days
- Olive oil (three parts) and essential oil of lavender (one part)
- Herbal shampoos or pomades
- A mixture of paw paw, thymol, and tea tree oil
- A combination of coconut oil, anise, and ylang ylang
- Other mixtures of essential oils
- RID Pure Alternative, a nontoxic, hypoallergenic, dye and fragrance-free product
- A spray containing phenethyl propionate, cedar oil, peppermint oil, and sodium lauryl sulfate (LiceFreee)
- Cocamide DEA (a lathering agent), triethanolamine (a local irritant), and disodium EDTA (a chelator), (SafeTek)is both a nontoxic pediculicide and a conditioner for combing out lice and nits

Cutting the hair or shaving the head may be effective. Aromatherapies also are available. Infested eyelashes and eyebrows should be treated with petroleum jelly for several days and the nits should be plucked off with tweezers or fingernails.

Body lice

Treatment for body lice is a thorough washing of the entire body and replacing infected clothing. Clothing and bedding should be washed at 140°F (60°C) and dried at high temperature, or dry-cleaned.

Pubic lice

A common herbal treatment for pubic lice consists of:

- Oil of pennyroyal (*Mentha pulegium*, 25%
- Oil of garlic (*Allium sativum*, 25%
- Distilled water, 50%

The mixture is applied to the pubic hair once a day for three days. Anyone with pubic lice should be tested for other sexually transmitted diseases.

Nit Removal

Neither alternative nor allopathic treatments will kill all lice nits. Hair and pubic lice nits must be removed manually to prevent re-infestation as the eggs hatch. Manual removal alone may effectively treat a lice infestation.

Before removing nits, one of the following procedures may be used:

- 50% vinegar rinse to loosen the nits
- wiping individual locks of hair from base to tip with a cloth soaked in vinegar
- 8% formic acid solution applied to the hair for 10 minutes, rinsed out, and towel-dried
- catching live lice with a comb, tweezers, fingernails, or by sticking them with double-sided tape
- enzymatic lice-egg remover

Furthermore:

- Hair should be clean, damp, and untangled
- Hair conditioner should not be used on hair treated allopathically
- Remove clothing and place a towel between the hair and shoulders
- Divide hair into square-inch (six sq.-cm.) sections. Clips or elastics can be used to divide long hair

Nits are manually removed with:

- Any fine-toothed comb, including pet flea combs
- A specialized nit comb (LiceMeister, LiceOut)
- A battery-powered vibrating or anti-static comb
- Tweezers
- Baby safety scissors
- Fingernails

To comb out nits:

- Comb along each hair section from scalp to tip
- Between each passing, dip the comb in water and wipe with a paper towel to remove lice and nits
- Hold the comb to the light to be sure it is clean
- If necessary, clean comb with a tooth or fingernail brush or dental floss
- Work under a good light, with a magnifying glass if necessary
- Do not rush. Long, thick hair may take an hour to comb out thoroughly
- Wash towels and clothing after combing
- Repeat at least twice a week for at least two weeks

Re-infestation

Re-infestation occurs often with all types of lice due to:

- Ineffective or incomplete treatment
- Chemical-resistant lice
- Failure to remove live nits
- Failure to treat all infected household members, playmates, or partners
- Failure to remove nits from clothing, bedding, towels, or other items
- Re-infestation from another source

Re-infestation with body or pubic lice can be prevented by washing underclothes, sleepwear, bedding, and towels in hot, soapy water and drying with high heat for at least 20 minutes. Clothing infected with body lice should be ironed under high heat. Sexual partners should be treated for public lice simultaneously and should re-examine themselves for several days.

To prevent head lice re-infestation:

- Repeat lice checks and nit removal daily until none are found
- Notify school, camp, or daycare, and parents of playmates
- Check and if necessary treat household members, playmates, schoolmates, school or daycare staff, and others in close contact with an infestation
- Treat combs and brushes with rubbing alcohol, Lysol, or soapy water above 130°F (54°C)
- Wash all bedding, clothing, headgear, scarves, and coats with soapy water at 130°F (54°C) and dry with high heat for at least 20 minutes
- Wash or vacuum stuffed animals and other toys
- Vacuum all helmets, carpets, rugs, mattresses, pillows, upholstery, and car seats
- Remove the vacuum cleaner bag after use, seal in a plastic bag, and place in the outside garbage
- Non-washable items should be dry cleaned or sealed in a plastic bag for up to four weeks
- Lice pesticide sprays for inanimate objects are toxic and are not recommended
- Repeat treatment if necessary

Allopathic treatment

All types of lice are treated allopathically with insecticidal lotions, shampoos, or cream rinses. However, experts disagree about the effectiveness and/or safety of pediculicides. Pediculicides do not kill nits, so nit removal and a second application in seven to 10 days may be necessary. Pediculicides can be poisonous if used improperly or too frequently and overuse can lead to the proliferation of chemically resistant lice. The residue may remain on the hair for several weeks and can cause skin or eye irritations.

Pediculicides should not be used:

- Near broken skin, eyes, or mucous membranes
- In the bathtub or shower

- By pregnant or nursing women or children under two

- By those with allergies, asthma, epilepsy, or some other medical conditions

Pyrethroids

All U.S. Food and Drug Administration (FDA)-approved non-prescription pediculicides contain relatively safe and effective pyrethroids. Insecticidal pyrethrins (0.33%) (RID, A-200) are extracts from chrysanthemum flowers. Permethrin (1%)(Nix) is a more stable synthetic pyrethrin. Pyrethroid pediculicides usually also contain 4% piperonyl butoxide.

To treat with pyrethroids:

- Apply for specified time, usually 10 minutes.

- Thoroughly rinse out.

- Do not wash hair for one or two days after treatment.

- Do not use cream rinse, hair spray, mousse, gels, mayonnaise, or vinegar before or within one week after treatment. These products may reduce pediculicide effectiveness

During the 1990s, as schools began requiring children to be lice and nit-free, the use of pyrethroids rose significantly and the FDA began receiving reports of ineffectiveness. The FDA ordered new labeling of pyrethroid pediculicides on the outside of the carton, in simpler language, and with more information, to take effect in 2005–2006. Permethrin sprays for treating mattresses, furniture, and other items are not recommended.

Other insecticides

Prescription insecticides are used when other lice treatments fail or cannot be used. These pesticides include:

- Malathion (0.5% in Ovide), a neurotoxic organophosphate, was withdrawn from the U.S. market due to an increase in malathion-resistant lice and re-introduced in 1999. It is foul-smelling and flammable. Sometimes infested clothing is treated with a 1% malathion powder

- Lindane (1% or higher) (Kwell), an organochloride neurotoxin, can induce seizures and death in susceptible people, even when used according to the directions. In 2003 the FDA required new labeling and a reduction in bottle size

- Ivermectin (Stromectol), an oral treatment for intestinal parasites, is effective against head lice but has not been approved for that use by the FDA

Infested eyelashes are treated with a thick coating of prescription petroleum ointment, applied twice daily for ten days.

Prognosis

Despite the presence of chemically resistant lice and the thoroughness required to prevent re-infestation, essentially all lice infestations can be eradicated eventually.

Prevention

Prevention of lice infestation depends on adequate personal hygiene and the following public health measures:

- Avoid sharing combs, brushes, hair accessories, hats, towels, or bedding

- Check hair and scalp weekly for lice and nits

- Limit sexual partners

Regular lice checks in schools and "no nit" re-entry policies have not been shown to be effective. The American Academy of Pediatrics, the Harvard School of Public Health, and the National Association of School Nurses recommend their elimination, although many healthcare professionals disagree.

Scientists have identified both the gene that enables head and body lice to digest blood and the gene that helps lice combat deadly infections, with the potential for new treatments and preventions for lice infestation.

Resources

BOOKS

Goldberg, Burton, et al. "Children's Health." *Alternative Medicine: The Definitive Guide.* 2nd ed. Berkeley, CA: Ten Speed Press, 2002.

Grossman, Leigh B. *Infection Control in the Child Care Center and Preschool.* Philadelphia: Lippincott Williams & Wilson, 2003.

PERIODICALS

Blenkinsopp, Alison. "Head Lice." *Primary Health Care* 13 (October 2003): 33–34.

Burgess, I. F. "Human Lice and Their Control." *Annual Review of Entomology* 49 (2004): 457.

Elston, D. M. "Drug-Resistant Lice." *Archives of Dermatology.* 139 (2003): 1061–1064.

Evans, Jeff "Pediatric Dermatology: Simple Methods Often Best: Lice, Mosquitoes, Warts." *Family Practice News.* 34 (January 15, 2004): 56.

Flinders, David C., and Peter De Schweinitz. "Pediculosis and Scabies." *American Family Physician* 69 (January 15, 2004): 341–352.

Heukelbach, Jorg, and Hermann Feldmeier. "Ectoparasites— The Underestimated Realm." *Lancet* 363 (March 13, 2004): 889–891.

Hunter, J. A., and S. C. Barker. "Susceptibility of Head Lice (*Pediculus humanus capitis*) to Pediculicides in Australia." *Parasitology Research* 90 (August 2003): 476–478.

Kittler, R., et al. "Molecular Evolution of *Pediculus humanus* and the Origin of Clothing." *Current Biology* 13 (August 19, 2003): 1414–1417.

"Recommendations Provided for Back-to-School Head Lice Problem." *Health & Medicine Week* October 6, 2003: 329.

Yoon, K. S., et al. "Permethrin-Resistant Human Head Lice, *Pediculus capitis*, and Their Treatment." *Archives of Dermatology* 139 (August 2003): 1061–1064.

Zepf, Bill. "Treatment of Head Lice: Therapeutic Options." *American Family Physician* 69 (February 1, 2004): 655.

OTHER

Lice. MayoClinic.com. August 5, 2002 [cited April 18, 2004]. http://www.mayoclinic.com/invoke.cfm?id= DS00368.

Lindane Shampoo and Lindane Lotion Questions and Answers. Center for Drug Evaluation and Research, U.S. Food and Drug Administration. April 15, 2003 [cited April 18, 2004]. http://www.fda.gov/cder/drug/infopage/lindane/lindaneQA.htm.

ORGANIZATIONS

American Academy of Dermatology (AAD). P.O. Box 4014, Schaumburg, IL 60168-4014. 847-330-0230. http://www.aad.org.

American Academy of Pediatrics (AAP). 141 Northwest Point Boulevard, Elk Grove Village, IL 60007-1098. 847-434-4000. kidsdocs@aap.org http://www.aap.org.

Centers for Disease Control and Prevention, National Center for Infectious Diseases, Division of Parasitic Diseases. 1600 Clifton Road, Atlanta, GA 30333. 404-639-3534. 800-311-3435. http://www.cdc.gov/ncidod/dpd/parasites/lice/default.htm.

National Pediculosis Association (NPA), Inc. 50 Kearney Road, Needham, MA 02494. 781-449-NITS. npa@headlice.org. http://www.headlice.org.

Rebecca J. Frey, PhD
Margaret Alic, PhD

Lichen *see* **Usnea**

Licorice

Description

Licorice, *Glycyrrhiza glabra*, is a purple and white flowering perennial, native of the Mediterranean region and central and southwest Asia. It is cultivated

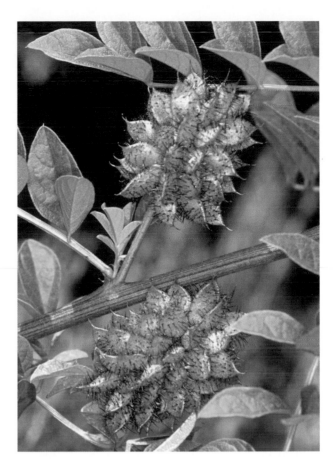

Common licorice. *(© blickwinkel / Alamy)*

widely for the sweet taproot that grows to a depth of four ft (1.2 m). Licorice is a hardy plant that thrives in full sun or partial shade and prefers rich, moist soil. It may grow to a height of 3-7 ft (1-2 m). The wrinkled, brown root has yellow interior flesh and is covered with a tangle of rootlets branching from the stolons. The aerial parts of the plant are erect and branching with round stems that become somewhat angular near the top. The leaves are alternate, odd, and pinnate, dividing into as many as eight pairs of oblong leaflets. Licorice blossoms in late summer. The sweet-pea like flowers grow in clusters forming in the angle where the stem joins the branch. The maroon colored seed pods are about 1-2 in (3-5 cm) long and contain one to six kidney-shaped seeds.

Licorice is a sweet and soothing herb that has been appreciated for its medicinal qualities for thousands of years. Hippocrates named the herb *glukos riza*, or sweet root. Several species of this member of the Leguminosae, or pea, family, are used medicinally. *Glycyrrhiza glabra*, also known as sweet wood or sweet licorice, is cited first in most herbals. Chinese licorice, *G. uralenis* or *G. viscida*, known as the peacemaker, was included in the Chinese classic herbal *Pen Tsao Ching* over 2,000 years ago, and is believed to promote longevity. An American variety, *G. lepidota* or wild licorice, was a common Native American remedy and was also used by early settlers. Dominican friars brought the herb to England in the sixteenth century. The abbess Hildegard of Bingen added licorice to her materia medica, and this well-loved herb was a favorite of German and English herbalists.

General use

The medicinal benefits of licorice root have been studied extensively, and its use in traditional medicine is well documented. Licorice is an expectorant, helpful in the treatment of upper respiratory tract catarrh. The root extract is demulcent, and commonly used as a component of many medicinal syrups and drops providing relief to a **sore throat** and for coughs. The glycoside glycyrrhizin, found in the root, is more than 50 times as sweet as sucrose. Glycyrrhizin, which becomes glycyrrhizic acid when ingested, has been credited with much of the pharmacological action of licorice. The herb is also effective as a mild laxative, cleansing the colon. Licorice is a liver tonic and is used as an anti-inflammatory medicine, useful in the treatment of arthritis. Along with other herbs, licorice is used to treat **muscle spasms**. It also acts to reduce stomach acid and relieves **heartburn**. Other active chemical constituents in licorice root include asparagine, flavonoids and isoflavonoids, chalcones, coumarins, sterols, and triterpenoid saponins. Studies have shown that licorice also stimulates the production of interferon.

Licorice preparations have been used in the healing of peptic ulcers. The demulcent action of the root extract coats and soothes the ulcerated tissue. Licorice also has a beneficial effect on the endocrine system and is helpful in treatment of problems with the adrenal gland, such as Addison's disease. Phytochemicals in the root act similarly to and stimulate the secretion of the body's natural adrenal cortex hormone, aldosterone. This sweet herb also has antibacterial action and is beneficial in treatment of **hypoglycemia**. Licorice increases bile flow and acts to lower blood **cholesterol** levels. Licorice root, when boiled to extract its sweetness, has been used traditionally in candy making. Commercially it is a flavoring in beer, soft drinks, and tobacco. Singers chew the root to ease throat irritation and to strengthen their voice. Many women's herbal formulas include licorice for its estrogenic properties as an aid to normalize and regulate hormone production during **menopause**; however, some recent studies indicate that licorice does not have the

---

KEY TERMS

Apoptosis—Cell suicide or self-destruction. Licorice contains a compound that induces apoptosis in some types of human cancer cells.

Decoction—A herbal extract prepared by boiling the plant material for some time.

Demulcent—A type of medication given to soothe the stomach lining or other irritated mucous membrane. Licorice extract can be used as a demulcent.

Expectorant—A substance or medication given to bring up phlegm or mucus from the respiratory tract.

Glycyrrhizin—A sweet-tasting compound in licorice root that has a number of beneficial effects on the cardiovascular and digestive systems.

Tincture—A herbal preparation made by soaking the roots, leaves, or other parts of the plant in alcohol or a mixture of alcohol and water.

---

estrogenic qualities that have been attributed to it. Licorice is frequently used in medicinal compounds with other herbs. In Chinese medicine, this herb is always used in compound, as it can minimize the bitter taste of some herbal components, and help to blend and harmonize the entire mixture.

More recently, licorice has been found to offer some protection against cardiovascular disease. A team of Israeli researchers found that licorice root extract added to the diet lowers blood cholesterol levels as well as the rate of oxidation in cardiovascular tissue.

Licorice also shows promise as a possible chemo-preventive against **cancer**. Glycyrrhizin, the glycoside credited with many of the beneficial effects of licorice, appears to inhibit the growth of cancer cells as well. In addition, a new polyphenol compound isolated from licorice root has been found to induce apoptosis, or self-destruction, in human prostate and breast tumor cells.

Preparations

The dried root is used in medicinal preparations. Harvest the taproot of three- to four-year-old plants in late autumn. Washed and dried, the root may be stored intact until needed for a preparation.

Decoction: Combine one teaspoonful of dried root, powdered or diced, for each cup of non-chlorinated water. Bring to boil, lower heat and simmer for 10-15 minutes. Dosage is three cups per day. Prepare fresh decoction daily.

Tincture: Combine one part dried root, powdered or diced, with five parts of brandy or vodka in a glass container. A 50/50 alcohol to water ratio is optimal. Seal the container with an airtight lid. Leave to macerate in a darkened place for two weeks. Shake daily. Strain the mixture through a cheesecloth or muslin bag and pour into a dark bottle for storage up to two years. Dosage is one to three milliliters of the tincture three times a day.

Precautions

People should avoid using licorice in large doses for long periods of time. This herbal remedy should be used for no longer than four to six weeks without medical advice. Pregnant women should not use the herb. Persons with high blood pressure or kidney disease should not use licorice, nor should those with cholestatic liver disorders or **cirrhosis**.

Side effects

Excessive use of the herbal extract may raise blood pressure, cause water retention, **headache**, and **potassium** loss; however, for persons on high potassium, low-sodium **diets**, this may not be a problem. Licorice taken in its natural form, such as chewing the root, may mitigate the side effect of water retention because of the high presence of the plant constituent asparagine. **Deglycyrrhizinated licorice** extract is commercially available for treatment of peptic ulcer and eliminates side effects possible with other licorice preparations.

Interactions

When licorice is used while taking thiazide diuretic medications, this may exacerbate potassium loss. Sensitivity to **digitalis** glycosides may increase with loss of potassium.

Resources

BOOKS

Blumenthal, Mark. *The Complete German Commission E Monographs, Therapeutic Guide to Herbal Medicines.* Massachusetts: Integrative Medicine Communications, 1998.

Bown, Deni. *The Herb Society of America, Encyclopedia of Herbs And Their Uses.* New York: D.K. Publishing, Inc., 1995.

Gladstar, Rosemary. *Herbal Healing for Women.* New York, Simon & Schuster, 1993.

Kowalchik, Claire, and William H. Hylton. *Rodale's Illustrated Encyclopedia of Herbs.* Pennsylvania: Rodale Press, 1987.

Mabey, Richard. *The New Age Herbalist.* New York: Simon & Schuster, Inc., 1998.

PERIODICALS

Amato, P., S. Christophe, and P. L. Mellon. "Estrogenic Activity of Herbs Commonly Used as Remedies for Menopausal Symptoms." *Menopause* 9 (March-April 2002): 145-150.

Fuhrman, B., N. Volkova, M. Kaplan, et al. "Antiatherosclerotic Effects of Licorice Extract Supplementation on Hypercholesterolemic Patients: Increased Resistance of LDL to Atherogenic Modifications, Reduced Plasma Lipid Levels, and Decreased Systolic Blood Pressure." *Nutrition* 18 (March 2002): 268-273.

Hsiang, C. Y., I. L. Lai, D. C. Chao, and T. Y. Ho. "Differential Regulation of Activator Protein 1 Activity by Glycyrrhizin." *Life Sciences* 70 (February 22, 2002): 1643-1656.

Rafi, M. M., B. C. Vastano, N. Zhu, et al. "Novel Polyphenol Molecule Isolated from Licorice Root (*Glycyrrhiza glabra*) Induces Apoptosis, G2/M Cell Cycle Arrest, and Bcl-2 Phosphorylation in Tumor Cell Lines." *Journal of Agricultural and Food Chemistry* 50 (February 13, 2002): 677-684.

Clare Hanrahan
Rebecca J. Frey, PhD

Licorice mint *see* **Agastache**

Light therapy

Definition

Light therapy, or phototherapy, is the administration of doses of bright light in order to treat a variety of sleep and mood disorders. It is most commonly used to re-regulate the body's internal clock and/or relieve **depression**.

Origins

Light, both natural and artificial, has been prescribed throughout the ages for healing purposes. Sunlight has been used medicinally since the time of the ancient Greeks; Hippocrates, the father of modern medicine, prescribed exposure to sunlight for a number of illnesses. In the late nineteenth and early twentieth centuries, bright light and fresh air were frequently prescribed for a number of mood and **stress** related disorders. In fact, prior to World War II, hospitals were regularly built with

Types of light therapy

Type	Description	Condition/disease
Back of knee	The area behind the knee, known as the popliteal region, contains photoreceptors that can adjust the body's circadian rhythms.	Seasonal affective disorder (SAD), jet lag
Colored	Different colored light has therapeutic effects on the body. Depending on the condition, the colored light can be projected as a beam on a specific area or as a floodlight that covers the whole body.	Used in conjunction with accupuncture (but they are not lasers), or on its own
Cold laser	Very low-intensity laser beams are directed at the body.	Used in laser acupunture to treat pain, stress tendinitis, etc.
Full spectrum, non - UV	Full spectrum light that does not emit UV rays.	Skin diseases, rashes, jaundice, and seasonal affective disorder (SAD)

(Illustration by Corey Light. Cengage Learning, Gale)

solariums, or sun rooms, in which patients could spend time recuperating in the sunlight.

In the 1980s, light therapy began to make an appearance in the medical literature as a treatment for **seasonal affective disorder**, or SAD. Today, it is widely recognized as a front-line treatment for the disorder.

Benefits

Light therapy is most often prescribed to treat seasonal affective disorder, a form of depression most often associated with shortened daylight hours in northern latitudes from the late fall to the early spring. It is also occasionally employed to treat such sleep-related disorders as **insomnia** and **jet lag**. Recently, light therapy has also been found effective in the treatment of such nonseasonal forms of depression as **bipolar disorder**. One 2001 study found that bright light reduced depressive symptoms 12–35% more than a placebo treatment in nine out of 10 randomized controlled trials.

When used to treat SAD or other forms of depression, light therapy has several advantages over prescription antidepressants. Light therapy tends to work faster than medications, alleviating depressive symptoms within two to 14 days after beginning light therapy as opposed to an average of four to six weeks with medication. And unlike antidepressants, which can cause a variety of side effects from **nausea** to concentration problems, light therapy is extremely well tolerated. Some side effects are possible with light but are generally not serious enough to cause discontinuation of the therapy.

There are several other different applications for light therapy, including:

- Full-spectrum/UV light therapy for disorders of the skin. A subtype of light therapy that is often prescribed to treat skin diseases, rashes, and jaundice.

- Cold laser therapy. The treatment involves focusing very low-intensity beams of laser light on the skin, and is used in laser acupuncture to treat a myriad of symptoms and illnesses, including pain, stress, and tendinitis.

- Colored light therapy. In colored light therapy, different colored filters are applied over a light source to achieve specific therapeutic effects. The colored light is then focused on the patient, either with a floodlight which covers the patient with the colored light, or

KEY TERMS

Dawn simulation—A form of light therapy in which the patient is exposed while asleep to gradually brightening white light over a period of an hour and a half.

Lux—The International System unit for measuring illumination, equal to one lumen per square meter.

Neurotransmitter—A chemical in the brain that transmits messages between neurons, or nerve cells.

Seasonal affective disorder (SAD)—A mood disorder characterized by depression, weight gain, and sleepiness during the winter months. An estimated 4–6% of the population of Canada and the northern United States suffers from SAD.

Serotonin—A neurotransmitter that is involved in mood disorders as well as transmitting nerve impulses.

with a beam of light that is focused on the area of the illness.

• Back of knee light therapy. A 1998 report published in the journal *Science* reported that the area behind the human knee known as the popliteal region contains photoreceptors that can help to adjust the body's circadian rhythms. The authors of the study found that they could manipulate circadian rhythms by focusing a bright light on the popliteal region. Further studies are needed to determine the efficacy of this treatment on disorders such as SAD and jet lag.

Description

Light therapy is generally administered at home. The most commonly used light therapy equipment is a portable lighting device known as a light box. The light box may be a full-spectrum box, in which the lighting element contains all wavelengths of light found in natural light (including UV rays), or it may be a bright light box, in which the lighting element emits non-UV white light. The box may be mounted upright to a wall, or slanted downwards towards a table.

The patient sits in front of the box for a prescribed period of time (anywhere from 15 minutes to several hours). For patients just starting on the therapy, initial sessions are usually only 10–15 minutes in length. Some patients with SAD undergo light therapy session two or three times a day, others only once. The time of day and number of times treatment is administered depends on the physical needs and lifestyle of the individual patient. If light therapy has been prescribed for the treatment of SAD, it typically begins in the fall months as the days begin to shorten, and continues throughout the winter and possibly the early spring. Patients with a long-standing history of SAD are usually able to establish a time-table or pattern to their depressive symptoms, and can initiate treatment accordingly before symptoms begin.

The light from a slanted light box is designed to focus on the table it sits upon, so patients may look down to read or do other sedentary activities during therapy. Patients using an upright light box must face the light source, and should glance toward the light source occasionally without staring directly into the light. The light sources in these light boxes typically range from 2,500–10,000 lux (in contrast, average indoor lighting is 300–500 lux; a sunny summer day is about 100,000 lux).

Light boxes can be purchased for between $200 and $500. Some healthcare providers and healthcare supply companies also rent the fixtures. This gives a patient the opportunity to have a trial run of the therapy before making the investment in a light box. Recently, several new light box products have become available. Dawn simulators are lighting devices or fixtures that are programmed to turn on gradually, from dim to bright light, to simulate the sunrise. They are sometimes prescribed for individuals who have difficulty getting up in the morning due to SAD symptoms. Another device known as a light visor is designed to give an individual more mobility during treatment. The visor is a lighting apparatus that is worn like a sun visor around the crown of the head. Patients with any history of eye problems should consult their healthcare professional before attempting to use a light visor.

Preparations

Full-spectrum light boxes do emit UV rays, so patients with sun-sensitive skin should apply a sun screen before sitting in front of the box for an extended period of time.

Precautions

Patients with eye problems should see an ophthalmologist regularly both before and during light therapy. Because UV rays are emitted by the light box, patients taking photosensitizing medications should consult with their healthcare provider before beginning treatment. In addition, patients with medical conditions that make them sensitive to UV rays should also be seen by a healthcare professional before starting phototherapy.

Patients beginning light therapy for SAD may need to adjust the length, frequency, and timing of their phototherapy sessions in order to achieve the maximum benefits. Patients should keep their healthcare provider informed of their progress and the status of their depressive symptoms. Occasionally, additional treatment measures for depression (i.e., antidepressants, herbal remedies, **psychotherapy**) may be recommended as an adjunct, or companion treatment, to light therapy.

Side effects

Some patients undergoing light therapy treatments report side effects of eyestrain, headaches, insomnia, **fatigue**, **sunburn**, and dry eyes and nose. Most of these effects can be managed by adjusting the timing and duration of the light therapy sessions. A strong sun block and eye and nose drops can alleviate the others. Long-term studies have shown no negative effects to eye function of individuals undergoing light therapy treatment.

A small percentage of light therapy patients may experience hypomania, a feeling of exaggerated, hyper-elevated mood. Again, adjusting the length and frequency of treatment sessions can usually manage this side effect.

Research and general acceptance

Light therapy is widely accepted by both traditional and complementary medicine as an effective treatment for SAD. The exact mechanisms by which the treatment works are not known, but the bright light employed in light therapy may act to readjust the body's circadian rhythms, or internal clock. Other popular theories are that light triggers the production of serotonin, a neurotransmitter believed to be related to depressive disorders, or that it influences the body's production of **melatonin**, a hormone that may be related to circadian rhythms. A recent British study suggests that dawn simulation, a form of light therapy in which the patient is exposed to white light of gradually increasing brightness (peaking at 250 lux after 90 min) may be even more effective in treating depression than exposure to bright light. Dawn simulation is started around 4:30 or 5 A.M., while the patient is still asleep.

Wide-spectrum UV light treatment for skin disorders such as **psoriasis** is also considered a standard treatment option in clinical practice. However, such other light-related treatments as cold laser therapy and colored light therapy are not generally accepted, since few or no scientific studies exist on the techniques.

Training and certification

Psychiatrists, psychologists, and other mental healthcare professional prescribe light therapy treatment for SAD. Holistic healthcare professionals and light therapists who specialize in this treatment are also available; in some states, these professionals require a license, so individuals should check with their state board of health to ensure their practitioner has the proper credentials. Light therapy for skin disorders should be prescribed by a dermatologist or other healthcare professional with expertise in skin diseases and light therapy treatment.

Resources

BOOKS

American Psychiatric Association. *Diagnostic and Statistical Manual of Mental Disorders*. 4th ed. Washington, DC: American Psychiatric Press, Inc., 1994.

Lam, Raymond, ed. *Seasonal Affective Disorder and Beyond: Light Treatment for SAD and Non-SAD Conditions*. Washington, DC: American Psychiatric Press, 1998.

Rosenthal, Norman. *Winter Blues: Seasonal Affective Disorder—What It Is and How to Overcome It*. New York: Guilford Press, 1998.

PERIODICALS

Eagles, John M. "SAD—Help Arrives with the Dawn" *Lancet* 358 (December 22, 2001): 2100.

Jepson, Tracy, et al. "Current Perspectives on the Management of Seasonal Affective Disorder." *Journal of the American Pharmaceutical Association*. 39 no. 6 (1999): 822–829.

Sherman, Carl. "Underrated Light Therapy Effective for Depression." *Clinical Psychiatry News* 29 (October 2001): 32.

ORGANIZATIONS

National Depressive and Manic Depressive Association. 730 Franklin Street, Suite 501, Chicago, IL 60610. (800) 826-3632. http://www.ndmda.org

Society for Light Treatment and Biological Rhythms. 824 Howard Ave., New Haven, CT 06519. Fax (203) 764-4324. http://www.sltbr.org. sltbr@yale.edu.

Paula Ford-Martin
Rebecca J. Frey, PhD

Ling zhi *see* **Reishi mushroom**

Linoleic acid

Description

Linoleic acid is a colorless to straw-colored liquid polyunsaturated fatty acid with the chemical formula ($C_{18}H_{32}O_2$) of the omega-6 series. Linoleic and another fatty acid, gamma-linolenic, or gamolenic, produce compounds called prostaglandins. Prostaglandins are substances found in every cell, are needed for the body's overall health maintenance, and must be replenished constantly. Linoleic acid is an essential fatty acid, which means that the body cannot produce it, so it must be obtained in the diet.

Linoleic acid is an important fatty acid, especially for the growth and development of infants. Fatty acids help to maintain the health of cell membranes, improve nutrient use, and establish and control cellular metabolism. They also provide the raw materials that help in the control of blood pressure, blood clotting, inflammation, body temperature, and other body functions. Fatty acids are consumed in the greatest quantities in the synthesis of fat. Although many people are encouraged to consume less fat in their **diets**, fat is still an important component of a healthy body. Fat stores the body's extra calories, helps insulate the body, and protects body tissues. Fats are also an important energy source during **exercise**, when the body depends on its calories after using up available carbohydrates. Fat helps in the absorption and transport through the bloodstream of the fat-soluble vitamins A, D, E, and K.

Conjugated linoleic acid (CLA) is a naturally occurring mixture of various isomers of linoleic acid with conjugated double bonds. The isomers of CLA have different shapes, functions, and benefits. CLA supplements, or fats containing CLA, generally contain a mixture of these isomers. Although CLA is present in many foods and can be synthesized from linoleic acid, it is made naturally in the stomach, especially in ruminant animals. (Ruminants are animals that regurgitate food and chew it, known as "chewing the cud." Cows and sheep are ruminants.) For this reason, CLA is found primarily in dairy and beef products, as well as other foods derived from ruminant animals. Many people have likely decreased their intake of CLA for two reasons. First, people in the 2000s are typically eating less beef and dairy fat in their diets. Second, many cattle are fed grain diets, which are lower in linoleic acid than the grass on which they would naturally feed, so there is less CLA in beef raised in the meat industry and in dairy foods. It is possible to increase the CLA in milk by adding a

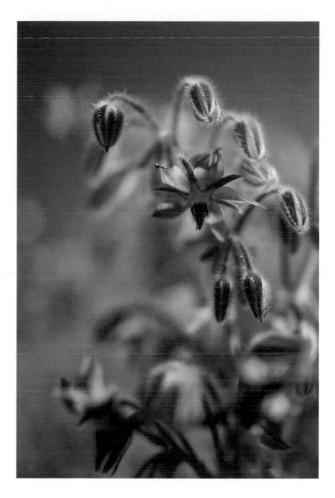

Borage is a source of linoleic acid. (© David Noton Photography / Alamy)

linoleic acid supplement to livestock feed. The supplement also increases lean tissue and decreases fat in the animals and induces dairy cattle to produce more milk.

Linoleic acid is found in **fish oil**, meat, milk, and other dairy products. It is also a constituent of many vegetable oils, including **evening primrose oil**, sunflower oil, and safflower oil. Commercially produced linoleic acid is used in margarine, animal feeds, emulsifying agents, soaps, and drugs.

General use

As mentioned, CLA supplements, or fats containing CLA, generally contain a mixture of CLA isomers. Plant oils, though they contain little CLA, are a rich source of linoleic acid. While linoleic acid may be taken as a supplement to help with certain conditions, the supplement will not necessarily increase CLA levels in the body.

Anticarcinogenic

One particular isomer in CLA, known as cis-9, trans-11, is linked to anticancer benefits. Studies with animals have shown CLA to reduce breast, prostate, stomach, colorectal, lung, and skin cancers. The CLA may slow the growth of cells that give rise to **cancer**. A human study has shown an association between linoleic acids and a decreased risk for **prostate cancer**. In addition, a study done in 2001 on human **breast cancer** cells grown in a laboratory medium showed that linoleic acid works to reduce tumor size through its effects on a gene that controls the rate of apoptosis, or cell self-destruction.

Cystic fibrosis

Infants with cystic fibrosis (CF) often have poor weight gain and growth and an inability to absorb fats. Some research suggests that infants with CF can benefit from formula with a high linoleic acid content because it optimizes **nutrition**, growth, and feeding efficiency.

Multiple sclerosis

Multiple sclerosis (MS) is a disease in which demyelination (loss of myelin sheath material) occurs. (The myelin sheath is a fatty substance that surrounds and insulates the axon of some nerve cells.) This condition leads to disruptions in nerve impulse transmission. Linoleic acid is believed to be helpful because myelin is composed of **lecithin**, which is made of linoleic and other fatty acids. Many diets recommended for MS patients include supplements. Patients supplementing with linoleic acid show a smaller increase in disability and reduced severity and duration of attacks than those with no linoleic acid supplement. Evening primrose oil is beneficial because of its specialized fatty-acid content, including linoleic acid. Doses of sunflower seed oil or evening primrose oil to provide 17 grams linoleic acid per day may be beneficial.

Pregnancy

One study indicated that low doses of linoleic acid and **calcium** can reduce the incidence of preeclampsia in high-risk women. (Preeclampsia is the development of **hypertension** with increased protein in the urine or accumulation of watery fluid in cells or tissues or both, due to pregnancy.) Another study showed, however, that linoleic acid consumption can have a negative effect on fetal growth. Pregnant women should talk to their doctors before taking linoleic acid or any other supplement.

Diet and nutrition

CLA helps regulate how the body accumulates and retains fat. It has been shown to reduce body fat, improve muscle tone, improve nutrient usage, and reduce the appetite by improving the way the body extracts energy from less food. These properties are useful for individuals trying to lose weight or tone muscles and also for people with nutrient absorption disorders and other digestive problems. The CLA isomer linked with reducing body fat and increasing lean muscle mass is trans-10, cis-12.

Skin care

Linoleic acid helps relieve flaky, itchy, or rough skin and maintain smooth, moist skin. A tablespoon of linoleic acid-rich foods or oils may be added on a daily basis to help improve and moisturize skin. Linoleic acid may also help with skin disorders such as atopic **eczema**. Evening primrose oil is taken to help with skin, hair, and nail repair.

Other uses

Animal research suggests that CLA supplementation may limit food allergy reactions and improve glucose tolerance. It is also used as a nutritional supplement for allergic respiratory disease, circulation, arthritis, and inflammatory problems. CLA is a potent antioxidant and may help reduce plaque formation in arteries and thus help prevent **heart disease**. Evening primrose oil helps to reduce arthritis **pain** and **depression**. It also helps to control diabetes, liver and kidney damage due to alcohol, and several symptoms of **premenstrual syndrome** (PMS).

Linoleic acid appears to have at least one negative effect on the human body, however. It appears to increase a person's risk of developing age-related **macular degeneration** (ARMD), a disease of the eye that leads to a progressive loss of vision and eventual blindness.

Preparations

Evening primrose oil is a fixed oil obtained from the seeds of *Oenothera biennis* or other spp. (Onagraceae). It contains about 72% linoleic acid and 9% gamolenic acid. Typical doses expressed as gamolenic acid are 320 or 480 mg daily, taken in two or three doses. Safflower oil is the refined fixed oil obtained from the seeds of the safflower, or false (bastard) **saffron**, *Carthamus tinctorius* (Compositae). It contains about 75% linoleic acid as well as various saturated fatty acids.

KEY TERMS

Age-related macular degeneration (ARMD)—An eye disease that appears to be related to high levels of linoleic acid in the body. ARMD is characterized by progressive and permanent loss of vision.

Apoptosis—The programmed self-destruction of a cell, which takes place when the cell detects some damage to its DNA. Apoptosis is sometimes called "cell suicide." The antitumor activity of linoleic acid is related to its effects on a gene that controls the rate of apoptosis.

Atopic eczema—Inflammation of the skin caused by allergic reaction.

Cystic fibrosis (CF)—A disorder of the exocrine glands that affects many organs of the body, especially the sweat glands and glands in the lungs and pancreas.

Isomers—Molecules that have the same molecular formula, but different configurations.

Multiple sclerosis (MS)—A disease caused by demyelination, or loss of myelin sheath material, which is essential in nerve impulse transmission.

Omega-6 fatty acid—A fatty acid with its first double bond at the sixth carbon in its carbon chain.

Phenothiazines—A parent compound for the synthesis of some antipsychotic compounds.

CLA is available in beef and dairy products, but to avoid eating too many fatty animal foods, supplements may be taken. CLA comes in capsules and softgels that range in potency from 600 to 1,000 mg. A specialist should be consulted to determine what is most appropriate.

Precautions

CLA appears to be safe and nontoxic at supplemental levels. However, using evening primrose oil as a supplement for linoleic acid can cause symptoms of undiagnosed temporal lobe **epilepsy** and should be used with caution in patients with a history of epilepsy.

Side effects

CLA may cause gastrointestinal upset in isolated cases, and evening primrose oil can cause minor gastrointestinal upset and **headache**.

Interactions

People who take epileptogenic drugs (drugs which cause epilepsy), in particular phenothiazines, may have interactions with evening primrose oil and should talk to their doctor before using a supplement.

Resources

BOOKS

Sebedio, J. L., W. W. Christie, and R. Adlof, eds. *Advances in Conjugated Linoleic Acid Research*, vol. 2. Champaign, IL: AOCS Press, 2006.

Williams, Lane. *Conjugated Linoleic Acid for Weight Loss*. Chapmanville, WV: Woodland Press, 2007.

Yurawecz, M. P., et al., eds. *Advances in Conjugated Linoleic Acid Research*, vol. 1. Champaign, IL: AOCS Press, 2006.

PERIODICALS

"Conjugated Linoleic Acid [Clarinol] Reduces Fat Mass in Specific Areas on the Body." *Inpharma* (April 21, 2007): 11.

Das, Undurti N. "Beneficial Actions of Polyunsaturated Fatty Acids in Cardiovascular Diseases: But How and Why?" *Current Nutrition & Food Science* (February 2008): 2–31.

Leaf, Alexander, Jing X. Kang, and Yong-Fu Xiao. "Fish Oil Fatty Acids as Cardiovascular Drugs." *Current Vascular Pharmacology* (January 2008): 1–12.

Logan, A. C. "Linoleic and Linolenic Acids and Acne Vulgaris." *British Journal of Dermatology* (January 2008): 201–202.

Rao, A. V., K. Andrews, and A. Logan. "A Double-Blind, Randomized-Controlled Trial of a Nutritional Supplement (abs+) Containing Conjugated Linoleic Acid (CLA) and Epigallocatechin-gallate (EGCG) in Human Weight Loss." *Journal of Herbs, Spices, & Medicinal Plants* (February 2007): 69–78.

Melissa C. McDade
Rebecca J. Frey, PhD
David Edward Newton, Ed.D.

Linseed *see* **Flaxseed**

Lipase

Definition

Lipase is an enzyme that is used by the body to break down dietary fats (lipids), especially triglycerides, into a form that can be absorbed in the intestines.

Description

Lipase is not found in foods; rather it is naturally manufactured in the pancreas. Small amounts are produced in the stomach and secreted in the saliva. The pancreas also makes two other groups of **digestive enzymes**: protease and amylase. The pancreas is a glandular organ near the stomach that secretes digestive juices into the small intestine and releases the hormones insulin, glucagon, and somatostatin into the bloodstream. Lipase appears in the blood together with another enzyme called amylase following damage to or diseases affecting the pancreas. It was once thought that abnormally high lipase levels were associated only with diseases of the pancreas. Other conditions are in the 2000s known to be associated with high lipase levels, especially kidney failure and intestinal obstruction. Diseases involving the pancreas, however, produce much higher lipase levels than diseases of other organs. Lipase levels in pancreatic disorders are often 5–10 times higher than normal.

Lipase levels are determined by a blood test. The lipase blood test is most often used in evaluating inflammation of the pancreas (**pancreatitis**), but it is also useful in diagnosing kidney failure, intestinal obstruction, **mumps**, and peptic ulcers. Doctors often order amylase and lipase tests at the same time to help distinguish pancreatitis from ulcers and other disorders in the abdomen. If the patient has acute (sudden onset) pancreatitis, the lipase level usually rises somewhat later than the amylase level—about 24–48 hours after onset of symptoms—and remains abnormally high for 5–7 days. Because the lipase level peaks later and remains elevated longer, its determination is more useful in late diagnosis of acute pancreatitis. However, lipase levels are not as useful in diagnosing chronic pancreatic disease.

Although fat digestion is not concentrated in the stomach, gastric lipase will digest egg yolk and cream in the stomach, since they are already emulsified fats. For fat to be digested properly, the liver needs to first emulsify the large fat molecules, and bile breaks it down to small droplets, allowing the lipase to start its work. Fat digestion in the small intestine is reliant on a pancreatic secretion called pancreatin containing lipase as well as protease and amylase. In some vegetarian **diets**, very little bile is produced since the liver is not stimulated to produce bile, with the result that the large fat molecules are not properly emulsified, making it difficult for the lipase to bind. This pattern leads to incomplete or reduced fat absorption. A shortage of lipase in the body may lead to high **cholesterol**, difficulty in losing weight, a tendency towards diabetes,

high urine sugar levels—which some believe can lead to arthritis, bladder problems, gall stones, **hay fever**, prostate problems, and heart problems. With too little lipase, the cell membranes' permeability is inefficient, and nutrients cannot enter the cell, while wastes cannot leave it. There is also a tendency among people suffering from lipase deficiency to have a problem with electrolyte balance. **Muscle spasms** and a spastic colon are also reported as symptoms of lipase deficiency. People suffering with a spastic colon may be lipase deficient as well as people with vertigo (Meniere's disease), which is **dizziness** made worse by movement.

General use

Lipase supplements, which usually contain protease enzymes and amylase, are used to treat people with pancreatic insufficiency, meaning the pancreas does not make enough of these enzymes to aid in food digestion. It is also used to treat **celiac disease** and gluten intolerance. It is used infrequently to treat **indigestion** caused by a deficiency of pancreatic enzymes. Several scientific studies have shown its effectiveness in treating pancreatic insufficiency, celiac disease, **irritable bowel syndrome**, and indigestion. There is a lack of scientific evidence that lipase is effective in treating other conditions. However, it is used by some healthcare professionals to help treat cystic fibrosis, Crohn's disease (chronic inflammation, usually of the lower intestinal tract), lactose intolerance, **rheumatoid arthritis**, and lupus.

Celiac disease and gluten intolerance

Celiac disease and gluten intolerance are basically the same condition. Gluten intolerance is the body's inability to break down or digest gluten and can range from mild to moderate. Celiac disease is a condition of the digestive system in which the body produces antibodies that attack the gluten. These antibodies damage the lining of the small intestine and interfere with the absorption of nutrients from food. It is in the severe range of gluten intolerance. As of 2007, the only treatment for celiac disease was a **gluten-free diet**. Gluten is primarily found in products that contains wheat, rye, barley, or oats. It helps to make bread rise and gives many foods a smooth, pleasing texture. In addition to the many obvious places gluten can be found in a normal diet, such as breads, cereals, and pasta, there are many hidden sources of gluten. These include ingredients added to foods to improve texture or enhance flavor and products used in food packaging. Gluten may even be present on surfaces used for food preparation or cooking. An estimated three million Americans have celiac disease but only about

3% of them have been diagnosed, according to the American Academy of Allergy, **Asthma**, and Immunology. Lipase, in combination with other pancreatic enzymes, enhances the benefits of a gluten-free diet for people with celiac disease and gluten intolerance.

Lipase is also used to treat pancreatic insufficiency, a condition in which food cannot be normally processed by the body, and insulin secretion may be inadequate. Studies have shown that taking 1.5 grams of 9X pancreatin with each meal can help people with pancreatic insufficiency to better digest food.

Preparations

Lipase supplements usually contain other enzymes that help digest carbohydrates and protein. In the United States, the supplement pancreatin contains lipase, amylase, and protease. A government standard is used to rate lipase supplements and is denoted as USP units. The standard government measurement for pancreatin is 25 USP units of amylase, 2 USP units of lipase, and 25 USP units of protolytic (protease) enzymes. So a lipase supplement that has a label indicating that it is "9X pancreatin" is nine times stronger than the government standard. Lipase supplements are usually made from enzymes found in animals, although there are a few supplements that use lipase and other pancreatic enzymes derived from plants.

Recommended dosage

Pancreatin supplements usually contain 6,000 LU (lipase activity units) of lipase. The recommended dosage for adults is one to two capsules or tablets three times a day. Dosages for children should be determined by a pediatrician.

Precautions

Lipase supplements should be taken under the supervision of a qualified health care professional. It should not be taken by pregnant women or women who are nursing without approval from their physician.

Side effects

There are no known adverse side effects associated with lipase supplements.

Interactions

Lipase can interact with the anti-obesity drug orlistat (Xenical). Studies have shown orlistat interferes with the activity of lipase supplements. Orlistate is prescribed to treat **obesity** and works by blocking the ability of lipase to break down fats. Also, the dietary

supplement betaine should not be taken with lipase supplements, since it can destroy lipase and other enzymes.

KEY TERMS

Celiac disease—A disorder caused by sensitivity to gluten that makes the digestive system unable to deal with fat.

Enzyme—Any complex chemical produced by living cells that is a catalyst for biochemical reactions.

Lupus—Either of two inflammatory diseases affecting connective tissue, one largely confined to the skin, the other affecting the joints and internal organs.

Pancreas—A large elongated glandular organ that is near the stomach and secretes juices into the small intestine and the hormones insulin, glucagon, and somatostatin into the bloodstream.

Pancreatitis—Inflammation of the pancreas.

Triglycerides—Natural fat found in human tissue that in high levels can increase the risk of heart disease and stroke.

Vertigo—Dizziness made worse by movement.

Resources

BOOKS

Parker, Philip M. *Familial Lipoprotein Lipase Deficiency—A Bibliography and Dictionary for Physicians, Patients, and Genome Researchers*. San Diego: Icon Group International, 2007.

Salleh, Abu Baker, et al., eds. *New Lipases and Proteases*. Hauppauge, NY: Nova Science, 2006.

PERIODICALS

Baer, Daniel M. "Clinical Utility of Amylase and Lipase." *Medical Laboratory Observer* (October 2005): 38(2).

Corbet, Kelly. "The Gluten Question: What You Need to Know." *Delicious Living* (October 2007): 49(3).

"Lipase, Serum." *CareNotes* (May 2007): N/A.

Luft, Friedrich C. "Lipoprotein Lipase and Heart Size." *Journal of Molecular Medicine* (February 2006): 109(3).

Rao, Bhaskar. "Elevated Serum Amylase and Lipase in Inflammatory Bowel Disease." *Internet Journal of Gastroenterology* (January 2005): N/A.

Serrano, Nicolas. "Increased Lipase Plasma Levels in ICU Patients: When Are They Critical?" *Chest* (January 2005): 7(4).

ORGANIZATIONS

American Academy of Allergy, Asthma, and Immunology, 555 E. Wells St., Suite 1100, Milwaukee, WI, 53202-3823, (414) 272-6071, www.aaaai.org.

National Institute of Diabetes and Digestive and Kidney Diseases, Bldg. 31, Room 9A06, 31 Center Dr., MSC 2580, Bethesda, MD, 20892, (800) 891-5390, http://www.niddk.nih.gov.

National Pancreas Foundation, 363 Boylston St., 4th Floor, Boston, MA, 02116, (866) 726-2737, http://www.pancreasfoundation.org.

Ken R. Wells

Live cell therapy *see* **Cell therapy**

Livingston-Wheeler therapy

Definition

Developed by Virginia Livingston-Wheeler, a U.S. medical doctor, this complex vaccine and nutrition-based **cancer** therapy assumed that cancer was caused by *Progenitor cryptocides*, a bacterium said to become active only when the body's immune system is weakened or stressed.

Origins

Livingston-Wheeler discovered *Progenitor cryptocides* during the 1940s. In the following decade, she formed her hypothesis that cancer is caused by this bacterium, and developed a vaccine against it. In 1969, she founded what became the Livingston Foundation Medical Center in San Diego. In the years since then, this center claimed to have treated thousands of patients.

Livingston-Wheeler died in 1990, but her clinic continued to offer the Livingston protocol to about 500 patients a year until the clinic closed in 2004.

Benefits

An analysis by Livingston-Wheeler showed an 82 percent survival rate among 62 of her patients with confirmed diagnoses of various cancers. Of those 62 patients, 37 survived three years or longer. A later, independent study, however, found no significant difference between survival rates among her patients and those at a university cancer center offering conventional therapy. This study, which included 78 pairs of patients, was published in a 1991 issue of the prestigious *New England Journal of Medicine*. The American Cancer Society concluded that no scientific evidence existed to support the claims that the Livingston-Wheeler therapy was an effective treatment for cancer. Although versions of the Livingston protocol were also offered to patients with lupus, arthritis, scleroderma, **allergies**, and stress-induced syndromes, the American Cancer Society also noted that no scientific evidence supported the therapy's use for those or any other diseases.

Description

The treatment was commenced during a 10-day period at the Livingston Foundation Medical Center in San Diego, and continued by the patient afterward at home. In addition to vaccines, the Livingston treatment also often employed vitamins, **digestive enzymes**, sheep spleen extract, liver extract, antibiotics, a vegetarian diet, and **detoxification**. Traditional drug therapy was also used, so long as it continued to enhance the body's immune system. A staff psychologist taught patients strategies for managing emotional trauma. In addition, visualization techniques were used to improve the immune response. The Livingston Center also offered a two-day annual "immunological diagnostic program" focused on preventative health.

Preparations

At the beginning of the 10-day program, patients underwent a physical examination and diagnostic tests including blood counts, electrolytes, chemistry, urinalysis, thyroid and liver function, tumor markers, and hormone levels.

Precautions

In a fact sheet on Livingston-Wheeler therapy, the U.S. National Cancer Institute strongly urged cancer patients "to remain in the care of qualified physicians who use accepted methods of treatment or who are participating in carefully conducted clinical trials (treatment studies). The use of unconventional methods may result in the loss of valuable time and the opportunity to receive potentially effective therapy and consequently reduce a patient's chance for cure or control of cancer." The U.S. Congressional Office of Technology Assessment (OTA) also warned, "As with any injection into the body of a foreign substance, the injection of the autogenous vaccine carries the associated risk of sepsis or anaphylaxis. Some risk of contamination in the preparation of the material is also possible, depending on the processes and procedures used to make and assure the sterility of the vaccines manufactured at the clinic." In addition, the OTA cautioned that "whole blood transfusion, even with directed donors' blood, carries a small risk of transmitting various infectious agents." and warned that injecting extracts of sheep liver and spleen, "carries certain risks associated with all types of cellular treatment."

Side effects

One University of Pennsylvania study found that self-reported quality of life among patients at the Livingston-Wheeler clinic was actually lower than among patients receiving conventional cancer care at the university's cancer center. Reported side-effects include malaise, slight **fever**, aching, tenderness at the site of vaccine injections, and appetite problems.

Research and general acceptance

In 1990, the Livingston clinic was ordered by California officials to stop using its vaccines on cancer patients, after a state panel of cancer experts and consumers concluded there was no conclusive scientific evidence proving they were safe and effective. The American Cancer Society also advised against the Livingston protocol. In addition, an article in CA: A Cancer Journal for Clinicians asserted that the premise for the Livingston-Wheeler treatment was faulty: the bacterium *Progenitor cryptocides* does not exist. It stated, "Careful research using modern techniques . . . has shown that there is no such organism and that Livingston-Wheeler has apparently mistaken several different types of bacteria, both rare and common, for a unique microbe."

Training and certification

The Livingston protocol and products were offered exclusively through the Livingston Foundation Medical Center in San Diego through its closure in 2004. During its operation, the center stated that it "is not affiliated with any other clinic, physician, research organization, or business entity anywhere in the world."

Resources

PERIODICALS

CA. "Unproven methods of cancer management: Livingston-Wheeler therapy." *CA: A Cancer Journal for Clinicians* 40 no. 2 (Mar/Apr 1990): 103–108.

Cassileth, B., E. Lusk, D. Guerry, A. Blake, W. Walsh, L. Kascius, and D. Schultz. "Survival and quality of life among patients receiving unproven as compared with conventional cancer therapy." *New England Journal of Medicine* 325 no. 15 (Oct. 10, 1991): 1103–1105.

ORGANIZATIONS

American Cancer Society. 1599 Clifton Rd. NE, Atlanta, GA 30329-4251, (800)227-2345. http://www.cancer.org/docroot/ETO/content/ETO_5_3X_Livingston-Wheeler_Therapy.asp?sitearea = ETO (accessed February 15, 2008).

David Helwig
Leslie Mertz, Ph.D.

Lobelia

Description

Lobelia inflata, also known as Indian tobacco, wild tobacco, pukeweed, emetic weed, **asthma** weed and gagroot, is native to North America and can commonly be found growing wild over much of the United States. Lobelia derives its name from Matthias de Lobel, a sixteenth-century Flemish botanist. The erect stem reaches a height of between 6 in (15 cm) and several feet. The many small blue flowers appear in midsummer and are visible through late fall. The stem is hairy, and the plant contains a milk-like sap.

Worldwide, there are more than 200 species of lobelia, growing predominantly in the temperate and tropical zones. Some species found at high elevations in mountainous areas of Asia and Africa may achieve a height of up to 15 ft (5.5 m). At the other end of the size spectrum, the dwarf lobelia (*Lobelia erina*) is sometimes cultivated as a small ornamental or hanging plant.

General use

This powerful plant has the distinction of being simultaneously a stimulant (for the respiratory system) and a general relaxant. This unusual combination may help account for the remarkably diverse assortment of ailments for which lobelia is used.

To begin with, lobelia is commonly associated with the treatment of lung-related ailments such as

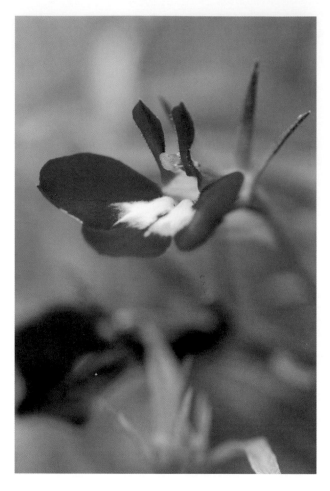

Edging Lobelia. *(© Arco Images / Alamy)*

KEY TERMS

Amphetamines—A group of drugs that stimulate the central nervous system. They are used medically to counteract depression, but are often used illegally as stimulants.

Beta-amyrin palmitate—A compound found in lobelia that has antidepressant properties.

Diuretic—A medication given to increase the body's output of urine.

Dopamine—A chemical in the brain that governs movement and emotions. Amphetamines trigger the release of dopamine, while lobeline opposes its effects.

Emetic—A medication given to induce vomiting.

Expectorant—A drug given to help bring up mucus or phlegm from the respiratory tract.

Hypokalemia—An abnormally low level of potassium in the bloodstream.

Lobeline—An alkaloid compound found in lobelia that resembles nicotine in its pharmacological effects. It has been studied by researchers in the field of tobacco addiction and drug abuse.

Methamphetamine—A form of amphetamine that is a potent stimulant of the central nervous system and is highly addictive. Slang terms for methamphetamine include "meth," "ice," "speed," and "chalk."

Nonsteroidal anti-inflammatory drugs (NSAIDs)—A term used for a group of pain-relieving medications that also reduce inflammation when used over a period of time. NSAIDs are often given to relieve the pain of osteoarthritis.

asthma, **bronchitis**, coughs, **pneumonia**, colds and flu, and other upper-respiratory problems.

Perhaps not surprisingly, then, this well-established medicinal plant has a special relationship with the (also long-established) practice of **smoking**. In some Native American cultures, lobelia was smoked as a treatment for lung diseases, which presumably led early European naturalists to dub the plant Indian tobacco. Considering the plant's value as an overall tonic for the lungs, this practice stands in marked contrast to contemporary use of tobacco (which many Native American cultures also used) as a plant to be smoked. Even more intriguingly, lobelia is commonly used as an aid to stopping smoking, sometimes in combination with **cramp bark**. One of the alkaloids in lobelia, lobeline, has effects on humans similar to those of nicotine and can be helpful in treating the symptoms of nicotine withdrawal. These same properties may perhaps also explain the use of the plant to treat hangovers and **alcoholism**. Recent research, however, has questioned the usefulness of lobeline in smoking cessation programs; a German study published in 2000 concluded that lobeline "cannot be recommended" as a treatment for nicotine dependence.

More recently, lobeline has attracted the attention of researchers as a possible treatment for methamphetamine addiction. Lobeline appears to oppose the action of dopamine, a brain chemical that regulates movement and emotion, and that is released by the effects of methamphetamine on the brain. Although reports published in 2001 and 2002 are promising, this use of lobeline has not yet reached the stage of clinical trials in humans.

Some Native Americans also used red lobelia to treat both intestinal **worms** and **syphilis**. Among the Shoshone of the American West, lobelia tea was brewed and used for its emetic and cathartic properties.

Lobelia is also commonly used as an emetic (i.e., to induce **vomiting**). This latter fact makes an interesting connection with the ancient "doctrine of signatures," which holds that a plant's appearance offers clues to its use: Lobelia inflata has been said to have "stomach-shaped" flowers.

Although it can be effective alone, lobelia is also commonly used in conjunction with other herbs. Among these are **coltsfoot**, **ephedra**, grindelia, lungwort, and **skullcap**.

In **homeopathy**, lobelia is used in ways similar to its herbal applications: more specifically, in cases of severe **nausea**, vomiting, asthma, **emphysema**, and dry **cough**, and in the treatment of **heart disease** (**angina** pectoris and cardialgia).

Externally, lobelia is used in connection with a variety of problems, including insect **bites** and poison ivy; **bruises**, **sprains** and arthritis; and ringworm.

Preparations

Lobelia is used both internally and externally, in various forms. The entire above-ground portion of the plant, including the seed pods, is harvested in late summer and fall, after it flowers. The leaves and seeds of the plant can be used to make a tincture. The dried herb can also be smoked or used as a tea. Prepared as a salve, it is appropriate for external use. All portions of the plant that are above ground are medicinally useful, including the stem.

Lobelia's chemical composition has been studied to a significant extent. It consists of various alkaloids (notably lobeline, as mentioned above), chelidonic acid, isolobeline, lobelic acid, lobeline, **selenium** and **sulfur**, among other substances.

Perhaps because of the plant's widespread and long-standing use for a diverse range of conditions, some of lobelia's pharmacological qualities have been investigated in the laboratory, including its action on the lungs and the antidepressant effect of a component isolated from the leaves known as beta-amyrin palmitate. A 1996 Russian study of 196 species of medicinal plants identified lobelia as being exceptionally high in **chromium** content, making it potentially useful for treating a chromium deficiency in humans.

Precautions

The effects of lobelia are unusually dose-specific; in other words, this plant can have widely varying effects—both in kind and intensity—depending on the amount taken. Herbal authorities differ markedly in their assessment of the plant's overall safety; some

consider it relatively harmless. On the other hand, the Food and Drug Administration (FDA) has issued warnings to consumers in 1993 and 1998 about the potentially dangerous side effects of lobelia, and the Australian government has declared it unsafe for human consumption.

As with any medicinal herb, users are advised to consult with qualified health-care professionals before attempting any form of self-treatment. People using any form of medication should make sure that all their caregivers are aware of any herbs they may also be taking.

More specifically, women who are either pregnant or nursing should not take lobelia. The herb is contraindicated in cases of heart disease, pneumonia, shock, stomach ulcers, ulcerative **colitis**, esophageal reflux, **diverticulitis**, and high blood pressure.

Reports of toxic effects of lobelia in children have led American pediatricians to warn people against giving the herb to children as a treatment for asthma. This warning is particularly urgent in areas of the Southwest where folk medicines containing lobelia are frequently used.

Some writers also report that lobelia sap is highly toxic to livestock.

Side effects

In small doses, lobelia can have a soothing, sedative effect. In larger doses, it induces vomiting. The plant's well-established use in connection with lung disorders is due, in part, to its expectorant effects.

In potentially toxic doses, lobelia produces nausea, pronounced weakness, sweating, speeding heartbeat (tachycardia), sensory disturbances and **diarrhea**. In some people, even very small doses can cause nausea and vomiting. Signs of an overdose of lobelia include profuse sweating, low blood pressure, convulsions, respiratory **depression**, paralysis, coma, and death.

Interactions

Lobelia has been reported to have adverse interactions with several groups of drugs. It may potentiate (intensify) the effects of medications given to control blood pressure. It interferes with the action of drugs given to control diabetes. Lobelia increases the risk of loss of **potassium** from the body (hypokalemia) if it is taken together with diuretics or corticosteroids. Aspirin and NSAIDs appear to increase the risk of toxic reactions to lobelia.

Resources

BOOKS

Balch, James F., MD. *Prescription for Nutritional Healing.* Garden City, N.Y.: Avery Publishing Group, 1997.

Hutchens, Alma R. *A Handbook of Native American Herbs.* Boston: Shambhala Publications, 1995.

PERIODICALS

Dwoskin, L. P., and P. A. Crooks. "A Novel Mechanism of Action and Potential Use for Lobeline as a Treatment for Psychostimulant Abuse." *Biochemical Pharmacology* 63 (January 15, 2002): 89-98.

Haustein, K. O. "Pharmacotherapy of Nicotine Dependence." *International Journal of Clinical Pharmacology and Therapeutics* 38 (June 2000): 273-290.

Mazur, L. J., L. De Ybarrondo, J. Miller, and G. Colasurdo. "Use of Alternative and Complementary Therapies for Pediatric Asthma." *Texas Medicine* 97 (June 2001): 64-68.

Miller, D. K., P. A. Crooks, L. Teng, et al. "Lobeline Inhibits the Neurochemical and Behavioral Effects of Amphetamine." *Journal of Pharmacology and Experimental Therapeutics* 296 (March 2001): 1023-1034.

Subarnas, A., Y. Oshima, and Y. Ohizumi. "An antidepressant principle of *Lobelia inflata L.* (Campanulaceae)." *Journal of Pharmaceutical Sciences* 81 (July 1992): 620-621.

ORGANIZATIONS

Office of Dietary Supplements (ODS), National Institutes of Health. 6100 Executive Boulevard, Room 3B01, MSC 7517, Bethesda, MD 20892. (301) 435-2920. www.ods.od.nih.gov.

United States Food and Drug Administration (FDA), Center for Food Safety and Applied Nutrition. 5100 Paint Branch Parkway, College Park, MD 20740. (888) SAFEFOOD. www.cfsan.fda.gov.

OTHER

U. S. Food and Drug Administration, Center for Food Safety and Applied Nutrition. *Illnesses and Injuries Associated with the Use of Selected Dietary Supplements.* Washington, DC: FDA/CFSAN, 1993. www.cfsan.fda.gov.

U. S. Food and Drug Administration, FDA Consumer, September-October 1998. *Supplements Associated with Illnesses and Injuries.* www.cfsan.fda.gov/~dms/fdsuppch.

Peter Gregutt
Rebecca J. Frey, PhD

Lockjaw *see* **Tetanus**

Lomatium

Description

The name lomatium generally refers to *Lomatium dissectum*, one of the numerous species and varieties of the *Lomatium* genus that is native to western North America. Lomatium is a member of the Apiaceae (carrot) family and grows in the northwestern United States and southwestern Canada. Like many wild plants that have attracted the attention of commercial interests, lomatium is presently threatened with extinction over parts of its range.

In the wild, lomatium grows in rocky soil and reaches a height of 3 ft (0.9 m). The entire lomatium plant is edible, and numerous Native American groups regarded the lomatium plant as a food source and medicinal remedy. For cultivation as an herbal remedy, lomatium roots are unearthed during the months between early spring and fall. Roots are washed and dried for several days. The roots are then sliced and allowed to dry again. When dried correctly, lomatium is said to keep its medicinal properties for 2–3 years. Lomatium's antimicrobial activity is due to the tetronic acids and glucoside of luteolin that it contains. Other ingredients include the resin, which causes rash in some people, and coumarins, which could possibly cause rash as well. The coumarins, however, are being investigated for their possible usefulness in treating HIV infection.

Lomatium is also known as Indian biscuit root, biscuit root, desert **parsley**, desert parsnip, fern-leafed lomatium, ferula dissoluta, Indian desert parsnip, Indian parsnip, leptaotaenia dissecta, tohza, toza, and wild carrot.

General use

Many Native American groups recognized the value of lomatium as a source of nourishment and medicinal remedy. Lomatium root was peeled, dried, and ground into flour to make sweet-tasting biscuits. Lomatium seeds were eaten raw or roasted, or ground into flour for baking.

Native Americans chewed on the root to treat a range of respiratory **infections**. Lomatium was used for conditions including cold, flu, **bronchitis**, tuberculosis, hay fever, **asthma**, and **pneumonia**. Lomatium was also used in a tobacco mixture. The herb was smoked during rituals, and healers used the smoke to treat respiratory infections. Lomatium was used when the Native Americans were exposed to tuberculosis and other diseases that Europeans brought to North America.

When the world faced the **influenza** pandemic of 1917–18, Americans tried remedies such as castor oil, tobacco, aspirin, and morphine. American herbalists recommended use of lomatium, and the remedy was used with reported success, especially in the Southwest.

KEY TERMS

Coumarins—A group of crystalline compounds found in lomatium that may be useful in treating HIV infection.

Infusion—A liquid extract of an herb prepared by steeping or soaking plant parts in water or another liquid.

Potentiate—To intensify the effects of another herb or prescription medication.

Tincture—A method of preserving herbs with alcohol or water.

Wildcrafting—The art of gathering or harvesting herbs or other plants from their native wild environment for human use.

Contemporary uses of lomatium

Lomatium is currently used as an antiviral remedy to treat colds, coughs, and infections. The herb is also known for boosting the immune system and reducing inflammation.

Lomatium can relieve chest **pain** and stomach upset that frequently accompany the flu. It has also been used for conditions such as asthma, **hay fever**, mononucleosis, infective bronchitis, **tuberculosis**, and the early stages of **tonsillitis**. Other uses of lomatium include treatment of skin infections, **cuts**, and sores. A health practitioner might recommend the use of lomatium for a person diagnosed with fibromyalgia, a muscular inflammatory condition. Causes of **fibromyalgia** are not known, but are thought by some to be connected to viruses. Symptoms include an impaired immune system, chronic pain, and **fatigue**.

The future of lomatium

Lomatium was among the plants placed on Montana's plant protection list in April 1999. The state enacted a law that placed a three-year moratorium on the wildcrafting of lomatium, wild echinacea, butterroot, and sundew that grow on state land. Wildcrafting is the harvesting of herbal plants in the wild. Plants like lomatium face the risk of becoming endangered because of increased popularity and usage of herbal remedies, and reduction of habitat due to development.

A moratorium on wildcrafting is one way to protect plants in the short term. Long-term solutions include habitat protection and cultivation of herbs in home gardens and on commercial farms. Several organizations, such as United Plant Savers (www. plantsavers.org), are intent on protecting medicinal plants in the wild and increasing their availability.

Preparations

Lomatium is available as an extract, as a tincture, and in capsule form. Fresh root extract in an alcohol solution is believed to be the most effective remedy.

Lomatium tea, an infusion, is made by pouring one cup of boiling water over 1–2 tsp. of the dried herb. The mixture is steeped for 25 minutes and then strained. Lomatium tea can be taken three times a day.

Lomatium contains a resin that can cause a painful rash in some people. To avoid this rash, people can use "lomatium isolates," which are extracts with the resins removed. The extract can be taken at a dosage of 1–3 ml each day. In tincture form, the daily dosage is generally 10–30 drops taken one to four times per day. Children who are ill with colds or flu can be given lomatium capsules.

Precautions

Before beginning herbal treatment, people should consult a physician or health practitioner. A knowledgeable herbalist can give advice about dosages. Consultation is important because high doses of lomatium can cause nausea and an itchy rash that covers the entire body. Lower doses can also cause rash in people who are sensitive to lomatium resin. A person should first take a small amount of tincture to test for a rash reaction. The rash will go away in one to six days after discontinuing use of lomatium.

Lomatium and other herbal remedies are not regulated by the United States Food and Drug Administration (FDA) in the same way that prescription drugs are regulated. This difference means that the effectiveness of lomatium has not been scientifically tested. In addition, supplements are not standard in their ingredients or dosages. Women who are pregnant or nursing should not use lomatium, because its safety for these conditions has not been determined.

Side effects

Although lomatium is generally believed to be safe, the herb has been reported to cause a skin rash. A high dosage of the herb may result in **nausea**.

Interactions

Lomatium has been reported to potentiate (intensify the effects of) two groups of drugs, anticoagulants (blood thinners) and immunostimulants (drugs given to boost the immune system).

Resources

BOOKS

Duke, James A. *The Green Pharmacy*. Emmaus, PA: Rodale Press, Inc., 1997.

Keville, Kathi. *Herbs for Health and Healing*. Emmaus, PA: Rodale Press, Inc., 1996.

Ritchason, Jack. *The Little Herb Encyclopedia*. Pleasant Grove, UT: Woodland Health Books, 1995.

Squier, Thomas Broken Bear, with Lauren David Peden. *Herbal Folk Medicine*. New York: Henry Holt and Company, 1997.

PERIODICALS

Lee, T. T., Y. Kashiwada, L. Huang, et al. "Suksdorfin: An Anti-HIV Principle from *Lomatium suksdorfii*, Its Structure-Activity Correlation with Related Coumarins, and Synergistic Effects with Anti-AIDS Nucleosides." *Bioorganic and Medicinal Chemistry* 2 (October 1994): 1051-1056.

McCutcheon, A. R., T. E. Roberts, E. Gibbons, et al. "Antiviral Screening of British Columbian Medicinal Plants." *Journal of Ethnopharmacology* 49 (December 1, 1995): 101-110.

ORGANIZATIONS

American Botanical Council. P.O. Box 201660, Austin, TX 78720.(512) 331-8868. http://www.herbalgram.org.

Herb Research Foundation. 1007 Pearl St., Suite 200, Boulder, CO 80302. (303) 449-2265. http://www.herbs.org.

Southwest School of Botanical Medicine. P. O. Box 4565, Bisbee, AZ 85603. (520) 432-5855. www.swsbm.com.

United Plant Savers. P.O. Box 98, East Barre, VT 05649. (802) 496-7053. Fax: (802) 496-9988. http://www.plantsavers.org.

OTHER

Cabrera, Chancel. "Uncommon Antibiotics: Usnea and Lomatium." Healthwell.com. http://www.healthwell.com.

Liz Swain
Rebecca J. Frey, PhD

Lomilomi

Definition

The term Lomilomi literally means "to break up into small pieces with the fingers." It is a type of healing massage that is traditionally practiced in the Hawaiian Islands. Lomilomi is also called "loving hands" massage.

Origins

This form of massage incorporates both physical and spiritual ritual components. Lomilomi originated in the South Pacific and is practiced mainly in the Hawaiian islands, although in the 2000s, lomilomi had grown in popularity and practitioners could also be found in most other states, as well as Australia, Canada, Japan, and the United Kingdom.

When Captain Cook and other European explorers disembarked on the islands of Polynesia, the indigenous people healed their aches and pains with therapeutic massage. Experts in lomilomi also knew how to use it in **childbirth** and to treat congestion, inflammation, rheumatism and other musculoskeletal disorders, **asthma**, and **bronchitis**. They also applied lomilomi to babies and children to strengthen them and mold their features for physical beauty.

In times past, lomilomi was practiced mainly among family members. There were various orders of medical priests, known as kahunas. The one who specialized in massage was the kahuna lomilomi. One member of the family would be trained by a village kahuna. This person would then pass the training on to the next generation. Kahunas trained practitioners in the physical aspects of massage, and they taught that an important aspect of the healing process is the transfer of positive thoughts from the lomilomi practitioner to the client in a way that channels energy, called mana or life force and releases a sense of well being. One goal of lomilomi is to unblock energy flow and allow it to move in a new direction. Unlike traditional lomilomi practitioners, some modern practitioners tend to concentrate more on the physical rather than the spiritual aspects of this therapy.

The best-known school for training lomilomi practitioners was run by Margaret Machado, known to her students as Aunty Margaret, on the island of Hawaii. Machado was born in the early 1900s and learned traditional lomilomi techniques from her grandfather. Her daughter, Nerita Machado, continued the family lomilomi teaching tradition.

Benefits

Lomilomi cleanses and relaxes the body, both physically and spiritually in order to achieve internal harmony. It increases circulation, relaxes tension spots, and relieves **pain**.

Description

A lomilomi massage generally begins with clients relaxing on a table and opening themselves to a healing state of mind. Some practitioners begin by using heated lomi stones to increase blood flow to certain areas of the body.

The traditional stroke of the lomilomi practitioner is out and away from the body. This touch is both deep and gentle, resembling in some ways **Swedish massage**. Unlike Swedish massage, however, lomilomi practitioners use their elbows and forearms and incorporate some vigorous deep tissue techniques. The forearm movement is typically applied across the grain of the long muscles of the back. There is no set pattern to the massage.

Sometimes lomi sticks are used to relieve facial tension or when deeper massage is needed in a specific part of the body. Lomilomi practitioners traditionally used indigenous oils prepared from coconut and leuki trees. The oil is worked into the skin in a rhythmic 1-2-3, 1-2-3, 1-2-3 movement. At its best, lomilomi releases healing energy that flows from the practitioner to the client.

Modern lomilomi massage varies in the length of time spent with the client time and may dispense with many of the traditional ritual preparations. Costs of this therapy are not typically covered by insurance. Many of the luxury resorts and spas in Hawaii have a practitioner trained in lomilomi on their staff.

Preparations

In traditional lomilomi, the client may drink herbal teas to cleanse the body internally before the massage. The body is also cleansed externally with red clay or salt. In some cases time is alternated between a steam hut and plunges in cold water to increase circulation before beginning the massage. Much of this preparation is dispensed with by modern practitioners.

Precautions

There are no particular precautions to be observed when receiving this therapy. Like many therapies, lomilomi is most effective when the client is in a receptive frame of mind to accept healing.

Side effects

No undesirable side effects had been reported as of 2008. Most clients report feel a reduction in **stress** and a general sense of well being. Others report specific relief of pains such as headaches and backaches.

Research and general acceptance

There are relatively few practitioners of lomilomi, so little controlled research had been done on its effectiveness as of the late 2000s. However, lomilomi has

---

KEY TERMS

Kahuna—A traditional Hawaiian village leader responsible for physical and spiritual healing; some specialize in herbs, others in massage.

---

been an accepted part of native Hawaiian culture for hundreds of years.

Training and certification

The Hawaiian Lomilomi Association offers certification to practitioners who have received training from any of their approved lomilomi instructors. There are three levels of certification, each of which requires an increased amount of instruction and supervised experience. These certification levels are certified lomilomi therapist, licensed lomilomi therapist, and lomilomi clinical practitioner. This last category requires a 10-year apprenticeship under an approved advanced master lomilomi practitioner and 20 years of experience. Hawaii also has licensing requirements that massage therapists are required to meet.

Resources

BOOKS

Chai, R. M. R. *Hawaiian Massage Lomilomi: Sacred Touch of Aloha.* Kailua, HI: Hawaiian Insights, 2007.

Chai, R. M. R. *Na Mo'olelo Lomilomi: The Traditions of Hawaiian Massage and Healing.* Honolulu, HI: Bishop Museum Press, 2005.

Kahalewai, Nancy S. *Hawaiian Lomilomi: Big Island Massage,* 2nd ed. Mountain View, HI: Island Massage, 2005.

Jim, Harry Uhane, and Garnette Arledge. *Wise Secrets of Aloha: Learn and Live the Sacred Art of Lomilomi.* San Francisco, CA: Weiser Books, 2007.

ORGANIZATIONS

Hawaiian Lomilomi Association, PO Box 2356, Kealakekua, HI, 96750-2356, http://www.hawaiilomilomi.com.

Tish Davidson, A. M.

Lou Gehrig's disease

Definition

Lou Gehrig's disease, or amyotrophic lateral sclerosis (ALS), is a neurodegenerative disease of unknown cause that breaks down tissues in the nervous system and affects the nerves responsible for movement. Its common name comes from the professional baseball player whose career was ended because of it.

Description

Lou Gehrig's disease is a disease of the motor neurons, those nerve cells reaching from the brain to the spinal cord (upper motor neurons) and the spinal cord to the peripheral nerves (lower motor neurons) that control muscle movement. In Lou Gehrig's disease, for unknown reasons, these neurons die, leading to a progressive loss of the ability to move virtually any of the muscles in the body. The disease affects "voluntary" muscles, those controlled by conscious thought, such as the arm, leg, and trunk muscles. Lou Gehrig's disease, in and of itself, does not affect sensation, thought processes, the heart muscle, or the "smooth" muscle of the digestive system, bladder, and other internal organs. Most sufferers retain function of their eye muscles, as well.

"Amyotrophic" refers to the loss of muscle bulk, a cardinal sign of ALS. "Lateral" indicates one of the regions of the spinal cord affected, and "sclerosis" describes the hardened tissue that develops in place of healthy nerves. Lou Gehrig's disease affects approximately 50,000 people in the United States, with about 5,000 new cases each year. The onset usually begins between the ages of 40 and 70, although younger onset is possible. Men have a slightly higher chance of developing the disease than women.

Causes and symptoms

Causes

The symptoms of Lou Gehrig's disease are caused by the death of motor neurons in the spinal cord and brain. Normally, these neurons convey electrical messages from the brain to the muscles to stimulate movement in the arms, legs, trunk, neck, and head. As motor neurons die, the muscles cannot be moved as effectively, and weakness results. In addition, lack of stimulation leads to muscle wasting, or loss of bulk. Involvement of the upper motor neurons causes spasms and increased tone in the limbs, and abnormal reflexes. Involvement of the lower motor neurons causes muscle wasting and twitching (fasciculations).

Although many causes of motor neuron degeneration have been suggested for Lou Gehrig's disease, none has yet been proven responsible. Results of recent research have implicated toxic molecular fragments known as free radicals. Some evidence suggests that a cascade of events leads to excess free radical production inside motor neurons, leading to their

death. Why free radicals should be produced in excess amounts is unclear, as is whether this excess is the cause or the effect of other degenerative processes. Additional agents within this toxic cascade may include excessive levels of a neurotransmitter known as glutamate, which may overstimulate motor neurons, thereby increasing free-radical production, and a faulty **detoxification** enzyme known as SOD–1, for superoxide dismutase type 1. The actual pathway of destruction is not known, however, nor is the trigger for the rapid degeneration that marks Lou Gehrig's disease. Further research may show that other pathways are involved, perhaps ones even more important than this one. Autoimmune factors or premature **aging** may play some role, as could viral agents or environmental toxins.

Two major forms of ALS are known: familial and sporadic. Familial Lou Gehrig's disease accounts for about 10% of all Lou Gehrig's disease cases. As the name suggests, familial Lou Gehrig's disease is believed to be caused by the inheritance of one or more faulty genes. About 15% of families with this type of Lou Gehrig's disease have mutations in the gene for SOD–1. SOD–1 gene defects are dominant, meaning only one gene copy is needed to develop the disease. Therefore, a parent with the faulty gene has a 50% chance of passing the gene along to a child. Sporadic Lou Gehrig's disease has no known cause. While many environmental toxins have been suggested as causes, to date no research has confirmed any of the candidates investigated, including aluminum and metal dental fillings. As research progresses, it is likely that many cases of sporadic Lou Gehrig's disease will be shown to have a genetic basis, as well. A third type, called Western Pacific Lou Gehrig's disease occurs in Guam and other Pacific islands. This form of the disease combines symptoms of both ALS and Parkinson's disease.

Symptoms

The earliest sign of Lou Gehrig's disease is most often weakness in the arms or legs, at first usually more pronounced on one side than the other. Loss of function is usually more rapid in the legs among people with familial Lou Gehrig's disease, and in the arms among those with sporadic Lou Gehrig's disease. Leg weakness may first become apparent by an increased frequency of stumbling on uneven pavement, or an unexplained difficulty climbing stairs. Arm weakness may lead to difficulty grasping and holding a cup, for instance, or loss of dexterity in the fingers.

Less often, the earliest sign of Lou Gehrig's disease is weakness in the *bulbar* muscles, those muscles in the mouth and throat that control chewing, swallowing, and speaking. A person with bulbar weakness may become hoarse or tired after speaking at length, or speech may become slurred.

In addition to muscle weakness, the other cardinal signs of Lou Gehrig's disease are muscle wasting and persistent twitching, which is known as fasciculation. These are usually noticed after weakness in muscles becomes obvious. Fasciculation is also common in people without the disease, and is virtually never the first sign of Lou Gehrig's disease.

While initial weakness may be limited to one region, Lou Gehrig's disease almost always progresses rapidly to involve virtually all the voluntary muscle groups in the body. Later symptoms include loss of the ability to walk, to use the arms and hands, to speak clearly or at all, to swallow, and to hold the head up. Weakness of the respiratory muscles makes breathing and coughing difficult, and poor swallowing control increases the likelihood of inhalation of food or saliva (aspiration). Aspiration increases the likelihood of lung infection, which is often the cause of death. With a ventilator and scrupulous bronchial hygiene, a person with Lou Gehrig's disease may live much longer than the average, although weakness and wasting will continue to erode any remaining functional abilities. Most people with Lou Gehrig's disease continue to retain function of the extraocular muscles that control movement of the eyes, allowing some communication to take place with simple blinks or through use of a computer–assisted device.

Diagnosis

The diagnosis of Lou Gehrig's disease begins with a complete medical history and physical exam, plus a neurological exam to determine the distribution and extent of weakness. An electrical test of muscle function, called an electromyogram, or EMG, is an important part of the diagnostic process. Various other tests, including blood and urine tests, x rays, and CT scans, may be done to rule out other possible causes of the symptoms, such as tumors of the skull base or high cervical spinal cord, thyroid disease, spinal arthritis, **lead poisoning**, or severe vitamin deficiency. Lou Gehrig's disease is rarely misdiagnosed following a careful review of all these factors.

Treatment

There is no cure for Lou Gehrig's disease, and no treatment that can significantly alter its course. There are many things that can be done, however, to help maintain quality of life and to retain functional ability even in the face of progressive weakness.

Two studies published in 1988 suggested that amino–acid therapies may provide some improvement for some people with Lou Gehrig's disease. While individual patient reports claim benefits for megavitamin therapy, herbal medicine, and removal of dental fillings, for instance, no evidence suggests that these offer any more than a brief psychological boost, often followed by a more severe letdown when it becomes apparent the disease has continued unabated. However, once the causes of Lou Gehrig's disease are better understood, alternative therapies may be researched more intensively. For example, if damage by free radicals turns out to be the root of most of the symptoms, antioxidant vitamins and supplements may be used more routinely to slow the progression of Lou Gehrig's disease. Or, if environmental toxins are implicated, alternative therapies with the goal of detoxifying the body may be of some use. In 2002, the Food and Drug Administration (FDA) granted approval for one company to begin trials on use of **creatine**, an amino acid dietary supplement, to treat ALS. Preliminary data from trials show that creatine might slow progression of Lou Gehrig's disease, but research remains to be completed before approval of the supplement for treatment of ALS.

A physical therapist works with the patient and family to implement **exercise** and stretching programs to maintain strength and range of motion, and to promote general health. Swimming may be a good choice for people with Lou Gehrig's disease, as it provides a low–impact workout to most muscle groups. One result of chronic inactivity is contracture, or muscle shortening. Contractures limit a person's range of motion, and are often painful. Regular stretching can prevent contracture.

An occupational therapist can help design solutions for movement and coordination problems, and provide advice on adaptive devices and home modifications. Speech and swallowing difficulties can be minimized or delayed through training provided by a speech-language pathologist. This specialist can also provide advice on communication aids, including computer-assisted devices and simpler word boards. Nutritional advice can be provided by a nutritionist. A person with Lou Gehrig's disease often needs softer foods to prevent jaw exhaustion or choking. Later in the disease, **nutrition** may be provided by a gastrostomy tube inserted into the stomach.

Allopathic treatment

As of early 2002, only one drug had been approved for treatment of Lou Gehrig's disease. Riluzole (Rilutek) appears to provide on average a three-month increase in life expectancy when taken regularly early in the disease, and shows a significant slowing of the loss of muscle strength. Riluzole acts by decreasing glutamate release from nerve terminals. Experimental trials of nerve growth factor have not demonstrated any benefit. No other drug or vitamin currently available has been shown to have any effect on the course of Lou Gehrig's disease. However, in 2002, researchers had identified how a common drug prescribed for **acne** could slow the progression of cell death in the brain that causes ALS. The drug, called minocycline, can safely be taken orally. Scientists are now working on a combination of minocycline with other drugs to better target a more powerful therapy for Lou Gehrig's disease patients.

Mechanical ventilation may be used when breathing becomes too difficult. Modern mechanical ventilators are small and portable, allowing a person with Lou Gehrig's disease to maintain the maximum level of function and mobility. Ventilation may be administered through a mouth or nose piece, or through a tracheostomy tube. This tube is inserted through a small hole made in the windpipe. In addition to providing direct access to the airway, the tube also decreases aspiration. While many people with rapidly progressing Lou Gehrig's disease choose not to use ventilators for lengthy periods, they are increasingly used to prolong life for a short time.

The progressive nature of Lou Gehrig's disease means that most patients will eventually require fulltime nursing care. This care is often provided by a spouse or other family member. While the skills involved are not difficult to learn, the physical and emotional burden of care can be overwhelming. Caregivers need to recognize and provide for their own needs, as well as those of the patient, to prevent **depression** and burnout. Throughout the disease, a support group can provide important psychological aid to the patient, and also act as a caregiver as they come to terms with the losses that Lou Gehrig's disease inflicts. Support groups are sponsored by both the Lou Gehrig's Disease Society and the Muscular Dystrophy Association.

Expected results

Lou Gehrig's disease usually progresses rapidly, and leads to death from respiratory infection within three to five years in most cases. The slowest disease progression is seen in those who are young and have their first symptoms in the limbs. About 10% of people with Lou Gehrig's disease live longer than eight years.

Prevention

There is no known way to prevent Lou Gehrig's disease or to alter its course.

Resources

BOOKS

Mitsumoto, Hiroshi and Forbes H. Norris Jr., eds. *Amyotrophic Lateral Sclerosis: A Comprehensive Guide to Management*. Demos Publications, 1996.

The Muscular Dystrophy Association. *When a Loved One Has ALS: A Caregiver's Guide*. Tucson, AZ: The Muscular Dystrophy Association, 1997.

PERIODICALS

"Creatine Granted Orphan Drug Designation." *Drug Topics* (April 15, 2002):HSE6.

The ALS Digest. http://http1.brunel.ac.uk:8080/~hssrsdn/alsig/alsig.htm.

"Research: Common Acne Antibiotic Minocycline Delays Progression of ALS." *Immunotherapy Weekly* (June 5, 2002):7.

The ALS Newsletter. Available from the Muscular Dystrophy Association.

ORGANIZATIONS

The ALS Association.21021 Ventura Blvd., Suite #321, Woodland Hills, CA 91364. (818) 340–7500.

The Muscular Dystrophy Association. 3300 East Sunrise Drive, Tucson, AZ 85718. (520) 529–2000 or (800) 572–1717. http://www.mdausa.org.

OTHER

With Strength and Courage: Understanding and Living with ALS. Videotape available from the Muscular Dystrophy Association.

Kathleen Wright
Teresa G. Odle

Low back pain

Definition

Low back **pain** (LBP) is a common complaint, second only to cold and flu as a reason why patients seek care from their family doctor. It may be a limited musculoskeletal symptom or caused by a variety of diseases and disorders that affect or extend from the lumbar (lower) spine. Low back pain is sometimes accompanied by **sciatica**, which is pain that involves the sciatic nerve and is felt in the lower back, the buttocks, the backs and sides of the thighs, and possibly the calves. More serious causes of LBP may be accompanied by **fever**, night pain that awakens a person from sleep, loss of bladder or bowel control, numbness, burning urination, swelling, or intense sharp pain.

Description

Low back pain is a symptom that affects 80% of Americans at some point in their life with sufficient severity to cause absence from work. It is a common reason for visits to primary care doctors, and is estimated to cost the U.S. economy more than $100 billion every year in lost wages, lost productivity, and direct healthcare costs. About one-third of the nation's disability-related costs are associated with LBP, a condition primarily affecting individuals between the ages of 30 and 50.

The most common cause of low back pain is lumbar strain. The structures of the normal lumbar region of the spine include the lumbar vertebrae, discs between each vertebrae, ligaments, muscles and muscle tendons, the spinal cord within the vertebrae and nerves extending outward from the spine through vertebral foramina (openings in the bone). The lumbar vertebrae are distinct from the cervical (neck area) and thoracic (upper back) vertebrae, being generally thicker for greater weight bearing support, and resting atop the sacrum (tailbone), the triangular shaped bone between the buttocks.

The discs between each vertebrae of the spine cushion and absorb the shock that might otherwise be transmitted through the spine. Occasionally, the discs may rupture or herniate outward through their fibrous sheath, or covering, putting pressure on the nerves. Nerve pressure on the sciatic nerve (sciatica) may be the cause of or add to LBP. Nerve pain from other local organs may also cause LBP, in which case diagnosis and treatment is more involved, usually much more serious, and may indicate a life-threatening condition.

Risks for low back pain are increased with fracture and **osteoporosis**, narrowing of the spinal canal within the vertebrae (stenosis), spinal curvatures, **fibromyalgia**, osteo- and **rheumatoid arthritis**, **pregnancy**, **smoking**, **stress**, age greater than 30, or disease or illness of the organs of the lower abdomen.

In addition to dividing low back pain into three categories based on duration of symptoms—acute, sub-acute or chronic—low back pain may be described in the following terms:

- Localized. In localized pain the patient feels soreness or discomfort when the doctor palpates, or presses on, a specific surface area of the lower back.
- Diffuse. Diffuse pain is spread over a larger area and comes from deep tissue layers.
- Radicular. The pain is caused by irritation of a nerve root and radiates from the area. Sciatica is an example of radicular pain.
- Referred. The pain is perceived in the lower back, but actually is caused by inflammation or disease elsewhere, such as the kidneys or other structures of or near the lower abdomen, including the intestines, appendix, bladder, uterus, ovaries or the testes.

Causes and symptoms

Acute and sub-acute pain

Lumbar strain or sprain is the most common cause of acute low back pain. The pain usually does not extend into the leg and usually occurs within 24 hours of heavy lifting or overuse of the back muscles. The pain is often localized and may be accompanied by **muscle spasms** or soreness to touch. The patient usually feels better when resting. Symptoms of acute LBP may be accompanied by stiffness (guarding), **constipation**, poor sleep and trouble finding a comfortable position, difficulties walking and other limits on normal range of motion.

Acute strain may follow a sudden movement, especially a lifting and simultaneous twisting motion; however, injury is usually preceded by overuse or lack of **exercise** and tone, especially of the opposing muscles (the abdominals, for example), improper use, long periods of sitting or standing in one position, poor vertebral alignments or conditions compromising **nutrition** of the supportive structures. Acute low back pain due to lumbar strain (approximately 60% of sufferers) usually resolves with a week with conservative therapies, including reducing but not eliminating all activity.

Sub-acute pain is associated with a duration of six to twelve weeks, by which time 90% of individuals experiencing low back pain and injury return to work. This category accounts for one-third of all disability-related costs. LBP persisting beyond three months is considered chronic.

Chronic pain

Chronic low back pain has several possible causes.

MECHANICAL. Chronic strain on the muscles of the lower back may be caused by **obesity**, pregnancy, or job-related stooping, bending, or other stressful postures. Construction, truck driving accompanied by vibration, jack hammering, sand blasting and other sources of chronic trauma strain to the back or nerve pressure may also contribute.

MALIGNANCY OR OTHER SERIOUS ILLNESS. Low back pain at night that is not relieved by lying down may be caused by a tumor in the cauda equina (the roots of the spinal nerves controlling sensation in and movement of the legs) or metastasized **cancer** that has spread to the spine from the prostate, breasts, or lungs. The risk factors for the spread of cancer to the lower back include a history of smoking, sudden weight loss, and age over 50. Kidney problems, such as **kidney stones**; ovarian and uterine problems, including fibroids; **endometriosis**; premenstrual water retention; and **ovarian cysts**; chronic constipation; sluggish or enlarged colon; benign tumors; bone **fractures**; aneurysm of the aorta; herpes zoster **shingles**; intra-abdominal infection or bleeding secondary to Coumadin therapy; osteomyelitis; **tuberculosis** of the spine (Pott's disease); and sepsis of the vertebral discs, all may be associated with pain to the lower back. Additional symptoms may include night sweats, being awakened at night by pain, weakness, numbness, muscle fatigue or poor coordination which progressively worsens, burning on urination, redness or swelling over the area of pain, changes in bowel or urinary patterns, and malaise.

ANKYLOSING SPONDYLITIS. Ankylosing spondylitis is a form of arthritis that causes chronic pain in the back. The pain is made worse by sitting or lying down and improves when the patient stands up. It is most commonly seen in males between the ages of sixteen and thirty-five. Ankylosing spondylitis is often confused with mechanical back pain in its early stages. Other symptoms include morning stiffness, a positive family history, and positive lab results for HLA-B27 antigen (an autoimmune marker), and an increased sedimentation (Sed) rate of the blood. This condition may have food allergy-related components, such as an allergy to wheat, worsened by drinking beer.

HERNIATED SPINAL DISC. Disc herniation is a disorder in which a spinal disc begins to bulge outward between the vertebrae. Herniated or ruptured discs are a common cause of chronic low back pain in adults. Pressure imposed on adjacent nerves results in pain that may worsen with movement, coughing, **sneezing**, or intra-abdominal strain, and may be accompanied by numbness of the skin in the area served by the nerve (dermatome). Deep tendon reflexes (DTRs) may be reduced, and the straight leg raising test may be positive. The crossed straight leg raising test, which is more specific to herniated disc, may also be positive.

PSYCHOGENIC. Back pain that is out of proportion to a minor injury or that is unusually prolonged may be associated with a somatoform disorder or other emotional disturbance. Psychosocial factors such as loss of work, job dissatisfaction, legal problems, and financial compensation issues are some of the non-organic factors that may be associated or causative. Psychogenic symptoms of LBP are usually diffuse, non-localized, and may include other stress related symptoms. A set of five tests called the Waddell tests may be used to help diagnose LBP of psychogenic origin.

Low back pain with leg involvement

Low back pain that radiates down the leg usually indicates involvement of the sciatic nerve. The nerve can be pinched or irritated by herniated discs, tumors of the cauda equina (the nerve roots of the spine), abscesses in the space between the spinal cord and its covering, spinal stenosis, and compression fractures. Some patients experience numbness or weakness of the legs, as well as pain. There may be spasming of muscles stimulated by the involved nerve and a positive leg raising test.

Diagnosis

The diagnosis of low back pain can be complicated. Most cases are initially evaluated by primary care physicians or other health practitioners, rather than by specialists.

Initial workup

PATIENT HISTORY. The doctor will ask the patient specific questions about the location of the pain, its characteristics, its onset, and the body positions or activities that make it better or worse. If the pain seems to be referred from other organs, the doctor may ask about a history of diabetes, peptic ulcers, kidney stones, urinary tract **infections**, heart murmurs, or other health issues. Age, family history, and previous medical history are also important. LBP in persons younger than 20 and older than 50 is apt to be associated with a more severe underlying condition or cause.

PHYSICAL EXAMINATION. The doctor will examine the patient's back and hips to check for conditions that require surgery or emergency treatment. The examination includes several tests that involve moving the patient's legs in specific positions to test for nerve root irritation or disc herniation. The flexibility of the lumbar vertebrae may be measured to rule out ankylosing spondylitis. Other physical tests include assessments of gait and posture, range of motion, and the ability to perform certain physical positions and coordinated movements. Reflex, sensory, and motor tests may help the clinician screen for referral to a specialist, as needed. Diagnostic tests may be used, especially with persisting, chronic pain. These tests may include x ray, CT scan, MRI, and electromyelographs (EMGs).

RED FLAGS. The presence of certain symptoms warrants a more rapid progress to deeper diagnostic examination as to cause. These serious symptoms include, but are not limited to the following:

- pain following violent injury, accident, or trauma
- constant pain that worsens
- upper spinal pain
- history of cancer
- being HIV positive
- history of steroid drug use or drug abuse
- development of an obvious structural deformity
- history of rapid weight loss
- unexplained fever or night sweats with back pain
- being under age 20 or over age 50

Treatment

A thorough differential diagnosis is important before any treatment is considered. There are times when alternative therapies may be most beneficial, and other times when more invasive treatments are needed.

Chiropractic

Chiropractic treats patients by manipulating or adjusting sections of the spine. It is one of the most popular forms of alternative treatment in the United States for relief of back pain caused by straining or lifting injuries and has been demonstrated through several rigorous randomized trials to be beneficial. Some osteopathic physicians, physical therapists, and naturopathic physicians also use spinal manipulation to treat patients with low back pain, along with work on soft tissue around the bones. Additional recommendations of shoe orthotics, exercise, cold packs to reduce and inhibit swelling immediately after injury, followed one to two days later by hot packs and cold packs to stimulate healing, **hydrotherapy**, and lifestyle adjustments may be recommended. Nutritional supplements known to be beneficial to joint repair and integrity, collagen support, and wound repair may also be recommended, including **glucosamine** sulfate, with or without **chondroitin**, methylsulfonylmethane(**MSM**), and a variety of mineral and vitamin cofactors.

Traditional Chinese medicine

Practitioners of **traditional Chinese medicine** treat low back pain with **acupuncture**, **acupressure**, massage, and the application of herbal poultices. They may also use a technique called **moxibustion**, which involves the use of glass cups, and heated air from a burning braid or stick of herb with a distinctive aroma.

Herbal medicine and anti-inflammatory enzymatic therapy

Herbal medicine uses a variety of antispasmodic and sedative herbs to help relieve low back pain due to spasm. For this purpose and easily available at a local health food store are herbs such as **chamomile** (*Matricaria recutita*), **hops** (*Humulus lupus*), passion flower (*Passiflora incarnata*), valerian (*Valeriana officinale*), and cramp bark (*Viburnum opulus*). **Bromelain** from pineapples has anti-inflammatory activity. Drinking fresh grape juice, preferably made from dark grapes, on a daily basis at a time other than mealtime, has also been found to be helpful. Minor backaches may be relieved with the application of a heating paste of **ginger** (*Zingiber officinale*) powder and water, allowed to sink in for 10 minutes and followed by an **eucalyptus** rub.

Aromatherapy with soothing **essential oils** of blue chamomile, birch, **rosemary**, and/or **lavender** can be effective when rubbed into the affected area after a hot bath.

Homeopathy

Homeopathic treatment for acute back pain consists of various applications of **Arnica** (*Arnica montana*); as an oil or gel applied topically to the sore area or oral doses alone or in prepackaged combination products, including other homeopathic remedies such as St. John's wort (*Hypericum perforatum*), Rhus tox (*Rhus toxicodendron*) and **Ruta** (*Ruta graveolens*). *Bellis perennis* may be recommended for deep muscle injuries.

Other remedies may be recommended based on the symptoms presented by the patient.

Body work and yoga

Massage and numerous other body work techniques can be very effective in treating low back pain. **Yoga**, practiced regularly and done properly, can be combined with **meditation** or imagery to both treat present and prevent future episodes of low back pain.

Allopathic treatment

All forms of treatment of low back pain are aimed either at symptom relief or to prevent interference with the processes of healing. None of these methods appears to speed up healing.

Acute pain

Acute back pain is treated with muscle relaxants or nonsteroidal anti-inflammatory drugs (NSAIDs), such as ibuprofen or aspirin. Applications of compresses using heat or cold also can be helpful to some patients. Acute LBP often resolves within a short time. Some patients may be prescribed opioid analgesics (pain relievers with codeine or codeine similars); however, statistics demonstrate no shortening of the healing period, as noted above. The use of muscle relaxants may increase risk of further damage, but they have been shown to be more effective than placebo (though no better than NSAIDS alone) in relieving acute pain. If the patient has not experienced some improvement after several weeks of treatment, the doctor will reinvestigate the cause of the pain.

Chronic pain

Patients with chronic back pain are treated with a combination of medications, physical therapy, and occupational or lifestyle modification. The medications given are usually NSAIDs, although patients with **hypertension**, kidney problems, or stomach ulcers are advised not take these drugs. Patients who take NSAIDs for longer than six weeks are advised to be monitored periodically for complications. Chronic pain, by definition longer than three months in duration, may also prompt a more thorough diagnostic analysis.

Physical therapy for chronic low back pain usually includes regular exercise for fitness and flexibility and massage or application of heat if necessary. Lifestyle modifications include quitting smoking, losing weight (if necessary), and evaluation of the patient's occupation or other customary activities. Good lift and bend mechanics may also be reviewed and counseled.

Patients with herniated discs may be treated surgically if the pain does not respond to medication. Vertebral fusion surgery may stiffen the spine; however, engineers of skyscrapers recognize the need of flexibility with height to preserve wind resistance: a fused spine may reduce capacity. Another surgical procedure known as kyphoplasty, involving guided penetration of the back and cemented repair, may be indicated in pain due to vertebral fracture. Patients with chronic low back pain sometimes benefit from pain management techniques, including **biofeedback**, acupuncture, and chiropractic manipulation of the spine. **Psychotherapy** is recommended for patients whose back pain is associated with a somatoform, **anxiety**, or depressive disorder.

Low back pain with leg involvement

Treatment of sciatica and other disorders that involve the legs may include NSAIDs. Patients with long-standing sciatica or spinal stenosis that do not respond to NSAIDs may be treated surgically. Although some doctors use cortisone injections in trigger points and vertebral facet joints to relieve the pain, this form of treatment is controversial. Also debated are benefits due to spinal traction and transcutaneous (through the skin) electrical nerve stimulation.

Expected results

The prognosis for most patients with acute low back pain is excellent. About 80% of patients recover completely in four to six weeks. The prognosis for recovery from chronic pain depends on the underlying cause.

Prevention

Low back pain due to muscle strain can be prevented by lifestyle choices, including regular physical exercise, weight control, avoiding smoking, and learning the proper techniques for lifting and moving heavy objects. Exercises designed to strengthen the muscles of the lower back and the opposing abdominals are also recommended. Simple actions can also help prevent low back pain, such as putting a small, firm cushion behind the lower back when sitting for long intervals; using a soft pillow for sleep that supports the lower neck without creating an unnatural angle for the head and shoulders; using a swiveling desk chair with a postural support or stool that maintains the knees at a higher level than the hips; standing on flexible rubber mats to avoid the impact of concrete floors at places of employment; and wearing supportive, soft-soled shoes and avoiding the use of high heels.

KEY TERMS

Ankylosing spondylitis—A type of arthritis that causes gradual loss of flexibility in the spinal column. It occurs most commonly in males between the ages of 16 and 35 and may be initiated by a food allergy component, such as an allergy to wheat.

Cauda equina—The nerve roots in the final portion of the spine, controlling movement and sensation in the legs. These nerve roots resemble a horse's tail.

Chiropractic—A method of treatment based on the interactions of the spine and the nervous system. Chiropractors adjust or manipulate segments of the patient's spinal column in order to relieve pain and increase the healthy flow of nerve energy.

Lumbar spine—The segment of the human spine above the pelvis that is involved in low back pain. There are five vertebrae, or bones, in the lumbar spine.

Osteoporosis—A condition found in older individuals in which bones decrease in density and become fragile and more likely to break. It can be caused by lack of vitamin D and/or calcium in the diet.

Placebo—A pill or liquid given during the study of a drug or dietary supplement that contains no medication or active ingredient. Usually study participants do not know if they are receiving a pill containing the drug or an identical-appearing placebo.

Radicular—Pain that is caused by compression or impingement at the root of a nerve.

Referred pain—Pain that is experienced in one part of the body but originates in another organ or area. The pain is referred because the nerves that supply the damaged organ enter the spine in the same segment as the nerves that supply the area where the pain is felt.

Sciatica—Pain caused by irritation of the sciatic nerve. Sciatica is felt in the lower back, the buttocks, the backs and sides of the upper legs, and sometimes the calves.

Spinal stenosis—Usually the result of arthritis of the spine, causing narrowing of the spinal canal in the lumbar vertebrae. The narrowing puts pressure on the roots of the sciatic nerve. It may cause sciatica, but not necessarily.

Resources

BOOKS

Hochschuler, Stephen. *Treat Your Back Without Surgery: The Best Nonsurgical Alternatives for Eliminating Back*

and Neck Pain, 2nd ed. Alameda, CA: Hunter House, 2002.

OTHER

"Back Pain." *Medline Plus* April 15, 2008 [cited April 18, 2008]. http://www.nlm.nih.gov/medlineplus/backpain.html.

"Low Back Pain." *American Academy of Orthopaedic Surgeons* September 2007 [cited April 18, 2008]. http://orthoinfo.aaos.org/.

"Low Back Pain Fact Sheet." *National Institute of Neurological Disorders and Stroke* April 11, 2008 [cited April 18, 2008]. http://www.ninds.nih.gov/disorders/backpain/detail_backpain.htm.

"Lower Back Pain (Lumbar Back Pain)." *MedicineNet.com* January 22, 2008 [cited April 18, 2008]. http://www.medicinenet.com/.

ORGANIZATIONS

American Academy of Orthopaedic Surgeons, 6300 North River Road, Rosemont, IL, 60018-4262, (847) 823-7186, http://www.aaos.org.

American Association of Naturopathic Physicians, 435 Wisconsin Ave. NW, Suite 403, Washington, DC, 20016, (202) 237-8150, (866) 538-2267, http://www.naturopathic.org.

American Chiropractic Association, 1701 Clarendon Blvd, Arlington, VA, 22209, (703) 276-8800, http://www.amerchiro.org.

American Holistic Medical Association, PO Box 2016, Edmonds, WA, 98020, (425) 967-0737, http://www.holisticmedicine.org.

American Physical Therapy Association, 1111 North Fairfax Street, Alexandria, VA, 22314-1488, (800) 999-APTA (2782), (703) 684-APTA (2782), http://www.apta.org.

Kathleen Wright
Katherine Nelson, N.D.
Tish Davidson, A. M.

Low blood sugar *see* **Hypoglycemia**

Lowfat diet *see* **Ornish diet**

Lumbar pain *see* **Low back pain**

Lung cancer

Definition

Lung **cancer** is a disease in which abnormal cells in the lung grow uncontrollably and form tumors. Cells from these tumors can enter the circulatory system and travel through the body to form tumors in new sites. Lung cancer is often fatal; only four in ten people with lung cancer live one year beyond the time of their diagnosis.

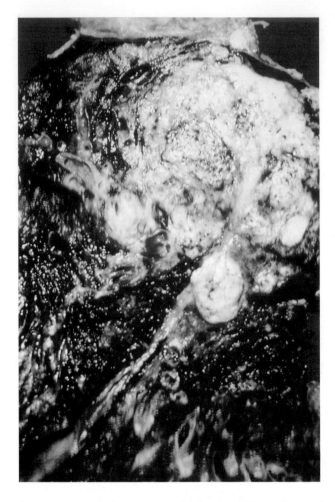

Cross section of a human lung with cancer. *(Science Source / Photo Researchers, Inc.)*

Description

There are two types of lung cancer, primary and secondary. Primary lung cancer originates in the lung. Primary lung cancer can further be divided into small cell lung cancer and non-small cell lung cancer, depending on how the cells look under the microscope. Secondary lung cancer is cancer that starts somewhere else in the body (for example, the breast or colon) and spreads (metastasizes) to the lungs.

Small cell lung cancer was formerly called oat cell cancer because the cells resemble oats in their shape. About one-fourth of all lung cancers are small cell cancers. This type of cancer is aggressive and spreads to other organs within a short time. It is found most often in people who are heavy smokers. Its treatment is different from the treatment of non-small cell lung cancers.

Non-small cell lung cancers account for 75% of lung cancers. There are three types of non-small cell

lung cancers. Although the cells of the non-small cell cancers look different, treatment of all three types is the same.

Incidence of lung cancer

Since 1987, lung cancer has been the leading cause of cancer death in both men and women in the United States. The American Cancer Society (ACS) estimated that in 2008 about 215,000 new cases of lung cancer would be diagnosed in the United States and approximately 162,000 Americans would die of the disease that year. Worldwide, more than one million new cases of lung cancer are diagnosed each year, 58% of which are in the developing world.

Lung cancer is usually diagnosed in people age 50 and older, with an average age at diagnosis being 60. Most lung cancer is not diagnosed until it is in an advanced stage. While in the United States the incidence of lung cancer has decreased among white men, it has steadily risen among African American men, and among both white and African American women. This change appears to be directly related to changes in the number of smokers in these groups.

Causes and symptoms

Lung cancer is most often caused by pollutants inhaled into the lungs over a long period. There are indications that genetic inheritance also plays a role in how susceptible different people are to these pollutants.

Smoking

Tobacco **smoking** (cigarettes, pipes, cigars) is the leading cause of lung cancer. Ninety percent of lung cancers can be prevented by completely avoiding tobacco use. Smoking **marijuana** cigarettes also is thought to be a risk factor for lung cancer, although it is difficult to obtain accurate information on marijuana use. Marijuana cigarettes have higher tar content than tobacco cigarettes. In addition, they are inhaled very deeply and the smoke is held in the lungs for a longer period than tobacco smoke.

Breathing in smoke from the environment (secondhand smoke) also increases the risk of lung cancer. In the twenty-first century many states have passed laws mandating smoke-free workplaces and public environments in order to protect non-smokers from secondhand smoke.

Exposure to asbestos and toxic chemicals

Repeated exposure to asbestos fibers, either at home or in the workplace, also is considered a risk factor for developing a specific type of rare lung cancer called mesothelioma. Studies show that compared to the general population, asbestos workers are seven times more likely to die from lung cancer. Asbestos workers who smoke increase their risk of developing lung cancer by 50 to 100 times. Besides asbestos, miners who are exposed to coal products or radioactive ores, such as uranium, and workers exposed to chemicals, such as arsenic, vinyl chloride, mustard gas, and other carcinogens, have a higher than average risk of contracting lung cancer.

Environmental contamination

Exposure to high levels of radon gas increases the risk of developing lung cancer. Radon is a naturally occurring radioactive gas that cannot be seen or smelled. It is produced by the breakdown of uranium. Outdoors, the tiny amounts of radon produced mix with the air and do not present a cancer risk. However, in the basements of some houses that are built over soil containing natural uranium deposits, radon may accumulate and reach dangerous levels. An inexpensive test can detect the presence of indoor radon. Having one's house tested for the presence of radon gas when buying or renting is a good idea and is required by law in some states to be done when a house is sold.

Manmade environmental pollution (e.g., auto exhaust fumes, industrial air pollution) also increases the risk of developing lung cancer. Studies have conclusively linked long-term exposure to fine-particle air pollution with lung cancer deaths. The risk of death from lung cancer is increased substantially for people living in heavily polluted metropolitan areas, particularly in the developing world where the rate of cigarette smoking also is high.

Other causes

Inflammation and scar tissue sometimes are produced in the lung by diseases such as silicosis and berylliosis. These diseases result from inhaling certain minerals, **tuberculosis**, and certain types of **pneumonia**. This scarring may increase the risk of developing lung cancer. Radiation therapy to the chest also increases the risk of lung cancer, especially in people who smoke.

Symptoms

Lung cancers tend to spread very early, but only about 15% are detected in early stages when they are most treatable. Many symptoms of lung cancer are similar to those caused by other diseases. The chance of early detection is improved by promptly seeking medical care if any of the following symptoms appear:

- a cough that does not go away
- chest pain
- shortness of breath
- persistent hoarseness
- swelling of the neck and face
- unintentional significant weight loss
- fatigue and loss of appetite
- bloody or brown-colored spit or phlegm (sputum)
- unexplained fever
- recurrent lung infections, such as bronchitis or pneumonia

If the lung cancer has spread to other organs, the patient may have other symptoms, such as headaches, bone **fractures**, **pain**, bleeding, or **blood clots**.

Diagnosis

Diagnosis begins with a detailed medical and life-style history to determine symptoms and assess risk factors. This assessment is followed by a complete physical examination. Among other checks, the doctor will examine the patient's throat to look for other possible causes of hoarseness or coughing and listen to the patient's breathing and the sounds made when the patient's chest and upper back are thumped (percussed). The physical examination usually is inconclusive.

Imaging tests

Based on symptoms and risk factors that give the doctor reason to suspect lung cancer, imaging tests are performed. These usually begin with a chest x ray that can show the presence of any masses in the lungs. Special imaging techniques, such as computed tomography (CT) scans or magnetic resonance imaging (MRI) scans, can provide more precise information about the size, shape, and location of any masses. A special type of computed tomography called spiral CT can detect lung cancer when tumors are smaller than a dime. Routine screening using spiral CT remains controversial because it produces a high number of false positives (detection of an abnormality that turns out not to be cancer). This results in additional unneeded tests and procedures. The National Lung Screening Trial, a large-scale trial of spiral CT technology to detect lung cancer in 50,000 smokers, was conducted between 2002 and 2008. Results, which were expected to be available by 2009, were anticipated to help to clarify whether using this CT spiral technology to routinely screen high-risk individuals produces accurate and cost effective results.

Positron emission tomography (PET) is a diagnostic tool that uses small amounts of radioactive glucose (sugar) to detect where cells are rapidly growing. Cancer cells grow faster than healthy cells and thus use more glucose. Radioactive glucose becomes concentrated in cancer cells and can be detected by special imaging techniques. This procedure is especially helpful in locating very early lung cancers and in determining where more advanced cancers have spread. Some facilities have equipment that performs a simultaneous PET and CT scan.

Sputum analysis

Sputum analysis involves microscopic examination of the cells that are either coughed up from the lungs or are collected through a special instrument called a bronchoscope. Sputum analyses can diagnose at least 30% of lung cancers, some of which are in the very earliest stages and do not show up on chest x rays. The sputum test does not, however, provide any information about the location of the tumor and must be followed by additional tests.

Lung biopsy

Lung biopsy is the definitive diagnostic tool for cancer. It can be performed in several different ways. The doctor can perform a bronchoscopy, which involves the insertion of a slender, lighted tube, called a bronchoscope, down the patient's throat and into the lungs. In addition to viewing the passageways of the lungs, the doctor can use the bronchoscope to obtain samples of the lung tissue. In another procedure known as a needle biopsy, the location of the tumor first is identified using a CT scan or MRI. The doctor then inserts a needle through the chest wall and collects a sample of tissue from the tumor. In a third procedure, known as surgical biopsy, the chest wall is opened and a part of or the entire tumor is removed. A doctor who specializes in the study of diseased tissue (a pathologist) examines the tumor samples to identify the cancer's type and stage.

Treatment

Alternative therapies do not replace conventional treatment but may complement it and improve the patient's quality of life. Before beginning any alternative therapy, lung cancer patients should consult their doctors concerning the appropriateness if treatment and its role in an overall cancer treatment plan. Appropriate alternative treatments may help prolong a patient's life, improve the quality of life, reduce the recurrence of tumors, prolong time in remission, or reduce adverse reactions to chemotherapy and radiation.

Dietary guidelines

The following dietary changes may help improve a patient's quality of life, as well as boost the immune function to better fight the disease. In general, these dietary guidelines are accepted by both alternative and conventional medical practitioners.

- Avoid fatty and spicy foods. A high-fat diet may be associated with increased risk of lung and other cancers. Also, lung cancer patients may have a hard time digesting greasy foods.
- Eat new and interesting foods. Tasty foods stimulate appetite so that patients can eat more and have the energy to fight cancer.
- Increase consumption of fresh fruits and vegetables. They are the best sources of antioxidants, vitamins, and minerals. Especially helpful are the yellow and orange fruits (orange, cantaloupes) and dark green vegetables.
- Eat more broccoli sprouts. These young sprouts are a good source of sulforaphane, a substance thought to help fight lung cancer.
- Eat many (5–6) small meals per day. Small meals are easier to digest.
- Establish a regular eating time and avoid eating around bedtime.
- Avoid foods containing preservatives or artificial coloring.
- Monitor weight and intake of adequate calories and protein.

Nutritional supplements

Many cancer-fighting claims are made for nutritional supplements. However, the effectiveness of some conventional anticancer drugs used to treat lung cancer can be reduced when patients take megadoses of **antioxidants** or other supplements. Free radicals damage DNA, and sometimes this damage leads to the development of cancer. In laboratory cell cultures and animal studies, antioxidants appear to slow the development of cancer. The results have been mixed in studies in which humans took antioxidant dietary supplements. In a large study of 29,000 men, when a beta-carotene dietary supplement, which the body converts into **vitamin A**, was taken by men who smoked, they developed lung cancer at a rate 18% higher and died at a rate 8% higher than men who were taking a placebo.

Another study that gave men dietary supplements of beta-carotene and vitamin A was stopped when researchers found the men receiving the beta-carotene had a 46% greater chance of dying from lung cancer than those who were given a placebo. Other large studies have shown either no or only slight protective effects against cancer. The position of the American Cancer Society, the National Cancer Institute, and several international health organizations is that antioxidants should come from a healthy diet high in fruits and vegetables and low in fat and not from dietary supplements. Cancer patients should check with their physicians before beginning any herbal or megadose vitamin or mineral therapy.

Most dietary supplements claim to help fight cancer by boosting the function of the immune system. A naturopath may recommend some of the following nutritional supplements to boost immune function and help fight tumor progression:

- Vitamins and minerals. Vitamins that are considered particularly beneficial to cancer patients include B-complex vitamins, especially vitamins B_6, along with vitamins C, D, E, and K. The most important minerals are calcium, chromium, copper, iodine, molybdenum, germanium, selenium, tellurium, and zinc. Many of these vitamins and minerals are strong antioxidants or cofactors for antioxidant enzymes. However, patients should not take megadoses of these supplements without first consulting their doctors. Significant adverse or toxic effects may occur at high dosages, which is especially true for the minerals.

- Other nutritional supplements may help fight cancer and support the body. They include essential fatty acids (fish or flaxseed oil), flavonoids, pancreatic enzymes (to help digest foods), hormones such as DHEA, melatonin, or phytoestrogens. Again, some of these supplements may interfere with specific conventional cancer treatments and should not be taken without consulting a physician knowledgeable about both conventional and alternative therapies.

Traditional Chinese medicine

Conventional treatment for lung cancer is associated with significant side effects. These adverse effects (such as **nausea**, **vomiting**, and **fatigue**) can be reduced with Chinese herbal preparations. Patients should consult an experienced herbalist who will prescribe remedies to treat specific symptoms that are caused by conventional cancer treatments.

Daily consumption of a soup used in **traditional Chinese medicine** is reported to have helped slow the progression of non-small cell lung cancer for patients with advanced stages of the disease. The soup consisted of herbs and vegetables containing natural ingredients that boost immunity and help fight tumors. Patients should check with their doctors and

with a licensed traditional Chine medicine specialist for more information. The soup does not prevent or reverse the disease, but may prolong survival.

Juice therapy

Juice therapy involves the consumption of the juice of raw fruit or vegetables. A person may drink juice preventively to stay healthy or to treat a medical condition such as cancer. Juice therapy may be helpful for patients with cancer. Advocates of **juice therapies** maintain that refraining from eating solid food boosts the body's ability to heal itself. Since the body is not spending time and energy on digesting complex high-fat food, it can concentrate on healing instead. Advocates also believe that all-juice **diets** can help the body eliminate toxins (poisons).

The most extreme form of juice therapy for cancer is the Gerson juice therapy diet. The **Gerson therapy** treatment is based on drinking freshly pressed vegetable and fruit juice every hour. During a typical day at a Gerson clinic, a person would drink 13 glasses of raw carrot/apple and green-leaf vegetable juices. Vegetarian meals of organically grown food are served. During treatment, the patient receives coffee enemas during the evening to detoxify the blood and tissues. This treatment is administered in only two clinics, one in California and the other in Mexico. Critics of the Gerson diet say that it has many dangerous side effects, including dehydration, electrolyte imbalance, **constipation**, infection, poor resistance to disease, excessive weight loss, inflammation of the colon, and in some cases even death and that it does not cure cancer.

Homeopathy

There is conflicting evidence regarding the effectiveness of **homeopathy** in cancer treatment. Because cancer chemotherapy may suppress the body's response to homeopathic treatment, homeopathy may not be effective during chemotherapy. Therefore, patients should wait until after chemotherapy to try this relatively safe alternative treatment.

Acupuncture

Acupuncture uses needles inserted into the body to stimulate or direct the meridians (channels) of energy flow. Acupuncture has not been shown to have any anticancer effects. However, for some individuals it is an effective treatment for nausea and other unpleasant side effects of chemotherapy and radiation.

Other treatments

Other alternative treatments include **stress** reduction, **meditation**, **yoga**, t'ai chi, and the use of **guided imagery**. These techniques help the individual cope with cancer and improve quality of life, but do not have any curative effects.

Allopathic treatment

Treatment for lung cancer depends on the type of cancer, its location, and its stage. Treating the cancer early is key. The most commonly used modes of treatment are surgery, radiation therapy, and chemotherapy. Often these treatments are used in combination.

Surgery

Surgery is not usually an option for small cell lung cancers because most have spread beyond the lung by the time they are diagnosed. Because non-small cell lung cancers are less aggressive, however; surgery sometimes can be used to treat them. The surgeon decides on the type of surgery depending on how much of the lung is affected. Surgery may be the primary method of treatment, or radiation therapy and/or chemotherapy may be used to shrink the tumor before surgery is attempted.

There are three different types of surgical operations:

- Wedge resection. This procedure involves removing a small part of the lung.
- Lobectomy. A lobectomy is the removal of one lobe of the lung. If the cancer is limited to one part of the lung, the surgeon will perform a lobectomy.
- Pneumonectomy. A pneumonectomy is the removal of an entire lung. If the surgeon feels that removal of the entire lung is the best option for curing the cancer, a pneumonectomy is performed.

The pain that follows surgery can be relieved by medications. A more serious side effect of surgery is the patient's increased vulnerability to bacterial and viral **infections**. Preventative antibiotics and sometimes antiviral medications are given after surgery.

Radiation therapy

Radiation therapy involves the use of high-energy rays to kill cancer cells. It is used either by itself or in combination with surgery or chemotherapy. There are two types of radiation treatments: external beam radiation therapy and internal (or interstitial) radiotherapy. In external radiation therapy, the radiation is delivered from a machine positioned outside the body. Internal radiation therapy uses a small pellet of radioactive materials placed inside the body in the area of the cancer.

Radiation therapy may produce such side effects as tiredness, skin **rashes**, upset stomach, and **diarrhea**. Dry or sore throats, difficulty in swallowing, and loss of hair in the treated area are all minor side effects of radiation. These may disappear either during the course of the treatment or after the treatment is over. The side effects and ways to minimize them should be discussed with the doctor.

Chemotherapy

Chemotherapy uses anticancer medications that are either given intravenously or taken by mouth (orally). These drugs enter the bloodstream and travel to all parts of the body, killing cancer cells that have spread to different organs. Chemotherapy is used as the primary treatment for cancers that have spread beyond the lung and cannot be removed by surgery. It also can be used in addition to surgery or radiation therapy to kill any remaining cancer cells.

Chemotherapy is tailored to each patient's needs. Most patients are given a combination of several different drugs. Besides killing the cancer cells, these drugs also harm normal cells. Hence, the dose has to be carefully adjusted to minimize damage to normal cells. Chemotherapy often has severe side effects, including nausea, vomiting, **hair loss**, **anemia**, weakening of the immune system, and sometimes **infertility**. Most of these side effects end when the treatment is over. Other medications can be given to lessen the unpleasant side effects of chemotherapy.

Expected results

If the non-small lung cancer is detected and appropriately treated before it has had a chance to spread to other organs, about 47% of patients survive five years or longer after the initial diagnosis. Less than 15% of lung cancers, however, are found at this early stage. The one-year survival rate for all lung cancers in 2008 is about 40%.

Prevention

Overwhelmingly, the most effective way to prevent lung cancer is to not smoke or to quit smoking if one has already started. Secondhand smoke should be avoided as much as possible. Appropriate precautions should be taken when working with cancer-causing substances (carcinogens). Monitoring the diet and eating well-balanced meals that consist of whole foods, vegetables, and fruits; eliminating toxins, exercising routinely, and weight reduction; testing houses for the presence of radon gas; and removing asbestos from buildings also are useful preventive strategies.

KEY TERMS

Antioxidant—A molecule that prevents oxidation. In the body antioxidants attach to other molecules called free radicals and prevent the free radicals from causing damage to cell walls, DNA, and other parts of the cell.

Biopsy—The surgical removal and microscopic examination of living tissue for diagnostic purposes.

Bronchoscope—A thin, flexible, lighted tube that is used to view the air passages in the lungs.

Carcinogen—Any substance capable of causing cancer.

Chemotherapy—Treatment of cancer with synthetic drugs that destroy the tumor either by inhibiting the growth of cancerous cells or by killing them.

Electrolyte—Ions in the body that participate in metabolic reactions. The major human electrolytes are sodium (Na^+), potassium (K^+), calcium (Ca^{2+}), magnesium (Mg^{2+}), chloride (Cl^-), phosphate ($HPO4^{2-}$), bicarbonate ($HCO3^-$), and sulfate ($SO4^{2-}$).

Free radical—A molecule with an unpaired electron that has a strong tendency to react with other molecules in DNA (genetic material), proteins, and lipids (fats), resulting in damage to cells. Free radicals are neutralized by antioxidants.

Lobectomy—Surgical removal of an entire lobe of the lung.

Pathologist—A doctor who specializes in the diagnosis of disease by studying cells and tissues under a microscope.

Placebo—A pill or liquid given during the study of a drug or dietary supplement that contains no medication or active ingredient. Usually study participants do not know if they are receiving a pill containing the drug or an identical-appearing placebo.

Pneumonectomy—Surgical removal of an entire lung.

Radiation therapy—Treatment using high energy radiation from x-ray machines, cobalt, radium, or other sources.

Sputum—Mucus or phlegm that is coughed up from the passageways of the lungs.

Stage—A term used to describe the size and extent of cancer.

Traditional Chinese medicine (TCM)—An ancient system of medicine based on maintaining a balance in vital energy or qi that controls emotions, spiritual, and physical wellbeing. Diseases and disorders result from imbalances in qi (the life force), and treatments such as massage, exercise, acupuncture, and nutritional and herbal therapy are designed to restore balance and harmony to the body

Wedge resection—Removal of only a small portion of a cancerous lung.

Resources

BOOKS

Henschke, Claudia I., and Peggy McCarthy. *Lung Cancer: Myths, Facts, Choices—and Hope.* New York: Norton, 2003.

Mayo Clinic Book of Alternative Medicine: The New Approach to Using the Best of Natural Therapies and Conventional Medicine. New York: Time Inc. Home Entertainment, 2007.

Parles, Karen. *100 Questions & Answers About Lung Cancer,* rev. ed Boston: Jones and Bartlett, 2005.

"Pulmonary Disorders: Tumors of the Lung." In *The Merck Manual of Diagnosis and Therapy,* 18th ed. Edited by Mark H. Beers, Robert S. Porter, and Thomas V. Jones. Whitehouse Station, NJ: Merck, 2007.

OTHER

"Lung Cancer." *MedicineNet.com.* September 11, 2007 [cited April 18, 2008]. http://www.medicinenet.com/lung_cancer/article.htm.

"Lung Cancer." *MedlinePlus.* March 14, 2008 [cited April 18, 2008]. http://www.nlm.nih.gov/medlineplus/lungcancer.html.

"What You Need to Know About Lung Cancer." *National Cancer Institute.* undated [cited April 18, 2008]. http://www.cancer.gov/cancertopics/wyntk/lung.

ORGANIZATIONS

American Cancer Society, 1599 Clifton Road NE, Atlanta, GA, 30329-4251, (800) ACS-2345, http://www.cancer.org.

American Holistic Medical Association, PO Box 2016, Edmonds, WA, 98020, (425) 967-0737, http://www.holisticmedicin.org.

American Lung Association, 61 Broadway, 6th Floor, New York, NY, 10006, (800) LUNG-USA, http://www.lungusa.org/.

LungCancer.org: A Program of Cancer Care, 275 Seventh Avenue, New York, NY, 10001, (212) 712-8400, (800) 813-4673, http://www.lungcancer.org.

National Cancer Institute Public Inquiries Office, 6116 Executive Blvd., Room 3036A, Bethesda, MD, 20892-8322, (800) 4-CANCER, http://www.cancer.gov.

Mai Tran
Teresa G. Odle
Tish Davidson, A.M.

Lupus *see* **Systemic lupus erythematoses**

Lutein

Definition

Lutein is one of only two **carotenoids** (the other is zeaxanthin) that are found in the human eye. Lutein is thought to protect against certain eye diseases and possibly against some cancers.

Description

Found in spinach, kale, turnip, collard, and mustard greens, summer squash, peas, broccoli, brussels sprouts, and yellow corn, as well as egg yolks, lutein is a nutrient with a number of potentially beneficial effects. It is a member of the carotenoid family, a group of chemicals related to **vitamin A**. While beta-carotene, the precursor of vitamin A, may be the most familiar carotenoid, there are almost 600 others whose effects had as of 2008 not been extensively studied. Aside from lutein, these include alpha-carotene, **lycopene**, zeaxanthin, and beta-cryptoxanthin.

In plants, carotenoids such as lutein help to give color to sweet potatoes, carrots, and other fruits and vegetables. In humans, lutein and zeaxanthin make up much of the pigment in the center of the retina (the macula), where vision sensitivity is greatest. While lutein is not considered an essential nutrient, studies suggest that it plays an important role in maintaining healthy vision and preventing or slowing eye diseases such as age-related **macular degeneration** (ARMD), **cataracts**, and retinitis pigmentosa. Getting adequate amounts of lutein may also decrease the risk of developing certain types of **cancer**.

Carotenoids such as lutein are **antioxidants** that react with free radicals. Molecules called free radicals form during normal cell metabolism and with exposure to ultraviolet light or toxins such as cigarette smoke. Free radicals cause damage by reacting with fats and proteins in cell membranes and genetic material. This process is called oxidation. Antioxidants are compounds that attach themselves to free radicals so that it is impossible for the free radical to react with, or oxidize, other molecules. In this way, antioxidants may protect cells from damage. Although lutein and other carotenoids have antioxidant activity in the laboratory, it is not clear how much they function as antioxidants in the body. Concentrated mainly in the lens and retina of the eye, lutein is thought to protect vision by neutralizing free radicals and by increasing the density of eye pigment. Lutein may also shield the eyes from the destructive effects of ultraviolet rays in sunlight by absorbing light in the blue wavelength range.

General use

Several well-controlled clinical trials have produced strong indications that lutein plays an important role in maintaining vision and preventing ARMD and cataracts, the two leading causes of vision loss in adults. It also appears to slow the progress of retinitis pigmentosa. Research is ongoing, and a list of clinical trials currently enrolling volunteers in studies using lutein to treat various eye diseases can be found at http://www.clinicaltrials.gov. There is no charge to the patient to participate in these studies.

Research also indicates that getting adequate amounts of lutein may decrease the risk of endometrial cancer in women. As of 2008, research was underway that continues to investigate the relationship between lutein cancer prevention.

Preparations

Typically the United States Institute of Medicine (IOM) of the National Academy of Sciences develops values called Dietary Reference Intakes (DRIs) for vitamins and minerals. The DRIs define the amount of a nutrient a person needs to consume daily and the largest daily amount from food or dietary supplements that can be taken without harm. The IOM has not as of 2008 developed any DRIs for lutein or other carotenoids because not enough scientific information was available and because no diseases had been identified as being caused by inadequate intake of any carotenoid. The IOM, the American Cancer Society, and the American Heart Association all recommend that people meet their need for antioxidants, including lutein, from a diet high in fruits, vegetables, and whole grains rather than from dietary supplements.

Egg yolks are the richest source and also contain a large amount of zeaxanthin, another carotenoid found in the eye. Other sources of lutein include corn, red seedless grapes, kiwi fruit, squash, and green vegetables

KEY TERMS

Age-related macular degeneration (ARMD)—A chronic, painless eye disease occurring in people over age 50 that damages the macula, or central part of the retina, causing irreversible loss of central vision.

Antioxidant—An organic substance that is able to counteract the damaging effects of oxidation in human and animal tissue. Lutein is an antioxidant.

Carotenoid—Any of a group of red and yellow pigments that are chemically similar to carotene. They are contained in animal fat and some plants.

Cataracts—The clouding of the eye lens, which under normal circumstances is clear.

Free radical—A molecule with an unpaired electron that has a strong tendency to react with other molecules in DNA (genetic material), proteins, and lipids (fats), resulting in damage to cells. Free radicals are neutralized by antioxidants.

Retina—The layer of light-sensitive cells located at the back of the eye.

Retinitis pigmentosa—A group of inherited disorders that affect the rod cells of the retina. Retinitis pigmentosa begins with loss of night vision, followed by gradual loss of peripheral vision, the development of tunnel vision, and finally blindness.

such as zucchini, spinach, collard greens, kale, leaf lettuce, celery, peas, broccoli, and leeks. Oranges and orange juice, tomatoes, and carrots also prove good sources of lutein. Getting too much lutein through food and drink is not considered a significant risk because the nutrient is only present in relatively small amounts in plant and animal foods.

Despite the fact that the optimum daily dosage of lutein has not been established with certainty, indications suggest that therapeutic dosages range from 5 to 30 mg per day, although 6 mg daily is generally considered adequate for cancer prevention and 10 mg daily for ARMD treatment or prevention. As a dietary supplement, lutein is available in capsule form.

Precautions

Lutein is not known to be harmful when taken in recommended dosages, although the long-term effects of taking lutein supplements were unknown as of 2008. Due to lack of sufficient medical study, lutein should be used with caution in children, women who are pregnant or breast feeding, and people with liver or kidney disease.

Side effects

When taken in recommended dosages, lutein is not known to be associated with any significant side effects.

Interactions

Lutein is not known to interact adversely with any drugs or dietary supplements; however, as of 2008, few studies of interactions had been conducted.

Resources

BOOKS

Challem, Jack, and Marie Moneysmith. *Basic Health Publications User&s Guide to Carotenoids & Flavonoids: Learn How to Harness the Health Benefits of Natural Plant Antioxidants*. North Bergen, NJ: Basic Health, 2005.

Krinsky, Norman, Susan T. Mayne, Helmut Sies, eds. *Carotenoids in Health and Disease*. New York: Marcel Dekker, 2004.

Mayo Clinic Book of Alternative Medicine: The New Approach to Using the Best of Natural Therapies and Conventional Medicine. New York: Time Inc. Home Entertainment, 2007.

PDR for Herbal Medicines, 4th ed. Montvale, NJ: Thomson Healthcare, 2007.

Weil, Andrew, *Natural Health, Natural Medicine*, rev. ed. New York: Houghton Mifflin, 2004.

OTHER

Higdon, Jane. "Carotenoids." *Linus Pauling Institute-Oregon State University* December 21, 2005 [cited April 19, 2008]. http://lpi.oregonstate.edu/infocenter/phytochemicals/carotenoids.

"Lutein and Its Role in Eye Disease." *National Eye Institute* [cited April 19, 2008]. http://www.nei.nih.gov/news/statements/lutein.asp.

Lutein Information Bureau [cited April 19, 2008]. http://www.luteininfo.com.

ORGANIZATIONS

Alternative Medicine Foundation, PO Box 60016, Potomac, MD, 20859, (301) 340-1960, http://www.amfoundation.org.

American Holistic Medical Association, PO Box 2016, Edmonds, WA, 98020, (425) 967-0737, http://www.holisticmedicin.org.

National Eye Institute, 2020 Vision Place, Bethesda, MD, 20892-3655, (301) 496-5248, http://www.nei.nih.gov.

Greg Annussek
Teresa Norris
Tish Davidson, A. M.

Lycium fruit

Description

Lycium fruit, sometimes called lycium berry, is used extensively in Chinese herbalism. The fruit are the berries of *Lycium chinense* and more commonly *Lycium barbarum*. The roots also have healing properties. Lycium is a shrub that grows to about 12 ft (4 m) in height. It grows wild on hillsides in the cooler regions of northern China and Tibet. However, it is also cultivated in almost all parts of China and in some other regions of Asia.

Lycium fruit is rich in carotene, vitamins B_1 and B_{12}, and **vitamin C**. The fruit also contains **amino acids** (the building blocks of proteins), **iron**, and trace elements essential to the body, including **zinc**, **copper**, **selenium**, **calcium**, and **phosphorus**. The bright red berries are usually harvested in late summer or early autumn. The roots are usually harvested in the spring, although they can be dug any time of the year. Berries and roots can be used either fresh or dried. Lycium is also called Chinese wolfberry. Its Chinese name is *Gou Qi Zi*.

General use

The first recorded use of lycium fruit as a medicinal herb is from the first century A.D. For thousands of years it has been used in China to promote a long, vigorous, and happy life. It is used as both a *jing* (yin) tonic for liver and kidney, and as a blood tonic. In the Chinese system of health, *jing* is an essential life substance. To remain healthy, yin aspects must be kept in balance with yang aspects. Ill health occurs when the energies and elements of the body are out of balance or in disharmony. Health is restored by taking herbs and treatments that restore this balance.

Lycium fruit is traditionally believed to have many different effects upon the body. In addition to being a general longevity herb, it is said to raise the spirits, fight **depression**, and increase cheerfulness. Berries are made into a blood tonic that is given for general weakness, to improve circulation, and increase the cells' ability to absorb nutrients. When blended with more yang herbs, lycium is used as a sexual tonic.

In Chinese medicine, the liver is associated with the function of the eyes. Lycium berries are used as a liver tonic to brighten the eyes, improve poor eyesight, treat blurred vision, sensitivity to light, and other general eye weaknesses.

One of the qualities ascribed to lycium root is that it said to cool the blood. It is used to reduce **fever** and to treat other conditions of what is referred to as excess heat. These include traditional uses to relieve excess sweating, stop **nosebleeds**, reduce **vomiting**, and treat **dizziness**. Some herbalists use a tea made of lycium root and *Scutellaria* (**skullcap** or *Huang Qin*) to treat **morning sickness** in pregnant women. Lycium is also used to treat certain types of coughs and **asthma**.

Modern herbalists use lycium roots to treat high blood pressure. There is some scientific basis for this treatment, since extracts from the root have been shown in laboratory experiments to relax the involuntary muscles, including artery muscles. This **relaxation** lowers blood pressure.

Other modern scientific studies have shown that extracts of lycium root can reduce fever, including fever associated with **malaria**. One Korean study looked at the effect extracts from the berries and roots had on the blood of mice that were exposed to whole body x rays. They concluded that the mice that received doses of root extract replaced leukocytes, erythrocytes, and thrombocytes faster than those that did not receive the extract. This effect may account for lycium's reputation for creating good health, vigor, and long life.

Since the mid 1990s, claims have been made by some researchers, mainly in China, that lycium extracts can inhibit the growth of **cancer** cells. As of 2007, according to Memorial Sloan-Kettering Cancer Center, "Despite claims by several marketers, the efficacy and safety of lycium products for cancer treatment in humans have not been established." Nevertheless, research continued on this herb.

Preparations

High-quality, fresh lycium fruit has thick flesh, few seeds, and a delicious sweet taste. It can be eaten raw on a daily basis to promote general health and happiness. Dried berries can be used just as raisins are in cooking. Herbalists also make a decoction from dried, chopped lycium berries. To treat eye problems, about 0.5 cup (100 ml) of decoction is consumed daily.

Roots are used either fresh or dried. About 0.5 cup (100 ml) of root decoction daily is given to reduce fevers. A tincture can also be made of the root. About 0.5 teaspoon (3 ml) diluted with water three times a day is taken for coughs.

Combinations

Lycium is regularly used in tonics and herbal formulas that treat blood deficiencies, poor kidney function, and liver depletion. Among these are lycium formula, a blood tonic that is intended to strengthen

KEY TERMS

Decoction—The liquid made from boiling an herb, then straining out the solid material.

Erythrocytes—Known as red blood cells, the ones that carry oxygen to every part of the body.

Leukocytes—Also called white blood cells, the ones that fight infection and boost the immune system.

Thrombocytes—Also called platelets, these help the blood to clot so that wounds can heal.

Tincture—An alcohol-based extract prepared by soaking plant parts.

Yang aspects—Qualities such as warmth, activity, and light, the opposite of yin aspects.

Yin aspects—Qualities such as cold, stillness, darkness, and passiveness, the opposite of yang aspects.

the entire body and brain. Lycium is an ingredient in rehmannia eight combination, a common *jing* tonic for older men and women that is said to regulate blood sugar and control diabetes, and a vision formula with the Chinese name of *Qi Ju Di Huang Wan* is made of lycium, chrysanthemum, and rehmannia.

Precautions

Chinese herbalists do not recommend lycium for people who have a fever due to infection or who have **diarrhea** or bloating. The safety of lycium during **pregnancy** has not been established.

Side effects

There are no reported side effects from taking lycium. Lycium has been used for centuries, both as a healing herb and as a food.

Interactions

Lycium is often used in conjunction with other herbs with no reported interactions. Lycium has also been found to enhance the action of the blood-thinning drug warfarin (Coumadin).

Resources

BOOKS

Chevallier, Andrew. *Herbal Remedies*. New York: DK Publishing, 2007.

Foster, Steven, and Rebecca Johnson. *National Geographic Desk Reference to Nature's Medicine*. Washington, DC: National Geographic Society, 2006.

PDR for Herbal Medicines, 4th ed. Montvale, NJ: Thomson Healthcare, 2007.

OTHER

"Lycium." Memorial Sloan-Kettering Cancer Center, updated April 14, 2007. http://www.mskcc.org/mskcc/html/69287.cfm (February 11, 2008).

ORGANIZATIONS

Alternative Medicine Foundation, PO Box 60016, Potomac, MD, 20859, (301) 340-1960, http://www.amfoundation.org.

American Association of Oriental Medicine, PO Box 162340, Sacramento, CA, 95816, (866) 455-7999, (914) 443-4770, http://www.aaaomonline.org.

Centre for International Ethnomedicinal Education and Research (CIEER), http://www.cieer.org.

Tish Davidson, A. M.

Lycopene

Description

Lycopene is a red, fat-soluble pigment found in vegetables, and most commonly found in tomatoes. It is one of a family of pigments called **carotenoids**. Carotenoids are naturally occurring pigments responsible for the brightly colored fall leaves and the vivid colors of flowers, fruits, and vegetables. In fruits and vegetables, these pigments range in hue from bright yellow in squash, to orange in carrots, to bright red in tomatoes and peppers.

Although the human body does not produce lycopene, it is readily available through the diet. Minor sources include guava, rosehip, watermelon, and pink grapefruit. However, about 85% of lycopene in the U.S. diet comes from tomatoes and tomato products such as juice, soup, sauce, paste, and ketchup. A diet rich in carotenoid-containing foods is associated with a variety of health benefits.

Once lycopene is absorbed in the body, it is deposited widely in the liver, lungs, prostate gland, colon, and skin. Its concentration in body tissues tends to be higher than most other carotenoids. Working as a powerful antioxidant, lycopene fights free radicals—highly reactive molecules that damage cell membranes, attack DNA, and cause disease. Studies have found that patients with HIV infection, inflammatory diseases, and high cholesterol levels (with and without lipid-lowering treatment) may have depleted lycopene serum (blood) levels. In contrast to other carotenoids, serum levels of lycopene are not usually reduced by

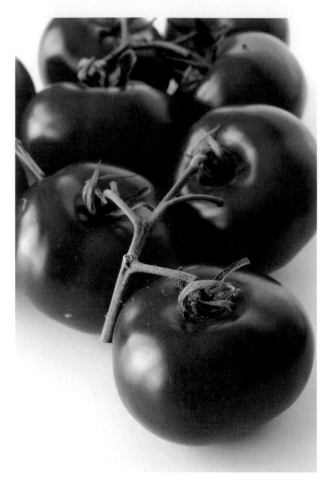

Tomatoes are a good source of lycopene. *(© Sorin Alexandru / Alamy)*

smoking or alcohol consumption but rather by increasing age.

General use

A number of studies have indicated that a lycopene-rich diet lowers the risk of certain chronic diseases such as cardiovascular disease, **cancer**, and age-related macular degeneration .

Cardiovascular disease

In its role as an antioxidant, lycopene prevents the oxidation of low-density liproprotein (LDH), the "bad" **cholesterol** that leads to **atherosclerosis** (hardening of the arteries) and coronary artery disease.

As serum lycopene levels rise, the levels of oxidized lipoprotein, protein, and DNA compounds go down, thus lowering the risk of heart disease. Individuals with high levels of lycopene are half as likely to

have a **heart attack** than those with low levels, according to one study.

Cancer

Researchers have found a strong relationship between lycopene intake and reduced risk of cancers of the prostate and pancreas. In several studies of these cancers, lycopene was the only carotenoid associated with risk reduction. In late 2001, the first clinical intervention trial of **prostate cancer** patients showed that supplementation with lycopene helped slow growth of prostate cancer. In fact, the spread of prostate cancer was reduced by 73%.

Consuming tomato products twice a week, as opposed to not at all, was associated with a reduced risk of prostate cancer of up to 34%, according to a study conducted by the Dana-Farber Cancer Institute. Of the 46 fruits and vegetables investigated, only tomato products showed a measurable association with reduced risk of prostate cancer. There is also medical evidence to suggest that a high intake of lycopene-rich tomato products is associated with a reduced risk of developing cancers of the lung, breast, cervix, and gastrointestinal tract.

Macular degeneration

Lycopene (as well as other carotenoids such as lutein and beta-carotene) may also help prevent macular degenerative disease, the leading cause of blindness in people over the age of 65. Lycopene is the only micronutrient whose serum level was shown to be inversely related to the risk of age-related **macular degeneration**.

In late 2001, a study showed that lycopene may also help relieve exercise-induced **asthma** symptoms.

Preparations

Although the major sources of lycopene for humans are tomatoes and tomato products, bioavailability from different food items varies considerably. Cooking fresh tomatoes with a source of fat, such as olive oil in spaghetti sauce, enhances the body's absorption of lycopene, since lycopene is fat-soluble. By heating the tomatoes, the bound chemical form of lycopene is converted into a form that is more easily digested. In fact, one study showed that lycopene is absorbed 2.5 times better from tomato paste than from fresh tomatoes.

Although no dietary guidelines have been established, research shows that drinking two cups (about 540 ml) of tomato juice per day provides about 40 mg of lycopene. This is the amount recommended to significantly reduce the oxidation of LDL cholesterol, according to one human dietary intervention study.

The approximate lycopene content of tomatoes and tomato products, based on an analysis by a number of laboratories (mg/100 g wet weight) are listed below.

- tomatoes, fresh (0.9–4.2)
- tomatoes, cooked (3.7)
- tomato sauce (6.2)
- tomato paste (5.4–150)
- tomato soup, condensed (8.0)
- tomato juice (5.0–11.6)
- sun-dried tomato in oil (46.5)
- pizza sauce, canned (12.7)
- ketchup (9.9–13.4)

Although lycopene is available in concentrated capsule form and in combination with other vitamins, such as **vitamin E** or multivitamin preparations, there is inadequate evidence to conclude that supplements are more beneficial than the lycopene consumed in foods. Since most of the health benefits of lycopene have been ascertained from studies of estimated dietary intake or blood concentrations, as of the year 2000, researchers recommend that individuals consume a diet rich in carotenoids and an array of fruits and vegetables rather than turning to lycopene supplements. The United States Department of Agriculture reported in 2001 that people intake an average of 10.9mg per day.

Precautions

There are no known precautions regarding lycopene itself. However, there are a number of indirect problems that may result from consuming excessive amounts of tomatoes or commercially prepared tomato products.

Although processed tomato products are the richest source of lycopene in the diet, ingesting tomatoes may aggravate certain health conditions. As a member of the nightshade variety of plants—which includes eggplants, potatoes, peppers, paprika, and tobacco—tomatoes have been strongly and consistently linked with certain forms of arthritis, particularly rheumatoid and **osteoarthritis**.

One theory maintains that the alkaloids (alkaline chemicals) in the nightshades are deposited in the connective tissue, stimulate inflammation, and then inhibit the formation of normal cartilage. As a result, joint cartilage continues to break down and is not replaced by new, healthy cartilage cells.

Another indirect precaution is that processed tomato products usually contain large amounts of **sodium**, unless the product is labeled low-sodium or salt-free. An excess amount of sodium in the diet can exacerbate high blood pressure.

Side effects

Although extensive research has not been conducted, there have been no reported side effects or toxicity associated with lycopene intake.

Interactions

Research into the interactions of lycopene with food, drugs, or diseases has not been conducted as of the year 2000.

Resources

PERIODICALS

Arab, Lenore and Susan Steck. "Lycopene and Cardiovascular Disease." *American Journal of Clinical Nutrition* (2000 suppl.): 1961S-1695S.
Bauer, Jeff. "A Tomato Antioxidant May Relieve Asthma." *RN* (October 2001):21.
Broiher, Kitty. "A Tomato a Day May Keep Cancer Away." *Food Processing* (April 1999): 58.
"Clinical Intervention Trial Finds Benefit of Lycopene." *Cancer Weekly* (November 27, 2001) :38.
Clinton, Steven K. "Lycopene: Chemistry, Biology, and Implications for Human Disease." *Nutrition Reviews* (February 1998): 35-51.
Edens, Neile K. "Representative Components of Functional Food Science." *Nutrition Today* (July 1999): 152.
McCord, Holly. "You say 'tomato' and I Say 'Terrific.'" *Prevention* (April 1995): 52.
Zoler, Mitchel L. "Lycopene May Reduce Prostate Cancer Tumor Grade." *Family Practice News* (May 1999): 28.

ORGANIZATIONS

American Heart Association, National Center. 7272 Greenville Avenue, Dallas, TX 75231. http://www americanheart.org.

National Cancer Institute. Public Inquiries Office. Building 31, Room 10A03, 31 Center Drive, MSC 2580, Bethesda, MD 20892. http://www.nci.nih.gov.

OTHER

Heinz Institute of Nutritional Sciences. http://www.lycopene.org.

Genevieve Slomski
Teresa Norris

Lycopodium

Description

Lycopodium (*Lycopodium clavatum*) is a perennial evergreen plant that grows in pastures, woodlands, heaths, and moors of Great Britain, Northern Europe, and North America. It has a slender stem that trails along the ground and vertical branches that grow to 3 to 4 in (7.5–10 cm). The plant belongs to the (*Lycopodiaceae* family and is related to mosses and ferns. It is often called **club moss**. Other names include wolf's claw, stag horn, witch meal, and vegetable sulfur.

The pale yellow pollen collected from the spores is used to make the homeopathic remedy called lycopodium. The pollen is odorless, water resistant, and highly flammable. For this reason, it used to be a component of fireworks. It was also formerly used to create a coating for pills and as a powder for medical gloves.

Early physicians used the plant to stimulate the appetite and to promote urination and the excretion of other body fluids. Lycopodium was also used in the treatment of flatulence, rheumatism, **gout**, lung ailments, and diseases of children and young girls. In the seventeenth century the pollen was used as an internal remedy for **diarrhea**, dysentery, and rheumatism. Externally, the pollen was a treatment for **wounds** and diseases of the skin such as **eczema**. The whole plant was used to heal kidney ailments.

General use

Lycopodium is prescribed by homeopaths for both acute and chronic ailments such as earaches, sore throats, digestive disorders, urinary tract difficulties, prostatitis, and eye conditions. The remedy acts on soft tissues, blood vessels, bones, joints, the liver, and the heart. This polychrest is also recommended in the treatment of back **pain**, **bedwetting**, fevers, **food poisoning**, mouth ulcers, **mumps**, colds, **muscle cramps**, **constipation**, coughs, cystitis, **gas**, **sciatica**, gout, skin conditions, and joint pain. It is often indicated in the

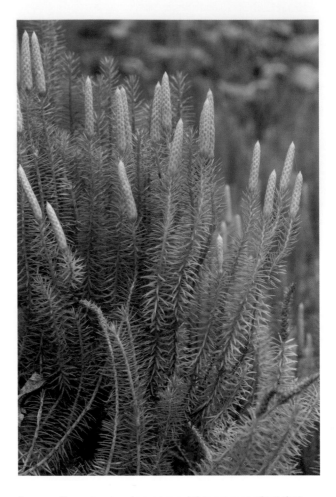

Lycopodium clavatum **is a perennial evergreen plant that grows in pastures, woodlands, heaths, and moors of Great Britain, Northern Europe, and North America.** *(Gregory K. Scott / Photo Researchers, Inc.)*

early stages of **pneumonia**. The levo-tetrahydropalmatine in lycopodium serratum preparations (also known as *Jin bu haun*) has sedative and analgesic properties.

According to homeopaths, lycopodium ailments are frequently the result of anger, horror, chagrin, disappointment, grief, fright, mental exertion, sexual excesses, overeating, or alcohol consumption. Typical lycopodium patients are alcoholic, timid, and fearful adults, irritable and domineering children, or intellectuals who are strong in mind but weak in body. The latter generally look older than they are and their hair becomes gray prematurely. Children who require lycopodium are prone to **tonsillitis**, gas, and bronchial **infections**. They have tantrums if they do not get their way and dislike naps, often kicking and screaming beforehand or upon waking.

Homeopaths may believe that patients likely to use lycopodium are predisposed to lung ailments, gas, and

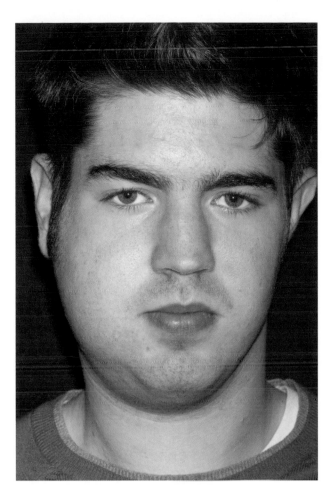

Lycopodium can aid in the treatment of mumps, pictured above. *(Dr. P. Marazzi / Photo Researchers, Inc.)*

gallstones. They have weak digestive systems and often suffer from dyspepsia, **colitis**, or gastro-enteritis. They become full soon after beginning a meal or have no appetite until eating, whereupon they become ravenous. They may crave sweets and dislike oysters, onions, cabbage, and milk. Their stomachs are often bloated, gassy, acidic, and sour, and are worse from cold drinks, beer, coffee, or fruit. They may become sleepy after eating.

Mentally these persons are irritable, restless, quarrelsome, sensitive, weepy, melancholy, and depressed. Other mental symptoms include dullness, confusion, poor memory, amnesia, anger, hypersensitivity to noise, sadness, and **anxiety** upon waking. They frequently suffer from performance anxiety and are nervous in social situations. They do not prefer the company of others and although they dread the presence of new persons, friends, or visitors, they are afraid to be alone.

Ailments are generally worse on the right side of the body, often traveling from right to left or from above downward. Symptoms are worse between 4:00 and 8:00 p.m. and worsen with cold food and drinks.

Exhaustion and illness may set in after much physical exertion. Symptoms are generally worse from cold conditions with the exception of head and spine symptoms, which are worse from warmth. Symptoms are better from open air, warm drinks, and motion.

Specific indications

Physical indications are hunger with sudden fullness, urine with a red sandy color, gas, **fatigue**, numbness of fingers or toes, and a trembling of the limbs. Liver ailments such as **cirrhosis**, **hepatitis**, fatty degeneration of the liver, and liver **cancer** warrant the use of this remedy.

Periodic headaches result from digestive disturbances. If lycopodium patients miss a meal, they may get a **headache**, which is relieved upon eating.

The **sore throat** that typically warrants using this remedy is sore on the right side, with swollen tonsils. The throat feels dusty and is better after swallowing warm drinks.

The cold indicative of lycopodium is accompanied by a headache, yellow mucous, and a stuffed, dry nose. The patient often has to breathe out of his mouth. The lycopodium **cough** is constant, deep and hollow. The chest is tight and the mucus that is expelled is salty, thick, and gray. The cough is worse in the evening.

Eye conditions may develop in which the eyes are inflamed and red and the eyelids are grainy.

When abdominal pains are present they are of a cutting, griping, clutching, or squeezing nature. Gas is accompanied by a bloated abdomen that relieved after passing gas and by wearing loose clothing. The gas is worse after eating.

Joint pains are typically tearing pains that start on the right side and move to the left side. The knee and finger joints are especially stiff. Pains are better from continued movement or warmth and worsened during **fever**, sitting still, and initial movement.

The typical lycopodium patient has a pale, sickly face that is often covered with skin eruptions. Eczema, **psoriasis**, **rashes**, herpetic eruptions, and brown and yellow spots on the skin are common.

Men may be impotent. Women often suffer from inflammation and pain of the ovaries and uterus. The pain generally affects the right ovary more than the left.

Preparations

The spores of the plant are gathered at the end of the summer. The pollen is extracted from the spores and diluted with milk sugar.

Lycopodium is available at health food and drug stores in various potencies in the form of tinctures, tablets, and pellets.

Precautions

If symptoms do not improve after the recommended time period, a homeopath or healthcare practitioner should be consulted. The recommended dose of lycopodium should not be exceeded.

In the United States, herbal remedies are considered dietary supplements, which are not standardized. Although it was regulated under the 1994 Dietary Supplement Health and Education Act (DSHEA), there are no safety reviews or FDA approved therapeutic uses for lycopodium. In addition, herbal remedies are not standardized and preparations of lycopodium can vary greatly. Therefore, it is important to read labels carefully and consult a physician before taking this or any other herbal supplement.

Side effects

Liver toxicity and hepatitis have been reported in several studies, with associated symptoms, including liver enlargement, **jaundice**, fever, fatigue, **nausea**, abdominal pain, and **itching**. Therefore, patients should consult their doctor before using this supplement, particularly if they have known or suspected liver disease.

Interactions

When taking any homeopathic remedy, it is advised to avoid **peppermint** products, coffee, or alcohol. These products may cause the remedy to be ineffective.

Lycopodium is incompatible with the remedy coffea. These remedies should not be taken simultaneously.

Resources

BOOKS

Gruenwald, Joerg. *PDR for Herbal Medicines,* 4th ed. Montvale, NJ: Thomson Healthcare, 2007.

PERIODICALS

Gola, Edyta M., Judith A. Jernstedt, and Beata Zagorska-Marek. "Vascular Architecture in Shoots of Early Divergent Vascular Plants, *Lycopodium clavatum* and *Lycopodium annotinum*." *New Phytologist* 174, no. 4 (June 2007): 774–786.

ORGANIZATIONS

Alternative Medicine Foundation, PO Box 60016, Potomac, MD, 20859, (301) 340-1960, http://www.amfoundation.org.

National Center for Complementary and Alternative Medicine, National Institutes of Health, 9000 Rockville Pike,, Bethesda, MD, 20892, (888) 644-6226, http://www.nccam.nih.gov.

Office of Dietary Supplements, National Institutes of Health, 6100 Executive Blvd., Room 3B01, MSC 7517, Bethesda, MD, 20892-7517, (301) 435-2920, http://ods.od.nih.gov.

Jennifer Wurges
Angela M. Costello

Lycopus

Defintion

Lycopus is a genus within the family *Lamiaceae* consisting of about a dozen species. The plant is also known by a number of common names, primarily bugleweed and gypsywort.

Description

Lycopus is somewhat similar in appearance to mint, although lacking in mint's characteristic taste and odor. It is a perennial herb that may grow to about two feet in height. It produces small white or pale purple flowers at the base of leaves. Leaves are bright green, lobed, and pointed. Its prefer habitat is moist soil or wetlands. The primary chemical components of lycopus include tannins, lithospermic acid, lycopine, flavone–glycosides, phenolic derivatives, essential oil, **magnesium** and resin. These components are responsible for the plant's somewhat bitter and astringent taste.

Humans have used lycopus since ancient times for a variety of purposes. Its common name of gypsywort is said to have come from an ancient practice by members of the Roma culture in Eastern Europe in which extracts of the plant were used to dye the skin in order to produce a shade similar to that of the Egyptians. Interest in the use of lycopus for medical purposes in the United States was apparently sparked by an article written in 1822 by J. Smyth Rogers and James M. Pendleton, "Observations on the Lycopus Virginicus, or *Bugleweed.*"

Herbalists and other practitioners use the leaves, stems, and flowers for their medicinal preparations.

Uses

The medicinal uses of lycopus have changed substantially over time. Traditionally it was used for a variety of purposes, including:

- treatment for coughs and sore throat
- as an astringent
- as a sedative or mild narcotic
- treatment of tuberculosis (consumption)
- treatment for heavy menstrual bleeding
- treatment for nosebleeds
- relief from anxiety

Modern medicinal applications of lycopus differ significantly from these traditional uses. Today, the plant is probably recommended most commonly for treatment of thyroid problems and palpitations. The herb is thought to be effective for these purposes because some of its components may reduce the activity of thyroid–stimulating hormone (TSH) and thyroxine, one of the primary hormones produced by the thyroid. Reduction of these hormones, in turn, is thought to relieve conditions of **hyperthyroidism**, which may be manifested in shaking and palpitations. The herb is also recommended, for this reason, for the treatment of Grave's disease, which is characterized by palpitations, shaking, and shortness of breath. The effectiveness of lycopus in the treatment of thyroid problems is less than that of synthetic drugs, but may be adequate to treat mild forms of the disorders.

Herbalists also suggest the use of lycopus for the treatment of a number of other diseases and disorders, including:

- cardiac problems
- dandruff
- as a sedative or mild narcotic
- excessive menstrual flow
- diuretic
- treatment for liver disorders
- breast and chest pain

As of 2008, the Natural Standard has found that "there is a lack of high–quality clinical trials investigating the safety and efficacy of bugleweed." The Natural Standard is an international research collaborative that collects and analyzes data on the safety and efficacy of complementary and alternative therapies

---

KEY TERMS

Astringent—A substance that dries tissue, producing a "puckered" appearance and feeling.

Diuretic—A substance that tends to increase urine flow.

Grave's disease—A condition produced by excessive production of thyroid hormones, characterized by and enlarged thyroid gland and protruding eyeballs.

Hyperthyroidism—A condition resulting from overproduction of thyroid hormones.

Hypothyroidism—A condition resulting from underproduction of thyroid hormones.

Side effects

Although lycopus may be safely used by people with hyperthyroidism, it should not be ingested by individuals with normal thyroid function or **hypothyroidism**. In such cases, reduction in thyroid function could result in serious health problems and, possibly, death. The herb should also not be used by pregnant women or women who are breast feeding. Since there are no long–term studies on the overall safety of lycopus preparations, the product should be taken only under the advice and care of a health care professional.

Interactions

Preparations of lycopus may interact with drugs used for the treatment of thyroid problems since they may magnify or diminish the effects of the allopathic treatment. In general, there has been relatively little research on the interaction among herbal products or between herbs and allopathic drugs. For this reason, care should be taken in combining the use of lycopus products with other herbal and allopathic remedies.

Resources

BOOKS

Gruenwald, Joerg, Thomas Brendler, and Christof Jaenicke, eds.. *PDR for Herbal Medicines,* 4th edition. London: Thomson Healthcare, 2007.

Juta, C. Rupert. *Modern Diseases and Disorders, and Homeopathy.* Charleston, S.C.: BookSurge Publishers, 2007.

Karalliedde, Lakshman, Rita Fitzpatrick, and Debbie Shaw. *Traditional Herbal Medicines: A Guide to Their Safer Use.* London: Hammersmith Press, 2007.

Mars, Brigitte. *The Desktop Guide to Herbal Medicine: The Ultimate Multidisciplinary Reference to the Amazing*

Realm of Healing Plants, in a Quick–study, One–stop Guide. Laguna Beach, Calif.: Basic Health Publications, 2007.

PERIODICALS

Beer, A. M., K. R. Wiebelitz, and H. Schmidt–Gayk. "Lycopus Europaeus (Gypsywort): Effects on the Thyroidal Parameters and Symptoms Associated with Thyroid Function." *Phytomedicine* (January 2008): 16–22.

Gibbons, S., et al. "Bacterial Resistance Modifying Agents from Lycopus Europaeus." *Phytochemistry* (January 2003): 83–87.

Vonhoff, C., et al. "Extract of Lycopus Europaeus L. Reduces Cardiac Signs of Hyperthyroidism in Rats." *Life Sciences* (February 2006): 1063–1070.

OTHER

Henriette's Herbal Homepage. "Lycopus.–Bugleweed." http://www.henrietteherbal.com/eclectic/kings/lycopus. html (February 17, 2008).

iHerb.com. "Bugleweed." http://healthlibrary.epnet.com/ GetContent.aspx (February 17, 2008).

Plants for a Future. "Lycopus virginicus–L." http:// www.pfaf.org/database/plants.php?Lycopus + virgini cus (February 17, 2008).

David Edward Newton, Ed.D

Lyme disease

Definition

Lyme disease, which is also known as Lyme borreliosis, is an infection transmitted by the bite of ticks carrying the spiral-shaped bacterium (spirochete) *Borrelia burgdorferi* (Bb). The disease was named for Old Lyme, Connecticut, the town where it was first diagnosed in 1975, after a puzzling outbreak of arthritis. The spiral-shaped bacterium was named for its discoverer, Willy Burgdorfer. The effects of this disease can be long-term and disabling, unless it is recognized and treated properly with antibiotics.

Description

Lyme disease is a vector-borne disease, which means it is delivered from one host to another. It is also classified as a zoonosis, which means that it is a disease of animals that can be transmitted to humans under natural conditions. In this case, a tick bearing the Bb organism literally inserts it into a host's bloodstream when it bites the host to feed on its blood. It is important, however, to note that neither Bb nor Lyme

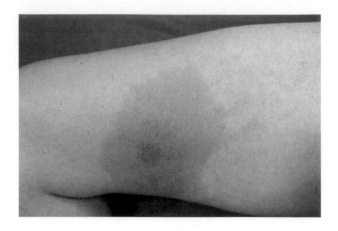

This Erythema migrans rash is one of the symptoms of Lyme disease, a common chronic disease in the United States and Europe. *(Adam Hart-Davis / Photo Researchers, Inc.)*

disease can be transmitted directly from one person to another.

In the United States, Lyme disease accounts for more than 90% of all reported vector-borne illnesses. It is a significant public health problem and continues in the late 2000s to be diagnosed in increasing numbers. The Centers for Disease Control and Prevention (CDC) attributes this increase to the growing size of the deer herd and the geographical spread of infected ticks rather than to improved diagnosis. In addition, some epidemiologists believe that the actual incidence of Lyme disease in the United States may be 5–10 times greater than that reported by the CDC. The reasons for this difference include the narrowness of the CDC's case definition as well as frequent misdiagnoses of the disease.

Controversy clouds the true incidence of Lyme disease because no test is definitively diagnostic for the disease, and many of its symptoms mimic those of so many other diseases. Cases of Lyme disease have been reported in 49 of the 50 states; however, 92% of the 17,730 cases reported to the CDC in 2000 were from only nine states (Connecticut, Rhode Island, New York, Pennsylvania, Delaware, New Jersey, Maryland, Massachusetts, and Wisconsin). The disease is also found in Scandinavia, continental Europe, the countries of the former Soviet Union, Japan, and China; in addition, it is possible that it has spread to Australia.

The risk for acquiring Lyme disease varies, depending on what stage in its life cycle a tick has reached. A tick passes through three stages of development—larva, nymph, and adult—each of which is dependent on a live host for food. In the United States, Bb is borne by ticks of several species in the genus *Ixodes*, which usually feed on the white-footed mouse and deer (and are often called deer ticks). In the summer, the larval ticks hatch from eggs laid in the ground and feed by attaching themselves to small animals and birds. At this stage they are not a problem for humans. It is the next stage—the nymph—that causes most cases of Lyme disease. Nymphs are very active from spring through early summer, at the height of outdoor activity for most people. Because they are still quite small (less than 2 mm in length), they are difficult to spot, giving them ample opportunity to transmit Bb while feeding. Although far more adult ticks than nymphs carry Bb, the adult ticks are much larger, more easily noticed, and more likely to be removed before the 24 hours or more of continuous feeding needed to transmit Bb.

Causes and symptoms

Lyme disease is a collection of effects caused by Bb. Once Bb gains entry to the body through a tick bite, it can move through the bloodstream quickly. Only 12 hours after entering the bloodstream, Bb can be found in cerebrospinal fluid (which means it can affect the nervous system). Treating Lyme disease early and thoroughly is important because Bb can hide for long periods within the body in a clinically latent state. That ability explains why symptoms can recur in cycles and can flare up after months or years, even over decades. It is important to note, however, that not everyone exposed to Bb develops the disease.

Lyme disease is usually described in terms of length of infection (time since the person was bitten by a tick infected with Bb) and whether Bb is localized or disseminated (spread through the body by fluids and cells carrying Bb). Furthermore, when and how symptoms of Lyme disease appear can vary widely from patient to patient. People who experience recurrent bouts of symptoms over time are said to have chronic Lyme disease.

Early localized Lyme disease

The most recognizable indicator of Lyme disease is a rash around the site of the tick bite. Often, the tick exposure has not been recognized. The area of rash eruption might be warm or itch. The rash—erythema migrans (EM)—generally develops within 3–30 days and usually begins as a round, red patch that expands. Clearing may take place from the center out, leaving a bull's-eye effect; in some cases, the center gets redder instead of clearing. The rash may look like a bruise on individuals with dark skin. Of those who develop Lyme disease, about 50% notice the rash; about 50% notice flu-like symptoms, including **fatigue**, **headache**, **chills**

and **fever**, muscle and joint **pain**, and lymph node swelling. However, a rash at the site can also be an allergic reaction to the tick saliva rather than an indicator of Lyme disease, particularly if the rash appears in *less* than three days and disappears only days later.

Late disseminated disease and chronic Lyme disease

Weeks, months, or even years after an untreated tick bite, symptoms can appear in several forms:

- fatigue, forgetfulness, confusion, mood swings, irritability, numbness
- neurologic problems, such as pain (unexplained and not triggered by an injury), Bell's palsy (facial paralysis, usually one-sided but may be on both sides), and a mimicking of the inflammation of brain membranes known as meningitis (fever, severe headache, stiff neck)
- arthritis (short episodes of pain and swelling in joints) and other musculoskeletal complaints

In the past, Lyme arthritis occurred in 60% of patients with Lyme disease, but as of 2006, this number dropped to 10%.

Less common effects of Lyme disease are heart abnormalities (such as irregular rhythm or cardiac block) and eye abnormalities (such as swelling of the cornea, tissue, or eye muscles and nerves).

Diagnosis

A clear diagnosis of Lyme disease can be difficult and relies on information the patient provides and the doctor's clinical judgment, particularly through elimination of other possible causes of the symptoms. Lyme disease may mimic other conditions, including **chronic fatigue syndrome** (CFS), **multiple sclerosis** (MS), and other diseases with many symptoms involving multiple body systems. Differential diagnosis (distinguishing Lyme disease from other diseases) is based on clinical evaluation with laboratory tests used for clarification, when necessary. A two-test approach is common to confirm the results. Because of the potential for misleading results (false-positive and false-negative), laboratory tests alone cannot establish the diagnosis.

Doctors generally know which disease-causing organisms are common in their geographic area. The most helpful piece of information is whether a tick bite or rash was noticed and whether it happened locally or while traveling. Doctors may not consider Lyme disease if it is rare locally, but will take it into account if a patient mentions vacationing in an area where the disease is commonly found.

Treatment

While antibiotics are essential in treating Lyme disease, many alternative therapies may minimize symptoms, improve the immune response, and help treat late disseminated or chronic disease. General nutritional guidelines include drinking plenty of fluids and eating cooked whole grains and fresh vegetables. The intake of sugar, fat, refined carbohydrates, and dairy products should be reduced. Alternative therapies used in treating Lyme disease include:

- Chinese medicine. Formulae used to treat systemic bacterial infections include Wu Wei Xiao Du Yin (Five-Ingredient Decoction to Eliminate Toxin), Yin Hua Jie Du Tang (Honeysuckle Decoction to Relieve Toxicity), and Huang Lian Jie Du Tang (Coptis Decoction to Relieve Toxicity). Inflammation at the site of infection may be treated externally with Yu Lu San (Jade Dew Extract) or Jin Huang San (Golden Yellow Powder). Specific Chinese herbs and treatments can be used for specific symptoms. For examples, for systemic bacterial infection, one may use honeysuckle flower, forsythia, isatidis, scutellaria, and phellodendron. Acupuncture and ear acupuncture treatments are also used.
- Herbals. Botanical remedies include Echinacea (*Echinacea* species) to clear infection and boost the immune system, goldenseal (*Hydrastis canadensis*) to clear infection and boost the immune system, garlic to clear bacterial infection, and spilanthes (*Spilanthes* species) for spirochete infections.
- Hydrotherapy. The joint pain associated with Lyme disease can be treated with hydrotherapy. Dull, penetrating pain may be relieved by applying a warm compress to the affected area. Sharp, intense pain may be relieved by applying an ice pack to the affected area.
- Imagery. The patient may treat Lyme disease by visualizing Bb as looking like ticks swimming in the bloodstream being killed by the flame of a candle.
- Probiotics. Probiotics is treatment with beneficial microbes either by ingestion or through a suppository. Probiotics can restore a healthy balance of bacteria to the body in cases in which long-term antibiotic use has caused diarrhea or yeast infection. Yogurt or *Lactobacillus acidophilus* preparations may be ingested.
- Supplements. Calcium and magnesium can be used for aches, chlorophyll to aide healing, vitamin C for bacterial infection and inflammation, bioflavonoids for joint inflammation and to boost the immune system, digestive enzyme for digestive problems, vitamin B complex to boost overall health, bromelain for inflammation, and zinc to boost the immune system and promote healing.

Allopathic treatment

For most patients, oral antibiotics (doxycycline or amoxicillin) are prescribed for 21 days. The doctor may have to adjust the treatment regimen or change medications based on the patient's response. Antibiotics can kill Bb while it is active, but not when it is dormant. When symptoms indicate nervous system involvement or a severe episode of Lyme disease, intravenous antibiotic (ceftriaxone) may be given for 14–30 days. Adults with late neurologic Lyme disease are often treated with intravenous ceftriaxone for a period of two to four weeks. Alternative treatments are intravenous cefotaxime or penicillin G.

Treatment for Lyme disease is a source of controversy. Some scientists believe that it is cured after a four-antibiotic regime and that further antibiotic treatment could result in drug allergy. Other researchers, however, believe that the B. burgdorferi may remain in a dormant state within human cells, necessitating another course of treatment.

Expected results

If aggressive antibiotic therapy is given early and the patient cooperates fully and sticks to the medication schedule, recovery should be complete. Only a small percentage of Lyme disease patients fail to respond or relapse (have recurring episodes). Most long-term effects of the disease result when diagnosis and treatment is delayed or missed. Co-infection with other infectious organisms spread by ticks in the same areas as Bb (babesiosis and ehrlichiosis, for instance) may be responsible for treatment failures or more severe symptoms. In certain cases, Lyme disease has been responsible for deaths, but that is rare. Most fatalities reported with Lyme disease involved patients co-infected with babesiosis.

Prevention

Vaccination withdrawn

A vaccine for Lyme disease known as LYMErix was available from 1998 to 2002, when it was removed from the U.S. market. The decision was influenced by reports that LYMErix may be responsible for neurologic complications in vaccinated patients. Researchers from Cornell-New York Hospital presented a paper at the annual meeting of the American Neurological Association in October 2002 that identified nine patients with neuropathies linked to vaccination with LYMErix. In April 2003, the National Institute of Allergy and Infectious Diseases (NIAID) awarded a federal grant to researchers at Yale University School of Medicine to develop a new vaccine against Lyme disease. As of 2008, the best prevention strategy was through minimizing risk of exposure to ticks and using personal protection precautions.

Minimizing risk of exposure

Precautions to avoid contact with ticks include moving leaves and brush away from living quarters. In highly tick-populated areas, each individual should be inspected at the end of the day to look for ticks. Most important are personal protection techniques when outdoors:

- Avoid walking through woods, shrubbery, or tall grasses.
- Use repellents containing DEET.
- Wear light-colored clothing to maximize ability to see ticks.
- Tuck pant legs into socks or boot top.
- Check children and pets frequently for ticks.

Minimizing risk of disease transmission

The two most important factors are removing the tick quickly and carefully, and seeking a doctor's evaluation at the first sign of Lyme disease. When in an area that may be tick-populated, follow these precautions:

- Although ticks are quite small, check for them, particularly in the area of the groin, underarm, behind ears, and on the scalp.
- Stay calm and grasp the tick as near to the skin as possible, using tweezers.
- To minimize the risk of squeezing more bacteria into the site of the bite, pull straight back steadily and slowly.
- Do not use petroleum jelly, alcohol, or a lit match to remove the tick.
- Place the tick in a closed container (for species identification later, should symptoms develop) or dispose of it by flushing it in a toilet.
- See a physician for any sort of rash or patchy discoloration that appears 3–30 days after a tick bite.

KEY TERMS

Babesiosis—A disease caused by protozoa of the genus *Babesia* characterized by a malaria-like fever, anemia, vomiting, muscle pain, and enlargement of the spleen. Babesiosis, like Lyme disease, is carried by a tick.

Bell's palsy—Facial paralysis or weakness with a sudden onset, caused by swelling or inflammation of the seventh cranial nerve, which controls the facial muscles. Disseminated Lyme disease sometimes causes Bell's palsy.

Blood-brain barrier—A blockade of cells separating the circulating blood from elements of the central nervous system (CNS); it acts as a filter, preventing many substances from entering the central nervous system.

Cerebrospinal fluid—Clear fluid found around the brain and spinal cord and in the ventricles of the brain.

Disseminated—Scattered or distributed throughout the body. Lyme disease that has progressed beyond the stage of localized EM is said to be disseminated.

Erythema migrans (EM)—A red skin rash that is one of the first signs of Lyme disease in about 75% of patients.

Lyme borreliosis—Another name for Lyme disease.

Probiotics—Treatment with beneficial microbes, either by ingestion or through a rectal or vaginal suppository, to restore a healthy balance of bacteria to the body.

Spirochete—A spiral-shaped bacterium. The bacteria that cause Lyme disease and syphilis, for example, are spirochetes.

Vector—An animal carrier that transfers an infectious organism from one host to another. The vector that transmits Lyme disease from wildlife to humans is the deer tick or black-legged tick.

Zoonosis (plural, zoonoses)—Any disease of animals that can be transmitted to humans under natural conditions. Lyme disease and babesiosis are examples of zoonoses.

Resources

PERIODICALS

Craig, David J., and Amy Sarah Clark. "Rash Judgment?" *Columbia Magazine* (Summer 2007). http://www.columbia.edu/cu/alumni/Magazine/Summer2007/contents.html (February 28, 2008).

Wormser, Gary P. "Early Lyme Disease." *New England Journal of Medicine* (2006): 2794–2801. http://www.uchc.edu/md/obgyn/Articles/2006/Sept/Early_Lyme_Disease_6_06.pdf (February 28, 2008).

OTHER

"Bell's Palsy." *National Institute of Neurological Disorders and Stroke* February 4, 2008. http://www.ninds.nih.gov/disorders/bells/bells.htm (February 28, 2008).

"Learn about Lyme Disease." *Centers for Disease Control and Prevention, Division of Vector-Borne Infectious Diseases.* http://www.cdc.gov/ncidod/dvbid/lyme/ (February 28, 2008).

ORGANIZATIONS

Centers for Disease Control and Prevention, 1600 Clifton Rd. NE, Atlanta, GA, 30333, (800) 311-3435, (404) 639-3311, http://www.cdc.gov.

Lyme Disease Foundation, One Financial Plaza, Hartford, CT, 06103, (800) 886-LYME , http://www. lyme.org.

Lyme Disease Network of NJ, 43 Winton R., East Brunswick, NJ, 08816, http://www.lymenet.org.

National Institute of Allergy and Infectious Diseases (NIAID), 31 Center Dr., Room 7A50 MSC 2520, Bethesda, MD, 20892, (301) 496-5717, http://www.niaid.nih.gov.

Belinda Rowland
Rebecca J. Frey, PhD
Rhonda Cloos, RN

Lymphatic drainage

Definition

Lymphatic drainage is a therapeutic method that uses massage-like manipulations to stimulate lymph movement. Lymph is the plasma-like fluid that maintains the body's fluid balance and removes bacteria. Combined with other techniques of complete decongestive physiotherapy, it is used to treat lymphedema, swelling in the limbs caused by lymph accumulation.

Origins

The use of massage and compression techniques to treat swollen arms and legs was pioneered by Alexander Von Winiwarter, a nineteenth-century surgeon from Belgium. These techniques were refined during the 1930s by Danish massage practitioner Emil Vodder into what is now known as manual lymph drainage. During the 1980s, German physician Michael Foldi combined lymph drainage with other techniques to develop complete decongestive physiotherapy, widely used in the treatment of lymphedema.

Benefits

Lymphatic drainage is said to beneficially effect the nervous, immune and muscular systems. Its primary purpose is the treatment of lymphedema, a condition that causes unattractive swelling of arms and legs and creates an environment ripe for infection.

Description

Lymphatic drainage is accomplished by gentle, rhythmic massage following the direction of lymph flow. Mild stretching movements are used on the walls of lymph collectors to redirect the flow away from blocked areas into other vessels that drain into the veins. This massage action is often combined with other elements of complex decongestive therapy, which include:

- bandages
- dietary changes
- skin and nail care to prevent infection
- therapeutic exercise
- special compression sleeves, stockings, and other garments
- patient-applied lymphatic drainage and bandaging techniques
- light-beam generators to stimulate lymphatic drainage

Precautions

Any patient who has undergone **cancer** surgery and experiences sudden swelling after lymphatic drainage should stop treatment and be examined by a medical doctor. Treatment should also be stopped if infection of the lymphatic vessels occurs. The U.S. National Lymphedema Network recommends that patients taking anticoagulants for vascular disease be first checked for **blood clots** using ultrasound or other technology, and followed closely during the treatment. Congestive heart failure patients who may not be able to tolerate excessive movement of lymph need close monitoring also. If any **pain** is associated with lymphatic drainage, the treatment should stop until either the source is discovered or the pain goes away.

Side effects

There are concerns that lymphatic drainage and associated techniques could cause cancer to spread in patients with recurrent or metastatic disease.

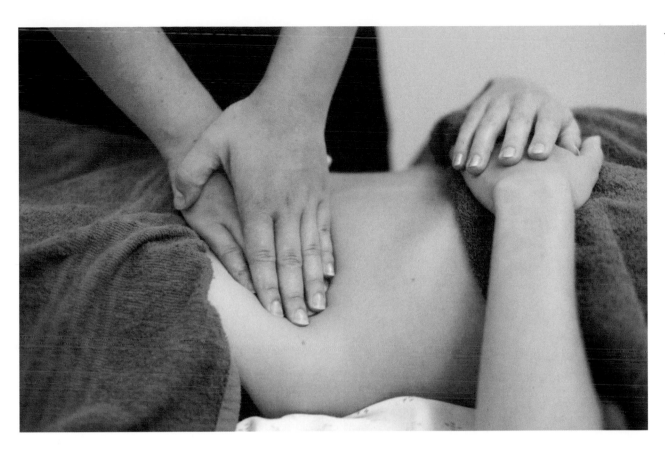

A therapist performs lymphatic drainage on a woman. *(© Arco Images / Alamy)*

Research and general acceptance

Lymphatic drainage has enjoyed widespread acceptance in Europe for several decades, and is gaining acceptance within the North American medical establishment.

Training and certification

Lymphatic drainage therapy procedures are most commonly done by osteopaths, chiropractors, physical therapists, occupational therapists, massage therapists, and nurses. Training is available from a number of institutions, and typically involves about 30–130 hours. The Florida-based Academy of Lymphatic Studies offers certification in manual lymph drainage and complete decongestive therapy.

Resources

National Lymphedema Network.Latham Square, 1611 Telegraph Avenue, Suite 1111, Oakland, CA 94612–2138. (800) 541–3259. www.lymphnet.org.

David Helwig

Lymphomas *see* **Hodgkin's disease**

Lysimachia

Description

Several different species of the plant known as lysimachia (genus *Lythrum*) exist. Lysimachia is in the Primulae family. The various species are known by a variety of common names, such as willow herb, purple willow herb, long purples, moneywort, rainbows, soldiers, creeping Jenny, and purple and yellow loosestrife. Other common names include flowering Sally and soldanella, trientalis, and alvet. It is also known through out the world as salicaire, braune, and rother. Lysimachia has no smell but a slightly bitter taste, with astringent properties.

Lysimachia is a perennial found throughout Europe, Russia, central Asia, Australia, and North America. It is an attractive, mainly low-growing plant, with a creeping habit, and deep taproots. Some species can grow to about 4 ft (1.2 m) high. It primarily grows in a damp habitat, preferring riversides and swamps. It flowers from June to August.

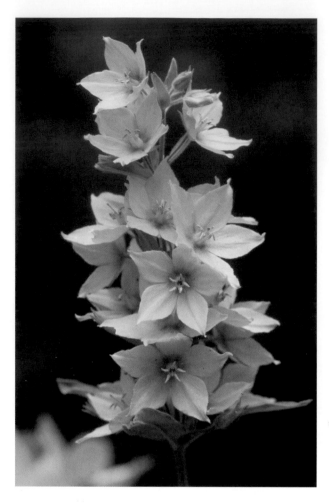

Lysimachia punctata. *(© Arco Images / Alamy)*

The flowers, which can be either yellow or purple, are quite eye-catching, and are generally about 1 in (2.54 cm) across, arranged in cone shaped clusters. The leaves of the loosestrife species are downy, yellowish, and about 1 in (2.54 cm) long, although in some species they can be 3-6 in (7.62-15.24 cm). The stems are square and hairy.

All species of lysimachia are commonly used as ornamental plants. They prefer shade, but all grow and multiply readily. Purple loosestrife is successful to such an extent that in parts of the United States, it has been declared a danger to wetlands, as it tends to quickly dominate and force out other species of local flora.

General use

Loosestrife was once widely employed as a medicinal herb, but it has become less popular in modern times. The different species have various medicinal uses, many of which are related to the plants' flavonoids, saponins and phenolic acids.

Yellow loosestrife

Lysimachia vulgaris is the largest of the lysimachia varieties, and is also known as willow herb, willow wort, and wood pimpernel. Its yellow flowers have red stems. Yellow loosestrife is generally larger than purple loosestrife. Yellow loosestrife has been recommended as an antidote to hemorrhage and excess **menstruation**. The smoke created by burning the plant can be used as an insect repellent. In other parts of the world, its smoke is also used to keep snakes away. In addition, it is credited with having a sedative effect, which may explain why some folk customs recommend its use for banishing discord. Loosestrife means "to tame strife." Yellow loosestrife is also used to make a yellow hair dye.

Purple loosestrife

Like other species of lysimachia, the whole herb of purple loosestrife is said to have astringent and demulcent properties. Herbalists say that it is unusual to find both these properties in any one herb.

Purple loosestrife has been used as a lymphatic cleanser. Many of its other properties are similar to those attributed to other species. It may be particularly valuable as a remedy for many of today's gastrointestinal (GI) tract diseases, such as Crohn's disease, **irritable bowel syndrome**, leaky gut syndrome, and others, as it is an effective cure for **diarrhea** and is also an effective anti-inflammatory, with healing properties.

It also has properties that enable it to lower blood-glucose levels, so herbalists consider it valuable as an adjunct to diabetes treatment.

Creeping jenny

Creeping jenny (*Lysimachia numularia*) is one of the smaller species of lysimachia, reaching only about 4 in (10.16 cm) in height. It is also known as money-wort, herb tuppence, string of sovereigns, wandering jenny, wandering sally, creeping charlie, and creeping john. Its leaves are smooth, and it is a leafy trailing plant. The stems may grow to about 4 ft (1.2 m) long. It has small bright yellow flowers that will last all summer if conditions are right.

Like yellow and purple loosestrife, it is known as a deterrent to vermin and insects when burned. In common folklore, it symbolizes peace.

It may be used as a decoction, ointment, or as a poultice for infected **wounds**.

Irish folklore

The various species of lysimachia are common to the British Isles, and are well known to folk medicine. In Irish folklore, lysimachia was known as *lus na s'iochana, earball cait'in,* and *cr'eachtach.* It was believed that its use would discourage bad feeling and discord between the inhabitants of a house. It was also used as a dye and as a medicinal tonic.

Herbalists consider lysimachia to be an effective antidote to diarrhea and have used it effectively to counter outbreaks of dysentery in Switzerland. It is said to be particularly suitable for treating diarrhea in infants. Other medicinal uses include leucorrhea, **tuberculosis**, fevers, liver disease, and even cholera and typhoid. It can also be used as an antiseptic, healing wash for wounds and sores. Made up into an ointment, it is said to be useful for fading scars.

Lysimachia has a reputation for healing eye ailments, and is said to be able to restore sight in certain conditions. Some practitioners say it is superior to **eyebright** for these purposes. It is recommended as a treatment for **macular degeneration**.

It can also be used as an antiseptic gargle to cure throat **infections** and is said to be good for quinsy, which is an infected and very painful throat condition. Loosestrife has astringent properties, and has been used in the leather-tanning process.

It is said to be useful for the treatment of **whooping cough** when boiled with wine or honey.

Preparations

The dried herb may be used as an infusion or decoction. Generally, the whole herb is used. It was once commonly made up into an ointment for the treatment of **cuts** and **bruises**.

To make a useful gargle or eyewash, herbalists recommend mixing half a teaspoon of salt into two cups of boiling water, adding 1-2 tsp of the dried herb or 1-2 tbsp if fresh. Once the mixture has steeped for 10–15 minutes, it is allowed to cool before use. The mixture should be kept covered if used as an eyewash, to avoid contamination.

Precautions

Purple loosestrife may be taken up to three times daily for short periods.

Side effects

Lysimachia tends to have a high tannin content, and because of this, it should not be used as a remedy

---

KEY TERMS

Decoction—An infusion allowed to boil to obtain a more concentrated liquid.

Demulcent—Soothing to the skin.

Infusion—Made up in the form of a tea.

Leukorrhea—Also known as yeast infection, a fungal infection of the vagina producing a thick white discharge.

Macular degeneration—Degeneration of the area of the eye that is responsible for vision, often comes with aging.

Poultice—A mixture of herbs or other substances applied to wounds and inflammations to draw out impurities and inflammation.

Quinsy—Acute inflammation of the tonsils and throat area that often results in abscesses.

---

over long periods of time, as it may lead to deficiencies in valuable minerals.

Interactions

Lysimachia is not known for its toxicity, and no records of any interaction have been found.

Resources

BOOKS

Chevallier, Andrew *Encyclopedia of Herbal Medicine: The Definitive Home Reference Guide to 550 Key Herbs with All Their Uses as Remedies for Common Ailments Complete Herbal*. New York: DK, 2006.

Hoffmann, David. *Medical Herbalism: The Science Principles and Practices Of Herbal Medicine.* Rochester, VT: Healing Arts Press, 2003.

Patricia Skinner
Leslie Mertz, Ph.D.

Lysine

Description

Lysine is an amino acid not produced by the body, but essential to the synthesis of protein molecules in the body. It is necessary for tissue repair and growth, and for producing antibodies, enzymes, and hormones.

Lysine is found in other protein sources, such as red meats, chicken, and turkey. Most individuals have an adequate intake of lysine from their normal diet. However, lysine levels may be low in vegetarians and low-fat dieters. Without enough lysine or any other of the eight essential **amino acids**, the body cannot build protein to sustain muscle tissue and carry out other essential body functions.

General use

The body uses L-lysine to synthesize protein. Since amino acid molecules are asymmetrical, each amino acid exists as both a right- and left-handed form, distinguished as D (for dextro, or right) and L (for levo, or left). As a supplement, L-lysine is used to treat the herpes simplex virus, help prevent **osteoporosis** and **cataracts**, and boost the immune system.

Herpes simplex virus remedy

In the 1950s, scientists discovered that foods containing certain amino acids could encourage or discourage the growth of the herpes virus. When added to the herpes virus, the amino acid **arginine** increases the growth of the virus. Lysine, by contrast, suppresses growth. Since the virus can cause cold sores, **canker sores**, and genital sores, L-lysine supplements increase the ratio of lysine to arginine in the body, preventing outbreak of the virus. Avoiding foods with arginine and eating foods with a higher lysine content helps alleviate the symptoms of the virus.

Foods containing arginine:

- legumes, especially soy
- fish and shellfish
- poultry
- spinach and seaweed
- nut and seed products

Foods containing lysine:

- fish and shellfish
- poultry
- red meats, especially game products
- eggs

Other uses

Lysine also promotes the body's absorption of **calcium**, helping to prevent osteoporosis. It slows the damage to the eyes caused by diabetes, and it may help prevent **atherosclerosis**. Since it is used to slow the growth of the herpes simplex virus, its antiviral properties may help treat **chronic fatigue syndrome**, **hepatitis**, and HIV.

KEY TERMS

Amino acid—An organic compound that contains both an amino (-NH$_2$) and carboxyl (-COOH) group. They are the constituents from which proteins are made.

Osteoporosis—A medical condition characterized by loss of bone mass, often leading to a greater risk for broken bones, especially in older women.

Preparations

L-lysine is best taken as a single supplement and not in combination with other amino acids. Such combinations are touted as nutritional supplements that build more muscle and are often used by athletes and bodybuilders. However, too much protein **strains** the functions of the liver and kidneys and can cause other health problems. The single supplement should be taken on an empty stomach because larger amounts of the amino acid can build up in the blood and brain, enhancing its health benefits. Supplements are best used by individuals suffering from a herpes outbreak or by vegetarians and low-fat dieters. Postmenopausal women can take lysine to encourage absorption of calcium by the body.

Precautions

Supplemental combinations of amino acids are not recommended to build muscle. Excessive build-up of protein in the body can cause kidney and liver problems.

Some consumers are sensitive or allergic to soybeans, a popular food used by vegetarians to replace the natural supply of lysine found in many meats. However, researchers have made progress in creating soybeans that are tolerated by consumers with those sensitivities by shutting off a gene in soybean seeds believed responsible for causing the **allergies**.

Side effects and interactions

As of 2008, no side effects or interactions had been identified.

Resources

BOOKS

Braverman, Eric R. *The Healing Nutrients Within: Facts, Findings, and New Research on Amino Acids*. Laguna Beach, CA: Basic Health, 2006.

Marshall, Keri. *User's Guide to Protein and Amino Acids*. Laguna Beach, CA: Basic Health, 2006.

Sahyun, Melville. *Proteins and Amino Acids in Nutrition.* Toronto: Richardson Press, 2007.

PERIODICALS

Benevenga, Norline J., and Kenneth P. Bleming. "Unique Aspects of Lysine Nutrition and Metabolism." *Journal of Nutrition* (June 2007): 1610S–1615S.

Singh, Betsy B., et al. "Safety and Effectiveness of an L-lysine, Zinc, and Herbal Based Product on the Treatment of Facial and Circumoral Herpes." *Alternative Medicine Review* (June 2005): 123–127.

OTHER

"Lysine." University of Maryland Medical Center. http://www.umm.edu/altmed/articles/lysine-000312.htm. (February 15, 2008).

Jacqueline L. Longe
Teresa G. Odle
David Edward Newton, Ed.D.

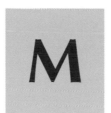

M

Ma huang *see* **Ephedra**

Mace *see* **Nutmeg**

Macrobiotic diet

Definition

A macrobiotic diet is part of a philosophy of life that incorporates the ancient Oriental concept of yin and yang. The diet itself consists mainly of brown rice, other whole grains, and vegetables. It requires foods to be cooked over a flame, rather than by electricity or microwave.

Origins

The term macrobiotics comes from two Greek words; *macro* (great) and *bios* (life). The macrobiotic diet is believed to have originated in nineteenth century Japan, with the teachings of Sagen Ishizuka, a natural healer. George Ohsawa (1893–1966), a Japanese teacher and writer, introduced macrobiotics to Europeans in the 1920s. Ohsawa claims to have cured himself of **tuberculosis** by eating Ishizuka's diet of brown rice, soup, and vegetables. The diet did not attract much attention in the United States until the mid-1960s, when Ohsawa's book *Zen Macrobiotics* was published and became a best seller, especially among the 1960s counterculture. The diet's popularity heightened when the macrobiotic philosophy was embraced by former Beatle John Lennon (1940–1980) and his wife, Yoko Ono (1933–). The macrobiotic diet has changed somewhat over the past forty years. Originally it recommended moving through stages of food elimination to achieve a diet that consisted almost solely of brown rice and water. These nutritionally unsafe dietary guidelines have mostly been replaced with a more moderate and balanced approach to eating.

Benefits

In the macrobiotic diet, foods are selected for their metaphysical qualities rather than their nutritional value. The regime, which is high in whole grains, vegetables, beans, and **soy protein**, has many of the same benefits as a vegetarian or vegan diet. Numerous scientific studies have shown that a diet of this type can significantly reduce the risk of diabetes, **heart disease**, **stroke**, and various cancers. The macrobiotic diet is rich in vitamins, high in dietary fiber, and low in fatty foods.

Description

In addition to its holistic approach to **nutrition**, macrobiotics applies these beliefs to life in general. Its philosophy recommends the following behaviors:

- eating two or three meals a day
- chewing each mouthful of food approximately 50 times to aid digestion and absorption of nutrients
- avoiding food for at least three hours before bedtime
- taking short baths or showers as needed, with warm or cool water
- consuming only organic foods
- using cast iron, clay pots, or stainless steel cookware
- cooking frequently with methods that use liquids (e.g. pressure cooking, boiling, steaming, soups, stews) instead of dry cooking methods (baking, broiling)
- eating nothing that is commercially processed and contains food additives
- taking no dietary supplements
- using grooming, cosmetic, and household products made from natural, non-toxic ingredients

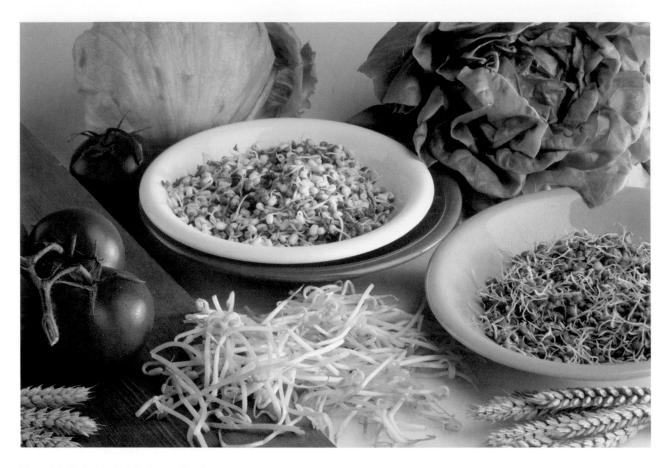

Macrobiotic food. *(© isifa Image Service s .r.o.)*

- wearing only cotton clothing and avoiding metallic jewelry
- spending as much time as possible in natural outdoor settings and walking at least 30 minutes daily
- doing such aerobic or stretching exercises as yoga, dance, or martial arts on a regular basis
- placing large green plants throughout the house to enrich the oxygen content of the air, and keeping windows open as much as possible to allow fresh air circulation
- avoiding food preparation with electricity or microwaves; using gas or wood stoves; and using only cast iron, stainless steel, or clay cookware
- avoiding television viewing and computer use as much as possible

The macrobiotic diet assigns yin and yang energies to foods. Yin represents female or cool, dark, inwardly focused energy. Yang represents male or warm, light, outwardly focused energy. In this ancient Asian philosophy, everything in the universe is assigned a yin or yang quality. For good mental and physical health and a harmonious life, yin and yang forces must be balanced. This balance must be reflected in the food the individual eats. Because environmental yin and yang forces change with the seasons, with climate, and time of day, the diet must also change with them.

Meat, fish, poultry, eggs, and hard cheeses are considered yang, while milk, cream, fruit juice, alcohol, and sugar are yin. The macrobiotic diet consists mainly of foods in the middle, such as brown rice and other whole grains, beans, vegetables, fruit, and nuts. The diet is flexible, and allows fish on occasion. Its flexibility enhances its appeal. The macrobiotic diet allows people to design their own food regimens based on their personal requirements, environment, and medical conditions.

One of the principles of the macrobiotic diet is that people should primarily eat organically grown foods native to their climate and area. The theory is that human health depends on the ability to adapt to changes in the environment. When people eat foods from a climate that differs from where they live, they lose that adaptability. Proponents of the macrobiotic diet claim that as society has moved away from its traditional ecologically based diet, there has been a corresponding rise in chronic illness. Therefore, for optimal health, the belief is that people need to return to a way of eating based on foods produced in their local environment, or at least grown in a climate that is similar to where they live.

Foods considered yang (contracted energy) last longer and can originate from a wide geographic area. Sea salt and sea vegetables are examples of yang foods. They can come from anywhere within the same hemisphere. Whole grains and legumes are also yang, and can originate anywhere within the same continent since they keep for a long time. Fresh fruits and vegetables are considered yin (expansive energy). Since they have a relatively short shelf life, they should be chosen only from those types that grow naturally within one's immediate area. According to macrobiotic beliefs, balance between yin and yang in diet and food helps achieve inner peace and harmony with one's self and the surrounding world.

Another aspect of the macrobiotic diet is that the type of foods eaten should change with the seasons. In the spring and summer, the food should be lighter, cooler, and require less cooking. This change is necessary because —according to the macrobiotic philosophy—the energy of fire is abundant in the form of sunlight and does not need to be drawn from cooked food. In the autumn and winter, the opposite is true.

The time of day also plays an important role in the macrobiotic diet since it relates to atmospheric energy levels. In the morning, when upward energy is stronger, breakfast should include light foods, such as a whole grain cooked in water. In the evening, when downward energy is stronger, the meal can be larger. Lunch should be quick and light, since afternoon energy is active and expansive.

In macrobiotics, it is believed that the dietary standards that are effective for one person may not work for another. These standards may change from day to day. Therefore, this diet requires a change in thinking from a static view of life to a dynamic one.

Many people are attracted to the diet because of claims that it can prevent or cure **cancer**. While no scientific studies support these claims, there are many people who believe the diet helped rid them of the disease when such conventional treatments as chemotherapy and radiation failed. Others use the diet to help treat diabetes, **hypertension**, arteriosclerosis, and other forms of heart disease. Many of the diet's supporters believe that these and other degenerative diseases occur because the body's yin and yang are out of balance, and that a macrobiotic diet helps restore this balance.

Macrobiotic foods

The primary food in the standard macrobiotic diet is whole cereal grains, including brown rice, barley, millet, rolled oats, wheat, corn, rye, and buckwheat. A small amount of whole grain pasta and breads is allowed. Grains should comprise about 50% of the food consumed.

Fresh vegetables should account for 20–30% of the diet. The most highly recommended vegetables include green cabbage, kale, broccoli, cauliflower, collard greens, carrots, parsnips, winter squash, bok choy, onions, **parsley**, daikon radishes, and watercress. Vegetables that should be eaten only occasionally include cucumber, celery, lettuce, and most herbs. Vegetables that should be avoided include tomatoes, peppers, potatoes, eggplant, spinach, beets, and summer squash.

About 10% of the diet should consist of beans and sea vegetables. The most suitable beans are azuki, chickpeas, and lentils. Tofu and tempeh are also allowed. Other beans can be eaten several times a week. Sea vegetables include nori, wakame, kombu, hiziki, arame, and agar-agar. Another 10% of the diet should include soups made with regular or sea vegetables.

Other permitted items include sweeteners such as barley malt, rice syrup, and apple juice; such seasonings as miso, tamari, soy sauce, rice or cider vinegar, **sesame oil**, tahini, and sea salt; occasional small amounts of seeds and nuts (pumpkin, sesame, sunflower, and almonds); and white-meat fish once or twice a week. Beverages allowed include tea made from twigs, stems, brown rice, and **dandelion** root, apple juice, and good-quality water without ice.

Items not allowed include meat, dairy products, fruits, refined grains, anything with preservatives, artificial flavorings and colorings or chemicals, all canned, frozen, processed, and irradiated foods, hot spices, **caffeine**, alcohol, refined sugar, honey, molasses, and chocolate.

Macrobiotic diet

Preparations

There are no specific procedures involved in preparing for the diet, except to change from a diet based on meat, sugars, dairy products, and processed foods, to one based primarily on whole grains, vegetables, and unprocessed foods. Some advocates of the macrobiotic diet recommend making the switch gradually rather than all at once.

Precautions

The macrobiotic diet does not include many fruits and vegetables that are important sources of nutrients and **antioxidants**, such as **vitamin C** and **beta carotene**. If followed rigidly, the diet can also be deficient in protein, **calcium**, **vitamin B$_{12}$**, folate, and **iron**. Individuals accustomed to a diet high in fat can experience sudden and drastic weight loss if they switch to a rigid macrobiotic diet. In its original form, the macrobiotic diet required foods to be slowly eliminated from the diet until only rice and beans were consumed. Carried to this extreme, the diet lacks significantly in necessary vitamins and nutrients.

A macrobiotic diet may worsen cachexia (malnutrition, wasting) in cancer patients. It is not recommended for people who have intestinal blockages, gluten-sensitive enteropathy (**celiac disease**), or cereal grain **allergies**. Children, pregnant women, and individuals with intestinal disorders, hypertension (high blood pressure), kidney disease, or malnutrition should consult their physician before starting a macrobiotic diet. A diet should never be a substitute for receiving appropriate medical treatment.

Side effects

There are no negative side effects associated with a macrobiotic diet in adults, other than such minor problems as **dizziness** in some people who experience rapid weight loss. Other, sometimes serious, side effects are possible if the diet is deficient in one or more vitamins or minerals.

Research and general acceptance

Like many alternative therapies, the macrobiotic diet is controversial and not generally embraced by allopathic medicine. Most of the controversy surrounds claims that the diet can cure cancer. These claims stem from anecdotal reports and are not substantiated by scientific research. The American Medical Association opposes the macrobiotic diet. The allopathic medical

---

KEY TERMS

Cachexia—General physical wasting and malnutrition, usually associated with such chronic diseases as cancer and AIDS.

Celiac disease—An intestinal disorder characterized by intolerance of gluten, a protein present in the grains of wheat, rye, oats, and barley.

Enteropathy—A disease of the intestinal tract.

Hypertension—Abnormally high blood pressure.

Hypocalcemia—Calcium deficiency in the blood.

Legumes—The fruit or seed of a family of plants, including beans and peas.

Scurvy—A disease characterized by loose teeth, and bleeding gums and mouth, caused by a lack of ascorbic acid (vitamin C) in the diet.

Tempeh—A dense high-fiber food product made from fermented soybeans.

Tofu—A high-protein curd made from soybeans, used in meat and dairy replacement products.

---

community is also concerned that people with such serious diseases as cancer may use the diet as a substitute for conventional treatment.

Scientific studies in the United States and Europe have shown that a strict traditional macrobiotic diet can lead to a variety of nutritional deficiencies, especially in protein, **amino acids**, calcium, iron, **zinc**, and ascorbic acid. These deficiencies can result in drastic weight loss, **anemia**, scurvy, and hypocalcemia. In children, a strict macrobiotic diet can cause stunted growth, protein and calorie malnutrition, and bone age retardation.

Training and certification

No special training or certification is required. There are, however, several institutes in the United States that offer courses in the macrobiotic philosophy and diet.

Resources

BOOKS

Aihara, Herman. *Basic Macrobiotics*. Oroville, CA: George Ohsawa Macrobiotic Foundation, 1998.

Bliss-Lerman, Andrea. *The Macrobiotic Community Cookbook*. New York: Avery, 2003.

Dente, Gerard, and Kevin J. Hopkins. *Macrobiotic Nutrition: Priming Your Body to Build Muscle and Burn Body Fat*. North Bergen, NJ: Basic Health Publications, 2004.

Kushi, Michio, and Alex Jack. *The Macrobiotic Path to Total Health: A Complete Guide to Naturally Preventing and Relieving More Than 200 Chronic Conditions and Disorders.* New York, NY: Ballantine Books, 2004.

Kushi, Michio, and Stephen Blauer. *The Macrobiotic Way: The Complete Macrobiotic Lifestyle Book.* Garden City Park, NY: Avery Penguin Putnam, 2004.

Kushi, Michio. *The Macrobiotic Approach to Cancer: Towards Preventing and Controlling Cancer With Diet and Lifestyle.* Garden City Park, NY: Avery Penguin Putnam, 2003.

Bliss-Lerman, Andrea. *Macrobiotic Community Cookbook.* Garden City Park, NY: Avery Penguin Putnam, 2003.

Pitchford, Paul. *Healing With Whole Foods: Asian Traditions and Modern Nutrition.* Berkeley, CA: North Atlantic Books, 2002.

Rivière, Françoise, *#7 Diet: An Accompaniment to Zen Macrobiotics,* 1st English ed. Chico, CA: George Ohsawa Macrobiotic Foundation, 2005.

PERIODICALS

"The Balance of Macrobiotics." *Natural Life* (January-February 2003): 9.

Kushi, Lawrence H., et al. "The Macrobiotic Diet in Cancer." *The Journal of Nutrition* (November 2001): 3056S-64S.

Kushi, Michio, and Alex Jack. "Cancer, Diet, and Macrobiotics: Relieving Cancer Naturally." *Share Guide* (September-October 2002): 18–19.

"Macrobiotic Diets Can be Healthful, but Not a Cancer Cure." *Environmental Nutrition* (November 2002): 7.

Priesnitz, Wendy. "Macrobiotics for Health." *Natural Life* (January-February 2004): 18.

OTHER

American Cancer Society. "Macrobiotic Diet." http://www.cancer.org/docroot/eto/content/ETO_5_3X_ Macrobiotic_Dict.aspAmerican Cancer Society, June 1, 2005.

Macrobiotics Online. http://www.macrobiotics.org&.[cited June 14, 2004].

Trevena, James and Kasia. "The Macrobiotic Guide." 2007. http://www.macrobiotics.co.uk/

ORGANIZATIONS

American Cancer Society, 1599 Clifton Road NE, Atlanta, GA, 30329-4251, 800 ACS-2345, http://www.cancer.org.

American Dietetic Association, 120 South Riverside Plaza, Suite 2000, Chicago, Illinois, 60606-6995, (800) 877-1600, http://www.eatright.org.

Kushi Institute, PO Box 7, Becket, MA, 01223, (800) 975-8744, (413) 623-8827, http://www.kushiinstitute.org.

National Center for Complementary and Alternative Medicine Clearinghouse, P. O. Box 7923, Gathersburg, MD, 20898, (888) 644-6226, TTY: (866) 464-3615, (866) 464-3616, http://nccam.nih.gov.

Ohsawa Macrobiotics, P.O. Box 3998, Chico, CA, 95927-3998, (530) 566-9765, (800) 232-2372, http://www.gomf.macrobiotic.net/Info.htm.

Ken R. Wells

Macular degeneration

Definition

Macular degeneration (MD) is the progressive deterioration of the macula, the light-sensitive cells of the central retina, at the back of the eye. The retina is the sensitive membrane (soft layer) of the eye that receives the image formed by the lens and is connected with the brain by the optic nerve. As these macular cells malfunction and die, central vision becomes gray, hazy, or distorted, and eventually is lost. Peripheral (away from the center) vision is unaffected.

Description

Millions of people suffer from MD and it accounts for about 12% of all blindness in the United States. The macula contains the highest concentration of photosensitive cells in the retina. These cells transform light into electrical signals that are sent to the brain for processing into vision. Fine detail vision and critical color vision are located in the macula. The macula depend on nutrient diffusion from the choroid layer, a region of several delicate vascular (pertaining to blood vessels) membranes or structures behind the retina and under the macula. Anything that interferes with this nutrient supply can lead to MD.

Age-related macular degeneration (AMD or ARMD) is by far the most common type of MD. One in six Americans develops AMD between the

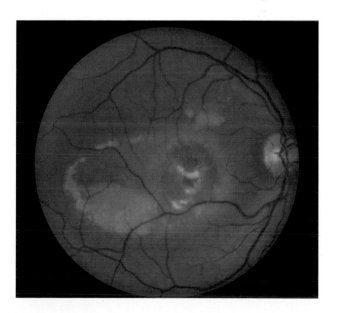

Macular degeneration. *(Jean-Luc Kokel / Photo Researchers, Inc.)*

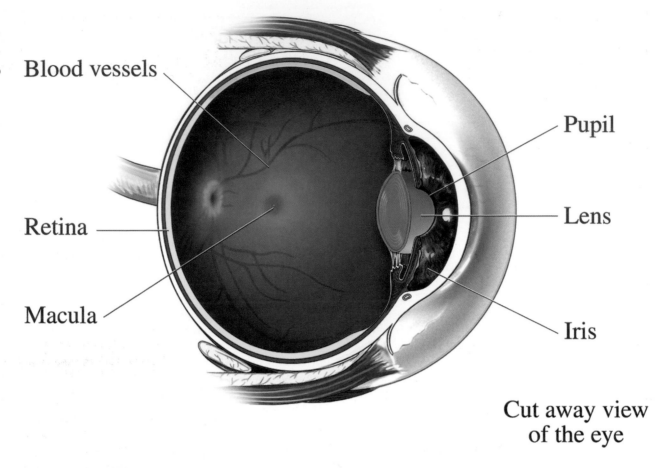

Blood vessels

Retina

Macula

Pupil

Lens

Iris

Cut away view
of the eye

Illustration of macular degeneration of the right eye, sagittal view. Macular degeneration is the progressive deterioration of the macula, which can lead to the loss of central vision. *(© PHOTOTAKE Inc. / Alamy)*

ages of 55 and 64 and one in three Americans over 75 has AMD. About 10% of those with AMD eventually suffer severe vision loss. The incidence of AMD is expected to triple by 2025, as the population ages. Whites and Asians are more susceptible than blacks. Women and those with lighter-colored eyes are somewhat more susceptible. AMD may occur in only one eye. However there is a very high likelihood that the other eye will be affected eventually.

About 90% of AMD is the dry form. Over time, the macula thins and the pigmented retinal epithelium, a dark-colored cell layer that supports the retina, is gradually lost. About 10% of dry AMD cases progress to the wet form. In a process called choroidal neovascularization (CNV), new blood vessels proliferate in the choroid and may invade the retina. These fragile vessels can leak blood and fluid into the retina, damaging or killing macular cells and resulting in scar tissue that interferes with vision. If untreated, the macula may be destroyed. Wet AMD progresses

more rapidly than dry AMD and severe vision loss typically occurs within two years.

Less common forms of MD include:

- juvenile macular degeneration (JMD), a group of inherited disorders affecting children and younger adults
- cystoid macular degeneration, the development of fluid-filled cysts (sacs) in the macular region, associated with aging, inflammation, or severe myopia (near-sightedness)
- diabetic macular degeneration
- retinal pigment epithelial detachment, a rare form of wet MD in which fluid leakage from the choroid causes the detachment or disappearance of the pigmented retinal epithelium

Causes and symptoms

Causes

Age-related macular degeneration (AMD) appears to result from a combination of hereditary,

KEY TERMS

Age-related macular degeneration (AMD, ARMD)— Macular degeneration that accompanies aging. The most common form of MD.

Amsler grid—A checkerboard pattern with a dot in the center that is used to diagnose MD.

Anthocyanosides—Flavonoid antioxidants from plant pigments that are particularly active in the eye.

Antioxidant—A substance that prevents oxidative damage, such as cellular damage caused by free radicals.

Carotenoid—A large class of red and yellow pigments found in some plants and in animal fat.

Choroid—The middle vascular layer of the eyeball, behind the retina.

Choroidal neovascularization (CNV)—The proliferation of new, fragile blood vessels in the choroid layer. Leakage from these vessels causes wet AMD.

Drusen—Yellowish-white fatty deposits on the retina, including the macula.

Electroretinogram—An instrument for measuring electrical signals from a point in the macula.

Fluorescein angiography—A method that uses a fluorescent dye for photographing blood vessels of the retina.

Free radical—A reactive atom or molecule with an unpaired electron. Oxygen free radicals can damage cells and their constituents.

Flavonoids—A group of chemical compounds naturally found in certain fruits, vegetables, teas, wines, nuts, seeds, and roots. Though not considered vitamins, they function nutritionally as biological response modifiers.

Indocyanin green angiography—A sensitive method for examining retinal blood vessels.

Lutein—An antioxidant carotenoid found in large quantities in dark-green, leafy vegetables such as spinach and kale. Lutein is deposited on the lens and macula of the eye where it protects cells from damage caused by ultraviolet and blue light.

Macula—An area of 0.1–0.2 in (3–5 mm) at the center of the retina that is responsible for sharp, central vision.

Omega-3 fatty acids.—Fatty acids from fish and vegetable oils that appear to protect against blood clots.

Ophthalmologist—A physician who specializes in eye diseases and disorders.

Ophthalmoscope—An instrument for examining the interior of the eyeball.

Optical coherence tomography (OCT) —A diagnostic method for imaging eye tissue.

Optometrist—A professional who examines eyes for visual acuity and prescribes eyeglasses or other visual aids.

Peripheral vision—Vision outside of the central vision.

Pigmented retinal epithelium—The dark-colored cell layer that supports the retina. It may thin or become detached with MD.

Photodynamic therapy (PDT)—A therapy that uses light-activated drugs to destroy rapidly-dividing cells or new blood vessels in the eye.

Retina—The nervous tissue membrane at the back of the eye, opposite the lens, that receives visual images and sends them to the brain via the optic nerve.

Visual acuity—Visual sharpness and resolving ability, usually measured by the ability to read numbers and letters.

Zeaxanthin—An antioxidant carotenoid that is the mirror image of lutein.

---

environmental, and metabolic factors. Over time, highly reactive free-oxygen radicals damage and destroy macular cells. Free radicals are produced by:

- bombardment of light on the macula, particularly long-term exposure to ultraviolet and blue light, including sunlight and sunlamps
- smoking, which increases the risk of AMD two- to four-fold
- a high-fat diet

The body's antioxidant systems that destroy free radicals become less effective with **aging**.

Factors that contribute to the hardening and blocking of the capillaries supplying the retina and lead to AMD include:

- smoking
- diets high in saturated fat and cholesterol
- low dietary consumption of antioxidants

The cause of choroidal neovascularization (CNV) in wet AMD is unknown. However many people with

AMD also have **cataracts** and cataract surgery increases the risk of dry AMD progressing to wet AMD.

Symptoms

AMD is painless, and in the early stages, the brain easily compensates for vision loss, particularly if AMD is restricted to one eye. Symptoms of AMD include:

• requiring more light for reading
• reduction, blurring, a blank spot, or loss of central vision while peripheral vision is unaffected
• difficulty recognizing faces
• visual distortions such as the bending of straight lines
• images appearing smaller
• changes in color perception or abnormal light sensations
• a decline of at least two lines in visual acuity as measured on a standard eye chart. For example, 20/20 vision declining to 20/80
• phantom visions, called "Charles Bonnet syndrome"

Diagnosis

Although vision loss is irreversible, early detection may halt or slow the progression of dry to wet AMD. However AMD is often fairly advanced by the time an ophthalmologist (a physician specializing in eye defects and diseases) is consulted. Tests for MD include:

• An Amsler grid, a checkerboard pattern with a black dot at the center. While staring at the dot with one eye, MD causes the straight lines to appear wavy or disappear or some areas to appear blank.
• A dilated eye exam whereby drops are used to dilate the pupils and a special magnifier called an ophthalmoscope shines a very bright light on the back of the lens to examine the retina. Gross macular changes, including scarring, thinning, or atrophy, may indicate MD. Numerous mid-sized yellow bumps called drusen, or one or more large drusen, can indicate intermediate-stage AMD. However, most people over age 42 have drusen in one or both eyes.
• Fluorescein or eye angiography, or retinal photography. An indicator dye is injected and photographs are taken to detect dye leakage from retinal blood vessels.
• Indocyanine green angiography examines choroid blood vessels that cannot be seen with fluorescein.
• Optical coherence tomography. Light waves are used to obtain cross-sectional views of eye tissue. This is easier and quicker than fluorescein angiography.

• An electroretinogram, whereby a weak or missing electrical signal from an illuminated point in the macula indicates MD.
• In a family history of MD suggesting hereditary juvenile macular degeneration (JMD), molecular genetic screening can reveal the presence of JMD-causing genes, facilitating early detection.

Treatment

Those with dry AMD should have a complete dilated eye examination at least once a year and use an Amsler grid daily to check for signs of wet AMD.

Diet

Dietary factors that can speed the progression from early-stage to advanced MD include:

• high fat consumption (70 gm versus 24 gm daily) triples the risk of advancement
• trans-fats consumption (4 gm versus 0.5 gm daily) doubles the risk
• consumption of commercial baked goods (two or more servings weekly) doubles the risk
• obesity doubles the risk of advancement

Foods containing omega-3 fats, such as nuts and fish, lower the risk of progression to advanced MD.

One study found that those with the highest dietary intake of **lutein** had a 57% lower risk for AMD. Foods high in lutein and zeaxanthin include:

• kale
• spinach
• mustard greens
• collard greens
• romaine lettuce
• leeks
• celery
• broccoli (cooked)
• peas
• corn
• zucchini
• yellow squash
• cucumbers
• orange bell peppers
• red grapes
• mangoes
• oranges

Many multi-vitamins also contain lutein.

Other factors for preventing AMD include:

- the use of sunglasses with UV protection
- maintaining normal blood pressure
- avoiding the risk factors, including smoking and secondhand smoke
- the use of supplemental estrogen by postmenopausal women is associated with a lower risk for AMD

Resources

BOOKS

Age-Related Macular Degeneration. San Francisco: American Academy of Ophthalmology, 2003.

Glaser, Bert, and Lester A. Picker. *The Macular Degeneration Sourcebook: A Guide for Patients and Families.* Omaha, NE: Addicus Books, 2002.

Gragoudas, Evangelos S., et al. *Photodynamic Therapy of Ocular Diseases.* Philadelphia: Lippincott Williams & Wilkins, 2004.

Holz, F. G., et al. *Age-Related Macular Degeneration.* Berlin: Springer, 2004.

Kondrot, Edward. *Healing the Eye the Natural Way: Alternative Medicine and Macular Degeneration.* 2nd ed. Carson City, NV: Nutritional Research Press, 2001.

Lim, Jennifer I., editor. *Age-Related Macular Degeneration.* New York: Marcel Dekker, 2002.

Loseliani, O. R., editor. *Focus on Macular Degeneration Research.* Hauppauge, NY: Nova Science, 2004.

Price, Ira Marc, and Linda Comac. *Living Well with Macular Degeneration: Practical Tips and Essential Information.* New York: New American Library, 2001.

Rosenthal, Bruce P., and Kate Kelly. *Focus on Macular Degeneration Research.* Hauppauge, NY: Nova Science, 2004.

PERIODICALS

"Ayes For Your Eyes." *Harvard Health Letter* (February 2004).

Friedman, E. "Update of the Vascular Model of AMD: Are Statins or Antihypertensives Protective?" *British Journal of Ophthalmology* 88 (February 2004): 161–63.

Hampton, Tracy. "Scientists Take Aim at Angiogenesis to Treat Degenerative Eye Diseases." *Journal of the American Medical Association* 291 (March 17, 2004): 1309–10.

Keegan, Lynn. "Age-Related Macular Degeneration and Nutrition." *Alternative Medicine Alert* 7 (February 2004): 16–21.

"Scaling Back on Fat in Foods, Especially Trans Fats, May Save Your Sight." *Environmental Nutrition* 27 (February 2004): 3.

Zarbin, M. A. "Current Concepts in the Pathogenesis of Age-Related Macular Degeneration." *Archives of Ophthalmology* 122 (April 2004): 598–614.

ORGANIZATIONS

American Macular Degeneration Foundation. P.O. Box 515, Northampton, MA 01061-0515. 888-MACULAR. 413-268-7660. amdf@macular.org. http://www.macular.org.

American Optometric Association. 243 North Lindbergh Blvd., St. Louis, MO 63141-7851. 314-991-4100. http://www.aoanet.org.

Macular Degeneration Foundation. P.O. Box 531313, Henderson, NV 89053. 888-633-3937. http://www.eyesight.org.

Macular Degeneration Partnership. 8733 Beverly Boulevard, Suite 201, Los Angeles, CA 90048-1844. 888-430-9898. 310-423-6455. http://www.amd.org.

OTHER

"Age-Related Macular Degeneration: What You Should Know." National Eye Institute. March 2004 [cited April 22, 2004]. http://www.nei.nih.gov/health/maculardegen/AMD_facts.htm.

"Macular Degeneration." *NWHRC Health Center.* National Women's Health Resource Center. March 4, 2004 [cited May 8, 2004]. http://www.healthywomen.org/.

Margaret Alic, Ph.D.

Magnesium

Description

The chemical element magnesium (Mg) has an atomic mass of 24.31 and atomic number 12. In its elemental form, magnesium is a silver-white metal with a density of 1.738 g/cm^3. In solution, it occurs as *cations* (positively charge ions). Magnesium is the fourth most abundant cation in the human body by weight, after **calcium**, **potassium**, and **sodium**. Ninety-nine percent of the body's magnesium is contained within its cells: about 60% in the bones, 20% in the muscles, 19% to 20% in the soft tissue, and 1% in the blood. Important to both **nutrition** and medicine, magnesium, like calcium and **phosphorus**, is considered a major mineral. Magnesium carbonate and magnesium sulfate have been used for centuries as a laxative. The name of the element comes from Magnesia, a city in Greece where large deposits of magnesium carbonate were discovered in ancient times.

Magnesium is an important element in the body because it activates or is involved in many basic processes or functions, including the following:

- as cofactor for over 300 enzymes
- oxidation of fatty acids
- activation of amino acids
- synthesis and breakdown of DNA
- neurotransmission

Recommended dietary allowance of magnesium

Age	mg/day
Children 0-6 mos.	30 (AI)
Children 7-12 mos.	75 (AI)
Children 1-3 yrs.	80
Children 4-8 yrs.	130
Children 9-13 yrs.	240
Boys 14-18 yrs.	410
Girls 14-18 yrs.	360
Men 19-30 yrs.	400
Women 19-30 yrs.	310
Men ≥ 31 yrs.	420
Women ≥ 31 yrs.	320
Pregnant women ≤ 18 yrs.	400
Pregnant women 19-30 yrs.	350
Pregnant women ≥ 31 yrs.	360
Breast feeding women ≤ 18 yrs.	360
Breast feeding women 19-30 yrs.	310
Breast feeding women ≥ 31 yrs.	320

Foods that contain magnesium

	mg
Cereal, 100% bran, 1/2 cup	129
Oat bran, 1/2 cup, dry	96
Halibut, cooked, 3 oz.	90
Almonds, roasted, 1 oz.	80
Cashew nuts, roasted, 1 oz.	75
Spinach, cooked, 1/2 cup	75
Swiss chard, cooked, 1/2 cup	75
Beans, lima, cooked, 1/2 cup	63
Shredded wheat, 2 biscuits	54
Peanuts, roasted, 1 oz.	50
Black-eyed peas, cooked, 1/2 cup	43
Brown rice, cooked, 1/2 cup	40
Beans, pinto, cooked, 1/2 cup	35

AI = Adequate Intake
mg = milligram

(Illustration by GGS Information Services. Cengage Learning, Gale)

- immune function
- interactions with other nutrients, including potassium, vitamin B$_6$, and boron

General use

Compounds of magnesium have a number of general uses, primarily in standard allopathic medicine, but also in some alternative therapies.

Nutrition

Good dietary sources of magnesium include nuts; dried peas and beans; whole grain cereals such as oatmeal, millet, and brown rice; dark green vegetables; bone meal; blackstrap molasses; **brewer's yeast**; and soy products. Dark green vegetables are important sources of magnesium because it is the central atom in the structure of chlorophyll. Drinking hard water or mineral water can also add magnesium to a person's diet.

Severe magnesium deficiency in a healthy person is unusual because normal kidneys are very efficient in keeping magnesium levels balanced. This condition, called *hypomagnesemia*, is usually caused either by disease (kidney disease, severe malabsorption, chronic **diarrhea**, **hyperparathyroidism**, or chronic **alcoholism**) or as a side effect of certain medications, most commonly diuretics, cisplatin (a **cancer** medication), and a few antibiotics. The symptoms of hypomagnesemia include disturbances of the heart rhythm, muscle tremors or twitches, seizures, hyperactive reflexes, and occasional personality changes (**depression** or agitation). A patient with hypomagnesemia may also produce Chvostek's sign, which is a facial spasm caused when the doctor taps gently over the facial nerve. This condition of painful intermittent muscle contractions and spasms is known as *tetany*. Hypomagnesemia can be treated with either oral or intravenous preparations containing magnesium.

Magnesium toxicity (hypermagnesemia) is rare because excessive amounts are usually excreted in the urine and feces. Most cases of hypermagnesemia are caused by overuse of dietary supplements containing magnesium. The symptoms of magnesium toxicity include central nervous system depression, muscle weakness, **fatigue**, and sleepiness. In extreme cases, hypermagnesemia can cause death. It can be treated with intravenous calcium gluconate along with respiratory support. Severe hypermagnesemia can be treated by hemodialysis or peritoneal dialysis.

Standard medical practice

DIAGNOSIS. The levels of magnesium in a patient's blood or body fluids can help diagnose several illnesses. A high magnesium level in the blood may indicate kidney failure, **hypothyroidism**, severe dehydration, Addison's disease, or overingestion of antacids containing magnesium. A low blood level of magnesium may indicate hypomagnesemia. Because 99% of the body's magnesium is contained in its cells, blood tests can measure only the approximately 1% of magnesium that is extra-cellular (circulating in the bloodstream), which makes it difficult to diagnose low magnesium levels in the body overall.

Fortunately, magnesium levels in urine can also aid diagnosis. High levels of urinary magnesium may indicate overconsumption of supplemental magnesium, overuse of diuretics, hypercalcemia (too much calcium in the body), hypophosphatemia (too little phosphate in the body), or metabolic acidosis (high blood acid levels). Low levels of magnesium in the urine may point to hypomagnesemia or hypocalcemia (too little magnesium or calcium in the body), an underactive parathyroid gland, or metabolic alkalosis (high blood alkaline levels).

TREATMENT. Compounds of magnesium are used to treat tachycardia (excessively rapid heartbeat) and low levels of electrolytes (chloride, potassium, and sodium). They help manage premature labor and can be given prophylactically to prevent seizures in toxemia of **pregnancy**. Magnesium sulfate is also effective in the treatment of eclampsia, a potentially fatal seizure condition in pregnant women.

Magnesium compounds help control seizures resulting from hypomagnesemia associated with alcoholism, **Crohn's disease**, or **hyperthyroidism**. Magnesium injections are also used to treat acute **asthma** attacks.

Magnesium preparations may be given as antacids in the treatment of peptic ulcers and hyperacidity. They are also given as laxatives for the short-term relief of **constipation** or to empty the patient's bowel prior to surgery or certain diagnostic procedures. Magnesium hydroxide is used to treat patients who have been poisoned by mineral acids or arsenic.

Magnesium in the form of magnesium sulfate is known as *Epsom salts*. It can be taken by mouth as a laxative but is also used externally to reduce tissue swelling, inflammation, and **itching** from insect **bites**, heat rash, or other minor skin irritations. Epsom salts can be applied to the affected skin or body part in moist compresses or dissolved in warm bath water.

Some research indicates that magnesium deficiency may contribute to **atherosclerosis** (hardening of the arteries), as well as to necrotizing enterocolitis (NEC), a sometimes-deadly inflammation that destroys the bowel in premature infants. Magnesium may also be useful in treating **attention-deficit hyperactivity disorder** (ADHD) and migraine headaches.

Alternative medicine

HOMEOPATHY. Phosphate of magnesia is a staple homeopathic remedy, called *Magnesia phosphorica*

(Mag. phos.) It is recommended for symptoms that are relieved by the application of warmth and gentle pressure, such as **hiccups** accompanied by **colic** in infants, menstrual cramps that are relieved when the woman bends forward, and abdominal **pain** without **nausea** and **vomiting**. Patients who benefit from *Mag. phos.* are supposedly less irritable or angry in temperament than those who need *Colocynthis* or *Chamomilla*.

NATUROPATHY. Naturopaths emphasize the importance of proper food selection and preparation to obtain an adequate supply of nutrients in the diet. They maintain that modern methods of agriculture promote overcropping and soil depletion, which they believe reduces the amount of magnesium (and other minerals) available from food grown in that soil. The processing and refining of wheat and rice, which discards the magnesium contained in the bran, **wheat germ**, or rice husks, also reduces the amount of magnesium in these foods. For these reasons naturopaths often recommend organic produce, which they believe contains higher levels of minerals, and suggest that they not be overcooked or boiled in too much water. In addition, this water, or "pot liquor," is often rich in magnesium that cooks out of the vegetables. It should not be discarded but saved for use in soups or stews.

Many naturopaths believe that the official government recommended daily allowance (RDA) of magnesium is too low. They think that it should be doubled to about 600 or 700 mg daily for adults. Many recommend the use of dietary supplements containing magnesium to make up the difference.

Naturopathic practitioners regard magnesium to be important in the relief or cure of the following conditions:

- Mitral valve prolapse: Magnesium deficiency may lower the body's ability to repair defective connective tissue, including defective mitral valves.

- Atherosclerosis.

- Certain psychological conditions, including apathy, decreased ability to learn, memory loss, and confusion.

- Kidney stones: Magnesium increases the solubility of certain calcium compounds that form kidney stones if they are not excreted in the urine.

- Hypertension: Hypertensive people often have lower levels of magnesium within their cells than people with normal blood pressure.

- Angina pectoris: Magnesium is thought to relax spastic arteries and help prevent arrhythmias.

Magnesium

- Osteoporosis: Many osteoporosis patients have low levels of magnesium in their bodies.
- Premenstrual syndrome (PMS) and menstrual cramps: Some women report relief from the symptoms of PMS when taking magnesium supplements.
- Naturopaths also treat asthma, epilepsy, autism, hyperactivity, chronic fatigue syndrome, noise-induced hearing loss, insomnia, and stress-related anxiety with supplemental magnesium.

Preparations

Dietary supplements

Naturopaths generally recommend supplemental magnesium for people with high blood **cholesterol**, postmenopausal women, women taking birth control pills, diabetics, people who eat a lot of fast food or other highly processed food, and people who drink alcohol. Many nutrition experts recommend supplements that contain a balanced ratio of calcium to magnesium, usually two parts of calcium to one of magnesium. People who increase their calcium intake should increase their dose of magnesium (and phosphate) as well because these supplements work together and complement each other.

Some naturopaths recommend taking magnesium in the form of magnesium aspartate or magnesium citrate, arguing that these compounds are more easily absorbed by the body than magnesium carbonate or magnesium oxide. Others prefer magnesium chelated with **amino acids**. Magnesium can also be obtained from herbal sources, such as red raspberries.

Standard medical preparations

Magnesium hydroxide is a common over-the-counter antacid, available as either a tablet or liquid. Most antacid tablets contain about 200 mg of magnesium hydroxide. Liquid magnesium hydroxide is sometimes called *milk of magnesia*. Magnesium carbonate works as a cathartic or laxative when combined with citric acid to produce magnesium citrate. It is often flavored with lemon or cherry to make it more pleasant to swallow. Magnesium sulfate (in the form of Epsom salts) is available over the counter, usually in half-pound or pound boxes. Epsom salts are small whitish or colorless crystals that dissolve easily in water and have a bitter or salty taste.

Magnesium for intravenous dosage is prepared as the sulfate in a 50% solution. In general, intravenous administration of magnesium is reserved for patients with such serious symptoms as seizures, preeclampsia or eclampsia of pregnancy, acute asthma attacks, or

severe cardiac arrhythmias. Magnesium sulfate can also be given by intramuscular injection.

Precautions

Preparations containing magnesium should not be given as laxatives to patients with kidney disease, nausea and vomiting, diarrhea, abdominal pain, rectal bleeding, symptoms of appendicitis, or symptoms of intestinal obstruction or perforation. In addition, these preparations should not be used routinely to relieve constipation, as individuals may become dehydrated, lose calcium from the body, or develop a dependence on them. Antacids containing magnesium should be used with caution in patients with kidney disease.

Side effects

Magnesium preparations taken internally may cause hypermagnesemia, especially with prolonged use; electrolyte imbalance; and abdominal cramps when taken as a laxative. Milk of magnesia occasionally produces nausea or diarrhea. There are no known side effects of Epsom salts when used externally.

Interactions

Milk of magnesia decrease the patient's absorption of chlordiazepoxide, digoxin, isoniazid, quinolones, and tetracycline antibiotics. Because it increases the gastrointestinal tract's mobility, magnesium can also decrease the absorption (and thereby the effectiveness) of many other drugs and supplements as well. Magnesium sulfate, if given intravenously, is incompatible with calcium gluceptate, clindamycin, dobutamine, polymyxin B sulfate, procaine, and sodium bicarbonate.

Resources

BOOKS

Nishizawa, Yoshiki, Hirotoshi Morii, and Jean Durlach, eds. *New Perspectives in Magnesium Research: Nutrition and Health.* New York: Springer, 2006.

Sircus, Mark. *Transdermal Magnesium Therapy.* Chandler, AZ: Phaelos Books and Mediawerks, 2007.

PERIODICALS

Tong, G. M., and R. K. Rude. "Magnesium Deficiency in Critical Illness." *Journal of Intensive Care Medicine* (January/February 2005): 3–17.

Khine, Khursheed, et al. "Magnesium (Mg) Retention and Mood Effects after Intravenous Mg Infusion in Premenstrual Dysphoric Disorder." *Biological Psychiatry* (February 2006): 327–333.

Ryder, Kathryn M., et al. "Magnesium Intake from Food and Supplements Is Associated with Bone Mineral Density in Healthy Older White Subjects." *Journal of the American Geriatrics Society* (November 2005): 1875–1880.

ORGANIZATIONS

American Association of Naturopathic Physicians, 4435 Wisconsin Ave. NW, Suite 403, Washington, DC, 20016, (866) 538-2267, http://www.naturopathic.org/.

Rebecca Frey
Teresa G. Odle
David Edward Newton, Ed.D.

Magnetic therapy

Definition

Magnetic therapy is the use of magnets to relieve **pain** in various areas of the body.

Origins

Magnetic therapy dates as far back as the ancient Egyptians. Magnets have long been believed to have healing powers associated with muscle pain and stiffness. Chinese healers as early as 200 B.C. were said to use magnetic lodestones on the body to correct unhealthy imbalances in the flow of *qi,* or energy. The ancient Chinese medical text known as *The Yellow Emperor's Canon of Internal Medicine* describes this procedure. The *Vedas,* or ancient Hindu scriptures, also mention the treatment of diseases with lodestones. The word "lodestone" or leading stone, came from the use of these stones as compasses. The word "magnet" probably stems from the Greek *Magnes lithos,* or "stone from Magnesia," a region of Greece rich in magnetic stones. The Greek phrase later became *magneta* in Latin.

Physiological reactions to positive and negative magnetic fields

Positive (stressful)

Increase in acid production

Depletes oxygen production

Cellular edema (water retention)

Produces insomnia, restlessness, wakefulness

Increases free radicals

Negative (anti-stressful)

Normalizes pH

Inhibits growth of microorganisms

Negates free radicals

Produces relaxation, rest, sleep

Increases oxygen production

(Illustration by Corey Light. Cengage Learning, Gale)

Sir William Gilbert's 1600 treatise, *De Magnete*, was the first scholarly attempt to explain the nature of magnetism and how it differed from the attractive force of static electricity. Gilbert allegedly used magnets to relieve the arthritic pains of Queen Elizabeth I. Contemporary American interest in magnetic therapy began in the 1990s, as several professional golfers and football players offered testimony that the devices seemed to cure their nagging aches and injuries.

Many centuries ago, the earth was surrounded by a much stronger magnetic field than it is today. Over the past 155 years, scientists have been studying the decline of this magnetic field and the effects it has had on human health. When the first cosmonauts and astronauts were going into space, physicians noted that they experienced bone **calcium** loss and **muscle cramps** when they were out of the Earth's magnetic field for any extended period of time. After this discovery was made, artifical magnetic fields were placed in the space capsules.

Benefits

Some of the benefits that magnetic therapy claims to provide include:

- pain relief
- reduction of swelling
- improved tissue alkalinization
- more restful sleep
- increased tissue oxygenation
- relief of stress
- increased levels of cellular oxygen
- improved blood circulation
- anti-infective activity

Description

There are two theories that are used to explain magnetic therapy. One theory maintains that magnets produce a slight electrical current. When magnets are applied to a painful area of the body, the nerves in that area are stimulated, thus releasing the body's natural painkillers. The other theory maintains that when magnets are applied to a painful area of the body, all the cells in that area react to increase blood circulation, ion exchange, and oxygen flow to the area. Magnetic fields attract and repel charged particles in the bloodstream, increasing blood flow and producing heat. Increased oxygen in the tissues and blood stream is thought to make a considerable difference in the speed of healing.

Preparations

There are no special preparations for using magnetic therapy other than purchasing a product that is specific for the painful area being treated. Products available in a range of prices include necklaces and bracelets; knee, back, shoulder and wrist braces; mattress pads; gloves; shoe inserts; and more.

Precautions

The primary precaution involved with magnetic therapy is to recognize the expense of this therapy. Magnets have become big business; they can be found in mail-order catalogs and stores ranging from upscale department stores to specialty stores. As is the case with many popular self-administered therapies, many far-fetched claims are being made about the effectiveness of magnetic therapy. Consumers should adopt a "let the buyer beware" approach to magnetic therapy. Persons who are interested in this form of treatment should try out a small, inexpensive item to see if it works for them before investing in the more expensive products.

Side effects

There are very few side effects from using magnetic therapy. Generally, patients using this therapy find that it either works for them or it does not. Patients using transcranial magnetic stimulation for the treatment of **depression** reported mild **headache** as their only side effect.

Research and general acceptance

Magnetic therapy is becoming more and more widely accepted as an alternative method of pain relief. Since the late 1950s, hundreds of studies have demonstrated the effectiveness of magnetic therapy. In 1997, a group of physicians at Baylor College of Medicine in Houston, Texas studied the use of magnetic therapy in 50 patients who had developed polio earlier in life. These patients had muscle and joint pain that standard treatments failed to manage. In this study, 29 of the patients wore a magnet taped over a trouble spot, and 21 others wore a nonmagnetic device. Neither the researchers nor the patients were told which treatment they were receiving (magnetic or nonmagnetic). As is the case with most studies involving a placebo, some of the patients responded to the nonmagnetic therapy, but 75% of those using the magnetic therapy reported feeling much better.

In another study at New York Medical College in Valhalla, New York, a neurologist tested magnetic therapy on a group of 19 men and women complaining of moderate to severe burning, tingling, or numbness in their feet. Their problems were caused by diabetes or other conditions present such as **alcoholism**. This group of patients wore a magnetic insole inside one of their socks or shoes for 24 hours a day over a two-month period, except while bathing. They wore a nonmagnetic insert in their other sock or shoe. Then for two months they wore magnetic inserts on both feet. By the end of the study, nine out of ten of the diabetic patients reported relief, while only three of nine non-diabetic patients reported relief. The neurologist in charge of the study believes that this study opens the door to additional research into magnetic therapy for diabetic patients. He plans a larger follow-up study in the near future.

In 2000, a federally funded study began at the University of Virginia. This study evaluated the effectiveness of magnetic mattress pads in easing the muscle pain, stiffness and **fatigue** associated with **fibromyalgia**.

Magnetic therapy is also being studied in the treatment of depression and for patients with **bipolar disorder**. A procedure called repeated transcranial magnetic stimulation has shown promise in treating this condition. In one study, patients with depression had a lower relapse rate than did those using electroconvulsive therapy. Unlike electroconvulsive therapy, patients using magnetic therapy did not suffer from seizures, memory lapses, or impaired thinking.

Progress continues on the study of magnets and the brain. In 2002, more than 2,000 patients had undergone transcranial magnetic stimulation (TMS) for treatment of depression at the University of South Carolina with promising preliminary results. TMS is less shocking to the brain than electroconvulsive therapy. Another study was testing the use of magnets for therapy of essential tremors. By using a control group with sham repetitive TMS, the researchers noted **tremor** improvement and no adverse effects from the magnet therapy. These applications of magnet therapy are still under study and are not approved by the Food and Drug Administration (FDA) but look promising.

Training and certification

There is no training or certification required for administering magnetic therapy. Magnetic therapy can be self-administered.

Resources

BOOKS

Lawrence, Ron, and Paul Rosch. *Magnet Therapy Book: The Pain Cure Alternative*. New York: Prima Publications, 1998.

PERIODICALS

Cole, Helene M. "Transcranial Magnetic Stimulation of the Cerebellum in Essential Tremor: A Controlled Study." *JAMA, The Journal of the American Medical Association* (June 19, 2002): 3061.

"Magnets for Pain Relief: Attractive but Unproven." *Tufts University Health and Nutrition Letter* (1999): 3.

"Magnets that Move Moods: New Treatment for Depression." *Newsweek* (June 24, 2002): 57.

Vallbona, C. "Evolution of Magnetic Therapy from Alternative to Traditional Medicine." *Physical Medicine Rehabilitation Clinics of North America*, 1999: 729-54.

Kim Sharp
Teresa G. Odle

Magnolia

Description

Many species of magnolia are used in both Eastern and Western herbalism. The Chinese have used the bark of *Magnolia officinalis*, called in Chinese *hou po* since the first century A.D. *M. officinalis* is a deciduous tree that grows to a height of 75 ft (22 m). It has large leaves surrounding a creamy white fragrant flower. The pungent aromatic bark is used in healing. Originally native to China where it grows wild in the mountains, *M. officinalis* is now grown as an ornamental for use in landscaping around the world.

Chinese herbalists also use the bud of *Magnolia liliflora* in healing. The Chinese name for magnolia flower is *xin yi hua*. In Chinese herbalism, magnolia bark and magnolia flower are considered different herbs with different properties and uses.

Western herbalists use other species of magnolia. These include *Magnolia virginiana, M, glauca, M. acuminate* and *M. tripetata*. Other names for magnolia

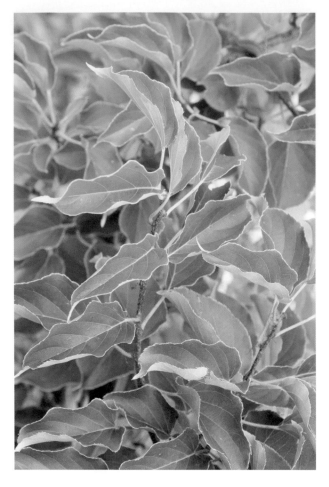

Magnolia vine. *(© Organica / Alamy)*

include white bay, beaver tree, swamp **sassafras** (not to be confused with other forms of sassafras used in the West), and Indian bark. The New World species of magnolia are smaller than their Asian counterparts, ranging in height from 6–30 ft (2–10 m). Both the bark and the root are used in **Western herbalism**.

General use

In Chinese herbalism, magnolia bark, *hou po*, is associated with the stomach, lungs, spleen, and large intestine. It is used to treat menstrual cramps, abdominal **pain**, abdominal bloating and **gas**, **nausea**, **diarrhea**, and **indigestion**. Injections of magnolia bark extract are said to cause muscle **relaxation**. It is also used in formulas to treat coughing and **asthma**. The bark is said to make the *qi* descend and is used for symptoms of disorders thought to move upward in the body.

Research suggests that compounds found in magnolia bark may have mild antibacterial and antifungal properties. These studies are in their preliminary stages, however, and have been limited to test tube research.

Magnolia flower, *xin yi hua*, is associated with the lungs. It is used to treat chronic respiratory **infections**, sinus infections, and lung congestion. Its main function is to open the airway. Little scientific research has been done on the magnolia flower.

Magnolia bark and root are also used occasionally in Western herbalism, although they are not major healing herbs. At one time, magnolia root was used to treat rheumatism, and was thought to be superior to quinine in treating **chills** and **fever**. It is not used much today. Russian herbalists use an oil extracted from the flowers and young leaves to treat **hair loss** and as an antiseptic on skin **wounds**. In homeopathic medicine a tincture of magnolia flower is a minor remedy for asthma and fainting.

Little recent scientific research has been done on magnolia in the West; however, Asian researchers have isolated a compound from *M. officinalis* known as honokiol. Honkiol is being studied for its ability to induce apoptosis, or cell self-destruction, in **cancer** cells. In Japan, honokiol is considered a useful in reducing **anxiety**; herbal preparations containing honokiol are prescribed as mild tranquilizers. Chinese researchers reported in 2007 that a mixture of honkiol and magnolol, another active ingredient in magnolia, acted as an antidepressant in rats.

Preparations

Magnolia bark is most commonly used with the following herbs:

- Agastache: for treatment of stomach flu and gastrointestinal upset
- Apricot seed and linum: for treatment of chronic constipation and hemorrhoids
- Bupleurum, inula and cyperus: for treatment of stress-related gastrointestinal disturbances All these formulas can be made into teas or are commercially available as pills or capsules.

Magnolia flower is most commonly used in xanthium and magnolia formula. It is used to relieve sinus congestion associated with a yellow discharge and to treat allergy symptoms such as runny nose. This formula can be made into a tea or is available in commercially produced capsules.

American herbalists dry magnolia bark and root and pound it into a powder or make a tincture that is taken several times daily. Russian herbalists soak the bark in vodka.

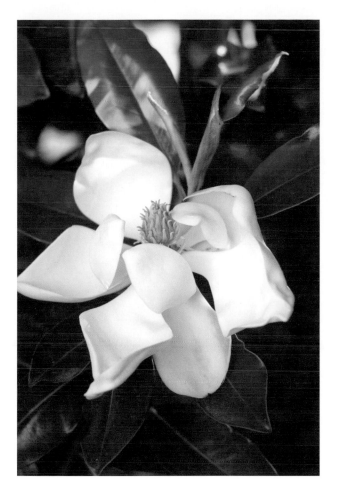

Magnolia flower. *(© D. Hurst / Alamy)*

Precautions

Chinese herbalists recommend that magnolia bark not be used by pregnant women and that magnolia flower be used with caution if the patient is dehydrated.

Side effects

There are no unwanted side effects reported with normal doses of any of the different uses of magnolia. Large quantities of magnolia preparations, however, have been reported to cause **dizziness**. In addition, allergic reactions to the pollen from magnolia trees are not unusual.

Interactions

In Chinese herbalism, both magnolia bark and flowers are often used in conjunction with other herbs with no reported interactions. There are no formal studies of its interactions with Western pharmaceuticals; however, there are anecdotal reports of harmful interactions between magnolia bark and prescription weight-loss medications. In addition, magnolia should not be taken together with any medications given to lower blood pressure, as it increases their effects.

Resources

BOOKS

Bensky, Dan, et al. *Chinese Herbal Medicine: Materia Medica,* 3rd ed. Seattle, WA: Eastland Press, 2004.

Chevallier, Andrew. *Herbal Remedies.* New York: DK Publishing, 2007.

PDR for Herbal Medicines, 4th ed. Montvale, NJ: Thomson Healthcare, 2007.

ORGANIZATIONS

Alternative Medicine Foundation. P. O. Box 60016, Potomac, MD 20859. (301) 340-1960. http://www.amfoundation.org.

American Association of Oriental Medicine. PO Box 162340, Sacramento, CA 95816. (866) 455-7999 or (914) 443-4770 http://www.aaaomonline.org.

American Holistic Medical Association. PO Box 2016 Edmonds, WA 98020. 425-967-0737. http://www.holisticmedicin.org.

Centre for International Ethnomedicinal Education and Research (CIEER). http://www.cieer.org.

OTHER

"Magnolia Bark Acts Like Antidepressant." *Chinese Medicine News. November 2007* [cited February 19, 2008]. http://chinesemedicinenews.com/2008/01/08/magnolia-bark-may-be-good-antidepressan.

Rebecca J. Frey, Ph. D.
Tish Davidson, A. M.

Maharishi Ayurveda *see* **Ayurvedic medicine**

Mai men dong *see* **Ophiopogon**

Maitake

Description

Maitake, *Grifola frondosa*, is a mushroom found growing wild in Japan and in forests in the eastern part of North America, where it grows on dying or already dead hardwood trees. The word *maitake* means "dancing mushroom" in Japanese; the mushroom was given this name because people were supposed to have danced for joy when they found it. It is also called "hen-in-the-woods" and can reach the size of a head of lettuce. Because maitake comes from the polypores group, it produces a bunch of leaf-like clumps that are intertwined. During Japan's feudal era, maitake was used as currency; the daimyo, or provincial nobles, would exchange maitake for its weight in silver from the shogun, the military ruler of Japan.

The mushroom is also cultivated in laboratories by growing a small amount of it on a sterile medium in a Petri dish. This culture is used to make what is called a spawn, which is then inoculated into production logs made from sawdust and grain. During the next 30 days, the spawn settles in and binds to the log. Then the logs are placed in temperature- and humidity-controlled mushroom houses until the mushrooms begin forming. They are then moved to a mushroom fruiting house. The entire procedure requires a period of 10–14 weeks.

Maitake's main ingredient is the polysaccharide beta-1.6-glucan, a complex carbohydrate substance high in sugar components bound together. The patented extracted form of this glucan is called the Maitake D-Fraction. Both terms can be used interchangeably. Two other components of maitake, named *fraction X* and *fraction ES*, were discovered by Harry Preuss, a medicine and pathology professor at Georgetown University Medical Center in Washington, DC.

General use

Although the Chinese and Japanese have used maitake in cooking and healing for many centuries, it is only in the last 20 years that studies have been conducted concerning its functions. Maitake's main functions are activating the immune system and acting as an antitumor agent. Maitake is known as an adaptogen and tonic, and as such it aids healthy people to keep their levels of blood sugar, blood pressure, **cholesterol**, and weight normal. The beta glucan in maitake is a *cell-surface carbohydrate*. This means that beta glucan aids cell communication in specific circumstances. As a polysaccharide, this glucan activates

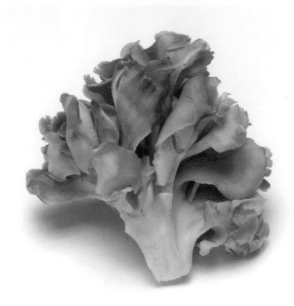

Maitake mushroom (Grifola frondosa). *(MIXA Co., Ltd. / Alamy)*

the white blood cells, called *macrophages*, which in turn devour microorganisms that produce disease, as well as tumors.

A 1995 study at Japan's Kobe Pharmaceutical University investigated the effects of maitake's D-fraction on **cancer** in mice. Results showed 73.3-45.5% reduction in breast, lung, liver and prostrate cancer growth, 25% reduction in **leukemia**, 33.3% reduction in stomach cancer and 0–16% in bone cancer. These benefits increased 4–13% when combined with traditional chemotherapy treatment, as well as reducing chemotherapy's side effects and making it work better in treating cancer. Researchers attribute this latter result to the X and ES fractions of the mushroom. More recent studies of the use of MD-fraction in treating cancer patients have also found that its effectiveness varies somewhat depending on the type of cancer; a higher proportion of patients with cancers of the breast, lung, or liver showed improvement than patients with leukemia or brain cancers.

Another study by the same group of researchers looked at maitake's D-fraction function of activating memory T-cells. In turn, these T-cells remember the cells that started the tumor growth and nail them for destruction. The study found that maitake both decreases cancer cells and prevents them from occurring elsewhere in the body. In addition to its antitumor effects, maitake extract appears to increase cellular immunity to cancer.

KEY TERMS

Adaptogen—A herb or herbal product that helps the body adapt to a broad range of life stresses.

Glucan—A complex sugar molecule consisting of smaller units of glucose.

Spawn—Grain, often rye or millet, that has been inoculated with mushroom spores and is used to grow mushrooms commercially.

Spore—The asexual reproductive body of a mushroom or other nonflowering plant.

Tonic—A medicine or herbal preparation that is given to strengthen and invigorate the body.

Cancer research on apoptosis is one of the main areas of study. This process of programmed cell death is found to kill not only cancer cells, but all cells. At the Department of Urology, New York Medical College, *in vitro* research by Hiroshi Tazaki and his team shows that the D-fraction can kill **prostate cancer** cells.

Preuss, who discovered the fraction X (anti-diabetic) and fraction ES (anti-hypertensive) components of maitake, conducted studies based on the hypothesis that such chronic diseases of **aging** as diabetes, **hypertension** and **obesity** are connected partly to glucose/insulin disorders. From his 1998 study, Preuss concluded that maitake could positively affect the glucose/insulin balance and prevent these age-related diseases. A study done at Georgetown University in 2002 found that an extract of maitake does indeed improve glucose/insulin metabolism in insulin-resistant mice.

Maitake's affect on liver and cholesterol were discovered in two more studies at Kobe Pharmaceutical University. A 1996 study on rats with hyperlipidemia were fed either cholesterol or dried powder containing 20% maitake mushroom. Results showed that maitake altered the metabolism of fatty acids by stopping fatty acid from increasing in the liver and fatty acid levels from rising in the blood serum.

Maitake can also decrease high blood pressure. In 1994, a study at New York's Ayurvedic Medical Center, hypertensive patients took maitake concentrate two times daily for a month. Results showed their blood pressure decreased from 5–20%.

Studies have also shown maitake can help **AIDS** patients. In *Mushrooms as Medicine*, two 1992 *in vitro* studies, one in Japan and one at the United States National Cancer Institute, showed that maitake both improves T-cell activity and kills HIV. One study,

using a sulfated maitake extract, stopped HIV killing T-cells by 97%. Another study, in 1996 at Memorial Sloan-Kettering Cancer Center in New York, looked at the functions of a variety of edible mushrooms, including maitake. Although the study showed that the information for mushrooms wasn't as strong as for vegetables, such as broccoli and cauliflower, the study also recommended that more research should be done regarding the use of mushrooms to treat serious diseases, such as cancer and AIDS.

In 1999, the U. S. Food and Drug Administration (FDA) granted Maitake Products approval to conduct a clinical study using maitake (in its patented D-fraction form) in people with advanced **breast cancer** and prostate cancer. The American Cancer Society (ACS) is less supportive of the claims made for maitake, stating in its guide to complementary and alternative treatments that "There is no scientific evidence that the maitake mushroom is effective in treating or preventing cancer in humans." The ACS points out that the Japanese studies of maitake have been done on mice, and that further research is necessary to show that the benefits also apply to humans.

Preparations

Maitake mushroom may be eaten fresh, made into a tea, taken as capsules, or taken as an alcohol extract.

When maitake mushroom is cooked, the taste is woodsy. The mushroom must be washed and soaked in water until it turns soft. It is sautéed in oil and used as a side dish, in stews, sauces, or in soups. Maitake mushrooms will keep from five to 10 days if properly stored in a paper bag in the refrigerator.

Dried maitake pieces may be made into a tea by using two to four grams per day, split into two preparations of tea. It is best to drink the tea between the morning and evening. To make the tea, it is first required to grind the dried maitake in a coffee grinder, then it is added to water, boiled and simmered from 20 minutes to four hours. Tea should be filtered before drinking. Grounds can be reused as long as they retain their color. Maitake can also be mixed with other tonic herbs, such as **green tea** or ginseng.

Capsules are available in 150-500 mg with a standardized D-fraction powder extract of 10 mg. They may be taken twice a day between meals or first thing in the morning. Dosage varies from one capsule of 150 mg to six capsules of 500 mg. It is best to consult with a health care provider for therapeutic doses. Taking maitake with **vitamin C** helps to increase maitake's absorption. Capsules should be stored in a cool dry place.

The FDA approved-for-clinical-study maitake products are available in D-fraction extracts of two to four ounce bottles, as well as capsules.

Precautions

Maitake is not recommended for children. Pregnant women and nursing women should consult a health care provider before taking maitake. People with such autoimmune diseases as lupus should avoid maitake. The mushroom stimulates the immune system, and their immune systems are already in overdrive.

Side effects

Side effects are rare and the only known one is possible loose bowels and stomach upset if the whole mushroom is eaten. To avoid this, take in capsule form.

Interactions

No interactions between maitake and prescription medications have been reported.

Resources

BOOKS

American Cancer Society (ACS). *ACS Guide to Complementary and Alternative Cancer Methods.* Atlanta, GA: American Cancer Society, 2001.

Balch, James F., MD, and Phyllis A. Balch, CNC. *Prescription for Nutritional Healing,* 2nd ed. Garden City Park, NY: Avery Publishing Group, 1997.

PERIODICALS

Haugen, Jerry and George B. Holcomb. "Specialty Mushrooms." *The Mushroom Growers' Newsletter*, Office of Communications, U.S.Department of Agriculture.

Inoue, A., N. Kodama, and H. Nanba. "Effect of Maitake (*Grifola frondosa*) D-Fraction on the Control of the T Lymph Node Th-1/Th-2 Proportion." *Biological and Pharmaceutical Bulletin* 25 (April 2002): 536-540.

Kodama, N., K. Komuta, and H. Nanba. "Can Maitake MD-Fraction Aid Cancer Patients?" *Alternative Medicine Review* 7 (June 2002): 236-239.

Manohar, V., N. A. Talpur, B. W. Echard, et al. "Effects of a Water-Soluble Extract of Maitake Mushroom on Circulating Glucose/Insulin Concentrations in KK Mice." *Diabetes, Obesity and Metabolism* 4 (January 2002): 43-48.

ORGANIZATIONS

Mushroom Council. 11875 Dublin Boulevard, Suite D-262, Dublin, CA 94568. (925) 556-5970. www.mushroom council.com.

U. S. Food and Drug Administration (FDA). 5600 Fishers Lane, Rockville, MD 20857. (888) 463-6332. www.fda.gov.

OTHER

"Maitake (*Grifola frondosa*)." Virtual Health 1998, HealthNotes Online. www.vitaminbuzz.com.

"Maitake Mushrooms." JHS Natural Products. www.jhsnp.com.

Sharon Crawford
Rebecca J. Frey, PhD

Malaria

Definition

Malaria is a serious infectious disease spread by certain mosquitoes. It is most common in tropical climates. It is characterized by recurrent symptoms of **chills**, **fever**, and an enlarged spleen. The disease can be treated with medication, but it often recurs. Malaria is endemic (occurs frequently in a particular locality) in many third world countries. Isolated, small outbreaks sometimes occur within the boundaries of the United States, with most of the cases reported as having been imported from other locations.

Description

Malaria is a growing problem in the United States. Although only about 1400 new cases were reported in the United States and its territories in 2000, many involved returning travelers. In addition, locally transmitted malaria has occurred in California, Florida, Texas, Michigan, New Jersey, and New York City. While malaria can be transmitted in blood, the American blood supply is not screened for malaria. Widespread malarial epidemics are far less likely to occur in the United States, but small localized epidemics could return to the Western world. As of late 2002, primary care physicians are being advised to screen returning travelers with fever for malaria, and a team of public health doctors in Minnesota is recommending screening immigrants, refugees, and international adoptees for the disease—particularly those from high-risk areas.

The picture is far more bleak, however, outside the territorial boundaries of the United States. A recent government panel warned that disaster looms over Africa from the disease. Malaria infects between 300 and 500 million people every year in Africa, India, southeast Asia, the Middle East, Oceania, and Central and South America. A 2002 report stated that malaria kills 2.7 million people each year, more than 75 percent of them African children under the age of five. It is predicted that within five years, malaria will kill about as many people as does **AIDS**. As many as half a billion people worldwide are left with chronic **anemia** due to malaria infection. In some parts of Africa, people battle up to 40 or more separate episodes of malaria in their lifetimes. The spread of malaria is becoming even more serious as the parasites that cause malaria develop resistance to the drugs used to treat the condition. In late 2002, a group of public health researchers in Thailand reported that a combination treatment regimen involving two drugs known as dihydroartemisinin and azithromycin shows promises in treating multidrug-resistant malaria in southeast Asia.

Causes and symptoms

Human malaria is caused by four different species of a parasite belonging to genus *Plasmodium*: *Plasmodium falciparum* (the most deadly), *Plasmodium vivax*, *Plasmodium malariae*, and *Plasmodium ovale*. The last two are fairly uncommon. Many animals can get malaria, but human malaria does not spread to animals. In turn, animal malaria does not spread to humans.

A person gets malaria when bitten by a female mosquito seeking a blood meal that is infected with the malaria parasite. The parasites enter the blood stream and travel to the liver, where they multiply. When they reemerge into the blood, symptoms appear. By the time a patient shows symptoms, the parasites have reproduced very rapidly, clogging blood vessels and rupturing blood cells.

Malaria cannot be casually transmitted directly from one person to another. Instead, a mosquito **bites** an infected person and then passes the infection on to the next human it bites. It is also possible to spread malaria via contaminated needles or in blood transfusions. This is why all blood donors are carefully screened with questionnaires for possible exposure to malaria.

It is possible to contract malaria in non-endemic areas, although such cases are rare. Nevertheless, at least 89 cases of so-called airport malaria, in which travelers contract malaria while passing through crowded airport terminals, have been identified since 1969.

The amount of time between the mosquito bite and the appearance of symptoms varies, depending on the strain of parasite involved. The incubation period is usually between eight and 12 days for falciparum malaria, but it can be as long as a month for the other types. Symptoms from some strains of *P. vivax* may

KEY TERMS

Arteminisinins—A family of antimalarial products derived from an ancient Chinese herbal remedy. Two of the most popular varieties are artemether and artesunate, used mainly in southeast Asia in combination with mefloquine.

Chloroquine—An antimalarial drug that was first used in the 1940s, until the first evidence of quinine resistance appeared in the 1960s. It is now ineffective against falciparum malaria almost everywhere. However, because it is inexpensive, it is still the antimalarial drug most widely used in Africa. Native individuals with partial immunity may have better results with chloroquine than a traveler with no previous exposure.

Mefloquine—An antimalarial drug that was developed by the United States Army in the early 1980s. Today, malaria resistance to this drug has become a problem in some parts of Asia (especially Thailand and Cambodia).

Quinine—One of the first treatments for malaria, quinine is a natural product made from the bark of the Cinchona tree. It was popular until being superseded by the development of chloroquine in the 1940s. In the wake of widespread chloroquine resistance, however, it has become popular again. Quinine, or its close relative quinidine, can be given intravenously to treat severe *Falciparum* malaria.

Sulfadoxone/pyrimethamine (Fansidar)—An antimalarial drug developed in the 1960s. It is the first drug tried in some parts of the world where chloroquine resistance is widespread. It has been associated with severe allergic reactions due to its sulfa component.

not appear until eight to 10 months after the mosquito bite occurred.

The primary symptom of all types of malaria is the "malaria ague" (chills and fever), which corresponds to the "birth" of the new generation of the parasite. In most cases, the fever has three stages, beginning with uncontrollable shivering for an hour or two, followed by a rapid spike in temperature (as high as 106°F [41.4°C]), which lasts three to six hours. Then, just as suddenly, the patient begins to sweat profusely, which will quickly bring down the fever. Other symptoms may include **fatigue**, severe **headache**, or **nausea** and **vomiting**. As the sweating subsides, the patient typically feels exhausted and falls asleep. In many cases, this cycle of chills, fever, and sweating occurs every other day, or every third day, and may last for between a week and a month. Those with the chronic form of malaria may have a relapse as long as 50 years after the initial infection.

Falciparum malaria is far more severe than other types of malaria because the parasite attacks all red blood cells, not just the young or old cells, as do other types. It causes the red blood cells to become very "sticky." A patient with this type of malaria can die within hours of the first symptoms. The fever is prolonged. So many red blood cells are destroyed that they block the blood vessels in vital organs (especially the brain and kidneys), and the spleen becomes enlarged. There may be brain damage, leading to coma and convulsions. The kidneys and liver may fail.

Malaria in **pregnancy** can lead to premature delivery, miscarriage, or stillbirth.

Certain kinds of mosquitoes belonging to the genus *Anopheles* can pick up the parasite by biting an infected human. (The more common kinds of mosquitoes in the United States do not transmit the infection.) This is true for as long as that human has parasites in his/her blood. Since strains of malaria do not protect against each other, it is possible to be reinfected with the parasites again and again. It is also possible to develop a chronic infection without developing an effective immune response.

Diagnosis

Malaria is diagnosed by examining blood under a microscope. The parasite can be seen in the blood smears on a slide. These blood smears may need to be repeated over a 72-hour period in order to make a diagnosis. Antibody tests are not usually helpful because many people developed antibodies from past **infections**, and the tests may not be readily available. A new laser test to detect the presence of malaria parasites in the blood was developed in 2002, but is still under clinical study.

Two new techniques to speed the laboratory diagnosis of malaria show promise. The first is acridine orange (AO), a staining agent that works much faster (3–10 min) than the traditional Giemsa stain (45–60 min) in making the malaria parasites visible under a microscope. The second is a bioassay technique that measures the amount of a substance called histadine-rich protein II (HRP2) in the patient's blood. It allows for a very accurate estimation of parasite development. A dip strip that tests for the presence of HRP2 in blood samples appears to be more accurate in diagnosing malaria than standard microscopic analysis.

Anyone who becomes ill with chills and fever after being in an area where malaria exists must see a doctor and mention their recent travel to endemic areas. A person with the above symptoms who has been in a high-risk area should insist on a blood test for malaria. The doctor may believe the symptoms are just the common flu virus. Malaria is often misdiagnosed by North American doctors who are not used to seeing the disease. Delaying treatment of falciparum malaria can be fatal.

Treatment

Traditional Chinese medicine

The Chinese herb qiinghaosu (the Western name is artemisinin) has been used in China and southeast Asia to fight severe malaria, and became available in Europe in 1994. It is usually combined with another antimalarial drug (mefloquine) to prevent relapse and drug resistance. It is not available in the United States and other parts of the developed world due to fears of its toxicity, in addition to licensing and other issues.

Western herbal medicine

A Western herb called **wormwood** (*Artemesia annua*) that is taken as a daily dose may be effective against malaria. Protecting the liver with herbs like **goldenseal** (*Hydrastis canadensis*), Chinese goldenthread (*Coptis chinensis*), and **milk thistle** (*Silybum marianum*) can be used as preventive treatment. These herbs should only be used as complementary to conventional treatment and not to replace it. Patients should consult their doctors before trying any of these medications.

Traditional African herbal medicine

As of late 2002, researchers were studying a traditional African herbal remedy against malaria. Extracts from *Microglossa pyrifolia*, a trailing shrub belonging to the daisy family (Asteraceae), show promise in treating drug-resistent strains of *P. falciparum*.

Allopathic treatment

Falciparum malaria is a medical emergency that must be treated in the hospital. The type of drugs, the method of giving them, and the length of the treatment depend on where the malaria was contracted and the severity of the patient's illness.

For all strains except falciparum, the treatment for malaria is usually chloroquine (Aralen) by mouth for three days. Those falciparum strains suspected to be resistant to chloroquine are usually treated with a combination of quinine and tetracycline. In countries where quinine resistance is developing, other treatments may include clindamycin (Cleocin), mefloquin (Lariam), or sulfadoxone/pyrimethamine (Fansidar). Most patients receive an antibiotic for seven days. Those who are very ill may need intensive care and intravenous (IV) malaria treatment for the first three days.

A patient with falciparum malaria needs to be hospitalized and given antimalarial drugs in different combinations and doses depending on the resistance of the strain. The patient may need IV fluids, red blood cell transfusions, kidney dialysis, and assistance breathing.

A drug called primaquine may prevent relapses after recovery from *P. vivax* or *P. ovale*. These relapses are caused by a form of the parasite that remains in the liver and can reactivate months or years later.

Another new drug, halofantrine, is available abroad. While it is licensed in the United States, it is not marketed in this country and it is not recommended by the Centers for Disease Control and Prevention in Atlanta.

Expected results

If treated in the early stages, malaria can be cured. Those who live in areas where malaria is epidemic, however, can contract the disease repeatedly, never fully recovering between bouts of acute infection.

Prevention

Preventing mosquito bites while in the tropics is one possible way to avoid malaria. Several researchers are currently working on a malarial vaccine, but the complex life cycle of the malaria parasite makes it difficult. A parasite has much more genetic material than a virus or bacterium. For this reason, a successful vaccine has not yet been developed. A new longer-lasting vaccine shows promise, attacking the toxin of the parasite and therefore lasts longer than the few weeks of those vaccines currently used for malaria prevention. However, as of late 2002, the vaccine had been tested only in animals, not in humans, and could be several years from use.

A newer strategy involves the development of genetically modified non-biting mosquitoes. A research team in Italy is studying the feasibility of this means of controlling malaria.

Malaria is an especially difficult disease to prevent by vaccination because the parasite goes through several life stages. One recent, promising vaccine appears to have protected up to 60% of people exposed to malaria. This was evident during field trials for the drug that were conducted in South America and Africa. It is not yet commercially available.

The World Health Organization has been trying to eliminate malaria for the past 30 years by controlling mosquitoes. Their efforts were successful as long as the pesticide DDT killed mosquitoes and antimalarial drugs cured those who were infected. Today, however, the problem has returned a hundredfold, especially in Africa. Because both the mosquito and parasite are now extremely resistant to the insecticides designed to kill them, governments are now trying to teach people to take antimalarial drugs as a preventive medicine and avoid getting bitten by mosquitoes.

Travelers to high-risk areas should use insect repellant containing DEET for exposed skin. Because DEET is toxic in large amounts, children should not use a concentration higher than 35%. DEET should not be inhaled. It should not be rubbed onto the eye area, on any broken or irritated skin, or on children's hands. It should be thoroughly washed off after coming indoors.

Those who use the following preventive measures get fewer infections than those who do not:
- Between dusk and dawn, remaining indoors in well-screened areas.
- Sleep inside pyrethrin or permethrin repellent-soaked mosquito nets.
- Wearing clothes over the entire body.

Anyone visiting areas where malaria is endemic should take antimalarial drugs starting one week before they leave the United States. The drugs used are usually chloroquine or mefloquine. This treatment is continued through at least four weeks after leaving the endemic area. However, even those who take antimalarial drugs and are careful to avoid mosquito bites can still contract malaria.

International travelers are at risk for becoming infected. Most Americans who have acquired falciparum malaria were visiting sub-Saharan Africa; travelers in Asia and South America are less at risk. Travelers who stay in air conditioned hotels on tourist itineraries in urban or resort areas are at lower risk than those who travel outside these areas, such as backpackers, missionaries, and Peace Corps volunteers. Some people in Western cities where malaria does not usually exist may acquire the infection from a mosquito carried onto a jet. This is called airport or runway malaria.

A 2002 report showed how efforts in a Vietnamese village to approach prevention from multiple angles resulted in a significant drop in malaria cases. Health workers distributed bednets treated with permethrin throughout the village and also made sure they were re-sprayed every six months. They also worked to ensure early diagnosis, early treatment, and annual surveys of villagers to bring malaria under control.

Resources

BOOKS

Desowitz, Robert S. *The Malaria Capers: More Tales of Parasites and People, Research and Reality*. New York: W.W. Norton, 1993.

"Extraintestinal Protozoa: Malaria." Section 13, Chapter 161 in *The Merck Manual of Diagnosis and Therapy*, edited by Mark H. Beers, MD, and Robert Berkow, MD. Whitehouse Station, NJ: Merck Research Laboratories, 1999.

Stoffman, Phyllis. *The Family Guide to Preventing and Treating 100 Infectious Illnesses*. New York: John Wiley & Sons, 1995.

PERIODICALS

Ambroise-Thomas P. "[Curent Data on Major Novel Anti-malarial Drugs: Artemisinin (qinghaosu) derivatives]". [Article in French]. *Bulletin of the Academy of National Medicine* 183, no.4 (1999): 797–780. Abstract.

Causer, Louise M, et al. "Malaria Surveillance—United States, 2000". *Morbidity and Mortality Weekly Report* (July 12, 2002): 9–15. Abstract.

Coluzzi, M., and C. Costantini. "An Alternative Focus in Strategic Research on Disease Vectors: The Potential of Genetically Modified Non-Biting Mosquitoes." *Parassitologia* 44 (December 2002): 131–135.

"Combination Approach Results in Significant Drop in Malaria Rates in Viet Nam." *TB & Outbreaks Week* (September 24, 2002): 17. Abstract.

Devi, G., V. A. Indumathi, D. Sridharan, et al. "Evaluation of ParaHITf Strip Test for Diagnosis of Malarial Infection." *Indian Journal of Medical Science* 56 (October 2002): 489–494.

Keiser, J., J. Utzinger, Z. Premji, et al. "Acridine Orange for Malaria Diagnosis: Its Diagnostic Performance, Its Promotion and Implementation in Tanzania, and the Implications for Malaria Control." *Annals of Tropical Medicine and Parasitology* 96 (October 2002): 643–654.

Kohler, I., K. Jenett-Siems, C. Kraft, et al. "Herbal Remedies Traditionally Used Against Malaria in Ghana: Bioassay-Guided Fractionation of *Microglossa pyrifolia* (Asteraceae)." *Zur Naturforschung* 57 (November-December 2002): 1022–1027.

Krudsood, S., K. Buchachart, K. Chalermrut, et al. "A Comparative Clinical Trial of Combinations of Dihydroartemisinin Plus Azithromycin and Dihydroartemisinin Plus Mefloquine for Treatment of Multidrug-Resistant *Falciparum* Malaria." *Southeast Asian Journal of Tropical Medicine and Public Health* 33 (September 2002): 525–531.

"Laser-based Malaria Test could be Valuable." *Medical Devices & Surgical Technology Week* (September 22, 2002):4.

Mack, Alison. "Collaborative Efforts Under Way to Combat Malaria." *The Scientist* 10 (May 12, 1997): 1, 6.

McClellan, S. L. "Evaluation of Fever in the Returned Traveler." *Primary Care* 29 (December 2002): 947–969.

"Multilateral Initiative on Malaria to Move to Sweden." *TB & Outbreaks Week* (September 24, 2002): 17.

Noedl, H., C. Wongsrichanalai, R. S. Miller, et al. "*Plasmodium falciparum*: Effect of Anti-Malarial Drugs on the Production and Secretion Characteristics of Histidine-Rich Protein II." *Experimental Parasitology* 102 (November-December 2002): 157–163.

"Promising Vaccine May Provide Long-Lasting Protection." *Medical Letter on the CDC & FDA* (September 15, 2002): 14.

Stauffer, W. M., D. Kamat, and P. F. Walker. "Screening of International Immigrants, Refugees, and Adoptees." *Primary Care* 29 (December 2002): 879–905.

Thang, H. D., R. M. Elsas, and J. Veenstra. "Airport Malaria: Report of a Case and a Brief Review of the Literature." *Netherlands Journal of Medicine* 60 (December 2002): 441–443.

ORGANIZATIONS

Centers for Disease Control Malaria Hotline. (770) 332–4555.

Centers for Disease Control Travelers Hotline. (770) 332–4559.

OTHER

Malaria Foundation. http://www.malaria.org.

Mai Tran
Teresa G. Odle
Rebecca J. Frey, PhD

Malignant lymphoma

Definition

Lymphomas are a group of cancers in which cells of the lymphatic system become abnormal and start to grow uncontrollably. Because there is lymph tissue in many parts of the body, lymphomas can start in almost any organ of the body.

Description

The lymphatic system is made up of ducts or tubules that carry lymph to all parts of the body. Lymph is a milky fluid that contains lymphocytes. These, along with monocytes and granulocytes make

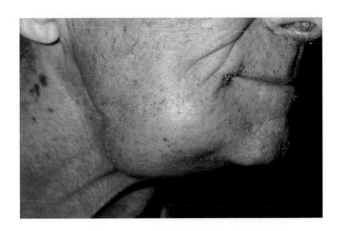

Swelling in the neck of a 70-year old woman with non-Hodgkin's type lymphoma, cancer of the lymph nodes. *(Dr. P. Marazzi / Photo Researchers, Inc.)*

up the leukocytes, or white blood cells, the infection-fighting and reparative bodies in the blood. Small pea-shaped organs found along the network of lymph vessels are called lymph nodes; their main function is to make and store lymphocytes. Clusters of lymph nodes are found in the pelvic region, underarm, neck, chest, and abdomen. The spleen (an organ in the upper abdomen), the tonsils, and the thymus (a small organ beneath the breastbone) are also part of the lymphatic system. Lymphocytes are held within the lymphoid tissue until they join the flow of lymph through the node. There are two main types of lymphocytes: the T cell and the B cell. Lymphomas develop from these two types. B-cell lymphomas are more common among adults, while among children, the incidence of T- and B-cell lymphomas are almost equal.

The T and the B cells perform different jobs within the immune system. When an infectious bacterium enters the body, the B cells make proteins called *antibodies,* which attach themselves to the bacteria, and flag them for destruction by other immune cells. The T cells help protect the body against viruses. When a virus enters a cell, it generally produces certain proteins that it projects onto the surface of the infected cell. T cells recognize these proteins and produce *cytokines* to destroy the infected cells. Some cytokines attract other cell types, which can digest the virus-infected cell. T cells can also destroy some types of **cancer** cells.

Lymphomas can be divided into two main types: Hodgkin's and non-Hodgkin's. There are at least 10 types of non-Hodgkin's lymphomas that are grouped (staged) by how aggressively they grow: slow growing (low grade), intermediate growing, and rapidly growing (high grade); and how far they spread.

Most non-Hodgkin's lymphomas begin in the lymph nodes; about 20% start in other organs, such as the lungs, liver or gastrointestinal tract. When lymphomas begin, malignant lymphocytes multiply uncontrollably and do not perform their normal functions, which affects the body's ability to fight **infections**. In addition, malignant cells may crowd the bone marrow, and, depending on the stage, prevent the production of normal red blood cells, white blood cells, and platelets. A low red blood cell count causes **anemia**, while a reduction in the number of platelets makes the person susceptible to excessive bleeding. Cancerous cells can also invade other organs through the circulatory system of the lymph, causing those organs to malfunction.

Causes and symptoms

The exact cause of non-Hodgkin's lymphomas is unknown. In general, males are at a higher risk than females, and the risk increases with age. Though it can strike people as young as 40, people between the ages of 60 and 69 are at the highest risk. In addition, the number of non-Hodgkin's cases has increased significantly in recent years, many of them due to the **AIDS** epidemic. (For reasons that are still poorly understood, AIDS patients have a higher likelihood of developing non-Hodgkin's lymphomas.)

People exposed to certain pesticides and ionizing radiation have a higher-than-average chance of developing this disease. For example, an increased incidence of lymphomas has been seen in survivors of the atomic bomb explosion in Hiroshima, and in people who have undergone aggressive radiation therapy. People who suffer from immune-deficient disorders, as well as those who have been treated with immune-suppressive drugs for heart or kidney transplants, and for conditions such as **rheumatoid arthritis** and autoimmune diseases, are at an increased risk for this disease. Some studies have shown a loose association between retroviruses, such as HTLV-I, and some rare forms of lymphoma. The Epstein-Barr virus has been linked to Burkitt's lymphoma in African countries. However, a direct cause-and-effect relationship has not been established.

The symptoms of lymphomas are often vague and nonspecific. Patients may experience loss of appetite, weight loss, **nausea**, **vomiting**, abdominal discomfort, and **indigestion**. The patient may complain of a feeling of fullness, which is a result of enlarged lymph nodes in the abdomen. Pressure or **pain** in the lower back is another symptom. In the advanced stages, the patient may have bone pain, headaches, constant coughing, and abnormal pressure and congestion in the face, neck, and upper chest. Some may have fevers and night sweats. In most cases, patients go to the doctor because of the presence of swollen glands in the neck, armpits, or groin area. Since all the symptoms are common to many other illnesses, it is essential to seek medical attention if any of the conditions persist for two weeks or more. Only a qualified physician can correctly diagnose if the symptoms are due to lymphoma or some other ailment.

Diagnosis

Like all cancers, lymphomas are best treated when found early. However, they are often difficult to diagnose. There are no screening tests available, and, since the symptoms are nonspecific, lymphomas are rarely recognized in their early stages. Detection often occurs by chance during a routine physical examination.

When the doctor suspects lymphoma, a thorough physical examination is performed and a complete medical history taken. Enlarged liver, spleen, or lymph nodes may suggest lymphomas. Blood tests will determine the cell counts and obtain information on how well the organs, such as the kidney and liver, are functioning.

A biopsy (microscopic tissue analysis) of the enlarged lymph node is the most definitive way to diagnose a lymphoma. Once the exact form of lymphoma is known, it is then staged to determine how aggressive it is, and how far it has spread. This information helps determine the appropriate treatment. The doctor may also perform a bone marrow biopsy. During this procedure, a cylindrical piece of bone—generally from the hip—and marrow fluid are removed. These samples are sent to the laboratory for examination. Biopsies may also be repeated during treatment to see how the lymphoma is responding to therapy.

Conventional imaging tests, such as x rays, computed tomography scans (CT scans), magnetic resonance imaging, and abdominal sonograms, are used to determine the extent of spread of the disease. *Lymphangiograms* are x rays of the lymphatic system. In this procedure, a special dye, called contrast medium, is injected into the lymphatic channels through a small incision (cut) made in each foot. The dye is injected slowly over a period of three to four hours. This dye clearly outlines the lymphatic system and allows it to stand out. Multiple x rays are then taken and any abnormality, if present, is revealed.

In rare cases a lumbar puncture (spinal tap) is performed to see if malignant cells are in the fluid that surrounds the brain. In this test, the physician inserts a needle into the epidural space at the base of the spine and collects a small amount of spinal fluid for microscopic examination.

Treatment

Non-Hodgkin's lymphoma is a life-threatening disease, and a correct diagnosis and appropriate treatment with surgery, chemotherapy, and/or radiation are critical to controlling the illness.

Acupuncture, **hypnotherapy**, and **guided imagery** may be useful tools in treating the pain of lymphomas. Acupuncture uses a series of thin needles placed in the skin at targeted locations known as *acupoints;* in theory, this harmonizes the energy flow within the body, and may help improve immune system function.

In guided imagery, patients create pleasant and soothing mental images that promote **relaxation** and improve their ability to cope with discomfort and pain. Another guided-imagery technique involves creating a mental picture of pain. Once the pain is visualized, patients can adjust the image to make it more pleasing, and thus more manageable.

Herbal remedies, such as Chinese herbs and mushroom extracts, may also lessen pain and promote relaxation and healing. Some herbs, such as **ginger**, are effective in the treatment of nausea caused by chemotherapy, and others, such as **astragalus**, help build the immune system. Check with an herbal practitioner before deciding on treatment. Depending on the preparation and the type of herb, the remedies may interfere with other prescribed medications. Naturally, any other activities that promote well-being, such as **exercise**, **stress** reduction, **meditation**, **yoga**, **t'ai chi**, and **qigong** will also benefit the patient. Proper **nutrition** and some specialized **diets** may help in recovering from lymphomas.

Allopathic treatment

Treatment options for lymphomas depend on the type of lymphoma and its stage. In most cases, treatment consists of chemotherapy, radiation therapy, or a combination of the two.

Chemotherapy uses anticancer drugs to kill cancer cells. In non-Hodgkin's lymphomas, combination therapy, which uses several drugs, has been found more effective than single-drug use. Treatment usually lasts about six months, but in some cases may be as long as a year. The drugs are administered intravenously (through a vein) or given orally. If cancer cells have invaded the central nervous system, then chemotherapeutic drugs may be instilled, through a needle in the brain or back, into the fluid that surrounds the brain. This procedure is known as intrathecal chemotherapy.

Radiation therapy, where high-energy ionizing rays are directed at specific portions of the body, such as the upper chest, abdomen, pelvis, or neck, is often used for treatment of lymphomas. External radiation therapy, where the rays are directed from a source outside the body, is the most common mode of radiation treatment.

Bone marrow transplantation is being tested as a treatment option when lymphomas do not respond to conventional therapy, or when the patient has had a relapse or suffers from recurrent lymphomas. There are two ways of doing bone marrow transplantation. In a procedure called *allogeneic* bone marrow transplant, the donor's marrow must match that of the patient. The donor can be a twin (best match), sibling, or not related at all. High-dose chemotherapy or radiation therapy is given to eradicate the lymphoma. The donor marrow is then given to replace the marrow destroyed by the therapy. In *autologous* bone marrow transplantation some of the patient's own marrow is harvested, chemically purged, and frozen. High-dose chemotherapy and radiation therapy are administered. The marrow that was harvested, purged, and frozen is then thawed and put back into the patient's body to replace the destroyed marrow.

A new option for lymphoma patients is *peripheral stem cell transplantation*. In this treatment, stem cells (immature cells from which all blood cells develop), that normally circulate in the blood are collected, treated to remove cancer cells, then returned to the patient in a process called *leukapheresis*. Researchers are exploring whether these cells can be used to restore the normal function and development of blood cells, rather than using a bone marrow transplant.

Expected results

Like all cancers, the prognosis for lymphoma patients depends on the stage of the cancer, and the patient's age and general health. When all the different types and stages of lymphoma are considered together, only 50% of patients survive five years or more after initial diagnosis. This is because some types of lymphoma are more aggressive than other types. The survival rate among children is definitely better than among older people. About 90% of children diagnosed with early-stage disease survive five years or more, while only 60-70% of adults diagnosed with low-grade lymphomas survive for five years or more. The survival rate for children with the more advanced stages is about 75-85%, while among adults it is 40-60%.

Prevention

Although the risk of developing cancer can be reduced by making wise diet and lifestyle choices, there is currently no known way to prevent lymphomas, nor are there special tests that allow early detection. Paying prompt attention to the signs and symptoms of this disease, and seeing a doctor if the symptoms persist, are the best strategies for an early diagnosis, which affords the best chance for a cure.

Resources

BOOKS

Dollinger, Malin, et al. *Everyone's Guide to Cancer Therapy.* Kansas City: Andrews McKeel Publishing, 1997.

Fauci, Anthony, et al., eds. *Harrison's Principles of Internal Medicine.* New York: McGraw-Hill, 1998.

Murphy, Gerald P. *Informed Decisions: The Complete Book of Cancer Diagnosis, Treatment, and Recovery.* New York: American Cancer Society, 1997.

PERIODICALS

"Alternative Cancer Therapies Popular Today." *Cancer.* 77, no. 6 (March 1996).

ORGANIZATIONS

American Cancer Society (National Headquarters). 1599 Clifton Road, N.E. Atlanta, GA 30329. (800) 227-2345. http://www.cancer.org.

Cancer Research Institute (National Headquarters). 681 Fifth Avenue, New York, NY 10022. (800) 992-2623. http://www.cancerresearch.org.

The Lymphoma Research Foundation of America, Inc. 8800 Venice Boulevard, Suite 207, Los Angeles, CA 90034. (310) 204-7040. http://www.lymphoma.org.

National Cancer Institute. 9000 Rockville Pike, Building 31, room 10A16, Bethesda, MD 20892. (800) 422-6237. http://www.nci.nih.gov.

Paula Ford-Martin

Malignant melanoma *see* **Skin cancer**

Mandarin orange peel *see* **Tangerine peel**

Manganese

Description

The chemical element manganese (Mn) has the atomic mass 54.938 and atomic number 25. Manganese is not to be confused with the somewhat better known element **magnesium**. Manganese is a trace mineral used by some people to help prevent bone loss and alleviate symptoms associated with **premenstrual syndrome** (PMS). It may have a number of other beneficial effects as well. While most of the body's mineral content is composed of such macrominerals as **calcium**, magnesium, and **potassium**, certain trace minerals are also considered essential in very tiny amounts to maintain health and ensure proper functioning of the body. They usually act as coenzymes, working in conjunction with proteins to facilitate important chemical reactions. Even without taking manganese supplements, people with an average diet consume somewhere between 2 and 3 mg of the mineral through food and drink. While most authorities agree that manganese is a vital micronutrient, it is not known for certain if taking extra amounts can be helpful in treating **osteoporosis**, menstrual symptoms, or other problems.

Manganese, which is concentrated mainly in the liver, skeleton, pancreas, and brain, is considered important because it is used to make several key enzymes in the body and activates others. One of the enzymes made from manganese is superoxide dismutase (SOD), an antioxidant facilitator. **Antioxidants** help to protect cells from damage caused by free radicals, the destructive fragments of oxygen produced as a byproduct during normal metabolic processes. As these rogue particles travel through the body, they cause damage to cells and genes by stealing electrons from other molecules, a process referred to as oxidation. Manganese may also have some anticancer activity as well as a number of other important functions. It is believed to play a role in **cholesterol** and carbohydrate metabolism, thyroid function, blood sugar control, and the formation of bone, cartilage, and skin. While the effects of a manganese-free diet had not been thoroughly studied in people as of 2008, animal experiments suggest that a lack of manganese can be unhealthy. Manganese deficiency in animals appears to have an adverse effect on the growth of bone and cartilage, brain function, blood sugar control, and reproduction. One study of dietary supplementation with manganese and other micronutrients in Mexican infants found that children who received the supplements grew faster and taller than a control group given a placebo. The authors concluded that growth

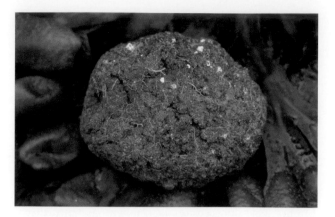

Manganese nodule. (© blickwinkel / Alamy)

retardation in children in developing countries is linked to manganese and other micronutrient deficiencies in the diet, among other factors.

General use

While considered necessary for general good health, manganese is also used for specific health concerns. Health food advocates have touted a number of possible benefits from using manganese supplements. Some conditions for which it has been recommended are:

- Alzheimer's disease
- anemia
- arthritis
- asthma
- cancers
- carpal tunnel syndrome
- chronic fatigue syndrome
- Chron's disease
- emphysema
- epilepsy
- Lyme's disease
- osteoporosis

As of 2008, research had produced only very limited evidence to support most of these claims. The strongest evidence appeared to involve the role of manganese in the development of strong bones. In a 2004 summary of scientific research on this point, the National Institute of Arthritis and Musculoskeletal and Skin Diseases concluded that manganese "helps certain enzymes and local regulators function properly" for optimal bone development and strength. Based on this conclusion, manganese is sometimes suggested as a possible treatment for osteoporosis, usually in combination with other trace minerals.

Recommended dietary allowance of manganese

Age	mg/day
Children 0-6 mos.	0.3 (AI)
Children 7-12 mos.	0.6 (AI)
Children 1-3 yrs.	1.2
Children 4-8 yrs.	1.5
Boys 9-13 yrs.	1.9
Girls 9-13 yrs.	1.6
Boys 14-18 yrs.	2.2
Girls 14-18 yrs.	1.6
Men ≥ 19 yrs.	2.3
Women ≥ 19 yrs.	1.8
Pregnant women	2.0
Breastfeeding women	2.6

Foods that contain manganese	mg
Tea, green, 1 cup	1.58
Pineapple, raw, 1/2 cup	1.28
Pecans, 1 oz.	1.12
Cereal, raisin bran, 1/2 cup	.94
Brown rice, cooked, 1/2 cup	.88
Spinach, cooked, 1/2 cup	.84
Tea, black, 1 cup	.77
Almonds, 1 oz.	.74
Bread, whole wheat, 1 slice	.65
Peanuts, 1 oz.	.59
Sweet potato, mashed, 1/2 cup	.55
Beans, navy, cooked, 1/2 cup	.51
Beans, lima, cooked, 1/2 cup	.48
Beans, pinto, cooked, 1/2 cup	.48

AI = Adequate Intake
mg = milligram

(Illustration by GGS Information Services. Cengage Learning, Gale)

A single, very small study conducted in 1993 suggested that manganese and calcium may be a potent team in alleviating menstrual symptoms and premenstrual syndrome (PMS). Researchers from the Grand Forks Human **Nutrition** Research Center, which is affiliated with the U. S. Department of Agriculture, examined how calcium and manganese affect menstrual symptoms in women in good health. Ten women with normal menstrual cycles were studied for about 170 days. The women received 587 or 1,336 mg of calcium a day with 1.0 or 5.6 mg a day of manganese. They filled out a Menstrual Distress Questionnaire during each cycle and the results were analyzed. Getting more calcium improved mood, concentration, and behavior, and also reduced menstrual **pain** and the water retention associated with the premenstrual phase. The role of manganese appeared to be important. Despite getting higher amounts of calcium, women who received lower amounts of manganese experienced more moodiness and pain prior to their periods. This study suggested that getting adequate amounts of calcium and manganese can help to reduce the pain and other symptoms associated with menstrual periods. The results of this study had not been confirmed, however, as of 2008.

Manganese may also be important for people with other diseases. Those with **epilepsy**, diabetes, and Perthes disease tend to have low levels of the mineral, which has led to suggestions that manganese may help to prevent or treat these disorders. Almost no research exists to support these contentions, however. A handful of animal studies have indicated that manganese may play a role in controlling seizures and blood sugar levels. Manganese may also decrease the risk of colon **cancer** by raising levels of the SOD enzyme, which has antioxidant effects.

Some people take manganese to help treat muscle **strains** or **sprains**, as well as **rheumatoid arthritis**, though there was as of 2008 no convincing scientific evidence to support these uses. Theoretically, manganese may act as an anti-inflammatory agent by boosting the activity of SOD.

Preparations

The optimum daily dosage of manganese has not been established with certainty. While there is no recommended daily allowance (RDA) or daily value (DV) for manganese, the U.S. government has established what is called an adequate intake level (AI) for certain nutrients. In adults over the age of 19, the AI for manganese is 2.3 mg/day for men and 1.8 mg/day for women. Adequate intake for children and adolescents varies with age and sex. Daily dosage ranges from 0.6 mg/day for both sexes from ages 7 to 12 months; 1.2 mg/day from age 1 to 3 years; 1.5 mg/day for ages 4 to 8; 1.9 mg/day for boys and 1.6 mg/day for girls age 9 to 13; and 2.2 mg/day for males and 1.6 mg/day for females age 14 to 18.

Even without taking supplements, most women get about 2.2 mg a day of manganese through their **diets**, while men consume about 2.8 mg. Vegetarians and people who consume large amounts of whole-grain foods may get as much as 10 to 18 mg a day. Some authorities believe it is better for people to avoid manganese supplements altogether and increase their intake of foods known to contain significant amounts of the mineral. Manganese-rich foods and drinks include peanuts, pecans, pineapples and pineapple juice, shredded wheat and raisin bran cereals, and oatmeal. Other good sources are rice; sweet potatoes; spinach; whole wheat bread; and lima, pinto, and navy beans. Meat, poultry, fish, and dairy products are considered poor sources. Getting too much manganese through food and drink is not considered a significant risk because the mineral is present only in small amounts in plants and animals.

Some people take as much as 50 to 200 mg of manganese for several weeks to help treat muscle sprains or strains, but the safety and effectiveness of taking dosages this high were unknown in the late 2000s.

Precautions

Manganese is not known to be harmful when taken in recommended dosages. Extremely high intake of the mineral, however, has resulted in cases of idiopathic **Parkinson's disease**. Some studies indicate that high levels of manganese alter the blood-brain barrier, lowering the **iron** content of blood plasma while allowing the iron content of cerebrospinal fluid to rise. These cases of manganese-induced parkinsonism are usually limited to miners who inadvertently breathe manganese-rich dust or people who drink contaminated water from wells. People who eat a manganese-rich diet are not considered at risk for these types of side effects. In fact, most foods high in manganese are believed to contribute to good health.

Side effects

When taken in recommended dosages, manganese is not associated with any bothersome or significant side effects.

Interactions

Manganese interacts with certain drugs and dietary supplements. People who take oral contraceptives or antacids may require higher intake of manganese. More of the mineral may be needed in people who also take **phosphorus**, fiber, **copper**, iron, **zinc**, magnesium, or calcium.

Resources

PERIODICALS

Greiffenstein, Manfred, and Paul Lees-Haley. "Neuropsychological Correlates of Manganese Exposure: A Meta-analysis." *Journal of Clinical and Experimental Neuropsychology* (February 2007): 113–126.

Gwiazda, Roberto, Roberto Lucchini, and Donald Smith. "Adequacy and Consistency of Animal Studies to Evaluate the Neurotoxicity of Chronic Low-Level Manganese Exposure in Humans." *Journal of Toxicology and Environmental Health: Part A* (January 2007): 594–605.

Klos, K. J., et al. "Neuropsychological Profiles of Manganese Neurotoxicity." *European Journal of Neurology* (October 2006): 1139–1141.

Wasserman, Gail A., et al. "Developmental Impacts of Heavy Metals and Undernutrition." *Basic & Clinical Pharmacology & Toxicology* (February 2008): 212–217.

OTHER

"Manganese: Health Information Summary." New Hampshire Department of Environmental Services, 2006. http://www.des.state.nh.us/factsheets/ehp/ard-ehp-15.htm. (February 15, 2008).

"Micronutrient Information Center: Manganese." Linus Pauling Institute, June 2007. http://lpi.oregonstate.edu/infocenter/minerals/manganese/. (February 15, 2008).

ORGANIZATIONS

NIH Osteoporosis and Related Bone Diseases National Resource Center, Bldg. 31, Room 4C02, 31 Center Dr.-MSC 2350, Bethesda, MD, 20892-2350, (301) 496-8190, http://www.niams.nih.gov/.

Greg Annussek
Rebecca J. Frey, PhD
David Edward Newton, Ed.D.

Mangosteen

Description

The mangosteen is the tree *Garcinia mangostana L.*. The tree is native to tropical Asia and is thought to have been first grown as a crop in Thailand or Burma. In the 2000s, mangosteens are cultivated mainly in Thailand, Burma, Kampuchea (Cambodia), Vietnam, Malaysia, and a few places in India and the Philippines.

Mangosteens are not hardy trees, and compared to many other species, they have a short lifespan. To survive, they need a tropical continuously warm, humid climate. Young trees die at temperatures below 45°F (7.2°C), and older trees do not survive temperatures above 100°F (37.8°C) or below 40°F (4.4°C). Mangosteens also require substantial amounts of water. They do best in areas with an annual rainfall of 50 inches (130 cm) or more and can survive in swampy conditions where their roots remain constantly wet. In dry spells they need daily irrigation. As a result of their environmental requirements, mangosteens have not done well as a commercial crop when introduced in such places as Hawaii, California, Florida, tropical Africa, the islands of the Caribbean, and tropical Central America.

Mangosteens grow slowly. It can take a tree 10–20 years to reach its full height of 20–80 feet (6–25 m). Trees have an outside layer of dark brown, flaky bark and an inside layer of bark that contains bitter latex. They produce thick, largish dark green leaves in the shape of elongated ovals. The fruit of the mangosteen is the only part of the plant used for food or in healing. Under the best conditions, trees do not bear fruit until they are six years old, and often they reach the age of 10–12 years before fruiting. Mangosteen fruit is produced asexually. There is no fertilization involved, and all fruit that comes from a single tree is genetically identical. This lack of genetic variation may explain why the tree has such rigorous environmental requirements and has not been successful when introduced outside its native range.

Mangosteen fruit is uniformly dark purple, round, and slightly smaller than a tennis ball. It has a hard rind (pericarp) that can be as much as 1 inch (2.5 cm) thick. The rind makes up about two-thirds of the weight of the fruit. Inside the rind are four to eight segments of soft, moist, white fruit. The taste is both acidic and sweet. Mangosteen fruit is considered highly desirable in the areas of Asia where it grows. The fresh fruit does not keep or travel well. U.S. law forbids the importation of fresh mangosteens from Asia into the continental United States because of concerns about contamination by insect pests. Small amounts of fruit from other locations are very sporadically available in some gourmet grocery stores. Some canned mangosteen fruit may be available in the United States, most often in grocery stores specializing in products from Southeast Asia. Despite having a name that sounds like the mango fruit, mangosteens and mangos are not closely related. In the areas where it grows, the mangosteen is also called mangostan, mangouste, mangostao, manggis, mang cut, mesetor, mangis, semtah, and sementah.

General use

Mangosteen fruit has two general uses, as food and as an herbal remedy. As food, mangosteens are usually eaten raw. They can also be canned or made into jam, but processing changes their flavor. Raw fruits are high in both acids and sugars, giving them their distinctive sweet-tart flavor. A 3.5 ounce (100 g) portion of flesh provides about 60 calories and is a good source of **potassium**.

Traditionally the rind of the mangosteen fruit has been used medicinally in Southeast Asia for several thousand years as part of both Ayurvedic and **traditional Chinese medicine**. Mangosteen is used to treat dysentery, **diarrhea**, cystitis (bladder inflammation), and **gonorrhea** (a sexually transmitted disease). Made into a lotion or paste, it is applied to the skin to treat skin **wounds** and diseases such as **eczema**. In the Philippines, the bark is used to treat **fever**, and in Malaysia the root is used to regulate **menstruation**.

In 2002, a Utah company began a mangosteen craze in the United States when it promoted a mangosteen-containing drink called XanGo. XanGo is a pasteurized dietary supplement beverage that promoters claim provides the nutritional value and health benefits of mangosteens. The contents of the beverage are proprietary and are not revealed, but the company has claimed the drink provides benefits against specific diseases.

As a dietary supplement, the production of XanGo is regulate in the United States under the 1994 Dietary Supplement Health and Education Act (DSHEA). At the time the act was passed, legislators believed that because many dietary supplements come from natural sources such as plants and have been used for hundreds of years by practitioners of complementary and alternative medicine(CAM), these products did not need to be as rigorously regulated as prescription and over-the-counter drugs used in conventional medicine. DSHEA regulates dietary supplements such as XanGo in the same way that food is regulated. Like food manufacturers, manufacturers of dietary supplements do not have to prove that a supplement is either safe or effective before it can be sold to the public. Nevertheless, dietary supplement manufacturers cannot claim that their products treat or cure specific diseases. In September 2006, the United States Food and Drug Administration (FDA) sent a letter of warning to the manufacturers of XanGo to stop making claims that XanGo treated or prevented specific diseases. The complete FDA letter can be found at the FDA Web site.

After the introduction of XanGo, dozens of health-promoting products claiming to contain mangosteen appeared on the market. These products claimed to treat bacterial **infections**, **fungal infections**, and skin infections; to promote wound healing; cure diarrhea; and prevent or cure **cancer** by killing cancer cells and acting as **antioxidants**. The basis for these claims was the presence of a group of compounds called xanthones that are found in the mangosteen fruit and the rind. Xanthone extracts have been shown in test tube and a few animal studies to have antibacterial, antifungal, and anti-inflammatory actions. In some laboratory experiments specific xanthones extracted from the mangosteen rind have killed certain cancer cells or slowed their growth. Extracts of the rind also have antioxidant properties.

Although xanthones, such as those found in mangosteen, seem to show potential health benefits in test-tube and animal studies, there is no evidence as of 2008 that these same effects will be carry over into humans, nor is there any indication of what dosage a human might need. There is also no evidence that any dietary supplements containing mangosteen offer any specific health benefits beyond their food value. Memorial Sloan-Kettering Cancer Center issued a statement in August 2007 saying that "There is no conclusive evidence regarding the efficacy and safety of mangosteen in treating cancer." This statement can be found at the center's Web site.

Preparations

Traditionally, mangosteen fruits are dried and the rind is ground into a powder that is used medicinally. Mixed with water mangosteen rind can be taken internally for diarrhea, or it can be made into a paste and applied to the skin. A decoction of the bark is taken internally to treat fever, and a decoction of the root is used to treat menstrual disorders.

As a dietary supplement, mangosteen is available primarily as a health beverage. These beverages are heat-treated (pasteurized) and usually contain other ingredients besides mangosteen juice. They are not equivalent to fresh mangosteen. Dried mangosteen is also incorporated into some lotions for external use. The mangosteen content of dietary supplements is not standardized, and as of the early 2000s there was no agreed-upon standard dosage of mangosteen. Because of the difficulty in cultivating and obtaining mangosteen, mangosteen dietary supplements tend to be expensive.

KEY TERMS

Antioxidant—A molecule that prevents oxidation. In the body antioxidants attach to other molecules called free radicals and prevent the free radicals from causing damage to cell walls, DNA, and other parts of the cell.

Ayurvedic medicine—A 5,000-year old system of holistic medicine developed on the Indian subcontinent. Ayurvedic medicine is based on the idea that illness results from a personal imbalance or lack of physical, spiritual, social, or mental harmony.

Decoction—A preparation made by boiling an herb, then straining the solid material out. The liquid is then taken internally as a drink.

Dietary supplement—A product, such as a vitamin, mineral, herb, amino acid, or enzyme, that is intended to be consumed in addition to an individual's diet with the expectation that it will improve health.

Traditional Chinese medicine (TCM)—An ancient system of medicine based on maintaining a balance in vital energy or qi that controls emotions, spiritual, and physical well being. Diseases and disorders result from imbalances in qi (the life force), and treatments such as massage, exercise, acupuncture, and nutritional and herbal therapy are designed to restore balance and harmony to the body.

Precautions

Individuals with diabetes should be careful when drinking mangosteen juice products because of their high sugar content.

Side effects

There are no known side effects of mangosteen. The fruit has been eaten for centuries and used medicinally without ill effects.

Interactions

Very little is known about how mangosteen products interact with pharmaceutical drugs or other herbal remedies. Nevertheless, because of their sugar content, mangosteen juice products may adversely affect individuals who take medication to control their blood sugar level. Mangosteen products also may interfere with the action of chemotherapy drugs.

Resources

PERIODICALS

Chen, L. G., L. L. Yang, and C. C. Wang. "Anti-inflammatory Activity of Mangostins from Garcinia Mangostana." *Food and Chemical Toxicology* 46, no. 2 (February 2008): 668–693.

Devi, Sampath, and K. Vijayaraghavan. "Cardioprotective Effect of Alpha-mangostin, a Xanthone Derivative from Mangosteen on Tissue Defense System Against Isoproterenol-induced Myocardial Infarction in Rats." *Journal of Biochemistry and Molecular Toxicology* 21, no. 6 (2007): 336–339.

Rassameemasmaung, S., A. Sirikulsathean, C. Amornchat, et al. "Effects of Herbal Mouthwash Containing the Pericarp Extract of Garcinia mangostana L on Halitosis, Plaque and Papillary Bleeding Index." *Journal of the International Academy of Peridontology.* 9, no. 1 (2007): 19–25.

Yeung, Simon. "Mangosteen for the Cancer Patient: Facts and Myths." *Journal of Integrated Oncology* 4, no. 3 (2006): 130–134.

OTHER

"About Herbs: Mangosteen." *Memorial Sloan-Kettering Cancer Center,* updated August 9, 2007. http://www.mskcc.org/mskcc/html/69295.cfm (February 11, 2008).

"The Mangosteen." *Mangosteen.com* August 8, 2007. http://www.mangosteen.com (February 11, 2008).

Tish Davidson, A. M.

Manic depression *see* **Bipolar disorder**

Manuka honey

Description

Manuka honey is the natural product of honeybees who gather nectar from the blossoms of the manuka bush *(Leptospermum scoparium)*, also known as tea tree. The manuka bush is a tropical evergreen shrub in the Myrtle family native to New Zealand and southeast Australia, and grows wild and abundantly throughout New Zealand. The honey it yields is darker and richer in taste than clover honey and has been found to contain unique antibiotic properties.

General use

From ancient times honey has been a valued folk remedy throughout the world. Honey has long been used in the diet and as a potent means of fighting infection. Honey is an effective anti-inflammatory and antioxidant. The Aboriginal Maori people, indigenous to New Zealand, used honey produced from the manuka bush as a medicinal treatment for stomach ailments and **wounds**. Manuka is a word from the Mauri language, and in Mauri traditional medicine, manuka honey has a reputation as a powerful antiseptic and healing salve.

Honey has been widely available and in continual use for thousands of years. The ancient physicians Dioscorides and Aristotle distinguished from various types of honey to find those best suited for treatment of specific ailments. Honey is in common use in modern times as a home-remedy for sore throats and coughs, as a treatment for **burns** and other external injuries, and in the diet as an immune boosting, infection preventative.

All honey has healing properties due primarily to the action of glucose oxidase, an enzyme secreted by worker bees into the nectar. When the honey is exposed to oxygen and applied to a damp surface, such as when applied to a wound, a chemical interaction releases hydrogen peroxide, which acts as a disinfectant. In addition, Honey is acidic with a high sugar but low water content, a combination that limits growth of micro-organisms that become dehydrated and unable to survive in the presence of honey. Although most bacteria and other microorganisms cannot grow or reproduce in honey, honey varies widely in its antibacterial and antimicrobial properties. This bioactivity of honey depends on many factors including the type of plant pollinated, and its location. Manuka honey from New Zealand is considered one of the most medicinally potent of the hundreds of types of honey available.

The particular healing qualities of manuka honey, and its very broad spectrum of antibiotic action, has been brought to wider attention due to the work of Professor Peter Molan, a New Zealand biochemist whose extensive investigations at Waikato University and the Waikato Honey Research Unit have demonstrated what he has termed "a unique manuka factor, or UMF." This factor works independently of and synergistically with the glucose oxidase action present in all honey to impart a higher level of antibiotic action. According to Molan, writing in 2008 on the blog site *Apitherapy News* "The currently used rating system, UMF, measures the actual antibacterial activity of each batch of honey, tested against Staphylococcus aureus, the species of bacteria that is the most common cause of wound infections.". Manuka honey is stable, and its healing properties are not diminished when exposed to light, heat, or air, or when stored for long periods of time.

Anecdotal evidence and reports from clinical practice of the healing qualities and therapeutic effectiveness of manuka honey include its success in the treatment of:

- abscesses
- Burns
- Conjunctivitis
- Dyspepsia
- Gastgroenteritis
- Periodontal disease
- Persistent wounds
- Pressure sores
- Stomach ulcers
- Strep throat
- Virus

Research

German researchers have identified the natural compound Methylglyoxal (MGO) as responsible for manuka honey's unique health-giving properties. Manuka honey has a significantly higher level of antibacterial activity when compared to other honeys, according to the researchers at the Institute of Food Chemistry in Dresden, Germany, who tested samples of New Zealand manuka honey compared with other commercially available honey. They found up to 100-fold higher amounts of MGO in the New Zealand manuka honey, with amounts ranging from 38 to 761 mg/kg. The antibacterial activity of manuka honey was detected even when the honey was diluted to 15-30 percent.

In 2006, the journal *Palative Medicine* reported on the success of daily applications of topical manuka honey applied to ulcers in three hospice patients whose sores were contaminated with the so-called superbug, *methicillin-resistant Staphylococcus aureus* (MRSA) that has been a significant health problem in hospitals and schools. Research at the University of Dresden shows that a minimum of 100mg/kg methylglyoxal (MGO) must be present in the manuka honey to inhibit *Staphylococcus aureus* and other harmful bacteria.

Manuka honey has demonstrated effectiveness against the streptococci bacterium present in **strep throat infections**. It is also effective against fungi, protozoa and other infectious organisms. It is useful as a topical antimicrobial for both chronic and acute wounds and burns, and has been shown effective for athlete's foot infections and ringworm.

Manuka honey has been found to be about twice as effective as other honey against *Eschericihia coli* and *Staphylococcus aureus*, the most common causes of infected wounds.

When taken internally, manuka honey gives a boost to the immune system and helps combat infections. Its dietary use may promote the rehydration of the body and reduce the duration of **diarrhea**, **vomiting** and upset stomach. Relief from stomach ulcers is possible through manuka honey's action against the *Helicobacter pylori* microbe found in stomach ulcers. Manuka honey has been demonstrated as beneficial in treatment of **acne**, cracked skin, sore gums, **indigestion**, and eye infections.

The acid-producing bacteria *Streptococcus mitis, Streptococcus sobrinus*, and *Lactobacillus caseii* found in the mouth, have demonstrated sharp reduction of acid production in laboratory tests, when antibacterial honey is present. Results of a 2004 pilot study of the effects of manuka honey on periodontal diseases such as gingivitis and plaque indicated that there were statistically "highly significant reductions" in plaque scores and the percentage of bleeding sites in the manuka honey group. Researchers reported no significant changes in the control group, and concluded that manuaka honey could be of therapeutic value in treatment of gingivitis and periodontal disease.

Though research on manuka honey has been going forward in New Zealand and elsewhere for the past two decades, more research needs to be done with randomized controlled trials to further substantiate the qualitative differences between manuka honey and other honey, and to provide further scientific confirmation of the anecdotal and clincical practice reports of the benefits of manuka honey.

Most of the available scientific evidence substantiates the wound healing properties of honey. According to biochemist Peter C. Molan of the University of Waikato in New Zealand, honey, and in particular manuka honey, acts effectively as a wound dressing in the following ways:

- Honey provides a protective barrier preventing cross-infections
- Honey maintains a moist healing environment
- Honey produces and provides controlled delivery of hydrogen peroxide
- Honey provides a rapid healing effect
- Honey saturated dressings do not stick to wounds
- Honey reduces scarring
- Honey inhibits the odor in healing wounds
- Honey facilitates the uptake of serum into the wound
- Honey has beneficial anti-inflammatory and antioxidant properties

Preparations

Wound healing

In 2007, the U.S. Food and Drug Administration approved a honey-impregnated wound-dressing product for wound and burn care. The "medical device" Medihoney is the trademarked brand marketed by the New Zealand based natural health company Comvita. Comvita controls a large share of production of New Zealand's manuka honey.

Manuka honey dressings can also be prepared at home. Wound treatment with sterilized manuka honey should begin first by cleansing the wound with a saline solution. Apply about one tablespoon of Manuka Honey to a sterile gauze and apply to the wound, covering with a few more layers of gauze on top of the first layer. Secure with paper tape to keep the dressing in place. The dressing should be changed every 24 hours until the wound is completely healed.

Internal use

Manuka honey can be introduced into the diet as a nutritious food, with anti-inflammatory and immune boosting benefits. For stomach or peptic ulcers, a more concentrated manuaka honey product can be taken a spoon at a time on an empty stomach, or spread on a small piece of bread about twenty minutes prior to a meal. Honey can be administered in spoon size doses to soothe sore throats and cold symptoms. In clinical settings, manuka honey has been used effectively as an ointment-like dressing beneath the eyelid to treat **conjunctivitis**.

Manuka honey is available commercially in various concentrations of the trade-marked UMF or "Unique Manuka Factor," as described by New Zealand researcher Professor Peter Molan. The more concentrated product is called "active manuka honey," and is available commercially from distributers throughout the world. Strengths range from UMF 5, said to be equivalent to a 5% solution of a standard antiseptic, to UMF 20, equivalent to a 20% solution.

Precautions

Researchers warn that untreated honey may carry a risk of botulism, and if applied to a wound may introduce the rare but deadly infection. Commercially available manuka honey is sterilized by gamma irradiation to eliminate the possible risk of introducing infection. The irradiation does not bring about loss of any of manuka honey's antibacterial activity, researchers say. Increasingly, sterilized honey dressings are now among the first line of treatment for early wound infections, and no adverse reactions have been noted, even in diabetic patients. There may be a mild stinging or burning sensation with topical application of honey due to its acidic content.

Resources

PERIODICALS

Alexander, Tania, "Sweet Wonder of Honey," *The Express* (UK), April 24, 2007.

Associated Press. "Honey Making a Medical Comeback." December 26, 2007. *MSNBC. Com Health News.* http://www.msnbc.msn.com/id/22398921/. Cited March 4, 2008.

Blaser, G, et al. "Effect of Medical Honey on Wounds Colonised or Infected With MRSA," *Journal of Wound Care.* (2007) 16: 325-28.

Chambers, John. "Topical Manuka Honey for MRSA Contaminated Skin Ulcers." *Palliative Medicine* (2006) 20, No.5: 557.

Dente, Karen, "Antibacterial Properties Could Make the Nectar an Effective Treatment for Sores that Refuse to Mend." *Los Angeles Times*, September 10, 2007.

English, H.K., et al. "The Effects of Manuka Honey on Plaque and Gingivitis: A Pilot Study." *Journal of the International Academy of Periodontology.* (2004) 6, No. 2: 63-7.

Jull, A, et al. "Randomized Clinical Trial of Honey-Impregnated Dressings for Venous Leg Ulcers." *British Journal of Surgery* (2008) 95: 175-82.

Kerwin, Mark. "Manuka Honey - Tasty Medicine From New Zealand." Down to Earth.Org. http://www.downtoearth.org/articles/print/p_manuka_honey.htm. Cited March 3, 2008.

Mavric, Elvira, et al. "Identification and Quantification of Methylglyoxal as the Dominant Antibacterial Constituent of Manuka." *Molecular Nutrition & Food Research.* (2008) 52.

Molan, Peter. "Molan: MGO Level Not Good Indicator of Honey's Antibacterial Activity," *Apitherapy News.* January 30, 2008. http://apitherapy.blogspot.com

Molan, P.C. "Manuka Honey As A Medicine." Honey Research Unit, University of Waikato, Hamilton, New zealand.

Patton, T., et al. "Use of a Spectrophotometric Bioassay for Determination of Microbial Sensitivity to Manuka Honey." *J. Microbiol. Meth.* (2006) 64: 84–95.

Trump, Eric Frederick. "Sweet Salve: Could Honey, an Ancient Remedy, Make a Comeback in Contemporary Wound Care?" *The Washington Post.* August 7, 2007. Washingtonpost.com.

Visavadia, Bhavin G., et al. "Manuka Hondy Dressing: An Effective Treatment for Chronic Wound Infections." *British Journal of Oral and Maxillofacial Surgery* (January 2008) 46, No. 1: 55-56.

Waikato Honey Research Unit. "What's Special About Active Manuka Honey?" http://bio.waikato.ac.nz/honey/special.shtml. Cited March 4, 2008.

OTHER

Manuka Honey.Com, Summer Glow Apiaries, Ltd. http://www.manukahoney.com.

Clare Hanrahan

Marigold *see* **Calendula**

Marijuana

Description

Marijuana (marihuana), *Cannabis sativa L.*, also known as Indian hemp, is a member of the Cannabaceae or hemp family, thought to have originated in the mountainous districts of India, north of the Himalayan mountains. The herb was referred to as "hempe" in A.D. 1000 and listed in a dictionary under that English name. Supporters of Pancho Villa (1878–1923) first called the mood-altering herb they smoked marijuana in 1895 in Sonora, Mexico. The term hashish is derived from the name for the Saracen soldiers, called *hashashins*, who ingested the highly potent cannabis resin before being sent out to assassinate enemies.

Two related species of cannabis are *C. ruderalis* and *C. indica*, a variety known as Indian hemp. Indian hemp grows to a height of about 4 ft (1.2 m) and the seed coats have a marbled appearance.

The species *C. sativa L.* has many variations, depending on the origin of the parent seed and the soil, temperature, and light conditions. These factors also affect the relative amounts of 9-tetrahydrocannabinol (THC) and cannabidiol, the chemicals present in varying amounts in cannabis that determine if the plant is primarily a fiber type or an intoxicant. Generally, the species grown at higher elevations and in hotter climates exude more resin and are more medicinally potent.

Marijuana is a somewhat weedy plant and may grow as high as 18 ft (5.4 m). The hairy leaves are arranged opposite one another on the erect and branching stem. Leaves are palmate and compound, deeply divided into five to seven narrow, toothed, and pointed leaflets. Male and female flowers are small and greenish in color and grow on separate plants. Male flowers grow in the leaf axils in elongated clusters. The female flowers grow in spike-like clusters. The resinous blossoms have five sepals and five petals. The male and female blossoms can be distinguished at maturity. The male plant matures first, shedding its pollen and dying after flowering. Female plants die after dropping the mature seeds. Marijuana produces an abundance of quickly germinating seeds. This hardy annual is wind pollinated and has escaped from cultivation to grow wild along roadsides, trails, stream banks, and in wayside places throughout the world. The plant matures within three to five months after the seed has been sown.

History

Marijuana has been cultivated for thousands of years. Cannabis was first described for its therapeutic use in the first known Chinese pharmacopoeia, the *Pen Ts'ao*. Cannabis was called a "superior" herb by the Emperor Shen-Nung (2737–2697 B.C.), who is believed to have authored the work. Cannabis was recommended as a treatment for many common ailments. Around that same period in Egypt, cannabis was used as a treatment for sore eyes. The herb was used in India in cultural and religious ceremonies and recorded in Sanskrit scriptural texts around 1400 B.C. Cannabis was considered a holy herb, and it was characterized as the "soother of grief," "the sky flyer," and "the poor man's heaven." Centuries later, around 700 B.C., the Assyrian people used the herb they called *Qunnabu* for incense. The ancient Greeks used cannabis as a remedy to treat inflammation, **earache**, and **edema**. Shortly after 500 B.C., the historian and geographer Herodotus recorded that the people known as Scythians used cannabis to produce fine linens. They called the herb *kannabis* and inhaled the "intoxicating vapor" that resulted when it was burned. By the year 100 B.C. the Chinese were using cannabis to make paper.

Cannabis use and cultivation migrated with the movement of traders and travelers, and knowledge of the herb's value spread throughout the Middle East,

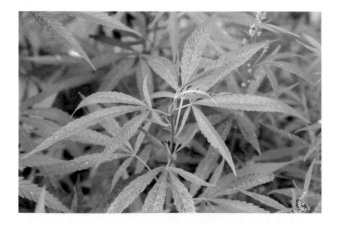

Marijuana plant. *(© Organica / Alamy)*

Eastern Europe, and Africa. Around A.D. 100, Dioscorides, a surgeon in the Roman Legions under the Emperor Nero, named the herb *Cannabis sativa* and recorded numerous medicinal uses. In the second century, the Chinese physician Hoa-Tho used cannabis in surgical procedures, relying on its analgesic properties. In ancient India, around 600, Sanskrit writers recorded a recipe for "pills of gaiety," a combination of hemp and sugar. By 1150, Moslems were using cannabis fiber in Europe's first paper production. This use of cannabis as a durable and renewable source of paper fiber continued for the next 750 years.

By the 1300s, government and religious authorities, concerned about the psychoactive effects on citizens consuming the herb, were placing harsh restrictions on its use. The Emir Soudon Sheikhouni of Joneima outlawed cannabis use among the poor. He destroyed the crops and ordered that offenders' teeth be pulled out. In 1484, Pope Innocent VIII outlawed the use of hashish, a concentrated form of cannabis resin. Cannabis cultivation continued, however, because of its economic value. A little more than a century later, Queen Elizabeth I issued a decree in England commanding that landowners holding 60 acres (24 ha) or more must grow hemp or pay a fine. Commerce in hemp, which was primarily valued for the strength and versatility of its fibers, was profitable and thriving. Hemp ropes and sails crossed the sea to North America with the explorers. By 1621, the British were growing cannabis in Virginia where cultivation of hemp was mandatory. In 1776, the Declaration of Independence was drafted on hemp paper. As president, both George Washington and Thomas Jefferson advocated hemp as a valuable cash crop. Jefferson urged farmers to grow the crop in place of tobacco. By the 1850s, hemp had become the third largest agricultural crop grown in North America. The United States Census of that year recorded 8,327 hemp plantations, each with 2,000 or more acres in cultivation. But the invention of the cotton gin was already bringing many changes, and cotton was becoming a prime and profitable textile fiber. More change came with the introduction of the sulfite and chlorine processes used to turn trees into paper. Restrictions on the personal use of cannabis as a mood-altering, psychoactive herb, were soon to come.

Controversy

The 1856 edition of the *Encyclopedia Britannica*, in its lengthy entry on hemp, noted that the herb "produces inebriation and delirium of decidedly hilarious character, inducing violent laughter, jumping and dancing." This inebriating effect of marijuana use has fueled controversy and led to restrictions that have surrounded marijuana use throughout history in many cultures and regions of the world. Cannabis use has been criminalized in some parts of the United States since 1915. Utah was the first state to criminalize it, followed by California and Texas. By 1923, Louisiana, Nevada, Oregon, and Washington had legal restrictions on the herb. New York prohibited cannabis use in 1927.

In 1937, the federal government passed the Marijuana Tax Act, prohibiting the cultivation and farming of marijuana. This bill was introduced to Congress by then-secretary of the Treasury Andrew Mellon, who was also a banker for the DuPont Corporation. That same year, the DuPont Chemical Company filed a patent for nylon, plastics, and a new bleaching process for paper. The 1937 Marijuana Transfer Tax Bill prohibited industrial and medical use of marijuana and classified the flowering tops as a narcotic. Restrictions on the cultivation and use of cannabis continued. Marijuana was categorized as an illegal narcotic, in the company of LSD, heroin, cocaine, and morphine. Nevertheless, illegal use continued. The FBI 1966 publication, *Uniform Crime Reports for the United States* reported that 641,642 Americans were arrested for marijuana offenses that year, with as many as 85% of these arrests for simple possession, rather than cultivation or commerce.

In a reversal of the state-by-state progression of criminalizing marijuana that led to the 1937 Marijuana Transfer Tax Bill, there is a movement underway, state by state, to endorse the legalized use of medical marijuana. By 1992, 35 states in the United States had endorsed referenda for medical marijuana. A growing body of scientific research and many thousands of years of folk use supported the importance of medical marijuana in treatment of a variety of illnesses, and the economic value of hemp in the textile, paper, and cordage industries has a long history.

Controversy and misinformation persists around this relatively safe and non-toxic herb. The World Health Organization, in a 1998 study, stated that the risks from cannabis use were unlikely to seriously compare to the public health risks of the legal drugs, alcohol and tobacco. Despite thousands of years of human marijuana use, not one death has been directly attributed to cannabis. The chief legitimate concern is the effect of **smoking** on the lungs. Cannabis smoke carries even more tars and other particulate matter than tobacco smoke, but the amount smoked is much less, especially in medical use.

General use

Every part of the cannabis plant, including buds, leaves, seeds, and root, has been used throughout the long history of this controversial herb. Despite persistent legal restrictions and criminal penalties for illicit use, marijuana continues to be widely used in the United States and throughout the world, both for its mood-altering properties and its proven medicinal applications. The conflicting opinions on the safety and effectiveness of cannabis in a climate of prohibition make any discussion of its beneficial uses politically charged.

Marijuana has analgesic, anti-emetic (anti-nausea), anti-inflammatory, sedative, anticonvulsive, and laxative actions. Clinical studies have demonstrated its effectiveness in relieving **nausea** and **vomiting** following chemotherapy treatments for **cancer**. The herb has also been shown to reduce intra-ocular pressure in the eye by as much as 45%, a beneficial action in the treatment for **glaucoma**. Cannabis has proven anticonvulsive action and may be helpful in treating **epilepsy**. Other research has documented an in-vitro tumor inhibiting effect of THC. Marijuana also increases appetite and reduces nausea and has been used with **AIDS** patients to counter weight loss and wasting that result from the disease. Several chemical constituents of cannabis have displayed antimicrobial action and antibacterial effects in research studies. The components CBC and d-9-tetra-hydrocannabinol have been shown to destroy and inhibit the growth of streptococci and staphylococci bacteria.

Cannabis contains chemical compounds known as cannabinoids. Different cannabinoids seem to exert different effects on the body after ingestion. Scientific research indicates that these substances have potential therapeutic value for **pain** relief, control of nausea and vomiting, and appetite stimulation. The primary active agent identified as of 2008 was THC. This chemical may constitute as much as 12% of the active chemicals in the herb and is said to be responsible for as much as 70 to 100% of the euphoric action, or high, experienced when ingesting the herb. The predominance of this mental lightness or euphoria depends on the balance of other active ingredients and the freshness of the herb. THC degrades into a component known as cannabinol, or CBN. This relatively inactive chemical predominates in marijuana that has been stored too long prior to use. Another chemical component, cannabidiol, known as CBD, has a sedative and mildly analgesic effect and contributes to a somatic heaviness sometimes experienced by marijuana users.

In the United States in the early twentieth century, cannabis was recommended for treatment of **gonorrhea**, **angina** pectoris (constricting pain in the chest due to insufficient blood to the heart), and choking fits. It was also used for **insomnia**, **neuralgia**, rheumatism, gastrointestinal disorders, cholera, **tetanus**, epilepsy, strychnine poisoning, **bronchitis**, **whooping cough**, and **asthma**. Other phytotherapeutic (plant-based therapeutic) uses include treatment of ulcers, cancer, **emphysema**, migraine, and **anxiety**.

The federal policy prohibits physicians from prescribing marijuana, even for seriously ill patients because of possible adverse effects, and the disputed belief that cannabis is dangerously addictive. Former U.S. attorney general Janet Reno warned that physicians in any state who prescribed marijuana could lose the privilege of writing prescriptions, be excluded from Medicare, and Medicaid reimbursement, and even be prosecuted for a federal crime, according to a 1997 editorial in the *New England Journal of Medicine*. Yet in 1996, California passed a law legalizing medical use of marijuana. By 2008, 35 states had passed legislation recognizing the medical value of marijuana and about one-third of those had either legalized or decriminalized medical use of the herb. The debate in the United States over medical use of the drug continued as of 2008. Some opponents believe that the movement to legalize marijuana for medicinal purposes is led by those who want the drug legalized for recreational purposes.

Preparations

Marijuana is ingested by smoking, which quickly delivers the active ingredients to the blood system. The dried herb is also variously prepared for eating. The essential oil consists of beta caryophyllenes, humules, caryophyllene oxide, alpha-pinenes, beta-pinenes, limonene, myrcene, and betaocimene. The oil expressed from the seeds is used for massage and in making salves used to relieve muscle strain. THC extract is available legally in some countries in capsule form.

Precautions

Marijuana is considered a Class I narcotic, and federal law in the United States has restricted its use since 1937. Penalties include fines and imprisonment in some states, but the herb has been decriminalized in others. California, for example, issues cards identifying medical marijuana users and allows them to purchase the drug openly at certain clinics.

Research has shown that cannabis acts to increase heart frequency by as much as 40 beats per minute. A study reported by the American Heart Association in February 2000 concluded that smoking marijuana can precipitate a **heart attack** in persons with pre-existing heart conditions. One hour after smoking marijuana, the likelihood of having a heart attack is four and one-half times greater than if the person had not smoked, according to the research. Marijuana also can cause a drop in blood pressure resulting in **dizziness**.

Marijuana use during **pregnancy** has been found to reduce the newborn's birth weight, a possible indication of problems. Pregnant and breastfeeding women should avoid using marijuana. Other research has shown that marijuana decreases male fertility and increases the number of abnormal sperm found in semen.

An additional health concern is the effect that marijuana smoking has on the lungs. Cannabis smoke carries more tars and other particulate matter than tobacco smoke. Long-term use is also associated with an increase in respiratory diseases such as bronchitis.

Studies have shown that motor coordination and driving ability can be impaired for up to eight hours after smoking marijuana. Individuals should avoid driving and using heavy machinery for several hours after using the herb.

Side effects

The *PDR for Herbal Medicine* reports that the most common side effect of marijuana use is psychotropic, as a euphoric state (pronounced gaiety, laughing fits) occurs almost immediately after smoking the herb. Long-term usage leads to a clear increase in tolerance for most of the pharmacological effects. Chronic use results in **laryngitis**, bronchitis, apathy, psychic decline, and disturbances of genital functions.

Some people may be hypersensitive to marijuana. They may experience paranoia or be allergic or sensitive to the plant. Chronic sinus **fungal infections** have been linked to chronic marijuana smoking. Clinical trials have shown that there is no decrease in cognitive function over time in moderate marijuana users when compared to non-users.

Interactions

Marijuana use may mask the perceived effects of alcohol and cocaine when the drugs are consumed together. Marijuana is said to exert a synergistic effect with other medicinal agents. When used with nitrous oxide it may enhance the nitrous oxide effect.

Marijuana use by individuals taking selective serotonin re-uptake inhibitors (SSRIs, used to treat **depression**) may develop manic symptoms. Use in

---

KEY TERMS

Edema—Swelling of a body tissue due to collection of fluids.

Glaucoma—An eye disorder caused by damage to the optic nerve resulting in vision loss. Glaucoma is usually accompanied by inflammation and increased pressure in the eye (intraocular pressure). There are several types that may develop suddenly or gradually.

Pharmacopeia—A book containing a list of medicinal drugs and their descriptions of preparation and use.

---

individuals taking tricyclic antidepressants can produce delirium and racing heart (tachycardia).

Resources

BOOKS

Boire, Richard, and Kevin Feeney. *Medical Marijuana Law.* Berkeley, CA: Ronin, 2006.

PDR for Herbal Medicines, 4th ed. Montvale, NJ: Thompson Healthcare, 2007.

Yarnell, Eric, and Karen Abascal. *Clinical Botanical Medicine,* 2nd rev. ed. Larchmont, NY: Mary Ann Liebert, 2008.

ORGANIZATIONS

Alternative Medicine Foundation, PO Box 60016, Potomac, MD, 20859, (301) 340-1960, http://www.amfoundation.org.

American Holistic Medical Association, PO Box 2016, Edmonds, WA, 98020, (425) 967-0737, http://www.holisticmedicin.org.

American Medical Marijuana Association, 17415 Ocean Dr., Fort Bragg, CA, 95437, http://americanmarijuana.org.

Centre for International Ethnomedicinal Education and Research (CIEER), http://www.cieer.org.

National Center for Complementary and Alternative Medicine Clearinghouse, PO Box 7923, Gaithersburg, MD, 20898, (888) 644-6226, http://nccam.nih.gov.

Clare Hanrahan
Teresa G. Odle
Tish Davidson, A.M.

Marsh mallow

Description

Marsh mallow (*Althaea officinalis*) is a perennial plant that grows in salt marshes, damp meadows, and on the banks of tidal rivers and seas. It originated in

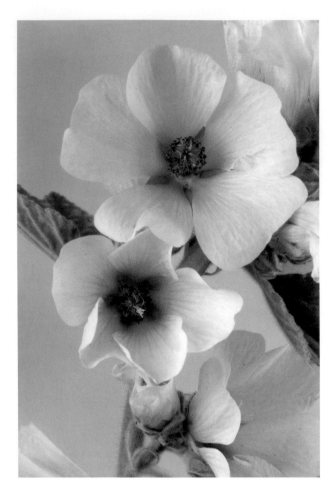

Marsh Mallow. *(© Arco Images / Alamy)*

countries adjoining the Caspian Sea, Black Sea, and in the eastern Mediterranean, and is native to Europe and western Asia. Marsh mallow is found in North America along the eastern seaboard.

The plant stems grow to a height of 3-4 ft (1-1.3 m) and have round, velvety leaves that are 2-3 in (5-7.5 cm) long. Pale pink or white flowers bloom in August or September, and the roots are thick and long. The whole plant is used medicinally. The leaves and flowers are picked when the flowers are blooming. The roots are harvested in the fall, but the plant must be two years old before the root is harvested.

The common name marsh mallow is derived from the environment in which it grows. The Latin name *Althaea* comes from the Greek word *altho*, which means to heal or to cure. The family name Malvaceae comes from the Greek word *malake*, meaning soft. Other names for marsh mallow include mallards, mauls, sweetweed, Schloss tea, and mortification root.

Marsh mallow's medicinal use dates back 2,000 years. Arabian doctors created a poultice from the leaves to treat inflammation. The father of medicine, Hippocrates, used marsh mallow to remedy **bruises** and blood loss. Dioscorides wrote about the beneficial properties of marsh mallow, while Horace praised the laxative properties of the leaves and roots. Roman doctors used marsh mallow for toothaches, insect **bites**, chilblains, and irritated skin. The Chinese, Egyptians, and Romans ate a variety of marsh mallow for food. The French eat the flowers and leaves in salads. Marsh mallow was used to soothe toothaches, insect bites, **indigestion**, and **diarrhea** in Europe during medieval times. Teething babies were often given marsh mallow root to provide comfort.

Nineteenth century doctors used the roots of marsh mallow to make a **sore throat** lozenge for children and adults. They combined the cooked juice of the root with egg whites and sugar and whipped the mixture into a meringue that later hardened into a candy. The marshmallows eaten today as sweet treats were derived from this candy, but no longer contain any herbal properties.

Marsh mallow contains starch, mucilage, pectin, oil, sugar, asparagin, phosphate of lime, glutinous matter, and cellulose. It is rich in **calcium, zinc, iron, sodium, iodine, vitamin B complex,** and **pantothenic acid**.

General use

The main therapeutic constituent of marsh mallow is mucilage, a spongy substance of the root that is composed of large sugar molecules. Mucilage's healing effect stems from its ability to support white blood cells against attacking microorganisms. When liquid is added to mucilage, it acquires a gel-like consistency. This gooey substance coats mucous membranes of the throat, mouth, stomach, and intestinal tract and provides relief from inflammation and **pain**. It also acts to expel phlegm from the lungs and to relax the bronchial tubes.

These anti-inflammatory and anti-irritant properties make marsh mallow a viable remedy for arthritis and joint pain; upper respiratory ailments such as **asthma**, **emphysema**, bronchial **infections**, coughs, sore throats, and lung congestion; inflamed kidneys and urinary tract disorders; and gastrointestinal disturbances including **Crohn's disease**, ulcers, **colitis**, diarrhea, dysentery, and stomach irritation.

The German Commission E has approved marsh mallow as a beneficial treatment for irritated and inflamed throat, pharyngeal, and gastric mucous membranes, and for dry coughs. Teas made from the root and leaf are licensed in Germany as standard medicinal teas. The root is also used as an ingredient in **cough** syrup and as a cough suppressant tea.

The British Herbal Compendium supports the use of marsh mallow for **gastroenteritis**, peptic and duodenal ulcers, colitis, and enteritis. In the United States, marsh mallow is an ingredient in dietary supplements and cough suppressants.

Marsh mallow provides external treatment for **cuts**, **wounds**, abscesses, **boils**, **burns**, and **varicose veins**. A gel created by adding water to finely chopped marsh mallow root may be applied to the affected area to reduce inflammation. A poultice containing **cayenne** and marsh mallow may relieve **blood poisoning**, **gangrene**, burns, bruises, and other wounds.

Preparations

Marsh mallow is available in whole bulk, tincture, and capsule forms. It can be taken internally as a tea, tincture, or capsule, or applied externally as an ointment or poultice.

A decoction may be made from the root to relieve congestion, sore throat, or dry cough. To create a decoction, 1-2 tsp of the finely chopped root is added to 1 cup of water and simmered for 10-15 minutes. The liquid is then cooled and strained. A person can drink 1 cup three times daily or as needed. An infusion can be made by steeping the crushed roots in cold water overnight. The infusion is then drunk as needed for symptomatic relief. For relief of an irritated kidney,

boiling water is poured over the flowers and leaves. The mixture is covered and steeped for three hours.

To make a poultice, the leaves and/or the powdered or crushed roots are steeped in water. The mixture is then applied externally to areas of inflamed skin, **eczema**, or **dermatitis**.

For capsules, 5-6 g may be taken daily or as recommended.

For a tincture, 5 ml may be taken three times daily or as recommended.

For insect bites, the leaves are rubbed on wasp or bee **stings** to alleviate pain, inflammation, and swelling.

For sore throat, the flowers are boiled in oil and water, cooled, and used as a gargle to relieve sore throat pain.

Precautions

Diabetics should take marsh mallow with caution since high doses may lower blood sugar levels.

Children and infants may take marsh mallow in low doses.

Side effects

There are no known side effects.

Interactions

Marsh mallow may slow the absorption of other drugs when taken simultaneously.

Resources

BOOKS

Lininger, D.C., Skye. *The Natural Pharmacy*. Virtual Health, LLC, 1998.
Time Life Books. *The Alternative Advisor*. Time Life Inc., 1997.

Jennifer Wurges

Martial arts

Definition

Martial arts cover a broad range of activities that involve fighting techniques, physical exercises, and methods of mental discipline, among other skills. Martial arts originated in the ancient cultures of Asia, and are used today around the world for self-defense, **exercise**, health, spiritual growth, law enforcement, and athletic competition.

Origins

Very few activities have as many legends and myths surrounding them as do martial arts. Hundreds of practices are included under the title of martial arts, and some of these were passed down in secrecy for many generations. Furthermore, martial arts developed in countries that have been historically isolated from the Western world. Thus, there are many conflicting theories and opinions concerning the origins of martial arts. What is known is that martial arts began in the ancient cultures of Asia, including China, India, and Japan. In both China and India, artifacts from 2,000 to 4,000 years old have been found with paintings of people striking possible martial arts poses. **Qigong**, one of the oldest systems that may be considered a martial art, is believed by some historians to be 5,000 years old or older, originating in ancient China. Some scholars trace the development of martial arts much later to the sixth century A.D. According to legend, that is when a Buddhist monk from India named Bodhidharma brought Buddhism, **yoga** exercises, and **meditation** techniques to the Shaolin Monastery in China.

Martial arts involve intellectual concepts as well as physical techniques, and have been influenced by many of the religious and philosophical systems of the East. The Taoist philosophy holds that the universe operates within laws of balance and harmony, and that people must live within the rhythms of nature. Martial arts cultivate these concepts of balance and adaptation to the natural flow of events. Buddhism is believed to have introduced breathing methods, meditation, and techniques of mental and spiritual awareness to the early founders of martial arts. Chinese Confucianism was concerned with ethical behavior in daily life, and martial arts often address these concerns. Some martial arts, such as **t'ai chi** and various kung fu methods, developed from qigong. Qigong, which means "energy cultivation," is a system designed to increase the flow of the body's *qi*, the universal life energy responsible for health and strength according to Chinese philosophy. **Traditional Chinese medicine** also incorporates concepts derived from martial arts to better the understanding of the body and health. Because therapeutic exercise is one of the major modalities of treatment in traditional Chinese medicine, some martial arts masters are also expert healers. There is, in fact, a subtype of qigong known as medical qigong in China, used to treat a wide range of diseases and disorders. Although most of the research in medical qigong has been conducted in China, some of this work has been translated into English. A video is available that presents the basic concepts of medical qigong.

KEY TERMS

Dojo—A martial arts school.

Meridian—Channel through which qi travels in the body.

Qi—Basic life energy according to traditional Chinese medicine.

Qigong—Chinese system of energy cultivation techniques.

Yin/Yang—Universal characteristics used to describe aspects of the natural world.

From China, martial arts spread to other Asian countries, and eventually arrived in Japan, where many new variations developed. Karate is the generic term for Japanese martial arts. Martial arts in Japan have been influenced by Zen Buddhism and by the samurai warrior tradition, which refined many weapons as well as methods of fighting. Some Japanese schools of instruction adopted the values of bushido, Japanese for "way of the warrior." This system insists on extreme physical and mental discipline, using martial arts as a means to spiritual enlightenment. Martial arts also flourished in Korea, Vietnam, and Thailand.

Martial arts were largely unknown to the Western world until after 1945, when a few American and British veterans of World War II brought back Japanese martial arts from occupied Japan. During the 1970s, there was a surge of interest in martial arts in America, due to several popular television shows and the charismatic actor Bruce Lee. With better communication and less secrecy among teachers, Chinese martial arts, including t'ai chi and qigong, have made their way to America. Today, there are martial arts schools all across America, and martial arts are a multi-billion dollar industry. Martial arts are a popular activity for self-defense, sport, exercise, **spirituality**, and health around the world. Present-day forms of martial arts include *kalarippayattu* in southern India, *escrima* in the Philippines, *pentjak silat* in Malaysia, *karate* in Okinawa, *aikido* in Japan, and *capoeira* in Brazil.

Benefits

Martial arts teach self-defense, and can improve confidence and self-esteem. When used as exercise, martial arts can improve balance, strength, stamina, flexibility, and posture. They also enhance weight loss and improve muscle tone. On the mental level, martial arts can teach **stress** management, improve concentration, and increase willpower. Some martial arts, such as qigong and t'ai chi, are used for longevity, disease prevention, and healing purposes, making them effective exercises for those with health conditions and for the elderly. Some teachers claim that martial arts can be used as spiritual practices, bringing balance, peace, and wisdom to dedicated practitioners.

Description

Basic concepts of martial arts

Many martial arts utilize basic concepts of traditional Chinese philosophy. Qi is the fundamental life energy of the universe. In the body, qi is the invisible vital force that sustains life. Qi is present in food, air, water, and sunlight. The breath is believed to account for the largest quantity of human qi, because the body uses air more than any other substance. All martial arts emphasize breathing techniques. Many movements and mental exercises are designed to improve the flow of qi in the body, which improves overall strength. There are many legends concerning martial arts masters who had such control of their qi that they could throw opponents across rooms merely by looking at them. Martial arts that focus on the development and use of qi are termed internal martial arts. In contrast, external martial arts focus on physical exercises, fighting methods, and the use of weapons. Many martial arts combine internal and external methods.

Qi travels through the body along channels of energy called meridians. On the meridians there are certain points (acupoints) where qi accumulates. Some martial arts teach defensive techniques that utilize the knowledge of these points on the body, which, if pressed in the correct manner, can be used to immobilize attackers. Martial arts also teach massage and exercise techniques that are designed to stimulate the energy flow along the meridians to improve health.

The concepts of yin and yang are also central to the martial arts. Yin and yang are the two separate but complimentary principles of the universe, which are always interacting, opposing, and influencing each other. Yin is associated with such qualities as cold, passivity, darkness, yielding, and inward movement. Yang is associated with heat, activity, light, assertiveness, outward movement, and so on. In martial arts, yin and yang movements are used to balance each other. For instance, a strong (yang) attack is taught to be met by a yin, or yielding, response. Martial arts cultivate an awareness and use of yin or passive qualities, which are ignored by many sports and fighting techniques. Another major yin/yang concept used in

martial arts is that the more one becomes familiar with violence, the more one learns to avoid and resist it. Some martial arts, such as aikido, teach peace as their ultimate lesson.

Types of martial arts

Although there are hundreds of different martial arts, many of them have more similarities than differences. Within the major categories, there are often many sub-schools and systems developed by different teachers. Martial arts are generally classified as soft or hard, internal or external, yin or yang, but they all need to embrace these complementary aspects. Internal arts such as qigong focus on yielding and inner strength. Hard arts such as karate focus on developing muscular power and speed, and the mastery of breaking and throwing techniques delivered with devastating impact.

Karate means "empty handed." This form of fighting originated on the Japanese island of Okinawa. Karate is now the general term for an entire group of Japanese martial arts. Karate emphasizes offensive and defensive moves, and avoids grappling and wrestling. Students are taught how to deliver quick, powerful blows with nearly every part of the body, including dangerous kicks with the legs. Karate also consists of hard styles and soft styles. Some schools teach "full contact" karate, for which students wear protective equipment to absorb the blows of actual fighting.

Kung fu means "skill" in Chinese, and is the generic term for a whole spectrum of martial arts methods that developed in China. In China, kung fu is called *wushu*. Kung fu consists of thousands of hard and soft techniques, taught for both offensive and defensive positions. Kung fu uses punching, kicking, grappling, and blocking moves in addition to the use of certain weapons. Kung fu may also emphasize internal methods to increase and improve qi energy.

Aikido is a relatively new martial art, developed in the 1930s by a Japanese teacher named Morihei Ueshiba (1883–1969). Ueshiba was a religious man who wanted to invent a martial art that emphasized non-aggression. In Japanese, aikido means "connecting with life energy." Aikido teaches students a variety of techniques to disarm an attacker, including such defense moves as blocks, escapes, grabs, and falling safely to the ground. Aikido also teaches internal methods of cultivating qi energy. Aikido has been called the "way of peace," because it teaches the philosophical ideals of love and harmony as ways of reducing conflict.

Judo means "gentle way" in Japanese and was developed as an educational tool by a teacher named

Jigoro Kano in the 1800s. Judo emphasizes such defensive moves as holds and grappling, and teaches students how to disarm attackers by applying pressure to specific sensitive points on the body. Judo is performed competitively in matches.

T'ai chi chuan, also called t'ai chi, consists of a sequence of flowing movements performed very slowly. These movements emphasize posture and the flow of the body's energy (qi). Although considered a martial art and consisting of fighting postures, tai chi is used more as a meditation and health technique. In China, millions of people, particularly the elderly, use tai chi daily to improve their health and flexibility. T'ai chi developed from qigong and shares many of the same concepts of energy cultivation, making it effective for healing and prevention of illness.

Jujitsu is a Japanese martial art that emphasizes flexibility, quickness, and fluidity of motion. It consists of kicking, punching, holding, and striking moves as well as the use of weapons. *Tae kwon do* is a Korean martial art that means "kick-punch-art." Tae kwon do consists of a variety of powerful kicking and punching techniques. *Kendo* is traditional Japanese sword fighting, teaching students how to use various weapons with agility, speed, and effectiveness. Kendo also emphasizes discipline and ethics.

A martial arts session

Most martial arts classes, held in schools called *dojos*, have similarities. Sessions begin with warm-up exercises and stretches. Then, depending on the school, certain exercises will be performed to improve strength, speed, and stamina. Sparring is often used, with students competing head to head. Some schools require students to stop short of striking one another, while other schools require students to wear equipment to protect them from authentic blows. Exercises for cooling down and for flexibility are performed at the end of class.

Most martial arts use the colored belt system to rank students, although colors and rankings can vary greatly among disciplines. In general, white belts signify beginners, brown belts represent intermediate students, and black belts are given to masters, with other colors in between.

Martial arts classes take between one to two hours. Some schools allow students to attend as many classes per week as they wish, while others limit the number of classes taken. Two to three classes per week are recommended. Schools often charge a monthly fee, ranging from $50 or more. Some schools charge a flat fee for training from beginner to expert. Many schools require students to regularly participate in competitions, and fees for these may begin at $25. Students are required to purchase uniforms and equipment as well. Uniforms may cost $100 or more, and protective equipment may cost roughly the same, depending on the practice.

Preparations

Prospective martial arts students should search for the style of martial arts that best meets their objectives. Students should attend classes at various schools (dojos), and should talk to students and teachers to find the right program. Finding a good instructor may be even more important than finding the right school. Students should search for instructors with such positive qualities as patience, knowledge, and strong communication skills. Prospective students should also search for schools with adequate facilities, including padded or sprung floors, full-length mirrors, and roomy practice spaces without obstructions.

Precautions

Martial arts can be dangerous. Students are often required to take blows and falls as part of the learning process, as well as to fight with weapons. Students should search for teachers and schools who teach these methods as safely as possible. People with health conditions and injuries should consult a physician before attempting a martial art, and should find a teacher familiar with their condition.

Training and certification

Martial arts teachers are usually certified with the achievement of an advanced black belt status. Many large schools of martial arts have organizations which oversee and certify the granting of belt ranks. The Aikido Association of America recognizes training programs and certifies ranking procedures.

The USA Karate Federation is the largest organization for certifying ranking systems and schools of karate. The Chinese Kung-Fu Wu-Su Association works with kung fu schools, ranking systems, and contests.

Resources

BOOKS

Cleary, Thomas. *The Japanese Art of War*. Boston: Shambhala, 1991.

Frantzis, Bruce. *The Power of Internal Martial Arts*. Berkeley, CA: North Atlantic, 1998.

Payne, Peter. *Martial Arts: The Spiritual Dimension*. New York: Thames and Hudson, 1981.

Stevens, John. *The Shambhala Guide to Aikido*. Boston: Shambhala, 1996.

PERIODICALS

Aikido Today. PO Box 1060, Claremont, CA 91711. (800) 445-AIKI.

Golden, Jane. "Qigong and Tai Chi as Energy Medicine." *Share Guide* (November-December 2001): 37.

Inside Kung Fu. PO Box 461621, Escondido, CA 92046. (800) 877-5528.

Johnson, Jerry Alan. "Medical Qigong for Breast Disease." *Share Guide* (November-December 2001): 109.

ORGANIZATIONS

Chinese Kung-Fu Wu-Su Association. 28 West 27th Street, New York, NY 10001. (212) 725-0535.

USA Karate Federation.1300 Kenmore Boulevard, Akron, OH 44314. (330) 753-3114.

Douglas Dupler
Rebecca J. Frey, PhD

Massage therapy

Definition

Massage therapy is the scientific manipulation of the soft tissues of the body for the purpose of normalizing those tissues and consists of manual techniques that include applying fixed or movable pressure, holding, and/or causing movement of or to the body.

Origins

Massage therapy is one of the oldest health care practices known to history. References to massage are found in Chinese medical texts more than 4,000 years old. Massage has been advocated in Western health care practices at least since the time of Hippocrates,

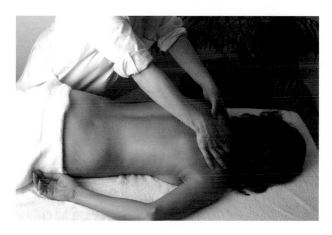

Woman having neck and shoulders massaged. *(© Bubbles Photolibrary / Alamy)*

the "Father of Medicine." In the fourth century B.C. Hippocrates wrote, "The physician must be acquainted with many things and assuredly with rubbing" (the ancient Greek term for massage was rubbing).

The roots of modern, scientific massage therapy go back to Per Henrik Ling (1776–1839), a Swede, who developed an integrated system consisting of massage and active and passive exercises. Ling established the Royal Central Gymnastic Institute in Sweden in 1813 to teach his methods.

Modern, scientific massage therapy was introduced in the United States in the 1850s by two New York physicians, brothers George and Charles Taylor, who had studied in Sweden. The first clinics for massage therapy in the United States were opened by two Swedish physicians after the Civil War period. Doctor Baron Nils Posse operated the Posse Institute in Boston and Doctor Hartwig Nissen opened the Swedish Health Institute near the Capitol in Washington, D.C.

Although there were periods when massage fell out of favor, in the 1960s it made a comeback in a different way as a tool for **relaxation**, communication, and alternative healing. Today, massage is one of the most popular healing modalities. It is used by conventional, as well as alternative, medical communities and is now covered by some health insurance plans.

Benefits

Generally, massage is known to affect the circulation of blood and the flow of blood and lymph, reduce muscular tension or flaccidity, affect the nervous system through stimulation or sedation, and enhance tissue healing. These effects provide a number of benefits:

- reduction of muscle tension and stiffness
- relief of muscle spasms
- greater flexibility and range of motion
- increase of the ease and efficiency of movement
- relief of stress and aide of relaxation
- promotion of deeper and easier breathing
- improvement of the circulation of blood and movement of lymph
- relief of tension-related conditions, such as headaches and eyestrain
- promotion of faster healing of soft tissue injuries, such as pulled muscles and sprained ligaments, and reduction in pain and swelling related to such injuries
- reduction in the formation of excessive scar tissue following soft tissue injuries
- enhancement in the health and nourishment of skin

- improvement in posture through changing tension patterns that affect posture
- reduction in stress and an excellent stress management tool
- creation of a feeling of well-being
- reduction in levels of anxiety
- increase in awareness of the mind-body connection
- promotion of a relaxed state of mental awareness

Massage therapy also has a number of documented clinical benefits. For example, massage can reduce **anxiety**, improve pulmonary function in young **asthma** patients, reduce psycho-emotional distress in persons suffering from chronic **inflammatory bowel disease**, increase weight and improve motor development in premature infants, and may enhance immune system functioning. Some medical conditions that massage therapy can help are: **allergies**, anxiety and **stress**, arthritis, asthma and **bronchitis**, **carpal tunnel syndrome** and other repetitive motion injuries, chronic and temporary **pain**, circulatory problems, **depression**, digestive disorders, tension **headache**, **insomnia**, myofascial pain, sports injuries, and temporomandibular joint dysfunction.

Description

Massage therapy is the scientific manipulation of the soft tissues of the body for the purpose of normalizing those tissues and consists of a group of manual techniques that include applying fixed or movable pressure, holding, and/or causing movement of or to the body. While massage therapy is applied primarily with the hands, sometimes the forearms or elbows are used. These techniques affect the muscular, skeletal, circulatory, lymphatic, nervous, and other systems of the body. The basic philosophy of massage therapy embraces the concept of *vis Medicatrix naturae*, which is aiding the ability of the body to heal itself, and is aimed at achieving or increasing health and well-being.

Touch is the fundamental medium of massage therapy. While massage can be described in terms of the type of techniques performed, touch is not used solely in a mechanistic way in massage therapy. One could look at a diagram or photo of a massage technique that depicts where to place one's hands and what direction the stroke should go, but this would not convey everything that is important for giving a good massage. Massage also has an artistic component.

Because massage usually involves applying touch with some degree of pressure and movement, the massage therapist must use touch with sensitivity in order to determine the optimal amount of pressure to use for each person. For example, using too much pressure may cause the body to tense up, while using too little may not have enough effect. Touch used with sensitivity also allows the massage therapist to receive useful information via his or her hands about the client's body, such as locating areas of muscle tension and other soft tissue problems. Because touch is also a form of communication, sensitive touch can convey a sense of caring—an essential element in the therapeutic relationship—to the person receiving massage.

In practice, many massage therapists use more than one technique or method in their work and sometimes combine several. Effective massage therapists ascertain each person's needs and then use the techniques that will meet those needs best.

Swedish massage uses a system of long gliding strokes, kneading, and friction techniques on the more superficial layers of muscles, generally in the direction of blood flow toward the heart, and sometimes combined with active and passive movements of the joints. It is used to promote general relaxation, improve circulation and range of motion, and relieve muscle tension. Swedish massage is the most commonly used form of massage.

Deep tissue massage is used to release chronic patterns of muscular tension using slow strokes, direct pressure, or friction directed across the grain of the muscles. It is applied with greater pressure and to deeper layers of muscle than Swedish, which is why it is called deep tissue and is effective for chronic muscular tension.

Sports massage uses techniques that are similar to Swedish and deep tissue, but are specially adapted to deal with the effects of athletic performance on the body and the needs of athletes regarding training, performing, and recovery from injury.

Neuromuscular massage is a form of deep massage that is applied to individual muscles. It is used primarily to release trigger points (intense knots of muscle tension that refer pain to other parts of the body), and also to increase blood flow. It is often used to reduce pain. Trigger point massage and **myotherapy** are similar forms.

Acupressure applies finger or thumb pressure to specific points located on the **acupuncture** meridians (channels of energy flow identified in Asian concepts of anatomy) in order to release blocked energy along these meridians that causes physical discomforts, and re-balance the energy flow. **Shiatsu** is a Japanese form of acupressure.

The cost of massage therapy varies according to geographic location, experience of the massage therapist, and length of the massage. In the United States, the average range is from $35-60 for a one hour session. Massage therapy sessions at a client's home or office may cost more due to travel time for the massage therapist. Most sessions are one hour. Frequency of massage sessions can vary widely. If a person is receiving massage for a specific problem, frequency can vary widely based on the condition, though it usually will be once a week. Some people incorporate massage into their regular personal health and fitness program. They will go for massage on a regular basis, varying from once a week to once a month.

The first appointment generally begins with information gathering, such as the reason for getting massage therapy, physical condition and medical history, and other areas. The client is asked to remove clothing to one's level of comfort. Undressing takes place in private, and a sheet or towel is provided for draping. The massage therapist will undrape only the part of the body being massaged. The client's modesty is respected at all times. The massage therapist may use an oil or cream, which will be absorbed into the skin in a short time.

To receive the most benefit from a massage, generally the person being massaged should give the therapist accurate health information, report discomfort of any kind (whether it's from the massage itself or due to the room temperature or any other distractions), and be as receptive and open to the process as possible.

Insurance coverage for massage therapy varies widely. There tends to be greater coverage in states that license massage therapy. In most cases, a physician's prescription for massage therapy is needed. Once massage therapy is prescribed, authorization from the insurer may be needed if coverage is not clearly spelled out in one's policy or plan.

Preparations

Going for a massage requires little in the way of preparation. Generally, one should be clean and should not eat just before a massage. One should not be under the influence of alcohol or non-medicinal drugs. Massage therapists generally work by appointment and usually will provide information about how to prepare for an appointment at the time of making the appointment.

Precautions

Massage is comparatively safe; however it is generally contraindicated, i.e., it should not be used, if a person has one of the following conditions: advanced heart diseases, **hypertension** (high blood pressure), **phlebitis**, thrombosis, embolism, kidney failure, **cancer** if massage would accelerate metastasis (i.e., spread a tumor) or damage tissue that is fragile due to chemotherapy or other treatment, infectious diseases, contagious skin conditions, acute inflammation, infected injuries, unhealed **fractures**, dislocations, **frostbite**, large hernias, torn ligaments, conditions prone to hemorrhage, and psychosis.

Massage should not be used locally on affected areas (i.e., avoid using massage on the specific areas of the body that are affected by the condition) for the following conditions: **rheumatoid arthritis** flare up, **eczema**, goiter, and open skin lesions. Massage may be used on the areas of the body that are not affected by these conditions.

In some cases, precautions should be taken before using massage for the following conditions: **pregnancy**, high fevers, **osteoporosis**, diabetes, recent postoperative cases in which pain and muscular splinting (i.e., tightening as a protective reaction) would be increased, apprehension, and mental conditions that may impair communication or perception. In such cases, massage may or may not be appropriate. The decision on whether to use massage must be based on whether it may cause harm. For example, if someone has osteoporosis, the concern is whether bones are strong enough to withstand the pressure applied. If one has a health condition and has any hesitation about whether massage therapy would be appropriate, a physician should be consulted.

Side effects

Massage therapy does not have side effects. Sometimes people are concerned that massage may leave them too relaxed or too mentally unfocused. To the contrary, massage tends to leave people feeling more relaxed and alert.

Research and general acceptance

Before 1939, more than 600 research studies on massage appeared in the main journals of medicine in English. However, the pace of research was slowed by medicine's disinterest in massage therapy.

Massage therapy research picked up again in the 1980s, as the growing popularity of massage paralleled the growing interest in complementary and alternative medicine. Well designed studies have documented the benefits of massage therapy for the treatment of acute and chronic pain, acute and chronic inflammation, chronic lymphedema, **nausea**, muscle spasm, various soft tissue dysfunctions, anxiety, depression, insomnia, and psycho-emotional stress, which may aggravate mental illness.

Premature infants treated with daily massage therapy gain more weight and have shorter hospital stays than infants who are not massaged. A study of 40 low-birth-weight babies found that the 20 massaged babies had a 47% greater weight gain per day and stayed in the hospital an average of six days less than 20 infants who did not receive massage, resulting a cost savings of approximately $3,000 per infant. Cocaine-exposed, preterm infants given massage three times daily for a 10 day period showed significant improvement. Results indicated that massaged infants had fewer postnatal complications and exhibited fewer stress behaviors during the 10 day period, had a 28% greater daily weight gain, and demonstrated more mature motor behaviors.

A study comparing 52 hospitalized depressed and adjustment disorder children and adolescents with a control group that viewed relaxation videotapes, found massage therapy subjects were less depressed and anxious, and had lower saliva cortisol levels (an indicator of less depression).

Another study showed massage therapy produced relaxation in 18 elderly subjects, demonstrated in measures such as decreased blood pressure and heart rate and increased skin temperature.

A combination of massage techniques for 52 subjects with traumatically induced spinal pain led to significant improvements in acute and chronic pain and increased muscle flexibility and tone. This study also found massage therapy to be extremely cost effective, with cost savings ranging from 15-50%. Massage has also been shown to stimulate the body's ability to naturally control pain by stimulating the brain to produce endorphins. **Fibromyalgia** is an example of a condition that may be favorably affected by this effect.

A pilot study of five subjects with symptoms of tension and anxiety found a significant response to massage therapy in one or more psycho-physiological parameters of heart rate, frontalis and forearm extensor electromyograms (EMGs) and skin resistance, which demonstrate relaxation of muscle tension and reduced anxiety.

Lymph drainage massage has been shown to be more effective than mechanized methods or diuretic drugs to control lymphedema secondary to radical mastectomy, consequently using massage to control lymphedema would significantly lower treatment costs. A study found that massage therapy can have a powerful effect upon psycho-emotional distress in persons suffering from chronic inflammatory bowel disease. Massage therapy was effective in reducing the frequency of episodes of pain and disability in these patients.

Massage may enhance the immune system. A study suggests an increase in cytotoxic capacity associated with massage. A study of **chronic fatigue syndrome** subjects found that a group receiving massage therapy had lower depression, emotional distress, and somatic symptom scores, more hours of sleep, and lower epinephrine and cortisol levels than a control group.

Training and certification

The generally accepted standard for training is a minimum of 500 classroom hours. Training should include anatomy, physiology, pathology, massage theory and technique, and supervised practice. Most massage therapists also take additional courses and workshops during their careers.

In the United States, massage therapists are currently licensed by states, the District of Columbia, and a number of localities. Most states require 500 or more classroom hours of training from a recognized training program and passing an examination.

A national certification program was inaugurated in June 1992 by the National Certification Board for Therapeutic Massage and Bodywork (NCBTMB). The NCBTMB program is accredited by the National Commission for Certifying Agencies, the chief outside agency for evaluating certification programs. Those certified can use the title Nationally Certified in Therapeutic Massage and Bodywork (NCTMB). Most states use the NCBTMB exam for their licensing exams.

A national accreditation agency, the Commission on Massage Therapy Accreditation, designed according to the guidelines of the U.S. Department of Education, currently recognizes about 70 training programs. The Accrediting Commission of Career Schools and Colleges of Technology and the Accrediting Council for Continuing Education and Training also accredit massage training programs.

Resources

BOOKS

Beck, Mark F. *Milady's Theory and Practice of Therapeutic Massage*. Milady Publishing, 1994.

Capellini, Steve. *Massage Therapy Career Guide for Hands-On Success*. Milady Publishing, 1998.

Downing, George. *The Massage Book*. New York: Random House, 1998.

Loving, Jean E. *Massage Therapy: Theory and Practice*. Appleton & Lange, 1998.

PERIODICALS

Field, T., W. Sunshine, M. Hernandez-Reif, and O. Quintino. "Chronic fatigue syndrome: massage therapy effects on depression and somatic symptoms in chronic fatigue syndrome." *J Chronic Fatigue Syndrome* (1997):43-51.

Ironson, G., T. Field, F. Scafidi, and M. Hashimoto. "Massage therapy is associated with enhancement of the immune system's cytotoxic capacity." *Int J Neuroscience* (February 1996):205-217.

Joachim, G. "The effects of two stress management techniques on feelings of well-being in patients with inflammatory bowel disease." *Nursing Papers* (1983):4, 5-18.

Kaarda, B., and O. Tosteinbo. "Increase of plasma beta-endorphins in connective tissue massage." *Gen pharmacology* (1989): 487-489.

Scafidi, F., T. Field, A. Wheeden, S. Schanberg, C. Kuhn, R. Symanski, E. Zimmerman, and E.S. Bandstra. "Cocaine exposed preterm neonates show behavioral and hormonal differences." *Pediatrics* (June 1996):851-855.

Weintraub, M. "Shiatsu, Swedish muscle massage, and trigger point suppression in spinal pain syndrome." *Am Massage Therapy J* Summer 1992; 31:3; 99-1 09.

ORGANIZATIONS

American Massage Therapy Association. www.amtamassage.org.

Elliot Greene

Mastitis *see* **Breastfeeding problems**

McDougall diet

Definition

The McDougall diet provides the structure of a low-fat, starch-based diet to promote a broad range of such health benefits as weight loss and the reversal of such serious health conditions as heart disease , without the use of drugs.

Origins

The McDougall diet began as a challenge to Dr. John McDougall by one of his patients. The patient simply asked him if he believed that diet is connected to the health problems he saw in his patients. At that time, McDougall believed the answer to this question was a definite no. The patient challenged him to ask his patients what they were eating, in order to see if there might be any relationship between their eating habits and their diseases. McDougall agreed, and the McDougall diet was born.

McDougall was a plantation physician based in the village of Honokaa, Hawaii. In his practice, he handled a variety of medical problems from delivering babies to performing brain surgery on accident victims. Although he felt a lot of satisfaction in saving people's lives, McDougall was bothered by his inability to help patients with such disease conditions as diabetes, heart disease, high blood pressure and strokes. He decided to further his education and took up another residency in internal medicine. During his internal medicine residency, McDougall did countless hours of research on the effects of diet and lifestyle on chronic illnesses. Unfortunately, the literature he read seemed to conflict with the approaches he was being taught in his residency.

McDougall began to change his own diet as he studied the literature. Over a period of a year, he began to cut out meat and dairy products and began to focus on eating more green and yellow vegetables, fruits, and whole grains. He noticed many improvements in his own health, such as lower weight, lower blood **cholesterol** levels, and lower blood pressure. The St. Helena Hospital and Health Center in Deer Park, California offered him an opportunity to present his diet program at their facilities in 1986.

Benefits

Many patients who have undertaken the McDougall diet have found an improvement in such conditions as:

- high blood pressure
- diabetes
- headaches
- constipation
- mild arthritis
- fatigue
- body odor
- oily skin
- allergies

Another possible benefit of the McDougall program is that patients may find themselves spending less for food. In addition, McDougall points to the possibility of saving considerable amounts of money by avoiding serious and costly health problems.

Description

The McDougall diet focuses on adopting a dietary regimen and lifestyle that encourages human beings' natural tendencies to be healthy. The program is based on proper foods, moderate **exercise**, adequate sunshine, clean air and water, and surroundings that promote psychological well-being.

Specifically, the McDougall diet is a very low-fat, starch-based program. Grains, fruits and such starchy plant foods as beans, corn, pastas, potatoes, and rice provide the major components of this diet. There are some fruits and vegetables used in this program that may be quite unfamiliar to the average person. Some of these include carambola, guava, persimmon, passion fruit, daikon, endive, fava beans, bok choy, kale, kohlrabi, taro root and watercress, to name a few. In addition, some of these foods are more easily obtained and less expensive in Hawaii than they might be in the upper Midwest or Canada.

Dairy products are not used in the McDougall diet. McDougall believes that many **allergies** and such conditions as post-nasal drip are related to people's use of dairy products.

Preparations

Patients should check with their physician before they begin this or any other diet and exercise program if they have any health problems such as **heart disease**, high blood pressure, diabetes, or arthritis. People who have a major health problem, or who are on medication, should request a doctor's examination before starting this program. This examination should include a complete history and thorough medical workup to use as a baseline evaluation for performance on this program.

McDougall recommends that patients spend some time evaluating their reasons for undertaking this program. Patients should determine how well they think they will be able to stick to the program for the initial 12 days as well as whether they can stay with the program for life. Examining any aspects of their lifestyle that are harmful to their health is also important. For example, **smoking** tobacco, drinking coffee, drinking alcohol, and the use of recreational drugs are all very damaging to anyone's health. Since few people can leave their normal environment for 12 days (as people do at the live-in McDougall diet program at the St. Helena Hospital and Health Center), they may find it stressful to work on these lifestyle problems at the same time they are making radical changes in their diet.

Those undertaking this program should also prepare family and friends for the changes this program will cause in their diet. They may find their families unwilling to change, and this fact will require a different approach to the program. On the other hand, McDougall points out that family members often decide to undertake the program themselves when they see the positive changes that result from the diet.

Before undertaking the program, patients will need to stock their pantry with new foods. They will also need to check the availability of the acceptable products in their local grocery and health food stores.

Precautions

Patients should not undertake this diet program without the advice of a physician if they have any health condition or are currently on medication.

Side effects

The primary negative side effect of the McDougall diet usually comes from **caffeine** withdrawal. Many people find they suffer from headaches while abstaining from caffeine. Although giving up caffeine is not required by the program, it is strongly recommended.

Research and general acceptance

There is extensive research about the effect of lifestyle and diet on various health conditions, although research on the McDougall diet specifically has not yet been released. Anecdotal evidence suggests, however, that significant improvement in some health problems can be achieved in a relatively short period of time.

Training and certification

The McDougall diet is self-administered. No training or certification is required.

Resources

BOOKS

McDougall, John A., M.D. *The McDougall Program: 12 Days to Dynamic Health*. New York: Penguin Group, 1990.

McDougall, John A., M.D. *The McDougall Program for Women: What Every Woman Needs to Know to Be Healthy for Life*. New York: Penguin Group, 1999.

ORGANIZATIONS

The McDougall Wellness Center. P.O. Box 14039. Santa Rosa, CA 95402. (707) 576-1654. http://www.crmcdougall.com

Kim Sharp

MCTs *see* **Medium-chain triglycerides**

Measles

Definition

Measles is a viral infection that causes an illness displaying a characteristic skin rash known as an exanthem. Measles is also sometimes called rubeola, five-day measles, or hard measles.

Description

Measles **infections** appear all over the world. Incidence of the disease in the United States is down to a record low and only 86 confirmed cases were reported in the year 2000. Of these, 62% were definitely linked to foreigners or international travel. Prior to the current effective immunization program, large-scale measles outbreaks occurred on a two to three year cycle, usually in the winter and spring. Smaller outbreaks occurred during the off-years. Babies up to about eight

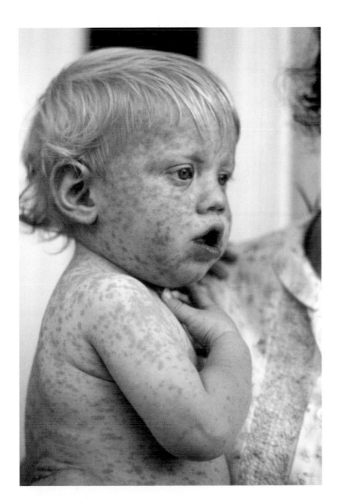

Small child with measles. (Lowell Georgia / Photo Researchers, Inc.)

months of age are usually protected from contracting measles, due to antibodies they receive from their mothers in the uterus. Once someone has had measles, he or she can never get it again.

Causes and symptoms

Measles is caused by a type of virus called a paramyxovirus. It is an extremely contagious infection, spread through the tiny droplets that may spray into the air when a person carrying the virus sneezes or coughs. About 85% of those people exposed to the virus will become infected with it. About 95% of those people infected with the virus will develop the illness. Once someone is infected with the virus, it takes about seven to 18 days before he or she actually becomes ill. The most contagious time period is the three to five days before symptoms begin through about four days after the characteristic measles rash has begun to appear.

The first signs of measles infection are **fever**, extremely runny nose, red, runny eyes, and a **cough**. A few days later, a rash appears in the mouth, particularly on the mucous membrane that lines the insides of the cheek. This rash consists of tiny white dots (like grains of salt or sand) on a reddish bump. These are called Koplik's spots, and are unique to measles infection. The throat becomes red, swollen, and sore.

A couple of days after the appearance of the Koplik's spots, the measles rash begins. It appears in a characteristic progression, from the head, face, and neck, to the trunk, then abdomen, and next out along the arms and legs. The rash starts out as flat, red patches, but eventually develops some bumps. The rash may be somewhat itchy. When the rash begins to appear, the fever usually climbs higher, sometimes reaching as high as 105°F (40.5°C). There may be **nausea**, **vomiting**, **diarrhea**, and multiple swollen lymph nodes. The cough is usually more problematic at this point, and the patient feels awful. The rash usually lasts about five days. As it fades, it turns a brownish color, and eventually the affected skin becomes dry and flaky.

Many patients (about 5–15%) develop other complications. Bacterial infections, such as ear infections, sinus infections, and **pneumonia** are common, especially in children. Other viral infections may also strike the patient, including **croup**, **bronchitis**, **laryngitis**, or viral pneumonia. Inflammation of the liver, appendix, intestine, or lymph nodes within the abdomen may cause other complications. Rarely, inflammation of the heart or kidneys, a drop in platelet count (causing episodes of difficult-to-control bleeding), or reactivation of an old **tuberculosis** infection can occur.

An extremely serious complication of measles infection is the inflammation and subsequent swelling of the brain. Called encephalitis, this can occur up to several weeks after the basic measles symptoms have resolved. About one out of every 1,000 patients develops this complication, and about 10–15% of these patients die. Symptoms include fever, **headache**, sleepiness, seizures, and coma. Long-term problems following recovery from measles encephalitis may include seizures and mental retardation.

A very rare complication of measles can occur up to 10 years or more following the initial infection. Called subacute sclerosing panencephalitis, this is a slowly progressing, smoldering, swelling, and destruction of the entire brain. It is most common among people who had measles infection prior to the age of two years. Symptoms include changes in personality, decreased intelligence with accompanying school problems, decreased coordination, and involuntary jerks and movements of the body. As the disease progresses, the patient becomes increasingly dependent, ultimately becoming bedridden and unaware of his or her surroundings. Blindness may develop, and the temperature may spike (rise rapidly) and fall unpredictably as the brain structures responsible for temperature regulation are affected. Death is inevitable.

Measles during **pregnancy** is a serious disease, leading to increased risk of a miscarriage or stillbirth. In addition, the mother's illness may progress to pneumonia.

Diagnosis

Measles is almost always diagnosed based on its characteristic symptoms, including Koplik's spots, and a rash that spreads from central body structures out towards the arms and legs. If there is any doubt as to the diagnosis, then a specimen of body fluids (mucus or urine) can be collected and combined with fluorescent-tagged measles virus antibodies. Antibodies are produced by the body's immune cells that can recognize and bind to markers (antigens) on the outside of specific organisms, in this case the measles virus. Once the fluorescent antibodies have attached themselves to the measles antigens in the specimen, the specimen can be viewed under a special microscope to verify the presence of the measles virus.

Treatment

There are a variety of general measures that can be taken to treat measles and help the patient feel more comfortable. These include:

- humidifying the air to ease cough
- drinking plenty of fluids to prevent dehydration
- keeping the room lights dim to relieve sensitivity to light
- getting plenty of rest
- eating nutritious and easily digestible food

Herbals and Chinese medicine

There are specific **acupuncture** and **acupressure** therapies for measles. The following herbals can also help relieve the symptoms associated with measles:

- Chamomile tea for restlessness.
- Echinacea plus goldenseal to clear infection, boost the immune system, and soothe skin and mucous membranes.
- A tea of lemon balm leaf, chamomile flower, peppermint leaf, licorice root, and elder flower to reduce fever and chills and increase perspiration.
- Ginger tea to reduce fever.
- Shiitake mushrooms to boost the immune system.
- Witch hazel (*Hamamelis virginiana*), chickweed (*Stellaria media*), or oatmeal baths to reduce itching.
- Eyebright (*Euphrasia officinalis*) eyewash to soothe eyes.
- Garlic to fight infection and boost the immune system.
- *Flos lonicerae* (10 g) and *Radix glycyrrhizae* (3 g) decoction to wash the mouth, eyes, and nose.

Supplements

Some studies have shown that children with measles encephalitis or pneumonia benefit from relatively large doses of **vitamin A**. Vitamin A may also heal mucous membranes. Bioflavinoids and **vitamin C** boost the immune system. **Zinc** promotes healing and is an immune system stimulant. Zinc can cause nausea and vomiting, and chronic use can cause low levels of **copper** and iron-deficiency **anemia**.

Homeopathy

Homeopathic remedies cater to the patient's specific symptoms. Remedies for common measles symptoms are listed. The patient can take 30x or 9c of the following remedies four times daily for two days:

- Apis mellifica: for swollen throat, breathing difficulty, and painful cough.
- Arsenicum album: for restlessness, feeling worse after midnight, and thirst.
- Belladonna: for high fever, red eyes, flushed face, headache, and swallowing difficulty.
- Gelsemium: for fever, droopy eyes, cough, feeling cold, and runny nose.
- Pulsatilla: for eye problems (tears, drainage, light sensitivity), dark red rash, thick yellow nasal discharge, and dry cough.

Allopathic treatment

There are no medications available to cure measles. Treatment is primarily aimed at helping the patient to be as comfortable as possible, and watching carefully so that antibiotics can be started promptly if a bacterial infection develops. Fever and discomfort can be treated with acetaminophen (Tylenol) or ibuprofen (Advil, Motrin, Nuprin). Children with measles should never be given aspirin, as this increases the risk of the fatal disease Reye's syndrome.

Expected results

The prognosis for an otherwise healthy, well-nourished child who contracts measles is usually quite good. In developing countries, however, death rates may reach 15–25%, as malnutrition, especially protein deficiency, for six months prior to the onset of measles increases the risk of death. Adolescents and adults usually have a more difficult course. Women who contract the disease while pregnant may give birth to a baby with a hearing impairment. Although only one in 1,000 patients with measles will develop encephalitis, 10–15% of those who do will die, and about another 25% will be left with permanent brain damage.

Prevention

Measles is a highly preventable infection. A very effective vaccine exists, made of live measles viruses that have been treated so they cannot cause infection. The important markers on the viruses are intact and cause the immune system to produce antibodies. In the event of a future infection with measles virus the antibodies will quickly recognize the organism and eliminate it. Measles vaccines are usually given at about 15 months of age. Prior to that age, the baby's immune system is not mature enough to initiate a reaction strong enough to ensure long-term protection from the virus. A repeat injection should be given at about 10 or 11 years of age. Outbreaks on college campuses have occurred among non-immunized or incorrectly immunized students.

Measles vaccine should not be given to a pregnant woman, however, in spite of the seriousness of gestational measles. The reason for not giving this particular vaccine during pregnancy is the risk of transmitting measles to the unborn child.

Surprisingly, new cases of measles began being reported in some countries—including Great Britain—in 2001 because of parents' fears about vaccine safety. The combined vaccine for measles, **mumps**, and **rubella** (MMR) was claimed to cause **autism** or bowel disorders in some children. However, the World Health Organization (WHO) says there is no scientific merit to these claims. The United Nations expressed concern that unwarranted fear of the vaccine would begin spreading the disease in developing countries, and ultimately in developed countries as well. Parents in Britain began demanding the measles vaccine as a separate dose and scientists were exploring that option as an alternative to the combined MMR vaccine. Unfortunately, several children died during an outbreak of measles in Dublin because they had not received the vaccine. Child mortality due to measles is considered largely preventable, and making the MMR vaccine widely available in developing countries is part of WHO's strategy to reduce child mortality by two-thirds by the year 2015.

Resources

BOOKS

Gershon, Anne. "Measles (Rubeola)." In *Harrison's Principles of Internal Medicine*, edited by Anthony S. Fauci, et al. New York: McGraw-Hill, 1998.

Stoffman, Phyllis. *The Family Guide to Preventing and Treating 100 Infectious Diseases*. New York: John Wiley and Sons, Inc., 1995.

"Viral Infections: Measles." Section 19, Chapter 265 in *The Merck Manual of Diagnosis and Therapy*, edited by Mark H. Beers, MD, and Robert Berkow, MD. Whitehouse Station, NJ: Merck Research Laboratories, 2002.

Ying, Zhou Zhong, and Jin Hui De. "Childhood Infections."
    In *Clinical Manual of Chinese Herbal Medicine and
    Acupuncture*. New York: Churchill Livingston, 1997.

PERIODICALS

Borton, Dorothy. "Keeping Measles at Bay: Use These Four
    Techniques to Stop the Spread." *Nursing* 27, no. 12
    (December 1997): 26.
Chiba, M. E., M. Saito, N. Suzuki, et al. "Measles Infection
    in Pregnancy." *Journal of Infection* 47 (July 2003): 40–44.
Hussey, Greg. "Managing Measles: Integrated Case Man-
    agement Reduces Disease Severity." *British Medical
    Journal* 314, no. 7077 (February 1, 1997): 316 + .
Jones, G., R. W. Steketee, R. E. Black, et al. "How Many
    Child Deaths Can We Prevent This Year?" *Lancet* 362
    (July 5, 2003): 65–71.
McBrien, J., J. Murphy, D. Gill, et al. "Measles Outbreak in
    Dublin, 2000." *Pediatric Infectious Disease Journal* 22
    (July 2003): 580–584.
"Measles—United States, 2000. (From the Centers for Disease
    Control and Prevention)." *Journal of the American Med-
    ical Association* 287, no. 9 (March 6, 2002): 1105–1112.
"Progress Toward Global Measles Control and Elimination,
    1990-1996." *Journal of the American Medical Associa-
    tion* 278, no. 17 (November 5, 1997): 1396 + .
Scott, L. A., and M. S. Stone. "Viral exanthems." *Derma-
    tology Online Journal* 9 (August 2003): 4.
Sur, D. K., D. H. Wallis, and T. X. O'Connell. "Vaccina-
    tions in Pregnancy." *American Family Physician* 68
    (July 15, 2003): 299–304.
"WHO: Vaccine Fears Could Lead to Unnecessary Deaths."-
    Medical Letter on the CDC & FDA (March 17, 2002): 11.

ORGANIZATIONS

American Academy of Pediatrics (AAP). 141 Northwest
    Point Boulevard, Elk Grove Village, IL 60007. (847)
    434-4000. http://www.aap.org.
Centers for Disease Control and Prevention. 1600 Clifton
    Rd., Atlanta, GA 30333. (404) 639-3311. http://www.
    cdc.gov.

OTHER

Zand, Janet. "Measles." *HealthWorld Online* [cited October
    2002]. http://www.healthy.net/library/books/smart/
    measles.htm.

Belinda Rowland
Teressa Odle
Rebecca J. Frey, PhD

Meditation

Definition

Meditation is a practice of concentrated focus
upon a sound, object, visualization, the breath, movement, or attention itself in order to increase awareness

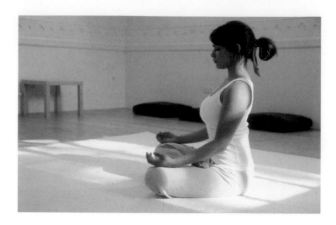

A young woman meditating. (© *Angela Hampton Picture Library /
Alamy*)

of the present moment, reduce **stress**, promote **relaxation**, and enhance personal and spiritual growth.

Origins

Meditation techniques have been practiced for
millennia. Originally, they were intended to develop
spiritual understanding, awareness, and direct experience of ultimate reality. The many different religious
traditions in the world have given rise to a rich variety
of meditative practices. These include the contempla-
tive practices of Christian religious orders, the Buddhist practice of sitting meditation, and the whirling
movements of the Sufi dervishes. Although meditation
is an important spiritual practice in many religious and
spiritual traditions, it can be practiced by anyone
regardless of their religious or cultural background
to relieve stress and **pain**.

As Western medical practitioners begin to understand the mind's role in health and disease, there has
been more interest in the use of meditation in medicine. Meditative practices are increasingly offered in
medical clinics and hospitals as a tool for improving
health and quality of life. Meditation has been used as
the primary therapy for treating certain diseases; as an
additional therapy in a comprehensive treatment plan;
and as a means of improving the quality of life of
people with debilitating, chronic, or terminal illnesses.

Benefits

Meditation benefits people with or without acute
medical illness or stress. People who meditate regularly
have been shown to feel less **anxiety** and **depression**.
They also report that they experience more enjoyment
and appreciation of life and that their relationships
with others are improved. Meditation produces a

KEY TERMS

Dervish—A member of the Sufi order. Their practice of meditation involves whirling ecstatic dance.

Mantra—A sacred word or formula repeated over and over to concentrate the mind.

Transcendental meditation (TM)—A meditation technique based on Hindu practices that involves the repetition of a mantra.

state of deep relaxation and a sense of balance or equanimity. According to Michael J. Baime, "Meditation cultivates an emotional stability that allows the meditator to experience intense emotions fully while simultaneously maintaining perspective on them." Out of this experience of emotional stability, one may gain greater insight and understanding about one's thoughts, feelings, and actions. This insight in turn offers the possibility to feel more confident and in control of life. Meditation facilitates a greater sense of calmness, empathy, and acceptance of self and others.

Meditation can be used with other forms of medical treatment and is an important complementary therapy for both the treatment and prevention of many stress-related conditions. Regular meditation can reduce the number of symptoms experienced by patients with a wide range of illnesses and disorders. Based upon clinical evidence as well as theoretical understanding, meditation is considered to be one of the better therapies for **panic disorder**, generalized anxiety disorder, **substance dependence** and abuse, ulcers, **colitis**, chronic pain, **psoriasis**, and dysthymic disorder. It is considered to be a valuable adjunctive therapy for moderate **hypertension** (high blood pressure), prevention of cardiac arrest (**heart attack**), prevention of **atherosclerosis** (hardening of arteries), arthritis (including **fibromyalgia**), **cancer**, **insomnia**, migraine, and prevention of **stroke**. Meditation may also be a valuable complementary therapy for **allergies** and **asthma** because of the role stress plays in these conditions. Meditative practices have been reported to improve function or reduce symptoms in patients with some neurological disorders as well. These include people with **Parkinson's disease**, people who experience **fatigue** with **multiple sclerosis**, and people with **epilepsy** who are resistant to standard treatment.

Overall, a 1995 report to the National Institutes of Health on alternative medicine concluded that, "More than 30 years of research, as well as the experience of a large and growing number of individuals and health care providers, suggests that meditation and similar forms of relaxation can lead to better health, higher quality of life, and lowered health care costs." A study of health care professionals published in 2002 indicates that the majority of physicians, nurses, and occupational therapists in the United States accept meditation as a beneficial adjunct to conventional medical or surgical treatments.

Description

Sitting meditation is generally done in an upright seated position, either in a chair or cross-legged on a cushion on the floor. The spine is straight yet relaxed. Sometimes the eyes are closed. Other times the eyes are open and gazing softly into the distance or at an object. Depending on the type of meditation, the meditator may be concentrating on the sensation of the movement of the breath, counting the breath, silently repeating a sound, chanting, visualizing an image, focusing awareness on the center of the body, opening to all sensory experiences including thoughts, or performing stylized ritual movements with the hands.

Movement meditation can be spontaneous and free-form or involve highly structured, choreographed, repetitive patterns. Movement meditation is particularly helpful for those people who find it difficult to remain still.

Generally speaking, there are two main types of meditation. These types are concentration meditation and mindfulness meditation. Concentration meditation practices involve focusing attention on a single object. Objects of meditation can include the breath, an inner or external image, a movement pattern (as in tai chi or **yoga**), or a sound, word, or phrase that is repeated silently (mantra). The purpose of concentrative practices is to learn to focus one's attention or develop concentration. When thoughts or emotions arise, the meditator gently directs the mind back to the original object of concentration.

Mindfulness meditation practices involve becoming aware of the entire field of attention. The meditator is instructed to be aware of all thoughts, feelings, perceptions, or sensations as they arise in each moment. Mindfulness meditation practices are enhanced by the meditator's ability to focus and quiet the mind. Many meditation practices are a blend of these two forms.

The study and application of meditation to health care has focused on three specific approaches: 1. transcendental meditation (TM); 2. The "relaxation response," a general approach to meditation developed by Dr. Herbert Benson; and 3. mindfulness meditation, specifically the program of mindfulness-based stress reduction (MBSR) developed by Jon Kabat-Zinn.

Transcendental meditation

TM has its origins in the Vedic tradition of India and was introduced to the West by Maharishi Mahesh Yogi. TM has been taught to somewhere between two and four million people. It is one of the most widely practiced forms of meditation in the West. TM has been studied many times; these studies have produced much of the information about the physiology of meditation. In TM, the meditator sits with closed eyes and concentrates on a single syllable or word (mantra) for 20 minutes at a time, twice a day. When thoughts or feelings arise, the attention is brought back to the mantra. According to Charles Alexander, an important TM researcher, "During TM, ordinary waking mental activity is said to settle down, until even the subtlest thought is transcended and a completely unified wholeness of awareness...is experienced. In this silent, self-referential state of pure wakefulness, consciousness is fully awake to itself alone..." TM supporters believe that TM practices are more beneficial than other meditation practices. A group of Australian researchers has recently recommended TM as a preventive strategy for **heart disease**.

The relaxation response

The relaxation response involves a similar form of mental focusing. Dr. Herbert Benson, one of the first Western doctors to conduct research on the effects of meditation, developed this approach after observing the profound health benefits of a state of bodily calm he calls "the relaxation response." In order to elicit this response in the body, he teaches patients to focus upon the repetition of a word, sound, **prayer**, phrase, or movement activity (including swimming, jogging, yoga, and even knitting) for 10–20 minutes at a time, twice a day. Patients are also taught not to pay attention to distracting thoughts and to return their focus to the original repetition. The choice of the focused repetition is up to the individual. Instead of Sanskrit terms, the meditator can choose what is personally meaningful, such as a phrase from a prayer.

Mindfulness meditation

Mindfulness meditation comes out of traditional Buddhist meditation practices. Psychologist Jon Kabat-Zinn has been instrumental in bringing this form of meditation into medical settings. In formal mindfulness practice, the meditator sits with eyes closed, focusing the attention on the sensations and movement of the breath for approximately 45–60 minutes at a time, at least once a day. Informal mindfulness practice involves bringing awareness to every activity in daily life. Wandering thoughts or distracting feelings are simply noticed without resisting or reacting to them. The essence of mindfulness meditation is not what one focuses on but rather the quality of awareness the meditator brings to each moment. According to Kabat-Zinn, "It is this investigative, discerning observation of whatever comes up in the present moment that is the hallmark of mindfulness and differentiates it most from other forms of meditation. The goal of mindfulness is for you to be more aware, more in touch with life and whatever is happening in your own body and mind at the time it is happening—that is, the present moment." The MBSR program consists of a series of classes involving meditation, movement, and group process. There are over 240 MBSR programs offered in health care settings around the world.

Meditation is not considered a medical procedure or intervention by most insurers. Many patients pay for meditation training themselves. Frequently, religious groups or meditation centers offer meditation instruction free of charge or for a nominal donation. Hospitals may offer MBSR classes at a reduced rate for their patients and a slightly higher rate for the general public.

Precautions

Meditation appears to be safe for most people. There are, however, case reports and studies noting some adverse effects. Thirty-three to 50% of the people participating in long silent meditation retreats (two weeks to three months) reported increased tension, anxiety, confusion, and depression. On the other hand, most of these same people also reported very positive effects from their meditation practice. Kabat-Zinn notes that these studies fail to differentiate between serious psychiatric disturbances and normal emotional mood swings. These studies do suggest, however, that meditation may not be recommended for people with psychotic disorders, severe depression, and other severe personality disorders unless they are also receiving psychological or medical treatment.

Side effects

There are no reported side effects from meditation except for positive benefits.

Research and general acceptance

The scientific study of the physiological effects of meditation began in the early 1960s. These studies

MAHARISHI MAHESH YOGI (1911–2008)

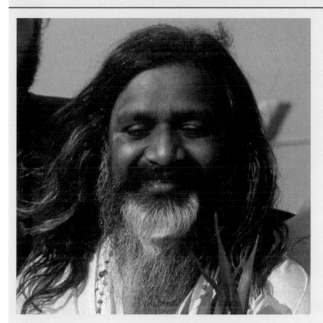

(Bernard Gotfryd/Hulton Archvie/Getty Images.)

Maharishi Mahesh Yogi was one of the most recognized spiritual leaders of the world. Almost single-handedly, the Maharishi (meaning great sage) brought Eastern culture into Western consciousness. He emerged in the late 1950s in London and the United States as a missionary in the cause of Hinduism, the philosophy of which is called Vedanta—a belief that "holds that God is to be found in every creature and object, that the purpose of human life is to realize the godliness in oneself and that religious truths are universal."

By 1967, the Maharishi became a leader among flower-children and an anti-drug advocate. The Maharishi's sudden popularity was helped along by such early fans as the Beatles, Mia Farrow, and Shirley MacLaine. These people, and many others, practiced Transcendental Meditation (TM), a Hindu-influenced procedure that endures in America to this day.

When the 1960s drew to a close, the Maharishi began to fade from public view. The guru still had enough followers, though, to people the Maharishi International University, founded in 1971. One of the main draws of Maharishi International University was the study of TM Sidha, an exotic form of Transcendental Meditation. Sidhas believe that group meditation can elicit the maharishi effect—a force strong enough to conjure world peace.

prove that meditation affects metabolism, the endocrine system, the central nervous system, and the autonomic nervous system. In one study, three advanced practitioners of Tibetan Buddhist meditation practices demonstrated the ability to increase "inner heat" as much as 61%. During a different meditative practice they were able to dramatically slow down the rate at which their bodies consumed oxygen. Preliminary research shows that mindfulness meditation is associated with increased levels of **melatonin**. These findings suggest a potential role for meditation in the treatment and prevention of breast and prostrate cancer.

Despite the inherent difficulties in designing research studies, there is a large amount of evidence of the medical benefits of meditation. Meditation is particularly effective as a treatment for chronic pain. Studies have shown meditation reduces symptoms of pain and pain-related drug use. In a four-year follow-up study, the majority of patients in a MBSR program reported "moderate to great improvement" in pain as a result of participation in the program.

Meditation has long been recommended as a treatment for high blood pressure; however, there is a debate over the amount of benefit that meditation offers. Although most studies show a reduction in blood pressure with meditation, medication is still more effective at lowering high blood pressure.

Meditation may also be an effective treatment for coronary artery disease. A study of 21 patients practicing TM for eight months showed increases in their amount of **exercise** tolerance, amount of workload, and a delay in the onset of ST-segment depression. Meditation is also an important part of Dean Ornish's program, which has been proven to reverse coronary artery disease.

Research also suggests that meditation is effective in the treatment of chemical dependency. Gelderloos and others reviewed 24 studies and reported that all of them showed that TM is helpful in programs to stop **smoking** and also in programs for drug and alcohol abuse.

Studies also imply that meditation is helpful in reducing symptoms of anxiety and in treating anxiety-related disorders. Furthermore, a study in 1998 of 37 psoriasis patients showed that those practicing mindfulness meditation had more rapid clearing of their skin condition, with standard UV light treatment, than the control subjects. Another study found that meditation decreased the symptoms of fibromyalgia; over half of the patients reported significant improvement. Research by a group of ophthalmologists indicates that nearly 60% of a group of patients being treated for **glaucoma** found meditation helpful in coping with their eye disorder. In addition, meditation was one of several stress management techniques used in a small study of HIV-positive men. The study showed improvements in the T-cell counts of the men, as well as in several psychological measures of well-being.

Training and certification

There is no program of certification or licensure for instructors who wish to teach meditation as a medical therapy. Meditation teachers within a particular religious tradition usually have extensive experience and expertise with faith questions and religious practices but may not have been trained to work with medical patients. Different programs have varied requirements for someone to teach meditation. In order to be recognized as an instructor of TM, one must receive extensive training. The Center for Mindfulness in Medicine, Health Care and Society at the University of Massachusetts Medical Center offers training and workshops for health professionals and others interested in teaching mindfulness-based stress reduction. The Center does not, however, certify that someone is qualified to teach meditation. The University of Pennsylvania program for Stress Management suggests that a person have at least 10 years of personal experience with the practice of mindfulness meditation before receiving additional instruction to teach meditation. Teachers are also expected to spend at least two weeks each year in intensive meditation retreats.

Resources

BOOKS

Astin, John A., et al. "Meditation." In *Clinician's Complete Reference to Complementary and Alternative Medicine*, edited by Donald Novey. St. Louis: Mosby, 2000.

Baime, Michael J. "Meditation and Mindfulness." In *Essentials of Complementary and Alternative Medicine*, edited by Wayne B. Jonas and Jeffrey S. Levin. New York: Lippincott, Williams and Wilkins, 1999.

Benson, Herbert, M.D. *The Relaxation Response.* New York: William Morrow, 1975.

Kabat-Zinn, John. *Full Catastrophe Living: Using the Wisdom of Your Body and Mind to Face Stress, Pain, and Illness.* New York: Dell, 1990.

Roth, Robert. *TM Transcendental Meditation: A New Introduction to Maharishi's Easy, Effective and Scientifically Proven Technique for Promoting Better Health.* Donald I. Fine, 1994.

PERIODICALS

King, M. S., T. Carr, and C. D'Cruz. "Transcendental Meditation, Hypertension and Heart Disease." *Australian Family Physician* 31 (February 2002): 164–168.

Rhee, D. J., G. L. Spaeth, J. S. Myers, et al. "Prevalence of the Use of Complementary and Alternative Medicine for Glaucoma." *Ophthalmology* 109 (March 2002): 438–443.

Schoenberger, N. E., R. J. Matheis, S. C. Shiflett, and A. C. Cotter. "Opinions and Practices of Medical Rehabilitation Professionals Regarding Prayer and Meditation." *Journal of Alternative and Complementary Medicine* 8 (February 2002): 59–69.

ORGANIZATIONS

Insight Meditation Society. 1230 Pleasant, St. Barre, MA 01005. (978) 355-4378. FAX: (978) 355-6398. http://www.dharma.org

Mind-Body Medical Institute. Beth Israel Deaconess Medical Center. One Deaconess Road, Boston, MA 02215. (617) 632-9525. http://www.mbmi.org

The Center for Mindfulness in Medicine, Health Care and Society. Stress Reduction Clinic. University of Massachusetts Memorial Health Care. 55 Lake Avenue North, Worcester, MA 01655. (508) 856-2656. Fax (508) 856-1977. jon.kabat-zinn@banyan@ummed.edu http://www.umassmed.edu/cfm

Linda Chrisman
Rebecca J. Frey, PhD

Mediterranean diet

Definition

The Mediterranean diet is based upon the eating patterns of traditional cultures in the Mediterranean region. Several noted nutritionists and research projects have concluded that this diet is one of the most healthful in the world in terms of preventing a variety of illnesses including **heart disease** and **cancer**, and increasing life expectancy.

Origins

The countries that have inspired the Mediterranean diet all surround the Mediterranean Sea. These cultures have eating habits that developed over thousands of years. In Europe, parts of Italy, Greece, Portugal, Spain, and southern France adhere to principles

Mediterranean diet

Frequency	Food	Tips
Monthly	Red meats	No more than a few times month
Weekly	Sweets	Opt instead for naturally sweet fresh fruit
	Eggs	Less than 4 per week, including those in processed foods
	Poultry	A few times a week. Take the skin off and choose white meat to lower fat intake
	Fish	A few times a week
Daily	Cheese and yogurt	Cheese and yogurt are good sources of calcium. Choose low-fat varieties
	Olive oil	The beneficial health effects of olive oil are due to its high content of monounsaturated fats and antioxidants. Olive oil is high in calories, consume in moderation to reduce calorie intake
	Fruits	At least a serving at every meal. A serving of fruit is a healthy option for snacks
	Vegetables	At least a serving at every meal. Choose a variety of colors
	Beans, legumes, nuts	Beans are a healthy source of protein, and are loaded with soluble fiber, which has been shown to lower blood cholesterol levels by five percent or more. Most nuts contain monounsaturated (heart-healthy) fat. A handful of nuts is a healthy option for snacks
	Whole grains, including breads, pasta, rice, couscous, and polenta	A grain is considered whole when all three parts—bran, germ and endosperm—are present. Substitute whole wheat for white bread, brown rice for white rice and whole-wheat flour when baking. Mix pasta, rice, couscous, polenta and potatoes with vegetables and legumes
	Water	At least 6 glasses daily
	Wine (in moderation)	The U.S. Department of Agriculture defines moderation as no more than a five-ounce glass of wine daily for women and up to 2 glasses (10 ounces) daily for men
	Physical activity	Thirty minutes of cardiovascular activity a day is recommended to get in shape, burn calories and boost the metabolism

Based on the Mediterranean diet pyramid. (Illustration by GGS Information Services. Cengage Learning, Gale)

of the Mediterranean diet, as do Morocco and Tunisia in North Africa. Parts of the Balkan region and Turkey follow the diet, as well as Middle Eastern countries like Lebanon and Syria. The Mediterranean region is warm and sunny, and produces large supplies of fresh fruits and vegetables almost year round that people eat many times per day. Wine, bread, olive oil, nuts, and legumes (beans and lentils) are other staples of the region, and the Mediterranean Sea has historically yielded abundant fish. The preparation and sharing of meals is a very important and festive part of Mediterranean culture as well, and Mediterranean cuisine is popular around the world for its flavors.

The first description of the traditional Mediterranean diet as it became followed in America was in a research study funded by the Rockefeller Foundation and published in 1953. The author was Leland Allbaugh, who carried out a study of the island of Crete as an underdeveloped area. Allbaugh noted the heavy use of olive oil, whole-grain foods, fruits, fish, and vegetables in cooking as well as the geography and other features of the island.

The Cretan version of the Mediterranean diet became the focus of medical research on the Mediterranean diet following the publication of Dr. Ancel Keys's Seven Country Study in 1980. Dr. Keys performed an epidemiological analysis of **diets** around the world. Epidemiology is the branch of public health that studies the patterns of diseases and their potential causes among populations as a whole. The Seven Countries Study is considered one of the greatest epidemiological studies ever performed. It was a systematic comparison of diet, risk factors for heart disease, and disease experience in men between the ages of 40 and 59 in eighteen rural areas of Japan, Finland, Greece, Italy, the former Yugoslavia, the Netherlands, and the United States from 1958 to 1970. (Women were not included as subjects because of the rarity of heart attacks among them at that time and because the physical examinations were fairly invasive). In addition to asking the subjects to keep records of their food intake, the researchers performed chemical analyses of the foods the subjects ate. It was found that the men living on the island of Crete—the location of Leland Allbaugh's 1953 study—had the lowest rate of heart attacks of any group of subjects in the study.

Several other studies have validated Keys' findings regarding the good health of people in the Mediterranean countries. The World Health Organization (WHO) showed in a 1990 analysis that four major Mediterranean countries (Spain, Greece, France, and Italy) have longer life expectancies and lower rates of heart disease and cancer than other European countries and America. The data are significant because the same Mediterraneans frequently smoke and don't have regular **exercise** programs like many Americans, which means that other variables may be responsible. Scientists have also ruled out genetic differences, because Mediterraneans who move to other countries tend to lose their health advantages. These findings suggest that diet and lifestyle are major factors.

The Mediterranean diet gained more notice when Dr. Walter Willett, head of the **nutrition** department at Harvard University, began to recommend it. Although low-fat diets were recommended for heart disease, Mediterranean groups in his studies had very high intakes of fat, mainly from olive oil. Willett and others proposed that the risk of heart disease could be reduced by increasing one type of dietary fat—monounsaturated fat. This is the type of fat in olive oil. Willett's proposal went against conventional nutritional recommendations to reduce all fat in the diet. It has been shown that unsaturated fats raise the level of HDL **cholesterol**, which is sometimes called "good cholesterol" because of its protective effect against heart disease. Willett has also performed studies correlating the intake of meat with heart disease and cancer.

Willett, other researchers at Harvard, and the WHO collaborated in 1994 and designed the Mediterranean Food Pyramid, which lists food groups and their recommended daily servings in the Mediterranean diet. These nutritionists consider their food groups a more healthful alternative to the food groups designated by the U.S. Department of Agriculture (USDA). The USDA recommends a much higher number of daily servings of meat and dairy products, which Mediterranean diet specialists attribute to political factors rather than sound nutritional analysis.

Benefits

Preventive health care

Most of the scientific research that has been done on Mediterranean diets concerns their role in preventing or lowering the risk of various diseases.

HEART DISEASE. Mediterranean diets became popular in the 1980s largely because of their association with lowered risk of heart attacks and **stroke**, particularly in men, following the publication of the Seven Countries study. Mediterranean diets are thought to protect against heart disease because of their high levels of **omega-3 fatty acids** even though blood cholesterol levels are not lowered.

ALZHEIMER'S DISEASE. A study published in *Annals of Neurology* in 2006 reported that subjects in a group of 2000 participants averaging 76 years of age who followed a Mediterranean-type diet closely were less likely to develop Alzheimer's than those who did not. Further study is needed, however, to discover whether factors other than diet may have affected the outcome.

ASTHMA AND ALLERGIES. A group of researchers in Crete reported in 2007 that the low rate of **wheezing** and allergic **rhinitis** (runny nose) on the island may be related to the traditional Cretan diet. Children who had a high consumption of nuts, grapes, oranges, apples, and tomatoes (the main local products) were less likely to suffer from **asthma** or nasal **allergies**. Children who ate large amounts of margarine, however, were more likely to develop these conditions.

METABOLIC SYNDROME. Research conducted at a clinic in Naples, Italy, suggests that Mediterranean diets lower the risk of developing and can even help in reversing the effects of metabolic syndrome, a condition associated with **insulin resistance** and an increased risk of heart disease and type 2 diabetes. The results from this clinic were corroborated by a study done at Tufts University in Massachusetts, which found that the symptoms of metabolic syndrome were reduced even in patients who did not lose weight on the diet.

Weight loss

Some population studies carried out in Mediterranean countries (particularly Italy and Spain) have found that close adherence to a traditional Mediterranean diet is associated with lower weight and a lower body mass index. Although there are relatively few studies of Mediterranean diets as weight-reduction regimens, a research team at the Harvard School of Public Health reported in 2007 that a Mediterranean-style diet is an effective approach to weight loss for many people. A major reason for its effectiveness is the wide variety of enjoyable foods permitted on the diet combined with a rich tradition of ethnic recipes making use of these foods—which makes it easier and more pleasant for people to stay on the diet for long periods of time.

Description

The Mediterranean diet has several general characteristics:

- The bulk of the diet comes from plant sources, including whole grains, breads, pasta, polenta (from corn), bulgur and couscous (from wheat), rice, potatoes, fruits, vegetables, legumes (beans and lentils), seeds, and nuts.
- Olive oil is used generously, and is the main source of fat in the diet as well as the principal cooking oil. The total fat intake accounts for up to 35% of calories.

Saturated fats, however, make up only 8% of calories or less, which restricts meat and dairy intake.

- Fruits and vegetables are eaten in large quantities. They are usually fresh, unprocessed, grown locally, and consumed in season.
- Dairy products are consumed in small amounts daily, mainly as cheese and yogurt (1 oz of cheese and 1 cup of yogurt daily).
- Eggs are used sparingly, up to four eggs per week.
- Fish and poultry are consumed only one to three times per week (less than 1 lb per week combined), with fish preferred over poultry.
- Red meat is consumed only a few times per month (less than 1 lb per month total).
- Honey is the principle sweetener, and sweets are eaten only a few times per week.
- Wine is consumed in moderate amounts with meals (1–2 glasses daily).

Preparations

Many Mediterranean cookbooks are available that can help with planning and preparing meals. A good first step is eliminating all oils, butter, and margarine and replacing them with olive oil. Meals should always be accompanied with bread and salads. Mediterranean fruits and vegetables are generally fresh and high in quality; American consumers may find equivalents by shopping in farmers' markets and health food stores that sell organic produce. Meat intake should be reduced and replaced by whole grains, legumes, and other foods at meals. The dairy products that are used should be yogurt and cheese instead of milk, which is not often used as a beverage by Mediterraneans.

Researchers have been quick to point out that there may be other factors that influence the effectiveness of the Mediterranean diet. Getting plenty of physical exercise is important, as is reducing **stress**. Researchers have noted that Mediterraneans' attitude toward eating and mealtimes may be a factor in their good health as well. Meals are regarded as important and joyful occasions, are prepared carefully and tastefully, and are shared with family and friends. In many Mediterranean countries, people generally relax or take a short nap (siesta) after lunch, the largest meal of the day.

Precautions

People who are making any major change in their dietary pattern in general should always consult their physician first. In addition, people who are taking monoamine oxidase inhibitors (MAOIs) for the treatment of **depression** should check with their doctor, as

these drugs interact with a chemical called tyramine to cause sudden increases in blood pressure. Tyramine is found in red wines, particularly aged wines like Chianti, and in aged cheeses.

People using a Mediterranean diet for weight reduction should watch portion size and monitor their consumption of olive oil, cheese, and yogurt, which are high in calories. Dieters may wish to consider switching to low-fat cheeses and yogurts.

Because olive oil is a staple of Mediterranean diets, consumers should purchase it from reliable sources. The safety of olive oil is not ordinarily a concern in North America; however, samples of olive oils sold in Europe and North Africa are sometimes found to be contaminated by mycotoxins (toxins produced by molds and fungi that grow on olives and other fruits). Some mycotoxins do not have any known effects on humans, but aflatoxin, which has been found in olive oil, is a powerful carcinogen and has been implicated in liver cancer.

Resources

BOOKS

Parker, Steven Paul, MD. *The Advanced Mediterranean Diet: Lose Weight, Feel Better, Live Longer.* Mesa, AZ: Vanguard Press, 2007.

Simopoulos, Artemis P., and Francesco Visioli, eds. *More on Mediterranean Diets.* New York: Karger, 2007.

Vegetarian Times Cooks Mediterranean. New York: William Morrow, 2000.

Willett, Walter, M.D. *Nutritional Epidemiology.* London: Oxford University Press, 1998.

PERIODICALS

Carollo, C., R. L. Presti, and G. Caimi. "Wine, Diet, and Arterial Hypertension." *Angiology* 58 (February-March 2007): 92–96.

Chatzi, L., G. Apostolaki, I. Bibakis, et al. "Protective Effect of Fruits, Vegetables, and the Mediterranean Diet on Asthma and Allergies among Children in Crete." *Thorax*, April 5, 2007.

Dalziel, K., L. Segal, and M. de Lorgeril. "A Mediterranean Diet Is Cost-Effective in Patients with Previous Myocardial Infarction." *Journal of Nutrition* 136 (July 2006): 1879–1885.

ORGANIZATIONS

Oldways Preservation and Exchange Trust (provides information on the diet), 45 Milk Street, Boston, MA, 02109, (617) 695-0600

Douglas Dupler

Medium-chain triglycerides

Description

Medium-chain triglycerides (MCTs) are a special class of fatty acids. Normal fats and oils contain long-chain fatty acids (LCTs). Compared to these fatty acids, MCTs are much shorter in length. Therefore, they resemble carbohydrates more than fat. As a result, they are more easily absorbed, digested, and utilized as energy than LCTs.

Medium-chain triglycerides are found naturally in milk fat, palm oil, and coconut oil. Commercial MCT oil, available as liquid and capsules, is obtained through lipid fractionation, the process in which MCTs are separated from other components of coconut oil. Medium-chain triglycerides were originally formulated in the 1950s as an alternative food source for patients who are too ill to properly digest normal fats and oils. The long chains of LCTs require a lot of bile acids and many digestive steps to be broken down into smaller units that can be absorbed into the bloodstream. Once in the bloodstream, they are absorbed by fat cells and stored as body fat. In contrast, the medium-chain triglycerides are more water-soluble and are able to enter the bloodstream quicker because of their shorter lengths. Once in the bloodstream, they are transported directly into the liver. Thus, MCTs are an immediately available source of energy and only a tiny percent is converted into body fat.

Medium-chain triglycerides were first used in the mid-1900s to reduce seizures with the help of the ketogenic diet. In the 1980s, MCTs became popular in sports as a substitute for normal dietary fats or oils. They quickly became a favorite energy source for many athletes, such as marathon runners, who participate in endurance sports. These athletes require a quick source of energy, which is readily supplied by carbohydrates. However, **diets** high in carbohydrates may cause rapid increase in insulin production, resulting in substantial weight gain, diabetes, and other health problems. Dietary fats or oils are not a readily available source of energy. In addition, they are believed to make the body fatter. MCT is also a form of fat; therefore, it is high in calories. Yet, unlike normal fats and oils, MCTs do not cause weight gain because they stimulate thermogenesis (the process in which the body generates energy, or heat, by increasing its normal metabolic, fat-burning rate). A thermogenic diet, which is high in medium-chain triglycerides, has been proposed as a type of weight loss regime.

General use

Endurance sport nutrition

Medium-chain triglycerides are often used by athletes to increase their endurance during sports or **exercise** regimes. MCTs are an immediate source of energy, and as such, the body can use them as an alternative energy source for muscle during endurance exercise. However, if consumed in moderate amounts (30 to 45 grams), MCTs are not very effective in either decreasing carbohydrate needs or in enhancing exercise endurance. Increased consumption may help. One study evaluated six athletes at different points during a 25-mile cycling trial. They were given either a medium-chain triglyceride beverage, a carbohydrate drink, or a combined MCT-carbohydrate mixture. The fastest speed was achieved when the athletes used the MCT-carbohydrate blend. The worst performance was associated with sport drinks containing MCT alone (without carbohydrate). Therefore, to gain significant increases in endurance, it is generally recommended

KEY TERMS

Endurance—The ability to sustain an activity over a period of time.

Hepatic encephalopathy—Brain and nervous system damage that occurs as a complication of liver disorders.

Ketones—The potentially toxic by-products of partially burned fatty acids that the body uses as an alternative fuel source when carbohydrates are not available.

Thermogenesis—The production of heat, especially within the body.

that an athlete consume at least 50 grams of MCTs per day in combination with some carbohydrates. However, dosages exceeding 30 grams often cause gastrointestinal upset, which can diminish an athlete's performance.

MCT products available in the market may have high water content or contain unwanted ingredients. Therefore, athletes should buy MCT-only products, and mix a small amount into carbohydrate soft drinks. Alternatively, they can purchase premixed MCT sport drinks, such as a brand known as SUCCEED.

Thermogenic diet

MCTs are popular among body builders because they help reduce carbohydrate intake, while allowing them ready access to energy whenever they need it. MCTs also have muscle-sparing effects. As a result, they can build muscles while reducing fats. However, this does not mean that these athletes will become healthier, because an improvement in body physique does not always correlate with higher fitness levels.

Pre-competition diet

Compared to carbohydrates, medium-chain triglycerides are a better and more efficient source of quick energy. They help conserve lean body mass because they prevent muscle proteins from being used as energy. Therefore, some athletes load up on medium-chain triglycerides the night before a competition. However, MCT intake should be raised gradually to allow the body to adapt to increasing MCT consumption. If MCT consumption abruptly increases, incomplete MCT metabolism may occur,

producing lactic acid in the body and a rapid rise of ketones in the blood, which can make the person ill.

Weight-loss diet

Studies have shown that MCT may increase metabolism, which is the rate that the body burns fat. It is believed that sustained increases in metabolic rate cause the body to burn more fat, resulting in weight loss. However, for any kind of meaningful weight loss, a person would have to consume more than 50% of total daily caloric intake in the form of medium-chain triglycerides.

Treatment of seizures

A ketogenic diet, or diet containing mostly medium-chain triglycerides, offers hope for those who have seizures that cannot be controlled by currently available drugs. Excessive consumption of MCTs produces ketones in the body; therefore, this type of diet is called a ketogenic diet. It has proven effective for some epileptic patients.

Nutritional supplements

MCTs are the preferred forms of fat for many patients with fat malabsorption problems. Many diseases cause poor fat absorption. For instance, patients with pancreatic insufficiency do not have enough pancreatic enzymes to break down LCTs. In children with cystic fibrosis, thick mucus blocks the enzymes that assist in digestion. Another fat absorption condition is short-bowel syndrome, in which parts of the bowel have been removed due to disease. Stressed or critically ill patients also have a decreased ability to digest LCTs. Unlike LCTs, medium-chain triglycerides are easily absorbed by patients with malabsorption conditions. These patients benefit most from oral preparations that contain MCTs as the primary source of fat (up to 85% of fat caloric intake). Several scientific studies have shown MCT to be effective in treating fat malabsorbtion, chronic **diarrhea**, and weight loss in patients with Acquired Immune Deficiency Syndrome (**AIDS**).

Many MCT products can be found in local health food stores or ordered through pharmacies. Before purchasing these products, patients should consult their doctors or registered dietitians for advice concerning appropriate dosage and use. MCT oil is not used for cooking. However, it can be used for tube feeding in critically ill patients. Healthy people may take it orally, by itself or mixed with water, juice, ice cream, or pudding.

Preparations

Available medium-chain triglyceride products include:

- MCT oil
- sports drinks
- energy bars
- meal replacement beverages

Precautions

- People with hepatic encephalopathy, brain and nervous system damage that occurs as a complication of liver disorders, should not take MCT.

- High consumption of medium-chain triglycerides can cause abdominal pain, cramps, and diarrhea.

- Long-term high-level MCT consumption is associated with increased risk of heart disease and other conditions. Even moderate consumption of medium-chain triglycerides can increase cholesterol and triglyceride levels. Therefore, no more than 10% of a person's diet should come from MCTs.

- Diabetic athletes and those with liver disease should not use MCT products.

- MCT oil should not completely replace all dietary fats, as this would result in a deficiency of other fatty acids— essential fatty acids— that the human body needs from food sources. To avoid essential fatty acid deficiencies, a person should also include omega-3 and omega-6 fatty acids in their diets. Good sources of omega-3 include fish, fish oils, or flaxseed oil. Omega-6 fatty acids are often found in vegetable oils and evening primrose oil . The omega-3 fats have several additional health benefits, such as alleviating inflammation and protecting the body against heart disease.

- A person should not take medium-chain triglyceride products on an empty stomach, as this may cause gastric upset.

- MCT oil is not for cooking. It is usually consumed in its uncooked form as sport bars, or mixed with a carbohydrate drink, protein shake, or other products.

- MCT oil leaches into plastic bags and containers. Therefore, non-plastic containers should be used for MCT oil storage.

Side effects

There are a few adverse effects associated with MCT use. Eating foods containing medium-chain triglycerides on an empty stomach often causes gastrointestinal upset. Regular consumption of MCTs may increase **cholesterol** and triglyceride blood levels.

Interactions

There have been no reported interactions between MCTs and other drugs.

Resources

BOOKS

Antonio, Jose, and Jeffery Stout. *Supplements for Endurance Athletes.* Champaign, IL: Human Kinetics, 2002.

Ivy, John, and Robert Portman. *The Performance Zone: Your Nutrition Action Plan for Greater Endurance and Sports Performance (Teen Health Series).* North Bergen, NJ: Basic Health Publications, Inc., 2004.

Ryan, Monique. *Sports Nutrition for Endurance Athletes.-* Boulder, CO: Velo Press, 2002.

Stapstrom, Carl E. *Epilepsy and the Ketogenic Diet: Clinical Implementation & the Scientific Basis.* Totowa, NJ: Humana Press, 2004.

PERIODICALS.

Donnell, S.C., et al. "The Metabolic Response to Intravenous Medium-Chain Triglycerides in Infants After Surgery." *Alternative Medicine Review* (February 2003): 94.

"Medium-Chain Triglycerides May Help Promote Weight Loss." *Obesity, Fitness & Wellness Week* (March 29, 2003): 5.

"Medium Chain Triglycerides." *Alternative Medicine Review* (October 2002): 418–20.

St-Onge, M.P., and P.J. Jones. "Physiological Effects of Medium-Chain Triglycerides: Potential Agents in the Prevention of Obesity." *Alternative Medicine Review* (June 2002): 260.

St-Onge, M.P., et al. "Medium-Chain Triglycerides Increase Energy Expenditure and Decrease Adiposity in Overweight Men." *Obesity Research* (March 2003): 395-402.

ORGANIZATIONS

American Dietetic Association (ADA) Consumer Information Hotline. (800)366-1655. http://www. eatright.org.

OTHER

Klein, Samuel. "Lipid Metabolism During Exercise." HealthWorld Online. Abstract from NIH Workshop: The Role of Dietary Supplements for Physically Active People. http://www.healthy.net.

PDRhealth.com article. "Medium-Chain Triglycerides." http://www.pdrhealth.com/drug_info/nmdrugprofiles/nutsupdrugs/med_0172.html.

Mai Tran

Melanoma *see* **Skin cancer**

Melatonin

Description

Melatonin is a hormone produced naturally in the pineal gland at the base of the brain. It is important in regulating sleep and may play a role in maintaining circadian rhythm, the body's natural time clock. The hypothalamus keeps track of the amount of sunlight that is taken in by the eye. The less sunlight, the more melatonin that is released by the pineal gland, thereby enhancing and regulating sleep. Melatonin can also be taken in an over-the-counter supplement sold mainly in health food stores and pharmacies.

General use

A variety of medical uses for melatonin have been reported, but in the late 2000s, its popularity resulted from its promotion as a sleep aid and a reducer of **jet lag**. However, medical experts caution that melatonin is not a harmless substance without risks. Natural melatonin production decreases with age, and the decrease is associated with some **sleep disorders**, particularly in the elderly.

A study conducted by the Institute of Medicine in 2005 found that 50 to 70 million Americans suffer from some kind of chronic sleep disorder that hinders their ability to function normally and adversely affects their health and longevity. The use of melatonin supplements became popular in the mid-1990s as a way of dealing with such sleep disorders. Numerous scientific studies have supported this practice, although there are a few studies that cast doubt on its effectiveness. People reporting the most benefit generally are those with mild and occasional **insomnia** and trouble falling asleep. Melatonin is not generally recommended for use on a regular basis since its long-term consequences are not known.

The second most popular use of melatonin is to ease the effects of jet lag, a physical condition caused by the disturbance of circadian rhythms, usually associated with air travel across several time zones. In its 2008 issue of the popular booklet *Health Information for International Travel*, the Centers for Disease Control and Prevention suggests that "limited evidence suggests melatonin is safe and well tolerated, and doses of 0.5 to 5 mg may promote sleep and decrease jet lag symptoms in travelers crossing five or more time zones."

As of 2008, questions remained about the efficacy of melatonin in treating sleep disorders and jet lag. In 2006, researchers at the University of Alberta, Canada, reported that their review of studies on melatonin conducted between 1999 and 2003 led them to conclude that "[t]here is no evidence that melatonin is effective in treating secondary sleep disorders or sleep disorders accompanying sleep restriction, such as jet lag and shift-work disorder."

Some researchers report that melatonin may be effective in reducing the effects of **aging**. In a 2007 study conducted by researchers at the University of Granada, Spain, mice whose diet included melatonin showed significantly fewer effects of aging than did a control group that received no melatonin. Further studies on the benefits, long-term effects, and proper dosage were being conducted through the National Institutes on Aging as of 2008.

In laboratory and animal experiments, melatonin appears to protect cells and boost the immune system. Melatonin supplementation is sometimes part of a holistic treatment regimen for people with HIV or **AIDS**. There have been no human trials that support this claim.

Preparations

Melatonin is available over the counter in varying doses of up to 3 mg per tablet. However, a fraction of this amount is required for insomnia, usually about 0.3 mg or less. Too much melatonin or taking it at the wrong time can interrupt normal circadian patterns. Melatonin is produced at its highest level in the pineal gland during darkness. Since melatonin occurs naturally in some foods, it can be sold as an over-the-counter dietary supplement. It is only one of two hormones (the other is **DHEA**) not regulated by the U.S. Food and Drug Administration (FDA). Natural, animal, and bovine melatonin supplements contain actual extracts from pineal glands. Synthetic melatonin is made from non-animal ingredients and is suitable for vegetarians. It is similar in molecular structure to melatonin produced in the human body.

The proper dosage of melatonin for various applications is not known, but it appears to differ greatly depending on the individual and extent of the sleep disorder. Persons starting the hormone should begin with a very low dose, 100 to 300 mcg (0.1–0.3 mg) or less and gradually increase the dosage if needed. Melatonin is quick-acting and should be taken about 30 minutes prior to bedtime. For jet lag, the general recommendation is 300 mcg just before boarding the flight and 1.5 mg after arrival before going to bed. Melatonin should not be taken during the day.

Researchers have long thought that melatonin is not available from any plant source. However, some

KEY TERMS

Circadian rhythm—The approximately 24-hour period, also known as the body's time clock, that regulates waking and sleeping periods.

Dehydroepiandrosterone (DHEA)—A hormone produced by the adrenal glands that is important in the synthesis of other hormones, especially estrogen and testosterone.

Estrogen—A hormone that stimulates development of female secondary sex characteristics.

Hypertension—Abnormally high blood pressure in the arteries.

Insomnia—A prolonged and usually abnormal inability to obtain adequate sleep.

Lymphoma—Cancer of the lymph nodes.

Pineal gland—A gland about the size of a pea at the base of the brain that is part of the endocrine system.

research showed that this view is not entirely correct. Studies have found that both cherries and walnuts contain small amounts of melatonin. The amounts of very small, however, amounting to no more than a few nanograms (billionths of a gram) of melatonin per gram of natural product. Anyone wanting to ingest melatonin from plants such as cherries or walnuts would, therefore, have to consume very large amounts of the plants.

Precautions

Women who are on estrogen or estrogen replacement therapy should not take melatonin without consulting their doctor. Since the safety of melatonin use during **pregnancy** has not been adequately studied as of 2008, women who are pregnant or breast feeding a child should not take melatonin. Also, women who are trying to get pregnant should avoid using it since some research suggests it may have a contraceptive effect. Studies in animals suggest melatonin can constrict blood vessels, which can raise blood pressure. Therefore, persons with **hypertension** or cardiovascular problems should consult with their doctor before taking the hormone. It is not recommended for people with lymphoma or **leukemia** and should not be used by children.

Side effects

Few studies have been done on the long-term effects or correct dosing of melatonin. In one study of melatonin, about 10% of patients said they experienced minor side effects such as nightmares, headaches, morning **hangover**, **depression**, and impaired sex drive.

Interactions

Melatonin should not be taken by people using certain antidepressants, such as a serotonin inhibitor (Prozac) or a monoamine oxidase inhibitor (Nardil). Interaction between melatonin and these types of antidepressants can cause a **stroke** or **heart attack**. Preliminary symptoms include confusion, sweating, shaking, **fever**, lack of coordination, elevated blood pressure, **diarrhea**, and convulsions.

Resources

BOOKS

Montilla, Pedro, and Isaac Tunez, eds. *Melatonin: Present and Future*. Hauppauge, NY: Nova Science, 2006.

Pandi-Perumal, S. R., and Daniel P. Cardinali, eds. *Melatonin: Biological Basis of Its Function in Health and Disease*. Hauppauge, NY: Nova Science, 2006.

Pandi-Perumal, S. R., and Daniel P. Cardinali, eds. *Melatonin: From Molecules to Therapy*. Hauppauge, NY: Nova Biomedical Books, 2007.

PERIODICALS

Pandi-Perumal, Seithikurippu R., et al. "Role of the Melatonin System in the Control of Sleep: Therapeutic Implications." *CNS Drugs* (December 2007): 995–1018.

Reilly, Thomas, et al. "Coping with Jet-lag: A Position Statement for the European College of Sport Science." *European Journal of Sport Science* (March 2007): 1–7.

Tekbas, Omer Faruk, et al. "Melatonin as an Antibiotic: New Insights into the Actions of this Ubiquitous Molecule." *Journal of Pineal Research* (March 2008): 222–226.

Tengattini, Sandra, et al. "Cardiovascular Diseases: Protective Effects of Melatonin." *Journal of Pineal Research* (January 2008): 16–25.

Wade, Alan, Nava Zisape, and Patrick Lemoine. "Prolonged-release Melatonin for the Treatment of Insomnia: Targeting Quality of Sleep and Morning Alertness." *Aging Health* (February 2008): 11–21.

ORGANIZATIONS

National Sleep Foundation, 1522 K St. NW, Suite 500, Washington, DC, 20005, (202) 347-3471, http://www.sleepfoundation.org.

Ken R. Wells
Teresa G. Odle
David Edward Newton, Ed.D.

Melissa officinalis see **Lemon balm**

Memory loss

Definition

Memory loss can be partial or total. Most memory loss occurs as part of the normal **aging** process, but memory loss may also occur as a result of severe emotional trauma or brain damage following disease or physical trauma. Memory loss can be described as amnesia, forgetfulness, or impaired memory.

Description

Memory is often classified as immediate (retention of information for a few seconds); short-term (retention of information for several seconds or minutes); and long-term (retention of information for days, weeks, or years). In short-term memory loss, patients can remember their childhood and past events but fail to remember events that happened in the previous few minutes. In long-term memory loss, patients are unable to recall events in the remote past.

Depending on the cause, memory loss can be sudden or gradual, and it can be permanent or temporary. Memory loss resulting from trauma to the brain is usually sudden and may be either permanent or temporary. By contrast, disease-related memory loss, such as in Alzheimer's disease, occurs gradually and is usually permanent. It is barely noticeable at first but progressively gets worse.

In most cases, memory loss is temporary and usually affects memories relating to a portion of a person's experience. However, severe physical brain trauma, such as that following a severe head injury, can cause total (global) memory loss. Some patients may temporarily lose memory and consciousness, then fully recover after the event.

Causes and symptoms

The following are common causes of memory loss:

- Aging. Even in people who do not have a disease associated with memory loss, the number of new nerve cells produced in the brain's hippocampus progressively decreases with age, and this decrease affects memory.
- Nutritional deficiency. Not enough thiamine (vitamin B_1), vitamin B_{12}, and/or protein contributes to memory loss.
- Depression. Depression can cause memory loss at any age. This is one of the main reasons for forgetfulness in the elderly. Depression-related memory loss is a treatable condition.
- Diseases. Memory loss can result from such chronic disease conditions as diabetes or hypothyroidism.
- Oxygen deprivation. Such conditions as severe head trauma, surgery, strokes, or heart attacks cause a sudden reduction of oxygen to the brain, which causes widespread death of nerve cells and significant memory loss.
- Structural abnormalities in or damage to the parts of the brain associated with memory formation. Two areas of the brain that are involved in memory formation are the hippocampus and the orbitofrontal cortex.
- Free-radical damage. Free-radical molecules are unstable and highly reactive molecules. These molecules destabilize other molecules around them, resulting in damage to the body at the molecular level. Free radicals can damage the blood-brain barrier, a membrane that separates the circulating blood and the brain. A weakened barrier may not be able to prevent toxic chemicals from entering the brain. Widespread brain damage, accelerated cell death, and memory loss occur as a result.
- Chemical poisoning. Daily exposure to toxic chemicals such as alcohol, tobacco, and illicit drugs (heroine, cocaine, and amphetamines) destroys brain cells at a rapid rate. Other environmental toxins, such as lead and mercury, can penetrate the blood-brain barrier. Once inside the brain, these heavy metals kill nerve cells. This action helps explain why exposure to heavy metals has been linked to memory and learning problems in children. Even though aluminum is not considered a heavy metal, its accumulation in the brain is believed to contribute to Alzheimer's disease.
- Central nervous system (CNS) infections and inflammation of the brain. Encephalitis (an inflammatory disease of the brain) can result in the death of nerve cells, which can lead to significant memory loss. CNS infections such as toxoplasmosis and neurosyphilis can also cause significant brain damage and memory loss.
- Stress. Emotional or physical stress stimulates the release of stress hormones such as cortisol and adrenaline. Constant exposure to stress hormones results in nerve-cell death and memory loss.
- Sensory overload. When a person is trying to do too many tasks or is worrying about too many things at the same time, the brain is overloaded with information and cannot process short-term memories. Therefore, if individuals are trying to remember a

lot of information, they may forget such details as where the car keys are or what appointments need to be kept.

- Low blood sugar. Nerve cells require glucose (sugar) to generate energy. If there is not enough glucose in the blood, nerve cells starve and die. Excessively low blood sugar can send a person into shock and/or into a coma.

- Genetic factors. A rare form of Alzheimer's disease is called early-onset familial AD. This form of the disease is inherited and usually strikes between the ages of 30 and 60. Most cases of Alzheimer's disease are described as "late-onset" because they do not occur until later in life. Although late-onset AD does not appear to be an inherited illness, scientists have identified a gene that may be involved. This gene's role is to make a protein known as apolipoprotein E, or ApoE. Although all people have this gene, about 15 percent of individuals have a certain form of the gene that increases the risk for AD. Scientists are also interested in the protein beta-amyloid, which is active in persons who have Alzheimer's disease. According to a study published in 2008, the protein is also very active in healthy young people. They believe the protein helps the brain delete unnecessary memories but causes problems in people with Alzheimer's disease because they lose memories faster than they make new ones. Studies were underway as of 2008 to search for possible other genetic risk factors. In addition, Down syndrome, which is caused by an abnormal form of human chromosome 21, is characterized by memory loss relatively early in life, often when individuals are in their 30s or 40s.

- Seizures. Prolonged seizures, such as in patients with epilepsy, can cause significant memory loss.

- Severe emotional trauma. Extreme emotional trauma has been associated with sudden amnesia. Dissociative amnesia is a type of amnesia that occurs when the brain splits off, or dissociates, extremely distressing memories from conscious recollection.

- Low estrogen levels in postmenopausal women. Women often report a significant decrease in memory function immediately following menopause.

Diagnosis

To find the underlying cause of memory loss, physicians obtain a detailed medical history, which documents the pattern, symptoms, and types of memory loss. They also inquire about contributing factors that may worsen or trigger memory loss. A routine physical and detailed neuropsychological examination with a focus on memory function is conducted. In addition, they may order several diagnostic tests.

Tests used to pinpoint the exact cause of memory loss include neuroimaging; electroencephalography (EEG) for patients with seizures; blood, cerebrospinal fluid, and tissue analysis to rule out specific diseases; and cognitive tests for gauging the patient's recent and remote (long-term) memory, and possibly the patient's attention span, judgment, and word comprehension as well. The most common brief test given to evaluate a person for memory loss and other aspects of cognitive function is the Mini-Mental Status Examination, or MMSE, which is also known as the Folstein.

Available neuroimaging techniques include computed tomography or CT scan, magnetic resonance imaging (MRI), positron emission tomography (PET), and single-photon emission computed tomography (SPECT). A CT scan can detect structural abnormalities, such as brain tumors or lesions. For detection of widespread loss of neurons associated with aging or degenerative diseases, an MRI, PET, or SPECT test can be performed. These tests can show the severity and extent of nerve damage. They can also help doctors pinpoint the cause of the memory loss. A PET scan is especially useful in that it allows doctors to track and record which memory centers are stimulated in a person's brain tissue while the person is functioning.

Treatment

Dietary guidelines

The following dietary changes are recommended to lower the risk of or slow memory loss:

- Reduce sugar intake.
- Avoid eating foods that contain such additives as artificial sweeteners, monosodium glutamate (MSG), preservatives, and artificial colors. These chemicals can accumulate in the body and become toxic, causing brain damage and memory loss.
- Eat organically grown foods. Pesticides and insecticides are toxic chemicals that can affect nerve function and cause memory loss.
- Limit alcohol intake and quit smoking.
- Do not use illicit drugs.
- Drink only filtered water to avoid toxic chemicals in the water system.
- Eat a low-fat, high-fiber diet with emphasis on fresh fruits and vegetables. Raw fruits and vegetables are the best sources of the vitamins, minerals, fiber, and antioxidants that the body needs for detoxifying. Antioxidants also protect and support brain function.

- Get enough protein. Protein is necessary to maintain healthy muscles, organs, and nerve cells; it also helps maintain blood sugar levels.
- Eat cold-water fish, which are a good source of omega-3 fatty acids. Omega-3 fats are believed to reduce the risk of strokes, blood clotting, and heart attacks. These are major causes of sudden memory loss in the elderly.

Nutritional supplements

The following nutritional supplements may help restore and maximize memory:

- L-Acetylcarnitine (LAC). Studies have shown that acetylcarnitine can improve memory function in the elderly. It may even reverse memory loss in some patients who have early Alzheimer's disease.
- Phosphatidylserine (100 mg three times per day). This supplement may help improve brain function in patients suffering from age-related memory loss and appears to be most effective for patients with milder symptoms.
- Vitamin E (400–800 IU per day). A strong antioxidant, vitamin E has been shown to promote memory performance.
- Omega-3 fatty acids. Flaxseed oil (1 tablespoon per day) and fish oil capsules are good sources of omega-3 fatty acids. Omega-3 enriched eggs are also beneficial.
- Thiamine (3–8 g per day). A vitamin B_1 deficiency can be treated with supplements. Thiamine/vitamin B_1 is an antioxidant that may improve mental function in Alzheimer's patients.
- Methylcobalamin (1,000 micrograms twice daily). Methylcobalamine is a supplemental form of cyanocobalamin, or vitamin B_{12}. Many Alzheimer's patients have been found to have a vitamin B_{12} deficiency.

Herbal therapy

Alternative medicine practitioners may recommend one or more of the following herbs to help reverse memory loss and/or improve mental performance:

- *Ginkgo biloba* extract (24% ginkgo flavonglycosides: 80 mg three times per day) is the herb most well-known as a memory booster. A study in 2002, however, indicated that gingko had no effect on memory or on concentration among generally healthy adults aged 60 to 82. Yet, several other studies demonstrated that ginkgo helps improve thinking and concentration in patients with Alzheimer's disease. Ginkgo is a strong antioxidant.
- Gotu kola (*Centella asiatica*: 70 mg taken twice daily). This herb is used to help improve memory by increasing blood circulation to the brain and by keeping blood vessels strong and healthy.
- Ginseng. Studies have shown that ginseng can improve memory and enhance learning ability. The recommended dosage of Korean ginseng is typically 3 to 9 **g** per day. Because ginseng may elevate blood pressure, patients with heart disease or high blood pressure should consult with their doctor before using this herb.
- Huperzine A. Huperzine A is isolated from a traditional Chinese medicine known as Qian Ceng Ta, which is made from a type of club moss (*Huperzia serrata*). It is sometimes recommended for treating dementia and for improving memory. Limited studied in China indicate that it is indeed useful in the treatment of memory loss due to dementia.
- Brahmi (*Bacopa monniera*). Brahmi is a herb native to India that is used in Ayurvedic medicine and Japanese medicine as a nerve tonic and treatment for insomnia. It is believed to improve a person's ability to retain new learning. Brahmi, which is sometimes called bacopa in Western countries, contains two compounds known as bacosides A and B. It is thought that these chemicals help to prevent memory loss by improving the efficiency of impulse transmission between nerve cells in the brain. An Australian study published in 2002 reported on the effects of brahmi on 76 human subjects. It showed that brahmi has a significant effect on people's ability to remember new information, although it does not affect a person's ability to retrieve information that was known prior to the experiment.

Allopathic treatment

The method of treatment for memory loss depends on underlying causes:

- Age. The elderly can be taught simple techniques to remember things better such as repeating a person's name several times, using word association, or jotting things down in a notebook.
- Depression. Depressed patients often show enhanced memory function after they are successfully treated for depression.
- CNS infections. Patients require effective antimicrobial treatment immediately to save them from death, significant brain damage, and profound memory loss.
- Trauma. Patients' memories usually return as they recover from the accident or injury. In some causes hypnosis is useful in helping patients retrieve traumatic memories without being overwhelmed by them.

KEY TERMS

Alzheimer's disease—A degenerative brain disease caused by physiological changes inside the brain. As a result, the patient experiences impaired memory and thought processes.

Antioxidant—Any substance that reduces the damage caused by oxidation, such as the harm caused by free radicals.

Bacosides—The name of two chemicals found in brahmi that are believed to aid memory by improving the efficiency of nerve impulse transmission.

Brahmi—A herb used in Ayurvedic and Japanese medicine that is believed to improve a person's ability to remember new information. Brahmi is also called bacopa.

Dissociation—A reaction to trauma in which the mind splits off certain aspects of the traumatic event from conscious awareness. Dissociation can affect the patient's memory, sense of reality, and sense of identity.

Dissociative amnesia—A disorder characterized by loss of memory for a period or periods of time in the patient's life.

Down syndrome—A genetic disorder caused by an extra human chromosome 21 (trisomy 21), characterized by mental retardation, muscular weakness, and folds over the patient's eyelids. Individuals with Down syndrome often begin to lose their memory in midlife.

Hippocampus—A horseshoe-shaped ridge in the brain that is part of the limbic system. The hippocampus is associated with the formation of short-term memory and with the sense of spatial orientation.

Mini-Mental Status Examination (MMSE)—A brief test of memory and cognitive function that is used to evaluate the presence and extent of memory loss and to monitor the effects of treatment for memory loss.

Neuron—A nerve cell that receives, processes, saves, and sends messages. It consists of an axon, a body, and dendrites.

- Alzheimer's disease (AD). Such medications as galantamine, rivastigmine, tacrine, or donepezil are often prescribed to improve memory and cognitive functions in patients with mild to moderate AD. Doctors may prescribe memantine to treat individuals with moderate to severe AD.

Expected results

A patient's prognosis depends on the underlying causes of his or her memory loss. Partial or complete recovery can be expected when the memory loss results from treatable causes such as **depression** or nutritional deficiencies. Patients with such degenerative nerve conditions as Alzheimer's disease, however, are expected to have a slow, irreversible decline of both memory and cognitive function. Medical treatment with memory-enhancing medications and long-term care are often required.

Prevention

A person can decrease or slow age-related memory loss by taking several steps. Keeping the mind active by continually learning new information is an important strategy in this regard. By eating healthy and nutritious foods, taking nutritional supplements and **antioxidants**, reducing stresses at home and at work, and avoiding environmental toxins, one can slow or even prevent memory loss.

Resources

BOOKS

Kandel, Eric. *In Search of Memory: The Emergence of a New Science of Mind.* New York: Norton, 2007.
Lorayne, Harry. *Ageless Memory: Secrets for Keeping Your Brain Young—Foolproof Methods for People Over 50.* New York: Black Dog & Leventhal, 2008.

PERIODICALS

Saey, Tina Hesman. "Alzheimer's Mystery Protein Unmasked." *Science News* (173, no. 12 (March 22, 2008): 189.

OTHER

"Alzheimer's Disease Fact Sheet." *National Institute on Aging, U.S. National Institutes of Health* October 26, 2007. http://www.nia.nih.gov/Alzheimers/Publications/adfact.htm. (April 12, 2008).

ORGANIZATIONS

Alzheimer's Disease Education & Referral (ADEAR) Center; The National Institute of Aging (NIA), PO Box 8250, Silver Spring, MD, 20907, (800) 438-4380, http://www.alzheimers.org.
American Psychiatric Association, 1000 Wilson Blvd., Suite 1825, Arlington, VA, 22209-3901, (703) 907-7300, http://www.psych.org.
NIH National Center for Complementary and Alternative Medicine; NCCAM Clearinghouse, 9000 Rockville Pike, Bethesda, MD, 20892, (888) 644-6226, http://nccam.nih.gov.

Mai Tran
Rebecca J. Frey, PhD
Leslie Mertz, Ph.D.

Ménière's disease

Definition

Ménière's disease is a condition characterized by recurrent vertigo (**dizziness**), **hearing loss**, and **tinnitus** (a roaring, buzzing, or ringing sound in the ears).

Description

Ménière's disease was named for the French physician Prosper Ménière, who first described the illness in 1861. It is an abnormality within the inner ear. A fluid called endolymph moves in the membranous labyrinth or semicircular canals within the bony labyrinth inside the inner ear. When the head or body moves, the endolymph moves, causing nerve receptors in the membranous labyrinth to send signals to the brain about the body's motion. A change in the volume of the endolymph fluid, or swelling or rupture of the membranous labyrinth is thought to result in Ménière's disease symptoms.

Causes and symptoms

Causes

The cause of Ménière's disease is unknown as of 2002; however, scientists are studying several possible causes, including noise pollution, viral **infections**, or alterations in the patterns of blood flow in the structures of the inner ear. Since Ménière's disease sometimes runs in families, researchers are also looking into genetic factors as possible causes of the disorder.

One area of research that shows promise is the possible relationship between Ménière's disease and **migraine headache**. Dr. Ménière himself suggested the possibility of a link, but early studies yielded conflicting results. A rigorous German study published in late 2002 reported that the lifetime prevalence of migraine was 56% in patients diagnosed with Ménière's disease as compared to 25% for controls. The researchers noted that further work is necessary to determine the exact nature of the relationship between the two disorders.

A study published in late 2002 reported that there is a significant increase in the number of CD4 cells in the blood of patients having an acute attack of Ménière's disease. CD4 cells are a subtype of T cells, which are produced in the thymus gland and regulate the immune system's response to infected or malignant cells. Further research is needed to clarify the role of these cells in Ménière's disease.

Another possible factor in the development of Ménière's disease is the loss of myelin from the cells

---

surrounding the vestibular nerve fibers. Myelin is a whitish fatty material in the cell membrane of the Schwann cells that form a sheath around certain nerve cells. It acts like an electrical insulator. A team of researchers at the University of Virginia reported in 2002 that the vestibular nerve cells in patients with unilateral Ménière's disease are demyelinated; that is, they have lost their protective "insulation." The researchers are investigating the possibility that a viral disease or disorder of the immune system is responsible for the demyelination of the vestibular nerve cells.

Symptoms

The symptoms of Ménière's disease are associated with a change in fluid volume within the labyrinth of the inner ear. Symptoms include severe dizziness or vertigo, tinnitus, hearing loss, and the sensation of **pain** or pressure in the affected ear. Symptoms appear suddenly, last up to several hours, and can occur as often as daily to as infrequently as once a year. A typical attack includes vertigo, tinnitus, and hearing loss; however, some individuals with Ménière's disease may experience a single symptom, like an occasional bout of slight dizziness or periodic, intense ringing in the ear. Attacks of severe vertigo can force the sufferer to have to sit or lie down, and may be accompanied by **headache**, **nausea**, **vomiting**, or **diarrhea**. Hearing

---

tends to recover between attacks, but becomes progressively worse over time.

Ménière's disease usually starts between the ages of 20 and 50 years; however, it is not uncommon for elderly people to develop the disease without a previous history of symptoms. Ménière's disease affects men and women in equal numbers. In most patients only one ear is affected but in about 15% both ears are involved.

Diagnosis

An estimated three to five million people in the United States have Ménière's disease, and almost 100,000 new cases are diagnosed each year. Diagnosis is based on medical history, physical examination, hearing and balance tests, and medical imaging with magnetic resonance imaging (MRI).

In patients with Ménière's disease, audiometric tests (hearing tests) usually indicate a sensory type of hearing loss in the affected ear. Speech discrimination, or the ability to distinguish between words that sound alike, is often diminished. In about 50% of patients, the balance function is reduced in the affected ear. An electronystagnograph (ENG) may be used to evaluate balance. Since the eyes and ears work together through the nervous system to coordinate balance, measurement of eye movements can be used to test the balance system. For this test, the patient is seated in a darkened room and recording electrodes, similar to those used with a heart monitor, are placed near the eyes. Warm and cool water or air are gently introduced into each ear canal and eye movements are recorded.

Another test that may be used is an electrocochleograph (EcoG), which can measure increased inner ear fluid pressure.

Treatment

Because there is no cure for Ménière's disease, most treatments are aimed at reducing its symptoms, especially tinnitus. General measures to mask the tinnitus include playing a radio or tape of white noise (low, constant sound). Exercising to improve blood circulation and reducing the intake of salt, alcohol, aspirin, **caffeine**, and nicotine may relieve Ménière's disease symptoms.

Ayurveda

Ayurvedic practitioners believe that tinnitus is a vata disorder. (Vata is one of three doshas, or body/mental types.) The patient can drink a tea prepared from 1 tsp of a mixture of **comfrey**, cinnamon, and **chamomile** two to three times a day. Yogaraj guggulu in warm water can be taken two or three times a day. Gentle massage of the mastoid bone (behind the ear) with warm **sesame oil** may help relieve tinnitus. Placing three drops of **garlic** oil into the affected ear at night may also be effective.

Homeopathy

Homeopathic remedies are chosen based on each patients specific set of symptoms. Salicylic acidum is indicated for patients who experience a roaring sound, deafness, and giddiness. **Bryonia** is recommended for patients with headache, a buzzing or roaring sound in the ear, and dizziness that is worsened by motion. Cocculus is indicated for those who experience dizziness and nausea. Conium is chosen for the patient who experiences light sensitivity and dizziness that is worsened by lying down. *Carbonium sulphuratum* is recommended for patients who experience a roaring with a tingling sensation and clogged ears. *Kali iodatum* is chosen for patients who have long-term ringing in the ears and no other symptoms. Theridion is indicated for patients who experience sensitivity to noise and dizziness with nausea and vomiting that is worsened by the slightest motion.

Other remedies

Other alternative medicine disciplines which have treatments to help relieve symptoms of Ménière's disease are:

- Acupuncture. The acupuncture ear points neurogate, kidney, sympathetic, occiput, heart, and adrenal may relieve dizziness associated with Ménière's disease. Chronic cases may be treated at the body points on the spleen, triple warmer, and kidney meridians. The World Health Organization (WHO) lists Ménière's disease as one of 104 conditions that can be treated effectively with acupuncture.

- Aromatherapy. The essential oils of geranium, lavender, and sandalwood may be added to bath water. Lavender or German chamomile oils may be used as massage oils.

- Body adjustments. Chiropractors or osteopaths may adjust the head, jaw, and neck to relieve movement restrictions that could affect the inner ear. Craniosacral therapists may gently move bones of the skull to relieve pressure on the head.

- Herbals. Ginkgo (*Ginkgo biloba*) improves circulation which may improve tinnitus and Ménière's disease. Ginkgo is a powerful antioxidant and blood thinner. Ginkgo relieves tinnitus in about half of the patients who use it. Fenugreek (*Trigonella foenum-graecum*) tea (steeped in cold water) stops cricket noises and ringing in the ears. Chamomile (*Matricaria recutita*) promotes relaxation and may help the patient to sleep.

- Reflexology. Working the cervical spine, ear, and neck points on the hands and feet and the points on the bottoms and sides of the big toes may relieve tinnitus.

- Relaxation techniques. Biofeedback, yoga, massage, and other stress-reduction techniques can promote relaxation and divert the patient's attention away from tinnitus. Stress can worsen tinnitus and bring on an attack of Ménière's disease so relaxation techniques can be beneficial.

- Supplements. Magnesium deficiency may cause tinnitus. Magnesium supplementation may relieve the tinnitus associated with Ménière's disease and protect the ears from damage resulting from loud sounds. Vitamin B_{12} supplementation has improved tinnitus in patients deficient in this vitamin. Other supplements recommended for the treatment of Ménière's disease include vitamins C, B_1, B_2, and B_6 and zinc.

- TENS. Transcutaneous electrical nerve stimulation reduced tinnitus in 60% of the Ménière's disease patients in a study of tinnitus sufferers. Patients received six to 10 treatments biweekly. A few of the study patients reported temporary or permanent worsening of tinnitus, however, the cause of the tinnitus in these patients was not specified.

Allopathic treatment

There is no cure for Ménière's disease, but medication, surgery, and dietary and behavioral changes can help control or improve the symptoms.

A special hearing aid is available which makes a soft noise to mask the ringing and other noises associated with Ménière's disease. This device does not interfere with hearing or speech.

Medications

Symptoms of Ménière's disease may be treated with a variety of oral medicine or through injections. Antihistamines, like diphenhydramine, meclizine, and cyclizine can be prescribed to sedate the vestibular system. A barbiturate medication like pentobarbital may be used to completely sedate the patient and relieve the vertigo. Anticholinergic drugs, like atropine or scopolamine, can help minimize nausea and vomiting. Diazepam has been found to be particularly effective for relief of vertigo and nausea in Ménière's disease. There have been some reports of successful control of vertigo after antibiotics (gentamicin or streptomycin) or a steroid medication (dexamethasone) are injected directly into the inner ear. Some researchers have found that gentamicin is effective in relieving tinnitus as well as vertigo.

A newer medication that appears to be effective in treating the vertigo associated with Ménière's disease is flunarizine, which is sold under the trade name Sibelium. Flunarizine is a **calcium** channel blocker and anticonvulsant that is presently used to treat **Parkinson's disease**, migraine headache, and other circulatory disorders that affect the brain.

Surgical procedures

Surgical procedures may be recommended if the vertigo attacks are frequent, severe, or disabling and cannot be controlled by other treatments. The most common surgical treatment is insertion of a small tube or shunt to drain some of the fluid from the canal. This treatment usually preserves hearing and controls vertigo in about one-half to two-thirds of cases, but it is not a permanent cure in all patients.

The vestibular nerve leads from the inner ear to the brain and is responsible for conducting nerve impulses related to balance. A vestibular neurectomy is a procedure where this nerve is cut so the distorted impulses causing dizziness no longer reach the brain. This procedure permanently cures the majority of patients and hearing is preserved in most cases. There is a slight risk that hearing or facial muscle control will be affected.

A labyrinthectomy is a surgical procedure in which the balance and hearing mechanism in the inner ear are destroyed on one side. This procedure is considered when the patient has poor hearing in the affected ear. Labyrinthectomy results in the highest rates of control of vertigo attacks, however, it also causes complete deafness in the affected ear.

Expected results

Ménière's disease is a complex and unpredictable condition for which there is no cure. The vertigo associated with the disease can generally be managed or eliminated with medications and surgery. Hearing tends to become worse over time, and some of the surgical procedures recommended, in fact, cause deafness.

Prevention

Because the cause of Ménière's disease is not definitely known as of 2002, there are no proven strategies for its prevention. **Stress** reduction and **relaxation** may prevent attacks of Ménière's disease. Wearing earplugs while exposed to loud sounds will help to prevent hearing damage and worsening of tinnitus.

Resources

BOOKS

"Ménière's Disease." *The Alternate Advisor: The Complete Guide to Natural Therapies and Alternative Treatments.* Edited by Robert. Richmond, VA: Time-Life Books, 1997.

The Merck Manual of Diagnosis and Therapy. 17th ed., edited by Mark H. Beers and Robert Berkow. Whitehouse Station, NJ: Merck Research Laboratories, 1999.

Pelletier, Kenneth R., MD. *The Best Alternative Medicine*, Part II, "CAM Therapies for Specific Conditions: Ménière's Disease." New York: Simon & Schuster, 2002.

PERIODICALS

Ballester, M., P. Liard, D. Vibert, and R. Hausler. "Ménière's Disease in the Elderly." *Otology and Neurotology* 23 (January 2002): 73–78.

Corvera, J., G. Corvera-Behar, V. Lapilover, and A. Ysunza. "Objective Evaluation of the Effect of Flunarizine on Vestibular Neuritis." *Otology and Neurotology* 23 (November 2002): 933–937.

Driscoll, C. L., et al. "Low-Dose Gentamicin and the Treatment of Ménière's Disease: Preliminary Results." *Laryngoscope* 107 (January 1997): 83–89.

Friberg, U., and H. Rask-Andersen. "Vascular Occlusion in the Endolymphatic Sac in Ménière's Disease." *Annals of Otology, Rhinology, and Laryngology* 111 (March 2002): 237–245.

Fung, K., Y. Xie, S. F. Hall, et al. "Genetic Basis of Familial Ménière's Disease." *Journal of Otolaryngology* 31 (February 2002): 1–4.

Ghosh, S., A. K. Gupta, and S. S. Mann. "Can Electrocochleography in Ménière's Disease Be Noninvasive?" *Journal of Otolaryngology* 31 (December 2002): 371–375.

Mamikoglu, B., R. J. Wiet, T. Hain, and I. J. Check. "Increased CD4+ T cells During Acute Attack of Ménière's Disease." *Acta Otolaryngologica* 122 (December 2002): 857–860.

Radtke, A., T. Lempert, M. A. Gresty, et al. "Migraine and Ménière's Disease: Is There a Link?" *Neurology* 59 (December 10, 2002): 1700–1704.

Saeed, Shakeel R. "Diagnosis and Treatment of Ménière's Disease." *British Medical Journal* 316 (January 1998): 368.

Spencer, R. F., A. Sismanis, J. K. Kilpatrick, and W. T. Shaia. "Demyelination of Vestibular Nerve Axons in Unilateral Méniè's Disease." *Ear, Nose and Throat Journal* 81 (November 2002): 785–789.

Steenerson, Ronald L., and Gaye W. Cronin. "Treatment of Tinnitus with Electrical Stimulation. *Otolaryngology-Head and Neck Surgery* 121 (November 1999): 511–513.

Yetiser, S., and M. Kertmen. "Intratympanic Gentamicin in Ménière's Disease: The Impact on Tinnitus." *International Journal of Audiology* 41 (September 2002): 363–370.

ORGANIZATIONS

American Academy of Otolaryngology-Head and Neck Surgery. One Prince Street, Alexandria, VA 22314. (703) 836-4444. http://www.entnet.org.

The Ménière's Network. 1817 Patterson Street, Nashville, TN 37203. (800) 545-4327. http://www. earfoundation.org.

Vestibular Disorders Association. P.O. Box 4467, Portland, OR 97208-4467. (800) 837-8428. http://www. vestibular.org.

Belinda Rowland
Rebecca J. Frey, PhD

Meningitis

Definition

Meningitis is a potentially fatal inflammation of the meninges, the thin, membranous covering of the brain and the spinal cord. Meningitis is most commonly caused by infection by bacteria, viruses, or

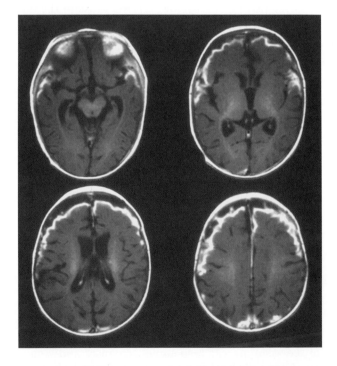

This composite of four contrast-enhanced MRI images shows H. Influenza meningitis. *(Living Art Enterprises, LLC / Photo Researchers, Inc.)*

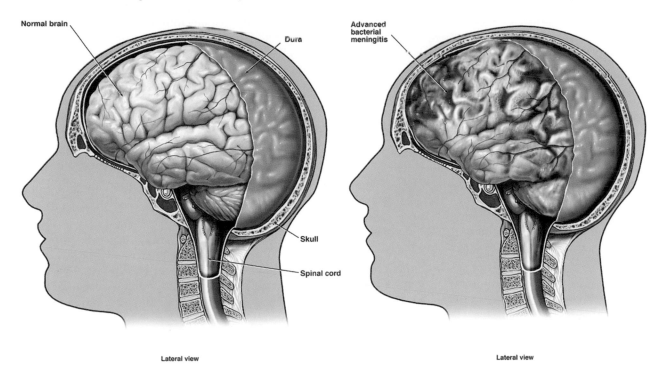

Normal Anatomy of Brain and Spinal Cord

Normal brain

Dura

Skull

Spinal cord

Lateral view

Brain with Bacterial Meningitis

Advanced bacterial meningitis

Lateral view

Illustration of bacterial meningitis in an adult. *(© PHOTOTAKE Inc. / Alamy)*

fungi, although it can also be caused by bleeding into the meninges, **cancer**, diseases of the immune system, and an inflammatory response to certain types of chemotherapy or other chemical agents. The most serious and the most difficult to treat types of meningitis tend to be those caused by bacteria.

Description

Meningitis is a particularly dangerous infection because of the very delicate nature of the brain. Brain cells are some of the only cells in the body that, once killed, will not regenerate themselves. Therefore, if enough brain tissue is damaged by an infection, then serious lifelong handicaps will remain.

In order to learn about meningitis, it is important to have a basic understanding of the anatomy of the brain. The meninges are three separate membranes, layered together, which encase the brain and spinal cord:

- The dura is the toughest, outermost layer, and is closely attached to the inside of the skull.

- The middle layer, the arachnoid, is important because of its involvement in the normal flow of the cerebrospinal

fluid (CSF), a lubricating and nutritive fluid that bathes both the brain and the spinal cord.

- The innermost layer, the pia, helps direct blood vessels into the brain.

- The space between the arachnoid and the pia contains CSF, which helps insulate the brain from trauma. Many blood vessels, as well as peripheral and cranial nerves course through this space.

CSF, produced within specialized chambers deep inside the brain, flows over the surface of the brain and spinal cord. This fluid serves to cushion these relatively delicate structures, as well as supplying important nutrients for brain cells. CSF is reabsorbed by blood vessels located within the meninges. A careful balance between CSF production and reabsorption is important to avoid the accumulation of too much CSF.

Because the brain is enclosed in the hard, bony case of the skull, any disease that produces swelling will be damaging to the brain. The skull cannot expand at all, so when the swollen brain tissue pushes up against the skull's hard bone, the brain tissue becomes damaged and the blood supply is compromised, and this tissue may ultimately die. Furthermore, swelling on the right side of the brain will not only cause pressure and damage to that side of the brain, but by taking up precious space within the tight confines of the skull, the left side of the brain will also be pushed up against the hard surface of the skull, causing damage to the left side of the brain, as well.

Another way that **infections** injure the brain involves the way in which the chemical environment of the brain changes in response to the presence of an infection. The cells of the brain require a very well-regulated environment. Careful balance of oxygen, carbon dioxide, sugar (glucose), **sodium**, **calcium**, **potassium**, and other substances must be maintained in order to avoid damage to brain tissue. An infection upsets this balance, and brain damage can occur when the cells of the brain are either deprived of important nutrients or exposed to toxic levels of particular substances.

The cells lining the brain's tiny blood vessels (capillaries) are specifically designed to prevent many substances from passing into brain tissue. This is commonly referred to as the blood-brain barrier. The blood-brain barrier prevents various substances that could be poisonous to brain tissue (toxins), as well as many agents of infection, from crossing from the blood stream into the brain tissue. While this barrier is obviously an important protective feature for the brain, it also serves to complicate treatment in the case of an infection by making it difficult for medications to pass out of the blood and into the brain tissue where the infection is located.

Causes and symptoms

The most common infectious causes of meningitis vary according to an individual's age, habits, living environment, and health status. While nonbacterial types of meningitis are more common, bacterial meningitis is more potentially life-threatening. Three bacterial agents are responsible for about 80% of all bacterial meningitis cases. These bacteria are *Haemophilus influenzae* type b, *Neisseria meningitidis* (causing meningococcal meningitis), and *Streptococcus pneumoniae* (causing pneumococcal meningitis).

In newborns, the most common agents of meningitis are those that are contracted from the newborn's mother, including Group B streptococci (becoming an increasingly common infecting organism in the newborn period), *Escherichia coli*, and *Listeria monocytogenes*. The highest incidence of meningitis occurs in babies under a month old, with an increased risk of meningitis continuing through about two years of age.

Older children are more frequently infected by bacteria, including *Haemophilus influenzae*, *Neisseria meningitidis*, and *Streptococcus pneumoniae*.

Adults are most commonly infected by either *S. pneumoniae* or *N. meningitidis*, with pneumococcal meningitis the more common. Certain conditions predispose to this type of meningitis, including **alcoholism** and chronic upper respiratory tract infections (especially of the middle ear, sinuses, and mastoids).

N. meningitidis is the only organism that can cause epidemics of meningitis. For instance, cases have been reported when a child in a crowded day care situation or a military recruit in a crowded training camp has fallen ill with meningococcal meningitis.

There have been case reports in recent years of meningitis caused by *Streptococcus bovis*, an organism that is ordinarily found in the digestive tract of such animals as cows and sheep; and *Pasteurella multocida*, an organism that usually infects rabbits. Other atypical

cases of meningitis include several caused by the anthrax bacillus. These cases have a high mortality rate.

Viral causes of meningitis include the herpes simplex virus, the **mumps** and **measles** viruses (against which most children are protected due to mass immunization programs), the virus that causes **chickenpox**, the **rabies** virus, and a number of viruses that are acquired through the **bites** of infected mosquitoes.

A number of medical conditions predispose individuals to meningitis caused by specific organisms. Patients with **AIDS** (acquired immunodeficiency syndrome) are more prone to getting meningitis from fungi, as well as from the agent that causes **tuberculosis**. Patients who have had their spleens removed, or whose spleens are no longer functional (as in the case of patients with sickle cell disease) are more susceptible to other infections, including meningococcal and pneumococcal meningitis.

The majority of meningitis infections are acquired by transmission through the blood. A person may have another type of infection (for instance, infection of the lungs, throat, or tissues of the heart) caused by an organism that can also cause meningitis. If this initial infection is not properly treated, the organism will continue to multiply, find its way into the blood stream, and be delivered in sufficient quantities to invade past the blood-brain barrier. Direct spread occurs when an organism spreads to the meninges from infected tissue next to or very near the meninges. This can occur, for example, with a severe, poorly treated ear or **sinus infection**.

Patients who suffer from skull **fractures** possess abnormal openings to the sinuses, nasal passages, and middle ears. Organisms that usually live in the human respiratory system without causing disease can pass through openings caused by such fractures, reach the meninges, and cause infection. Similarly, patients who undergo surgical procedures or who have had foreign bodies surgically placed within their skulls (such as tubes to drain abnormal amounts of accumulated CSF) have an increased risk of meningitis.

Organisms can also reach the meninges via an uncommon but interesting method called intraneural spread. This involves an organism invading the body at a considerable distance away from the head, spreading along a nerve, and using that nerve as a sort of ladder into the skull, where the organism can multiply and cause meningitis. Herpes simplex virus is known to use this type of spread, as is the rabies virus.

The classic symptoms of meningitis (particularly of bacterial meningitis) include **fever**, **headache**, **vomiting**, sensitivity to light (photophobia), irritability,

severe **fatigue** (lethargy), stiff neck, and a reddish purple rash on the skin. Untreated, the disease progresses with seizures, confusion, and eventually coma.

A very young infant may not show the classic signs of meningitis. Early in infancy, a baby's immune system is not yet developed enough to mount a fever in response to infection, so fever may be absent. However, checking an infant's temperature to see if it is high or low could be an indication. Some infants with meningitis have seizures as their only identifiable symptom. Similarly, debilitated elderly patients may not have fever or other identifiable symptoms of meningitis.

Damage due to meningitis occurs from a variety of phenomena. The action of infectious agents on the brain tissue is one direct cause of damage. Other types of damage may be due to the mechanical effects of swelling and compression of brain tissue against the bony surface of the skull. Swelling of the meninges may interfere with the normal absorption of CSF by blood vessels, causing accumulation of CSF and damage from the resulting pressure on the brain. Interference with the brain's carefully regulated chemical environment may cause damaging amounts of normally present substances (carbon dioxide, potassium) to accumulate. Inflammation may cause the blood-brain barrier to become less effective at preventing the passage of toxic substances into brain tissue.

Diagnosis

A number of techniques are used when examining a patient suspected of having meningitis to verify the diagnosis. Certain manipulations of the head (lowering the head, chin towards chest, for example) are difficult to perform and painful for a patient with meningitis.

The most important test used to diagnose meningitis is the lumbar puncture (LP), commonly called a spinal tap. Lumbar puncture involves the insertion of a thin needle into a space between the vertebrae in the lower back and the withdrawal of a small amount of CSF. The CSF is then examined under a microscope to look for bacteria or fungi. Normal CSF contains set percentages of glucose and protein. These percentages will vary with bacterial, viral, or other causes of meningitis. For example, bacterial meningitis causes a smaller than normal percentage of glucose to be present in CSF, as the bacteria are essentially "eating" the host's glucose, and using it for their own **nutrition** and energy production. Normal CSF should contain no infection-fighting cells (white blood cells), so the presence of white blood cells in CSF is another indication of meningitis. Some of the withdrawn CSF is also put into special lab dishes to allow growth of the suspected infecting organism, which can then be identified more easily. Special immunologic and serologic tests may also be used to help identify the infectious agent.

In rare instances, CSF from a lumbar puncture cannot be examined because the amount of swelling within the skull is so great that the pressure within the skull (intracranial pressure) is extremely high. This pressure is always measured immediately upon insertion of the LP needle. If it is found to be very high, no fluid is withdrawn because doing so could cause herniation of the brain stem. Herniation of the brain stem occurs when the part of the brain connecting to the spinal cord is thrust through the opening at the base of the skull into the spinal canal. Such herniation will cause compression of those structures within the brain stem that control the most vital functions of the body (breathing, heart beat, consciousness). Death or permanent debilitation follows herniation of the brain stem.

Treatment

Because meningitis is a potentially deadly condition, doctors should be contacted immediately for diagnosis and treatment. Alternative treatments should be used only to support the recovery process following appropriate antibiotic treatments, or used concurrently with antibiotic treatments.

General recommendations

Patients should be well rested in bed, preferably in a darkened room. They should be given lots of fluids and nutritious foods. Patients should avoid processed foods and those with high fat and sugar content. Fats are difficult to digest in severely ill patients; sugar tends to depress the immune system and impede recovery process. Patients should also take **vitamin A** (up to 10,000 IU per day), B-complex vitamins (up to 1,500 mg per day), and **vitamin C** (up to 2 g per day) to help keep the body strong and prevent future infections. Additionally, the patient may consider taking other **antioxidants**, **essential fatty acids** (EFAs), and/or participate in therapies, such as **massage therapy** and movement therapies (e.g., **t'ai chi**).

Other treatments

Alternative therapies, such as **homeopathy**, **traditional Chinese medicine**, and Western herbal medicine may help patients regain their health and build up their immune systems. The recovering individual, under the direction of a professional alternative therapist, may opt to include mushrooms into his or her diet to stimulate immune function. Contact an experienced herbalist or homeopathic practitioner for specific remedies.

Allopathic treatment

Antibiotics are the first line of treatment for bacterial meningitis. In recent years, however, doctors have turned to such newer medications as vancomycin or the fluoroquinolones to treat bacterial meningitis because strains of *S. pneumoniae* and *N. meningitidis* have emerged that are resistant to penicillin and the older antibiotics. Because of the effectiveness of the blood-brain barrier in preventing the passage of substances into the brain, medications must be delivered directly into the patient's veins (intravenously) at very high doses. Antiviral drugs (acyclovir) may be helpful in shortening the course of viral meningitis, and antifungal medications are available as well. Patients who develop seizures will require medications to halt the seizures and prevent their return.

Expected results

Viral meningitis is the least severe type of meningitis, and patients usually recover with no long-term effects from the infection. Bacterial infections, however, are much more severe, and progress rapidly. Without very rapid treatment with the appropriate antibiotic, the infection can swiftly lead to coma and death in less than a day's time. While death rates from meningitis vary depending on the specific infecting organism, the overall death rate is just under 20%.

The most frequent long-term effects of meningitis include deafness and blindness, which may be caused by the compression of specific nerves and brain areas responsible for the senses of hearing and sight. Some patients develop permanent seizure disorders, requiring lifelong treatment with antiseizure medications. Scarring of the meninges may result in obstruction of the normal flow of CSF, causing abnormal accumulation of CSF. This may be a chronic problem for some patients, requiring the installation of shunt tubes to drain the accumulation regularly.

Some cases of sudden and unexplained death in adults have been attributed to rapidly developing meningitis.

Prevention

Prevention of meningitis primarily involves the appropriate treatment of other infections an individual may acquire, particularly those that have a track record of seeding to the meninges (such as ear and sinus infections). Preventive treatment with antibiotics is sometimes recommended for the close contacts of an individual who is ill with meningococcal or *H. influenzae* type b meningitis. A meningococcal vaccine exists, and is sometimes recommended to individuals who are traveling to very high risk areas. A vaccine for *H. influenzae* type b is now given to babies as part of the standard array of childhood immunizations.

Resources

BOOKS

"Meningitis." *The Medical Advisor: The Complete guide to Alternative & Conventional Treatments. Home Edition.* Richmond, VA: Time Life Inc., 1997.

Ray, C. George. "Central Nervous System Infections." In *Sherris Medical Microbiology: An Introduction to Infectious Diseases,* edited by Kenneth J. Ryan. Norwalk, CT: Appleton and Lange, 1994.

Swartz, Morton N. "Bacterial Meningitis." In *Cecil Textbook of Medicine,* edited by J. Claude Bennett and Fred Plum. Philadelphia: W.B. Saunders, 1996.

PERIODICALS

Aronin, S. I. "Current Pharmacotherapy of Pneumococcal Meningitis." *Expert Opinion on Pharmacotherapy* 3 (February 2002): 121–129.

Black, M., and D. I Graham. "Sudden Unexplained Death in Adults Caused by Intracranial Pathology." *Journal of Clinical Pathology* 55 (January 2002): 44–50.

Green, B. T., K. M. Ramsey, and P. E. Nolan. "*Pasteurella multocida* Meningitis: Case Report and Review of the Last 11 Years." *Scandinavian Journal of Infectious Disease* 34 (2002): 213–217.

Meissner, Judith W. "Caring for Patients With Meningitis." *Nursing* (July 1995): 50 + .

Schuchat, Anne, et al. "Bacterial Meningitis in the United States in 1995." *New England Journal of Medicine* (October 2, 1997).

Tasyaran, M. A., O. Deniz, M. Ertek, and K. Cetin. "Anthrax Meningitis: Case Report and Review." *Scandinavian Journal of Infectious Diseases* 34 (2002): 66–67.

Tunkel, A. R., and W. M. Scheld. "Treatment of Bacterial Meningitis." *Current Infectious Disease Reports* 4 (February 2002): 7–16.

Vilarrasa, N., A. Prats, M. Pujol, et al. "*Streptococcus bovis* Meningitis in a Healthy Adult Patient." *Scandinavian Journal of Infectious Diseases* 34 (2002): 61–62.

ORGANIZATIONS

American Academy of Neurology. 1080 Montreal Avenue, St. Paul, MN 55116. (612) 695-1940. http://www.aan.com

Meningitis Foundation of America. 7155 Shadeland Station, Suite 190, Indianapolis, IN 46256-3922. (800) 668-1129. http://www.musa.org/welcome.htm

Mai Tran
Rebecca J. Frey, PhD

Menopause

Definition

Menopause represents the irreversible end of ovulation and **menstruation**. Technically menopause refers to the final menstrual period after which a woman can no longer conceive children. Nevertheless, menopause is not an abrupt event, but a gradual process that involves many physical and hormonal changes before fertility ceases. Menopause is not a disease that needs to be treated, but a natural result of **aging**. However, the changes that occur during the time surrounding menopause can cause symptoms of widely varying severity that a women may wish to treat. Women have many options for managing these symptoms.

Description

Perimenopause is the time surrounding menopause. It can last for several years, and many women have irregular periods and other changes during this time. Although it is not easy to pinpoint when menopause begins, doctors agree that it is complete when a woman has not had a menstrual period for a full year.

There is no method to determine when the ovaries will begin to scale back, but a woman can get a general idea of when she will experience menopause based on her family history, body type, and lifestyle. A woman is likely to enter menopause at about the same age as her mother and sisters. Women who are smokers are more likely to begin menopause earlier than non-smokers. Women who began menstruating early will not necessarily stop having periods early. Eight out of every 100 women stop menstruating before age 40. At the other end of the spectrum, five out of every 100

Signs and symptoms of menopause

- Changes in periods (they may be shorter or longer, heavier or lighter, or have more or less time in between)
- Hot flashes
- Night sweats
- Trouble sleeping through the night
- Vaginal dryness
- Mood changes
- Hair loss or thinning on the head, more hair growth on the face

Although menopause itself is the time of a woman's last period, symptoms can begin several years before that in a stage called peri-menopause. Menopause and peri-menopause affect every woman differently. (*Illustration by GGS Information Services. Cengage Learning, Gale*)

continue to have periods until they are almost 60. The average age of menopause is 51.

Causes and symptoms

Once a woman enters puberty, her body releases one of the more than 400,000 eggs (ova) that are stored in her ovaries, about every 28 days in response to the interaction of several hormones. Blood supply to the womb (uterus) increases, and the lining of the uterus thickens in anticipation of receiving a fertilized egg. If the egg is not fertilized, the level of progesterone, the hormone mainly responsible for this uterine thickening, drops, and the uterine lining is sloughed off along with some blood. This menstrual flow is visible evidence ovulation has occurred.

By the time a woman reaches her late 30s or 40s, her ovaries begin to produce less of the female hormones estrogen and progesterone and to release eggs less regularly. As the levels of hormones fluctuate, the menstrual cycle begins to change. Some women may have longer periods with heavy flow followed by shorter cycles and very little bleeding. Others will begin to miss periods entirely. These irregular menstrual cycles make it more difficult for a woman to become pregnant. The gradual decline of estrogen also causes a wide variety of changes in tissues that respond to estrogen including the vagina, vulva, uterus, bladder, urethra, breasts, bones, heart, blood vessels, brain, skin, hair, and mucous membranes. Less immediately, the long-term lack of estrogen can make a woman more vulnerable to **osteoporosis**.

The most common symptom of perimenopause include:

- changes in the menstrual cycle
- hot flashes
- night sweats
- insomnia
- mood swings and increased irritability
- memory or concentration problems
- vaginal dryness
- heavy bleeding
- fatigue
- depression
- changes in the thickness and texture of hair
- headaches
- heart palpitations
- sexual disinterest
- urinary changes
- weight gain

Diagnosis

The clearest indication of menopause is the absence of a period for one full year. If it has been at least three months since a woman's last period, a follicle-stimulating hormone (FSH) test might be helpful in determining whether menopause has occurred. FSH levels rise steadily as a woman ages. The FSH test alone cannot be used as proof that a woman has entered early menopause. A better measure of menopause is to determine the levels of FSH, estrogen, progesterone, testosterone, and related hormones at mid-cycle. These tests are not routinely performed as most women can recognize the symptoms of perimenopause and menopause. They can, however, be helpful diagnostic tests in younger women who are showing symptoms of perimenopause.

Treatment

Decisions about if and how to treat symptoms associated with perimenopause should be made by a woman and her health care provider after taking into consideration her medical history and current research findings. Some women report success in using natural remedies to treat the unpleasant symptoms of menopause, although alternative therapies have only received significant attention in the United States in the last decade or so. Debate continues until scientific studies can prove these treatments' effectiveness on menopausal symptoms.

For women nearing menopause, alternative medical practitioners and traditional healthcare professionals generally recommend a diet high in fresh fruits, fresh vegetables, whole grains, nuts, seeds, and fresh vegetable juices and low in sugary treats and fats, especially animal fats. Calorie and portion control becomes more important as metabolism slows. Because a decrease in estrogen accelerates bone loss, women should make sure they get enough **calcium**. Most often a calcium supplement is recommended in addition to dairy products that provide calcium. Women generally need less **iron** after menopause because they no longer bleed monthly.

Herbs

Herbs have been used to relieve menopausal symptoms for centuries. In reasonable quantities, many herbs are relatively safe. Often adverse reactions to herbs come not from the herbs themselves, but from contaminants. Because the United States Food and Drug Administration (FDA) does not regulate herbal products as strictly as pharmaceutical medicines, contamination, mislabeling, or accidental overdose is possible. Herbs should be purchased from a recognized company or through a qualified herbal practitioner. Herbal practitioners recommend a dose based on a woman's history, body size, lifestyle, diet, and reported symptoms. Women who choose to take herbs for menopausal symptoms should learn as much as possible about herbs and work with a qualified practitioner such as an herbalist, a traditional Chinese doctor, or a naturopathic physician.

The following list of herbs include those that herbalists recommend to treat menopausal symptoms:

- black cohosh (*Cimicifuga racemosa*): >): hot flashes and other menstrual complaints
- black currant (*Ribes migrum*): breast tenderness
- chaste tree/chasteberry (*Vitex agnus-castus*): hot flashes, excessive menstrual bleeding, moodiness
- chickweed (*Stellaria media*): hot flashes
- evening primrose oil (*Oenothera biennis*): mood swings, irritability, breast tenderness
- fennel (*Foeniculum vulgare*): hot flashes, digestive gas, bloating
- flaxseed (*Linum usitatissimum*): excessive menstrual bleeding, breast tenderness, and other symptoms, including dry skin and vaginal dryness
- ginkgo (*Ginkgo biloba*): memory problems
- ginseng (*Panax ginseng*): hot flashes, fatigue, vaginal thinning
- hawthorn (*Crataegus laevigata*): memory problems, fuzzy thinking
- horsetail (*Equisetum arvense*): osteoporosis
- lady's mantle (*Alchemilla vulgaris*): excessive menstrual bleeding
- Licorice (*Glycyrrhiza glabra*) root: general menopausal symptoms
- Mexican wild yam (*Dioscorea villosa*) root: vaginal dryness, hot flashes, general menopause symptoms
- motherwort (*Leonurus cardiaca*): night sweats, hot flashes
- oat straw (*Avena sativa*): mood swings, anxiety
- passionflower (*Passiflora incarnata*): insomnia, pain
- raspberry leaf (*Rubus idaeus*): normalizes hormonal system
- sage (*Salvia officinalis*): mood swings, headaches, night sweats
- skullcap (*Scutellaria lateriflora*): insomnia
- sesame oil (*Sesamum orientale*): vaginal dryness (applied topically)
- valerian (*Valeriana officinalis*): insomnia
- violet (*Viola odorata*): hot flashes.

Natural estrogens (phytoestrogens)

Phytoestrogens are estrogen compounds found in plants. Proponents of plant estrogens (including soy products) believe that plant estrogens are better than synthetic estrogens, but science has not yet proved this. The results of small preliminary trials suggest that the estrogen compounds in soy products (soy is very high in plant estrogens) can relieve the severity of **hot flashes** and lower **cholesterol**. In one study at Bowman-Gray Medical School in North Carolina, women were able to ease their menopausal symptoms such as hot flashes by eating a large amount of fruits, vegetables, and whole grains, together with 4 oz of tofu four times a week. However, no one has shown that plant estrogens can provide these benefits without causing the same negative side effects as estrogen replacement therapy. In addition, it is difficult to judge how much estrogen is in various plant products as there is no requirement for standardization. Many women believe that natural or plant-based means harmless. In large doses, phytoestrogens can promote the abnormal growth of cells in the uterine lining. Unopposed estrogen of any type can lead to an increased risk of **cancer**.

Several studies have shown that a **black cohosh** extract (Remifemin) relieved menopausal symptoms as well as or better than estrogen and that it showed the greatest promise among alternative treatments. In a 2007 study conducted at the University of Pennsylvania and published in *International Journal of Cancer*, Remifemin was also shown to reduce the risk of **breast cancer**. The United States Office of Dietary Supplements considers the evidence from studies of black cohosh promising but cautions that the long-term safety of this herb has not been established and recommends that if women choose to use black cohosh extract, they do so for no more than six months.

Flaxseeds also are a good source of phytoestrogens. Other sources include **red clover** leaf, **licorice**, wild yam, chickpeas, pinto beans, lima beans, and pomegranates. In 2003, red clover leaf was thought to offer relief for hot flashes, but in two short clinical trials, it failed to demonstrate hot flash relief.

Homeopathy

Women interested in homeopathic remedies for menopausal symptoms should consult a homeopathic physician. The following homeopathic remedies are often recommended to alleviate specific groups of symptoms:

- lachesis: hot flashes, irritability, talkativeness, tightness around abdomen, dizziness, fainting

- sepia: bleeding between periods, chilliness, tearfulness, withdrawal from loved ones, sinking feeling in stomach
- pulsatilla: tearfulness, thirstless, feels better with others, avoids heat, hot flashes, varicose veins, hemorrhoids
- sulfur: philosophical personality, feeling hot, itching and burning of vagina and rectum
- lycopodium: low self esteem, bloated after eating, infrequent menstruation, low blood sugar, weak digestion, belching
- *Argentum nitricum:* gas, indigestion, craving for sweets and chocolate, panic attacks, fear of crossing bridges
- Magnesium phosphoricum: severe cramping
- transitional formula: hot flashes, night sweats, insomnia, skin-crawling sensation
- women's formula: perimenopause, PMS, irregular cycles, infertility, absent or excessive bleeding, menopausal discomfort
- vital formula: anxiety, headaches, palpitations, PMS, mood swings

Yoga

Many women find that **yoga** can ease menopausal symptoms. Yoga focuses on helping women unite the mind, body, and spirit to create balance. Because yoga has been shown to balance the endocrine system, some experts believe it may affect hormone-related problems. Studies have found that yoga can reduce **stress**, improve mood, boost a sluggish metabolism, and slow the heart rate. Specific yoga positions deal with particular problems, such as hot flashes, mood swings, vaginal and urinary problems, and other pains.

Exercise

Exercise helps ease hot flashes by lowering the amount of circulating FSH and by raising endorphin levels (which drop during a hot flash). Even exercising 20 minutes three times a week can significantly reduce hot flashes. Weight bearing exercises help to prevent osteoporosis. Regular exercise also provides many health benefits unrelated to menopause.

Acupuncture

This ancient Asian art involves placing very thin needles into different parts of the body to stimulate the system and unblock energy. It is usually painless and has been used for many menopausal symptoms including **insomnia**, hot flashes, and irregular periods. Practitioners believe that **acupuncture** can facilitate the opening of blocked energy channels, allowing the life force energy (chi) to flow freely. This allows the menopausal woman to keep her energy moving. Blocked energy usually increases the symptoms of menopause.

Acupressure and massage

Therapeutic massage involving **acupressure** can bring relief from a wide range of menopause symptoms by placing finger pressure at the same meridian points on the body that are used in acupuncture. There are more than 80 different types of massage, including foot **reflexology**, **Shiatsu** massage, and **Swedish massage**, but they all are based on the idea that boosting the circulation of blood and lymph benefits health. Breast massage (rubbing **castor oil** or olive oil on the breasts for five minutes three times a week) is claimed to help balance hormone levels, help the uterus contract during menstruation, and prevents cramping pains.

Biofeedback

Some women have been able to control hot flashes through **biofeedback**, a painless technique that helps a person train her mind to control her body. A biofeedback machine provides information about body processes (such as heart rate) as the woman relaxes her body. Using this technique, it is possible to control the body's temperature, heart rate, and breathing.

Other treatments

Therapeutic touch, an energy-based practice, may relieve menopausal symptoms. Cold compresses on the face and neck can ease hot flashes. Sound or **music therapy** may relieve stress and other menopausal symptoms. **Prayer** or **meditation** can help improve coping ability.

Dietary supplements

Women should discuss the use of dietary supplements with their health care provider. Some supplements interfere with the action of traditional pharmaceuticals and herbal remedies. Other supplements are harmful in large quantities. Supplementation with calcium, **vitamin D**, **vitamin K**, **boron**, **manganese**, **magnesium**, and phosphorous may aid in preventing osteoporosis. **Vitamin E** supplementation may reduce hot flashes and risk of **heart disease**.

Allopathic treatment

When a woman enters menopause, her levels of estrogen drop and symptoms, such as hot flashes and vaginal dryness, begin. Before 2002, many physicians treated these symptoms with hormone replacement therapy (HRT). HRT treats these symptoms by increasing estrogen and progesterone levels enough to suppress symptoms. However, in the summer of 2002, preliminary results from a large Women's Health Initiative study were released that showed HRT could have significantly harmful effects (harmful enough that the study was stopped early). The study found that a combination of estrogen and progestin (a form of progesterone) HRT caused the following when compared to a placebo (no hormones):

- increased risk of heart attack, stroke, and blood clots
- increased risk of invasive breast cancer
- increased risk of dementia
- decreased risk of colorectal cancer
- decreased risk of bone fractures

Treatment with estrogen alone produced the following results:

- no change in the risk of heart attacks
- increased risk of stroke and blood clots
- unclear changes in the risk of breast cancer
- no change in the risk of colorectal cancer
- decreased risk of bone fractures
- no data available on changes in risk of dementia

At the time the results of the Women's Health Initiative became available, about 9 million American women were using HRT. Most physicians now no longer routinely recommend HRT to treat menopausal symptoms. Nevertheless, under certain circumstances when symptoms associated with menopause are so severe as to interfere with activities of daily life, a short course of HRT may be prescribed. Some doctors believe that short-term use of estrogen for those women with severe symptoms of hot flashes or night sweats is a sensible choice as long as they do not have a history of breast cancer. However, other doctors believe that in almost all cases the risks of HRT outweigh the benefits. The decision should be made by a woman and her doctor after taking into consideration her medical history and situation. Women who choose to take hormones should have an annual mammogram, breast exam, and pelvic exam and should report any unusual vaginal bleeding or spotting (a sign of possible **uterine cancer**).

Postmenopausal treatment for osteoporosis

Raloxifene (Evista, Keoxifene) is a drug that is used to treat osteoporosis (bone loss) in postmenopausal women. It does not increase the risk breast cancer, although it may increase breast tenderness. It may also worsen hot flashes and cause uterine bleeding. It is not a treatment for symptoms associated with

KEY TERMS

Endometrium—The lining of the uterus that is shed with each menstrual period.

Estrogen—Female hormone produced by the ovaries and released by the follicles as they mature. Responsible for female sexual characteristics, estrogen stimulates and triggers a response from at least 300 tissues, and may help some types of breast cancer to grow. After menopause, the production of the hormone gradually stops.

Follicle-stimulating hormone (FSH)—The pituitary hormone that stimulates the ovary to mature egg capsules (follicles). It is linked with rising estrogen production throughout the cycle. An elevated FSH (above 40) indicates menopause.

Hormone—A chemical messenger secreted by a gland that is released into the blood, and that travels to distant cells where it exerts an effect.

Hormone replacement therapy (HRT)—The use of estrogen and progesterone to replace hormones that the ovary no longer supplies. HRT is no longer used as long-term therapy for postmenopausal women.

Hot flash—A wave of heat that is one of the most common perimenopausal symptoms, triggered by the hypothalamus' response to estrogen withdrawal.

Hysterectomy—Surgical removal of the uterus.

Ovary—One of the two almond-shaped glands in the female reproductive system responsible for producing eggs and the hormones estrogen and progesterone.

Phytoestrogen—An estrogen-like substance produced by plants.

Placebo—a pill or liquid given during the study of a drug or dietary supplement that contains no medication or active ingredient. Usually study participants do not know if they are receiving a pill containing the drug or an identical-appearing placebo.

Progesterone—The hormone that is produced by the ovary after ovulation to prepare the uterine lining for a fertilized egg.

Testosterone—Male hormone produced by the testes and (in small amounts) in the ovaries. Testosterone is responsible for some masculine secondary sex characteristics such as growth of body hair and deepening voice.

Uterus—The female reproductive organ that contains and nourishes a fetus from implantation until birth. Also known as the womb.

menopause. Several other drugs are also available to help reduce the risk of **fractures** in postmenopausal women with osteoporosis. In 2002, the FDA approved teriparatide (Forteo) for the treatment of osteoporosis. Ibandronate (Boniva) and alendronate (Fosamax) are also used to treat osteoporosis in postmenopausal women.

Testosterone replacement

The ovaries also produce a small amount of male hormones (about 300 micrograms), which decrease slightly as a woman enters menopause. Most women never need testosterone replacement. Testosterone can improve the libido, and decrease **anxiety** and **depression**. Adding testosterone is especially beneficial to women who have had hysterectomies. Testosterone also eases breast tenderness and helps prevent bone loss. Side effects include mild **acne** and some facial hair growth.

Expected results

Menopause is a natural condition of aging. Some women have no problems with menopause, while others notice significant unpleasant symptoms. Results of allopathic and alternative treatments vary from one woman to another.

Prevention

Menopause cannot be prevented, although some of the symptoms can be relieved by the treatments listed above.

Resources

BOOKS

Boston Women's Health Book Collective. *Our Bodies, Ourselves: Menopause.* New York: Simon & Schuster, 2006.

Jones, Marcia. *Menopause for Dummies,* 2nd ed. Indianapolis, IN: Wiley Pub., 2006.

Lee, John R. and Virginia Hopkins. *What Your Doctor May Not Tell You About Menopause: The Breakthrough Book on Natural Hormone Balance.* New York: Warner Books, 2004.

Manson, JoAnn E. and Shari Bassuk. *Hot Flashes, Hormones, & Your Health.* New York: McGraw-Hill, 2007.

Northrup, Christiane. *The Wisdom of Menopause: Creating Physical and Emotional Health and Healing During the Change,* rev. ed. New York: Bantam Books, 2006.

Wingert, Pat and Barbara Kantrowitz. *Is It Hot in Here? Or Is It Me?: The Complete Guide to Menopause.* New York: Workman Pub., 2006.

OTHER

"Hormone Therapy News." April 3, 2007 [cited February 19, 2008, 2008]. *National Women's Health Network.* http://www.nwhn.org/hrt_statement_apr3-07.

"Menopause" *Federation of Feminist Women's Health Centers.* October 5, 2007 [cited February 19, 2008, 2008]. http://www.fwhc.org/menopause/index.htm.

"Menopause Infocenter" *Holistic Online.* [cited February 19, 2008]. http://www.holisticonline.com/remedies/hrt/hrt_home.htm.

"Menopause Online" *Menopause Online.* [cited February 19, 2008]. http://www.menopause-online.com.

ORGANIZATIONS

American Holistic Medical Association, PO Box 2016, Edmonds, WA, 98020, (425) 967-0737, http://www.holisticmedicin.org.

American Menopause Foundation, Inc, Empire State Bldg., 350 Fifth Ave., Ste. 2822, New York, NY, 10118, (212) 714- 2398, http://www.americanmenopause.org.

Federation of Feminist Women's Health Centers, 14220 Interurban Ave South #140, Seattle, WA, 98168, http://www.fwhc.org/menopause.

National Women's Health Network, 514 10th Street NW, Suite 400, Washington, DC, 20004, (202) 628-7814, http://www.nwhn.org.

North American Menopause Society, PO Box 94527, Cleveland, OH, 44101, (216) 844-8748, http://www.menopause.org.

Belinda Rowland
Teresa G. Odle
Tish Davidson, A. M.

Menstrual cramps *see* **Dysmenorrhea**

Menstruation

Definition

Menstruation is the monthly discharge through the vagina of the blood and tissues that are laid down in the uterus in preparation for **pregnancy**.

Description

The cyclic production of hormones that culminates in the release of a mature egg (ovum) is called the menstrual cycle, which begins during puberty and ends at **menopause**. The first menstrual cycle is called menarche. Hormones that control the menstrual cycle are produced by the hypothalamus, pituitary gland, and ovaries. The beginning of a menstrual cycle is marked by the maturation of an egg in an ovary and preparation of the uterus (womb) to establish pregnancy. Menstruation occurs when pregnancy has not been achieved.

The menstrual cycle is divided into four phases and is, on average, 28 days long (21–45 days). The onset of menstruation, called a period, monthly, menses, or menstrual period, begins a new menstrual cycle and is considered day one. This first phase usually lasts five days. Menstruation occurs in response to drops in the level of the hormone progesterone. It is estimated that a woman has 500 menstrual periods in her lifetime.

The second phase of the menstrual cycle is called the follicular or proliferative phase. The ovary, in response to increasing levels of follicle stimulating hormone, begins the egg maturation process. Although 10–20 eggs begin to develop within follicles of the ovaries, usually only one egg reaches maturity. Follicles are clusters of cells that encase a developing egg, hence the name "follicular phase." Developing follicles release the hormone estrogen that stimulates the lining of the uterus, called the endometrium, to grow (proliferate) in preparation to receive an embryo (an egg that has been fertilized and begun dividing) and establish pregnancy. This phase usually lasts through day 13.

The ovulation phase occurs in response to a surge in luteinizing hormone and is marked by the release of a mature egg from the follicle. Ovulation usually occurs on day 14.

The fourth phase is called the luteal, secretory, premenstrual, or postovulatory phase, and usually lasts from days 15–28. During this phase, the empty follicle, now called the corpus luteum, releases the hormone progesterone which further prepares the uterus for implantation of an embryo. The endometrium thickens because of cell growth, changes in blood vessels and glands, and increases in fluid. If pregnancy does not occur, the fall in progesterone levels initiates the onset of a new menstrual cycle. However, if pregnancy does occur, progesterone levels remain high, and the endometrium is not shed.

In the United States, menstruation typically begins at 12.8 years of age in Caucasian girls and 12.4 years of age for African American girls. Factors that help to dictate the age at which menarche occurs include race, mother's age at menarche, nutritional status, body fat, as well as climate and elevation. Studies have shown that a body fat level of 17% is necessary for menstruation to begin.

Women who live together or work in close proximity tend to find that their cycles begin to coincide. During the menstrual cycle, the body releases hormones called pheromones, which may signal surrounding women's cycles to begin.

Puberty signals the maturation of a young woman's reproductive hormones. As a girl reaches puberty, the pituitary gland in the brain starts to produce the hormones that signal the ovaries to begin functioning. The interaction between these hormones and the hormones estrogen and progesterone causes the lining of the uterus to swell and thicken in anticipation of a fertilized egg. If the egg is not fertilized, the lining is discharged through the vagina, resulting in menstrual bleeding.

Menstrual problems

Women may experience menstrual cycles that fall outside the norm as described above. Menstrual problems include missing a period; change in the length of the cycle; changes in the flow, color, or consistency of menstrual blood; and extreme **pain** or other menstrual symptoms.

Women may also experience emotional distress or wide mood swings during the luteal phase of the menstrual cycle. The fourth edition of the *Diagnostic and Statistical Manual of Mental Disorders*, or DSM-IV, lists premenstrual dysphoric disorder (PMDD) in an appendix of criteria sets for further study. To meet full criteria for PMDD, a patient must have at least five out of 11 emotional or physical symptoms during the week preceding the menses for most menstrual cycles over the previous 12 months. Although the DSM-IV definition of PMDD as a mental disorder is controversial because of fear that it could be used to justify prejudice or job discrimination against women, there is evidence that a significant proportion of premenopausal women suffer emotional distress or impairment in job functioning in the week before their menstrual period. One group of researchers estimates that 3–8% of women of childbearing age meet the strict DSM-IV criteria for PMDD, with another 13–18% having symptoms severe enough to interfere with their normal activities.

Causes and symptoms

Menstruation is not an illness, but a normal part of the menstrual cycle. However, menstrual problems do occur, and are due to varying causes.

Amenorrhea

Amenorrhea, the absence of menstruation, can be either primary or secondary. Primary amenorrhea is failure to menstruate by age 16 years in girls who have normal puberty or two years after sexual maturation has occurred. Primary amenorrhea may be caused by genetic disorders, hormonal imbalance, brain defects, or physical abnormality of the reproductive organs. In 2003, a group of researchers reported on a new genetic mutation associated with primary amenorrhea. In addition, certain systemic diseases may delay puberty and menstruation. Delayed menstruation may occur in athletes, especially gymnasts, ballerinas, and long-distance runners because of insufficient body fat. Amenorrhea associated with athletic training and professional dance is a growing health concern, however, because it often occurs together with eating disorders and a loss of bone mass that can lead to early **osteoporosis**.

Secondary amenorrhea refers to the absence of menstruation after an interval of normal menstruation. It is identified as not menstruating for three months in females with irregular menstrual cycles, six months in females with normal menstrual cycles, and 18 months in females who had just started menstruating. Secondary amenorrhea can be caused by pregnancy, weight loss, excessive **exercise**, breast feeding, disease, or menopause. Menopause takes place when the ovaries stop producing estrogen, causing periods to become irregular and then stop. It generally occurs when a woman is between 48 and 52 years of age.

Dysfunctional and abnormal uterine bleeding

Dysfunctional uterine bleeding is excessive or irregular bleeding from the uterus. It is caused by uncontrolled estrogen production that leads to excessive build up of the endometrium.

Abnormal uterine bleeding is excessive bleeding during menstruation, frequent bleeding, and/or irregular bleeding. Abnormal bleeding can be caused by fibroids (noncancerous uterine growths), **endometriosis** (when endometrium spreads outside of the uterus), uterine **infections**, **hypothyroidism**, clotting problems, intrauterine devices (IUD), or **cancer**.

Dysmenorrhea

Dysmenorrhea is painful and difficult menstruation. Studies have found that 60–92% of adolescents suffer from dysmenorrhea. It usually begins six to 12 months following menarche. Symptoms may be severe enough to cause missed work or school and prevent participation in normal activities. Risk factors for developing dysmenorrhea may include long menstrual periods, **obesity**, early age at menarche, **smoking**, and alcohol use.

Primary dysmenorrhea is believed to be caused by high levels of prostaglandins (fatty acids that stimulate

muscle contractions, among other activities) which cause painful uterine **muscle spasms**. Symptoms of primary dysmenorrhea occur when bleeding starts and may include moderate to severe menstrual pain (cramping, spasmodic, and labor-like or a dull ache), **nausea**, **vomiting**, **headache**, **fatigue**, **low back pain**, thigh pain, and **diarrhea**.

Secondary dysmenorrhea is caused by conditions such as endometriosis, abnormalities of the pelvic organs, **pelvic inflammatory disease**, fibroids, **ovarian cysts**, tumors, **inflammatory bowel disease**, and salpingitis (inflammation of the fallopian tube). Symptoms of secondary dysmenorrhea usually occur a few days before bleeding starts. The symptoms depend upon the specific cause of dysmenorrhea, but pain is the hallmark symptom.

A study released in 2003 found that oral contraceptives did not impact the mood of most women during the premenstrual timeframe. The study found that, among those taking oral contraceptives, mood declined in women who had a history of **depression** and that mood improved in women with early-onset premenstrual disturbances of mood as well as those with painful menstruation.

Heavy periods

Many women experience heavy menstrual bleeding during their periods, called menorrhagia. Heavy periods cause more blood loss than normal periods or may last longer than seven days. Women suffering from menorrhagia may lose up to 92% of their total fluid and tissue in the first three days of their cycle. Heavy menstruation is common in young girls who have just started their periods.

Menorrhagia is often caused by a failure to ovulate, which leads to a deficiency of progesterone. Without progesterone, the uterine lining becomes unstable and periods tend to be longer and unpredictable. Toxins in the bloodstream tend to settle in the endrometrial tissue. When this tissue is shed each month, so are the toxins. Heavy periods may be a toxin-excretion technique.

A deficiency in **vitamin A** or **iron**, or hypothyroidism may also cause heavy periods. Painful heavy periods may be linked to endometriosis, fibroids, pelvic inflammatory disease, or the use of an intrauterine device (IUD). A single heavy period that takes place later in the cycle may be a miscarriage.

Tampon use

Many women use tampons to absorb their monthly flow. There has been much controversy over the safety of tampons. The use of high-absorbency tampons has been shown to cause **toxic shock syndrome** (TSS), a bacterial infection caused when tampons left in too long create tiny breaks in the vaginal lining and allow bacteria to enter the blood stream. Symptoms of TSS are high **fever**, rash, muscle and joint aches, and diarrhea. In the 2000s TSS has become uncommon, but women have died from it.

To reduce the risk of TSS, the United States Food and Drug Administration (FDA) recommends that women use the lowest absorbency tampon required to meet their needs. It is also suggested that tampons be left in for no longer than four to eight hours. Alternatives to tampons are sanitary pads, reusable menstrual collection cups, and washable cloth pads.

One controversy was sparked in the early 1990s over the use of dioxin in tampons. Dioxin is a chemical byproduct of bleach that is a carcinogen. Tampons in the United States are bleached with chlorine during production so they will have a fresher appearance. Research conducted using monkeys showed that dioxin exposure may be linked to endometriosis.

In 1992, an investigation revealed that FDA scientists had found trace amounts of dioxin in some tampons. Further FDA research determined that the tampons subsequently manufactured were produced in a dioxin-free process. However, trace amounts of dioxin may be absorbed from the air, water, or ground. These levels are generally nondetectable and, according to the FDA, do not pose a health risk.

Premenstrual syndrome

Premenstrual syndrome (PMS) is a condition that occurs during the premenstrual phase of the menstrual cycle. The cause is unclear but theories include: abnormal hormone levels, other biochemical abnormalities, inappropriate diet, nutrient deficiencies, psychological factors, or a combination of many factors.

Emotional and mental symptoms include fatigue, mood swings, irritability, nervousness, confusion, depression, tearfulness, and **anxiety**. Physical symptoms are bloating, discomfort, breast tenderness, cravings, weight gain, **acne**, change in bowel movements, joint pains, and **dizziness**.

Other menstrual problems

• A missed period can be caused by pregnancy, stress, increased exercise, emotions, grief, and illness, among others.

• Metrorrhagia is bleeding in between normal episodes of menstruation. It may be caused by ovulation, hormonal factors, cervical lesions, or uterine cancer.

• Polymenorrhoea is bleeding associated with menstrual cycles that are shorter than 21 days. It may be caused by hormonal or ovulatory problems.

• Oligomenorrhea is infrequent menstruation with 35 days to six months between menstrual cycles. Researchers discovered that women with a menstrual cycle of 40 days or longer are twice as likely as women with average-length cycles to develop type II (adult-onset) diabetes mellitus. It is thought that long or highly irregular menstrual cycles may be associated with insulin resistance.

Diagnosis

Menstrual problems can be diagnosed and treated by gynecologists. Most menstrual problems would be diagnosed by taking a detailed medical history (with an emphasis on menstrual history) and performing a physical exam, which would include a pelvic exam. Pelvic exams have two components: the manual exam and the speculum exam. During the manual exam, the doctors insert one or two fingers into the vagina and press their other hand on the lower abdomen to feel the uterus and ovaries. A speculum exam involves inserting a speculum (a metal or plastic tool for opening the vagina) to allow viewing of the vagina and cervix, and to obtain smears for Pap testing (sampling of cervical cells) or culture if an infection is suspected.

Ultrasound exam, in which internal organs are visualized using sound waves, may be performed. Abnormal findings from the examination and laboratory tests may warrant laparoscopy in which a thin, wand like instrument is inserted into an incision in the navel to visualize abdominal organs.

Urine tests may be performed to diagnose pregnancy or infection. Blood tests to determine hormone levels, as well as other blood parameters, may be performed. Patient history and physical exam findings may suggest specific illnesses that would require additional laboratory testing.

The patient may be asked to fill out a diary in which daily menstrual symptoms are recorded over a period of three to six months. In some cases, the patient may be referred to a psychiatrist for evaluation for PMDD.

Treatment

There are many alternative treatments for menstrual problems. Because menstrual difficulties may be due to a serious condition, patients should consult a doctor before self-treating.

Diet

Phytoestrogens are estrogen-like compounds produced by certain plants. Food sources of phytoestrogens include soy products, flaxseeds, chick peas, pinto beans, french beans, lima beans, and pomegranates. Phytoestrogens can lighten menstruation and lengthen menstrual cycles. By contrast, researchers have found that women who were fed soy-based formulas in infancy instead of cow's milk are more likely to report heavy menstrual bleeding and painful periods in adult life.

PMS symptoms may be relieved by avoiding **caffeine**, sugar, salt, white flour, red meat, dairy, butter, monosodium glutamate (MSG), fried foods, and processed foods during the two weeks prior to menstruation. Foods that help to fight PMS include steamed green vegetables, salad, beans, grains, and fruit. To obtain **essential fatty acids** (omega-3 and omega-6) women can eat flaxseeds, sesame seeds, pumpkin seeds, salmon, mackerel, and tuna.

Herbal remedies and Chinese medicine

A variety of herbal remedies may alleviate symptoms associated with menstrual problems. These include:

- black cohosh (*Cimicifuga racemosa*): mood swings, tension, establishing ovulation (an important source of phytoestrogens). The German Commission E, however, states that women should not take black cohosh for menstrual problems for longer than six months because of the risk of side effects.
- black haw (*Viburnum prunifolium*): cramps
- chamomile (*Matricaria recutita*): mood swings, tension, and cramps
- cramp bark (*Viburnum opulus*): cramps
- dandelion (*Taraxacum dang gui*): fluid retention and bloating
- dong quai (*Benincasa cerifera*): PMS symptoms, cramps, irregular cycles, heavy bleeding, or bleeding in between cycles
- fenugreek (*Trigonella foenum-graecum*): irregular bowel movements
- feverfew (*Chrysanthemum parthenium*): headaches and PMS symptoms
- ginger (*Zingiber officinale*): cramps, irregular cycles, heavy bleeding, or bleeding in between cycles
- goldenseal (*Hydrastis canadensis*): heavy bleeding
- horsetail (*Equisetum arvense*): heavy bleeding

- licorice: PMS symptoms
- milk thistle (*Silybum marianum*) extract: heavy bleeding
- nettle (*Urtica dioica*) extract: heavy bleeding
- peppermint (*Mentha piperita*): mood swings and tension
- raspberry tea: cramps, irregular cycles, heavy bleeding, or bleeding in between cycles
- red clover (*Trifolium pratense*): phytoestrogen source
- rosemary (*Rosmarinus officinalis*): cramps
- shepherd's purse (*Capsella bursa–pastoris*): heavy bleeding
- St. John's wort (*Hypericum perforatum*): depression associated with PMS
- valerian (*Valeriana officinales*): mood swings and tension
- vitex: PMS symptoms
- wild yam: phytoestrogen source
- yarrow (*Achillea millefolium*): cramps

Supplements

The following supplements may treat menstrual problems:

- Calcium deficiency may be associated with PMS.
- Iron supplementation can treat anemia.
- Magnesium pidolate supplementation reduced dysmenorrhea symptoms by up to 84%, especially on days two and three.
- Niacin may help to relieve cramps.
- Omega-3 fatty acids deficiency is associated with dysmenorrhea pain (in one small study, patients taking omega-3 fatty acids had lower pain scores).
- Thiamine (vitamin B_1) cured dysmenorrhea in 87% of the patients for up to two months after treatment.
- Vitamin A may be useful to treat heavy bleeding in women who have vitamin A deficiencies.
- Vitamin B complex may help hormonal function, prevent anemia, reduce water retention, and relieve stress.
- Vitamin E may reduce mood swings and menstrual cramps.

Other treatments

Other treatments for menstrual problems include:

- Acupressure. Acupressure can relieve pain, reduce stress, and improve circulation.
- Acupuncture. This treatment is associated with improvement or cure of dysmenorrhea and PMS and decreased use of pain medications. A National Institutes of Health

(NIH) panel concluded that acupuncture may be a useful treatment for menstrual cramps. A study released in 2008 found that acupuncture is an effective treatment for patients suffering from dysmenorrhea. In the study, acupuncture was associated with improvements in both pain and quality of life.

- Aromatherapy. Massage with essential oils: rose, ylang-ylang, bergamot, and/or geranium oils for mood swings; lavender, sandalwood, and clary sage oils for menstrual cramps; and chamomile, cypress, melissa, lavender, and jasmine oils for irregular menstruation or amenorrhea.
- Biofeedback. Weekly biofeedback therapy for 12 weeks led to significant reduction in PMS symptoms.
- Chiropractic. Spinal manipulation may help to ease cramps.
- Exercise. Regular, moderate aerobic exercise reduces or eliminates menstrual pain, improves PMS, reduces the amount of menstrual bleeding, reduces the risk for endometriosis, and reduces cyclic breast pain and cysts. Yoga stretching can relieve back and thigh pain.
- Homeopathy. Homeopathic remedies include: lachesis or sepia for PMS, cimicifuga, colocynthis, or magnesia phosphorica for cramps, and pulsatilla or aconitum for irregular menstruation or amenorrhea.
- Hydrotherapy. Soaking in a hot tub or using a moist heating pad relaxes uterine muscles which relieves cramping.
- Reflexology. Ear, hand, and foot reflexology led to a significant decrease in PMS symptoms that lasted for several months following treatment.
- Transcutaneous electric nerve stimulation (TENS). In four small studies using TENS for the treatment of dysmenorrhea, 42%–60% of the patients experienced at least moderate relief of symptoms. TENS worked faster than naproxen and there was less need for NSAIDs.

Allopathic treatment

The treatment for amenorrhea depends upon the cause. Primary amenorrhea may require hormonal therapy.

Patients with dysfunctional or abnormal uterine bleeding may be prescribed iron supplements to treat **anemia**. Naproxen **sodium** (Aleve) reduces excessive blood loss. Oral contraceptives are often prescribed to treat abnormal bleeding. High doses of estrogens may cause vomiting, which means that anti-emetics (drugs to prevent vomiting) may also be necessary. Excessive bleeding may require hospitalization for observation and treatment.

KEY TERMS

Amenorrhea—Lack of menstruation.

Dysmenorrhea—Painful menstruation.

Endometrium—The lining of the uterus that is shed during menstruation.

Follicle—The cluster of cells that surround the developing egg.

Hormones—Chemical messengers that control the events associated with the menstrual cycle.

Menarche—The first menstrual period or the establishment of the menstrual function.

NSAIDs—Nonsteroidal anti–inflammatory drugs such as ibuprofen and naproxen.

Oligomenorrhea—Scanty or infrequent menstrual periods.

Phytoestrogens—Estrogen-like compounds derived from plants.

Toxic shock syndrome (TSS)—A potentially serious bacterial infection associated with the use of tampons to absorb menstrual flow.

Uterus—The organ that carries and provides nutrition to a developing baby. Also called the womb.

Primary dysmenorrhea is usually successfully treated with nonsteroidal anti-inflammatory drugs (NSAIDs); aspirin is not strong enough to be effective. NSAIDs are numerous and include ibuprofen (Advil, Motrin, Nuprin), Naproxen (Aleve), and fenamates (Meclomen). Oral contraceptives (birth control pills) may be used if NSAIDs fail. Treatment of secondary dysmenorrhea involves treating the causative condition and may involve medications or surgery.

Because the cause(s) of PMS are unclear, treatment usually focuses on relieving symptoms. A study released in 2007 found that both acetaminophen and ibuprofen were effective in treating the pain associated with menstruation. Ibuprofen was found to be the more potent pain reliever.

With regard to PMDD, medications that have been reported to be effective in treating it include the tricyclic antidepressants and the selective serotonin reuptake inhibitors (SSRIs). Effective treatments other than medications include cognitive **behavioral therapy** (CBT), aerobic exercise, and dietary supplements containing **calcium, magnesium**, and vitamin B_6.

Expected results

Most menstrual problems can be successfully treated using conventional or alternative treatments.

Prevention

Avoiding sodium and caffeine may reduce some menstrual symptoms. Regular moderate aerobic exercise or **yoga** is often beneficial for menstruation difficulties. Getting yearly pelvic exams and Pap smears help to identify problems before they become advanced.

Resources

BOOKS

PERIODICALS

Dawood, Yusoff, and Firyal S. Khan-Dawood. "Clinical Efficacy and Differential Inhibition of Menstrual Fluid Prostaglandin F2a in a Randomized, Double-Blind, Crossover Treatment with Placebo, Acetaminophen, and Ibuprofen in Primary Dysmenorrhea." *American Journal of Obstetrics & Gynecology* 196, no. 1 (January 2007): 35.

Witt, Claudia M. et al. "Acupuncture in Patients with Dysmenorrhea: A Randomized Study on Clinical Effectiveness and Cost-Effectiveness in Usual Care." *American Journal of Obstetrics & Gynecology* 198, no. 2 (February 2008): 166.

ORGANIZATIONS

American College of Obstetricians and Gynecologists (ACOG), 409 Twelfth St. SW, PO Box 96920, Washington, DC, 20090-6920, http://www.acog.org.

American Psychiatric Association (APA), 1400 K St. NW, Washington, DC, 20005, (888) 357-7924, http://www.psych.org.

Feminist Women's Health Center, 106 East E St., Yakima, WA, 98901, (509) 575-6473 x112, http://www.fwhc.org.

National Women's Health Network, 514 Tenth St. NW, Suite 400, Washington, DC, 20004, (202) 628-7814, http://www.womenshealthnetwork.org.

Belinda Rowland
Rebecca J. Frey, PhD
Rhonda Cloos, RN

Mercurius vivus

Description

Mercurius vivus is the Latin name for a homeopathic remedy made from elemental mercury. The English word quicksilver is a literal translation of the Latin. Although Samuel Hahnemann, the founder of homeopathic medicine, also formulated a soluble preparation of mercury that he called *Mercurius solubilis*, most contemporary American homeopaths regard these two preparations as essentially the same remedies and use them to treat the same symptom profiles.

General use

Homeopathic medicine operates on the principle that "like heals like." This means that a disease can be cured by treating it with substances that produce the same symptoms as the disease, while also working in conjunction with the homeopathic law of infinitesimals. In opposition to traditional medicine, the law of infinitesimals states that the *lower* a dose of curative, the more effective it is. To achieve a low dose, the curative is diluted many, many times until only a tiny amount remains in a huge amount of the diluting liquid.

The homeopathic *Materia Medica* indicates that, *Mercurius vivus* is the remedy of choice for acute disorders of the skin and mucous membranes characterized by severe inflammation with pus formation and possibly areas of broken or raw skin. Disorders with this symptom profile include:

- eye infections with discharges of pus
- bacterial infections with pus behind the eardrum
- sore throats with open patches of skin and pus formation
- urinary tract infections
- diseases of the skin such as herpes and boils

Other disorders that are treated with *Mercurius vivus* include backache, **chickenpox**, colds, **diarrhea**, **influenza**, **indigestion**, mouth ulcers, and **toothache** accompanied by heavy salivation.

The general symptoms that would suggest *Mercurius vivus* treatment to a homeopath include heavy, foul-smelling perspiration, foul-smelling breath and **body odor**, and copious, drooling salivation. *Mercurius vivus* patients are easily irritated by temperature or other environmental changes, and they are comfortable only within a narrow range of moderate circumstances. They tend to tremble or shake, are generally weak, and easily tired by activity. These patients are slow to respond to treatment and infected parts of the body take a long time to heal and often appear severely diseased.

A female *Mercurius vivus* patient is likely to have heavy periods with painful cramps and **anxiety**. A nursing mother will produce milk that has a bad taste to the infant. A male patient may have burning

pain on urination accompanied by thick mucus or pus from the urethra. The inflammatory sensations associated with *Mercurius vivus* symptoms are present throughout the body. The mouth and gums are typically sore and inflamed, and the patient may complain of a metallic taste in the mouth. The gums may ooze blood when touched, and the patient often has lost several teeth. If the patient has a **headache**, it will have a burning quality. The *Mercurius vivus* patient may also have feelings of gnawing or burning in the chest and abdomen. There may be little appetite for food, but often an intense thirst or desire for cold drinks.

In **homeopathy**, certain remedies are thought to be especially effective in people with specific personality and physical traits. The mental and psychological symptoms of *Mercurius vivus* patients include restlessness, an agitated quality, and a tendency toward impatience and willfulness. The patient may jabber or chatter rather than talking at a normal pace and may act on impulse. These impulses sometimes lead to violence; *Mercurius vivus* patients may act out suicidal or murderous thoughts. Other personality traits of the *Mercurius vivus* patient are quarrelsomeness and dissatisfaction.

In homeopathic practice, the circumstances or factors that make the patient feel better or worse are considered as important a part of the symptom profile as the physical indications. These circumstances, which include weather, time of day, level of activity, light or noise, body position, sleeping patterns, etc., are known as modalities. With *Mercurius vivus* patients, the modalities that make the patient's condition worse include temperature extremes, open air, drafts, a warm bed, evening, being touched, lying on the right side, feeling sweaty, or eating something sweet. Those that make the patient feel better include moderate temperatures, dry weather, and sitting up while at rest.

Preparations

There are two homeopathic dilution scales, the decimal (x) scale with a dilution factor of 1:10 and the centesimal (c) scale with a dilution factor of 1:100. The most common form of *Mercurius vivus* preparation on the market is 30c or 30x tablets, although the remedy is also available in liquid form. The abbreviation 30c means that one part of mercury has been diluted with 99 parts of water or alcohol. This process of dilution, along with vigorous shaking of the remedy, has been repeated 30 times to achieve the desired potency. A potency of 30x means that one part of the medicine is mixed with nine parts of alcohol or water; thus 30x means that this decimal dilution has been repeated 30 times. In homeopathic practice, the strength of the remedy is in inverse proportion to the amount of chemical or plant extract in the alcohol or water; thus a 30c preparation of *Mercurius vivus* is considered a much higher potency than a 30x preparation. The tablet form of a homeopathic remedy is made by pouring the diluted liquid over sugar pills.

Precautions

Taken by itself, mercury is poisonous to humans and can cause irreversible damage to the nervous system even if the patient survives. Other symptoms of **mercury poisoning** include burning thirst, swelling and discoloration of the membranes lining the mouth, abdominal pain, bloody diarrhea, and shock. Samuel Hahnemann's interest in accidental poisonings from medicines that were commonly used in the eighteenth century is one reason why mercury was one of the first substances that he studied. Since ancient times, mercury had been used for medicinal purposes to cleanse **fever** victims of toxins. In the modern world, however, mercury poisoning is more likely to result accidentally from breathing metallic vapors given off in certain industrial processes rather than from mercury-based medicines. Standard homeopathic preparations of *Mercurius vivus* are so dilute that they are highly unlikely to cause mercury poisoning even if the patient takes a sizable overdose.

Side effects

Homeopathic remedies rarely have side effects in the usual sense of the phrase because they are so dilute. On the other hand, a homeopathic remedy may sometimes appear to be making a patient's symptoms temporarily worse as part of the healing process. This worsening is called an aggravation. Aggravations are regarded by homeopaths as an indication that the remedy is effectively stimulating the patient's body to heal itself. *Mercurius vivus* patients appear to be more likely to experience aggravations than patients given other remedies.

Interactions

Homeopathic preparations are so dilute that the chances of their interacting with conventional prescription medications are minimal to nonexistent. On the other hand, a typical homeopathic *Materia Medica* will include some brief notes about the interactions of some remedies. The action of *Mercurius vivus* is thought to be intensified by **belladonna**, **silica**, and *Hepar sulphuricum*.

KEY TERMS

Aggravation—In homeopathy, a temporary worsening or intensification of the patient's symptoms prior to improvement and healing.

Materia medica—A Latin phrase that means "the materials of medicine." In homeopathy, a *materia medica* is a book that lists the various homeopathic remedies together with the symptoms that they treat.

Modality—A factor or circumstance that makes a patient's symptoms better or worse. Modalities include such factors as time of day, room temperature, external stimuli, the patient's level of activity, sleep patterns, etc.

Resources

BOOKS

Chernin, Dennis. *The Complete Homeopathic Resource for Common Illnesses.* Berkeley, CA: North Atlantic Books, 2006.

Cummings, Stephen, and Dana Ullman. *Everybody's Guide to Homeopathic Medicines.* 3rd ed. rev. New York: Tarcher, 2004.

ORGANIZATIONS

Alternative Medicine Foundation. P. O. Box 60016, Potomac, MD 20859. (301) 340-1960. http://www.amfoundation.org.

American Institute of Homeopathy. 801 N. Fairfax Street, Suite 306, Alexandria, VA 22314 (888) 445-9988. http://homeopathyusa.org.

National Center for Homeopathy. 801 N. Fairfax St., Suite 306, Alexandria, VA 22314. (703) 548-7790. http://www.homeopathic.org/contact.htm.

OTHER

"Mercurius Vivus" *ABC Homeopathy.* [cited February 19, 2008]. http://abchomeopathy.com/r.php/Merc.

"British Homeopathic Library." *Hom-Inform.* [cited February 19, 2008]. http://www.hom-inform.org.

Rebecca Frey, Ph. D.
Tish Davidson, A. M.

Mercury poisoning

Definition

Mercury poisoning occurs when a person has ingested, inhaled, or had skin or eye contact with the toxic (poisonous) heavy metal mercury and suffers damage to the nervous system and other systems of the body. Mercury, which has the chemical symbol of Hg, is liquid at room temperature, like a few other elements. Because it easily converts to a gas, it is extremely volatile. There are three forms of mercury circulating throughout the environment, and all three forms are toxic to humans and many other living organisms to varying degrees.

Elemental mercury, also known as quicksilver, is mercury in its metallic (solid) elemental form. Elemental mercury is also referred to as mercury-zero. It is frequently found in the home in glass thermometers. It is also found in fluorescent light bulbs, thermostats, some pesticides, switches, preservatives, some paints, and in some dental amalgam fillings—although there are often mercury-free options available. In the past, according to a State of Michigan publication *Mercury Poisoning,* it was used as the active ingredient in ointments, animal worming medicines, antiseptics, disinfectants, diuretics and fungicides. As of 2008, the publication states, it is present in seed fungicides, anti-slime fungicides used by the pulp and paper industries, by-products of burning coal, mining tailings (residue), and wastes from chlorine-alkali industries. In its solid state, elemental mercury is less toxic than some of its other forms, but it is still very volatile. The most toxic effect of elemental mercury occurs when its extremely dangerous vapor is inhaled, which is most likely to occur in an industrial setting.

Elemental mercury can be converted by bacteria into a charged ion (an electrically charged atom or group of atoms) known as mercury-two. There are two dangerous aspects to this form. First, unlike elemental mercury, it readily dissolves in water and combines with other ions to form new compounds. Second, bacteria can change mercury-two into one of mercury's most toxic organic compounds, methylmercury, which is capable of being dissolved in water and thus finds its way into the food chain, where it enters fish and other animals. Large, long-lived fish such as swordfish are most likely to have high levels of methylmercury. The mercury found in fish can be dangerous for a developing fetus, for babies, and young children. It can be passed to infants through breast milk. Breastfeeding women, pregnant women, and women who may become pregnant are advised by the United States Food and Drug Administration (FDA) to avoid eating large, long-lived fish such as shark and swordfish, and to limit other fish consumption to an average of 12 ounces a week (an average portion of fish is about six ounces). The FDA also recommends that the fish eaten be varied regularly and that the same type of fish or shellfish not be eaten more than once a week.

Inorganic mercury takes the form of various compounds known as mercuric salts. Mercuric salts are used in various folk medicines, particularly in some Chinese herbal preparations and in some Mexican remedies. Exposure to mercuric salts over a long term can cause kidney and nerve damage.

Description

Many people do not take the risk of mercury poisoning seriously because they have played with elemental or liquid mercury or broken thermometers containing mercury without experiencing negative health effects. While these "small" mercury exposures can appear to be free of detectable health consequences, even a small spill can have serious effects, including hospitalization and even death, if improperly cleaned up, if there is poor ventilation, or the mercury is exposed to heat. It is extremely important, therefore, that any mercury spill, even a small one, be properly cleaned up. If not, the home, school, or workplace may be contaminated. Poisoning from elemental mercury is most likely to occur during inhalation of mercury vapors. The danger lies in the fact that after it is inhaled into the lungs in vapor form, mercury passes into the blood stream. The person who inhales mercury requires immediate medical treatment.

Inhalation of mercury vapor might happen in a factory where mercury is used. Most small household spills of elemental mercury are not dangerous if cleaned up correctly. Elemental mercury usually passes right through the body if swallowed, so this is usually not poisonous to a person with a healthy digestive system. Elemental mercury is not easily absorbed by the skin, so touching elemental mercury is usually not enough to cause poisoning. But if elemental mercury is spilled in the home, from a broken thermometer or fluorescent light, for example, it must be correctly and carefully cleaned up. It should not be swept up with a broom or vacuumed because doing so can break the mercury into small particles and spread it. Spilled mercury should be sucked up with an eyedropper, scooped up with paper, or picked up with sticky tape. Then the mercury should be sealed in three layers of plastic bags and disposed of according to local hazardous waste procedures. Any clothes or rags that have been exposed to mercury should also be discarded, rather than washed in a washing machine, which would further spread the mercury. The area of the spill should be ventilated for several days.

Inorganic mercury, or mercury salts, have long been used in folk medicines. Exposure to inorganic mercury through folk medicines can cause poisoning, which can lead to kidney damage, tissue death, and nerve damage. Calomel, or mercurous chloride, and cinnabar, or mercuric sulfide, are two common toxic inorganic mercury compounds that should not be ingested. Folk medicines containing calomel, cinnabar, or other mercuric salts should also not be used on the skin.

Several Chinese herbal medicines have been identified as containing dangerous amounts of mercury and arsenic. These are usually prepared as an herbal ball. Known Chinese herbal medicines to avoid are: An Gong Niu Huang Wan, Da Huo Luo Wan, Niu Huang Chiang Ya Wan, Niu Huang Chiang Hsin Wan, Ta Huo Lo Tan, Tsai Tsao Wan, and Dendrobium Moniliforme Night Sight Pills.

Poisoning from organic mercury is perhaps the most troubling form of mercury exposure. Organic mercury is widespread in the environment, and there is a lot of debate about how it can most safely and cost-effectively be cleaned up. Some mercury finds its way into the atmosphere naturally, from volcanoes for example. But much of the mercury that finds its way into the food supply comes from industrial pollution. Mercury is emitted by power plants that burn fossil fuel and travels through the air. It deposits in bodies of water, where it is first taken up by plankton (floating animal and plant life). Fish that feed on plankton accumulate organic mercury in their bodies, and fish that eat those fish accumulate even more. This process, called bioaccumulation, concentrates the mercury in animals at the top of the food chain.

Because mercury can travel great distances through the air, the problem of mercury pollution affects all of North America and is a global environmental issue. As of 2008, the debate continued on how much mercury is safe and how it should be regulated. In the United States, the Environmental Protection Agency (EPA) is responsible for monitoring mercury emissions. In 2004, the EPA promulgated new rules on mercury emissions, which were criticized by some politicians and environmental groups as too lenient. The FDA, the United States government agency responsible for food safety, revised its findings on the mercury in fish several times during the early 2000s.

Some studies suggest that mercury exposures of up to four times the limits in the FDA guidelines may be safe for people. There are many health benefits to eating fish, and the mercury level in any individual fish meal may vary greatly. Most states in the United

States post warnings on consuming fish or certain types of fish caught in lakes and streams. Specific bodies of water or specific species of fish may have been found to be more dangerous than others. People who fish for sport or for subsistence should check with local government agencies about warnings for eating local fish.

Causes and symptoms

Common home products that contain elemental mercury, such as lights, thermostats, thermometers, and appliances are not dangerous to humans unless they are broken, mercury is released, and there is exposure to mercury vapors because of improper cleanup.

In June 1997, Karen Wetterhahn, 48, a Dartmouth College **cancer** research scientist whose specialty was dangerous heavy metals, died of dimethylmercury poisoning, ten months after she spilled one to several drops of it on her rubber gloves while she was studying how mercury prevents cells from repairing themselves. Tests after the spill revealed that the mercury could pass quickly through the rubber latex gloves without damaging them. Three months after the spill, Wetterhahn experienced two episodes of **nausea** and **vomiting**. Two months later, she began losing her balance and having speaking and hearing difficulties. At the time she was hospitalized, tests showed 80 times the lethal dose of mercury in her blood. She then went into a coma and died. The chairman of the Dartmouth chemistry department, John S. Winn, explained that although methylmercury looks like water, it is three times as dense and is readily absorbed by the body. He also said that about 100 laboratories around the world work with dimethylmercury. Dartmouth officials in a letter to the American Chemical Society urged those who work with dimethylmercury to wear neoprene gloves with long cuffs and to have frequent blood and urine testing.

In 1963, a new filling for dental cavities, non-gamma-two amalgam, was introduced as a solution to conventional amalgam being prone to corrosion and mechanical weakness. Non-gamma-two amalgam quickly caught on, despite the fact that it caused a much-increased mercury emission, and replaced conventional amalgam. In the early 1980s, dentists were regularly using elemental mercury amalgam for dental fillings. However, dentists and other health professionals who had turned to holistic or alternative medicine began to publicize the toxicity of amalgam fillings and advocate their replacement with a non-toxic composite material. One study reported that people with amalgam filings had mercury vapors in their mouths that were nine times greater than people without the filings. If the person with the amalgam filing chewed, the level of vapor increased six-fold, giving the people with amalgam filings vapor levels that were 54 times greater than those without amalgam filings. The level continued to increase as the people brushed their teeth or after they drank hot beverages. Although these findings may seem extreme, they come from only one study. The American Dental Association (ADA) has not found sufficient evidence of the dangers of amalgam fillings to recommend against them. Starting January 1, 2008, Norway banned the use of amalgam fillings in most circumstances. This ban, however, pertained to environmental effects of mercury, not concerns about the safety of the fillings.

Environmental mercury can be extremely dangerous. Walter Crinnion described the effects of the pollution of Minamata Bay in Japan by methylmercury and the neurotoxicity suffered by inhabitants of the area that came to be known Minamata disease: ataxia (lack of normal coordination of voluntary muscles), speech impairment, constriction of visual fields, hypoesthesia (reduced capacity to feel sensation), dysarthria (slurred, slow speech from inability to coordinate mouth muscles), hearing impairment, and sensory disturbances. As the mercury contamination spread, these symptoms did also. Forty years after the spill and almost 30 years since a fishing ban was put into effect in the area, problems continued predominantly in the fishing villages. Males complained of stiffness, poor ability to feel sensation, hand tremors, **dizziness**, loss of **pain** sensation, cramping, atrophy (wasting away) of upper arm muscles, arthralgia (pain in the joints), **insomnia**, and lumbago (back pain). Females had significantly higher complaints of leg tremors, **tinnitus** (ringing in the ears or head), loss of touch sensation, atrophy of leg muscles, and muscular weakness.

The symptoms of poisoning from inorganic mercury may include nausea and vomiting, abdominal pain, bloody **diarrhea**, and decreased urination. If inorganic mercury is applied to the skin, the skin may eventually redden or discolor. Skin contact with inorganic mercury can lead to nerve damage. The symptoms of nerve damage are weakness, numbness, and tingling.

The symptoms of poisoning from organic mercury include **fatigue**, **headache**, **depression**, memory problems, **hair loss**, tremors, and/or a metallic taste in the mouth. These symptoms are also caused by many other common conditions, so organic mercury poisoning can be difficult to diagnose. The doctor will ask the individual questions about possible workplace, home, or dietary exposure to mercury to help make a diagnosis.

Diagnosis

Measurement of mercury in the urine is the recommended method of diagnosing metallic and inorganic mercury poisoning. Organic mercury cannot be measured by urinalysis because it does not leave the body in urine. If the urine collection cannot be done over 24 hours, spot urine samples should be collected at the same time each day.

Extent of exposure to organic mercury, including methylmercury and metallic and inorganic mercury, can be measured by a blood test. Unexposed people usually have less than 2 µg/100mL of mercury in their blood. Early effects of toxicity are indicated when the blood concentration exceeds 3 µg/100 mL.

Treatment

It is worth noting that some herbal and folk treatments for health problems can be a source of mercury. The herbal preparations listed under the "Description" heading above are known to have large concentrations of inorganic mercury. A person prescribed a Chinese herbal ball preparation may want to ask the practitioner about mercury and be alert for symptoms of mercury exposure. Some Mexican skin creams and stomach remedies may also be sources of mercury.

Fish oil supplements are a popular non-prescription treatment used by many people who hope to lower the risk of **heart disease**, lower **cholesterol** levels, and improve mental function. Because in the United States, the manufacture of nutritional supplements is not regulated like pharmaceuticals are, fish oil supplements may vary greatly from maker to maker and so exposure to organic mercury from fish oil supplements is not readily quantifiable. It makes most sense for a person taking fish oil supplements to determine—if necessary by contacting the manufacturer directly—what kinds of fish are used for the oil, and if mercury levels have been tested for that brand.

Alternative treatment—by a naturopathic physician, a holistic medical doctor or osteopathic physician, or a homeopathic practitioner—is based on physical examination, biochemical testing, and an extensive history, including a history of family illness. After the doctor evaluates all of this information, treatment may include a comprehensive diet tailored to the individual patient; vitamins, minerals, enzymes, **amino acids** and or homeopathic remedies tailored to the individual; removal of toxins from patient's environment and diet; removal of amalgam fillings; necessary **chiropractic** adjustments; counseling; supplementary physical treatment; **stress** reduction and proper **exercise**; a stress-free home with help, if needed; a **detoxification**

program; use of a sauna; and chelation, a recognized treatment for **heavy metal poisoning**, the intravenous injection of ethylenediamine tetraacetic (EDTA) that will chemically bind with the heavy metal and allow it to be removed from the body in the urine.

Allopathic treatment

A person diagnosed with mercury poisoning may be prescribed a drug that binds the mercury and thus helps the body excrete it quickly. The body naturally excretes metallic and inorganic mercury in the urine even without treatment. A doctor may recommend that a person diagnosed with mercury poisoning avoid eating any fish or shellfish. Further monitoring of blood and urine can determine whether mercury levels are falling. The nervous system, mouth, lungs, eyes and skin, target organs for exposure, should also be periodically checked.

Expected results

For adults, small levels of mercury poisoning typically constitute a reversible problem. The body can rid itself of mercury if the exposure to mercury is halted. Symptoms such as fatigue and memory problems seem to go away as mercury levels fall. However, large doses of mercury can cause permanent organ, brain, and neurological damage, or be fatal. For children and developing fetuses, even very low levels of mercury poisoning can cause long-term neurological problems. Mercury exposure before birth has been linked to lower intelligence and delays in learning motor skills.

Prevention

Avoiding mercury is the best way to prevent mercury poisoning. Folk remedies that may contain mercury should not be consumed or rubbed on the skin. People should follow local guidelines about eating fish caught in local waters and should follow federal guidelines for consumption of commercial fish. Much of the scientific literature on long-term exposure to mercury from fish is still mixed, and consumers should try to stay up to date on the FDA recommendations for consumption.

Resources

BOOKS

Eisler, Ronald. *Mercury Hazards to Living Organisms.* Boca Raton, FL: CRC/Taylor & Francis, 2006.

Harmon, Daniel E. *Fish, Meat, and Poultry: Dangers in the Food Supply.* New York: Rosen Central, 2008.

National Wildlife Federation *Poisoning Wildlife: The Reality of Mercury Pollution.* Reston, VA: National Wildlife Federation, 2006.

PERIODICALS

Morrissey, Michael T. "Mercury in Seafood: Facts and Discrepancies." *Food Technology* (August 2006): 132.

Saldana, M., et al. "Diet-related Mercury Poisoning Resulting in Visual Loss." *British Journal of Ophthalmology* 90, no. 11 (November 2006): 1432–1435.

Strom, Sean M. "Total Mercury and Methylmercury Residues in River Otters from Wisconsin." *Archives of Environmental Contamination and Toxicology* 54, no. 3 (April 2008): 546–555.

Ruth Ann Carter
Helen Davidson

Mesoglycan

Description

Mesoglycan is a mucopolysaccharide complex that is extracted from calf aorta or synthetically created and taken in pill or capsule form as a dietary supplement. Mucopolysaccharides are long molecular chains of sugar. They are used by the body in the building of connective tissues, such as cartilage, tendons, and ligaments. The substance is related to the blood-thinning drug heparin, and the supplements **glucosamine** and **chondroitin**. Both are used to treat joint pain and arthritis.

General use

Aortic glycosaminoglycans and mucopolysaccharides such as mesoglycan are used to treat diseases of blood vessels, joints, and cartilage such as:

- atherosclerosis
- varicose veins
- phlebitis
- hemorrhoids
- arthritis
- bursitis
- headaches
- ulcers
- angina
- allergies

There is some evidence that mucopolysaccharides and the related aortic glycosaminoglycans may slow the development of **atherosclerosis** (hardening of the arteries) by lowering **cholesterol** levels in the blood. In one study, a group of men with early atherosclerosis was given a 200 mg daily dose of aortic glycosaminoglycans, while another group received no treatment. After 18 months, the layering of the vessel lining in the untreated group was 7.5 times greater than in the treated group.

Heparan sulfate and dermatan sulfate are the two main components of mesoglycan. These substances have a protective effect on the walls of blood vessels.

Mesoglycan is an active ingredient found in the aloe vera plant. There have been studies that have found mesoglycan to be effective in treating inflammation, AIDS, and **cancer**. One clinical trial conducted in the 1980s showed that **AIDS** patients who took oral mucopolysaccharides showed a 70% improvement in their symptoms.

Mucopolysaccharides have also been shown to reduce inflammation in diseases such as arthritis, gastric reflux, and ulcerative **colitis**. There is also evidence suggesting that mesoglycan can slow the progression of arthritic diseases.

Preparations

Dosage ranges from 24-200 mg per day for one to six months, depending on the condition being treated. In a study patients with deep vein thrombosis, a dosage of 72 mg per day was found to be effective. An oral dosage of mesoglycan of 72-96 mg per day for 10-13 weeks has been used to treat hyperlipidemia. A dosage of 24-50 milligrams per day is used to treat patients with arterial disease.

Initially, mesoglycan and other mucopolysaccharides were only available through injections. They are now available in oral form.

Some common names for preparations containing mucopolysaccharides include chondroitin and glucosamine. Glucosamine stimulates the production of glycosaminoglycans and proteoglycans, the building blocks of cartilage. If the body does not produce enough glucosamine on its own, the joints can dry out, crack, or wear away completely. If the joints have no protection from glucosamine, they can become swollen, inflamed, and very painful, a common condition known as **osteoarthritis**.

Researchers believe that taking glucosamine can help the body stimulate its own production of protective cartilage around joints. Combining glucosamine together with chrondroitin is thought to increase the overall effectiveness, although some practitioners prescribe glucosamine alone.

Precautions

Mesoglycan and other aortic glycosaminoglycans are basically compounds found naturally in the body, so they are generally considered to be safe to take, even in large quantities. There is some ability, however, for aortic glycosaminoglycans to reduce blood clotting. Maximum safe dosages for young children, pregnant or nursing women, or in those with liver or kidney disease have not been determined.

The Dietary Supplement Health and Education Act of 1994 permits the marketing of a product labeled as a "dietary supplement" without the approval of any government agency as long as the labeling includes a disclaimer stating that it has not been evaluated by the Food and Drug Administration (FDA), and that the product is not intended to diagnose, treat, or prevent any disease. Purity of dietary supplements cannot be guaranteed. Because of this, consumers should **exercise** caution when using any dietary supplement and be sure to discuss the use of dietary supplements with their physician or health practitioner. Currently, the only known medical condition that precludes the use of mesoglycan is hemorrhagic disease.

Side effects

In many studies, mesoglycan was found to be tolerated well. Gastrointestinal discomfort and **nausea** are side effects sometimes reported. With intramuscular injections of mesoglycan, injection site reactions may occur.

Interactions

If you are taking any type of prescription or other medication that decreases blood clotting such as coumadin (warfarin), heparin, trental (pentoxifylline) or aspirin, do not use aortic glycosaminoglycans or mucopolysaccharides without the advice of a physician.

Resources

BOOKS

The Columbia Encyclopedia. 6th ed., New York: Columbia University Press, 2000.

PERIODICALS

Lotti T., I. Ghersetich, C. Comacchi, and J. Jorizzo. "Cutaneous Small-Vessel Vasculitis." *Journal of the American Academy of Dermatology.* (1998): 1-38.

"Glucosamine for Arthritis." *The Medical Letter on Drugs and Therapeutics.* (1997): 91-92.

OTHER

"Mesoglycan." Micromedex Database. (December 1999).

Kim Sharp

Metabolic therapies

Definition

Metabolic therapies differ considerably according to practitioner; however they typically involve a belief that **cancer** and certain other diseases are caused by imbalances in a patient's metabolism. These imbalances are caused by accumulations of toxins in the body. Treatment involves removing these toxins and strengthening the immune system and biochemical processes.

Origins

The origins of metabolic therapies are as varied as the therapies themselves. One of the best-known proponents was Harold Manners, a biology professor who claimed in 1977 to have cured cancer in mice using injected laetrile, **vitamin A**, and **digestive enzymes**. Manner left the academic world and started a clinic in Tijuana, Mexico before he died in 1988.

Benefits

In addition to cancer, metabolic therapies have also been used against arthritis, **multiple sclerosis**, and other diseases believed linked to metabolic imbalances.

Description

Metabolic therapies are an eclectic and controversial mix of treatment protocols, including the following:

- American biologics: Abstinence from caffeine, sugar and refined carbohydrates, as well as excess animal protein; enemas and colonic irrigation; laetrile; embryonic live cell therapy involving adrenal and cerebral tissues; vitamin C and other dietary supplements.
- Evers therapy: Laetrile; magnetic field therapy; hyperbaric oxygen; diet; Eversol chelation therapy; shark cartilage; Koch vaccination; injections of frozen thymus and other cells; detoxification.

- Gerson therapy: Low-salt vegan diet; hourly intake of fresh fruit and vegetable juices; three or four coffee enemas a day; dietary supplements including thyroid extracts, pancreatin, pepsin, niacin, and potassium.
- Issels' whole body therapy: Removal of mercury dental fillings and infected teeth; vaccines; organic diet with acidophilus support; abstinence from coffee, tea, tobacco; hyperthermia (provoking a fever to strengthen the immune system); hemotogenic oxidation therapy (to stimulate an immune response within the blood); informal psychotherapy.
- Kelley-Gonzalez diet: Individualized diet, often including large quantities of raw fruits, juices, raw and steamed vegetables, cereals, and nuts; abstinence from red meat, white sugar, chicken, refined grain products, and soy; freeze-dried pancreatic enzymes; frequent coffee enemas and laxative purging; as many as 150 dietary supplements a day.
- Manner metabolic diet therapy: Laetrile; enzymes; daily coffee enemas; vitamins, minerals, and other supplements; direct injections of enzymes into tumors; psychological counseling.
- Revici therapy: Intravenous doses of selenium, oxygen, copper, calcium, and other substances intended to balance body chemistry.

Precautions

Generally the controversial and unproven nature of these therapies, combined with the seriousness of the diseases they are intended to treat, make the ongoing involvement of a competent medical professional strongly advisable. One major drawback to trying alternative cancer therapies is that opportunities may be lost for timely application of other, more effective therapies.

Side effects

Concern has been expressed that patients on some metabolic **diets** may risk electrolyte imbalances or even death. Further concern exists about the safety of enzyme injections and the toxicity of megavitamin

therapy. Laetrile has been linked to life-threatening cyanide toxicity.

Research and general acceptance

Most metabolic therapies for cancer are well outside the comfort zone of traditional medical practitioners. Some proponents have experienced considerable opposition from regulators and law-enforcement officials.

Training and certification

Metabolic therapies are usually offered in small medical clinics that have developed their own treatment protocols. A number of these clinics are clustered in northwestern Mexico, just a few miles from the United States border. There, practitioners are easily accessible to visiting Americans, yet outside the jurisdiction of United States regulators.

Resources

ORGANIZATIONS

American Cancer Society. 1599 Clifton Road, N.E., Atlanta, GA 30329. (800) 227–2345.

David Helwig

Methionine

Description

Methionine ($C_5H_{11}NO_2S$) is an essential, sulfur–containing amino acid. It is the source of **sulfur** for numerous compounds in the body, including the **amino acids** cysteine and taurine. The body uses sulfur in the development of hair follicles and to promote healthy hair, skin, and nail growth. Sulfur also increases the liver's production of **lecithin** (which reduces **cholesterol**), reduces liver fat, protects the kidneys, helps the body to excrete heavy metals, and reduces bladder irritation by regulating the formation of ammonia in the urine. Methionine is a lipotropic—a nutrient that helps prevent fat accumulation in the liver, and usually helps detoxify metabolic wastes and toxins.

S–adenosyl–L–methionine (SAM, or SAMe) is an active compound made from methionine and adenosine triphosphate (ATP), an enzyme found in muscle tissue. SAMe is manufactured within the body and is found in almost every tissue, but it can also be made synthetically. It acts as a methyl donor in a variety of biochemical pathways. Methylation reactions are essential for the **detoxification** of harmful products of metabolism, and the synthesis of numerous physiological agents including neurotransmitters, cartilage, and **glutathione**. (Glutathione is a chemical that plays an important role in biological oxidation–reduction processes, and as a coenzyme. It can combine with toxic substances to form water soluble compounds that can be excreted through the kidneys.)

Methionine is considered essential because it cannot be manufactured in the body and must be obtained through diet. This particular amino acid is found only in meat, fish, eggs, and dairy products. Natural and synthetic methionine supplements are available, as well as supplements containing SAMe.

General use

Acetaminophen overdose

Methionine is used to treat acetaminophen (paracetamol) poisoning that may result in liver damage. Preparations containing both methionine and acetaminophen have been formulated for use in situations where overdose may occur.

Arthritis

Most people with arthritis rely on continuous doses of non–steroidal, anti–inflammatory drugs (NSAIDs) such as ibuprofen, aspirin, and naproxen for **pain** relief. SAMe has several advantages over these standard painkillers. It provides effective pain relief and has fewer side effects than these drugs. Users are generally able to tolerate SAMe better than they can other drugs, which is a significant issue for arthritis sufferers. While NSAIDs can cause gastrointestinal bleeding, SAMe can protect against injury to the stomach. Another advantage is that SAMe may actually have a protective effect on joints and even repair cartilage.

Depression

SAMe is beneficial for most forms of **depression**. In Europe, SAMe is prescribed more often than any other type of antidepressant. Many studies have shown SAMe to be as effective as other antidepressant drugs. It works more quickly and has fewer side effects. SAMe may boost the activity of several brain chemicals involved in mood, such as norepinephrine, dopamine, and serotonin.

Liver function

Methionine levels help determine the liver's concentration of sulfur–containing compounds and SAMe improves and normalizes liver function. SAMe is used in Europe in the treatment of **cirrhosis** and liver damage caused by alcohol. It is essential for the production of glutathione. Methionine itself has a protective effect on glutathione and prevents depletion during toxic overload, which can protect the liver from the damaging effects of toxic compounds.

Through methylation, SAMe is able to inactivate estrogens to prevent estrogen–induced cholestasis (suppressed bile flow) in pregnant women and those on oral contraceptives. It also increases membrane fluidity, restoring several factors that promote bile flow. Treatment with SAMe can also help decrease serum bilirubin (pigment in the blood that can cause **jaundice**) in patients with Gilbert's syndrome, a condition characterized by a chronically elevated serum bilirubin level.

Neurological disorders

SAMe improves the binding of neurotransmitters to receptor sites in the brain. It is essential for the regeneration of neuron axons following injury, and for the formation of myelin sheaths (a fatty substance) that surround axons. Alzheimer's and Parkinson's patients have very low levels of SAMe, and methionine may help treat some symptoms of **Parkinson's disease**.

Persons with **AIDS** have low levels of methionine, which may explain some of the nervous system deterioration that can occur to cause symptoms such as **dementia**. Methionine may improve memory recall in persons with AIDS–related nervous system degeneration, and SAMe may be used in the treatment of HIV–related motor and sensory changes in the extremities.

Low levels of methionine in pregnant women are related to an increased risk of neural tube defects (NTDs) in the fetus. Neural tube defects are caused by the failure of the neural tube to close properly during the formation of the central nervous system in the developing embryo. Mothers whose methionine intake is adequate during the period from three months prior to conception through the first trimester of **pregnancy** have a significantly lowered risk of having a baby with a neural tube defect.

Other uses

In Europe, SAMe has been used in clinical studies to treat **anxiety, schizophrenia**, demyelination diseases, and dementia. Oral doses of methionine have also been given to lower urinary pH and to help in the treatment of liver disorders. SAMe's ability to inactivate estrogens supports the use of methionine in conditions of presumed estrogen excess such as PMS.

Methionine in combination with several **antioxidants** may reduce pain and recurrences of attacks of **pancreatitis** (inflammation of the pancreas). SAMe also improves the symptoms of **fibromyalgia** patients, who suffer from chronic muscle pain, non–restorative sleep, and profound **fatigue**.

Cancer researchers are also studying the role of methionine in a special diet for patients diagnosed with colon cancer.

Preparations

Amino acid requirements vary according to body weight. Most average–size adults require approximately 800–1,000 mg of methionine per day. Infants require five times that amount, and children need twice that amount. Dosage rates of SAMe for conditions such as depression, fibromyalgia, liver ailments, migraines, and **osteoarthritis** are 200–400 mg, two or three times per day. Before taking SAMe supplementation, a physician or qualified health practitioner should be consulted.

The usual oral dose of methionine for acetaminophen poisoning is 2.5 g every four hours for four doses starting less than 10–12 hours after acetaminophen ingestion. It may also be given intravenously.

Precautions

Homocysteine is an amino acid that the liver produces after ingesting methionine. Increased methionine intake, in the presence of inadequate intake of **folic acid**, vitamin B_6, and **vitamin B_{12}**, may increase the homocysteine in the blood and increase the risk of **heart disease**, or **stroke**. A doctor should be consulted to determine if any nutrient supplementation is needed.

Homocystine is the amino acid formed by the oxidation of homocysteine; homocystinuria is an inherited disorder in which there is excess homocystine in the plasma that is excreted in the urine. People with homocystinuria may benefit from a diet low in methionine, and should consult a physician before taking a supplement.

Patients with acidosis (condition of increased acidity in body fluids) or established liver insufficiency should not take methionine, and it should be used with caution in patients with severe liver disease.

A person who is already taking prescription medications for depression should not attempt to take SAMe, since it increases the efficiency of these medications. Those suffering from bipolar (manic–depressive) disorders should not take SAMe, since its antidepressant

---

KEY TERMS

Amino acids—Raw materials used by the body to manufacture proteins, which are vital components of all human cells.

Antioxidant—A substance that inhibits oxidation of another substance, such as low–density lipoprotein (LDL). LDL can cause plaque build–up and hardening of the arteries.

Methionine—An essential sulfur–containing amino acid, found in protein foods.

Methylation—The process by which a methyl group ($-CH_3$) is added to some compound, ion, or other chemical species.

Neural tube defects (NTDs)—A group of birth defects caused by failure of the neural tube to close completely during the formation of the baby's central nervous system. Recent research indicates that methionine deficiency in pregnant women increases the risk of NTDs in their newborns.

SAMe—An active compound made from methionine and adenosine triphosphate (ATP), an enzyme found in muscle tissue.

---

properties may induce or heighten the manic phase of this condition.

Women who are healthy and eat a well–balanced diet do not require methionine supplementation during pregnancy or while breastfeeding. They should talk to their doctors before using any kind of supplement.

Side effects

No toxic dosage of methionine has been determined, but it may cause **nausea**, **vomiting**, drowsiness, and irritability in moderate amounts. Supplementation of up to 2 g methionine daily for long periods of time has not produced any serious side effects.

Interactions

There are no well–known drug interactions with methionine.

Resources

BOOKS

Methionine–A Medical Dictionary, Bibliography, and Annotated Research Guide to Internet References. San Diego: ICON Health Publications, 2004.

PERIODICALS

Koc, Ahmeti, and Vadim Gladyshev. "Methionine Sulfoxide Reduction and the Aging Process." *Annals of the New York Academy of Sciences* (April 2007): 383–396.

Mischoulon, David, and Maurizio Fava. "Role of S–adenosyl–L–methionine in the Treatment of Depression: A Review of the Evidence." *American Journal of Clinical Nutrition* (November 2002): 1158S–1161S.

Shippy, R. Andrew, et al. "S–adenosylmethionine (SAM–e) for the Treatment of Depression in People Living with HIV/AIDS." *BMC Psychiatry* (November 2004): 38–43.

Tchantchou, F., et al. "S–adenosyl Methionine: A Connection between Nutritional and Genetic Risk Factors for Neurodegeneration in Alzheimer's Disease." *Journal of Nutrition, Health, and Aging* (November–December 2006): 541–544.

Van Brummelen, R., and D. du Toit. "L–methionine as Immune Supportive Supplement: A Clinical Evaluation." *Amino Acids* (July 2007): 157–163.

OTHER

MayoClinic.com. "SAMe." http://www.mayoclinic.com/health/same/NS_patient–same (February 18, 2008).

VitaminStuff.com. "Methionine." http://www.vitaminstuff.com/methionine.html (February 18, 2008).

Wikipedia. "S–adenosyl Methionine." http://en.wikipedia.org/wiki/S–adenosylmethionine (February 18, 2008).

Melissa C. McDade
Rebecca J. Frey, PhD

Methylcobalamin *see* **Vitamin B$_{12}$**

Mexican yam

Description

Mexican yam is one of some 850 species of yam in the Dioscoreaceae family. It is a perennial plant with twisting, climbing vines that grows in warm tropical climates. There are also some twists and turns related to this plant's identity and its use as a herbal remedy.

The wild yam (*Dioscorea villosa*) is a climbing plant that is native to the southeast United States and Canada. Such wild yam species as *Dioscorea floribunda* as well as *Dioscorea villosa* are native to Mexico. These plants are used for the herbal preparations known as Mexican yam and Mexican wild yam. Mexican wild yam also grows in the southeastern United States and Appalachia.

An extract of this plant is used as a herbal remedy called Mexican yam, wild yam, and Mexican wild yam. It is sold as a "natural hormone" cream and oral remedy.

Mexican wild yam is also known as **colic** root, China root, rheumatism root, devil's bones, and yuma.

There is another twist to this plant's identity. Although the Mexican yam has fleshy edible roots, this is not the yam that people associate with Thanksgiving dinner. That yam is actually the sweet potato, a vegetable that is the root of a trailing plant. It is a member of the morning glory family. The identification of the sweet potato as a yam is can be traced to the pre-Civil War era of slavery in the United States. The sweet potato reminded slaves from sub-Saharan Africa of the yam plants in their homeland.

General use

Mexican yam has long had a reputation as a woman's herb. During the eighteenth and nineteenth centuries, wild yam was used to treat menstrual **pain** and conditions related to childbirth . Pregnant women used wild yam to combat nausea , ease aching muscles, and prevent miscarriages.

Wild yam was also used as a colic remedy. Furthermore, the plant's anti-inflammatory properties were thought to be effective in the treatment of rheumatoid arthritis.

Most of those uses were forgotten after Japanese researchers in 1936 discovered that wild yam contained diosgenin, a chemical that scientist Russell Marker used in the 1940s to create synthetic progesterone and the hormone **DHEA**.

Synthetic progesterone

Marker worked with species of Mexican yams. Others used his technique for manufacturing progesterone to develop such products as the birth control pill and steroid drugs. During the 1990s, companies began marketing Mexican yam products as a source of natural progesterone and DHEA.

Mexican yam products are also advertised as treatments for menstrual problems and **osteoporosis**. They are sometimes recommended for hormone replacement therapy during menopause, and sometimes the natural hormones are said to slow down the aging process. In addition, Mexican yam and wild yam products are said to boost progesterone effects that fall during the last half of the month. A rise in hormones could help a woman conceive.

This marketing, in terms of the progesterone content and the results, has drawn criticism for misleading consumers. Herbal expert Varro Tyler described this campaign as a "wild yam scam" in his book, *Tyler's Honest Herbal.*

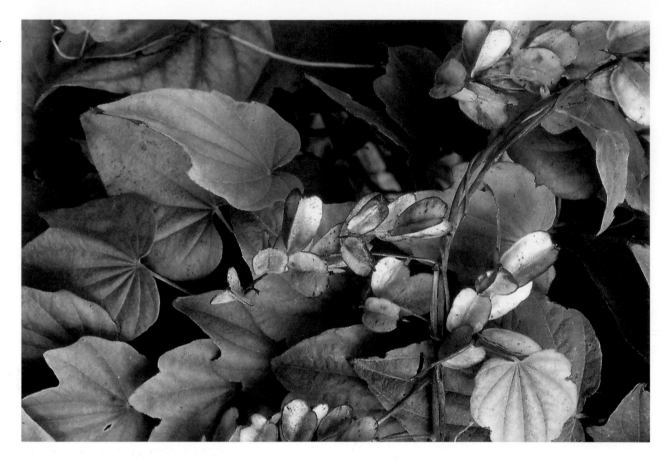

Mexican yam. *(©PlantaPhile, Germany. Reproduced by permission.)*

Contemporary uses of Mexican yam

Although Mexican yam cream does not provide natural progesterone, the herb can be used for cramping conditions like menstrual pain. It can help to build up good **cholesterol** levels while alleviating poor circulation, nervousness and restlessness. In addition, wild yam root tea has been suggested as a means of increasing a woman's ability to conceive.

Preparations

Mexican yam cream is marketed with the promise that it is natural progesterone. The cream is applied to the skin based on a woman's condition. Dosages are based on the outcome expected.

Mexican yam's other uses

Mexican yam is sold as a powdered herb, liquid extract, tincture, and in capsule form. While there are general dosage recommendations for wild yam, instructions on commercial packages should be followed since product strength can vary.

Wild yam tea, which is also known as an infusion, is made by pouring 1 cup (240 mL) of boiling water over 1–2 tsp (1.5–2.5 g) of the dried herb. The mixture is steeped for 10–15 minutes and then strained. Wild yam tea can be drunk three times a day.

A tincture of wild yam in an alcohol solution can be taken 3–4 times a day. A single dosage consists of 2–3 mL (approximately 1.2 tsp) of wild yam.

Wild yam capsules contain the dried root. The average dosage is 1–2 pills, taken three times daily.

Mexican yam combinations

Mexican yam can be combined with other herbs to treat a range of conditions. The following conditions can be treated by these combination remedies:

- Menstrual cramps can be treated with a tea made with wild yam and cramp bark. Those herbs can also be blended into a tea with such herbs as motherwort, fresh oats, and chamomile.

- Relief for rheumatoid arthritis may come from a combination of wild yam and black cohosh.

- For kidney stones, wild yam can be combined in a tea with such herbs as cramp bark, hydrangea root, and yarrow.

Precautions

Mexican wild yam is safe if taken within prescribed therapeutic dosages, according to the *PDR (Physician's Desk Reference) for Herbal Medicines*. The book draws on the findings of Germany's Commission E, a government agency that studies herbal remedies for approval as over-the-counter drugs. An English version of the German Commission E *Monographs* was published in 1997.

Pregnant and nursing women, as well as patients with hormone imbalances, **depression**, or hormone-sensitive cancers should avoid wild yam unless they are under the guidance of a clinical herbalist or physician.

Furthermore, although wild yam root tea has been suggested as a method for a woman to become pregnant, the herb should not be used during the last half of a menstrual period.

Side effects

Large doses of Mexican yam may produce **nausea**. There is also a risk of poisoning.

Interactions

There are no known interactions when Mexican yam is taken with standard medications, other herbs, or dietary supplements.

Resources

BOOKS

Duke, James A. *The Green Pharmacy*. Emmaus, PA: Rodale Press, Inc., 1997.

Keville, Kathi. *Herbs for Health and Healing*. Emmaus, PA: Rodale Press, Inc., 1996.

PDR for Herbal Medicines. Montvale, NJ: Medical Economics Company, 1998.

Ritchason, Jack. *The Little Herb Encyclopedia*. Pleasant Grove, UT: Woodland Health Books, 1995.

Tyler, Varro, and Steven Foster. *Tyler's Honest Herbal*. Binghamton, NY: The Haworth Herbal Press, 1999.

ORGANIZATIONS

American Botanical Council. P.O. Box 201660. Austin TX, 78720. (512) 331-8868. http://www.herbalgram.org.

Herb Research Foundation. 1007 Pearl St., Suite 200. Boulder, CO 80302. (303) 449-2265. http://www.herbs.org.

Liz Swain

Middle ear infection *see* **Ear infection**

Migraine headache

Definition

Migraine is a type of **headache** marked by severe head **pain** lasting several hours or more.

Description

Migraine is an intense and often debilitating type of headache. The term *migraine* is derived from the Greek word *hemikrania*, meaning "half the head," because the classic migraine headache affects only one side of the person's head. Migraines affect as many as 24 million people in the United States, and are responsible for billions of dollars in lost work, poor job performance, and direct medical costs. Approximately 18% of women and 6% of men experience at least one migraine attack per year. Currently, one American in 11 now suffers from migraines, more than three times as many are women, with most of them being between the ages of 30 and 49. Migraines often begin in adolescence, and are rare after age 60.

Two types of migraine are recognized. Eighty percent of migraine sufferers experience "migraine without aura" (common migraine). In "migraine with aura," or classic migraine, the pain is preceded or accompanied by visual or other sensory disturbances, including hallucinations, partial obstruction of the visual field, numbness or tingling, or a feeling of heaviness. Symptoms are often most prominent on one side of the head or body, and may begin as early as 72 hours before the onset of pain.

Causes and symptoms

Causes

The physiological basis of migraine has proved difficult to uncover. There are a multitude of potential triggers for a migraine attack, and recognizing one's own set of triggers is the key to prevention.

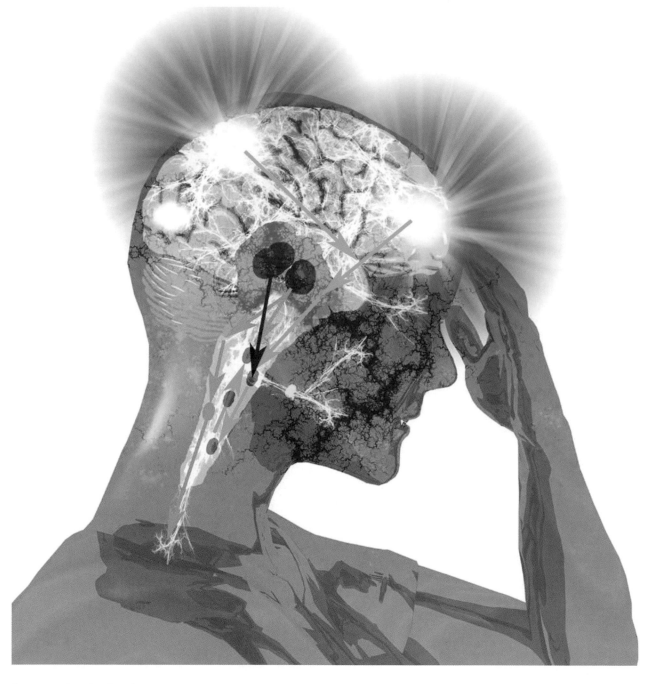

Anatomy of a migraine. Sensory triggers cause the thalamus to interact with the trigeminal nucleus and nerve (red arrow) and dilate blood vessels in face and brain. Pain signals sent to the brainstem nuclei (green arrows). The hypothalamus may also send signals to the brainstem and gut to induce pain, nausea, and vomiting (blue arrows). *(© PHOTOTAKE Inc. / Alamy)*

PHYSIOLOGY. The most widely accepted hypothesis of migraine suggests that a migraine attack is precipitated when pain-sensing nerve cells in the brain (called nociceptors) release chemicals called neuropeptides. At least one of the neurotransmitters, substance P, increases the pain sensitivity of nearby nociceptors. This process is called sensitization.

Other neuropeptides act on the smooth muscle surrounding cranial blood vessels. This smooth muscle regulates blood flow in the brain by relaxing or contracting, thus dilating (enlarging) or constricting the enclosed blood vessels. At the onset of a migraine headache, neuropeptides are thought to cause muscle **relaxation**, allowing vessel dilation and

KEY TERMS

Aura—A group of visual or other sensations that precedes the onset of a migraine attack.

Autogenic training—A form of self-hypnosis developed in Germany that appears to be beneficial to migraine sufferers.

Coenzyme Q$_{10}$—A substance used by cells in the human body to produce energy for cell maintenance and growth. It is being studied as a possible preventive for migraine headaches.

Nociceptor—A specialized type of nerve cell that senses pain.

Transcutaneous electrical nerve stimulation (TENS)—A treatment in which a mild electrical current is passed through electrodes on the skin to stimulate nerves and block pain signals.

increased blood flow. Other neuropeptides increase the leakiness of cranial vessels, allowing fluid leak, and promote inflammation and tissue swelling. The pain of migraine is thought to result from this combination of increased pain sensitivity, tissue and vessel swelling, and inflammation. The aura seen during a migraine may be related to constriction in the blood vessels that dilate in the headache phase.

GENETICS. Susceptibility to some types of migraine is inherited. A child of a migraine sufferer has as much as a 50% chance of developing migraines. If both parents are affected, the chance rises to 70%. In 2002, a team of Australian researchers identified a region on human chromosome 1 that influences susceptibility to migraine. It is likely that more than one gene is involved in the inherited forms of the disorder. Many cases of migraine, however, have no obvious familial basis. It is likely that the genes that are involved set the stage for migraine, and that full development requires environmental influences, as well.

Two groups of Italian researchers have recently identified two loci on human chromosomes 1 and 14 respectively that are linked to migraine headaches. The locus on chromosome 1q23 has been linked to familial hemiplegic migraine type 2, while the locus on chromosome 14q21 is associated with migraine without aura.

TRIGGERS. A wide variety of foods, drugs, environmental cues, and personal events are known to trigger migraines. It is not known how most triggers set off the events of migraine, nor why individual migraine sufferers are affected by particular triggers but not others.

Common food triggers include:

- alcohol
- caffeine products, as well as caffeine withdrawal
- chocolate
- foods with an extremely high sugar content
- dairy products
- fermented or pickled foods
- citrus fruits
- nuts
- processed foods, especially those containing nitrites, sulfites, or monosodium glutamate (MSG)

Environmental and event-related triggers include:

- stress or time pressure
- menstrual periods, menopause
- sleep changes or disturbances, including oversleeping
- prolonged overexertion or uncomfortable posture
- hunger or fasting
- odors, smoke, or perfume
- strong glare or flashing lights

Drugs that may trigger migraine include:

- oral contraceptives
- estrogen replacement therapy
- Theophylline
- Reserpine
- Nifedipine
- Indomethicin
- Cimetidine
- oversuse of decongestants
- analgesic overuse
- benzodiazepine withdrawal

Symptoms

Migraine without aura may be preceded by elevations in mood or energy level for up to 24 hours before the attack. Other pre-migraine symptoms may include **fatigue**, **depression**, and excessive yawning.

Aura most often begins with shimmering, jagged arcs of white or colored light progressing over the visual field in the course of 10–20 minutes. This may be preceded or replaced by dark areas or other visual disturbances. Numbness and tingling are common, especially of the face and hands. These sensations may spread, and may be accompanied by a sensation of weakness or heaviness in the affected limb.

Migraine pain is often present only on one side of the head, although it may involve both, or switch sides during attacks. The pain is usually throbbing, and may range from mild to incapacitating. It is often accompanied by **nausea** or **vomiting**, painful sensitivity to light and sound, and intolerance of food or odors. Blurred vision is also common.

The pain tends to intensify over the first 30 minutes to several hours, and may last from several hours to a day, or longer. Afterward, the affected person is usually weary, and sensitive to sudden head movements.

Diagnosis

Ideally, migraine is diagnosed by a careful medical history. Unfortunately, migraine is underdiagnosed because many doctors tend to minimize its symptoms as "just a headache." According to a 2003 study, 64% of migraine patients in the United Kingdom and 77% of those in the United States never receive a correct medical diagnosis for their headaches.

So far, laboratory tests and such imaging studies as computed tomography (CT scan) or magnetic resonance imaging (MRI) scans have not been useful for identifying migraine. However, these tests may be necessary to rule out a brain tumor or other structural causes of migraine headache in some patients.

Treatment

At the onset of symptoms, the migraine sufferer should seek out a quiet, dark room and attempt to sleep. Placing a cold, damp cloth or a cold pack on the forehead may help. Additionally, tying a headband tightly around the head can relieve migraines.

Migraine headaches are often linked with food **allergies** or intolerances. Identification and elimination of the offending food or foods can decrease the frequency of migraines and/or alleviate these headaches altogether.

Alternative treatments for migraine include:

- Acupressure. Pressing on the Gates of Consciousness (GB 20) points can relieve migraine.
- Acupuncture. A National Institutes of Health (NIH) panel concluded that acupuncture may be a useful treatment for headache.
- Aromatherapy. The essential oil rosemary eases migraine pain.
- Autogenic training. Autogenic training is a form of self-hypnosis developed in Germany in the 1930s that has been shown in several studies to relieve the pain of migraine.
- Cognitive behavior therapy.
- Herbals. Valerian (*Valeriana officinalis*), passionflower (*Passiflora incarnata*), feverfew (*Chrysanthemum parthe-*

nium), ginger, ginkgo (*Ginkgo biloba*), goldenseal (*Hydrastis canadensis*), hawthorn (*Crataegus oxyacantha*), linden, wood betony (*Stachys officinalis*), skullcap (*Scutellaria lateriflora*), or cramp bark (*Viburnum opulus*) may relieve migraines.

- Hydrotherapy. Contrast showers, in which a short hot shower is followed by a longer cold shower, may halt an oncoming migraine. A hot enema can temporarily relieve migraine pain.
- Naturopathy. Migraine headaches are one of the most common reasons for consulting naturopathic practitioners. Naturopaths typically treat migraine with a combination of nutritional therapy and mind/body techniques.
- Relaxation techniques. Meditation, yoga, hypnosis, visualization, breathing exercises, or progressive muscular relaxation may halt the progression of a migraine.
- Supplements. Clinical studies have shown that vitamin B_2 (riboflavin), magnesium, 5-HTP, or melatonin can reduce the severity of migraines.
- Transcutaneous electrical nerve stimulation (TENS).

Allopathic treatments

Nonsteroidal anti-inflammatory drugs (NSAIDs) acetaminophen (Tylenol), ibuprofen (Motrin), and naproxen (Aleve) are helpful for early and mild headache. Excedrin Migraine is a combination product that is indicated for migraine headache.

More severe or unresponsive attacks may be treated with ergotamine (botulinum toxin), dihydroergotamine, sumatriptan (Imitrex), beta-blockers and **calcium** channel-blockers, antiseizure drugs, antidepressants (SSRIs), meperidine, or metoclopramide. Some of these drugs are also available as nasal sprays, intramuscular injections, or rectal suppositories when vomiting prevents taking the drug by mouth.

Sumatriptan and other triptan drugs (zolmitriptan, rizatriptan, naratriptan, almotriptan, and frovatriptan) should not be taken by people with any kind of vascular disease because they cause coronary artery narrowing. Otherwise these drugs have been shown to be very safe.

Continued use of some antimigraine drugs can lead to "rebound headache," marked by frequent or chronic headaches, especially in the early morning hours. Rebound headache can be avoided by using antimigraine drugs under a doctor's supervision, with the minimum dose necessary to treat symptoms. Tizanidine (Zanaflex) has been reported to be effective in treating rebound headaches when taken together with an NSAID.

Expected results

Most people can control migraines through recognizing and avoiding triggers, and by using effective treatments. Some people with severe migraines do not respond to preventive or drug therapy. Migraines usually wane in intensity by age 60 and beyond.

Prevention

The frequency of migraine headaches may be lessened by avoiding triggers. It is useful to track these triggers by keeping a headache journal.

One substance that is being studied as a possible migraine preventive is **coenzyme Q$_{10}$**, a compound used by cells to produce energy needed for cell growth and maintenance. Coenzyme Q$_{10}$ has been studied as a possible complementary treatment for **cancer**. Its use in preventing migraines is encouraging and merits further study.

A study published in early 2003 reported that three drugs currently used to treat disorders of muscle tone are being explored as possible preventive treatments for migraine. They are botulinum toxin type A (Botox), baclofen (Lioresal), and tizanidine (Zanaflex). Early results of open trials of these medications are positive.

Anti-epileptic drugs, which are also known as anticonvulsants, are also being studied as possible migraine preventives. As of 2003, **sodium** valproate (Epilim) is the only drug approved by the Food and Drug Administration (FDA) for prevention of migraine. Such newer anticonvulsants as gabapentin (Neurontin) and topiramate (Topamax) are presently being evaluated as migraine preventives.

A natural preparation made from butterbur root (*Petasites hybridus*) has been sold in Germany since the 1970s as a migraine preventive under the trade name Petadolex. Petadolex has been available in the United States since December 1998 and has passed several clinical safety and postmarketing surveillance trials.

Other possible preventive measures include: eating at regular times, not skipping meals, reducing the use of **caffeine** and pain-relievers, restricting physical exertion (especially on hot days), and keeping regular sleep hours, but not oversleeping. Other measures include:

- Aerobic exercise, which can reduce the frequency of migraines.
- Biofeedback thermal control was found to be as effective as medications in preventing migraines.
- Celery juice consumed twice daily may help to prevent migraines.
- Feverfew was shown to reduce the severity and frequency of migraines. This herb should not, however, be used during pregnancy or by people taking blood-thinning medications.
- Ginger may help prevent migraines.
- Pulsing electromagnetic fields. A preliminary study found that pulsing electromagnetic fields reduced the frequency of migraines.
- Relaxation techniques can reduce migraine frequency.
- Supplementation with magnesium and riboflavin was shown to prevent migraines.

Resources

BOOKS

American Council on Headache Education. *Migraine: The Complete Guide*. New York: Dell, 1994.

"Migraine." Section 14, Chapter 168 in *The Merck Manual of Diagnosis and Therapy*, edited by Mark H. Beers, MD, and Robert Berkow, MD. Whitehouse Station, NJ: Merck Research Laboratories, 1999.

Pelletier, Kenneth R., MD. *The Best Alternative Medicine*, Part II, "CAM Therapies for Specific Conditions: Headaches." New York: Simon & Schuster, 2002.

PERIODICALS

Bendtsen, L. "Sensitization: Its Role in Primary Headache." *Current Opinion in Investigational Drugs* 3 (March 2002): 449–453.

Corbo, J. "The Role of Anticonvulsants in Preventive Migraine Therapy." *Current Pain and Headache Reports* 7 (February 2003): 63–66.

Danesch, U., and R. Rittinghausen. "Safety of a Patented Special Butterbur Root Extract for Migraine Prevention." *Headache* 43 (January 2003): 76–78.

Diamond, S., and R. Wenzel. "Practical Approaches to Migraine Management." *CNS Drugs* 16 (2002): 385–403.

Freitag, F. G. "Preventative Treatment for Migraine and Tension-Type headaches : Do Drugs Having Effects on Muscle Spasm and Tone Have a Role?" *CNS Drugs* 17 (2003): 373–381.

Lea, R. A., A. G. Shepherd, R. P. Curtain, et al. "A Typical Migraine Susceptibility Region Localizes to Chromosome 1q31." *Neurogenetics* 4 (March 2002): 17–22.

Lipton, R. B., A. I. Scher, T. J. Steiner, et al. "Patterns of Health Care Utilization for Migraine in England and in the United States." *Neurology* 60 (February 11, 2003): 441–448.

Marconi, R., M. De Fusco, P. Aridon, et al. "Familial Hemiplegic Migraine Type 2 is Linked to 0.9Mb Region on Chromosome 1q23" *Annals of Neurology* 53 (March 2003): 376–381.

Pryse–Phillips, William E.M., et al. "Guidelines for the Nonpharmacologic Management of Migraine in Clinical Practice." *Canadian Medical Association Journal* 159 (July 14, 1998): 47–54.

Rozen, T. D., M. L. Oshinsky, C. A. Gebeline, et al. "Open Label Trial of Coenzyme Q$_{10}$ as a Migraine Preventive." *Cephalalgia* 22 (March 2002): 137–141.

Sheftell, F. D., and S. J. Tepper. "New Paradigms in the Recognition and Acute Treatment of Migraine." *Headache* 42 (January 2002): 58–69.

Sinclair, Steven. "Migraine Headaches: Nutritional, Botanical and Other Alternative Approaches." *Alternative Medicine Review* 4 (1999): 86–95.

Soragna, D., A. Vettori, G. Carraro, et al. "A Locus for Migraine Without Aura Maps on Chromosome 14q21.2-q22.3." *American Journal of Human Genetics* 72 (January 2003): 161–167.

Stetter, F., and S. Kupper. "Autogenic Training: A Meta-Analysis of Clinical Outcome Studies." *Applied Psychophysiology and Biofeedback* 27 (March 2002): 45–98.

Tepper, S. J., and D. Millson. "Safety Profile of the Triptans." *Expert Opinion on Drug Safety* 2 (March 2003): 123–132.

ORGANIZATIONS

American Council for Headache Education. 19 Mantua Road, Mt. Royal, NJ 08061. (609) 423-0043 or (800) 255-2243. http://www.achenet.org

National Headache Foundation. 428 West St. James Place, Chicago, IL 60614. (773) 388-6399 or (800) 843-2256. http://www.headaches.org

U. S. Food and Drug Administration (FDA). 5600 Fishers Lane, Rockville, MD 20857. (888) 463-6332. http://www. fda.gov.

OTHER

"Migraine." *American Medical Association.* (cited December 2002). http://www.ama-assn.org/special/migraine.

Belinda Rowland
Rebecca J. Frey, PhD

Milk thistle

Description

Milk thistle (*Silybum marianum* or *Cardus marianum*) is a plant used for treating liver disorders, breastfeeding problems, and other illnesses. The active ingredient of the herb, silymarin, is found in the ripe seeds of the plant. The milk thistle plant has a long stem, green leaves with white spots, and pink to purple spiky flowered head (which true to its name, resembles a thistle). The plant is native to Europe and grows in the wild in the United States and South America. Other common names for the plant include Mary thistle, St. Mary thistle, Marian thistle, and lady's thistle.

The medicinal benefits of milk thistle have been valued for more than 2,000 years. Written records

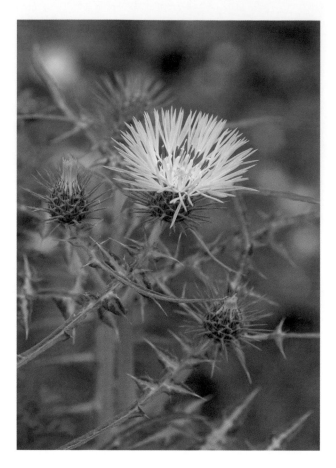

Milk Thistle. *(© blickwinkel / Alamy)*

show that as early as the first century, Romans were using the plant as a liver-protecting agent. The plant was also frequently used throughout the Middle Ages, and it is in the herbal literature of this period that the medicinal properties of milk thistle seeds are first noted. Nicholas Culpepper, a British herbalist, wrote about the value of the herb in treating diseases of the liver and spleen in the late eighteenth century, and by the end of the next century, records show that American physicians were also prescribing the substance. Silymarin was first isolated from the milk thistle plant by German scientists in the 1960s.

The leaves and stem of the milk thistle plant are edible, and can be used in salads or eaten raw. The plant was cultivated as a vegetable in Europe through the end of the nineteenth century.

General use

Milk thistle is prescribed for a number of medicinal uses, including liver disease treatment and prevention, HIV treatment, lactation problems, gallbladder disorders, mushroom poisoning, and **psoriasis**, a chronic skin disease characterized by reddish patches.

Liver disease

Milk thistle is thought to promote the growth of new liver cells, and to prevent toxins from penetrating through healthy liver cells by binding itself to the cell membranes. It is prescribed for **cirrhosis**, **hepatitis**, and other liver disorders. Several clinical studies have demonstrated that individuals with cirrhosis who take daily doses of milk thistle extract have a lower mortality rate than those who took a placebo (or sugar pill). While further research needs to be completed, a 2001 article reports that clinical trials show that milk thistle (at 140 mg three times per day) did indeed improve survival among cirrhosis patients.

In addition, milk thistle may have a protective effect on the liver, and is sometimes prescribed for patients who take medications that can cause liver damage (e.g., Thorazine, Haldol), or those who are exposed to liver-damaging substances such as lead. A large, controlled trial sponsored by the National Center for Complementary and Alternative Medicine (NCCAM) and the National Institutes of health (NIH) of milk thistle's medicinal value in the treatment of hepatitis and liver injury was scheduled to begin in the year 2000.

HIV treatment

Milk thistle is sometimes prescribed for HIV-positive patients to protect the liver from diseases such as hepatitis and from the hepatotoxic effects of other medications prescribed for HIV treatment.

Lactation problems

Milk thistle is frequently prescribed for breast-feeding mothers to promote increased breast milk secretion. Although the herb is considered safe for nursing mothers, it should be acquired from a reputable source and prescribed by an herbalist, naturopathic physician, or other healthcare professional familiar with its use.

Cancer prevention

The active chemical components of the milk thistle, silymarin (a complex of flavonoids) and its constituent, silibin, act as **antioxidants**. These substances have been shown to slow cell growth in some types of **cancer**.

Gallbladder disorders

Milk thistle may prevent inflammation of the gallbladder ducts and clear up **jaundice**.

Death cap mushroom poisoning

Milk thistle is the only known antidote for death cap mushroom (*Amanita phalloides*) poisoning. Ingesting this deadly mushroom can destroy the liver by shutting down protein production in liver cells. Milk thistle neutralizes these toxins and protects the liver. Milk thistle may also be helpful in acetaminophen overdosage.

Psoriasis

Because the liver neutralizes certain toxins associated with psoriasis attacks, milk thistle is believed to help prevent psoriasis outbreaks by promoting proper liver function.

Several other dermatological uses for the herb are currently under investigation. The antioxidant properties of the herb may have a healing effect on skin **wounds** and **burns**. Milk thistle has also been proposed as a cosmetic agent to retain skin tone and quality. Further studies are needed to prove the efficacy of the herb for these applications.

Preparations

Milk thistle is available in seed form, in capsules, and in extracts and tinctures. A tincture is an herbal preparation made by diluting the herb in alcohol. Tinctures of milk thistle can be taken in 1 or 2 ml doses three times a day.

Milk thistle seed has a low level of water solubility, so infusions (or teas) made from the herb are weaker than milk thistle tinctures and extracts. An infusion of milk thistle can be prepared by pouring a cup of boiling water over one teaspoon of seeds that have been ground to a fine texture. After the mixture steeps for 10-20 minutes, the herb is strained out and the mixture can be drunk. Instead of straining, the herb can also be placed into an infuser ball, tea bag, or a piece of cheesecloth or muslin and removed after steeping. Individuals can drink two to three cups of the infusion daily.

Milk thistle seed can also be taken by mouth in a dose of 1 tsp of fresh ground seeds daily. The herb should always be stored in an airtight container in a cool location away from bright light to maintain its potency.

Precautions

Individuals who suspect they have a liver disorder should always seek care from a healthcare professional.

Milk thistle should always be obtained from a reputable source that observes stringent quality control procedures and industry-accepted good manufacturing practices. Consumers should look for the designations "U.S.P." (*U.S. Pharmacopeia*) or "NF" (*National Formulary*) on milk thistle labeling. Herbal preparations prepared under USP or NF guidelines meet nationally recognized strength, quality, purity, packaging, and labeling standards as recommended by the U. S. Food and Drug Administration (FDA).

Botanical supplements are regulated by the FDA; however, they currently do not have to undergo any approval process before reaching the consumer market, and are classified as nutritional supplements rather than drugs. Legislation known as the Dietary Supplement Health and Education Act (DSHEA) was passed in 1994 in an effort to standardize the manufacture, labeling, composition, and safety of botanicals and supplements, and in January 2000, the FDA's Center for Food Safety and Applied **Nutrition** (CFSAN) announced a 10-year plan for establishing and implementing these regulations by the year 2010.

Pregnancy

Milk thistle is considered safe to use during **pregnancy** and in women who breastfeed. However, there are currently no long-term studies on use of the herb during pregnancy or lactation. A woman should speak with her healthcare practitioner before taking any herbs and/or medications during pregnancy.

Side effects

Milk thistle may cause mild **nausea** and **diarrhea**, or loose stools. The herb may also cause an allergic reaction in some individuals, particularly those with known **allergies** to plants in the Asteraceae family (thistles, daisies, artichokes). No other widely reported side effects are known when milk thistle is taken in proper therapeutic dosages. However, people with chronic medical conditions should consult with their healthcare professionals before taking the herb.

Interactions

There are no reported negative interactions between milk thistle and other medications and herbs, although certain drugs with the same therapeutic properties as milk thistle may enhance the effect of the herb. Again, individuals should consult their healthcare provider if they are taking other medications concurrently with milk thistle.

Resources

BOOKS

Medical Economics Corporation. *The PDR for Herbal Medicines*. Montvale, NJ: Medical Economics Corporation, 1998.

Hoffman, David. *The Complete Illustrated Herbal*. New York: Barnes & Noble Books, 1999.

PERIODICALS

Tyler, Varro. "This weed is a potent healer; protect your body from environmental toxins with milk thistle." *Prevention* 50, no. 1 (October 1998):79.

Walsh, Nancy. "Milk Thistle for Liver Disease (Alternative Medicine: An Evidence-Based Approach." *Internal Medicine News* (January 1, 2002): 10.

ORGANIZATIONS

Office of Dietary Supplements. National Institutes of Health. Building 31, Room 1B25, 31 Center Drive, MSC 2086, Bethesda, Maryland 20892-2086. (301) 435-2920 Fax: (301) 480-1845. http://odp.od.nih.gov/ods.

Paula Ford-Martin
Teresa Odle

Mind/body medicine

Definition

Mind/body medicine, also known as behavioral medicine, is the field of medicine concerned with the ways that the mind and emotions influence the body and physical health.

Origins

There was a time not long ago when Western medicine believed that health depended solely upon the physical mechanisms of the body. That is, a person is made up only of physical and chemical reactions that can be measured and manipulated scientifically. The notion that the mind and body live in separate compartments, so to speak, goes back to certain philosophers of classical antiquity. This concept of mind/body separation was also present in such religious groups as the Gnostics and some sects on the fringes of medieval Christianity. The scientific version of this split between mind and body is generally traced back to the seventeenth-century French philosopher Rene Descartes, whose thinking aided the development of science. It has taken a lot of time and research, three centuries after Descartes, for mainstream medicine to begin to accept that the mind plays a major role in health and disease.

The idea that the mind and body interact is not new, however. It can be traced to the Wisdom literature in the Old Testament and to Hippocrates, the father of Western medicine. The ancient Hebrews attributed some physical illnesses to grief or anger. Hippocrates believed that health depends upon a balance of the body, mind and environment, and that disease is caused by imbalances in these areas. As modern science progressed, the mind and emotions became neglected, since researchers found it difficult to measure and quantify mental states with the scientific methods and equipment that were so highly valued.

In the early 1900s, Harvard physiologist Walter Cannon coined the term "fight-or-flight response" for the body's reaction to threats, a response that causes increases in heart rate, blood pressure, blood sugar, muscle tension and respiration. During the 1950s, Hans Selye of McGill University pioneered research in what he called **stress**. Selye determined that the fight-or-flight response could be triggered by psychological factors as well as by physical threats. Stress includes having fight-or-flight reactions in situations where there is no immediate threat except mental perceptions and worries. Stress is not necessarily negative, except when people fail to cope with it effectively. Selye's work laid the groundwork for researchers to determine that stress and reactions to it play an integral role in health and disease.

Other mind/body relationships became apparent to medical researchers. The so-called **placebo effect** has been studied by doctors and psychologists for years. In clinical experiments, people who are given

inert substances made to look like medicines, such as sugar pills, often experience the same improvements as those patients who are given real medications. It is estimated that nearly one out of every three patients improves with medication simply because of the placebo effect, and not because of the drug itself. Researchers have also noted that some conditions and illnesses have no physical explanations. Doctors termed these conditions psychosomatic illnesses, as they seem to be caused by the psyche, or mind.

Researchers then theorized that certain personality types are susceptible to particular conditions. For instance, "Type A" personalities tend to be aggressive, ambitious, and always rushed. They tend to cope with stress by getting angry and upset. Researchers have found that these personalities are more prone to **heart disease**, high blood pressure, and other stress-related conditions. "Type B" personalities are those who cope with stressful situations with communication and balance instead of anger and aggression, and have been found to be less prone to stress-related conditions. Researchers have added a "Type C" personality, who tends to suppress emotions and has trouble with self-expression. Some clinicians have proposed a link between suppressed emotions and the development of **cancer**.

In the past few decades, researchers have begun to unravel the complex ways in which the mind and body interact. Many findings have demonstrated that the mind and body are intimately interconnected. Medical science has shown that the nervous system works closely with the immune system, systems that were at one time believed to be separate. Nerve endings have been found that connect directly to important components of the immune system called lymph nodes. This connection demonstrates that there is a physical link between the mind and the immune system. Studies have also shown that thoughts and emotions alone can influence the activity of immune system cells.

In the 1970s, Dr. Herbert Benson at Harvard Medical School discovered what he called the "relaxation response." Benson observed that trained **yoga** specialists (yogis) could control bodily functions that had previously been believed to be autonomic, or beyond the control of the mind. During **meditation**, these yogis could reduce their heart rates, blood pressure, metabolism, body temperature, and other physiological processes to surprising levels. Other people who were then taught meditation were able to reach deep states of **relaxation** and calmness as well. This relaxation response, as Benson termed it, is essentially the opposite of the fight-or-flight response. The relaxation response reduces blood pressure, respiration, heart rate, oxygen consumption, muscle tension, and other bodily processes that are elevated by stress. Researchers soon began to theorize that if stress could have harmful effects on health, then the relaxation response might have the opposite effect. It wasn't long before the Harvard Mind/Body Medical Institute was founded, and other major medical clinics followed by integrating mind/body practices and studies into their health programs. A new field opened up in academic medicine called **psychoneuroimmunology** (PNI), which is the study of how the mind and nervous system affect the immune system. Studies have since shown that the mind and emotions play roles in many diseases, including cancer, diabetes, heart disease, gastrointestinal problems, and **asthma**.

In 1993, Dr. David Eisenberg wrote in the *New England Journal of Medicine* about a study that showed that one out of every three adults in America had used some form of unconventional medicine. Of those alternative treatments, mind/body practices were used most often. The popular PBS series by journalist Bill Moyers, called *Healing and the Mind*, brought mind/body medicine into millions of homes. Dr. Benson of Harvard claims that mind/body medicine should no longer be considered alternative. Despite the acclaim and success, however, there is still resistance to the simple idea that the mind is an important part of health, and many mainstream doctors still adhere to the belief that medicine is just a matter of "drugs killing bugs."

Benefits

Mind/body therapies have shown promise in treating cancer, heart disease, **hypertension**, asthma, and mental illness. They have been used as effective complementary therapies alongside such conventional treatments as surgery and chemotherapy. Mind/body therapies have also been shown to increase quality of life, reduce **pain**, and improve symptoms for people with chronic diseases and health conditions. They may also help control and reverse certain diseases, particularly those that are stress-related. By reducing stress, mind/body therapies may even prevent many diseases. Another benefit of mind/body therapies is that they pose very little risk. Some are inexpensive, and most have few side effects.

Description

There are many alternative techniques that draw upon the interconnections between mind and body. These include **art therapy**, assertiveness training, autogenic training, bioenergetics, **biofeedback**, **breath therapy**, mental imagery, dance and **movement therapy**, dreamwork, Gestalt therapy, group therapy, hypnosis, meditation, mindfulness training, Jungian psychoanalysis, postural integration, **prayer** and faith healing, progressive relaxation, psychodrama, **psychotherapy**, Reichian therapy, support groups, and yoga. Some of the most widely used techniques are meditation, mindfulness training, biofeedback, breath therapy, hypnosis, mental imagery, and movement therapies, which are discussed below.

Costs can vary widely for mind/body treatments, depending on the type and the medical training of the practitioner. Many insurance companies will reimburse some mind/body treatments and training sessions; consumers should be aware of their insurance provisions.

Meditation

There are many forms of meditation, but they all have the same goal, which is to calm and focus the mind. As beginning meditators find out, however, calming and clearing the mind of thoughts and worries is easier said than done. When performed on a regular basis, meditation is an efficient way of promoting the relaxation response. Meditation is used to ease the discomfort of many health problems, including stress-related conditions, chronic pain, panic disorders, tension headaches, and asthma. A 2002 report stated research shows that transcendental meditation can reduce hardening of the arteries, eventually helping reduce risk of **heart attack** and **stroke**.

Meditation can be practiced anywhere, but a quiet and peaceful setting is recommended. Meditators should sit or lie in a comfortable position. Sitting with the spine as straight as possible without straining is the most commonly recommended position. Breathing during meditation should be deep, calm and slow. The meditator may concentrate on the breath or on a still object such as a flower or candle flame. The meditator often may repeat a soft sound, word, or phrase, known as a mantra. Mantras can be affirmative statements, prayers, or humming sounds. The goal of the meditator is to concentrate deeply in order to reduce the amount of thinking, and to calm the worries and thoughts that typically fill the mind. When thoughts or distractions arise, the meditator should allow them to pass without directing attention toward them.

Meditation should be done twice a day, for 20 minutes at a time, preferably at consistent times to develop discipline. It can be learned from books or tapes, but instruction is widely available and recommended, as beginners can find properly meditating and quieting the mind to be difficult at first.

Mindfulness training

This form of mental discipline was made popular by Dr. Jon Kabat-Zinn, a psychologist at the University of Massachusetts Medical Center, who has written some popular books on mind/body medicine. Kabat-Zinn uses mindfulness training to help patients deal with chronic illnesses and pain. Mindfulness training is also good for stress-related conditions, and those undergoing difficult treatments like surgery or chemotherapy. Practitioners of mindfulness claim it helps them experience more pleasure and less stress in their everyday activities.

Mindfulness training originates from a Buddhist practice called *vipassana*. Its basic idea is that deep awareness of the present moment is the essential discipline. Lack of awareness and attention can lead to stress and bad health habits. To be mindful is to participate fully in whatever one is doing at the present moment, whether reading, walking, working, eating, exercising, relaxing, etc. When a person pays full attention to the present moment without judgment, then worries about the past and future tend to disappear, and stress levels are also significantly reduced.

Mindfulness training teaches that painful situations and emotions should be experienced with full attention as well, which helps people to confront and accept them. Mindfulness training also uses techniques like the body scan, in which the patient focuses full attention on each part of the body in succession.

This technique helps people become more aware of their bodies and learn to control their reactions to stress, change, and illness.

Biofeedback

Biofeedback uses special instruments that measure and display heart rate, perspiration, muscle tension, brain wave activity, body temperature, respiratory patterns, and other indicators of stress and physiological activity. Patients can observe their measurements and learn to consciously control functions that were previously unconsciously controlled. Biofeedback also helps people learn how to initiate the relaxation response quickly and effectively.

Biofeedback is used to treat hypertension, stress-related headaches, migraine headaches, attention-deficit disorder, and diabetes. Biofeedback is used often in physical therapy to rehabilitate damaged nerves and muscles. It is also an approved treatment for a vascular disorder called **Raynaud's syndrome**. Patients with this syndrome experience blanching and numbness in their hands and feet in response to cold or emotional stress. A 2002 study showed that biofeedback helped children with a disease called vesicoureteral reflux (an abnormal backflow or urine from the bladder to the ureter) learn to correct reflux. This helped the children avoid surgery and prolonged antibiotic therapy.

Breath therapy

Breath therapy works on the premise that breathing plays a central role in the body and mind. People who are under stress tend to breathe rapidly and shallowly, whereas slow and deep breathing has been shown to reduce stress and promote the relaxation response. In **Ayurvedic medicine** and **traditional Chinese medicine**, the breath is considered the most important metabolic function. In yoga, there is a science of breathing techniques known as pranayama, which is designed to reduce stress and promote health.

Breath therapy is often used in conjunction with meditation and other mind/body techniques. It can be learned from books and tapes, or can be learned from a yoga or mind/body specialist. It is an inexpensive treatment, and once learned can be practiced easily anywhere.

Hypnosis

Hypnosis is deeply focused attention that brings about a trance state that is somewhere between waking and sleeping. During hypnosis, the mind is very open to suggestion. Mental imagery is often used in conjunction with hypnosis to maximize positive thinking and healing.

Hypnosis, or **hypnotherapy**, is used to reduce stress, **anxiety**, and pain, and help patients suffering from chronic diseases. It is also used to assist people in overcoming bad health habits, and addictions to nicotine, alcohol and drugs. Some dentists use hypnosis to help patients relax during dental procedures. Research continues to show the benefits of hypnosis. In 2002, a summary of recent studies included one that evaluated the effectiveness of self–hypnosis for patients undergoing angioplasty and other medical procedures. They required half the sedation of patients in control groups, and their procedures took less time. Pregnant adolescents who were counseled on hypnosis needed less anesthesia during delivery, needed less pain medication after delivery, and left the hospital sooner than patients in the control groups. Hypnosis is best performed by trained hypnotherapists, who can teach techniques of self-hypnosis to the patient.

Mental imagery

This technique uses the imagination to stimulate healing responses in the body, as studies have shown that the imagination can cause the same activity in the brain and immune system as real events. Patients are taught to imagine places or situations in which they have felt happy, healthy, or safe. Patients can also focus on images that increase confidence, reduce stress, and promote healing. Cancer patients are taught to imagine that their immune cells are eliminating cancer cells from their bodies. Heart attack sufferers are taught to imagine their hearts getting healthy and strong. Women can mentally rehearse **childbirth**, and patients imagine themselves successfully going through surgery as preparation for the real event.

Mental imagery has shown promise treating immune system problems, and is used often in cancer treatment and **AIDS** cases. It has been used to treat **irritable bowel syndrome** and asthma. Mental imaging techniques are also used in conjunction with many other mind/body techniques like meditation and hypnosis, as it is an efficient means of promoting positive mental attitudes. Mental imaging techniques can be learned from books, audiotapes, videos, and from professional therapists and teachers.

Movement therapy

Movement routines such as **dance therapy** have been shown to have a significant mind/body element. In these therapies, which also include **martial arts**, yoga, and tai chi, strict routines of physical movements are designed to involve high levels of mental concentration and awareness of the body. Movement therapies are good for people who have trouble sitting still for meditation, and are an excellent way of improving physical strength and mental health at the same time.

Precautions

Mind/body practices are safe and have few side effects. They should not, however, be relied upon solely when other medical care is required, particularly for serious conditions like heart disease, cancer, or diabetes. Consumers should also seek out reliable and properly trained practitioners, particularly in those practices and states for which certification is not required by law.

Research and general acceptance

Because of its increasing acceptance by mainstream medicine, mind/body medicine has been the subject of intense research. Studies have shed new light on everything from the minute interactions of the immune and nervous systems to the effective results of individual therapies like meditation and **guided imagery**. Other studies have indicated relationships between stress and disease. Some eye-opening results have been observed as well, such as studies that have shown that cancer and heart disease patients utilizing mind/body techniques had significantly longer survival rates on average than those patients who did not use mind/body therapies. Despite increasingly proven benefits to mind–body medicine, few health plans pay for the treatments.

Training and certification

Training programs and certification criteria tend to vary with individual therapies and states.

The Biofeedback Certification Institute of America lists certified biofeedback practitioners. Address: 10200 W. 44th Ave., Suite 304. Wheatridge, CO 80033. (303) 420-2902.

The American Society of Clinical Hypnosis is the largest organization for certifying hypnotherapists. Address: 2200 East Devon Ave., Suite 291. Des Plaines, IL 60018. (708) 297-3317.

The Wellness Community provides information on support groups organized throughout the country. Address: 2716 Ocean Park Blvd., Suite 1040. Santa Monica, CA 90405. (310) 314-2555.

The Academy for Guided Imagery provides resources for mental imaging treatments. Address: PO Box 2070. Mill Valley, CA 94942. (800) 726-2070.

ANDREW WEIL (1942–)

Dr. Andrew Weil, a Harvard-educated physician, adds credibility and expertise to the natural healing methods he espouses in his best-selling books, on his Internet Web site, in his talk show appearances, and in his popular audio CD of music and meditation. Weil's *Spontaneous Healing* spent more than a year on the best-seller list, and his 1997 book, *Eight Weeks to Optimum Health*, also was a runaway best-seller. Perhaps the best-known proponent of naturalistic healing methods, Weil has been trying to establish a field he calls integrative medicine. He is director of Tucson's Center for Integrative Medicine, which he founded in 1993. In 1997, he began training doctors in the discipline at the University of Arizona, where he teaches.

After getting his bachelor's degree in botany from Harvard University, Weil applied for admission to Harvard Medical School in 1964. During his second year, he led a group of students who argued they could succeed better studying on their own than going to classes; in fact, the group got higher scores on their final exams than their classmates. After graduating from Harvard Medical School, he volunteered at the notorious counter-cultural Haight-Asbury Free Clinic in San Francisco, CA. Later in 1969, Weil got a job in Washington, DC, with the National Institute of Mental Health's Drug Studies Division. From 1971 to 1975, he traveled extensively in South America and Africa, soaking up information about medicinal plants, shamanism, and natural healing techniques. He never returned to the practice of conventional medicine.

His approach to alternative medicine is eclectic, mingling traditional medicine with herbal therapy, acupuncture, homeopathy, chiropractic, hypnotism, cranial manipulation, and other alternative healing methods. Though his books discuss the benefits of everything from healing touch to herbal cures, Weil doesn't dismiss the benefits of standard Western medicine when appropriate.

The Vipassana Meditation Center is a resource for those interested in mindfulness training and meditation. Address: PO Box 24. Shelbourne Falls, MA 01370. (413) 625-2160.

Resources

BOOKS

Benson, Herbert, MD. *The Relaxation Response.* New York: Random House, 1992.

Borysenko, Joan. *Minding the Body, Mending the Mind.* New York: Bantam, 1988.

Cousins, Norman. *Head First: The Biology of Hope and the Healing Power of the Human Spirit.* New York: Viking, 1990.

Goleman, Daniel, and Joel Gurin, eds. *Mind/Body Medicine.* Yonkers, NY: Consumer Reports Books, 1993.

Kabat-Zinn, Jon. *Full Catastrophe Living: Using the Wisdom of Your Body and Mind to Face Stress, Pain, and Illness.* New York: Dell, 1990.

PERIODICALS

Advances: The Journal of Mind-Body Health. 9292 West KL Ave. Kalamazoo, MI 49009. (616) 375-2000.

"Hypnosis: Theory and Application Part II." *Harvard Mental Health Letter* (June 2002).

Jesitus, John. "Mind and Body Medicine: Putting Mind Over Health Matters (Feature Story)." *Managed Healthcare Executive* (April 2002): 33.

Morain, Claudia. "Biofeedback Speeds Resolution of Reflux in Children." *Urology Times* (April 2002): 23.

"Research Briefs: Meditation Reduces Atherosclerosis." *GP* (May 13, 2002):4.

ORGANIZATIONS

The Mind/Body Medical Institute. Deaconess Hospital. 1 Deaconess Road. Boston MA 02215.

Center for Mind-Body Medicine. 5225 Connecticut Ave. NW, Suite 414. Washington, DC 20015. (202) 966-7338.

Center for Attitudinal Healing. 19 Main Street. Tiburon, CA 94920. (415) 435-5022.

Douglas Dupler
Teresa G. Odle

Mindfulness meditation *see* **Meditation**

Mistletoe

Description

Mistletoe is a parasitic evergreen plant that lives on trees such as oaks, elms, firs, pines, apples, and elms. The parasitic plant has yellowish flowers; small, yellowish green leaves; and waxy, white berries. There are many species of this plant in the Viscacea and Loranthacea plant families. European mistletoe (*Viscum album*) and American mistletoe (*Phoradendron leucarpum*) are used as medical remedies. In addition to Europe and North America, mistletoe is also found in Australia and Korea.

Mistletoe berries are poisonous to cats and other small animals. There is, however, some debate about

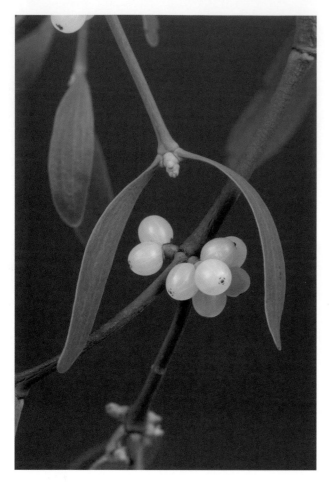

Mistletoe. *(© Holt Studios International Ltd. / Alamy)*

how toxic the berries are to humans, and there is controversy about whether it is safe to use mistletoe as a remedy. Mistletoe is also known as mystyldene, all-heal, bird lime, golden bough, and devil's fuge.

General use

Mistletoe is known popularly as the plant sprig that people kiss beneath during the Christmas season. That custom dates back to pagan times when, according to legend, the plant was thought to inspire passion and increase fertility.

In the centuries since then, mistletoe has acquired a reputation as a nearly all-purpose herbal remedy. In the seventeenth century, French herbalists prescribed mistletoe for nervous disorders, epilepsy, and the spasms known as the St. Vitus dance.

Mistletoe has also been used in folk medicine as a digestive aid, heart tonic, and sedative. It was used to treat arthritis, hysteria and other mental disturbances,

amenorrhea, **wounds**, asthma, bed wetting, infection, and to stimulate glands.

For centuries, mistletoe also served as a folk medicine treatment for **cancer**, and the plant is currently used in Europe to treat tumors. Iscador is an extract of the European mistletoe plant that is said to stimulate the immune system and kill cancer cells. It reportedly reduces the size of tumors and improves the quality of life. One team of researchers in France has found evidence that mistletoe extracts increase the efficiency of the body's natural killer cells in destroying cancer cells. A German study published in 2002 indicates that Iscador does indeed inhibit tumor growth. Another recent German case study of an 80-year-old woman with metastasized **breast cancer** documented that the patient lived for 41 months after first being given Iscador, with good quality of life. Iscador is one brand name of the mistletoe extract in Europe, and other brand names include Helixor and Eurixor.

Other contemporary uses of mistletoe include treatment of rheumatism, **anxiety**, migraine headaches, dizziness, high blood pressure, relief of spasms, **asthma**, rapid heartbeat, **diarrhea**, hysteria, and amenorrhea. Research continues on the use of mistletoe to treat **AIDS** patients.

There are some differences among the species. American mistletoe is said to cause a rise in blood pressure, while its European counterpart is believed to lower blood pressure.

Although mistletoe appears to be a multipurpose remedy, there is disagreement among medical experts about the safety and effectiveness of this herb. The number of possible interactions with other medications described below indicates that mistletoe should be used with caution.

Preparations

In alternative medicine, the leaves, twigs, and sometimes the berries of mistletoe are used. In Europe, mistletoe remedies range from tea made from mistletoe leaves to injections of Iscador. While European research indicates that mistletoe is safe and effective, sources in the United States maintain that the berries are poisonous and that the herb can cause liver damage.

Since mistletoe has not been tested by the United States Food and Drug Administration (FDA), many experts urge caution until more research is completed. European research includes work completed by Germany's Commission E, a governmental agency that studies herbal remedies for approval as over-the-counter drugs. An English version of the German Commission E monographs was published in 1997 and was the basis for the *PDR (Physicians' Desk Reference) for Herbal Medicines.*

Home remedies

Mistletoe tea may be taken for high blood pressure, asthma, epilepsy, nervousness, diarrhea, hysteria, whooping cough, amenorrhea, vertiginous attacks, and chorea. The tea is prepared by adding 1 tsp (5 g) of finely cut mistletoe to 1 cup (250 ml) of cold water. The solution is steeped at room temperature for 12 hours and then strained. Up to 12 cups of tea may be consumed each day.

Mistletoe wine is prepared by mixing 8 tsp (40 g) of the herb into 34 oz (1 L) of wine. After three days, the wine can be consumed. Three to four glasses of medicinal wine may be consumed each day.

Mistletoe must be stored away from light and kept above a drying agent.

Cancer treatment

Iscador, the European extract, may be injected before surgery for cancers of the cervix, ovary, breast, stomach, colon, and lung. Cancer treatments can take several months to several years. The treatment is given by subcutaneous injection, preferably near the tumor. Iscador may be injected into the tumor, especially tumors of the liver, cervix, or esophagus.

The dosage of Iscador varies according to the patient's age, sex, physical condition, and type of cancer. The treatment usually is given in the morning three to seven days per week. As treatment continues, the dosage may be increased or adjusted.

European cancer research has been conducted since the 1960s, and most has involved European mistletoe. However, researchers believe there may be some similar active components in other species. In the United States, some cancer patients may qualify for participation in clinical trials of Iscador.

Advocates of Iscador believe it can stimulate the immune system, kill cancer cells, inhibit the formation of tumors, and extend the survival time of cancer patients. They maintain that mistletoe can help prevent cancer and serve as companion therapy for standard cancer treatments. They also think that mistletoe could possibly repair the DNA that is decreased by chemotherapy and radiation.

In general, however, American researchers are skeptical about European claims regarding mistletoe as an effective cancer remedy. The latest information summary on mistletoe extracts, updated in May 2002 and available from the National Cancer Institute web site, states that "There is no evidence from well-designed clinical trials that mistletoe or any of its components are effective treatments for human cancer."

AIDS treatment

Mistletoe extract has been used to combat AIDS. In 1998 European studies, Iscador injections were used to improve the immune response. Experts reported from early results that when patients were given Iscador, no additional progression of HIV was seen. The combination of Iscador with standard therapy could be potentially beneficial, but more research is needed.

In 1996, the first United States patent was issued for T4GEN, a pharmaceutical version of the mistletoe extract. ABT Global Pharmaceutical of Irvine, California (the patent owner) has developed the synthetic version to be tested and potentially approved as a drug by the FDA. As of summer 2000, there have been no further announcements about T4GEN research.

Precautions

Opinions are sharply divided on how safe and effective the herb is as a home remedy and in the treatment of conditions like cancer and AIDS. There is controversy about which parts of the plants are poisonous. Although the berries are classified as poisonous in the United States, some sources say that eating berries is only dangerous for babies, and only if handfuls are consumed. Pregnant or breast-feeding women, however, should not use the plant.

According to a report from the **Hepatitis** Foundation International, mistletoe is toxic to the liver. However, the *PDR for Herbal Medicines* advises that there are no health hazards when mistletoe is taken properly and in designated therapeutic dosages. Other sources state that mistletoe's toxicity could cause cardiac arrest.

People considering mistletoe should consult with their doctor or practitioner. Until there is definitive proof otherwise, there is a risk that the herbal remedies will conflict with conventional treatment.

Herbal experts including Varro Tyler advise against using mistletoe as a beverage or home remedy until more definitive research is completed. Tyler, a respected pharmacognosist, is the coauthor of the *Tyler's Honest Herbal*.

Side effects

Mistletoe may be potentially toxic to the liver. For people diagnosed with hepatitis, use of an herb like mistletoe may cause additional liver damage. However, advocates of mistletoe point out that the herb has been tested in Europe. That research indicated less severe side effects. Mistletoe extracts can produce **chills**, **fever**, **headache**, chest **pain**, and orthostatic circulatory disorders.

Commercial mistletoe extracts may produce fewer side effects. The body temperature may rise and there may be flu-like symptoms. The patient may experience **nausea**, abdominal pain, and (if given the extract injection) inflammation around the injection sight. In a slight number of cases, allergy symptoms have resulted.

Interactions

Mistletoe shouldn't be used by people who take monoamine oxidase (MAO) inhibitor antidepressants like Nardil. Potential reactions include a dangerous rise in blood pressure and a lowering of blood **potassium** levels (hypokalemia). In addition, mistletoe appears to interfere with the action of antidiabetic medications; to increase the activity of diuretics; and to increase the risk of a toxic reaction to aspirin or NSAIDs. Cancer patients considering mistletoe treatment should first consult with their doctor or practitioner.

Resources

BOOKS

Albright, Peter. *The Complete Book of Complementary Therapies*. Allentown, PA: People's Medical Society, 1997.
The Burton Goldberg Group. *Alternative Medicine: The Definitive Guide*. Fife, WA: Future Medicine Publishing, 1995.
Collinge, William. *The American Holistic Health Association Complete Guide to Alternative Medicine*. New York: Warner Books, 1996.
Gottlieb, Bill. *New Choices in Natural Healing*. Emmaus, PA: Rodale Press, Inc., 1995.
Medical Economics Company. *PDR for Herbal Medicines*. Montvale, NJ: 1998.
Time-Life Books Editors. *The Alternative Advisor*. Alexandria, VA: Time-Life Books, 1997.
Tyler, Varro, and Steven Foster. *Tyler's Honest Herbal*. Binghamton, NY: The Haworth Herbal Press, 1999.

PERIODICALS

Kroz, M., F. Schad, B. Matthes, et al. "Blood and Tissue Eosinophilia, Mistletoe Lectin Antibodies and Quality of Life in a Breast Cancer Patient Undergoing Intratumoral and Subcutaneous Mistletoe Injection." [in German] *Forschende Komplementarmedizin und Klassische Naturheilkunde* 9 (June 2002): 160-167.
Maier, G., and H. H. Fiebig. "Absence of Tumor Growth Stimulation in a Panel of 16 Human Tumor Cell Lines by Mistletoe Extracts in Vitro." *Anticancer Drugs* 13 (April 2002): 373-379.
Mengs, U., D. Gothel, and E. Leng-Peschlow. "Mistletoe Extracts Standardized to Mistletoe Lectins in Oncology: Review on Current Status of Preclinical Research." *Anticancer Research* 22 (May-June 2002): 1399-1407.
Tabiasco, J., et al. "Mistletoe Viscotoxins Increase Natural Killer Cell-Mediated Cytotoxicity." *European Journal of Biochemistry* 269 (May 2002): 2591-2600.

ORGANIZATIONS

American Botanical Council. P.O. Box 201660, Austin, TX 78720. (512) 331-8868. http://www.herbalgram.org.
Herb Research Foundation. 1007 Pearl St., Suite 200, Boulder, CO 80302. (303) 449-2265. http://www.herbs.org.
National Cancer Institute (NCI). NCI Public Inquiries Office, Suite 3036-A, 6116 Executive Boulevard, MSC8322, Bethesda, MD, 20892.(800) 422-6237. www.nci.nih.gov/cancerinfo/pdq/cam/mistletoe.

Liz Swain
Rebecca J. Frey, PhD

Monkshood *see* **Aconite**

Mononucleosis

Definition

Infectious mononucleosis is caused by the Epstein-Barr virus, which in teenagers and young adults may result in acute symptoms that last for several weeks. **Fatigue** and low energy can linger for several months.

Remedies for mononucleosis

Therapy	Description	Target symptom
Aromatherapy	Add lavender or eucalyptus to a warm bath	Fatigue
Herbal medicine	Echinacea; yarrow or edler flower tea	Fight infection and fever, strengthen immune system
Home remedies	Rest, drink fluids; gargle with salt water; and massage lower back	Fatigue, dehydration, and sore throat
Mind/body	Meditation, biofeedback, and guided imagery	Stress-induced fatigue
Diet	Eat fresh fruits and vegetables. Avoid caffeine, sugars, and animal proteins	Strengthen immune system and increase energy
Yoga	Cobra pose	Fatigue

(Illustration by Corey Light. Cengage Learning, Gale)

Description

Infectious mononucleosis (IM), also called mono or glandular **fever**, is commonly transmitted among teenagers and young adults by kissing; hence, it is sometimes called the kissing disease.

By age 35 to 40, approximately 95% of the population has been infected with the Epstein-Barr virus (EBV) that causes IM. Although anyone can develop mononucleosis, primary (first) **infections** commonly occur in young adults between the ages of 15 and 35. Symptoms of IM are particularly common in teenagers. In the developed world, 15 to 20% of people are infected during adolescence and about half of these teens become ill. Among adults, 30 to 50% of those contracting IM become ill. Males and females are equally susceptible, and in the United States whites are 30 times more likely than blacks to contract IM.

Typically IM runs its course in about four weeks. However, people with weakened or suppressed immune systems, such as **AIDS** or organ-transplant patients, are especially vulnerable to potentially serious complications from mononucleosis.

Following IM, the EBV remains dormant (latent) in a few cells in the throat and blood for the remainder of one's life. Periodically the virus may reactivate and be transmitted through saliva; however, IM symptoms rarely reoccur.

Causes and symptoms

Causes

Infectious mononucleosis is caused by the first infection with the Epstein-Barr virus, also called herpes virus 4. It is one of the most common human viruses and is endemic throughout the world. EBV is a member of the herpes family of DNA viruses. This family of viruses includes those that cause cold sores, **chickenpox**, and **shingles**. Most people are infected with multiple strains of EBV. The different EBV strains are found in separate parts of the body: the circulating lymphocytes (white blood cells), cell-free blood plasma, or the oral cavity.

EBV is spread by contact with viral-infected saliva through coughing, **sneezing**, kissing, or the sharing of items such as drinking glasses, eating utensils, straws, toothbrushes, or lip gloss. However, EBV is not highly contagious, and household members have only a very small risk of infection unless there is direct contact with infected saliva.

Symptoms

Less than 10% of children under age ten develop symptoms with EBV infection. The incubation period after exposure to EBV is generally about four to six weeks. An infected person can transmit EBV during this period and for as long as five months after symptoms disappear.

The first symptoms of IM are usually general weakness and extreme fatigue. An infected person may require 12 to 16 hours of sleep daily prior the development of other symptoms. IM symptoms are similar to cold or flu symptoms:

- Fever and chills occurs in about 90% of IM cases. EBV is most contagious during this stage of the illness.
- An enlarged spleen, causing pain in the upper left of the abdomen, occurs in about 50 to 60% of infections.
- Sore throat and/or swollen tonsils occurs in less than 50% of mononucleosis infections.
- Swollen lymph glands (nodes) in the neck, armpits, and/or groin develop in less than 50% of infections.
- Jaundice (yellowing of the skin and eyes) develops in more than 20% of patients, depending on age, and indicates an inflamed or enlarged liver.
- A red skin rash, particularly on the chest, occurs in about 5% of infections.

Acute symptoms include the following:

- loss of appetite
- stomach pain and/or nausea
- muscle soreness and/or joint pain
- headache
- chest pain
- coughing
- rapid or irregular heartbeat These acute symptoms usually last one to two weeks.

Splenic enlargement generally peaks during the fourth week after symptoms appear and then subsides. However, an enlarged spleen may rupture in 0.1 to 0.2% of cases, causing sharp **pain** on the left side of the abdomen. Additional symptoms of a ruptured spleen include light-headedness, a fast heart rate, and difficulty breathing. Splenic rupture most often occurs within the first three weeks and is the most common cause of death from mononucleosis. It requires immediate medical attention and may require emergency surgery to stop the bleeding.

There are other rare—but potentially life-threatening—complications of mononucleosis:

- Neurological complications affecting the central nervous system may develop in 1 to 2% of infections. Bell's palsy is a temporary condition caused by weakened or paralyzed facial muscles on one side of the face.
- The heart muscle may become inflamed.
- A significant number of the body's red blood cells or platelets may be destroyed and there may be reduced numbers of circulating red and white blood cells.

Diagnosis

A variety of conditions can produce symptoms similar to those of IM; however, if cold or flu-like symptoms persist for longer than two weeks, mononucleosis may be suspected. Mononucleosis is usually diagnosed by a blood test called a mono spot test that measures antibodies to EBV. Antibodies may not be detectable until the second or third week after the onset of symptoms. The antibodies peak between weeks two and five and can persist at low levels for up to a year.

About 90% of IM cases show a positive mono spot. Infants and young children do not make the type of antibodies that are measured by the mono test. If the mono spot is inconclusive, additional blood tests may be performed that measure an increase in the overall number of white blood cells or an increase in abnormal-appearing lymphocytes that make antibodies against EBV. Other tests can identify at least six specific types of EBV antibodies that may be present in the blood.

Treatment

The most effective treatment for infectious mononucleosis is rest, followed by a gradual return to normal activities. If the spleen is enlarged, all contact sports, heavy lifting, and jarring activity such as cheerleading, should be avoided until the enlargement has subsided completely. Since mononucleosis can involve the liver, it is important not to consume alcohol.

Although there is no cure for mononucleosis, alternative remedies may help the body to fight the infection and relieve symptoms. Medical practitioners recommend eating four to six small daily meals of unprocessed foods, fresh fruits, and vegetables. It is important to drink plenty of water. Meat, sugar, saturated fats, and caffeinated and decaffeinated drinks should be avoided. Gargling with salt water (one half teaspoon in one cup of warm water) or sucking on lozenges may relieve a **sore throat**.

Vitamins A, B-complex, and C, and **magnesium**, **calcium**, and **potassium** supplements can boost the immune system and increase energy levels.

Herbals

Herbal remedies may help treat mononucleosis, although they are unproven:

- astragalus (*Astragalus membranaceus*) for physical weakness
- cleavers (*Galium* species) to cleanse the lymphatic system

- echinacea (*Echinacea augustifolia*) to boost the immune system
- elder (*Sambucus nigra*) flower to reduce fever
- garlic to fight viral infection
- goldenseal (*Hydrastis canadensis*) to relieve sinus congestion
- slippery elm bark and licorice can be gargled to soothe a sore throat
- St. John's wort (*Hypericum perforatum*) to relieve anxiety and depression
- vervain (*Verbena officinales*) to relieve anxiety and depression and treat jaundice
- wild indigo (*Baptisia tinctoria*) to cleanse the lymphatic system
- yarrow (*Achillea millefolium*) to reduce fever

Other remedies

The following treatments may help relieve symptoms of mononucleosis:

- Acupressure point Lung 6 may boost lung function and the immune system.
- Aromatherapy with bergamot, eucalyptus, and lavender essential oils may relieve fatigue and other symptoms.
- Chinese medicine uses acupuncture and Xiao Chai Hu Wan (Minor Bupleurum pills) in combination with other herbs.
- Homeopathic physicians choose remedies based on a patient's specific symptoms.
- Relaxation techniques such as biofeedback, visualization, meditation, and yoga can reduce fatigue by relieving stress.

Allopathic treatment

Acetaminophen (Tylenol) or ibuprofen (Advil, Motrin) may relieve symptoms of IM. Aspirin should not be given to children or teens because it has been linked to the development of Reye's syndrome, a potentially fatal illness.

Although antibiotics are ineffective for treating EBV, a sore throat from mononucleosis can be complicated by a streptococcal infection, **sinus infection**, or an **abscess** or pocket of infection on the tonsils. Such bacterial infections can be treated with antibiotics. A five-day course of corticosteroid anti-inflammatory medications (Prednisone) occasionally is prescribed for breathing difficulties caused by swollen tonsils or lymph nodes in the neck or throat.

KEY TERMS

Antibody—A specific protein produced by the immune system in response to a specific antigen such as a foreign protein.

Endemic—A disease that is always prevalent in a particular location.

Epstein-Barr virus (EBV)—An endemic DNA-containing herpes virus that causes infectious mononucleosis.

Immune system—The body system that recognizes and eliminates foreign pathogens and materials.

Lymph glands or nodes—The filtering components of the lymphatic system that can swell during infection.

Lymphatic system—The vessels, nodes, and organs that carry the clear lymph fluid, containing lymphocytes and other white blood cells, throughout the body and that filter the blood to remove dead cells and other debris.

Lymphocytes—White blood cells that are involved in the immune response, including antibody-producing cells.

Reye's syndrome—A very rare, often-deadly, childhood condition that can occur after a viral infection.

Spleen—A large lymphatic organ, located just under the left rib cage, that filters the blood.

Prognosis

Most people with IM begin to return to their normal daily routines within two to three weeks, but it may take up to six months for normal energy levels to return.

A large study suggested that EBV infection increases the risk for Hodgkin lymphoma, a highly treatable **cancer** of the lymphatic system. About one-third of Hodgkin tumors contain EBV and about one in 1,000 young adults with mononucleosis develop the cancer, typically about four years after IM.

The development of two other rare types of cancer—Burkitt's lymphoma and nasopharyngeal carcinoma—appears to be associated with EBV. There also is some evidence that people with high levels of antibodies against EBV are at a higher risk of developing **multiple sclerosis**.

Prevention

Even though IM is not highly contagious, there is no way to completely avoid infection with EBV. In the majority of cases, IM is without symptoms. Furthermore, EBV can be transmitted long after the symptoms of infection are gone and, indeed, periodically throughout the remainder of life. Good hygiene, particularly hand washing and the habit of not sharing toothbrushes or eating utensils may help prevent EBV infection.

Resources

BOOKS

Hoffmann, Gretchen. *Mononucleosis.* New York: Marshall Cavendish Benchmark, 2006.

Tselis, Alex, and Hal B. Jenson, eds. *Epstein-Barr Virus.* New York: Taylor & Francis, 2006.

Umar, Constantine S. *New Developments in Epstein-Barr Virus Research.* New York: Nova Science, 2006.

PERIODICALS

Arias, Donya C. "Vaccine for Mono Showing Promise." *Nation's Health* 38, no. 1 (February 2008): 13.

White, P. D. "What Causes Prolonged Fatigue After Infectious Mononucleosis—and Does it Tell Us Anything About Chronic Fatigue Syndrome?" *Journal of Infectious Diseases* 196, no. 1 (July 1, 2007): 4–6.

ORGANIZATIONS

National Institute of Allergy and Infectious Diseases, National Institutes of Health. 6610 Rockledge Drive, MSC 6612, Bethesda, MD, 20892-6612, (866) 284-4107, http://www.niaid.nih.gov.

Margaret Alic, PhD

Morinda citrifolia *see* **Noni**

Morning sickness

Definition

Morning sickness is the **nausea** and **vomiting** experienced during **pregnancy**, particularly in the first trimester. Although it is called morning sickness, it can and usually does occur at any time of the day or night.

Description

Morning sickness is characterized by extreme nausea and vomiting. It varies widely in intensity; some women experience only minor stomach upset for a very brief time period, while others become so ill that they have difficulty keeping food and fluids down and functioning normally.

In the majority of women, morning sickness symptoms subside toward the end of the first trimester

---

(at 12–14 weeks). However, some women continue to experience nausea well into the second trimester, and some mothers of multiples (twins, triplets, etc.) may have morning sickness throughout their pregnancy.

Causes and symptoms

The exact cause of morning sickness is unknown, but several factors are thought likely to contribute to the illness, including:

- Hormones. The pregnancy hormone hCG enters the bloodstream in high levels in the first trimester of pregnancy. These high hormone levels may trigger activity in the nausea and vomiting center of the brain, which is located in the brainstem.

- Muscle relaxation in the digestive tract. During pregnancy, the muscles of the gastrointestinal tract relax, slowing the digestion somewhat and possibly contributing to nausea.

- Heightened sense of smell. Pregnant women experience a heightened sense of smell during pregnancy that can transform unpleasant odors into unbearable, nausea-producing scents.

- Excessive salivation. The phenomena ptyalism, or excess saliva, is another symptom of pregnancy that can cause nausea in some women.

- Postnasal drip. Many pregnant women experience postnasal drip and/or nasal congestion, triggered by high levels of estrogen in their bloodstream. Estrogen increases the blood flow throughout the body, including the mucous membrane of the nose. This postnasal drip contributes to upset stomach in many pregnant women.

Diagnosis

Because it is such a common occurrence, morning sickness is easily diagnosed in pregnant women. A healthcare practitioner should question the patient about her pregnancy symptoms during each prenatal visit. In women who are visiting their healthcare providers because of unexplained nausea, morning sickness is sometimes the first symptom or sign of pregnancy.

Nausea and vomiting accompanied by abdominal **pain** may indicate a more serious problem than simple

---

morning sickness, such as gall bladder or pancreatic disease. Women who experience pain symptoms in conjunction with their nausea should contact their healthcare provider or an emergency medical facility immediately.

Treatment

There are a number of remedies for morning sickness. These include:

- Eat small, frequent meals. When the stomach is empty, it produces acid that irritates the stomach lining. In addition, an empty stomach can cause low blood sugar, which can also cause nausea.

- Eat foods high in proteins and complex carbohydrates. Protein foods (e.g., eggs, cheese, and yogurt) and complex carbohydrates (e.g., whole-grain breads and cereals, dried beans and peas, and baked potatoes) discourage stomach upset and are also beneficial to both mother and baby.

- Avoid foods and beverages that do not sound appealing. Pregnant women usually experience at least one food aversion. The more appetizing a food appears to be, the more likely it is to stay down.

- Stay hydrated. Dehydration can worsen nausea, so pregnant women should drink plenty of fluids. If a woman has an aversion to fluids, she can eat foods with a high water content, such as watermelon, grapes, and other fruits.

- Try a vitamin B$_6$ supplement. Vitamin B$_6$ reduces nausea in some women, and is not harmful in recommended doses during pregnancy. Women should consult their healthcare practitioner before taking supplements.

- Eat or drink ginger. Ginger (*Zingiber officinale*) settles the stomach for some women. Ginger tea and foods made with ginger (such as ginger snaps) are usually available at grocery or health food stores.

- Try an herbal infusion. An infusion, or tea, of two parts black horehound (*Ballota nigra*), one part meadowsweet (*Filipendula ulmaria*), and one part chamomile (*Chamaemelum nobile*), taken three times a day, can soothe morning sickness for some women. Women should always consult their healthcare practitioner before taking herbal remedies during pregnancy.

- Wear sea bands. Sea bands are elastic bands worn around the wrists which place pressure on the inner wrist, an acupressure point for controlling nausea. They are usually used for controlling carsickness and seasickness.

- Keep the mouth fresh. Mints and regular tooth brushing can decrease excess saliva. Using a mouth rinse and/or brushing the teeth after vomiting is a good idea to control tooth decay and lessen stomach upset.

- Stay well rested. Fatigue and stress can make morning sickness worse.

Allopathic treatment

Some women with extreme cases of morning sickness may develop a condition known as hyperemesis gravidarium (excessive vomiting during pregnancy). These women are at risk for dehydration and insufficient weight gain, and may require bed rest and intravenous **nutrition** and fluids if vomiting cannot be controlled.

Several antiemetic, or antivomiting, medications are available for pregnant women. Antiemetic medication should always be prescribed by a physician familiar with its use and with the patient's medical history. Antiemetics may be contraindicated (or not recommended) for patients with certain medical conditions. They may also interact with other medications.

Expected results

Morning sickness treatments have varying success. Some women will find one or more remedies that can completely cure their nausea, while others may remain sick throughout their pregnancy. In addition, women expecting two or more babies usually experience heightened morning sickness due to the higher level of pregnancy hormones in their bodies, and may suffer from nausea and vomiting for a longer time than women with a single pregnancy. However, for the majority of pregnant women, nausea stops or at least diminishes by the end of the first trimester.

Prevention

The best cure for preventing bouts of nausea is to eat frequently. Many women find that eating six small meals or snacks a day (morning, mid-morning, noon, afternoon, evening, and bedtime) prevents stomach upset. Getting adequate rest can also help to keep morning sickness at bay.

Resources

BOOKS

Eisenberg, Arlene et al. *What to Expect When You're Expecting.* 2d ed. New York: Workman Publishing Company, 1996.

Hoffman, David. *The Complete Illustrated Herbal.* New York: Barnes & Noble Books, 1999.

Paula Ford-Martin

Mosquito plant *see* **Pennyroyal**

Motherwort

Description

Motherwort (*Leonurus cardiaca*) is a perennial plant native to Europe and temperate parts of central Asia. It has been introduced into North America and now grows wild there. A different species, called Chinese motherwort (*Leonurus heterophyllus*), is used by Chinese herbalists in many of the same ways as *Leonurus cardiaca* is used in the West.

Motherwort grows mainly in poor soil or on wastelands, although it is sometimes cultivated in gardens. The plant grows to about 3 ft (1 m) tall. It has a stem that is often red-violet in color and hairy. The hairy, palm-shaped leaves are a dull green, with the upper surface darker than the under surface. The small flowers range from white to pink to red depending on the plant. flowers and leaves are dried and used medicinally. The leaves are at their most potent when harvested just after the plant flowers. Motherwort is also the source of a dark green dye. The plant has astringent properties and an unpleasant smell. Other names for motherwort include lion's tail, lion's ear, throw-wort, heartwort, and *yi mu cao*.

General use

Motherwort has a long history of traditional uses in many different cultures. The Latin name, *cardiaca* refers to the heart, and motherwort has traditionally been used to treat heart-related conditions. These include nervous heart complaints such as palpitations, cardiac arrhythmia (irregular beat), and fast heartbeat. It has also been used as a general tonic to strengthen the heart and to treat cardiac insufficiency. Modern herbalists continue to prescribe motherwort for these conditions.

Motherwort is also used as a mild general sedative, as a calming agent, and as a treatment for **epilepsy**. Scientists have isolated many different active compounds in motherwort. Leonurine and stachydine, both found in the herb, have been show to lower blood pressure and calm the central nervous system in studies using laboratory animals and animal hearts. Scientific investigation into the central nervous system and cardiac effects of motherwort is ongoing with mixed results. As of 2008, the German Federal Health Agency's Commission E, established in 1978 to independently review and evaluate scientific literature and case studies pertaining to herb and plant medications, had found that there is adequate evidence to suggest that motherwort is effective in the

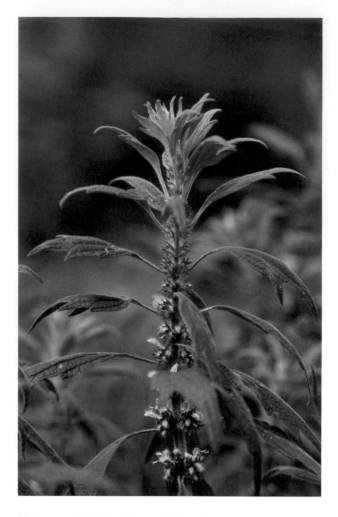

Motherwort. (© Petra Wegner / Alamy)

treatment of nervous heart complaints and thyroid dysfunction.

Motherwort is also used to treat female conditions related to **menstruation** and **childbirth**. The herb is often given to stimulate menstruation when it is absent (**amenorrhea**) or irregular and delayed (**dysmenorrhea**). At childbirth it is taken to aid labor, and after childbirth it is given to help the uterus relax and return to normal. There appear to be no scientific studies that specifically relate to the effects of motherwort on the reproductive system, so these traditional uses of the herb can be neither confirmed nor denied. Other Western uses of motherwort include treatment for **asthma**, **hyperthyroidism**, flatulence (**gas**), and **insomnia**. It is also used externally as a douche for **vaginitis**.

Chinese herbalists use Chinese motherwort to treat problems of the heart, liver, and kidneys. In addition to the heart and reproductive uses known to Western herbalists, Chinese practitioners use motherwort to treat water retention, in conjunction with other herbs, such as **hawthorn**, to prevent **stroke** and to treat certain kinds of **eczema**. Some Chinese researchers have reported that Chinese motherwort, *Leonurus heterophyllus*, can prevent **blood clots**. Motherwort is an ingredient in several common Chinese herbal formulas, including leonuris and achyranthes.

Motherwort is also used occasionally in homeopathic medicine for the treatment of heart conditions, flatulence, and overactive thyroid (hyperthyroidism).

Preparations

Motherwort is normally prepared by adding about 1 tsp of leaves to 1 cup (8 oz or 250 ml) of boiling water. The resulting infusion is taken twice a day. This infusion has a bitter and unpleasant taste. Honey, lemon, or other flavorings may be added to make its taste more acceptable. Motherwort is also available as a tincture. The normal dose is 2–6 ml daily.

Precautions

Pregnant women should not take motherwort because of its effects on the uterus. Women who have heavy menstrual flow should also avoid motherwort. Anyone who has a heart disorder or who is taking any medication for a heart condition should consult a doctor before taking motherwort. People who are taking medication for thyroid disorders should also consult a doctor before using this herb.

Side effects

Motherwort has a long history of use without any negative side effects being reported when the herb is taken internally as an infusion or tincture. However, some people break out in a rash when handling motherwort leaves.

Interactions

There has been little scientific study of the interaction of motherwort and pharmaceuticals. As noted above, however, people who are taking medications for heart, thyroid, or other serious medical conditions should consult a doctor before taking motherwort.

The herb has been used in herbal mixtures for centuries without any known herbal interactions.

Resources

BOOKS

Bensky, Dan, et al.*Chinese Herbal Medicine: Materia Medica,* 3rd ed. Seattle, WA: Eastland Press, 2004.

Chevallier, Andrew. *Herbal Remedies*. New York: DK Publishing, 2007.

Cummings, Stephen, and Dana Ullman. *Everybody's Guide to Homeopathic Medicines.* 3rd ed. rev. New York: Tarcher, 2004.

Foster, Steven and Rebecca Johnson. *National Geographic Desk Reference to Nature's Medicine*. Washington, DC: National Geographic Society, 2006.

PDR for Herbal Medicines, 4th ed. Montvale, NJ: Thomson Healthcare, 2007.

ORGANIZATIONS

Alternative Medicine Foundation, P. O. Box 60016, Potomac, MD, 20859, (301) 340-1960, http://www.amfoundation.org.

American Association of Oriental Medicine, PO Box 162340, Sacramento, CA, 95816, (866) 455-7999, (914) 443-4770, http://www.aaaomonline.org.

American Holistic Medical Association, PO Box 2016, Edmonds, WA, 98020, (425) 967-0737, http://holisticmedicine.org.

Centre for International Ethnomedicinal Education and Research (CIEER), http://www.cieer.org.

National Center for Homeopathy, 801 N. Fairfax St., Suite 306, Alexandria, VA, 22314, (703) 548-7790, http://www.homeopathic.org/contact.htm.

Tish Davidson, A. M.

Motion sickness

Definition

Motion sickness is a condition characterized by uncomfortable sensations of **dizziness**, **nausea**, and **vomiting** that people experience when their sense of balance and equilibrium is disturbed by constant motion. Riding in a car, aboard a ship or boat, or riding on a swing all cause stimulation of the vestibular system and visual stimulation that often lead to discomfort. While motion sickness can be bothersome, it is not a serious illness, and can be prevented.

Description

Motion sickness is a common problem, with nearly 80% of the general population suffering from it at one time in their lives. People with migraine headaches or Ménière's syndrome, however, are more likely than others to have recurrent episodes of motion sickness. Researchers at the Naval Medical Center in San Diego, California, reported in 2003 that 70% of research subjects with severe motion sickness had abnormalities of the vestibular system; these abnormalities are often found in patients diagnosed with migraines or **Ménière's disease**.

While motion sickness may occur at any age, it is more common in children over the age of two, with the majority outgrowing this susceptibility.

When looking at why motion sickness occurs, it is helpful to understand the role of the sensory organs. The sensory organs control a body's sense of balance by telling the brain what direction the body is pointing, the direction it is moving, and if it is standing still or turning. These messages are relayed by the inner ears (or labyrinth), the eyes, the skin pressure receptors, such as in those in the feet, and the muscle and joint sensory receptors (which track what body parts are moving). The central nervous system (the brain and spinal cord), is responsible for processing all incoming sensory information.

Motion sickness and its symptoms surface when conflicting messages are sent to the central nervous system. An example of this is reading a book in the back seat of a moving car. The inner ears and skin receptors sense the motion, but the eyes register only the stationary pages of the book. This conflicting information may cause the usual motion sickness symptoms of dizziness, nausea, and vomiting.

Causes and symptoms

While all five of the body's sensory organs contribute to motion sickness, excess stimulation to the vestibular system within the inner ear (the body's "balance center") has been shown to be one of the primary reasons for this condition. Balance problems, or vertigo, are caused by a conflict between what is seen and how the inner ear perceives it, leading to confusion in the brain. This confusion may result in higher heart rates, rapid breathing, nausea, and sweating, along with dizziness and vomiting. There are people who suffer from constant motion sickness. Names for these conditions vary, such as positional dizziness.

Pure optokinetic motion sickness is caused solely by visual stimuli; that is, by what is seen. The optokinetic system is the reflex that allows the eyes to move when an object moves. Many people suffer when they view rotating or swaying images, even if they are standing still. Optokinetic motion sickness is of particular concern to the civilian aviation industry as well as to military aerospace programs. In the United States, both the Federal Aviation Agency (FAA) and the National Aeronautics and Space Administration (NASA) have research programs for the prevention and treatment of optokinetic motion sickness.

Additional factors that may contribute to the occurrence of motion sickness include:

- Poor ventilation lowers a person's threshold for experiencing motion.
- Anxiety or fear also lowers the threshold.
- Food. Physicians recommend avoiding heavy meals of spicy or greasy foods before and during a trip.
- Alcohol. A drink is often thought to help calm the nerves, but in this case it could upset the stomach further. A hangover for the next morning's trip may also lead to motion sickness.
- Pregnancy. Susceptibility in women to vomiting during pregnancy appears to be related to motion sickness, although the precise connections are not well understood.

- Genetic factors. Research suggests that some people inherit a predisposition to motion sickness. This predisposition is more marked in some ethnic groups than in others; one study published in 2002 found that persons of Chinese or Japanese ancestry are significantly more vulnerable to motion sickness than persons of British ancestry.

Often viewed as a minor annoyance, some travelers are temporarily immobilized by motion sickness, and a few continue to feel its effects for hours and even days after a trip (the "mal d'embarquement" syndrome). For those with constant motion sickness, it may not stop at all.

Diagnosis

Most cases of motion sickness are mild and self-treatable disorders. If symptoms such as dizziness become chronic, a doctor may be able to help alleviate the discomfort by looking further into a patient's general health. Questions regarding medications, head injuries, recent **infections**, and other questions about the ear and neurological system will be asked. An examination of the ears, nose, and throat, as well as tests of nerve and balance function, may also be completed.

Severe cases of motion sickness symptoms, and those that become progressively worse, may require additional specific tests. Diagnosis in these situations deserves the attention and care of a doctor with specialized skills in diseases of the ear, nose, throat, equilibrium, and neurological system.

Treatment

Alternative treatments for motion sickness have become widely accepted as a standard means of care. They include herbal therapy, **acupressure**, and **homeopathy**.

Herbal therapy

Ginger (*Zingiber officinale*) in its various forms is often used to calm the stomach, and it is now known that the oils it contains (gingerols and shogaols) appear to relax the intestinal tract in addition to mildly depressing the central nervous system. Some of the most effective forms of ginger include the powdered, encapsulated form; ginger tea prepared from sliced ginger root; or candied pieces. All forms of ginger should be taken on an empty stomach when treating motion sickness.

Acupressure

Placing manual pressure on the Neiguan or Pericardium-6 **acupuncture** point (located about three finger-widths above the wrist on the inner arm), either by acupuncture, acupressure, or a mild, electrical pulse, has shown to be effective against the symptoms of motion sickness. Elastic wristbands sold at most drugstores are also used as a source of relief due to the pressure they place in this area. Pressing the small intestine 17 (just below the earlobes in the indentations behind the jawbone) may also help in the functioning of the ear's balancing mechanism.

Homeopathy

There are several homeopathic remedies that work specifically for motion sickness. They include *Cocculus, Petroleum, Ipecacuanha,* and *Tabacum.*

Traditional Chinese medicine

In **traditional Chinese medicine**, cases of chronic motion sickness would be considered a "wind" disorder because it is an abnormality movement as the wind causes. Herbs and acupuncture may treat this.

Allopathic treatment

There are a variety of medications to help ease the symptoms of motion sickness, and most of these are available without a prescription. Known as over-the-counter (OTC) medications, it is recommended that these be taken 30-60 minutes before traveling to prevent motion sickness symptoms, as well as during an extended trip.

Drugs

The following OTC drugs consist of ingredients that have been considered safe and effective for the treatment of motion sickness by the Food and Drug Administration:

- Marezine (and others). Includes the active ingredient cyclizine and is not for use in children under age six years.
- Benadryl (and others). Includes the active ingredient diphenhydramine and is not for use in children under age six years.
- Dramamine (and others). Includes the active ingredient dimenhydrinate and is not for use in children under age two years.
- Bonine (and others). Includes the active ingredient meclizine and is not for use in children under age 12 years.

Each of these active ingredients, including such other antiemetics as cinnarizine, are antihistamines whose main side effect is drowsiness. Caution should be used when driving a vehicle or operating machinery, and alcohol should be avoided when taking any drug for motion sickness. Medications for motion sickness may also cause **dry mouth** and occasional blurred vision. People with **emphysema**, chronic **bronchitis**, **glaucoma**, or difficulty urinating due to an enlarged prostate should not use these drugs unless directed by their physician.

The side effects of cinnarizine and the other antihistamine antiemetics indicate that they should not be used by members of flight crews responsible for the control of aircraft or for other tasks that require sustained attention and alertness.

Longer trips may require a prescription medication called scopolamine (Transderm Scop). Scopolamine gel is most effective when smeared on the arm or neck and covered with a bandage. In chronic cases, such antiseizure drugs as clonazepam (Klonopin) are used.

Another prescription drug that is sometimes given for motion sickness is ondansetron (Zofran), which was originally developed to treat nausea associated with **cancer** chemotherapy. Unlike cyclizine, ondansetron appears to be safe for use in children under the age of six.

Several newer antiemetic medications are under development. The most promising of these newer drugs is a class of compounds known as neurokinin-1 (substance P) antagonists. The neurokinins are being tested for the control of nausea following cancer chemotherapy as well as nausea related to motion sickness. In March 2003 the Food and Drug Administration (FDA) approved the first of this new class of antiemetic drugs. Known as aprepitant, it is sold under the trade name Emend.

Expected results

While there is no cure for motion sickness, its symptoms can be controlled or even prevented. Most people respond successfully to the variety of treatments, or avoid the unpleasant symptoms through prevention methods.

Prevention

Because motion sickness is easier to prevent than treat once it has begun, the best treatment is prevention. The following steps may help deter the unpleasant symptoms of motion sickness before they occur:

- Avoiding reading while traveling, and choosing a seat that faces forward.
- Always riding where the eyes may see the same motion that the body and inner ears feel. Safe positions include the front seat of the car while looking at distant scenery; the deck of a ship where the horizon can be seen; and sitting by the window of an airplane. The least motion on an airplane is in a seat over the wings and the worst is in the tail section.
- Maintaining a fairly straight-ahead view.
- Eating a light meal before traveling, or avoiding food altogether.
- Avoiding conversation with another traveler who is having motion sickness.
- Taking a motion sickness medication at least 30–60 minutes before travel begins, or as recommended by a physician.
- Learning to live with the condition. Even those who frequently endure motion sickness can learn to travel by anticipating the conditions of their next trip. Research also suggests that increased exposure to the stimulation that causes motion sickness may help decrease its symptoms on future trips.

Resources

BOOKS

Blakely, Brian W., and Mary-Ellen Siegel. "Peripheral Vestibular Disorders." In *Feeling Dizzy: Understanding and Treating Dizziness, Vertigo, and Other Balance Disorders.* New York: Macmillan, 1995.

"Motion Sickness." In *The Medical Advisor: The Complete Guide to Alternative & Conventional Treatments.* Richmond, VA: Time-Life, Inc., 1996.

Pelletier, Dr. Kenneth R. *The Best Alternative Medicine.* New York: Simon and Schuster, 2002.

PERIODICALS

Black, F. O. "Maternal Susceptibility to Nausea and Vomiting of Pregnancy: Is the Vestibular System Involved?" *American Journal of Obstetrics and Gynecology* 185 (May 2002)(Supplement 5): S204-S209.

Bos, J. E., W. Bles, and B. de Graaf. "Eye Movements to Yaw, Pitch, and Roll About Vertical and Horizontal Axes: Adaptation and Motion Sickness." *Aviation, Space, and Environmental Medicine* 73 (May 2002): 434-444.

Hamid, Mohamed, MD, PhD, and Nicholas Lorenzo, MD. "Dizziness, Vertigo, and Imbalance." *eMedicine*, 17 September 2002. http://emedicine.com/neuro/topic693.htm.

Harm, D. L., and T. T. Schlegel. "Predicting Motion Sickness During Parabolic Flight." *Autonomic Neuroscience* 31 (May 2002): 116-121.

Hoffer, M. E., K. Gottshall, R. D. Kopke, et al. "Vestibular Testing Abnormalities in Individuals with Motion Sickness." *Otology and Neurotology* 24 (July 2003): 633–636.

Keim, Samuel, MD, and Michael Kent, MD. "Vomiting and Nausea." *eMedicine*, 29 April 2002. http://emedicine.com/aaem/topic476.htm.

Liu, L., L. Yuan, H. B. Wang, et al. "The Human Alpha(2A)-AR Gene and the Genotype of Site -1296 and the Susceptibility to Motion Sickness." [in Chinese] *Sheng Wu Hua Xue Yu Sheng Wu Wu Li Xue Bao (Shanghai)* 34 (May 2002): 291-297.

Loewen, P. S. "Anti-Emetics in Development." *Expert Opinion on Investigational Drugs* 11 (June 2002): 801-805.

Nicholson, A. N., et al. "Central Effects of Cinnarizine: Restricted Use in Aircrew" *Aviation, Space, and Environmental Medicine* 73 (June 2002): 570-574.

O'Brien, C. M., G. Titley, and P. Whitehurst. "A Comparison of Cyclizine, Ondansetron and Placebo as Prophylaxis Against Postoperative Nausea and Vomiting in Children." *Anaesthesia* 58 (July 2003): 707–711.

Patel, L., and C. Lindley. "Aprepitant—A Novel NK1-Receptor Antagonist." *Expert Opinion in Pharmacotherapy* 4 (December 2003): 2279–2296.

ORGANIZATIONS

Civil Aerospace Medical Institute. P. O. Box 20582, Oklahoma City, OK 73125. (202) 366-4000. www.cami.jccbi.gov.

National Aeronautics and Space Administration, Office of Biological and Physical Research. www.spaceresearch.nasa.gov.

Vestibular Disorders Association. PO Box 4467, Portland, OR 97208-4467. (800) 837-8428. http://www.teleport.com/veda.

Mai Tran
Rebecca J. Frey, PhD

Mountain grape *see* **Barberry**

Movement therapy

Definition

Movement therapy refers to a broad range of Eastern and Western movement approaches used to promote physical, mental, emotional, and spiritual well-being. Some forms of movement therapy that combine deep-tissue manipulation and postural correction with movement education are also known as bodywork therapies.

Origins

Movement is fundamental to human life. In fact movement is life. Contemporary physics tells us that the universe and everything in it is in constant motion. We can move our body and at the most basic level our body is movement. According to the somatic educator Thomas Hanna, "The living body is a moving body— indeed, it is a constantly moving body." The poet and philosopher Alan Watts eloquently states a similar view, "A living body is not a fixed thing but a flowing event, like a flame or a whirlpool." Centuries earlier, the great Western philosopher Socrates understood what modern physics has proven, "The universe is motion and nothing else."

Since the beginning of time, indigenous societies around the world have used movement and dance for individual and community healing. Movement and song were used for personal healing, to create community, to worship, to ensure successful crops, and to promote fertility. Movement is still an essential part of many healing traditions and practices throughout the world.

Western movement therapies generally developed out of the realm of dance. Many of these movement approaches were created by former dancers or choreographers who were searching for a way to prevent injury, attempting to recover from an injury, or who were curious about the effects of new ways of moving. Some movement therapies arose out of the fields of physical therapy, psychology, and bodywork. Other movement therapies were developed as way to treat an incurable disease or condition.

Eastern movement therapies, such as **yoga**, **qigong**, and **t'ai chi** began as a spiritual or self-defense practices and evolved into healing therapies. In China, for example, Taoist monks learned to use specific breathing and movement patterns in order to promote mental clarity, physical strength, and support their practice of **meditation**. These practices, later known as qigong and t'ai chi, eventually became recognized as ways to increase health and prolong life.

Benefits

The physical benefits of movement therapy include greater ease and range of movement, increased balance, strength and flexibility, improved muscle tone and coordination, joint resiliency, cardiovascular conditioning, enhanced athletic performance, stimulation of circulation, prevention of injuries, greater longevity, **pain** relief, and relief of rheumatic, neurological, spinal, **stress**, and respiratory disorders. Movement therapy can also be used as a meditation practice to quiet the mind, foster self-knowledge, and increase awareness. In addition, movement therapy is beneficial in alleviating emotional distress that is expressed through the body. These conditions include eating disorders, excessive clinging, and **anxiety** attacks. Since movements are related to thoughts and feelings, movement therapy can also bring about changes in attitude and emotions.

KEY TERMS

Bodywork—A term that covers a variety of therapies that include massage, realignment of the body, and similar techniques to treat deeply ingrained stresses and traumas carried in the tissues of the body.

Equine-facilitated therapy—Another term for therapeutic riding.

Qigong—A traditional form of Chinese energy therapy that includes physical exercises, breathing techniques, postures, and mental discipline. Internal qigong refers to exercises practiced to maintain one's own health and vitality; external qigong refers to the transfer of energy from a qigong master to another person for healing purposes. External qigong is also known as medical qigong.

T'ai chi—A Chinese system of meditative physical exercise, characterized by slow methodical circular and stretching movements.

Yoga—A method of joining the individual self with the divine, universal spirit, or cosmic consciousness. Physical and mental exercises are designed to help achieve this goal, also called self-transcendence or enlightenment. On the physical level, yoga postures, called asanas, are designed to tone, strengthen, and align the body. On the mental level, yoga uses breathing techniques (pranayama) and meditation (dyana) to quiet, clarify, and discipline the mind.

People report an increase in self-esteem and self-image. Communication skills can be enhanced and tolerance of others increased. The physical openness facilitated by movement therapy leads to greater emotional openness and creativity.

Movement therapy is being studied more intensively as a useful adjunct to rehabilitation programs for victims of **stroke** or spinal cord injuries. Actor Christopher Reeves, who was paralyzed in a 1995 accident just below the two top vertebrae in his neck, recovered feeling throughout most of his body and took small steps in a swimming pool. Reeves credited his improvement, which many doctors considered impossible, to exercising five hours every day. Some neuroscientists studied Reeves and other patients with spinal cord injuries to test the hypothesis that movement itself can cause damaged nerves to regenerate.

Another important benefit of movement therapy that is increasingly recognized by mainstream as well as alternative practitioners is social support. Many people, particularly those suffering from **depression** related to physical illness or other forms of stress, find that taking a yoga class or other group form of movement therapy relieves feelings of loneliness and isolation. People who have taken therapeutic riding have reported that the positive relationship they develop with their horse helps them relate better to other animals and to people.

Description

There are countless approaches to movement therapy. Some approaches emphasize awareness and attention to inner sensations. Other approaches use movement as a form of **psychotherapy**, expressing and working through deep emotional issues. Some approaches emphasize alignment with gravity and specific movement sequences, while other approaches encourage spontaneous movement. Some approaches are primarily concerned with increasing the ease and efficiency of bodily movement. Other approaches address the reality of the body "as movement" instead of the body as only something that runs or walks through space.

The term movement therapy is often associated with **dance therapy**. Some dance therapists work privately with people who are interested in personal growth. Others work in mental health settings with autistic, brain injured and learning disabled children, the elderly, and disabled adults.

Laban movement analysis (LMA), formerly known as Effort-Shape is a comprehensive system for discriminating, describing, analyzing, and categorizing movements. LMA can be applied to dance, athletic coaching, fitness, acting, psychotherapy, and a variety of other professions. Certified movement analysts can "observe recurring patterns, note movement preferences, assess physical blocks and dysfunctional movement patterns, and the suggest new movement patterns." As a student of Rudolf Laban, Irmgard Bartenieff developed his form of movement analysis into a system of body training or reeducation called Bartenieff fundamentals (BF). The basic premise of this work is that once the student experiences a physical foundation, emotional, and intellectual expression become richer. BF uses specific exercises that are practiced on the floor, sitting, or standing to engage the deeper muscles of the body and enable a greater range of movement.

Authentic movement (AM) is based upon Mary Starks Whitehouse's understanding of dance, movement, and depth psychology. There is no movement instruction in AM, simply a mover and a witness. The mover waits and listens for an impulse to move and then follows or "moves with" the spontaneous movements that arise. These movements may or may not be visible to the witness. The movements may be in response to an emotion, a dream, a thought, pain, joy, or whatever is being experienced in the moment. The witness serves as a compassionate, non judgmental mirror and brings a "special quality of attention or presence." At the end of the session the mover and witness speak about their experiences together. AM is a powerful approach for self development and awareness and provides access to preverbal memories, creative ideas, and unconscious movement patterns that limit growth.

Gabrielle Roth (5 Rhythms movement) and Anna Halprin have both developed dynamic movement practices that emphasize personal growth, awareness, expression, and community. Although fundamentally different forms, each of these movement/dance approaches recognize and encourage our inherent desire for movement.

Several forms of movement therapy grew out of specific bodywork modalities. **Rolfing** movement integration (RMI) and Rolfing rhythms are movement forms which reinforce and help to integrate the structural body changes brought about by the hands-on work of Rolfing (structural integration). RMI uses a combination of touch and verbal directions to help develop greater awareness of one's vertical alignment and habitual movement patterns. RMI teacher Mary Bond says, "The premise of Rolfing Movement Integration . . . is that you can restore your structure to balance by changing the movement habits that perpetuate imbalance." Rolfing rhythms is a series of lively exercises designed to encourage awareness of the Rolfing principles of ease, length, balance, and harmony with gravity.

The movement education component of **Aston-Patterning** bodywork is called neurokinetics. This movement therapy teaches ways of moving with greater ease throughout every day activities. These movement patterns can also be used to release tension in the body. Aston fitness is an **exercise** program which includes warm-up techniques, exercises to increase muscle tone and stability, stretching, and cardiovascular fitness.

Rosen method movement (an adjunct to Rosen method bodywork) consists of simple fun movement exercises done to music in a group setting. Through gentle swinging, bouncing, and stretching every joint in the body experiences a full range of movement. The movements help to increase balance and rhythm and create more space for effortless breathing.

The movement form of **Trager psychophysical Integration** bodywork, Mentastics, consists of fun, easy swinging, shaking, and stretching movements. These movements, developed by Dr. Milton Trager, create an experience of lightness and freedom in the body, allowing for greater ease in movement. Trager also worked successfully with polio patients.

Awareness through movement, the movement therapy form of the **Feldenkrais** method, consists of specific structured movement experiences taught as a group lesson. These lessons reeducate the brain without tiring the muscles. Most lessons are done lying down on the floor or sitting. Moshe Feldenkrais designed the lessons to "improve ability . . . turn the impossible into the possible, the difficult into the easy, and the easy into the pleasant."

Ideokinesis is another movement approach emphasizing neuromuscular reeducation. Lulu Sweigart based her work on the pioneering approach of her teacher Mabel Elsworth Todd. Ideokinesis uses imagery to train the nervous system to stimulate the right muscles for the intended movement. If one continues to give the nervous system a clear mental picture of the movement intended, it will automatically select the best way to perform the movement. For example, to enhance balance in standing, Sweigart taught people to visualize "lines of movement" traveling through their bodies. Sweigart did not train teachers in ideokinesis but some individuals use ideokinetic imagery in the process of teaching movement.

The Mensendieck system of functional movement techniques is both corrective and preventative. Bess Mensendieck, a medical doctor, developed a series of exercises to reshape, rebuild and revitalize the body. A student of this approach learns to use the conscious will to relax muscles and releases tension. There are more than 200 exercises that emphasize correct and graceful body movement through everyday activities. Unlike other movement therapy approaches this work is done undressed or in a bikini bottom, in front of mirrors. This allows the student to observe and feel where a movement originates. Success has been reported with many conditions including **Parkinson's disease**, muscle and joint injuries, and repetitive strain injuries.

The **Alexander technique** is another functional approach to movement therapy. In this approach a teacher gently uses hands and verbal directions to subtly guide the student through movements such as sitting, standing up, bending and walking. The Alexander technique emphasizes balance in the neck-head relationship. A teacher lightly steers the students head into the proper balance on the tip of the spine while the student is moving in ordinary ways. The student learns to respond to movement demands with the whole body, in a light integrated way. This approach to movement is particularly popular with actors and other performers.

Pilates or physical mind method is also popular with actors, dancers, athletes, and a broad range of other people. Pilates consists of over 500 exercises done on the floor or primarily with customized exercise equipment. The exercises combine sensory awareness and physical training. Students learn to move from a stable, central core. The exercises promote strength, flexibility, and balance. Pilates training is increasingly available in sports medicine clinics, fitness centers, dance schools, spas, and physical therapy offices.

Many approaches to movement therapy emphasize awareness of internal sensations. Charlotte Selver, a student of somatic pioneer Elsa Gindler, calls her style of teaching sensory awareness (SA). This approach has influenced the thinking of many innovators, including Fritz Perls, who developed gestalt therapy. Rather than suggesting a series of structured movements, visualizations, or body positions, in SA the teacher outlines experiments in which one can become aware of the sensations involved in any movement. A teacher might ask the student to feel the movement of her breathing while running, sitting, picking up a book, etc. This close attunement to inner sensory experience encourages an experience of body-mind unity in which breathing becomes less restricted and posture, coordination, flexibility, and balance are improved. There may also be the experience of increased energy and aliveness.

Gerda Alexander Eutony (GAE) is another movement therapy approach that is based upon internal awareness. Through GAE one becomes a master of self-sensing and knowing which includes becoming sensitive to the external environment, as well. For example, while lying on the floor sensing the breath, skin or form of the body, one also senses the connection with the ground. GAE is taught in group classes or private lessons which also include hands-on therapy. In 1987, after two years of observation in clinics throughout the world, GAE became the first mind-body discipline accepted by the World Health Organization (WHO) as an alternative health-care technique.

Kinetic awareness developed by dancer-choreographer Elaine Summers, emphasizes emotional and physical inquiry. Privately or in a group, a teacher sets up situations for the student to explore the possible causes of pain and movement restrictions within the body. Rubber balls of various sizes are used as props to focus attention inward, support the body in a stretched position and massage a specific area of the body. The work helps one to deal with chronic pain, move easily again after injuries and increase energy, flexibility, coordination, and comfort.

Body-mind centering (BMC) was developed by Bonnie Bainbridge Cohen and is a comprehensive educational and therapeutic approach to movement. BMC practitioners use movement, touch, **guided imagery**, developmental repatterning, dialogue, music, large balls, and other props in an individual session to meet the needs of each person. BMC encourages people to develop a sensate awareness and experience of the ligaments, nerves, muscles, skin, fluids, organs, glands, fat, and fascia that make up one's body. It has been effective in preventing and rehabilitating from chronic injuries and in improving neuromuscular response in children with **cerebral palsy** and other neurological disorders.

Continuum movement has also been shown to be effective in treating neurological disorders including spinal chord injury. Developed by Emilie Conrad and Susan Harper, continuum movement is an inquiry into the creative flux of our body and all of life. Sound, breath, subtle and dynamic movements are explored that stimulate the brain and increase resonance with the fluid world of movement. The emphasis is upon unpredictable, spontaneous or spiral movements rather than a linear movement pattern. According to Conrad, "Awareness changes how we physically move. As we become more fluid and resilient so do the mental, emotional, and spiritual movements of our lives."

More recently, a form of movement therapy that involves horses has gained fresh attention. It is variously known as therapeutic riding or equine-assisted therapy. Therapeutic riding originated with a Swedish horsewoman who lost her ability to walk when she contracted polio in 1946, and was determined to recover by returning to horseback riding. She eventually won a silver medal in the 1952 Olympics. Therapeutic riding programs allow persons with physical, psychological, or learning disabilities to gain self-esteem and social growth as well as improved balance, body awareness, and physical strength.

Such Eastern movement therapies as yoga, t'ai chi, and qigong are also effective in healing and preventing a wide range of physical disorders, encouraging emotional stability, and enhancing spiritual awareness. There are a number of different approaches to yoga. Some emphasize the development of physical strength, flexibility, and alignment. Other forms of yoga emphasize inner awareness, opening, and meditation.

Precautions

Persons who are seriously ill, acutely feverish, or suffering from a contagious infection should wait until they have recovered before beginning a course of movement therapy. As a rule, types of movement therapy that involve intensive manipulation or stretching of the deeper layers of body tissue are not suitable for persons who have undergone recent surgery or have recently suffered severe injury. With regard to emotional or psychiatric disturbances, persons who are recovering from abuse or receiving treatment for any post-traumatic syndrome or dissociative disorder should consult their therapist before undertaking a course of movement therapy. While movement therapy is often recommended as part of a treatment plan for these disorders, it can also trigger flashbacks or dissociative episodes if the movement therapist is unaware of the client's history. It is always best to consult with a knowledgeable physician, physical therapist, or mental health therapist before a course of movement therapy.

Research and general acceptance

Although research has documented the effects of dance therapy, qigong, t'ai chi, yoga, Alexander technique, awareness through movement (Feldenkrais), and Rolfing, other forms of movement therapy have not been as thoroughly researched.

Training and certification

Training and certification vary widely with each form of movement therapy. Many approaches require several years of extensive training and experience with the particular movement form. Movement therapies that are also considered forms of bodywork have an umbrella national certification board, listed below under Resources. Therapeutic riding programs are accredited by the North American Riding for the Handicapped Association (NARHA), which also credentials riding instructors.

Resources

BOOKS

Halprin, Anna. *Dance as a Healing Art: Returning to Health Through Movement and Imagery*. Life Rhythm, 1999.

Hartley, Linda. *Wisdom of the Body Moving: An Introduction to Body-Mind Centering*. Berkeley, CA: North Atlantic Press, 1995.

Knaster, Mirka. *Discovering the Body's Wisdom*. New York, NY: Bantam Books, 1996.

Pelletier, Kenneth R., MD. *The Best Alternative Medicine, Part I: Sound Mind, Sound Body*. New York: Simon & Schuster, 2002.

PERIODICALS

Bagnall, A. M., P. Whiting, R. Richardson, and A. J. Sowden. "Interventions for the Treatment and Management of Chronic Fatigue Syndrome/Myalgic Encephalomyelitis. (Effectiveness Bulletin)." *Quality and Safety in Health Care* 11 (September 2002): 284-288.

Batty, G. David, and I-Min Lee. "Physical Activity for Preventing Strokes: Better Designed Studies Suggest That It is Effective." *British Medical Journal* 325 (August 17, 2002): 350-351.

Cottingham, John T., and Jeffrey Maitland. "Integrating Manual and Movement Therapy With Philosophical Counseling for Treatment of a Patient With Amyotrophic Lateral Sclerosis: A Case Study That Explores the Principles of Holistic Intervention." *Alternative Therapies Journal* (March 2000): 120-128.

Crandall, Melissa. "Healing Horses." *ASPCA Animal Watch* 22 (Winter 2002): 21-25.

Shute, Nancy. "A Super Feeling." *U. S. News & World Report*, September 23, 2002, 58.

Stanten, Michele, and Selene Yeager. "Kinder, Gentler Workouts: These No-Sweat Exercises Offer More Than Just Relaxation." (Fitness News). *Prevention* 54 (July 2002): 74-75.

Vidrine, M., P. Owen-Smith, and P. Faulkner. "Equine-Facilitated Group Psychotherapy: Applications for Therapeutic Vaulting." *Issues in Mental Health Nursing* 23 (September 2002): 587-603.

ORGANIZATIONS

American Yoga Association. www.americanyogaassociation.org.

Canadian Taijiquan Federation. P.O. Box 421, Milton, Ontario L9T 4Z1. www.canadiantaijiquanfederation.ca.

Feldenkrais Guild of North America. 3611 S.W. Hood Avenue, Suite 100, Portland, OR 97201. (800) 775-2118 or (503) 221-6612. Fax: (503) 221-6616. www.feldenkrais.com.

The Guild for Structural Integration. 209 Canyon Blvd. P.O. Box 1868. Boulder, CO 80306-1868. (303) 449-5903. (800) 530-8875. www.rolfguild.org.

International Association of Yoga Therapists (IAYT). 4150 Tivoli Avenue, Los Angeles, CA 90066.

North American Riding for the Handicapped Association (NARHA). P. O. Box 33150, Denver, CO 80233. (303) 452-1212 or (800) 369-RIDE. www.narha.org.

Patience T'ai Chi Association. 2620 East 18th Street, Brooklyn, NY 11235. (718) 332-3477. www.patiencetaichi.com.

Qigong Human Life Research Foundation. PO Box 5327. Cleveland, OH 44101. (216) 475-4712.

The Society of Teachers of the Alexander Technique. www.stat.org.uk.

The Trager Institute. 21 Locust Avenue, Mill Valley, CA 94941-2806 (415) 388-2688. Fax: (415) 388-2710. www.trager.com.

OTHER

National Certification Board for Therapeutic Massage and Bodywork. 8201 Greensboro Drive, Suite 300. McLean, VA 22102. (703) 610-9015.

NIH National Center for Complementary and Alternative Medicine (NCCAM) Clearinghouse. P. O. Box 8218, Silver Spring, MD 20907-8218. TTY/TDY: (888) 644-6226. Fax: (301) 495-4957. Web site: http://www.nccam.nih.gov.

Linda Chrisman
Rebecca J. Frey, PhD

Moxibustion

Definition

Moxibustion is a technique used in traditional Chinese medicine in which a stick or cone of burning mugwort, *Artemesia vulgaris*, is placed over an inflamed or affected area on the body. The cone is placed on an acupuncture point and burned. The cones is removed before burning the skin. The purpose is to stimulate and strengthen the blood and the life energy, or *qi*, of the body.

Origins

The actual Chinese character for **acupuncture** literally translates into "acupuncture-moxibustion." More than 3,000 years ago, during the Shang Dynasty in China, hieroglyphs of acupuncture and moxibustion were found on bones and tortoise shells, meaning

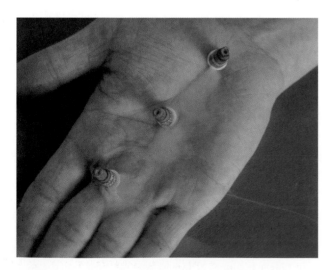

Moxibustion hand acupuncture for stomach, kidneys and chest. (© PHOTOTAKE Inc. / Alamy)

the practice precedes that date. The root word, "moxa" is actually derived from the Japanese.

Benefits

Moxibustion is used for people who have a cold or stagnant condition. The moxa stick is burned to warm up the blood and qi that are not circulating well. It is particularly known for its ability to turn breech presentation babies into a normal head-down position that is considered safer during **childbirth**. In a 1998 study published in the *Journal of the American Medical Association*, 75% of the pregnant women in the study had breech fetuses that turned in the normal position. Moxibustion significantly increases fetal movements in pregnant women. Moxibustion is also used to treat inflammations. For example, if treating a patient with tendinitis, the moxa stick is burned over the elbow area. It is also highly regarded for menstrual cramps, where the stick is waved over the abdominal area. Often, the cramps disappear immediately.

Moxa on acupuncture points is frequently done with acupuncture treatment for many kinds of ailments. The treatment brings warmth and helps strengthen the activity of the blood.

Description

Moxibustion is the burning of **mugwort** over inflamed and affected areas of the body. The mugwort can come in sticks that closely resemble the circumference and length of a cigar. Moxa cones can also be burned. The mugwort, called *Ai Ye* in **traditional Chinese medicine**, is positioned over acupuncture points to stimulate the qi and blood. In breech presentation babies, the acupoint BL 67, located on the outside of the little toe, is stimulated. For menstrual cramps, the meridian called the Ren Channel, the center line of the lower abdomen, is treated. Moxibustion is almost always used in conjunction with acupuncture, as a complementary technique. In Japan, there are practitioners who are separately licensed to practice as specialists in moxibustion. It is used for a wide variety of ailments, depending on the patient's needs and history. Therefore, it is difficult to cite costs and length of the treatment. For menstrual cramps, moxibustion can be used once. For breech presentation, the turning may occur during the treatment. Similar to acupuncture, it is sometimes covered by insurance and workers' compensation. Patients can be taught how to treat themselves, and moxa sticks are easily purchased.

Preparations

Because patients who undergo moxibustion treatment are also getting acupuncture, it is sometimes

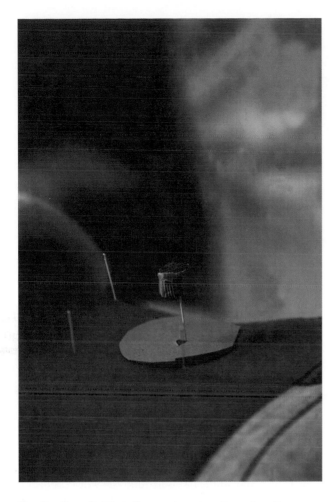

Moxibustion. *(© Photo Researchers, Inc. Reproduced by permission.)*

recommended to consult a physician prior to this therapy.

Precautions

Moxibustion is specifically used for patients with a cold or stagnant constitution. Therefore, if any patient has too much heat, they should not undergo moxibustion treatment. An expert practitioner can advise patients in these matters.

Side effects

Because moxibustion often includes the burning of **smoking** mugwort sticks, patients who have respiratory problems should avoid the use of smoking moxa sticks. Smokeless moxa sticks are available, and patients who have respiratory difficulties may opt for this method. There is also the occasional report of external **burns** if the moxa stick is held too close to the patient, although this is rare.

Research and general acceptance

Moxibustion has been used in traditional Chinese medicine for centuries, and as a result, it is widely accepted in Asia. It is gaining popularity in the west, in particular, for its ability to turn breech presentation babies. Several studies in the *Journal of the American Medical Association* have praised the use of this therapy.

Training and certification

Although moxibustion alone does not require a particular licensing or accreditation process, because it is used with acupuncture, the practitioner must have an acupuncture license in the United States.

Resources

BOOKS

Cheng, Kinnong. *Chinese Acupuncture and Moxibustion.* China Books and Periodicals, 2000.

Cui Yongqiang. *Test: Chinese Acupuncture and Moxibustion.* China Publishing and Trading, 1993.

Fei, X., and M. Jianhua. *Acupuncture and Moxibustion.* IOS Press, 2000.

Cheng, Dan-An et al. *Acupuncture and Moxibustion Formulas and Treatments.* China Books and Periodicals, Blue Poppy Press, 1996.

PERIODICALS

Cardini, Francesco, and Huang Weixing. "Moxibustion for Correction of Breech Presentation: A Randomized Controlled Trial." *Journal of the American Medical Association* (Nov 11, 1998).

ORGANIZATIONS

American Association of Oriental Medicine. 433 Front Street, Catasauqua, PA 18035. (888) 500-7999. aaom1@aol.com. http://www.aam.org.

OTHER

About.com. http://altmedicine.about.com/health/altmedicine/library/weekly/blatherpm.htm?rnk=rl&terms=moxibustion.

Nanjng University of Traditional Chinese Medicine. http://www.njutcm.edu.cn/index.html.

Katherine Y. Kim

MS *see* **Multiple sclerosis**

MSM

Description

Methylsulfonylmethane, or MSM, is also known as methyl sulfone and dimethylsulfone ($DMSO_2$). It is a sulfur-bearing compound that exists naturally in many fruits, vegetables, grains, and animals, including humans. Its presence and activity was discovered while working with its parent compound, DMSO, of which it is an oxidized metabolite (hence the O_2 designation). Although 55,000 papers have been written on DMSO, research on MSM has been more limited. A wide range of therapeutic benefits are attributed to it, along with a high degree of safety, and a low degree of toxicity. Actor James Coburn, crippled by **rheumatoid arthritis**, praised MSM's **pain** relieving benefits.

The history of MSM, as derived from DMSO, includes the following highlights:

- DMSO was first synthesized in a nineteenth century Russian lab, and was investigated for its usefulness as a solvent (a dissolver of other substances).

- British scientist Lovelock, working with red blood cells and cryogenics—the science of "alive freezing," reported DMSO as a uniquely helpful agent.

- Stanley Jacob, M.D., an American working in the 1950s to perfect kidney transplants, found Lovelock's report on cryogenic uses of DMSO, and met with DMSO chemist researcher, Robert Herschler, Ph.D.

- Drs. Jacob and Herschler discovered that DMSO, in addition to being useful in transplant surgery, facilitated delivery of other medications through the skin into the body, and that it had significant pain relieving and anti-inflammatory properties. They also discovered an undesirable effect of DMSO—a fishy taste and body odor.

- DMSO was approved for veterinary use (1970) in the treatment of joint and muscle related problems.

- In Russia (1973), prescription DMSO began use for the treatment of pain related to autoimmune disorders, arthritis, and diabetic ulcers. (One source reports as of 1999, more than 125 countries are using DMSO more safely and less expensively than drugs used for the same conditions in the United States.)

- In 1978, DMSO was approved by the United States Food and Drug Administration (FDA) for human use in the treatment of interstitial cystitis only, a painful inflammatory condition affecting many women.

- With lagging FDA approval, Herschler continued research and discovered that approximately 15% of DMSO turns into MSM in the body, and that the MSM metabolite produced the pain-relieving and anti-inflammatory benefits without the unpleasant odor side effect.

- Since that time, Drs. Jacob and Herschler, and others by anecdote, have found MSM to be clinically helpful in treating many more conditions, and that it is extremely safe, and has no known toxicity.

MSM occurs naturally in some foods including cow's milk (its highest source). One source specifies the presence of MSM—in descending order—in unpasteurized cow's milk, coffee, tomatoes, tea, Swiss chard, beer, corn, and **alfalfa**. Some reports say that natural levels of MSM decline with age. Dr. Herschler believes that the average diet is deficient in MSM because of the foods that are eaten or the way in which they are prepared. However, other sources refute the need for supplementing **sulfur** in the form of MSM, claiming that dietary sources of sulfur are sufficient. Sulfur-containing foods include cabbage, Brussels sprouts, broccoli, cauliflower (these are all known as cruciferous vegetables), sunflower seeds, **garlic**, onions, asparagus, avocados, beans, peas, mustard, horseradish, lentils, soybeans, and yogurt. Dietary sources of the three sulfur-containing amino acids—methionine, cystine, and cysteine—include meat, fish, poultry, eggs, milk, cheeses, and nuts, The cruciferous vegetables are reported to contain other sulfur compounds in addition to the sulfur-bearing **amino acids**. Nevertheless, many anecdotes cite the benefit of supplementing the diet with MSM.

General use

Because of its yellow color, the ancients named sulfur "the sun carrier." Sulfur is the fourth most common mineral in the human body. Through the ages, its curative uses have motivated many pilgrimmages to hot springs and sulfur baths around the world. Sulfur's uses within the human body are numerous. In many tissues, it is important in biological processes including nerve signal transmission, facilitative enzymatic processes, insulin production, carbohydrate metabolism regulation, **detoxification**, and waste removal.

MSM, with a 34% bio-availablility of sulfur according to one source, is reported to be useful in treating musculoskeletal, respiratory, circulatory, eliminative, autoimmune, and degenerative disorders. One of the most widely reported benefits is the relief of pain, inflammation, and **muscle spasms**, especially when related, but not limited to, **osteoarthritis** and autoimmune disorders such as lupus, scleroderma, and rheumatoid arthritis. MSM is said to reduce and improve the quality of scar tissue; promote improved healing of joints, tendons, ligaments and collagen support structures; soften, renew and strengthen the skin; and increase blood flow. It is reported to improve mucus membranes, thereby reducing food and airborne allergic reactions, and symptoms related to **asthma** and **emphysema**; improve vascular smooth muscle growth, reducing the risk of coronary artery disease; and improve athletic performance by reducing lactic acid effects, strengthening muscle elasticity and suppleness, and enhancing **fatigue** recovery times. It is reported to have an antiparasitic effect, especially against the parasite giardia. Another reported benefit is its tonic effect on the bowels, which increases peristalsis (waves of motion that move food along the digestive tract). This benefit is helpful to the elderly, those with sluggish colons, and those addicted to laxatives. At least one report noted possible anticancer activity.

Preparations

MSM is commonly available in these forms: powder, capsule, lotion, or gel. By itself, the powder is said to have a bitter taste. Users are advised to put the prescribed amount on the forward part of the tongue, followed by a large glass of water. In this way, the powder is dissolved in the stomach, and its bitter taste is not registered by the taste buds, which are located on the back of the tongue. Plenty of water throughout the day is also advised, due to its detoxifying action.

Suggested dosages range widely, from one to three grams daily, and up to 18 grams daily with medical supervision. One report suggests taking from two to six grams daily; the optimal dose depends on body size, age, and the severity of the condition being treated. Dr. Jacob recommends that, "A couple of grams a day would be a good general dosage," and higher doses may be useful to achieve a therapeutic effect. An example of a higher dose is three to four grams, taken for relief of allergy symptoms.

The elderly may benefit with as little as one tenth of a gram (100 mg) daily, up to five grams. Encapsulated preparation dosage recommendations may vary according to how many other ingredients—glucosamine sulfate or **chondroitin**, for example—are included in the preparation. Recommended amounts for topical applications of gel or lotion may also vary. Some sources advise adding an extra amount of powder to a gel or lotion for enhanced effect.

Precautions

MSM has blood thinning effects; therefore caution and consultation with a healthcare professional is especially advised when using medications such as warfarin (commonly known as Coumadin), aspirin, herbals such as ginkgo (**Ginkgo biloba**), and other supplements such as fish and flax oils, which contain Omega-3. An essential fatty acid, Omega-3 also has blood thinning properties.

Product purity is another concern. There are precautions against contamination by other ingredients including bacteria or DMSO, a chemical solvent that is not approved for use by the FDA. One company's product was recalled due to bacterial contamination. However, no related injuries were reported.

Dilution of the more expensive MSM product with less expensive bulk filler ingredients like Epsom salts, is a caution to buyers. ConsumerLab, LLC, lists many of these products on their Web site, with additional ingredients and test findings.

One product reported that it achieved "GRAS" (generally regarded as safe) status. The named product, as others, may derive mainly from pine tree lignan. A plant cell wall constituent, lignan facilitates the transport of nutrients up and down the stem or tree trunk. MSM may therefore facilitate movement and metabolism of other drugs, supplements, or nutrients within the body. Several reports caution that the sulfur of MSM must not be confused with sulfa drugs or with sulfites used as food preservatives. Some persons demonstrate allergic reaction to one or both of these.

Several sources report that few well-designed human studies have been conducted or reported. This factor contributes to the charge that MSM is unproven, while the array of anecdotal testimony points to the contrary.

Side effects

Side effects include gastrointestinal disturbance, such as **diarrhea**; **headache**; decreased ability to fall asleep (may occur if taken at bedtime); skin that is softer; nails that are thicker; and hair that is harder. Some reports have claimed that diarrhea or GI disturbances such as hyperacidity, **nausea**, and inflammation that are part of a **stress** response prior to taking MSM may clear "dramatically" by using MSM.

Interactions

Favorable interactions

Two sources report syngergistic interactions that reduced swelling and scarring in trauma patients, involving combinations of MSM and **vitamin C**. This occurred with additional use of the digestive proteins for starch and cellulose (amylase and cellulase, respectively), fats (**lipase**), sugars (sucrase, maltase and lactase), and **bromelain** (from pineapples). The addition of **glucosamine** HCL is reported to improve MSM effects when used for osteoarthritis.

Unfavorable interactions

Unfavorable interactions may include blood thinning medications such as Coumadin (warfarin), aspirin, and fish or flax (Omega-3) oil. One source reports studies involving prevention, regression, and promotion of tumor growth. Unfavorable interactions between MSM and chemotactic or chemopreventive agents may exist. The counsel of a knowledgeable healthcare professional is advised.

Resources

BOOKS

Jacob, M.D., Stanley W., Ronald M. Lawrence M.D., Ph.D., and Martin Zucker. *The Miracle of MSM, the Natural Solution for Pain.* New York: Penguin Putnam, 1999.

OTHER

Challem, Jack. "MSM and DMSO." *The Nutrition Reporter.* November 25, 2000. [Cited May 13, 2004]. http://www. thenutritionreporter.com/MSM and DMSO.html.

Consumer Labs, LLC. *Product Review: Joint Supplements (Glucosamine, Chondroitin and MSM)* November 2, 2003. [Cited May 13, 2004]. http://www.consumerlab. com/results/gluco.asp.

"Eye and Nasal Drops." *Ophthalmology Times* September 15, 2001. [Cited May 13, 2004] http://galenet.gale group.com/servlet/HWRC.

Lang, Kerry L. *Methylsulfonylmethane (MSM).* June 17, 2001. [Cited May 13, 2004] http://www.quackwatch. org/01QuackeryRelatedTopics/DSH/msm.htm.

"Lignisul MSM achieves GRAS status." *Nutraceuticals World.* May 2003. [Cited May 13, 2004] http://gale-net.galegroup.com/servlet/HWRC.

"Methylsulfonylmethane (MSM)." *Alternative Medicine Review.* November 2003. [Cited May 13, 2004] http:// galenet.galegroup.com/servlet/HWRC.

"MSM to Quell Arthritis Symptoms." *Tufts University Health & Nutrition Letter* January 2002. [Cited May 13, 2004] http://galenet.galegroup.com/servlet/HWRC.

Nature doctor. *MSM—MethylSulfonylMethane.* [Cited May 13, 2004] http://www.pages.prodigy.net/naturedoctor/ msm.html.

"Sulfur (MSM)." [Cited May 13, 2004] http://www.all-nat ural.com/msm.html.

"What is MSM?" *MSM Information Center* [Cited May 13, 2004] http://www.health-n-energy.com/msminfo.htm.

Katherine E. Nelson, N.D.

Mugwort

Description

Mugwort (*Artemisia vulgaris*) also known as common artemisia, felon herb, St. John's herb, chrysanthemum weed, sailor's tobacco, and moxa is a perennial member of the Compositae family, and a close relative of **wormwood** (*Artemisia absinthium L.*). Mugwort's generic name is from that of the Greek moon goddess Artemis, a patron of women. Mugwort has long been considered an herbal ally for women with particular benefit in regulating the menstrual cycle and easing the transition to **menopause**. The common name may be from the old English word *moughte* meaning "moth," or *mucgwyrt*, meaning "midgewort," referring to the plant's folk use to repel moths and other insects.

Mugwort has a long history of folk tradition and use. Anglo-Saxon tribes believed that the aromatic mugwort was one of the nine sacred herbs given to the world by the god Woden. It was used as a flavoring additive to beer before **hops** (*Humulus lupulus*) became widely used. Mugwort is considered a magical herb, with special properties to protect road-weary travelers against exhaustion. The Romans planted mugwort by roadsides where it would be available to passersby to put in their shoes to relieve aching feet. St. John the Baptist was said to have worn a girdle of mugwort when he set out into the wilderness. Some of the magic in mugwort is in its reputed ability to induce prophetic and vivid dreams when the herb is placed near the bed or under the sleeper's pillow. In Pagan ceremony, a garland or belt of mugwort is worn while dancing

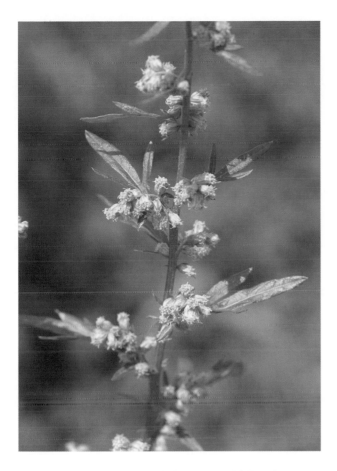

Mugwort (Artemisia vulgaris). (© blickwinkel / Alamy)

General use

Mugwort leaf and stem are used medicinally. Mugwort acts as a bitter digestive tonic, uterine stimulant, nervine, menstrual regulator, and antirheumatic. The volatile oil of mugwort includes thujone, linalool, borneol, pinene, and other constituents. The herb also contains hydroxycoumarins, lipohilic flavonoids, vulgarin, and triterpenes.

Mugwort acts as an emmenagogue, an agent that increases blood circulation to the pelvic area and uterus and stimulates **menstruation**. It is a useful remedy for painful and irregular menstruation. A compress of the herb has been used to help promote labor and assist with expulsion of the afterbirth. A mild infusion of mugwort is useful as a digestive stimulant. It is helpful in cases of mild **depression** and nervous tension. The herb also may stimulate the appetite. A weak infusion of mugwort has sedative properties that may quiet restlessness and **anxiety**. Its antispasmodic action may relieve persistent **vomiting**, and has been used in the treatment of **epilepsy**. Mugwort added to bath water is an aromatic and soothing treatment for relief of aches in the muscles and joints. In a clinical trial, crushed fresh mugwort leaves applied to the skin were shown to be effective in eradicating **warts**. Taken as an infusion, mugwort is helpful in ridding the system of pinworm infestation. Dried mugwort leaf also acts as a natural tinder, useful in holding a smoldering fire. The dried herb has also been smoked as a nicotine-free tobacco. A species of mugwort (*A. douglasiana*), common in the southwestern United States, was used by some western Native Americans as a prevention for poison **oak** rash. The fresh mugwort leaf was rubbed over areas of exposed skin before walking into poison oak habitat. The two plants often grow near one another.

In Chinese medicine mugwort, known as *Ai ye* or *Hao-shu* is highly valued as the herb used in **moxibustion**, a method of heating specific **acupuncture** points on the body to treat physical conditions. Mugwort is carefully harvested, dried and aged, then it is shaped into a cigar-like roll. This "moxa" is burned close to the skin to heat the specific pressure points. It has been used in this way to alleviate rheumatic pains aggravated by cold and damp circumstances. Mugwort has also been used in various size cones that are places on the skin directly or on top of an herb or some salt and burned. In Japan, some practitioners only use moxa for treatment.

A study published in the *Journal of the American Medical Association* reported on the successful use of moxibustion in reversing breech birth positions. The study found that 75% of 130 fetuses had reversed their

around the fire during summer solstice celebrations. The herb is then thrown into the fire to ensure continued protection throughout the coming year.

Mugwort is a tall and hardy European native with stout, angular, slightly hairy stems tinged with a purple hue. Leaves, which may be as long as 4 in (10 cm), are deeply divided with numerous lance-shaped, pointed segments, which may be toothed or entire. They are arranged alternately along the erect, grooved stem and are a dark green on top and pale green with downy hairs on the underside. Mugwort has a pungent aroma when the leaves are crushed. In late summer the small reddish-yellow disk flowers cluster in long spikes at the top of the plant. Mugwort may reach to 6 ft (2 m) or more in height. This tenacious herb has naturalized throughout North America and may be found growing wild in rocky soils, along streams and embankments, and in rubble and other waste places, particularly in the eastern United States. In some areas, including North Carolina and Virginia, mugwort is characterized as a noxious, alien weed. Mugwort root is about 8 in (20 cm) long with many thin rootlets. It spreads from stout and persistent rhizomes.

KEY TERMS

Antioxidant—Any substance that reduces the damage caused by oxidation, such as the harm caused by free radicals.

Artemisinin—An antimalarial agent derived from an ancient Chinese herbal remedy. Two of the most popular varieties are artemether and artesunate, used mainly in Southeast Asia in combination with mefloquine.

Emmenagogue—A type of medication that brings on or increases a woman's menstrual flow.

Mugwort-spice syndrome—A type of food allergy that occurs in people who are sensitized to mugwort, celery, carrots, and other spices. It often takes the form of a skin rash.

Tonic—Characterized by tonus, a state of partial contraction that is maintained at least in part by a continuous bombardment of motor impulses.

Volatile oil—The fragrant oil that can be obtained from a plant by distillation. The word "volatile" means that the oil evaporates in the open air.

position after moxibustion treatment of the mother. The technique is said to stimulate the acupuncture point known as BL67, located near the toenail of the fifth toe, stimulating circulation and energy flow and resulting in an increase in fetal movements.

In Chinese medicine, mugwort is ingested to stop excessive or inappropriate menstrual bleeding.

Mugwort has also been used in Brazilian folk medicine as a remedy for stomach ulcers. Researchers have found that the plant contains **antioxidants** which help to explain its protective effects on gastric tissues.

More recently, mugwort has attracted attention as the source of a natural compound, artemisinin, which has been shown to have antimalarial properties. Artemisinin is a promising natural remedy for **malaria** because of its low toxicity and its effectiveness against drug-resistant mutations of the malaria parasite. In addition to its effectiveness in treating malaria, artemisinin is also being tested as a possible anticancer drug. A group of researchers in Mississippi has shown that artemisinin is toxic to several different types of human **cancer** cells.

Preparations

Mugwort is harvested just as the plant comes into flower, before the blossoms are fully open. The leaves

are removed from the stalks and dried on paper-lined trays in a light, airy room, away from direct sunlight. The flowerheads should be dried intact and the dried herb stored in clearly-labeled, tightly-sealed, dark glass containers.

For infusion, 1 oz of fresh mugwort leaf, less if dried, is placed in a warmed glass container. One pint of fresh, nonchlorinated boiling water is added to the herb. The mixture is covered to prevent loss of volatile oils. The tea should be infused for five to 10 minutes. A mild infusion is best. After straining, it is recommended to drink two cups of mugwort tea per day. Use should be discontinued after six days.

Four ounces of finely-cut fresh or powdered dry herb can be combined with 1 pt of brandy, gin, or vodka, in a glass container. The alcohol should be enough to cover the plant parts and have a 50/50 ratio of alcohol to water. The mixture should be kept in a dark place for about two weeks, shaking several times each day. It can then be strained and stored in a tightly capped, dark glass bottle. Dosage recommendations vary, with some herbalists cautioning against ingestion of mugwort in medicinal preparations.

In **traditional Chinese medicine**, the herb is burned slightly in a pan before simmering with other herbs to stop menstrual bleeding.

Precautions

Mugwort should be avoided during **pregnancy** and lactation. The herb is a uterine stimulant. Women should avoid its use during lactation as the chemical constituent thujone may be passed to the baby through the mother's milk. Mugwort should no be ingested if uterine inflammation or pelvic infection is present.

Side effects

High doses of mugwort may cause liver damage, **nausea**, and convulsions.

Some people develop a **contact dermatitis**, or allergic skin rash, if they are in contact with mugwort and certain other spices. This food allergy has been called the mugwort-spice syndrome, or sometimes the mugwort-celery-spice syndrome. Other foods and spices that are part of this syndrome include carrots, paprika, curry, cumin, birch, and pepper. In addition, mugwort pollen has been reported to cause **asthma** in susceptible children.

Interactions

People who are allergic to mugwort are also highly likely to be allergic to **chamomile** and should not take preparations made from either herb.

Resources

BOOKS

Culpeper, Nicholas. *Culpeper's Complete Herbal & English Physician*. IL: Meyerbooks, 1990.

Foster, Steven, and Duke, James A. *Peterson Field Guides, Eastern/Central Medicinal Plants*. NY: Houghton Mifflin Company, 1990.

Mabey, Richard. *The New Age Herbalist*. New York: Simon & Schuster, Inc., 1988.

Ody, Penelope. *The Complete Medicinal Herbal*. New York: Dorling Kindersley, 1993

Palaise, Jean. *Grandmother's Secrets, Her Green Guide to Health From Plants*. NY: G.P. Putnam's Sons, 1974.

PDR for Herbal Medicines. Montvale, NJ: Medical Economics Company, 1998.

PERIODICALS

Anliker, M. D., S. Borelli, and B. Wuthrich. "Occupational Protein Contact Dermatitis from Spices in a Butcher: A New Presentation of the Mugwort-Spice Syndrome." *Contact Dermatitis* 46 (February 2002): 72-74.

Bibi, H., D. Shosheyov, D. Feigenbaum, et al. "Comparison of Positive Allergy Skin Tests Among Asthmatic Children from Rural and Urban Areas Living Within Small Geographic Area." *Annals of Allergy, Asthma and Immunology* 88 (April 2002): 416-420.

Bilia, A. R., D. Lazari, L. Messori, et al. "Simple and Rapid Physico-Chemical Methods to Examine Action of Antimalarial Drugs with Hemin: Its Application to *Artemisia annua* Constituents." *Life Sciences* 70 (January 4, 2002): 769-778.

Galal, A. M., S. A. Ross, M. A. Elsohly, et al. "Deoxyartemisinin Derivatives from Photooxygenation of Anhydrodeoxydihydroartemisinin and Their Cytotoxic Evaluation." *Journal of Natural Products* 65 (February 2002): 184-188.

Moneret-Vautrin, D. A., M. Morisset, P. Lemerdy, et al. "Food Allergy and IgE Sensitization Caused by Spices: CICBAA Data (Based on 589 Cases of Food Allergy)." *Allergie et immunologie (Paris)* 34 (April 2002): 135-140.

Repetto, M. G., and S. F. Llesuy. "Antioxidant Properties of Natural Compounds Used in Popular Medicine for Gastric Ulcers." *Brazilian Journal of Medicine and Biological Research* 35 (May 2002): 523-534.

ORGANIZATIONS

American College of Allergy, Asthma, and Immunology. 85 West Algonquin Road, Suite 550, Arlington Heights, IL 60005. (847) 427-1200. www.acaai.org.

Herb Research Foundation. 1007 Pearl Street, Suite 200, Boulder, CO 80302. (303) 449-2265. www.herbs.org.

OTHER

Grieve, Mrs. M. "A Modern Herbal, Mugwort." Botanical.com. http://www.botanical.com/botanical/mgmh/m/mugwor61.html.

Hoffmann, David L. "Mugwort." *Health World Online*. http://www.healthy.net.

Clare Hanrahan
Rebecca J. Frey, PhD

Mullein

Description

Mullein (*Verbascum thapsus*) also known as great mullein, is a dramatic biennial herb of the Scrophulariaceae or figwort family. The family name of this European native may have derived from the word scrofula, a disease that is now understood to be a form of **tuberculosis**. In Ireland mullein was widely cultivated as a remedy for tuberculosis. The seed is said to have arrived on the North American continent in the dirt used as ballast in old sailing vessels. At least five species of mullein have naturalized in North America. This sturdy and adaptive herb is found on roadsides, rocky and gravely banks, and in marginal areas throughout the world. It thrives in full sun and adapts well to arid conditions. The seeds of this hardy plant, particularly *V. blattaria*, may remain viable as long as 70 years.

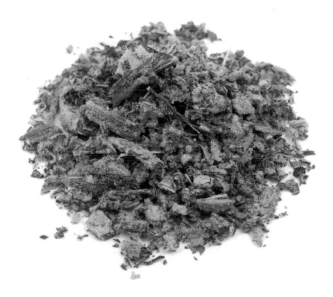

Mullein (Verbascum thapsus). *(© Geoffrey Kidd / Alamy)*

Mullein is known by many names reflecting the numerous medicinal and practical uses people have found for this beneficial wayside herb throughout its long association with human communities. Among the common names for mullein are flannel leaf, beggar's blanket, velvet plant, feltwort, tinder plant, candlewick plant, witch's candle, Aaron's rod, lady's **foxglove**, donkey's ears, hag's taper, candlewick plant, torches, and Quaker rouge. This last name was given because the leaves were sometimes used as a natural rouge rubbed vigorously on the cheeks to give a rosy glow, particularly among young women whose cultures have shunned cosmetics. Mullein has been known for centuries as Gordolobo in Mexico, where it was used by the Nahuatl and other indigenous cultures long before the coming of the conquistadors. Gordolobo is still sold in medicinal herbs stands throughout Mexico as a remedy for **hemorrhoids** and **varicose veins** as well as throat ailments.

Like many plants of European origin, mullein was credited with power over witches and evil spirits. It was considered one of 23 important healing herbs in medieval Jewish medical practice. Mullein's large stalk was used as a ceremonial torch as far back as ancient Rome. Stripped of its leaves and dipped in tallow, the cylindrical spike could hold a flame when carried aloft from place to place. One name for mullein is miner's candle. During the 1849 California gold rush, the mine shafts were aglow with mullein torches carried by the prospectors. The leaves were used as tinder to start fires, or as a smudge, burned over the embers of Native American campfires. The smoke was inhaled to relieve pulmonary congestion. Mullein leaf, which some tribes called "big tobacco," was mixed with nicotine leaf and smoked to relieve **asthma**. The leaves were boiled to make a hot poultice to treat **gout** and painful joints. Mullein's thick, soft leaves lined the shoes of many common folk during the winter months to provide extra warmth. The leaves were also warmed over a hot rock and fitted to the foot to relieve **fatigue**. Figs were wrapped in the leaves to ripen and keep, and the flowers were used to add blonde highlights to the hair, or soaked in oil to make ear drops.

Mullein's branching, spindle-shaped root produces a low-lying basal rosette of broadly lance-shaped leaves in the first year of growth. Dense and downy white hairs give mullein's light-green leaves a soft texture somewhat like the fine pile of velvet. These leaves winter over from the first year's growth. They may reach 15-20 in (38-50 cm) in length and 8 in (20 cm) across. In its second season mullein transforms, reaching skyward with a single, pithy and fibrous stem stout enough hold itself erect when in full leaf.

Small yellow, five-petaled blossoms each form a golden cup and encircle the upper few feet of the stem, opening randomly. The usually solitary stem, which may grow to 10 ft (3 m) high, is sometimes branched. The leaves clasp the stem, growing alternately, and are increasingly smaller toward the top of the stem, an arrangement that facilitates the flow of rain water to the roots.

General use

The flowers, leaves, and root of mullein have been used as healing remedies for centuries. Mullein leaf and flower were listed as an official medicine in the United States *National Formulary* from 1916 to 1936. The plant contains mucilage, triterpene saponins, volatile oil, flavonoids, and bitter glycosides. The efficacy of these compounds in the quantity found in mullein is questioned by at least one researcher. However, in the realm of folk medicine, practiced for centuries, mullein is valued as a demulcent, emollient, antispasmodic, astringent, diuretic, vulnerary, and expectorant. Mullein is approved by the German Commission E, an advisory panel for herbal medicine, for treatment of respiratory catarrh. Studies have confirmed the anti-inflammatory action of mullein. Mullein tea, made from the flowers and leaf, is a beneficial remedy for **bronchitis**, **sore throat**, **tonsillitis**, dry coughs, and hoarseness. The flowers have bactericidal and sedative properties and are generally considered more medicinally potent than the leaves. Their bactericidal activity was confirmed by researchers at Clemson University, who reported in 2002 that mullein extracts are effective against several species of disease bacteria, including *Staphylococcus aureus*, *Staphylococcus epidermidis*, *Escherichia coli*, and *Klebsiella pneumoniae*.

An oil extract of mullein flowers relieves **earache**, and the blossom tea can ease **headache pain** and promote sleep. The fresh leaves, traditionally boiled in milk and consumed daily, are an Irish folk remedy for tuberculosis. When this mixture is applied externally in poultice form, it is helpful in the treatment of **boils**, carbuncles, skin ulcers, chilblains, and hemorrhoids.

Preparations

Mullein leaves should be harvested before the herb is in blossom, leaving at least two thirds of the foliage on the plant. The flowers should be harvested just as they open. Blossoms are short-lived and drop easily from the plant. Roots are best harvested in the fall of the year. Leaves and blossoms should be dried in a single layer on paper-lined trays in a light, warm, and airy room out of direct sunlight. The medicinal

KEY TERMS

Antispasmodic—A drug or other substance that relieves mild cramping or muscle spasms.

Catarrh—Inflammation of a mucous membrane, especially of the nose and air passages.

Chilblains—Redness and swelling of the skin often accompanied by burning, itching, and blisters. A condition caused by excessive exposure to the cold.

Demulcent—A gelatinous or oily substance that has a protective or soothing influence on irritated mucous membranes.

Diuretic—An herbal preparation or medication given to increase urinary output.

Expectorant—A drug that promotes the discharge of mucus from respiratory system.

Mucilage—A gummy, gelatinous substance found in the stems of borage that is useful for treating throat irritations.

properties of the flowers are diminished if they lose their color, so care should be taken in the drying process.

Oil extraction: Combine one cup of mullein blossoms in one-half cup of olive oil in a glass double boiler over low flame. Heat slowly for about three hours. Strain with cheesecloth to remove all plant parts. Pour the oil into small, dark glass bottles, tightly sealed and clearly labeled for storage. A cold extraction can also be prepared. Cover flowers in olive oil in a glass container with a lid and set aside on a sunny windowsill to steep for seven to 10 days. Strain before storing in dark glass bottles.

Infusion: Place 2 oz of finely cut fresh (less if dried) mullein leaf and blossom in a warmed glass container. Bring 2.5 cups of fresh, nonchlorinated water to the boiling point, add it to the herbs. Cover. Infuse the tea for about 10 minutes. Strain carefully, as mullein's fine hairs are an irritant. The blossoms are sweeter to the taste than the leaf. The prepared tea will store for about two days in the refrigerator. Drink three cups a day.

Syrup: Using fresh blossoms and leaves, prepare a strong infusion of mullein. Combine the infusion with a 50/50 mixture of honey and brown sugar. Use 24 oz of sweetener for each 2.5 cups of the herbal infusion. Heat mixture in a glass or enamel pot; stir frequently as the mixture thickens. Cool and pour into a clearly labeled glass bottles. Refrigerate for storage. Take 1 tsp of syrup three times a day, or every two hours if needed for chronic coughs.

Precautions

The seeds of some species of mullein are considered toxic. The seeds of the species *N. phlomoides* contains a type of poisonous saponin and are slightly narcotic. They have been used to intoxicate fish to make them easier to catch. The Clemson researchers, however, found that mullein extract has this effect on fish only at high concentrations.

Although mullein is safe to use by itself, it is sometimes mixed with such other herbs as **comfrey**, **echinacea**, Irish moss, **yarrow**, **garlic**, or ginseng in a variety of commercial herbal preparations. The Food and Drug Administration (FDA) has issued consumer warnings about thirteen different herbal syrups, powders, capsules, or other dietary supplements containing mullein since 1999. Because the FDA classifies herbal preparations as dietary supplements and does not subject them to the approval process that prescription drugs must pass, consumers should purchase herbs and herbal products only from established manufacturers. People who would like to try mullein as an alternative remedy for sore throats might want to use the herb by itself first before trying herbal mixtures.

Side effects

There have been isolated case reports of people developing **contact dermatitis** (allergic skin rash) from mullein plants.

Interactions

Mullein has been reported to inhibit the effectiveness of antidiabetic drugs. It intensifies the effects of muscle relaxants and lithium. Persons taking prescription diuretics should consult a physician before taking mullein, as it may interact with the prescription drugs to cause a loss of **potassium** from the body.

Resources

BOOKS

Duke, James A., Ph.D. *The Green Pharmacy*. Emmaus, PA: Rodale Press, 1997.

McIntyre, Anne. *The Medicinal Garden*. New York: Henry Holt and Company, 1997.

Ody, Penelope. *The Complete Medicinal Herbal*. New York: Dorling Kindersley, 1993.

PDR for Herbal Medicines. Montvale, NJ: Medical Economics Company, 1998.

Prevention's 200 Herbal Remedies. Emmaus, PA: Rodale Press, Inc., 1997.

Thomson, William A. R. *Medicines From The Earth.* SF: Harper & Row, 1983.

Tyler, Varro E., Ph.D. *Herbs of Choice.* New York: Pharmaceutical Products Press, 1994.

Tyler, Varro E., Ph.D. *The Honest Herbal.* New York: Pharmaceutical Products Press, 1993.

Weiss, Gaea, and Shandor Weiss. *Growing & Using The Healing Herbs.* NY: Wings Books, 1992.

PERIODICALS

Ertle, Lynn. "Mullein the Maligned." *The Herb Quarterly* (Summer) 1977.

Lev, E. "Some Evidence for the Use of Doctrine of Signatures in the Land of Israel and Its Environs During the Middle Ages." [in Hebrew] *Harefuah* 141 (July 2002): 651-655.

Turker, A. U., and N. D. Camper. "Biological Activity of Common Mullein, a Medicinal Plant." *Journal of Ethnopharmacology* 82 (October 2002): 117-125.

ORGANIZATIONS

Herb Research Foundation. 1007 Pearl St., Suite 200, Boulder, CO 80302. (303) 449-2265. www.herbs.org.

Southwest School of Botanical Medicine. P. O. Box 4565, Bisbee, AZ 85603. (520) 432-5855. www.swsbm.com.

United States Food and Drug Administration (FDA), Center for Food Safety and Applied Nutrition. 5100 Paint Branch Parkway, College Park, MD 20740. (888) SAFEFOOD. www.cfsan.fda.gov.

Clare Hanrahan
Rebecca J. Frey, PhD

Multiple chemical sensitivity

Definition

Multiple chemical sensitivity—also known as MCS syndrome, environmental illness, idiopathic environmental intolerance, chemical **AIDS**, total allergy syndrome, or simply MCS—is a disorder in which a person develops symptoms from exposure to chemicals in the environment. With each incidence of exposure, lower levels of the chemical will trigger a reaction and the person becomes increasingly vulnerable to reactions triggered by other chemicals.

Medical experts disagree on the cause of the syndrome, and as to whether MCS is a clinically recognized illness. In a 1992 position statement that remained unchanged as of early 2000, the American Medical Association's Council on Scientific Affairs did not recognize MCS as a clinical condition due to a lack of accepted diagnostic criteria and controlled studies on the disorder. A more recent discussion of methodological problems in published studies of MCS, as well as recommendations for patient care, may be found in the 1999 position paper on MCS drafted by the American College of Occupational and Environmental Medicine (ACOEM). As of 2003, however, many researchers in Europe as well as the United States regard MCS as a contemporary version of neurasthenia, a concept first introduced by a physician named George Miller Beard in 1869.

Description

Multiple chemical sensitivity typically begins with one high-dose exposure to a chemical, but it may also develop from long-term exposure to a low level of a chemical. Chemicals most often connected with MCS include: formaldehyde; pesticides; solvents; petrochemical fuels such as diesel, gasoline, and kerosene; waxes, detergents, and cleaning products; latex; tobacco smoke; perfumes and fragrances; and artificial colors, flavors, and preservatives. People who develop MCS are commonly exposed in one of the following situations: on the job as an industrial worker; residing or working in a poorly ventilated building; or living in conditions of high air or water pollution. Others may be exposed in unique incidents.

Because MCS is difficult to diagnose, estimates vary as to what percentage of the population develops MCS. However, most MCS patients are female. The median age of MCS patients is 40 years old, and most experienced symptoms before they were 30 years old. There is also a large percentage of Persian Gulf War veterans who have reported symptoms of chemical sensitivity since their return from the Gulf in the early 1990s.

Causes and symptoms

Chemical exposure is often a result of indoor air pollution. Buildings that are tightly sealed for energy conservation may cause a related illness called **sick building syndrome**, in which people are thought to develop symptoms from chronic exposure to airborne environmental chemicals such as formaldehyde from the furniture, carpet glues, and latex caulking. A person moving into a newly constructed building, which has not had time to degas (or air out), may experience the initial high-dose exposure that leads to MCS.

The specific biochemical and physiological mechanisms in humans that lead to MCS are not well understood. A recent hypothesis, however, suggests that MCS is the end result of four different mechanisms of sensitization acting to reinforce one

KEY TERMS

Capsaicin—A colorless, bitter compound that is present in cayenne and gives it its heat.

De-gas—To release and vent gases. New building materials often give off gases and odors and the air should be well circulated to remove them.

Neurasthenia—Nervous exhaustion; a disorder with symptoms of irritability and weakness, commonly diagnosed in the late 1800s.

Sick building syndrome—An illness related to multiple chemical sensitivity in which a person develops symptoms in response to chronic exposure to airborne environmental chemicals found in a tightly sealed building.

another. Further research is required to test this hypothesis.

The symptoms of MCS vary from person to person and are not chemical-specific. Symptoms are not limited to one physiological system, but primarily affect the respiratory and nervous systems. Symptoms commonly reported are **headache**, **fatigue**, weakness, difficulty concentrating, short-term **memory loss**, **dizziness**, irritability and **depression**, **itching**, numbness, burning sensation, congestion, **sore throat**, hoarseness, shortness of breath, **cough**, and stomach pains.

One commonly reported symptom of MCS is a heightened sensitivity to odors, including a stronger emotional reaction to them. A Japanese study published in late 2002 reported that patients diagnosed with MCS can identify common odors as accurately as most people, but regard a greater number of them as unpleasant.

One test that has been devised to evaluate patients with MCS is the capsaicin inhalation test. Capsaicin is an alkaloid found in hot peppers that is sometimes used in topical creams and rubs for the treatment of arthritis. When inhaled, capsaicin causes coughing in healthy persons as well as those with **allergies** that affect the airway; however, persons with MCS cough more deeply and frequently than control subjects when given a dose of capsaicin. Although the test is not diagnostic in the strict sense, it has been shown to be an effective way of identifying patients with MCS.

Diagnosis

Multiple chemical sensitivity is a twentieth-century disorder, becoming more prevalent as more human-

made chemicals are introduced into the environment in greater quantities. It is especially difficult to diagnose because it presents no consistent or measurable set of symptoms and has no single diagnostic test or marker. For example, a 2002 study of PET scans of MCS patients found no significant functional changes in the patients' brain tissues. Physicians are often either unaware of MCS as a condition, or refuse to accept that MCS exists. They may be unable to diagnose it, or may misdiagnose it as another degenerative disease, or may label it as a psychosomatic illness (a physical illness that is caused by emotional problems). Their lack of understanding generates frustration, **anxiety**, and distrust in patients already struggling with MCS. However, a new specialty of medicine is evolving to address MCS and related illnesses: occupational and environmental medicine. A physician looking for MCS will take a complete patient history and try to identify chemical exposures.

Some MCS patients may be helped by a psychologic evaluation, particularly if they show signs of panic attacks or other anxiety disorders. It is known that many patients with MCS suffer from comorbid depression and anxiety. In addition, MCS patients appear to have high rates of mood disorders compared to **asthma** patients as well as normal test subjects.

A 1999 consensus statement signed by 34 physicians and MCS researchers and published in the *Archives of Environmental Health* lists six criteria for MCS diagnosis:

- The MCS symptoms are chronic.
- The symptoms are reproducible with repeated chemical exposure.
- Low levels of chemical exposure trigger symptoms.
- Symptoms occur with multiple, unrelated chemicals.
- Symptoms improve when the chemicals are removed.
- Symptoms involve multiple organ systems.

Treatment

The most effective treatment for MCS is to avoid the chemicals that trigger the symptoms. Avoidance becomes increasingly difficult as the number of offending chemicals increases; things as seemingly harmless as air freshener devices, scented soaps, and perfume can trigger serious reactions in MCS patients. Individuals with MCS often remain at home where they are able to control the chemicals in their environment. In many cases, it may be recommended that an individual turn one room in his or her home, usually the bedroom, into an environmentally safe haven by removing all known chemical irritants and furnishing it with 100% natural materials. The isolation that is a necessary part of treatment for MCS patients limits their abilities to work and socialize, so supportive counseling is often appropriate.

Many MCS patients undergo food-allergy testing and testing for accumulated pesticides in the body to learn more about their condition and what chemicals to avoid. Eliminating foods with artificial colors and flavors, preservatives, monosodium glutamate, and other additives can help to lessen MCS symptoms, as can choosing pesticide-free, organically grown fruits and vegetables.

Some MCS patients find relief with **detoxification** programs of **exercise** and sweating, and chelation of heavy metals. **Acupuncture** can give added support to any treatment program for MCS patients. **Yoga**, massage, and **aromatherapy** may be helpful in relieving **stress** symptoms associated with MCS. However, great care should be taken when selecting aromatherapy oils for MCS patients, and the practice is best left to a trained aromatherapist familiar with MCS. **Essential oils** should be verified as 100% unadulterated and nonchemically extracted. If a negative reaction results from the use of a particular oil, the MCS patient should stop using it immediately and consult his or her healthcare professional.

A number of herbs may be prescribed to treat the symptoms of MCS. They should also be prescribed and selected with great care, especially in those patients who suffer from known food allergies. Herbs should be recommended by a trained herbalist or naturopathic healthcare professional, and small sample doses may be administered before trying full dosage strength in order to check for an allergic reaction. **Milk thistle** (*Silybum marianum*) can be useful for cleansing the liver after chemical damage.

Allopathic treatment

Some doctors may recommend antihistamines, analgesics, and other medications to combat the symptoms of MCS. Care must be taken in prescribing these substances, as they may provoke a reaction in some MCS patients.

Expected results

Once MCS sets in, sensitivity continues to increase and a person's health continues to deteriorate. Strictly avoiding exposure to triggering chemicals for a year or more may improve health.

Prevention

Multiple chemical sensitivity is difficult to prevent because even at high-dose exposures, different people react differently. Ensuring adequate ventilation in situations with potential for acute high-dose or chronic low-dose chemical exposure, as well as wearing the proper protective equipment in industrial situations, will minimize the risk.

Resources

BOOKS

American Psychiatric Association. *Diagnostic and Statistical Manual of Mental Disorders*, 4th edition, text revision. Washington, DC: American Psychiatric Association, 2000.

Gibson, Pamela. *Multiple Chemical Sensitivity: A Survival Guide*. Oakland, CA: New Harbinger Publications, 2000.

Hu, Howard, and Frank E. Speizer. "Specific Environmental and Occupational Hazards." In *Harrison's Principles of Internal Medicine*. 14th ed., edited by Anthony S. Fauci, et al. New York: McGraw-Hill, 1998.

"Multiple Chemical Sensitivity Syndrome." Section 21, Chapter 287 in *The Merck Manual of Diagnosis and Therapy*, edited by Mark H. Beers, MD, and Robert Berkow, MD. Whitehouse Station, NJ: Merck Research Laboratories, 1999.

PERIODICALS

Bornschein, S., C. Hausteiner, A. Drzezga, et al. "PET in Patients With Clear-Cut Multiple Chemical Sensitivity (MCS)." *Nuklearmedizin* 41 (December 2002): 233–239.

Bornschein, S., C. Hausteiner, T. Zilker, and H. Forstl. "Psychiatric and Somatic Disorders and Multiple Chemical Sensitivity (MCS) in 264 'Environmental Patients'." *Psychological Medicine* 32 (November 2002): 1387–1394.

Caccappollo-vanVliet, E., K. Kelly-McNeil, B. Natelson, et al. "Anxiety Sensitivity and Depression in Multiple Chemical Sensitivities and Asthma." *Journal of Occupational and Environmental Medicine* 44 (October 2002): 890–901.

Johansson, A., O. Lowhagen, E. Millqvist, and M. Bende. "Capsaicin Inhalation Test for Identification of Sensory Hyperreactivity." *Respiratory Medicine* 96 (September 2002): 731–735.

Ojima, M., H. Tonori, T. Sato, et al. "Odor Perception in Patients with Multiple Chemical Sensitivity." *Tohoku Journal of Experimental Medicine* 198 (November 2002): 163–173.

Pall, M. L. "NMDA Sensitization and Stimulation by Peroxynitrite, Nitric Oxide, and Organic Solvents as the Mechanism of Chemical Sensitivity in Multiple Chemical Sensitivity." *FASEB Journal* 16 (September 2002): 1407–1417.

Schafer, M. L. "On the History of the Concept Neurasthenia and Its Modern Variants Chronic-Fatigue-Syndrome,

Fibromyalgia and Multiple Chemical Sensitivities" [in German] *Fortschritte der Neurologie-Psychiatrie* 70 (November 2002): 570–582.

Ternesten-Hasseus, E., M. Bende, and E. Millqvist. "Increased Capsaicin Cough Sensitivity in Patients with Multiple Chemical Sensitivity." *Journal of Occupational and Environmental Medicine* 44 (November 2002): 1012–1017.

ORGANIZATIONS

American Academy of Environmental Medicine. P.O. Box CN 1001-8001, New Hope, PA 18938. (215) 862-4544.

American College of Occupational and Environmental Medicine (ACOEM). 1114 North Arlington Heights Road, Arlington Heights, IL 60004. (847) 818-1800. www.acoem.org.

OTHER

"Multiple Chemical Sensitivities: Idiopathic Environmental Intolerance." Position Statement by the American College of Occupational and Environmental Medicine (ACOEM), April 26, 1999. www.acoem.org/position/statements.asp?CATA_ID=46.

Paula Thivierge
Rebecca J. Frey, PhD

Symptoms of multiple sclerosis

Symptoms

Numbness in one or more limbs, typically occurring on one side of the body at a time, or on the bottom half of the body.

Tingling in one or more limbs and chest

Tremors, or unsteady gait

Lack of muscular coordination

Blurred vision, double vision, or loss of vision (often in one eye at a time, with pain during eye movement

Incontinence

Exhaustion and weakness in limbs/Fatigue

Dizziness

Electric-shock sensations that occur with certain head movements

(Illustration by Corey Light. Cengage Learning, Gale)

Multiple sclerosis

Definition

Multiple sclerosis is a chronic, degenerative disease of the central nervous system (CNS). The CNS is comprised of the brain and the spinal cord. In the CNS, the nerves are covered by a protective layer called the myelin sheath. Myelin helps keep the nerve healthy. It also improves nerve conduction. In multiple sclerosis, inflammation causes the nerves to gradually lose this myelin cover. This repeated inflammation and erosion leads to scarring (sclerosis), which impairs the nerve's ability to conduct impulses. Eventually, even the nerves themselves are affected. Because the nervous system controls and coordinates a number of body functions, patients with MS gradually lose a variety of functions, including memory and the ability to see, speak or walk.

Description

Multiple sclerosis is a chronic debilitating disease that affects as many at 350,000 in the United States alone (2.5 million worldwide). Most patients are first diagnosed of the disease at age 20-40. However, the disease may appear as early as age 12 or as late as age 50. MS strikes women earlier in life. Women are also affected more frequently than men and whites more often than other races.

Causes and symptoms

The causes of multiple sclerosis are still unknown, although many factors are suspected. In the United States, whites are diagnosed with MS twice as often as blacks or Hispanics. Asians are the least affected. There is some consensus, however, that the following factors may contribute to the development of multiple sclerosis:

- *Genetic heredity.* Family members of multiple sclerosis patients have a 1 in 50 chance of having MS; the odds for people without an affected family member are 1 in 1,000. If an identical twin is diagnosed with MS, the remaining twin has a 1 in 3 chance of becoming affected as well. Recent research has shown that several autoimmune diseases, including MS, share a common genetic link. In other words, patients with MS might share common genes with family members that have other autoimmune diseases like systemic lupus, rheumatoid arthritis, and others.

- *Viral infection.* Most MS patients have high levels of antibodies to measles and other viruses. Therefore, multiple sclerosis may be the body's delayed immune reaction to viruses such as measles, *Herpes simplex*, rubella, and parainfluenza. A 2001 study also suggested that Epstein-Barr virus, the virus that causes mononucleosis, probably increases risk of MS.

- *Autoimmune reaction*. Scientists know that MS is an autoimmune disorder, an illness in which the body attacks its own myelin as if it were a foreign substance. Although research has identified which immune cells are responsible and how they are activated, no one knows what causes the immune system to begin this attack.

- *Geography*. Countries in the temperate zones (above 40°) such as Northern Europe, North America, Australia, and New Zealand have significantly higher incidence of multiple sclerosis than countries in the tropics. In the United States, people who live below the 37th parallel develop MS at a rate of 57–78 cases per 100,000 people. Those who live above the line have a prevalence rate of 110–140 cases per 100,000 people.

- *Diet*. Studies have shown that populations at high risk of developing multiple sclerosis tend to consume a lot of dairy products and animal fats. On the contrary, in countries such as Japan, people eat few dairy products but consume lots of fish, soy-rich foods, and seeds, which are good sources of essential fatty acids. The incidence rates in these countries are very low. Thus, essential fatty acid deficiency due to excessive consumption of saturated fats may contribute to the development of multiple sclerosis.

Diagnosis

In order to determine whether or not a patient has multiple sclerosis, doctors often rely on the Schumacher criteria:

- Patient's symptoms indicate neurological damage in more than one areas.
- Patient's symptoms have worsened for more than six months.
- There are at least two events (each lasting for more than one day) separated by at least one month.
- Neurological exam of the patient shows abnormal central nervous system function.
- Symptoms reflect damage in the white matter of the CNS only.
- Patient is older than 10 but less than 50 years old.
- Patient does not have stroke, lupus, or any disease that may have similar symptoms.

A diagnosis of multiple sclerosis is made when patient's symptoms fit Schumacher's criteria and

---

neurological exams, MRI, and laboratory results also show corresponding abnormalities. In 2001, a panel convened by the National Multiple Sclerosis Society wrote new diagnostic criteria for MS, the first update in about 20 years. The new criteria formally recommend MRI and outline how doctors should use the results of tests like cerebral spinal fluid analysis.

MS symptoms vary significantly in terms of severity, intensity and duration. Sensory symptoms are the first warning signs. Many patients notice color distortion, blurred or double vision, and temporary blindness. Their senses of smell, hearing, touch, and taste are also affected. They experience muscle weakness and difficulty walking, as well as **muscle spasms** and numbness, tingling, or prickling ("pins and needles") sensations called *paresthesias*. As the disease progresses, sudden partial or complete paralysis of the arms or legs is common, as are an inability to speak clearly, move without tremors, or hear clearly. Mental functions are also affected. Patients can not concentrate or remember as clearly as before. They often become depressed. They may laugh or cry uncontrollably. As conditions worsen, they lose control of bodily functions. Some patients find that hot weather exacerbates their symptoms. Cold baths or air conditioning may help during these periods. There are also periods, called remissions, in which patients are free of symptoms; remission can be complete or partial.

While there is a rare, rapidly progressing form of MS that can be fatal in as little as a few days or weeks,

MS generally affects the quality of life more than it diminishes life expectancy. Most patients can look forward to decades of life after diagnosis. Many are able to continue to live a relatively normal life for at least 20 years after onset, although some patients become disabled within a few months of being diagnosed. In addition, because MS patients are frequently forced into immobility and spend a lot of time sitting in wheelchairs, they are susceptible to such common complications of the disabled as urinary tract **infections**, skin ulcers, pneumonia, or pulmonary embolism (blood clot in the lung) in addition to side effects from prescribed drugs.

Treatment

Nutritional therapy

Many multiple sclerosis patients follow a low-fat diet developed by Dr. Roy Swank, who recommends his diet to slow down disease progression. The following are his recommendations:

- Consume no more than 10 g of saturated fat per day.
- Limit polyunsaturated fat consumption to 50 g or less per day.
- Take 1 tbsp of cod liver oil per day to supplement essential fatty-acid intake. Cod liver oil is a good source of omega-3 fatty acid, one of the two essential fatty acids.
- Consume adequate amount of protein in the diet, preferably plant protein such as soy, beans, seeds, and nuts.
- Eat more fish, a good source of omega-3 fatty acid. Swank recommends having fish three or more times per week. Omega-3 fatty acid is believed to support myelin production and improve nerve function.

In addition to following the Swank diet, Dr. Michael Murray and Dr. Joseph Pizzorno, the authors of the book *Encyclopedia of Natural Medicine* also recommend the following nutritional supplements:

- *Flaxseed oil.* Murray and Pizzorno recommend replacing the fish oil in Swank's diet with flaxseed oil because the latter can provide both omega-3 and omega-6 fatty acids. Omega-6 fats, studies have shown, also help alleviate MS symptoms.
- *Antioxidants* such as selenium , vitamin C, and vitamin E. Patients with multiple sclerosis often have antioxidant deficiency.
- *Vitamin B_{12}.* MS patients often lack Vitamin B_{12}, and correcting this deficiency is believed to help decrease myelin destruction.

Exercise and physical therapy

Almost any form of **exercise** or **movement therapy** is beneficial for MS patients. For patients too weak to exercise alone, a massage or assisted physical therapy should be helpful to improve circulation to the limbs and promote well-being. Those that are less restricted may find **t'ai chi**, **qigong**, **yoga**, martial arts, conventional cardiovascular exercise, and/or water aerobics helpful.

Other treatments

Other alternative treatments such as aromatherapy (body massage with **rosemary** or juniper **essential oils**) and **hydrotherapy** (hot or cold baths used to treat affected areas, also a program of exercise performed in water) may also improve muscle strength in MS patients. Chinese herbs, especially ginseng, are also helpful in managing the disease. Wearing a cooling vest may also help, according to a 2001 study. The vest cools patients (without affecting their temperatures) and also appears to promote production of white cell nitrous oxide, which may play a role in MS.

Allopathic treatment

Standard treatment consists of an exercise program, diet modification, and medication. Three relatively new drugs may be prescribed: beta-interferon A (Avonex), which can limit the progressions of disability; beta-interferon-B (Betaseron), which reduces the number and severity of relapses; and Glatiramer acetate (Copaxone), which helps prevent relapse in patients with the relapsing-remitting (RR) type of MS. (These are patients who have a period of time with no or few symptoms [remission] following acute exacerbations [relapse] of disease.) All are administered by injection. These drugs have significant side effects including **fever**, tiredness, weakness, chills, muscle aches and inflammation at injection sites. Avonex may be better tolerated than Betaseron.

For symptomatic treatment of muscle spasm, Baclofen is most effective; its dosage must be carefully tailored to specific patient's needs. An implantable infusion pump that delivers the drug directly into the spinal cord can be used for patients with severe spasticity. Diazepam (valium) is sometimes given together with baclofen to increase its effectiveness. Alternative antispastic drugs are tizanidine and dantrolene. Steroids such as methylprednisolone and prednisone are also sometimes used to treat flare-ups.

Expected results

Patients whose symptoms worsen quickly right after diagnosis, those who have significant impairment in muscle movement or brain functions at onset and who have very abnormal magnetic resonance imaging (MRI) results at the beginning have poor prognosis. On the other hand, patients who recover quickly after the initial symptoms or those who experience only sensory impairment for five years or more after diagnosis often are able to maintain work longer and live longer than those with chronic progressive multiple sclerosis.

Prevention

There is no way to prevent the onset of multiple sclerosis, though a diet low in saturated fat may be helpful.

Resources

BOOKS

Burton Golberg Group. "Multiple Sclerosis." In *Alternative Medicine: The Definitive Guide*. Tiburon, CA: Future Medicine Publishing, Inc., 1999.

Holland, Nancy J., T. Jock Murray, and Stephen C. Rheingold. *Multiple Sclerosis: A Guide for the Newly Diagnosed*. New York, NY: Demos Vermande, 1996.

Murray, Michael T., and Joseph E. Pizzorno. "Multiple Sclerosis." In *Encyclopedia of Natural Medicine. Revised 2nd ed.* Rocklin, CA: Prima Publishing, 1998.

Rudick, Richard A. "Multiple Sclerosis and Related Conditions." In *Cecil Textbook of Medicine, 21st ed.* W.B. Saunders Company, 2000.

PERIODICALS

Acherio, Alberto, et al. "Epstein-Barr Virus Antibodies and Risk of Multiple Sclerosis: A Prospective Study." *JAMA, The Journal of the American Medical Association.*286; no. 24 (December 26, 2001):3083-3086.

Moran, M. "Autoimmune Diseases Could Share Common Genetic Etiology."*American Medical News.*44; no. 38: (October 8, 2001):38.

Vastag, B. "New Diagnostic Criteria for MS Issued." *JAMA, The Journal of the American Medical Association.*286; no. 14(October 10, 2001):1703.

"Wearing Colling Vest Helps Improve Symptoms." *Pain and Central Nervous System Week.*(October 6, 2001).

ORGANIZATIONS

Multiple Sclerosis Association of America (MSAA). 706 Haddonfield Road. Cherry Hill, NJ 08002-2652. (800) LEARN-MS(532-7667) Fax: (609) 661-9797. http://www.msaa.com.

Multiple Sclerosis Foundation, Inc. (MSF). 6350 North Andrews Avenue. Fort Lauderdale, FL 33309. (800) 441-7055 Fax: (954) 938-8708.

National Multiple Sclerosis Society (NMSS). 733 3rd Avenue. New York, NY 10017-3288. (800) 344-4867 or (212) 986-3240. http://www.nmss.org.

OTHER

Lazoff, Marjorie, MD. "Multiple Sclerosis." *Emedicine.com* http://www.emedicine.com/emerg/topic321.htm

Mai Tran
Teresa Odle

Mum *see* **Chrysanthemum flower**

Mumps

Definition

Mumps is a relatively mild short-term viral infection of the salivary glands that usually occurs during childhood. Typically, mumps is characterized by a painful swelling of both cheek areas, although the person could have swelling on one side or no perceivable swelling at all. The salivary glands are also called the parotid glands; therefore, mumps is sometimes referred to as an inflammation of the parotid glands (epidemic parotitis). The word mumps comes from an old English dialect word that means lumps or bumps within the cheeks.

Description

Mumps is a very contagious infection that spreads easily in such highly populated areas as day care centers and schools. Although not as contagious as **measles** or **chickenpox**, mumps was once quite common.

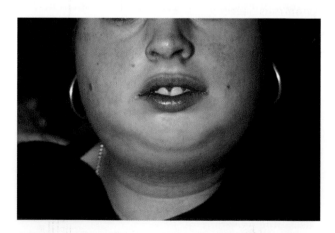

Mumps is an acute generalized virus infection, commonly causing enlargement of the salivary glands, especially the parotid gland. *(© Hercules Robinson / Alamy)*

Prior to the release of a mumps vaccine in the United States in 1967, approximately 92% of all children had been exposed to mumps by the age of 15. In these pre-vaccine years, most children contracted mumps between the ages of four and seven. Mumps epidemics came in two to five year cycles. The greatest mumps epidemic was in 1941 when approximately 250 cases were reported for every 100,000 people. In 1968, the year after the live mumps vaccine was released, only 76 cases were reported for every 100,000 people. By 1985, less than 3,000 cases of mumps were reported throughout the entire United States, which works out to about 1 case per 100,000 people. The reason for the decline in mumps was the increased usage of the mumps vaccine. However, 1987 noted a five-fold increase in the incidence of the disease because of the reluctance of some states to adopt comprehensive school immunization laws. Since then, state-enforced school entry requirements have achieved student immunization rates of nearly 100% in kindergarten and first grade. In 1996, the Centers for Disease Control and Prevention (CDC) reported only 751 cases of mumps nationwide, or, in other words, about one case for every five million people.

Causes and symptoms

The paramyxovirus that causes mumps is harbored in the saliva and is spread through **sneezing**, coughing, and other direct contact with another person's infected saliva. Once the person is exposed to the virus, symptoms generally become noticeable in 14–24 days. Initial symptoms include **chills**, **headache**, loss of appetite, and a lack of energy. However, an infected person may not experience these initial symptoms. Swelling of the salivary glands in the face (parotitis) generally occurs within 12–24 hours of the above symptoms. Accompanying the swollen glands is **pain** on chewing or swallowing, especially with acidic beverages, such as lemonade. A **fever** as high as 104°F (40°C) is also common. Swelling of the glands reaches a maximum on about the second day and usually disappears by the seventh day. Once a person has contracted mumps, he or she becomes immune to the disease, despite how mild or severe symptoms may have been.

While the majority of cases of mumps are uncomplicated and pass without incident, some complications can occur. Complications are, however, more noticeable in adults who get the infection. In 15% of cases, the covering of the brain and spinal cord becomes inflamed (**meningitis**). Symptoms of meningitis usually develop within four or five days after the first signs of mumps. These symptoms include a stiff

KEY TERMS

Autism—A developmental disability that appears early in life, in which normal brain development is disrupted and social and communication skills are retarded, sometimes severely.

Encephalitis—Inflammation of the brain, usually caused by a virus. The inflammation may interfere with normal brain function and may cause seizures, sleepiness, confusion, personality changes, weakness in one or more parts of the body, and even coma.

Epidemic parotitis—The medical name for mumps.

Immunoglobulin G (IgG)—Immunoglobulin type gamma, the most common type found in the blood and tissue fluids.

Meningitis—An infection or inflammation of the membranes that cover the brain and spinal cord. It is usually caused by bacteria or a virus.

Orchitis—Inflammation of one or both testes, accompanied by swelling, pain, fever, and a sensation of heaviness in the affected area.

Paramyxovirus—A genus of viruses that includes the causative agent of mumps.

Parotitis—Inflammation and swelling of one or both of the parotid salivary glands.

neck, headache, **vomiting**, pain with bending or flexing the head, and a lack of energy. Mumps meningitis is usually resolved within seven days, and damage to the brain is exceedingly rare.

Mumps infection can spread into the brain causing inflammation of the brain (encephalitis). Symptoms of mumps encephalitis include the inability to feel pain, seizures, and high fever. Encephalitis can occur during the parotitis stage or one to two weeks later. Recovery from mumps encephalitis is usually complete, although complications, such as seizure disorders, have been noted. Only about 1 in 100 patients with mumps encephalitis dies from the complication.

About one-quarter of all post-pubertal males who contract mumps can develop a swelling of the scrotum (orchitis) about seven days after the parotitis stage. Symptoms include marked swelling of one or both testicles, severe pain, fever, **nausea**, and headache. Pain and swelling usually subside after 5–7 days, although the testicles can remain tender for weeks.

Girls occasionally suffer an inflammation of the ovaries, or oophoritis, as a complication of mumps, but this condition is far less painful than orchitis in boys.

As of late 2002, some researchers in Europe are studying the possibility that mumps increases a person's risk of developing **inflammatory bowel disease** (IBD) in later life. This hypothesis will require further research, as present findings are inconclusive.

Diagnosis

When mumps reaches epidemic proportions, diagnosis is relatively easy on the basis of the physical symptoms. The doctor will take the child's temperature, gently palpate (touch) the skin over the parotid glands, and look inside the child's mouth. If the child has mumps, the openings to the ducts inside the mouth will be slightly inflamed and have a "pouty" appearance. With so many people vaccinated today, a case of mumps must be properly diagnosed in the event the salivary glands are swollen for reasons other than viral infection. For example, in persons with poor oral hygiene, the salivary glands can be infected with bacteria. In these cases, antibiotics are necessary. Also in rare cases, the salivary glands can become blocked, develop tumors, or swell due to the use of certain drugs, such as **iodine**. A test can be performed to determine whether the person with swelling of the salivary glands actually has the mumps virus.

Researchers in London have reported the development of a bioassay for measuring mumps-specific IgG. This test allows a doctor to check whether an individual patient is immune to mumps, and allow researchers to measure the susceptibility of a local population to mumps in areas with low rates of vaccination.

Treatment

Nutritional therapy

Nutritional therapy may alleviate pain and aid healing. A nutritionist or naturopath may recommend the following:

- drinking lots of fluids to replace fluid loss
- eating only such easy-to-digest foods as soups, broth or bland foods
- taking multivitamin/mineral supplement to help boost the immune function

Homeopathy

A number of homeopathic remedies can be used in the treatment of mumps. For example, **belladonna**

may be useful for flushing, redness, and swelling. **Bryonia** (wild **hops**) may be useful for irritability, lack of energy, or thirst. **Phytolacca** (poke root) may be prescribed for extremely swollen glands. A homeopathic physician should always be consulted for appropriate doses for children, and remedies that do not work within one day should be stopped. A homeopathic preparation of the mumps virus can also be used prophylactically or as a treatment for the disease.

Herbal therapy

Several herbal remedies may be useful in helping the body recover from the infection or may help alleviate the discomfort associated with the disease. **Echinacea** (*Echinacea* spp.) can be used to boost the immune system and help the body fight the infection. Other herbs taken internally, such as cleavers (*Galium aparine*), **calendula** (*Calendula officinalis*), and phytolacca (poke root), target the lymphatic system and may help to enhance the activity of the body's internal filtration system. Since phytolacca can be toxic, it should only be used by patients under the care of a skilled practitioner. Topical applications are also useful in relieving the discomfort of mumps. A cloth dipped in a heated mixture of vinegar and **cayenne** (*Capsicum frutescens*) can be wrapped around the neck several times a day. Cleavers or calendula can also be combined with vinegar, heated, and applied in a similar manner.

Acupressure

Acupressure can be used effectively to relieve pain caused by swollen glands. The patient can, by using the middle fingers, gently press the area between the jawbone and the ear for two minutes while breathing deeply.

Allopathic treatment

When mumps occurs, the illness is usually allowed to run its course. The symptoms, however, are treatable. Because of difficulty swallowing, the most important challenge is to keep the patient fed and hydrated. The individual should be provided a soft diet, consisting of cooked cereals, mashed potatoes, broth-based soups, prepared baby foods, or foods put through a home food processor. Aspirin, acetaminophen, or ibuprofen can relieve some of the pain due to swelling, headache, and fever. Avoiding fruit juices and other acidic foods or beverages that can irritate the salivary glands is recommended, as is avoiding dairy products that can be hard to digest. In the event of complications, a physician should be contacted at once. For example, if orchitis occurs, a physician should be called. Also, supporting the scrotum in a cotton bed on an adhesive-tape bridge between the thighs can minimize tension. Ice packs are also helpful.

Expected results

When mumps is uncomplicated, the prognosis for full recovery is excellent. In rare cases, however, a relapse occurs after about two weeks. Complications can also delay complete recovery.

Prevention

A vaccine exists to protect against mumps. The vaccine preparation (MMR) is usually given as part of a combination injection that helps protect against measles, mumps, and **rubella**. MMR is a live vaccine administered in one dose between the ages of 12-15 months, 4-6 years, or 11-12 years. Persons who are unsure of their mumps history and/or mumps vaccination history should be vaccinated. Susceptible health care workers, especially those who work in hospitals, should be vaccinated. Because mumps is still prevalent throughout the world, susceptible persons over age one who are traveling abroad would benefit from receiving the mumps vaccine.

The mumps vaccine is extremely effective, and virtually everyone should be vaccinated against this disease. There are, however, a few reasons why people should *not* be vaccinated against mumps:

- Pregnant women who contract mumps during pregnancy have an increased rate of miscarriage, but not birth defects. As a result, pregnant women should not receive the mumps vaccine because of the possibility of damage to the fetus. Women who have had the vaccine should postpone becoming pregnant for three months following vaccination.

- Unvaccinated persons who have been exposed to mumps should not get the vaccine, as it may not provide protection. The person should, however, be vaccinated if no symptoms result from exposure to mumps.

- Persons with minor fever-producing illnesses, such as an upper respiratory infection, should not get the vaccine until the illness has subsided.

- Because mumps vaccine is produced using eggs, individuals who develop hives, swelling of the mouth or throat, dizziness, or breathing difficulties after eating eggs should not receive the mumps vaccine.

- Persons with immune deficiency diseases and/or those whose immunity has been suppressed with anti-cancer drugs, corticosteroids, or radiation should not receive the vaccine. Family members of immunocompromised

people, however, should get vaccinated to reduce the risk of mumps.

- The CDC recommends that all children infected with human immunodeficiency disease (HIV) who are asymptomatic should receive an MMR vaccine at 15 months of age.

The mumps vaccine has been controversial in recent years because of concern that its use was linked to a rise in the rate of childhood **autism**. The negative publicity given to the vaccine in the mass media led some parents to refuse to immunize their children with the MMR vaccine. One result has been an increase in the number of mumps outbreaks in several European countries, including Italy and the United Kingdom.

In the fall of 2002, the *New England Journal of Medicine* published a major Danish study disproving the hypothesis of a connection between the MMR vaccine and autism. A second study in Finland showed that the vaccine is not associated with aseptic meningitis or encephalitis as well as autism. Since these studies were published, American primary care physicians have once again reminded parents of the importance of immunizing their children against mumps and other childhood diseases.

Resources

BOOKS

"Viral Infections: Mumps." Section 19, Chapter 265 in *The Merck Manual of Diagnosis and Therapy*, edited by Mark H. Beers, MD, and Robert Berkow, MD. Whitehouse Station, NJ: Merck Research Laboratories, 1999.

Zand, Janet, Allan N. Spreen, and James B. LaValle. "Mumps." *Smart Medicine for Healthier Living*. Garden City Park, NY: Avery Publishing Group, 1998.

PERIODICALS

Gabutti, G., M. C. Rota, S. Salmaso, et al. "Epidemiology of Measles, Mumps and Rubella in Italy." *Epidemiology and Infection* 129 (December 2002): 543–550.

Kimmel, S. R. "Vaccine Adverse Events: Separating Myth From Reality." *American Family Physician* 66 (December 1, 2002): 2113–2120.

Madsen, K. M., A. Hviid, M. Vestergaard, et al. "A Population-Based Study of Measles, Mumps, and Rubella Vaccination and Autism." *New England Journal of Medicine* 347 (November 7, 2002): 1477–1482.

Makela, A., J. P. Nuorti, and H. Peltola. "Neurologic Disorders After Measles-Mumps-Rubella Vaccination." *Pediatrics* 110 (November 2002): 957–963.

McKie, A., D. Samuel, B. Cohen, and N. A. Saunders. "A Quantitative Immuno-PCR Assay for the Detection of Mumps-Specific IgG." *Journal of Immunological Methods* 270 (December 1, 2002): 135–141.

Nielsen, S. E., O. H. Nielsen, B. Vainer, and M. H. Claesson. "Inflammatory Bowel Disease—Do Microorganisms

Play a Role?" [in Danish] *Ugeskrift for laeger* 164 (December 9, 2002): 5947–5950.

Pugh, R. N., B. Akinosi, S. Pooransingh, et al. "An Outbreak of Mumps in the Metropolitan Area of Walsall, UK." *International Journal of Infectious Diseases* 6 (December 2002): 283–287.

ORGANIZATIONS

American Academy of Pediatrics (AAP). 141 Northwest Point Boulevard, Elk Grove Village, IL 60007. (847) 434-4000. http://www.aap.org.

Centers for Disease Control and Prevention. 1600 Clifton Rd., NE, Atlanta, GA 30333. (800) 311-3435, (404) 639-3311. http://www.cdc.gov

OTHER

Recommended Childhood Immunization Schedules, United States, 1995. June 16, 1995, Volume 44, RR-5. Can be purchased from Superintendent of Documents, U. S. Government Printing Office, Washington, DC 20402-9325. (202) 783-3238.

Update: Vaccine Side Effects, Adverse Reactions, Contraindications, and Precautions. September 6, 1996, Volume 45, RR-12. Can be purchased from Superintendent of Documents, U. S. Government Printing Office, Washington, DC 20402-9325. (202) 783-3238.

Mai Tran
Rebecca J. Frey, PhD

Muscle spasms & cramps

Definition

Muscle spasms and cramps are spontaneous, often painful muscle contractions.

Description

Most people are familiar with the sudden **pain** of a muscle cramp. The rapid, uncontrolled contraction, or spasm, happens unexpectedly. Sometimes it can happen during or following athletic activity or a workout. It can also happen with either no stimulation or some trivially small one. The muscle contraction and pain last for several minutes, and then slowly ease. Cramps may affect any muscle, but are most common in the calves, thighs, feet, and hands. While painful, they are harmless, and in most cases, not related to any underlying disorder. Nonetheless, cramps and spasms can be manifestations of many neurological or muscular diseases.

The terms cramp and spasm are often used interchangeably. They can be somewhat vague because they are sometimes used to also include types of abnormal muscle activity other than sudden painful contraction. These include stiffness at rest, slow muscle **relaxation**, and spontaneous contractions of a muscle at rest (fasciculation or clonism). Fasciculation is a type of painless muscle spasm, marked by rapid, uncoordinated contraction of many small muscle fibers that people often describe as a sort of "muscle fluttering." For a physician, a critical part of diagnosis is to distinguish these different meanings and to allow the patient to describe the problem as precisely as possible.

Causes and symptoms

Normal voluntary muscle contraction begins when electrical signals are sent from the brain through the spinal cord along nerve cells called motor neurons. These include both the upper motor neurons within the brain and the lower motor neurons within the spinal cord and leading out to the muscle. At the muscle, chemicals released by the motor neuron stimulate the internal release of **calcium** ions from stores within the muscle cell. These calcium ions then interact with proteins within the muscle cell, causing chains of the proteins actin and myosin to slide past one another with a ratchet-like motion. This motion pulls their fixed ends closer, thereby shortening the cell and, ultimately, contracting the muscle itself. Recapture of calcium and unlinking of actin and myosin allows the muscle fiber to return to its resting length (i.e., relax).

Abnormal contraction may be caused by abnormal activity at any stage in this process. Certain mechanisms within the brain and the rest of the central nervous system monitor the length of the muscles and help regulate contraction. Interruption of these mechanisms can cause spasm. Motor neurons that are overly sensitive may fire below their normal thresholds. The muscle membrane itself may be hypersensitive, causing contraction without stimulation. Calcium ions may not be recaptured quickly enough, causing prolonged contraction.

Interruption of brain mechanisms and overly sensitive motor neurons may result from damage to the nerve pathways. Possible causes include **stroke**, **multiple sclerosis**, **cerebral palsy**, neurodegenerative diseases, trauma, spinal cord injury, and such nervous system poisons as strychnine, **tetanus** toxin, and certain insecticides. Nerve damage may lead to a prolonged or permanent muscle shortening called contracture. However, most muscle spasms are not caused by disease, but more commonly by physical activity or **stress**.

KEY TERMS

Actin—A protein that functions in muscular contraction by combining with myosin.

Fasciculation—Small involuntary muscle contractions visible under the skin.

Motor neuron—A nerve cell that specifically controls and stimulates voluntary muscles.

Myosin—A protein found in muscle tissue that interacts with another protein called actin during muscle contraction.

Myotonia—The inability to normally relax a muscle after contracting or tightening it.

Changes in muscle responsiveness may be due to or associated with:

- Prolonged exercise. Relaxation of a muscle actually requires energy to be expended. The energy is used to recapture calcium and to unlink the actin and myosin. This causes the muscles fibers to lengthen because the unlinked chains slide back to their resting positions. Normally, sensations of pain and fatigue signal that it is time to slow down or stop. Resting allows the muscles to restore their supplies of energy. Ignoring or overriding those warning signals can lead to such severe energy depletion that the muscle cannot be relaxed, causing a cramp. For example, this is why long distance runners may cramp up after a run. The lack of blood flow deprives the muscles of their source of energizing oxygen and nutrients and removal of fatigue causing waste. Rigor mortis, the stiffness of a corpse within the first 24 hours after death, is also due to this phenomenon.

- Using a muscle inappropriately. Muscle cramps in such sports as golf or tennis are sometimes caused by an incorrect grip on the club or racket, or an incorrect swing.

- Anemia adversely effects blood flow to the muscles and can cause cramping and spasms.

- Dehydration and salt depletion. This may be brought on by protracted vomiting or diarrhea, or by copious sweating during prolonged exercise, especially in high temperatures. Loss of fluids and salts—especially sodium, potassium, magnesium, and calcium—can disrupt ion balances in both muscle and nerves. This can prevent them from responding and recovering normally, and can lead to a cramp.

- Metabolic disorders that affect the energy supply in muscle. These are inherited diseases in which particular muscle enzymes are deficient. They include deficiencies of myophosphorylase (McArdle's disease), phosphorylase b kinase, phosphofructokinase, phosphoglycerate kinase, and lactate dehydrogenase.

- Myotonia. Myotonia is a condition that causes stiffness due to delayed relaxation of the muscle, but does not cause the spontaneous contraction usually associated with cramps. However, many patients with myotonia do experience cramping from exercise. Symptoms of myotonia are often worse in the cold. Myotonias include myotonic dystrophy, myotonia congenita, paramyotonia congenita, and neuromyotonia.

- Vascular disease, such as arteriosclerosis, Reynaud's disease, and diabetic vasculopathy, decreases blood flow to muscles, which can cause cramping.

- Exposure to cold can also decrease blood flow, resulting in cramping and muscle spasms.

Fasciculations may be due to **fatigue**, cold, medications, metabolic disorders, nerve damage, or neurodegenerative disease, including amyotrophic lateral sclerosis. Most people experience brief, mild fasciculations from time to time, usually in the calves.

The pain of a muscle cramp is intense, localized, and often debilitating. Coming on quickly, it may last for minutes and fade gradually. Contractures develop more slowly, over days or weeks, and may be permanent if untreated. Fasciculations may occur at rest or after muscle contraction, and may last several minutes.

Diagnosis

Abnormal contractions are diagnosed through a careful medical history, physical and neurological examination, and electromyography of the affected muscles. Electromyography records electrical activity in the muscle during rest and movement.

Treatment

Most cases of simple cramps require no medical treatment. However, because cramps hurt, a person suffering a cramp will want to stop the cramp. An effective method for stopping a cramp involves contracting the muscle that causes the opposite action of the cramping muscle. This technique requires some training and knowledge of muscular anatomy, so it may be more effective if done by a therapist. Gently and gradually stretching and massaging the affected muscle may ease the pain and hasten recovery.

A massage technique that can work is applying broad pressure on the cramping muscle. Applying ice can help if cramps persist. Fluid and salt replacement, by drinking water or properly prepared "sports drinks," and/or eating fruits and salads bearing **sodium**, **potassium**, **magnesium**, and calcium (bananas are a good source) can also help.

Cramps may be treated or prevented with gingko (*Ginkgo biloba*) or Japanese quince (*Chaenomeles speciosa*). Supplements of **vitamin B₁₂**, folate, **vitamin E**, **niacin**, calcium, and magnesium may also help. Taken at bedtime, they may help to reduce the likelihood of night cramps.

Guided imagery, relaxation, and **meditation** may all help lessen the pain associated with muscle cramps and spasms and may also dissipate the cramp or spasm.

Allopathic treatment

More prolonged or regular cramps may be treated with drugs such as carbamazepine, phenytoin, or quinine. Treatment of underlying metabolic or neurologic disease, where possible, may help relieve symptoms. Identified **anemia** can be treated with **iron** supplementation.

Prevention

The likelihood of developing cramps may be reduced by eating a healthy diet with appropriate levels of minerals, and getting regular **exercise** and adequate rest to build up energy reserves in muscle. Exercise should be accompanied by a proper stretching program. Avoiding exercising in extreme heat helps prevent heat cramps. Heat cramps can also be avoided by drinking ample amounts of water before prolonged exercise in hot weather. For intense activity over one hour, drinking fluid containing some sodium plus 4–8% carbohydrate in the form of sugars (glucose or sucrose) or starch (maltodextrin) is useful. Fluid temperature should be cool (45–55°F or 7.2–12.8°C). Taking a warm bath before bedtime may increase circulation to the legs and reduce the incidence of nighttime leg cramps.

Resources

BOOKS

Bradley, Walter G., et al. *Neurology in Clinical Practice*. 2nd ed. Woburn, MA: Butterworth-Heinemann, 1995.

PERIODICALS

Horton, John F., David M. Lindsay, and Brian R. Macintosh. "Abdominal Muscle Activation of Elite Male

Golfers with Chronic Low Back Pain." *Medicine and Science in Sports and Exercise* 33 (October 2001): 1647–1654.

Elliot Greene
Rebecca J. Frey, PhD

Music therapy

Definition

Music therapy is a technique of complementary medicine that uses music prescribed in a skilled manner by trained therapists. Programs are designed to help patients overcome physical, emotional, intellectual, and social challenges. Applications range from improving the well being of geriatric patients in nursing homes to lowering the **stress** level and **pain** of women in labor. Music therapy is used in many settings, including schools, rehabilitation centers, hospitals, hospices, nursing homes, community centers, and sometimes even in the home.

Origins

Music has been used throughout human history to express and affect human emotion. In biblical accounts, King Saul was reportedly soothed by David's harp music, and the ancient Greeks expressed thoughts

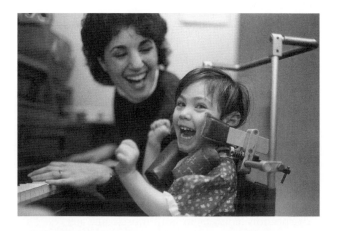

A music therapist with a disabled child. (*Abraham Menashe / Photo Researchers, Inc.*)

about music having healing effects as well. Many cultures are steeped in musical traditions. It can change mood, have stimulant or sedative effects, and alter physiologic processes such as heart rate and breathing. The apparent health benefits of music to patients in Veterans Administration hospitals following World War II lead to it being studied and formalized as a complementary healing practice. Musicians were hired to continue working in the hospitals. Degrees in music therapy became available in the late 1940s, and in 1950, the first professional association of music therapists was formed in the United States. The National Association of Music Therapy merged with the American Association of Music Therapy in 1998 to become the American Music Therapy Association.

Benefits

Music can be beneficial for anyone. Although it can be used therapeutically for people who have physical, emotional, social, or cognitive deficits, even those who are healthy can use music to relax, reduce stress, improve mood, or to accompany **exercise**. There are no potentially harmful or toxic effects other than the risk that listening to loud music poses by contributing to hearing loss. Music therapists help their patients achieve a number of goals through music, including improvement of communication, academic strengths, attention span, and motor skills. They may also assist with **behavioral therapy** and pain management.

Physical effects

Brain function physically changes in response to music. The rhythm can guide the body into breathing in slower, deeper patterns that have a calming effect. Heart rate and blood pressure are also responsive to the types of music that are listened to. The speed of the heartbeat tends to speed or slow depending on the volume and speed of the auditory stimulus. Louder and faster noises tend to raise both heart rate and blood pressure; slower, softer, and more regular tones produce the opposite result. Music can also relieve muscle tension and improve motor skills. It is often used to help rebuild physical patterning skills in rehabilitation clinics. Levels of endorphins, natural pain relievers, are increased while listening to music, and levels of stress hormones are decreased. This latter effect may partially explain the ability of music to improve immune function. A 1993 study at Michigan State University showed that even 15 minutes of exposure to music could increase interleukin-1 levels, a consequence which also heightens immunity.

Mental effects

Depending on the type and style of sound, music can either sharpen mental acuity or assist in **relaxation**. Memory and learning can be enhanced, and this used with good results in children with learning disabilities. This effect may also be partially due to increased concentration that many people have while listening to music. Better productivity is another outcome of an improved ability to concentrate. The term "Mozart effect" was coined after a study showed that college students performed better on math problems when listening to classical music.

Emotional effects

The ability of music to influence human emotion is well known, and is used extensively by moviemakers. A variety of musical moods may be used to create feelings of calmness, tension, excitement, or romance. Lullabies have long been popular for soothing babies to sleep. Music can also be used to express emotion nonverbally, which can be a very valuable therapeutic tool in some settings.

Description

Goals

Music is used to form a relationship between the therapist and the patient. The music therapist sets goals on an individual basis, depending on the reasons for treatment, and selects specific activities and exercises to help the patient progress. Objectives may include development of communication, cognitive, motor, emotional, and social skills. Some of the techniques used to achieve this are singing, listening, instrumental music, composition, creative movement, **guided imagery**, and other methods as appropriate. Other disciplines may be integrated as well, such as dance, art, and psychology. Patients may develop musical abilities as a result of therapy, but this is not a major concern. The primary aim is to improve the patient's ability to function.

Techniques

Learning to play an instrument is an excellent musical activity to develop motor skills in individuals with developmental delays, brain injuries, or other motor impairment. It is also an exercise in impulse control and group cooperation. Creative movement is another activity that can help to improve coordination, as well as strength, balance, and gait. Improvisation facilitates the nonverbal expression of emotion. It encourages socialization and communication about feelings as well. Singing develops articulation, rhythm, and breath control. Remembering lyrics and melody is an exercise in sequencing for **stroke** victims and others who may be intellectually impaired. Composition of words and music is one avenue available to assist the patient in working through fears and negative feelings. Listening is an excellent way to practice attending and remembering. It may also make the patient aware of memories and emotions that need to be acknowledged and perhaps talked about. Singing and discussion is a similar method, which is used with some patient populations to encourage dialogue. Guided Imagery and Music (GIM) is a very popular technique developed by music therapist Helen Bonny. Listening to music is used as a path to invoke emotions, picture, and symbols from the patient. This is a bridge to the exploration and expression of feelings.

Music and children

The sensory stimulation and playful nature of music can help to develop a child's ability to express emotion, communicate, and develop rhythmic movement. There is also some evidence to show that speech and language skills can be improved through the stimulation of both hemispheres of the brain. Just as with adults, appropriately selected music can decrease stress, **anxiety**, and pain. Music therapy in a hospital environment with those who are sick, preparing for surgery, or recovering postoperatively is appropriate and beneficial. Children can also experience improved self-esteem through musical activities that allow them to succeed.

Newborns may enjoy even greater benefits from music. Premature infants experience more rapid weight gain and an earlier discharge from the hospital than their peers who are not exposed to music. There is also anecdotal evidence of improved cognitive function in premature infants from listening to music.

Music and rehabilitation

Patients with brain damage from stroke, traumatic brain injury, or other neurologic conditions have been shown to exhibit significant improvement as a result of music therapy. This is theorized to be partially the result of entrainment, which is the synchronization of movement with the rhythm of the music. Consistent practice leads to gains in motor skill ability and efficiency. Cognitive processes and language skills often benefit from appropriate musical intervention.

Music and the elderly

The geriatric population can be particularly prone to anxiety and **depression**, particularly in nursing home residents. Chronic diseases causing pain are also not uncommon in this setting. Music is an excellent outlet to provide enjoyment, relaxation, relief from pain, and an opportunity to socialize and reminisce about music that has had special importance to the individual. It can have a striking effect on patients with **Alzheimer's disease**, even sometimes allowing them to focus and become more responsive for a time. Music has also been observed to decrease the agitation that is so common with this disease. One study shows that elderly people who play a musical instrument are more physically and emotionally fit as they age than their nonmusical peers.

Music and psychiatric disorders

Music can be an effective tool for treating the mentally or emotionally ill. **Autism** is one disorder that has been particularly researched. Music therapy has enabled some autistic children to relate to others and have improved learning skills. **Substance abuse**, **schizophrenia**, paranoia, and disorders of personality, anxiety, and affect are all conditions that may be benefited by music therapy. In these groups, participation and social interaction are promoted through music. Reality orientation is improved. Patients are helped to develop coping skills, reduce stress, and express their feelings.

In the treatment of psychotic disorders, however, the benefits of music therapy appear to be limited. One study of patients diagnosed with schizophrenia or schizoaffective psychosis found that while music therapy improved the patients' social relationships, these benefits were relatively short-lived.

Music and hospice care

Pain, anxiety, and depression are major concerns with patients who are terminally ill, whether they are in hospice or not. Music can provide some relief from pain, through release of endorphins and promotion of relaxation. It can also provide an opportunity for the patient to reminisce and talk about the fears that are associated with death and dying. Music may help regulate the rapid breathing of a patient who is anxious, and soothe the mind. The Chalice of Repose project, headquartered at St. Patrick Hospital in Missoula, Montana, is one organization that attends and nurtures dying patients through the use of music, in a practice they called music-thanatology by developer Therese Schroeder-Sheker. Practitioners in this program work to relieve suffering through music prescribed for the individual patient.

Music and gynecologic procedures

Research has proven that women require less pharmaceutical pain relief during labor if they make use of music. Listening to music that is familiar and associated with positive imagery is the most helpful. During early labor, music will promote relaxation. Maternal movement is helpful to get the baby into a proper birthing position and dilate the cervix. Enjoying some "music to move by" can encourage the mother to stay active for as long as possible during labor. The rhythmic auditory stimulation may also prompt the body to release endorphins, which are a natural form of pain relief. Many women select different styles of music for each stage of labor, with a more intense, or faster-moving piece feeling like a natural accompaniment to the more difficult parts of labor. Instrumental music is often preferred.

The benefits of music therapy during **childbirth** have also been shown to apply to other surgical procedures. Women who have listened to music tapes during gynecologic surgery have more restful sleep following the procedure and less postoperative soreness.

Precautions

Patients making use of music therapy should not discontinue medications or therapies prescribed by other health providers without prior consultation.

Research and general acceptance

There is little disagreement among physicians that music can be of some benefit for patients, although the extent of its effects on physical well-being is not as well acknowledged in the medical community. Acceptance of music therapy as an adjunctive treatment modality is increasing, however, due to the growing diversity of patient populations receiving music therapy. Research has shown that listening to music can decrease anxiety, pain, and recovery time. There are also good data for the specific subpopulations discussed. A therapist referral can be made through the AMTA.

Training and certification

Music therapists are themselves talented musicians; they also study the ways in which music can be applied to specific groups and circumstances. Coursework includes classes regarding music history and performance, behavioral science, and education. The American Music Therapy Association dictates what classes must be included in order for a music therapy program to be certified. There are approximately 70 colleges with approved curricula. A six-month internship follows the completion of the formal music therapy program, and the graduate is then able to take a national board exam to gain certification.

Resources

BOOKS

Campbell, Don. *The Mozart Effect*. Avon Books, 1997.

Cassileth, Barrie. *The Alternative Medicine Handbook*. W. W. Norton & Co., Inc., 1998.

Dillard, James, and Terra Ziporyn. *Alternative Medicine for Dummies*. IDG Books Worldwide, Inc., 1998.

Sears, William, and Martha Sears. *The Birth Book*. Little, Brown & Co., 1994.

Woodham, Anne, and David Peters. *Encyclopedia of Healing Therapies*. DK Publishing, Inc., 1997.

PERIODICALS

Good, M., J. C. Anderson, M. Stanton-Hicks, et al. "Relaxation and Music Reduce Pain After Gynecologic Surgery." *Pain Management Nursing* 3 (June 2002): 61-70.

Gregory, D. "Four Decades of Music Therapy Behavioral Research Designs: A Content Analysis of *Journal of Music Therapy* Articles." *Journal of Music Therapy* 39 (Spring 2002): 56-71.

Hayashi, N., Y. Tanabe, S. Nakagawa, et al. "Effects of Group Musical Therapy on Inpatients with Chronic Psychoses: A Controlled Study." *Psychiatry and Clinical Neuroscience* 56 (April 2002): 187-193.

Magee, W. L., and J. W. Davidson. "The Effect of Music Therapy on Mood States in Neurological Patients: A Pilot Study." *Journal of Music Therapy* 39 (Spring 2002): 20-29.

Robinson, A. "Music Therapy and the Effects on Laboring Women." *Kentucky Nurse* 50 (April-June 2002): 7.

Standley, J. M. "A Meta-Analysis of the Efficacy of Music Therapy for Premature Infants." *Journal of Pediatric Nursing* 17 (April 2002): 107-113.

ORGANIZATIONS

American Music Therapy Association, Inc. 8455 Colesville Road, Suite 1000 Silver Spring, ML 20910. (301) 589-3300. http://www.musictherapy.org.

The Chalice of Repose Project at St. Patrick Hospital, 312 East Pine Street, Missoula, MT 59802. (406)329-2810 Fax: (406)329-5614. http://www.saintpatrick.org/chalice/.

Judith Turner
Rebecca J. Frey, PhD

Myocardial infarction *see* **Heart attack**

Myocarditis *see* **Heart disease**

Myopia

Definition

Myopia is the medical term for nearsightedness. People with myopia see objects more clearly when they are close to the eye, while distant objects appear blurred or fuzzy. Reading and close-up work may be clear, but distance vision is blurry.

Description

Myopia affects about 30% of the population in the United States. To understand myopia it is necessary to have a basic knowledge of the main components involved in the eye's focusing system: the cornea, lens, and retina. The cornea is a tough, transparent, dome-shaped tissue that covers the front of the eye (not to be confused with the white, opaque sclera). The cornea lies in front of the iris (the colored part of the eye). The lens is a transparent, double-convex structure located behind the iris. The retina is a thin membrane that lines the rear of the eyeball. Light-sensitive retinal cells convert incoming light rays into electrical signals that are sent along the optic nerve to the brain, which then interprets the images. In people with normal vision, parallel light rays enter the eye and are bent by the cornea and lens (a process called refraction) to focus precisely on the retina, providing a crisp, clear image. In the myopic eye, the focusing power of the cornea (the major refracting structure of the eye) and the lens is too great with respect to the length of the eyeball. Light rays are bent too much, and they converge in front of the retina. This results in what is called a refractive error. In other words, an overly focused, fuzzy image is sent to the brain.

There are many types of myopia. Some common types include:

- physiologic
- pathologic
- acquired

By far the most common, physiologic myopia develops sometime between the ages of five to 10 years and gradually progresses until the eye is fully grown. This may include refractive myopia (cornea and lens-bending properties are too strong) and axial myopia (the eyeball is too long). Pathologic myopia is a far less common abnormality. This condition begins as physiologic myopia, but rather than stabilizing, the eye continues to enlarge at an abnormal rate (progressive myopia). This more advanced type of myopia may lead to degenerative changes in the eye, or degenerative myopia. Acquired myopia occurs after infancy. This condition may be seen in association with uncontrolled diabetes and certain types of **cataracts**. Antihypertensive drugs and other medications can also affect the refractive power of the lens.

Causes and symptoms

Myopia is said to be caused by an elongation of the eyeball. This means that the oblong (as opposed to normal spherical) shape of the myopic eye causes the cornea and lens to focus at a point in front of the retina. A more precise explanation is that there is an inadequate correlation between the focusing power of the cornea and lens and the length of the eye.

Myopia is considered to be primarily a hereditary disorder, meaning that it runs in families. People are generally born with a small amount of **hyperopia** (farsightedness), but as the eye grows this decreases and myopia does not become evident until later. Because of this, it is sometimes argued that myopia is not inherited, but acquired. Some eyecare professionals believe that a tendency toward myopia may be inherited, but the actual disorder results from a combination of environmental and genetic factors. Environmental factors include close work, **stress**, and eye strain.

The symptoms of myopia are blurred distance vision, eye discomfort, squinting, and eye strain.

Diagnosis

The diagnosis of myopia is typically made during the first several years of elementary school when a teacher notices a child having difficulty seeing the chalkboard, reading, or concentrating. The teacher or school nurse often recommends an eye exam by an ophthalmologist or optometrist. An ophthalmologist—M.D. or D.O. (Doctor of Osteopathy)—is a medical doctor trained in the diagnosis and treatment of eye problems. Ophthalmologists also perform eye surgery. An optometrist (O.D.) diagnoses and manages and/or treats eye and visual disorders. In many states,

KEY TERMS

Accommodation—The ability of the lens to change its focus from distant to near objects and vice versa. It is achieved through the action of the ciliary muscles that change the shape of the lens.

Cornea—The clear, dome-shaped outer covering of the eye that lies in front of the iris and pupil. The cornea lets light into the eye.

Diopter (D)—A unit of measure for describing the refractive power of a lens.

Laser-assisted in-situ keratomileusis (LASIK)—A procedure that uses a cutting tool and a laser to modify the cornea and correct moderate to high levels of myopia (nearsightedness).

Lens—The transparent, elastic, curved structure behind the iris (colored part of the eye) that helps focus light on the retina. Also refers to any device that bends light waves.

Ophthalmologist—A physician who specializes in the anatomy and physiology of the eyes and in the diagnosis and treatment of eye diseases and disorders.

Optic nerve—A bundle of nerve fibers that carries visual messages from the retina in the form of electrical signals to the brain.

Optometrist—A health care professional who examines and tests the eyes for disease and treats visual disorders by prescribing corrective lenses and/or vision therapy. In many states, optometrists are licensed to use diagnostic and therapeutic drugs to treat certain ocular diseases.

Orthokeratology—A method of reshaping the cornea using a contact lens. It is not considered a permanent method to reduce myopia.

Peripheral vision—The ability to see objects that are not located directly in front of the eye. Peripheral vision allows people to see objects located on the side or edge of their field of vision.

Photorefractive keratectomy (PRK)—A procedure that uses an excimer laser to reshape the cornea and permanently correct nearsightedness (myopia).

Radial keratotomy (RK)—A surgical procedure involving the use of a diamond-tipped blade to make several spoke-like slits in the peripheral (non-viewing) portion of the cornea to improve the focus of the eye and correct myopia by flattening the cornea.

Refraction—The turning or bending of light waves as the light passes from one medium or layer to another. In the eye it means the ability of the eye to bend light so that an image is focused onto the retina. Also used to describe the determination and measurement of the eye's focusing system by an optometrist or ophthalmologist.

Refractive eye surgery—A general term for surgical procedures that can improve or correct refractive errors of the eye by permanently changing the shape of the cornea.

Retina—The inner, light-sensitive layer of the eye containing rods and cones. The retina transforms the image it receives into electrical signals that are sent to the brain via the optic nerve.

Visual acuity—Sharpness or clearness of vision.

---

optometrists are licensed to use diagnostic and therapeutic drugs.

A patient's distance vision is tested by reading letters or numbers on a chart posted a set distance away (usually 20 ft, or 6 m). The doctor has the patient view images through a variety of lenses to obtain the best correction. The doctor also examines the inside of the eye and the retina. An instrument called a slit lamp is used to examine the cornea and lens. The eyeglass prescription is written in terms of diopters (D), which measure the degree of refractive error. Mild to moderate myopia usually falls between -1.00D and -6.00D. Normal vision is commonly referred to as 20/20 to describe the eye's focusing ability 20 ft away from an object. For example, 20/50 means that a myopic person must be 20 ft away from an eye chart to see what a normal person can see at 50 ft (15 m). The larger the bottom number, the greater the myopia.

Treatment

Nutritional therapy

The following nutritional supplements may help improve vision:

- Vitamin A: essential vitamin for healthy eyes.
- Bioflavonoids. These plant chemicals can help myopic people see better, especially at night.
- Zinc: may improve night vision.
- Ginkgo extract: increases blood supply to the eye. It may help prevent deterioration in vision.

Eye exercises

Some eye care professionals recommend exercises to help improve circulation, reduce eye strain, and relax the eye muscles. The **Bates method** is a common set of exercises. It is possible that by combining exercises with changes in behavior, the progression of myopia may be slowed or prevented. Alternative treatments include: visual therapy (also referred to as vision training or eye exercises); discontinuing close work; reducing eye strain (taking a rest break during periods of prolonged near vision tasks); and wearing bifocals to decrease the need to accommodate when doing close-up work.

Acupuncture

Acupuncture, by acting on eye muscles, causes changes in the shape of the eyeball and thus, may be able to correct nearsightedness. Approximately 10 sessions followed by daily eye exercises are needed to see significant and prolonged results.

Allopathic treatment

People with myopia have three main options for treatment: eyeglasses, contact lenses, and for those who meet certain criteria, refractive eye surgery.

Eyeglasses

Eyeglasses are the most common method used to correct myopia. Concave glass or plastic lenses are placed in frames in front of the eyes. The lenses diverge the light rays so they focus further back, directly upon the retina, producing clear distance vision.

Contact lenses

Contact lenses are a second option for treatment. Contact lenses are extremely thin round discs of plastic that are worn on the eye in front of the cornea. Contact lenses offer several benefits over glasses, including: better vision, less distortion, clear peripheral vision, and cosmetic appeal. In addition, contacts don't steam up from changes in temperature or perspiration.

Refractive eye surgery

Recommended for people who find glasses and contact lenses inconvenient and uncomfortable, refractive eye surgery improves myopic vision by permanently changing the shape of the cornea so light rays focus properly on the retina. These procedures are performed on an outpatient basis and generally take 10-30 minutes. There are three types of corrective surgeries available as of 1998: (1) radial keratotomy, (2) photorefractive keratectomy, and (3) laser-assisted in-situ keratomileusis (LASIK). Each of these surgery techniques changes rapidly in price and effectiveness. Patients should investigate the procedures and ask many questions of their doctors or others who have had the procedures before having them done.

RADIAL KERATOTOMY. Radial keratotomy (RK), the first of these procedures made available, is considered the riskiest. The surgeon uses a delicate diamond-tipped blade, a microscope, and microscopic instruments to make several spoke-like, "radial" incisions in the non-viewing (peripheral) portion of the cornea. The slits surgically alter the curve of the cornea, making it flatter, which may improve the focus of images onto the retina.

PHOTOREFRACTIVE KERATECTOMY. Photorefractive keratectomy (PRK) involves the use of a computer to measure the shape of the cornea. Using these measurements, the surgeon applies a computer-controlled laser to make modifications to the cornea. The PRK procedure flattens the cornea by vaporizing small amounts of tissue from the cornea's surface. Photorefractive keratectomy can be used to treat mild to moderate forms of myopia. The cost is approximately $2,000 per eye.

LASER-ASSISTED IN-SITU KERATOMILEUSIS. Laser-assisted in-situ keratomileusis (LASIK) is the newest of these procedures. It is recommended for moderate to severe cases of myopia. A variation on the PRK method, LASIK uses lasers and a cutting tool called a microkeratome to form a circular flap on the cornea. The flap is flipped back to expose the inner layers of the cornea. The cornea is treated with a laser to change the shape and focusing properties, then the flap is replaced.

Myopia treatments under research include corneal implants and permanent, surgically placed contact lenses.

Expected results

Glasses and contact lenses can (but not always) bring vision to 20/20. Refractive surgery can make permanent improvements for the right myopic candidate. Ophthalmologists continue to improve upon and develop new techniques to correct myopia. Alternative treatments have not been widely studied.

Prevention

Myopia is generally considered a hereditary condition, which means that it runs in families. From this perspective there is nothing that can be done to prevent this disorder. However, because the percentage of people with myopia in the United States has steadily increased over the last 50 years, some believe that the condition results from a combination of genetic and environmental factors. If this is true, then it may be possible to prevent or control myopia by reducing close work, reading and working in good light, maintaining good **nutrition**, and practicing visual therapy (when recommended). In fact, a 2002 study showed that children's **diets** high in starches may be adding to the high prevalence of myopia. Diets high in refined starches from breads and cereals increase insulin levels, which in turn affect development of the eyeball. Increasing protein consumption has been shown to slow the progression of myopia in children.

Eye strain can be prevented by using sufficient light for reading and close work, and by wearing corrective lenses as prescribed. Everyone should have regular eye exams to see if the prescription has changed or if any other problems have developed. This is particularly important for people with high (degenerative) myopia who may be at a greater risk of developing retinal detachments or other problems.

Resources

BOOKS

Birnbaum, Martin H. *Optometric Management of Nearpoint Vision Disorders*. Boston: Butterworth-Heinemann, 1993.

Curtin, Brian J. *The Myopias: Basic Science and Clinical Management*. Philadelphia: Harper & Row, 1985.

Rosanes-Berrett, Marilyn B. *Do You Really Need Eyeglasses?* Barrytown, NY: Station Hill Press, 1990.

The Burton Goldberg Group. "Vision Disorders." *Alternative Medicine: The Definitive Guide*. Tiburon, CA: Future Medicine Publishing, Inc., 1999.

"Vision Disorders." *Reader's Digest Guide to Medical Cures & Treatments*. Canada: The Reader's Digest Association, Inc., 1996.

Zinn, Walter J., and Herbert Solomon. *Complete Guide to Eyecare, Eyeglasses, and Contact Lenses*. Hollywood, FL: Lifetime Books, 1996.

PERIODICALS

Carey, Benedict. "Goodbye Glasses: New Surgery Can Deliver Sharp Vision to the Nearsighted-Without a Single Cut of the Scalpel (Photorefractive Keratotomy)." *Health* 10 (September 1996): 46.

"Catching Your Eye (Photorefractive Keratotomy Evaluation.)" *People's Medical Society Newsletter* 15 (August 1996): 6.

Fox, Douglas. "Blinded by Bread: Are Diets High in Starch Making Kids Short-Sighted?." *New Scientist* (April 6, 2002): 9–11.

"Insight on Eyesight: Seven Vision Myths: Blind Spots About Vision Can Cause Needless Worry, Wasted Effort, and Unnecessary Treatment." *Consumer Reports on Health* 9 (April 1997): 42.

"9 Ways to Look Better: If You Want to Improve Your Vision—Or Just Protect What You Have—Try These Eye Opening Moves." *Men's Health* 13 (Jan.-Feb. 1998): 50.

Schwartz, Leslie. "Visionquest (Use of Lasers in Treatment of Nearsightedness or Myopia)." *Shape* 16 (March 1997): 28.

ORGANIZATIONS

American Academy of Ophthalmology. P.O. Box 7424, San Francisco, CA 94120-7424. (415) 561-8500. http://www.eyenet.org.

American Optometric Association. 243 N. Lindbergh Blvd., St. Louis, MO 63141. (314) 991-4100. http://www.aoanet.org.

Myopia International Research Foundation. 1265 Broadway, Room 608, New York, NY 10001. (212) 684-2777.

National Eye Institute. NIH Bldg. 31, 9000 Rockville Pike, Bethesda, MD 20892. (301) 496-5248. http://www.nei.nih.gov.

Mai Tran
Teresa G. Odle

Myotherapy

Definition

Myotherapy is a method intended to relieve **pain**, and is based on the application of pressure at trigger points throughout the body. Trigger points are defined as hypersensitive locations in the muscles that cause pain in response to undue **stress**. They may be caused by occupational or other injuries as well as by disease, physical stress, and emotional stress. Trigger points rarely occur in the same location where the pain is felt. Myotherapy is founded on the notion that relief of tension in the muscle followed by revitalization of the relieved muscle through stretching, promotes healing and reduces the disposition of the muscle and the nerve to cause further pain.

Origins

Myotherapy developed out of trigger-point therapy, a method of pain relief developed by Dr. Janet Travell. Fitness expert Bonnie Prudden built on Travell's method to investigate certain parallels that she perceived between the injection of pain relievers into nerve locations in trigger-point therapy and the potential to relieve pain similarly through external physical pressure on the nerve points. She spent approximately four years investigating and experimenting with the idea. During that time, she studied anatomy and developed a new pain-relief therapy that she named myotherapy. Its name is derived from the Greek prefix "myo," meaning muscle. Within 10 years, she had established a certified training program for myotherapy technicians.

Benefits

Myotherapy is claimed to be effective in eliminating 95 percent of all physical pain associated with muscular discomfort and to be successful in patients suffering from many types of head, back, and **neck pain**. It is also used to relieve the discomfort of **carpal tunnel syndrome**, **fibromyalgia**, and arthritis, and to reduce swelling in patients who have **multiple sclerosis**.

In addition, some athletes seek myotherapy to experience enhanced physical performance.

Description

Myotherapy is used to eliminate pain and swelling through the application of pressure at strategically located nerve sites called trigger points. Unlike many other techniques to alleviate **muscle spasms**, myotherapy is not based on topical or internal medication.

Myotherapy treatment is a two-step process. The therapist first locates and diffuses the trigger points of pain by applying pressure to those locations. This process is designed to relieve the pain and also to relax the muscles associated with the specific discomfort. Secondly, the patient undergoes a series of exercises during the therapy session to progressively stretch the muscles that have been relaxed by the pressure therapy. Therapy generally continues for fewer than 10 sessions.

The age of the patient who undergoes myotherapy is significant only in determining the number of trigger points that might cause muscle pain. Because practitioners believe trigger points accumulate over time, they expect older patients to usually have developed more trigger points.

Preparations

As with most treatments, patients should have a physical examination done by a qualified doctor or technician before undergoing this pain-relief technique. Patients should seek clearance for treatment from a general practitioner (M.D.), osteopath (D.O.), doctor of podiatric medicine (D.P.M.), doctor of **chiropractic** (D.C.), doctor of **naturopathic medicine** (N.M.D.), registered nurse practitioner (R.N.P.), or physical therapist (P.T.) before myotherapy treatment. Patients

---

KEY TERMS

Trigger points—Hypersensitive muscle locations that cause pain in response to undue stress.

---

who undergo myotherapy to relieve the discomfort of **temporomandibular joint syndrome** (TMJ) or other facial pain should consult a dentist (D.D.S.) for a clearance examination. Preparatory examination is necessary to determine that no structural anatomical problem is causing the pain, because problems of this nature require medical treatment that cannot be replaced by myotherapy.

To benefit fully from myotherapy, adherents note that the patient should have a positive attitude and willingness to give up any emotional investment in the pain syndrome. They assert that myotherapy requires full commitment to the therapy sessions and an attitude of self-healing to bring about relief.

Precautions

To facilitate recuperation from pain relief, myotherapy patients are advised to involve a relative, friend, or other trusted acquaintance who can learn the technique as well as the patient's personal pressure points. This buddy system allows the patient to renew the effects of the myotherapy sessions in the event of a relapse.

Side effects

Myotherapy has no known side effects. For anatomical pathology patients, however, medical attention is necessary before seeking myotherapy treatment. This examination is crucial in order to eliminate any physical abnormalities that may be the source of the patient's discomfort.

Athletes who gain enhanced performance following myotherapy may consider the improvement a positive side effect.

Research and general acceptance

Many myotherapists operate as self-employed practitioners in private clinics. In addition, certified myotherapists hold positions in hospitals, doctors' offices, dental offices, and clinics.

Training and certification

Certified myotherapists undergo a two-year program of education and training in preparation for certification. After the completion of the training

BONNIE PRUDDEN (1914-)

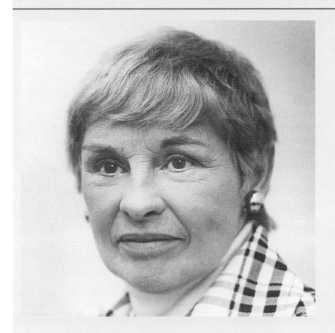

(AP/Wide World Photos. Reproduced by permission.)

Fitness expert Bonnie Prudden was born on January 29, 1914, in New York City. She attended Columbia University Extension School, Grand Central School of Art, and Weidman-Humphrey School of Dance. Prudden served as the director of both the ski patrol and Red Cross disaster units in New York State from 1939–1949. She founded and directed the Institute for Physical Fitness in White Plains, New York in 1950.

Prudden came to the attention of the American public in 1955 after she used the Kraus-Weber test to assess the physical fitness levels of children worldwide. Prudden's test results revealed that 58% of American children were unfit and scored worse than the children of underdeveloped nations. She presented her test results to President Dwight Eisenhower, and her actions ultimately inspired what has come to be called the President's Council on Physical Fitness and Sport.

During the era before videotape, Prudden released six exercise recordings and authored 19 books on fitness. She hosted the first nationally televised exercise show and established physical fitness programs at schools, hospitals, and other institutions. Prudden, the mother of two daughters, was credited with inventing the first pre- and post-natal exercise programs for women. Additionally, over 500,000 babies learned rudimentary water skills as a result of her mother and baby, swim and gym classes.

Prudden altered her focus in 1976 when she discovered the theory of myotherapy, the use of applying pressure to trigger points in the body to lessen muscle spasms and pain and to improve circulation. In 1979, after some investigation, she established the Bonnie Prudden Two-year School of Physical Fitness and Myotherapy. She explained the basics of myotherapy in her 1980 book, *Pain Erasure,* and later published *Bonnie Prudden's Complete Guide to Pain-Free Living,* followed by *Fitness Guide for the After 50 Crowd.* Additionally she presented seminars on the topic.

Bonnie Prudden has received many honors, including a Safety Award from Eastern Amateur Ski Association and a Service to Youth Award from Young Men's Christian Association.

regimen, the candidate must pass a board examination in order to receive official recognition as a Certified Bonnie Prudden Myotherapist. The training sessions total 1,300 hours prior to the board-certification examination. To retain myotherapist credentials, a program of continuing education involving 45 hours of enrichment and update training on a bi-annual basis is required.

Resources

BOOKS

Prudden, Bonnie. *Pain Erasure.* New York: M. Evans and Company, Inc., 2002.

Davies, Clair and Amber Davies. *The Trigger Point Therapy Workbook: Your Self-Treatment Guide for Pain Relief.* Second edition. Oakland, CA: New Harbinger Publications, 2004.

ORGANIZATIONS

Bonnie Prudden Myotherapy(r). P.O. Box 65240. Tucson, AZ 85728. (800)221-4634. http://www.bonnieprudden.com (accessed February 15, 2008).

Gloria Cooksey
Leslie Mertz, Ph.D.

Myrrh

Description

Myrrh (*Commiphora molmol,C. abyssinica,* or *C. myrrha*) is a close relative and member of the Burseraceae family, native to the eastern Mediterranean, Ethiopia, the Arabian peninsula, and Somalia. Myrrh

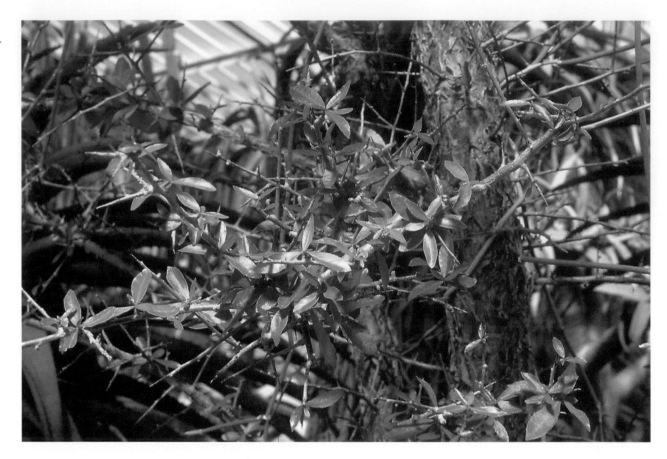

Myrrh. *(©PlantaPhile, Germany. Reproduced by permission.)*

is a shrubby desert tree known variously as gum, myrrh tree, guggal gum, guggal resin, didin, and didthin. Myrrh is an Arabic word meaning bitter. The highly valued aromatic gum resin of myrrh has a bitter, pungent taste and a sweet, pleasing aroma. A particularly treasured variety of myrrh is known as *karam* or Turkish myrrh.

Myrrh grows to a height of about 9 ft (2.7 m). The light gray trunk is thick and the main branches are knotted with smaller branches protruding at a right angle and ending in sharp spines. The hairless, roughly toothed leaves are divided into one pair of small, oval leaflets with a larger, terminal leaflet. The yellow-red flowers grow on stalks in an elongated and branching cluster. The small brown fruit is oval, tapering to a point.

During the time of the Egyptian pharaoh Thutmose III, around the fifteenth century B.C., the pharaoh's aunt, Queen Hatshepsut, sent an expedition to Africa and the "Land of Punt" where myrrh trees were abundant. The Queen wanted to please the god Amon by surrounding his temple with living myrrh trees. The

mission was successful and the story of the expedition was depicted on the walls of the temple built to enclose the Queen's tomb. According to legend Queen Hatshepsut was promised "life, stability and satisfaction . . . forever" by the well-pleased god, and the revered myrrh tree was introduced to the Egyptian people.

Myrrh has been used since ancient times in incense, perfumes, and holy ointments. The Egyptians used myrrh in embalming compounds and burned pellets of myrrh to repel fleas. Archeological evidence indicates that myrrh was carried in small pouches that wealthy persons hung around the neck for fragrance. The Ebers Papyrus, believed to have been found in the necropolis outside Thebes, provides evidence of Egyptian medicinal use of myrrh. This ancient document contains as many as 800 medicinal recipes using such plants as myrrh, **peppermint**, **aloe**, **castor oil**, and numerous other herbs in common use today. Myrrh was mentioned in the bible as a component of the bitter solution offered to the crucified Jesus during Roman times. The herb was traditionally mixed with wine and offered to prisoners prior to execution to ease **pain**.

The use of myrrh medicinally was recorded in China in A.D. 600 during the Tang Dynasty. Myrrh is used today in Chinese medicine to treat **wounds**, relieve painful swelling, and to treat menstrual pain due to blood stagnation. Myrrh is called *mo yao* in China.

Myrrh was a highly valued commodity for commerce on ancient spice routes, and is woven into legend and myth. In Syrian legend the myrrh tree is named for the daughter of Thesis, a Syrian king. She was transformed by the gods into a myrrh tree to escape her father's murderous wrath.

General use

Myrrh is the sweet-smelling oleo-gum resin that naturally exudes from wounds or **cuts** in the stems and bark of several species of this shrubby desert tree. This sap forms a thick, pale yellow paste as it seeps out. It then hardens into a mass about the size of a walnut, taking on a reddish-brown color. The volatile oil contained in the resin consists of sesquiterpenes, triterpenes, and mucilage. The tannin content gives myrrh its astringent action. Powdered myrrh has been endorsed by the German advisory Commission E as a beneficial treatment for mild inflammations in the throat and mouth. Myrrh acts as a broad-spectrum antiseptic and can be applied directly to sores and wounds.

Taken internally in tincture or capsule form, myrrh is a beneficial treatment for loose teeth, gingivitis, and bad breath. The tincture may also be applied directly to a tooth to relieve tooth ache. It is antifungal, and has been used to treat **athlete's foot** and candida. Some research indicates that myrrh is effective in reducing **cholesterol** levels. It is a tonic remedy said to relax smooth muscles, increase peristaltic action, and stimulate gastric secretions. The myrrh resin has antimicrobial properties and acts to stimulate macrophage activity in the blood stream. The herb is being studied for its potential as an anticancer medication. Taken internally in tincture or capsule form, myrrh is useful for relieving gastric distress and as an expectorant, though this folk application has not been confirmed by experimental evidence. Myrrh is burned as incense and used to repel mosquitoes. It is also a component in healing salves used in veterinary medicine. In Chinese medicine, it is used for wounds, **bruises**, and bleeding.

Preparations

Myrrh is available in capsule, powder, and tincture form. It is pulverized into powder, and prepared as a tincture. It is found combined with other ingredients in dental powders, mouthwash preparations, and toothpaste. Myrrh is used as fragrance in cosmetics, perfumes, and soaps, and as flavoring in foods.

Tincture: Four ounces of powdered myrrh are combined with 1 pt of brandy, gin, or vodka in a glass container, with enough alcohol to cover the herb. A 50/50 ratio of alcohol to water is generally recommended. The mixture should be placed away from light for about two weeks, and shaken several times each day. Strain and store in a tightly capped, dark glass bottle. A standard dose is 1 or 2 ml of the tincture three times a day.

Essential oil: Myrrh's essential oil is pale yellow to amber in color. It is obtained by steam distillation. The essential oil is commercially available from numerous sources. It is said to be beneficial when used as a chest rub to treat **bronchitis**, and externally in diluted form on ulcers and wounds.

Gargle: One teaspoon of dry, powdered myrrh should be combined with 1 tsp of boric acid. One pint of boiling water is poured over the mixture and steeped for 30 minutes, then strained. This mixture is a good gargle preparation, according to herbalist John Lust.

Precautions

Myrrh should be avoided during **pregnancy** and should not be administered to children. It should be kept away from the eyes and mucous membranes and out of children's reach.

Side effects

According to the *PDR For Herbal Medicine*, "No health hazards or side effects are known in conjunction with the proper administration of designated therapeutic dosages."

Interactions

No interactions are reported.

Resources

BOOKS
Elias, Jason, and Shelagh Ryan Masline. *The A to Z Guide to Healing Herbal Remedies.* Lynn Sonberg Book Associates, 1996.
Foster, Steven and James A. Duke. *Peterson Field Guides, Eastern/Central Medicinal Plants.* Boston-New York: Houghton Mifflin Company, 1990.
Kowalchik, Claire, and William H. Hylton. *Rodale's Illustrated Encyclopedia of Herbs.* Pennsylvania: Rodale Press, 1987.

Lust, John. *The Herb Book*. NY: BantamBooks, 1974.
Magic And Medicine of Plants. The Reader's Digest Association, Inc. 1986.
Ody, Penelope. *The Complete Medicinal Herbal*. New York: Dorling Kindersley, 1993.
PDR for Herbal Medicines. New Jersey: Medical Economics Company, 1998.
Tyler, Varro E., Ph.D. *The Honest Herbal*. New York: Pharmaceutical Products Press, 1993.

OTHER

"Myrrh Essential Oil for Aromatherapy." *Nature's Sunshine Products*. http://www.herbs4u.com/oils_myrrh.html.

Mrs. M. Grieve. "A Modern Herbal, Myrrh." *Botanical. com*. http://ww.botanical.com/botanical/mgmh/m/myrrh-66.html.
"Myrrh (Commiphora molmol)." *MotherNature.com*. http://ww.mothernature.com/ency/Herb/Myrrh.asp.
"Bridges for Peace." *Gold, Frankincense, and Myrrh*. http://www.serve.com/Bridges/dfjevery1295.htm.

Clare Hanrahan

Myrtle *see* **Periwinkle**

Nail problems *see* **Ingrown nail**

Narcolepsy

Definition

Narcolepsy is a neurological disorder characterized by uncontrollable episodes of sleepiness during the day. Episodes can last from a few seconds to more than an hour and can significantly interfere with daily activities.

Description

People with narcolepsy often fall asleep suddenly, anywhere at any time, even in the middle of a conversation. They may sleep for just a few seconds or for up to a half hour, and then reawaken feeling alert until they fall asleep again. The condition affects 135,000 Americans. **Sleep apnea** (difficulty in breathing while sleeping) is the leading cause of excessive daytime sleepiness. Narcolepsy is the second leading cause.

The attacks of sleepiness that are the hallmark of this condition may be mildly inconvenient or deeply disturbing. Some people continue to function during the sleep episodes, even talking and putting things away, but will reawaken with no memory of what they had been doing while briefly asleep.

Narcolepsy is related to the dreaming part of sleep known as rapid eye movement (REM) sleep. Normally, people fall asleep for about 90 minutes of non-REM sleep followed by REM sleep. However, people with narcolepsy enter REM sleep immediately; then, after reawakening, REM sleep recurs inappropriately throughout the day.

Causes and symptoms

Scientists believe narcolepsy is caused by a deficiency of the brain cells that make a substance called hypocretin; genetics are a factor in the condition, as well. Hypocretin, which is secreted by the hypothalamus, is responsible for enhancing wakefulness. Researchers are unsure why the hypocretin-secreting neurons are destroyed in some individuals; one possibility is that a person's immune system is a factor.

Cross-ethnic studies indicate significant variations in the prevalence of narcolepsy in different countries, with the Japanese having a very high rate and Israeli Jews one of the lowest in the world. One study of five European countries found that the prevalence of narcolepsy is higher in the United Kingdom and Germany than in Italy, Portugal, and Spain.

In the late 1990s, three independent research groups discovered a neuropeptide system in the hypothalamus, a gland in the brain that regulates body temperature and appetite. The discovered system, which was called the hypocretinergic system, regulates sleep and wakefulness. The nerve cells, or neurons, in this part of the hypothalamus secrete substances known as hypocretins or orexins, which regulate the sleep/wake cycle in humans. There are two of these compounds, known as orexin-A and orexin-B, or as hypocretin-1 and hypocretin-2. As of 2002, narcolepsy was thought to be an orexin deficiency syndrome; that is, it develops when a person's hypothalamus does not secrete enough orexins to keep the person from falling asleep at inappropriate times. Samples of cerebrospinal fluid taken from patients with narcolepsy contain little or no orexins. MRI scans of these patients indicate that there is some loss of brain tissue in the hypothalamus itself, suggesting that the neurons responsible for secreting orexins have died.

Symptoms of narcolepsy typically appear during adolescence; however, studies have shown that they may also begin in childhood. The disorder itself may not be diagnosed for many years after the first appearance of symptoms. The primary symptom is an overwhelming feeling of **fatigue**, together with sleep attacks that may occur with or without warning. About 75% of patients also experience cataplexy, a sudden loss of muscle control lasting a few seconds to 30 minutes resulting in physical collapse without any loss of consciousness. Episodes of narcolepsy can be triggered by emotions such as laughter, fear, or anger. Other symptoms include sleep paralysis and hypnogogic (vivid) hallucinations as the person wakes up or falls asleep. Some patients may also have trouble staying asleep at night.

Diagnosis

If a person has both excessive daytime sleepiness and cataplexy, narcolepsy can be diagnosed on the basis of patient history alone. Lab tests, however, can confirm a diagnosis. Tests at a **sleep disorders** clinic include an overnight polysomnogram (sleep monitored with electrocardiography, video, and respiratory parameters) followed by a multiple sleep latency test, which measures sleep onset and how quickly REM sleep occurs. In narcolepsy, sleep latency is usually less than five minutes. First REM period latency is also abnormally short.

A genetic blood test can reveal certain antigens in people who have a tendency to develop narcolepsy. Positive blood test results suggest, but do not prove, the existence of narcolepsy.

As of 2002, the diagnosis of narcolepsy could be confirmed by taking a sample of the patient's cerebrospinal fluid by a spinal tap and testing it for the presence of hypocretin-1. Patients with narcolepsy have no hypocretin-1 in their spinal fluid.

Treatment

Several short naps scheduled throughout the day may help relieve some of the sleepiness associated with narcolepsy. The botanical remedy **yohimbe** (*Pausinystalia yohimbe*) may also be useful in promoting alertness. As with any herbal preparation or medication, individuals should check with their healthcare professional before taking the remedy to treat narcolepsy.

Allopathic treatment

Patients can be treated with amphetamine-like stimulant drugs (Dexedrine) to control drowsiness and sleep attacks. The symptoms of abnormal REM sleep (cataplexy, sleep paralysis, and hypnogogic hallucinations) are treated with antidepressants.

In the 2000s nonamphetamine wake-promoting drugs were available to treat narcolepsy. These medications lack the unpleasant side effects of amphetamines, particularly jitteriness and **anxiety**. Modafinil (Provigil) is the most commonly prescribed of the psychostimulants. Modafinil is believed to stimulate the

---

KEY TERMS

Cataplexy—A symptom of narcolepsy in which there is a sudden episode of muscle weakness triggered by emotions. The muscle weakness may cause the person's knees to buckle or the head to drop. In severe cases, the patient may become paralyzed for a few seconds to minutes.

Hypnogogic hallucinations—Dream-like auditory or visual hallucinations that occur while falling asleep.

Hypocretins—Chemicals secreted in the hypothalamus that regulate the sleep/wake cycle.

Hypothalamus—A gland in the forebrain that controls heartbeat, body temperature, thirst, hunger, body temperature and pressure, blood sugar levels, and other functions.

Orexin—Another name for hypocretin, a chemical secreted in the hypothalamus that regulates the sleep/wake cycle. Narcolepsy is sometimes described as an orexin deficiency syndrome.

Sleep paralysis—An abnormal episode of sleep in which the patient cannot move for a few minutes, usually occurring on falling asleep or waking up. Often found in patients with narcolepsy.

---

neurons in the brain that are responsible for a person's wakefulness.

Patients who do not like taking high doses of stimulants may choose to nap every couple of hours to relieve daytime sleepiness and take smaller doses of stimulants.

Expected results

Narcolepsy can be a devastating disease that impairs a person's ability to work, play, and engage in meaningful activities. In severe cases, an inability to work and drive can interfere with daily life, leading to **depression** and a loss of independence. Drug treatments can ease symptoms but will not cure the disease. Narcolepsy is not a degenerative disease, and patients are not expected to develop new neurologic symptoms. Lifespan is normal if common sense is exercised regarding such hazards as automobile accidents.

Resources

PERIODICALS

Chen, Infei. "From Faithful Dogs and Difficult Fish: Insight into Narcolepsy." *New York Times* (October 23, 2007).

ORGANIZATIONS

Narcolepsy Network, 10921 Reed Hartman Highway, Cincinnati, OH, 45242, (513) 891-3522, http://www.web sciences.org/narnet/.

National Sleep Foundation, 1522 K St. NW, Suite 500, Washington, DC, 20005, (202)347-3471, http://www sleepfoundation.org.

Stanford Center for Narcolepsy, Stanford University School of Medicine, 701-B Welch Rd., Room 146, Palo Alto, CA, 94304, (650) 725-6517, http://www-med.stanford. edu/school/Psychiatry/narcolepsy.

Paula Ford-Martin
Rebecca J. Frey, PhD
Rhonda Cloos, RN

> ## KEY TERMS
>
> **Medicine bundle**—A leather bag or animal skin in which a Native American healer carries herbs, stones, and various ritual objects as a sign of his or her healing powers.
>
> **Peyote**—One of the dried tops of the mescal cactus. Peyote contains mescaline, a hallucinogen that is sometimes used in Native American healing ceremonies.
>
> **Shaman**—In certain indigenous tribes or groups, a person who acts as an intermediary between the natural and supernatural worlds. Shamans are regarded as having the power or ability to cure illnesses.

Native American medicine

Definition

According to Ken "Bear Hawk" Cohen, "Native American medicine is based on widely held beliefs about healthy living, the repercussions of disease-producing behavior, and the spiritual principles that restore balance." These beliefs are shared by all tribes; however, the methods of diagnosis and treatment vary greatly from tribe to tribe and healer to healer.

Origins

The healing traditions of Native Americans have been practiced in North America since at least 12,000 years ago and possibly as early as 40,000 years ago. Although the term Native American medicine implies that there is a standard system of healing, there are approximately 500 nations of indigenous people in North America, each representing a diverse wealth of healing knowledge, rituals, and ceremonies.

Many aspects of Native American healing have been kept secret and are not written down. The traditions are passed down by word of mouth from elders, from the spirits in vision quests, and through initiation. It is believed that sharing healing knowledge too readily or casually will weaken the spiritual power of the medicine.

There are, however, many Native American healers who recognize that writing down their healing practices is a way to preserve these traditions for future generations. Many also believe that sharing their healing ways and values may help all people to come into a healthier balance with nature and all forms of life.

Benefits

Native American medicine can benefit anyone who sincerely wishes to live a life of wholeness and balance. These benefits may be physical, emotional, or spiritual. There is, however, the understanding that "the diseases of civilization," or white man's diseases, often need white man's medicine. In those cases, Native American medicine can be an important part of an integrative approach to healing. For example, the most successful programs for treating alcohol addiction in Native communities have combined Western approaches to psychological counseling, social work, and traditional Native American healing practices.

Such inherited conditions as birth defects or retardation are not easily treatable with Native American medicine. Native healers also believe that some illnesses are the result of a patient's behavior. Sometimes they will not treat a person because they do not want to interfere with the life lessons the patient needs to learn. Other illnesses are not treated because they are "callings" or initiation diseases. Native healer Medicine Grizzly Bear Lake explains, "The calling comes in the form of a dream, accident, sickness, injury, disease, near-death experience, or even actual death."

Description

Native American medicine is based upon a spiritual view of life. A healthy person is someone who has a sense of purpose and follows the guidance of the Great Spirit. This guidance is written upon the heart of every person. To be healthy, a person must be committed to a path of beauty, harmony, and balance. Gratitude, respect, and generosity are also considered to be essential for a healthy life. Ken Cohen writes, "Health means restoring the body, mind, and spirit to balance and wholeness: the balance of life energy in the body; the balance of ethical, reasonable, and just behavior; balanced relations within family and community; and harmonious relationships with nature."

Theories of disease causation and even the names of diseases vary from tribe to tribe. Diseases may be thought to have internal or external causes or sometimes both. According to Cherokee medicine man Rolling Thunder, negative thinking is the most important internal cause of disease. Negative thinking includes not only negative thoughts about oneself but also feelings of shame, blame, low self-esteem, greed, despair, worry, **depression**, anger, jealousy, and self-centeredness. Johnny Moses, a Nootka healer, says "No evil sorcerer can do as much harm to you as you can do to yourself."

Diseases have external causes too. "Germs are also spirits," according to Shabari Bird of the Lakota Nation. A person is particularly susceptible to harmful germs if they live an imbalanced life, have a weak constitution, engage in negative thinking, or are under a lot of **stress**. Other people or spirits may also be responsible for an illness. Another external source of disease is environmental poisons. These poisons include alcohol, impure air, water, and some types of food.

Native American healers believe that disease can also be caused by physical, emotional, or spiritual trauma. These traumas can lead to mental and emotional distress, loss of soul, or loss of spiritual power. In these cases the healer must use ritual and other ways to physically return the soul and power to the patient. Some diseases are caused when people break the "rules for living." These rules may include ways of showing respect for animals, people, places, ritual objects, events, or spirits.

Native American healers have several different techniques for diagnosing an illness. These may include a discussion of one's symptoms, personal and family history, observation of non-verbal cues like posture or tone of voice, and medical divination. More important than the particular technique is the healer's intuition, sensitivity, and spiritual power.

There is no typical Native American healing session. Methods of healing include **prayer**, chanting, music, smudging (burning **sage** or aromatic woods), herbs, laying-on of hands, massage, counseling, imagery, **fasting**, harmonizing with nature, dreaming, sweat lodges, taking hallucinogens (e.g., peyote), developing inner silence, going on a shamanic journey, and ceremony. Family and community are also important in many healing sessions. Sometimes healing

happens quickly. Sometimes a long period of time is needed for healing. The intensity of the therapy is considered to be more important than the length of time required. Even if the healing happens quickly, however, a change in life style is usually required in order to make the healing last.

A medicine bundle may also be used in Native American healing. The medicine bundle is a bag made of leather or an animal pelt in which the healer carries an assortment of ritual objects, charms, herbs, stones, and other healing paraphernalia. The bundle is a concrete token of the medicine power that the spirits have given the healer, either for healing in general or for healing a particular illness. The bundles vary according to clan, tribe, and individual.

Native American medicine is not covered by insurance unless perhaps the practitioner is a licensed health care provider. Most Native healers do not charge a set fee for their services. Healing is considered to be "a gift from the Great Spirit." Gifts to the healer are welcomed, however. The offering of a gift "ensures success of treatment because healing spirits appreciate generosity." Gifts may include groceries, cloth, money, or another personal expression of respect and appreciation. Frequently the only gift that is required is a pouch of tobacco.

Preparations

The medicine person tells the patient what preparations are necessary before the healing ceremony.

Precautions

A medicine person is essential to ensure safe healing through Native American medicine. People with **hypertension** should watch themselves during a sweat lodge ceremony for a possible increase in blood pressure. People with **asthma** may have difficulty when sage or cedar is used in a ceremony. People who are claustrophobic may find the close, hot, dark environment of a sweat lodge overwhelming.

Side effects

Some herbs may cause **vomiting**, **nausea**, or **diarrhea**. From the Native American point of view these reactions are usually welcomed and considered a form of purging or cleansing of the physical body.

Research and general acceptance

There has been no formal scientific research conducted on Native American healing practices. Medicine people do not write down their practices out of fear that they might be misused by people who are not trained in their sacred ways. The most prominent users of this form of medicine are Native Americans or others who want a spiritually based approach to medicine.

Training and certification

Native American medicine has been passed down by word of mouth for thousands of years. Healing power can come from one's ancestors, another healer, or through training and initiation. Generally, healers train under one primary mentor. Today, however, with the ease of long-distance travel and communication, many healers have several mentors. Training as a medicine person is a long process that requires strength, sacrifice and patience. Denet Tsosi, a Navajo medicine man, said that it took him six years to learn one of the chants.

Resources

BOOKS

Beck,P. V., and A. L. Walters. *The Sacred: Ways of Knowledge, Sources of Life.* Tsaile (Navajo Nation), AZ: Navajo Community College Press, 1977.

Cohen, Ken. *Honoring the Medicine: Native American Healing.* New York: Ballantine, 1999.

Cohen, Ken "Bear Hawk". "Native American Medicine." In *Essentials of Complementary and Alternative Medicine,* ed.Wayne B. Jonas, M.D. and Jeffrey S. Levin, Ph.D, M.P.H. New York: Lippincott Williams and Wilkins, 1999.

Krippner, Stanley, and P. Welch. *Spiritual Dimensions of Healing.* New York: Irvington Publishers, 1992.

Lyon, William S. *Encyclopedia of Native American Healing.* New York: W. W. Norton and Co., 1998.

Mehl-Madrona, Lewis, M.D. *Coyote Medicine: Lessons from Native American Healing.* New York: Fireside, 1997.

Nauman, Eileen. "Native American Medicine". In *Clinician's Complete Reference to Complementary and Alternative Medicine,* ed. Donald W. Novey, M.D. St. Louis, MO: Mosby, 2000.

ORGANIZATIONS

American Indian Science and Engineering Society (AISES). 5661 Airport Blvd. Boulder, CO 80301-2339. (303) 939-0023. Fax: (303) 939-8150. aisehq@spot.colorado.edu. http://www.colorado.edu/aises.

The Buffalo Trust. P.O. Box 89. Jemez Springs, NM 87025-0089. (505) 829-3635. Fax: (505) 829-3450. natachee@aol.com.

Cultural Survival. 96 Mount Auburn St. Cambridge, MA 02138. (617) 441-5400. Fax (617) 441-5417. csinc@cs. org. http://www.cs.org.

Dine College, Office of Continuing Education. P.O. Box 731. Tuba City, AZ 86045. (520) 283-6321. Fax (520) 283-4590. nccce@crystal.ncc.cc.nm.us.

Linda Chrisman

Natrum muriaticum

Description

Natrum muriaticum is the homeopathic remedy commonly known as table salt or **sodium** chloride. Salt is the second most common substance in nature, water being the first. Salt is an important component in regulating the balance of body fluids. Salt is a constituent in both body fluids and tissues. Excessive salt intake inhibits proper absorption of nutrients and weakens the nervous system, while a lack of salt creates a lack of fluid, resulting in an emaciated and withered appearance.

Salt was not extensively used for medicinal purposes until the time of Samuel Hahnemann, the father of **homeopathy**. While ancient physicians did employ salt in the treatment of liver enlargement and other swellings,

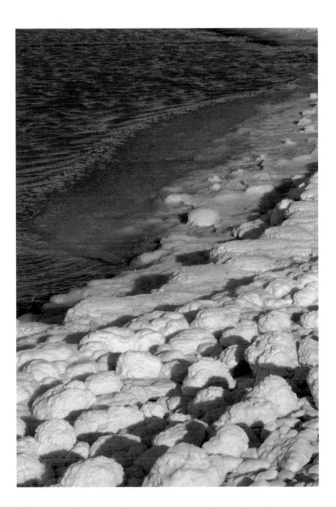

Natrum muriaticum, also known as sodium chloride, seen here as crystallized salt deposits beside China's Dead Sea, Xinjiang. (© *Natural Visions / Alamy*)

salt had little medicinal value until Hahnemann's studies of the remedy in the early nineteenth century.

Natrum muriaticum (*Nat. mur.*) is a slow acting remedy that responds well to chronic ailments. It is seldom prescribed for acute conditions, and then only when symptoms specific to the remedy are present. This polychrest is a very powerful and deep acting remedy and makes long lasting changes, often continuing to bring about results for several years.

Nat. mur. increases production of red blood cells and albumin, a protein found in animal and vegetable tissues. It does not cure by supplying the amount of salt that the body needs, but acts to alter and restore the tissues of the body so they can assimilate the body's needs for salt from food. By bringing the body into a state of health, *Nat. mur.* reduces the patient's susceptibility to colds, fevers, and other ailments.

General use

Nat. mur. ailments typically come about as a result of emotional excitement, trauma, bad news, grief, disappointed love, fright, suppression of emotions, sexual excess, and head injuries. Exposure to the sun and intake of alcohol or salt may also cause *Nat. mur.* ailments. These conditions may weaken the immune system and create illness.

This remedy is frequently indicated in emaciated persons, teething children, persons who are congested and catch cold easily, the elderly, or awkward, pubescent girls who suffer from headaches and menstrual irregularities. *Nat. mur.* children are frequently serious. They dislike excessive physical contact and hate to be teased. These children often have frightening dreams about being robbed.

Nat. mur. is indicated when the following remedy picture is present. The patient's face is pale and waxy and her body has an emaciated appearance. Her face and hair may be oily, while the lips and corners of the mouth are dry and cracked. She is weak, both in body and mind, and is absent-minded and forgetful. The mucous from bodily discharges has the constituency of egg whites. A craving for salty, sour, or bitter foods is present, as is an aversion to bread, fats, or rich foods. The patient is thirsty for cold drinks even though she is constantly chilly and suffers from a lack of vital heat. She is sensitive to light touch and pressure. Cold sores on the lips or mouth may appear frequently, often as a result of suppressed emotions or as a companion to **fever**. The body may exude a sour smell. Hangnails are prevalent. Complaints are better from open air, but worse from warmth or heat.

Mentally she is depressed, sad, easily startled, sensitive, anxious, irritable, restless, angry, moody, nervous, easily offended, and indifferent. She dwells on past occurrences and is fearful of crowds, of an impending situation or calamity, thunderstorms, or being robbed. The patient wishes to be alone and demonstrates introverted behavior. To avoid being hurt she may avoid intimacy. She is very emotional but does not like to express her emotions in public and retires to the safety of her own home to cry. Her emotions are exaggerated and her moods often alternate radically. She may appear to desire consolation, but when it is offered she becomes angry or rejects it. She acts in a hasty or rushed manner and cannot urinate in public.

Symptoms are generally worse in the morning around 10 A.M., at night, from the cold, the heat of summer, sun exposure, open air, consolation, suppression of sweat, physical and mental exertion, lying on the left side, after eating, from noise, from pressure or touch, and before, after, and during **menstruation**. Symptoms are better from bathing in cold water, lying down, from sweating, or through rest.

Specific indications

Nat. mur. patients frequently suffer from digestive ailments, oftentimes from the suppression of emotions. The stomach is distended with **gas**, there is a slowness of bowel function, and digestion takes a long time. Other indications include stomach **pain, heartburn**, liver pain two or three hours after eating, excessive hunger and thirst, a constant need to urinate, an aversion to bread, and a craving for salty, sour, and bitter foods. An empty feeling in the stomach may occur at 10 A.M. Symptoms are often relieved upon eating. The patient is frequently constipated. When stools do occur, they are dry and hard and often difficult to expel. They may be preceded by rumbling in the abdomen and flatulence. *Nat. mur.* is a good remedy for **indigestion** caused by the consumption of rich food, which often causes green, watery **diarrhea**. Symptoms are worse from eating starchy food.

The *Nat. mur.* woman is greatly affected by her menstrual cycle. Her mental symptoms are increased before menstruation, and she may suffer from headaches, **nausea**, skin eruptions, weakness, back pains, heart palpitations, and pains in her abdomen and loins. She is discontented and lacks enjoyment of any kind. Her cycle is either early or late. After the menstrual flow has stopped, the woman may still suffer from **depression**, **headache**, or cramps.

The headaches typical of *Nat. mur.* are centered in the forehead and temples, although they may occur at the back of the head. Headaches are often caused by emotional excitement, grief, anger, head injuries, eye strain, **anemia**, or malnutrition. The pain is of a bursting or throbbing nature. The headache is accompanied by nausea, **vomiting**, **dry mouth**, and extreme thirst. The eyes are sore and watery. The headache is worse from 10 A.M. to 3 P.M., after eating, light, noise, motion, mental strain, lying down, and during menstruation. It is often relieved by sweating.

The **cough** is dry, hacking, and irritating. It is worse during fever, and may be accompanied by a bursting headache. Involuntary urination may occur while coughing or **sneezing**.

The cold is accompanied by watery eyes, postnasal drip, thirst, stuffy nose, dry lips, sneezing, and white mucus. The patient may lose his sense of smell and taste. The same symptoms occur in **hay fever**.

The fever is hot and burning. The patient is chilled and may be nauseous, sleepy, restless, and dazed. His face is flushed and he may talk without stopping. He is also excessively thirsty.

The **sore throat** is dry and burning. The voice is hoarse and the patient can only swallow liquids. There may be a sensation described as a lump in the throat.

Preparations

The homeopathic remedy is created by dissolving sodium chloride in hot, boiling water. The mixture is then filtered and crystallized through evaporation. The resulting substance is then dissolved in water and succussed to create the final preparation.

Natrum muriaticum is available at health food and drug stores in various potencies in the form of tinctures, tablets, and pellets.

Precautions

If symptoms do not improve after the recommended time period, a homeopath or healthcare practitioner should be consulted.

The recommended dose of *Nat. mur.* should not be exceeded.

Side effects

There are no known side effects, although individual aggravations may occur.

Interactions

When taking any homeopathic remedy, use of **peppermint** products, coffee, or alcohol should be avoided. These products may cause the remedy to be ineffective.

Resources

BOOKS

Cummings, Stephen, M.D., and Dana Ullman, M.P.H. *Everybody's Guide to Homeopathic Medicines.* New York, NY: Jeremy P. Tarcher/Putnam, 1997.

Kent, James Tyler. *Lectures on Materia Medica.* Delhi, India: B. Jain Publishers, 1996.

Jennifer Wurges

Natural hormone replacement therapy

Definition

Natural hormone replacement therapy (NHRT) is the use of non-synthetic, bio-identical hormones (estrogens, progesterone, and/or testosterone), derived from plants), to treat hormone imbalances and deficiencies. The first oral contraceptive pill was originally derived from Dioscorea species, wild yam; later soy was used as the precursor for oral contraceptive hormones.

Origins

Chinese medicine has made use of phytohormones for thousands of years. Natural progesterone was first crystallized from plants in 1938. NHRT was developed in the late 1970s and became available commercially in the early 1980s. By 1989 micronized (very finely ground) progesterone was developed for better absorption into the bloodstream. The use of NHRT has increased as women have become increasingly dissatisfied with conventional hormone replacement therapy (HRT) because of ineffectiveness, side effects, and/or growing concerns about risks, especially breast and **uterine cancer** risk.

KEY TERMS

Androgen—Sex hormones that are predominant in males.

Andropause—Midlife hormonal changes in men.

Bioavailability—The amount of a substance that can enter the bloodstream and be utilized effectively by the body.

Bioidentical—Molecules that are identical in chemical formulae and similar or identical in chemical structures, actions, and effects to naturally occurring biological molecules.

Compounding pharmacy—A pharmacy that uses bulk materials to fill prescriptions according to a physician's formulation; a formulating pharmacy.

Dehydroepiandrosterone (DHEA)—A hormone precursor to testosterone, estrogen, and other hormones.

Diosgenin—A phytohormone extracted from Mexican yams that is used to make natural progesterone.

Estrogen—A class of steroid hormones that are predominant in females. The term often refers to the three major estrogens: estriol, estradiol, and estrone.

Follicle-stimulating hormone (FSH)—A hormone that stimulates the development of egg follicles in the ovaries, egg maturation, and the production of estrogen.

Isoflavone—A phytoestrogen found in soybeans and other plants that sometimes is used as an estrogen supplement.

Menopause—The permanent cessation of menstruation; also called the change of life or climacteric.

Micronized—A crystal that is ground to a very fine powder.

Osteoporosis—A disease in which bone is lost and new bone formation is slowed. It usually occurs in older people, particularly postmenopausal women.

Phytohormones—Steroid hormones found in plants, including phytoestrogens and phytoandrogens.

Premenstrual syndrome (PMS)—Symptoms including lower back and abdominal pain, nervous irritability, and/or breast tenderness, occurring during the week prior to the onset of menstruation.

Progesterone—An important hormone, particularly in women, that declines sharply during menopause.

Receptor—A cell-surface molecule that binds a specific hormone to produce a specific biological effect.

Stigmasterol—A plant steroid that is extracted from soybeans and used to produce natural human hormones.

Testosterone—A steroid hormone that is predominant in males.

Benefits

NHRT often alleviates symptoms of hormone imbalances and deficiencies that may occur at any stage of life after puberty. In particular, NHRT is used to support hormone balance in the body during and after **menopause**, when estrogens, progesterone and testerone decline. It also is used in men to treat andropause that often affects middle-aged men as testosterone levels fall. Menopausal and andropausal symptoms often subside within months to years without any treatment. The symptoms also often improve after one to three months of NHRT use.

Low levels of estrogen, progesterone, and testosterone may be associated with chronic diseases of **aging**.

- heart disease
- bone loss and osteoporosis
- cancer
- digestive problems
- high cholesterol levels
- Alzheimer's disease

Some researchers claim that NHRT may slow the aging process and help prevent:

- fibroblastic or lumpy breasts
- heart disease
- osteoporosis
- cancer

Reported benefits of testosterone NHRT therapy in men include:

- increased muscle mass and lower body fat
- increased sex drive
- increased energy levels
- improved concentration and productivity

Description

Human sex hormones

The major steroid sex hormones—estrogen, progesterone, and testosterone—control gender and the aging process. They help maintain health and have profound effects on emotions and behavior. Cells throughout the body have receptor molecules on their surfaces that bind specific hormones. Receptor-binding causes a series of reactions within the cell that are specific for the hormone and cell type.

In the human body **cholesterol** is converted into pregnenolone, which is converted into both progesterone and dehydroepiandrosterone (**DHEA**). These hormones, in turn, can be converted into estrogens, testosterone, and other hormones.

High levels of sex hormones are produced in the developing fetus and then almost disappear until puberty. Estrogen and progesterone are at high levels during the reproductive years and are extremely high during **pregnancy**. With aging, the levels of sex hormones decline. When ovulation ceases at menopause, progesterone production drops to very low levels. Estrogen and progesterone have opposing effects in the body, balancing each other. At various times in their lives, many women experience hormone imbalances or sudden changes in hormone levels. During menopause the ratio of estrogen to progesterone may increase. During andropause the ratio of testosterone to estrogen may decline.

Although the body produces many forms of estrogen, the term usually refers to the three major types:

- Estriol is the weakest estrogen.
- Estradiol is the most active estrogen. Nearly every cell in the body has estradiol receptors, making it extremely important for cell and organ function.
- Estrone is made from testosterone derivatives in fat cells of postmenopausal women.

The body also produces several different types of testosterone.

NHRT hormones

The hormones used in NHRT are considered to be "bioidentical" to human sex hormones. The chemical formulae of NHRT hormones are identical to the corresponding hormones produced in the human body. They are very similar or identical to human hormones in their chemical structures, modes of action, and interactions with cell-surface receptors and other hormones. Receptors do not distinguish between the body's own hormones and natural hormones. Therefore natural hormones do not compete with endogenous hormones for receptor sites; rather they supplement and balance the endogenous hormones. In contrast, the synthetic hormones used in conventional HRT are processed and synthesized from chemicals or animal products and are not chemically or biologically identical to human hormones. Synthetic hormones can compete with or replace the body's own hormones because some receptors mistake them for endogenous hormones.

Prescription-strength natural hormones usually are produced from stigmasterol extracted from soybeans. They are chemically altered so as to be bioidentical to human forms such as progesterone or the human estrogens. Progesterone and testosterone may be micronized for NHRT. Over-the-counter (OTC) natural progesterone creams usually are derived from diosgenin extracted from the giant **Mexican yam**. NHRT hormones are manufactured for pharmaceutical companies that make standard-dosage medications and for compounding or formulating pharmacies that make up individualized medications.

Testosterone is often supplied as DHEA. Pharmaceutical-grade DHEA is available without a prescription.

NHRT delivery

Natural estriol, estradiol, estrone, and progesterone are available as:

- oral capsules
- oral tablets
- gel caps
- lozenges, drops, or sprays that are absorbed through the mucous membranes under the tongue
- transdermal creams and gels applied to the skin
- injectable solutions
- suppositories
- implants

Estradiols are available as skin patches (Estraderm, Vivelle, Climera) that slowly and continuously release estrogen through the skin into the bloodstream, bypassing the liver. The patches are worn at all times and changed once or twice per week.

Oil-based micronized oral progesterone appears to be most-readily utilized by the body, since the oil protects the progesterone from stomach acids. Some research suggests that a natural vitamin-E base (tocopherol) is more effective and least toxic. Mineral-oil-based preparations may not be effectively absorbed and/or metabolized.

Testosterone as DHEA is available as:

- oral tablets
- lozenges
- transdermal or vaginal creams
- patches

NHRT creams and gels are absorbed rapidly through the skin in areas with high blood flow, such as the lower neck, upper chest, inner wrists, or hands. Lower dosages are used for NHRT creams and gels because they are absorbed into the bloodstream more efficiently than oral NHRT. Transdermal preparations bypass the gastrointestinal tract and the liver where side effects are more likely to occur. With creams and gels, individual dosages can be adjusted easily, according to symptom relief. Low-dosage natural progesterone creams are available without a prescription. However, absorption of transdermals is highly variable between patients. Those with dry skin, poor circulation, etc. absorb less transdermally. Studies also show that transdermal delivery of hormones may result if very high blood levels over time. More research is need in this area, but for this reason some physicians do not prefer transdermal delivery forms.

Some NHRTs mix highly concentrated estrogen, progesterone, and sometimes testosterone in a propylene glycol base for rapid absorption through the skin. Only one to four drops are required daily, costing as little as $70 per year.

Forms of NHRT

Typical NHRTs include:

- estradiol gel applied daily
- micronized ethinyl estradiol (Estrace) as 0.3–2.5-mg daily tablets
- estriol (80%) and estradiol (20%) as 1.25- or 2.3-mg twice-daily tablets (Biestrogen)
- estriol (80%), estradiol (10%), and estrone (10%), as a 2.5–5% gel applied daily (Triest), or as 1.25- or 2.5-mg, twice-daily tablets (Triestrogen)
- micronized progesterone as 50-, 100-, or 200-mg peanut-oil-based tablets or capsules (oral micronized progesterone, Prometrium)
- micronized progesterone as a 5% cream (percutaneous progesterone cream) or gel
- combined NHRT as 1.25-mg Triestrogen tablets and oral micronized progesterone (50–100 mg), twice daily
- oral micronized testosterone as 1.25–5-mg tablets

- micronized testosterone as a 1% cream or gel (Androgel), applied to the inner thigh or scrotum once or twice daily

Vaginal creams, tablets, and rings are not significantly absorbed into the bloodstream. However they can be useful for treating menopausal symptoms such as urinary problems, vaginal dryness, and thinning of the vaginal wall, which can cause painful intercourse. Vaginal NHRTs include:

- micronized estriol cream, 0.5 mg per g of base (Estriol)
- micronized estradiol cream, 1 mg per g of base (Estrace)
- estradiol as a silicone ring with a 2-mg reservoir, changed every 90 days (Estring)
- progesterone gel, 4 or 8% (Crinone)

Most effective NHRTs require a prescription and may be covered by insurance.

Women's symptoms & NHRT

The dosages and duration of NHRT vary according to response, as determined by symptom relief. Dosages in women may be cycled to correspond to the menstrual cycle.

Symptoms of hormone imbalance in teenagers and young women with normal menstrual cycles include:

- acne
- mood swings
- stress syndromes
- night sweats
- sleep disturbances
- premenstrual syndrome (PMS)

A typical NHRT is micronized progesterone cream, 4–6 mg per kg (2.2 lb) body weight, rubbed daily on the neck, upper chest, and inner wrists, for the entire month or for two weeks prior to **menstruation**, depending on symptoms. It is not used on the face in the presence of **acne**.

Symptoms of hormone imbalances in women in their twenties and thirties with normal menstrual cycles, in addition to the above, may include:

- occasional or postpartum (after giving birth) depression
- infertility
- bloating from salt and fluid retention
- migraine headaches
- breast tenderness
- decreased attention span
- weight gain
- food cravings

Typical NHRTs for three months to one year:

- micronized progesterone cream, 4-6 mg per kg (2.2 lb) body weight, daily
- estradiol, 6–8 µg per kg body weight.

In addition to the above symptoms, hormone imbalances in premenopausal women (aged 35 to over 40), with regular or irregular menstruation, may cause:

- sleep disorders
- hair loss
- hot flashes
- depression
- loss of libido
- digestive problems
- anxiety

Typical NHRTs for three months to one year:

- Micronized progesterone, 4–6 mg per kg (2.2 lb) body weight, daily
- Estradiol, 7–9 micro;g per kg (2.2 lb) body weight, daily

NHRT may be particularly appropriate for perimenopausal symptoms in women aged 40–55. Their symptoms can be similar to those listed above, but may be more pronounced. Menstruation may have ceased or cycles may be irregular. Typical NHRTs:

- micronized progesterone cream, 5–7 mg per kg (2.2 lb) body weight
- estradiol, 6–9 µg. per kg (2.2 lb) body weight
- testosterone cream, 10 µg per kg (2.2 lb) body weight, applied to the labia and around the clitoris

Daily NHRT is continued for two to four months, followed by a five-day break.

Menopausal and postmenopausal women (usually aged 55 or older) may have, in addition to any of the above symptoms:

- bone loss
- cardiac disease
- urinary incontinence

Typical NHRTs:

- micronized progesterone cream, 5–7 mg per kg (2.2 lb) body weight, daily
- estradiol, 6–9 µg per kg (2.2 lb) body weight, daily.

Men's symptoms and NHRT

Symptoms of low testosterone levels or hormone imbalances in andropausal men are very similar to those in women. Additional symptoms may include:

- fatigue
- nighttime urination
- impotence or decreased ability to maintain an erection
- decrease in muscle-building ability
- inability to lose weight

A natural androgen replacement protocol, lasting 3–14 months, might consist of:

- pine pollen, 0.5–5 gm, once or twice daily; a one-quarter-teaspoon tincture, three times daily; 5–10 gm daily in warm milk, in Chinese and Korean medicine
- David's lily flower, one-quarter-teaspoon tincture, twice daily
- Panax/tienchi ginseng tincture, one-third teaspoon daily
- nettle root (*Urtica dioica*), 300–1,200 mg daily
- tribulus (*Tribulus terrestris*), 250–500 mg standardized extract as pills or tablets, three times per day
- pregnenolone, a primary steroid hormone (prohormone) in men and women, 5–50 mg daily
- androstenedione (andro), 50–100 mg, one to three times per day, as a pill dissolved under the tongue
- androstenediol (andiol, 4-andiol, androdiol), 100 mg once or twice daily
- DHEA, 25–50 mg daily
- zinc, 20–40 mg daily
- celery juice, daily from three fresh stalks
- a diet high in oatmeal, corn, and pine nuts

Zinc is required for the transformation of **androstenedione** to testosterone. Zinc preparations usually include **copper** to prevent copper depletion.

Ginseng as an androgen replacement:

- Asian ginseng as 1–9 gm daily tablets
- Asian white (20–40 drops) and Kirin or dark red (5–20 drops) as a daily tincture
- Asian ginseng combined with tienchi (*Panax pseudoginseng*), one to one, one-third teaspoon daily in water
- Siberian ginseng

Foods & supplements

Most researchers believe that the human body cannot utilize the phytoestrogens in soy or the progesterone in yams; nor can the body transform these phytohormones into biologically available hormones. However some researchers believe that phytoestrogens called isoflavones (genistein and daidzein) found in soy can serve as short-term estrogen supplements. **Soy protein** in a low-fat diet reduces the risk of **heart disease** and isoflavones may help prevent bone loss. Isoflavones are found in tofu, tempeh, and soy drinks but not in soy oil.

Wild Mexican yam creams may contain phytoestrogens; however they are ineffective as progesterone supplements because they contain only a progesterone precursor which is inactive in the human body.

Phytoandrogens have been reported to increase androgen levels and the androgen-to-estrogen ratio in men. Foods containing high levels of phytoandrogens:

- celery
- parsnips
- corn
- oats (*Avena sativa*)
- garlic (*Allium sativum*)
- onions
- pine nuts

Foods that lower androgen levels and suppress androgenic activity in men include:

- licorice
- black cohosh (*Cimicifuga racemosa*), which is very high in estrogen and sometimes used to treat hot flashes in menopausal women
- hops, one of the most powerful estrogenic foods
- grapefruit, which interferes with removal of estrogen from the body

Preparations

Blood hormone levels may be measured before and/or during NHRT:

- Follicle-stimulating hormone (FSH): high FSH levels indicate low sex hormone production and menopause.
- Estrogen blood tests measure how much of one type of estrogen is circulating in the blood and the total amount present in the bloodstream. However most estrogen in the body is bound to other molecules or cell receptors and cannot be measured.

Other tests include:

- Saliva hormone testing: inexpensive as performed by mail-order laboratories or with home test kits
- Urine testing reveals how much hormone is excreted through the kidneys over a 24-hour period. It is expensive and may be difficult to interpret.
- Yearly bone mineral density tests for those using NHRT to improve bone density
- Annual pelvic ultrasounds can be used to monitor the effectiveness of NHRT. These tests are inexpensive and enable the physician to view the thickness of the uterine

lining and the shape of the ovaries, both of which are affected directly by estrogen and progesterone. Pelvic ultrasound also can detect and monitor ovarian cysts that may develop with hormone therapies.

Testosterone and/or DHEA levels in the blood or saliva are monitored regularly when DHEA is used in NHRT. However hormone levels are constantly changing and most tests reflect only the measurable hormone present at a single point in time.

Precautions

Although they are approved by the U. S. Food and Drug Administration, natural hormones are not regulated as drugs. Most large manufacturers use standardized labeling and dosages of active ingredients. Nevertheless, the bioavailability—the amount of active ingredient that enters the bloodstream and can be utilized effectively—is not known for most NHRTs. The results of oral NHRT may be inconsistent since many factors can affect their bioavailability. Although many OTC products are labeled as natural hormones, they contain very low concentrations and their bioavailability is unknown. They may be useful if only a small amount of hormone supplementation is required.

NHRTs, especially androgen replacement, have not been well-studied. There have been no clinical safety trials. It is not known whether NHRT carries risks similar to some HRTs, including increased risk for **breast cancer**, coronary heart disease, **stroke**, and pulmonary embolism (a blood clot in an artery of the lung). Androgen replacement therapies should not be used by adolescent males.

Some synthetic hormone products may be labeled as "natural" because they are synthesized from naturally occurring substances. For example, synthetic estrogen is manufactured from the urine of pregnant horses. Some prescription hormones contain bioidentical estrogen but synthetic progesterone.

Side effects

There have been very few reports of side effects from NHRT in women. Since the estrogens used in NHRT are bioidentical to human estrogens and tend to be weaker than the synthetic estrogens used in HRT, they are expected to have fewer side effects. Furthermore, NHRT can be halted and resumed at any time without side effects.

Natural androgen replacement therapy may cause irritability and other side effects in men, particularly in coffee-drinkers. Ginseng has many side effects and should be used with caution. Very high zinc intake also can have numerous side effects.

Research and general acceptance

The few research studies that have included NHRT have had positive results. NHRT practitioners claim that it is safer and more effective than HRT.

Training and certification

Most NHRTs are available only as prescriptions from a medical or naturopathic physician or nurse practitioner. Most doctors who use NHRT rely on personal research and the experiences of their patients.

Resources

BOOKS

Buhner, Stephen Harrod. *Vital Man: Natural Health Care for Men at Midlife*. New York: Avery, 2003.

Northrup, Christiane. *The Wisdom of Menopause*. New York: Bantam, 2001.

Schwartz, Erika. *The Hormone Solution*. New York: Warner, 2002.

Schwartz, Erika. *The 30-Day Natural Hormone Plan: Look and Feel Young Again—Without Synthetic HRT*. New York: Warner, 2004.

PERIODICALS

Karmon, Eran. "'Natural' Alternative to Hormone Replacement Therapy Replaces Woman's Estrogen." *Knight Ridder Tribune Business News* (August 21, 2002): 1.

Ward, Elizabeth M. "Health Concerns at Menopause: HRT Vs. Natural Remedies for Relief." *Environmental Nutrition* 25, no. 1 (January 2002): 1.

Watt, P. J., et al. "A Holistic Programmatic Approach to Natural Hormone Replacement." *Family and Community Health* 26 (January–March 2003): 53–63.

ORGANIZATIONS

American Menopause Foundation. 350 Fifth Ave., Suite 2822, New York, NY 10118. (212) 714-2398. http://www.americanmenopause.org.

National Women's Health Information Center. 8550 Arlington Blvd., Suite 300, Fairfax, VA 22031. (800) 994-9662. http://www.4woman.gov.

Natural Woman Foundation. 8539 Sunset Blvd, No. 135, Los Angeles, CA 90069. (888) 489-6626. Chriscoprd@aol.com. http://www.naturalwoman.org.

North American Menopause Society. P.O. Box 94527, Cleveland, OH 44101. 440-442-7550. info@menopause.org. http://www.menopause.org.

OTHER

"Alternative Therapies for Managing Menopausal Symptoms." National Center for Complementary and Alternative Medicine. August 2, 2002 [cited April 27, 2004]. http://nccam.nci.nih.gov/health/alerts/menopause.

Margaret Alic, PhD

Natural hygiene diet

Definition

The natural hygiene diet is a system of healthy living whereby moral, physical, and environmental pollution is strictly avoided, and natural healthy food is chosen in preference over processed food. The principle is to provide everything the body needs to be healthy, and to avoid anything that may hinder health and well being.

Origins

Actually, early in the twentieth century, there were similar "natural hygiene" movements or health culture societies advocating exercise, the consumption of healthy foods, and massage. The American Natural Hygiene Society was founded in 1948, and as such is the oldest and largest natural hygiene organization in the world. The Society publishes the *Health Science* magazine. The British Natural Hygiene Society was founded in 1959 by Keki Sidhwa and two other natural hygienists. Their magazine, *Hygienist,* which is published quarterly, was started in 1959, making it the oldest natural hygiene publication. Both organizations aim to educate and inform, and they can also recommend practitioners and clinics.

Benefits

This regime is designed to cleanse the body of all toxic matter, so that it is free to work, instead of being hampered by stored wastes that reduce the efficiency of the human organism. Together with improved nutrition, this should bring about a complete transformation for most people. Less sleep may be needed, and there should be a general feeling of increased well being and energy, which will almost certainly help the individual to make better and more productive use of his or her time.

It is possible that an improvement may be noticed in powers of recall; many people complain of loss of memory in our time, and this may be due to a combination of **stress** and a toxic body system.

Proponents say improvement in symptoms of conditions such as arthritis, migraine, hypoglycemia, diabetes, and more can be expected. In addition, the principles of natural hygiene often lead to unexpected benefits, such as improvements in the appearance and texture of skin, and the condition of hair and fingernails, the disappearance of eye bags, and less body odor.

KEY TERMS

Denatured—Changed from its natural state and robbed of nutrients.

Hypoglycemia—A condition characterized by abnormally low levels of glucose in the blood.

Description

The term "natural hygiene" refers more to a way of life than merely to a diet. For some time, proponents have asserted that their recommendations can provide the foundation for a healthy, fulfilling life that is disease-free and emotional ennui that have become commonplace in so-called modern society. These, and many other diseases of modern life, are due to the multi-faceted pollution of ourselves and our planet, and a denatured diet. Together, it is considered that they cause poisoning and the stifling of the body's natural strength and vitality. Natural hygienists reason that since the body "constructs itself" after the fertilization of the ovum, it must also have powers of repair and renewal in order to maintain the organism, if given the right conditions.

Natural hygiene concerns every aspect of a human being's life, because everything—the physical, the spiritual, and the moral—affects the well being of the individual and society. The theory is that people should obey their natural instincts, and that only when they have achieved perfect health, will they be able to achieve their full potential as human beings.

Natural hygienists believe that mankind is naturally good and virtuous, but will not display these traits unless they are following all the principles of healthy lifestyle. The theories of natural hygiene, they claim, if properly adhered to will allow mankind to achieve supreme heights of achievement at all levels of his being.

If given the right circumstances and facilities, the human body, believed to be perfect in its creation, will be able to preserve itself in an optimum state, and efficiently perform repairs when needed, quickly returning to a state of total well being. The prerequisites for total well being are pure air, pure water, sufficient rest and sleep, and uncontaminated food of a high quality that will provide all the necessary nutrients in a readily available form. In addition to these, satisfactory human companionship should be sought, as well as protection from extreme cold and extreme heat, sunshine, sufficient exercise, a purpose in life, and in general, an atmosphere conducive to all that is good concerning human life.

An essential concept of natural hygiene is that to be healthy is normal, and healing is a biological process that cannot be bought. The same natural laws apply whether one is sick or well, and that which makes a well person sick can never make a sick person well. Allopathic medicine, in treating merely the symptoms of disease, in many instances actually worsens the condition in the long run.

A simple example of this would be the administering of laxatives to a patient suffering from **constipation**, as opposed to finding the underlying cause of the constipation. With time, laxatives cause the bowels to become even more sluggish, and so the cycle continues. Natural hygiene aims to correct the cause.

The first step, when embarking on a regime of natural hygiene, is to rid the body of accumulated toxins. There are many aspects to be taken into account for this procedure. Usually, the first to be considered is the gastrointestinal tract, but in addition, the skin, liver, gallbladder, lymphatic system, lungs, kidneys, and bladder all need to be detoxified in order to facilitate perfect functioning of the human organism. Although cleansing is of major concern, natural hygiene therapists caution that it is also very important to ensure that the body has access to fresh, clean air, clean water, and good food while the **detoxification** is in process, so that the body can rebuild itself. They warn that cleansing without rebuilding will weaken a body and its immune system.

There are many variations on this, but basically this consists of **fasting** the body at some time, and feeding it mainly fruits and vegetables that will have a dual effect of cleansing and rebuilding. Usually, food combining is an important aspect of the **nutrition** of natural hygiene, and requires that a protein food is never eaten with a starch food. They should be taken at different meals with a minimum of four hours between each meal. Fruit is recommended to be eaten by itself, but since it digests quickly only half an hour need pass before other food can be consumed.

To follow the natural hygiene way of living at home, the only expenses that will be incurred are the cost of **organic food**, which can be more expensive than ordinary food. However, if patients feel that they would benefit from a trip to a natural hygiene clinic, information can be obtained from some natural hygiene organizations.

Preparations

Those wishing to treat themselves in accordance with natural hygiene principles are required to follow a mainly raw diet that includes all the nutrients and enzymes that will help to flush toxins from the body, while at the same time building health. However, it is wise to consult a natural hygienist before beginning treatment.

There are special formulas for speeding the elimination of toxins, which can be obtained from practitioners who specialize in natural hygiene. Information regarding these treatments can be obtained from various national organizations.

Precautions

When undertaking a cleansing diet, it is important not to impose anything too harsh on the body. If an individual is suffering from acute toxicity, it may be better advised to proceed slowly and cautiously with the process of detoxification, particularly if the patient is continuing as normal with his/her everyday life.

Side effects

There are few side affects associated with the practice of natural hygiene. Some may experience what is known as a "healing crisis" while the body is throwing off toxins. Symptoms may include headaches, **nausea**, or sensitivity. These symptoms are transient, and may normally be relieved with herbal teas, a walk in the fresh air, or by simply lying in a darkened room for a while.

Under very rare circumstances, an individual may have such a toxic condition that it would be dangerous for him/her to undertake cleansing without assistance. When the body is subjected to poisons, whether in their food, in the air, or from the water they drink, the body attempts to deal with them in such a way that they will cause the least harm to the body. Thus, they may be stored in the liver, or in fatty deposits under the skin.

When a person who has poisons stored in such a way undergoes a fast, or undertakes some other method to flush poisons from the body, sometimes the flushing causes large amounts of toxins to enter the blood system at the same time. Without proper supervision or consultation, and without the correct step being taken, the results could possibly be fatal.

Research and general acceptance

There is a large body of research to support the theories of natural hygienists, although most of it is not accepted by allopathic practitioners. General belief exists that detoxification can improve the effectiveness of many healing therapies. Though many nutritionists see numerous health benefits in eating natural foods and greater amounts of fruits and vegetables, they may warn against eating large amounts of any particular kind of food. For example, eating too many fruits and vegetables at one time can cause **diarrhea**. Fasting may be dangerous for some individuals—those with weakened immune systems, the elderly, or pregnant women. It may also cause muscle weakness and **dizziness** in healthy individuals.

However, many people continue to seek assistance from clinics dispensing some form of natural hygiene and are satisfied with the results. Keki Sidhwa, the president of the British Natural Hygiene Society, has records covering many years of successful treatment of his patients, where many leave from his clinic days or weeks later in a better state of health.

Training and certification

The American College of Health Science awards degrees up to PH.D. standard, but these are not yet accredited by mainstream education in the United States. Practitioners must be members of one of the national associations.

Resources

BOOKS

Diamond, Marilyn, and Harvey Diamond. *Fit For Life II*. New York: Warner Books Inc. 1989.

PERIODICALS

Hunter, Beatric Trum. "Improving the Quality of One's Life (Book Corners)." *Townsend Letter for Doctors and Patients* (July 2002): 131.

ORGANIZATIONS

The American Natural Hygiene Society. PO Box 30630, Tampa, FL 33630 813–855–6607. anhs@anhs.org ANHS. http://www.anhs.org.

The British Natural Hygiene Society. Shalimar, 3 Harold Grove, Frinton on Sea, Essex, England, CO13 9BD. 011-44-1255 672823. http://members.rotfl.com/bnhs.

OTHER

Holistic Healing Webpage. http://www.holisticmed.com/ detox/dtx–intro.txt.

Living Nutrition. http://www.livingnutrition.com/articles/ art–1.html.

Patricia Skinner
Teresa G. Odle

Naturopathic medicine

Definition

Naturopathic medicine is a branch of medicine in which a variety of natural medicines and treatments are used to heal illness. It uses a system of medical diagnosis and therapeutics based on the patterns of chaos and organization in nature. Naturopathy is founded on the premise that people are naturally healthy, and that healing can occur through removing obstacles to a cure and by stimulating the body's natural healing abilities. The foundations of health in natural medicine are diet, **nutrition**, **homeopathy**, physical manipulation, **stress** management, and **exercise**.

Naturopaths are general practitioners who treat a wide variety of illnesses. They believe in treating the "whole person"—the spirit as well as the physical body—and emphasize preventive care. They often recommend changes in diet and lifestyle to enhance the health of their patients.

Origins

People have always seen connections between diet and disease; many therapies are built around special **diets**. Naturopathy began in the eighteenth and nineteenth centuries, as the industrial revolution forced many people into unhealthy lifestyles, and the European custom of "taking the cure" at natural spas became popular. Benedict Lust, who believed deeply in natural medicine, organized naturopathy as a formal system of healthcare in the 1890s. By the early 1900s, it was flourishing.

The first naturopaths in the United States emphasized the healing properties of a nutritious diet, as did a number of their contemporaries. In the early twentieth century, for instance, John Kellogg, a physician and vegetarian, opened a sanitarium that used such healing methods as **hydrotherapy**, often prescribed by today's naturopaths. His brother Will produced such health foods as corn flakes and shredded wheat. The Post brothers helped make naturopathic ideas popular and emphasized the value of whole grains over highly refined ones. Together with one of their employees, C. W. Post, they eventually went on to start the cereal companies that bear their names.

In the early 1900s, most states licensed naturopaths as physicians. There were 20 medical schools of naturopathic medicine. From early on, naturopathic physicians were considered "eclectic," since they drew on a variety of natural therapies and traditions for treating their patients.

In the 1930s, naturopathy dramatically declined for several reasons. Allopathic medicine finally stopped using such therapies as bloodletting and heavy metal poisons as curative compounds. New therapies were more effective and less toxic. Allopathic medical schools became increasingly well-funded by foundations with links to the emerging drug industry. In

---

KEY TERMS

Clinical nutrition—The use of diet and nutritional supplements as a way to enhance health and prevent disease.

Cryosurgery—Freezing and destroying abnormal cells.

Herb—In naturopathy, a plant or plant derivative or extract prescribed for health or healing.

Homeopathy—A holistic system of treatment developed in the eighteenth century. It is based on the idea that substances that produce symptoms of sickness in healthy people will have a curative effect when given in very dilute quantities to sick people who exhibit those same symptoms. Homeopathic remedies are believed to stimulate the body's own healing processes.

Hydrotherapy—The use of water (hot, cold, steam, or ice) to relieve discomfort and promote physical well-being. Also called water therapy.

Physical manipulation—The use of deep massage, spinal alignment, and joint manipulation to stimulate tissues.

Ultrasound—A painless and non-invasive procedure in which sound waves are bounced off the kidneys. These sound waves produce a pattern of echoes that are then used by a computer to create pictures of areas inside the kidney (sonograms).

---

addition, allopathic physicians became much more organized and came to wield considerable political clout. Naturopathy has experienced a resurgence over the last 20 years, however. The lay public is aware of the connections between a healthful diet and lifestyle and avoiding chronic disease. In addition, conventional medicine is often unable to treat these chronic diseases. Patients are now health care consumers, and will seek their own resolution to health problems that cannot be resolved by conventional physicians. As a result, even medical groups that once considered naturopathy ineffective are now beginning to accept it.

Benefits

Naturopathic medicine is useful for treating chronic as well as acute diseases. It is sometimes used in conjunction with allopathic care to enhance wellness and relieve chronic symptoms, such as **fatigue** and **pain**. A naturopath treats a wide range of health problems, ranging from back pain to **depression**.

A naturopathic physician will spend extra time interviewing and examining the patient to find the underlying cause for a medical problem. Emotional and spiritual symptoms and patterns are included in the assessment. The naturopath often spends more time educating patients in preventive health, lifestyle, and nutrition than most M.D.s.

Description

Naturopathic medicine modalities include a variety of healing treatments, such as diet and clinical nutrition, homeopathy, **botanical medicine**, soft tissue and spinal manipulation, ultrasound, and therapeutic exercise. A naturopath provides complete diagnostic and treatment services in such specialties as obstetrics and pediatrics. Some are also licensed midwives.

Naturopaths consider health to be not just the absence of disease, but complete physical, mental and social well being. Naturopathic physicians often say that diseases must be healed not just by suppressing symptoms, but by rooting out the true cause. Symptoms are actually viewed as the body's natural efforts to heal itself and restore balance.

A typical office visit to a naturopath takes about an hour. During the first visit, the doctor will ask detailed questions about the patient's symptoms, lifestyle, history of illness, and state of his or her emotions. The naturopath will take a complete medical history, and may order lab tests such as urine and blood tests. A naturopath may talk with the patient about the possible causes for an illness—poor diet, life stresses, occupational dangers, and mental, emotional, and spiritual problems. Naturopaths believe that even widely varying symptoms can sometimes be traced to one underlying cause. Often environmental or metabolic toxins or serious stress bring on an illness.

As with most doctors, treatment by a naturopath can range from one office visit to many. Some acute illnesses can be alleviated with one or two visits. Other chronic diseases need regular weekly or monthly attention. Clinical care provided by naturopathic physicians are covered by insurance in a number of states in the United States.

Preparations

There are about 1,500 naturopathic physicians in the United States practicing as of 2004; nearly 80% of these practitioners entered the profession following the revival of interest in naturopathy in the late 1970s. Consumers can find naturopaths by contacting the American Association of Naturopathic Physicians (AANP) or logging on to their web site. Naturopaths

recommended by the AANP have met requirements for state licensure and have taken a national exam that qualifies them to practice. Qualified naturopaths can also be found through the local branch of the national or state association of naturopathic physicians. It is sometimes useful to request names from another health care provider who knows naturopathic practitioners in the community.

Precautions

A good naturopath is always willing to work with the patient's other physicians or health care providers. To avoid drug interactions and to coordinate care, it is important for a patient to inform his or her allopathic doctor about supplements prescribed by a naturopath.

Many naturopaths give childhood vaccinations, but some do not. If a parent is concerned about immunizations, it is best to go to an allopathic doctor for vaccinations.

Naturopaths are not licensed to perform major surgery, or prescribe narcotics and antidepressant drugs. They must also consult an oncologist when treating a **cancer** patient.

Side effects

Although naturopathic remedies are derived from natural sources and pose much less risk than allopathic drugs do, there are certain side effects associated with the use of some herbal preparations. One problem they can pose is through interactions with prescription medicines. It is important for a patient to inform his or her allopathic physician about any natural remedies or herbs prescribed by a naturopath.

It is also important to note that the U.S. Food and Drug Administration (FDA) considers medicinal herbs to be dietary supplements, not drugs; as a result, they are not subject to the same regulations as prescription medications. Because herbal remedies come from natural sources, the active ingredients may not always be in the same concentration from bottle to bottle, since plants naturally vary. To guard against using too little or too much of a natural remedy, patients should use herbs and supplements recommended by a naturopath or those produced by well-respected companies.

Research and general acceptance

Medical research in naturopathy has increased dramatically in the United States within the last 10 years. Naturopathic research often employs case histories,

BENEDICT LUST (1872–1945)

German healer, Benedict Lust, is credited with naming the natural medical technique of naturopathy. He was married to Louisa Lust who was a student of another naturopathy pioneer, Arnold Rikli.

Benedict, who was born in Germany in 1872, immigrated to the United States in 1892 but returned to his native Germany when he contracted tuberculosis. In Germany he met Father Sebastian Kneipp who treated and cured Lust using hydrotherapy. Lust subsequently returned to the United States as Kneipp's representative to publicize the cure. He founded the Water Cure Institute in New York City and established Kneipp Societies throughout the United States.

Lust acquired degrees in osteopathy and medicine and drew from his combined knowledge to devise the healing art of naturopathy. In 1901 he organized the Naturopathic Society of America, and he founded the American School of Naturopathy. He purchased the rights to the term naturopathy from John H. Scheel in 1902 and publicized himself as a naturopath. Lust's school initially offered a two-year, post-graduate curriculum and later expanded into a four-year residential program. The school received a charter in 1905 and, thereafter, awarded degrees in naturopathy and chiropractic. Lust established a second school devoted to teaching the principles of massage and physiotherapy. Additionally he offered home-study courses in naturopathy and started a magazine about naturopathy.

Lust later reorganized the Naturopathic Society of America at the national level, calling the group the American Institute of Naturopathy. Likewise in 1919, he combined the independent Kneipp Societies into a unified group, called the American Naturopathic Association (ANA). In 1921 the ANA elected Lust to a lifetime term as president of the society. Benedict Lust, a staunch proponent of natural healing and natural food remedies, championed the cause of the naturopath and spent much of his lifetime battling the American Medical Association for legitimacy.

summaries of practitioners' clinical observations, and medical records. Some studies by naturopaths in the United States have also met today's scientific gold standard; they were double-blind and placebo-controlled. Much naturopathic research has also been done in Germany, France, England, India, and China.

Some mainstream medical practitioners remain distrustful of naturopathy, however. Such problems as health-food store employees without naturopathic credentials giving health-related advice to customers, or occasional rare cases of **infections** caused by naturopathic injections, continue to damage the reputation of this form of alternative medicine.

Single-treatment studies

Research in naturopathy tends to focus on single treatments used by naturopaths, rather than naturopathy as a whole. In 1998, an extensive review of such single-treatment studies found that naturopathic healing methods were effective for 15 different medical conditions, including **osteoarthritis**, **asthma**, and middle ear infections. A study of 8,341 men in with damaged heart muscles in 1996 revealed that supplementation with **niacin**, a B vitamin, was associated with an 11% reduced risk of mortality over 15 years. In 1996, a study showed **St. John's wort** was effective as prescription antidepressants in relieving depression, and had fewer side effects.

Women's health

Naturopathic studies have also demonstrated benefits in the arena of women's health issues. In recent years, more women than men have been drawn to naturopathy because of its holistic emphasis, its tradition of relative equality between practitioner and patient, and its philosophy of eclecticism and freedom of choice in healing methods. In one classic 1993 study, women with **cervical dysplasia** or abnormal Pap smears were treated by naturopaths with topical applications of herbs and dietary supplements. These medications included Bromelian, an enzyme from the pineapple; **bloodroot**; marigold; **zinc** chloride; and suppositories made from herbal and nutritional ingredients, such as **echinacea**, **vitamin A**, and **vitamin E**. Thirty-eight of the 43 women in the study had normal Pap smears and normal tissue biopsies after treatment. The study concluded that these protocols might benefit the health of patients undergoing more traditional treatments for cervical dysplasia, such as cryosurgery.

Other more recent research has documented the benefits of such nutritional foods as soy in relieving **hot flashes** and vaginal dryness. Nutritional supplements prescribed by naturopaths to enhance women's health during **menopause** have also proven effective; in general, naturopathy appears to be as useful as conventional medicine for treating menopausal symptoms. Research shows vitamin E supplements are helpful for

50% of postmenopausal women with thinning vaginal tissue. Studies also reveal that **bioflavonoids** with **vitamin C** and gamma-oryzanol, a substance taken from rice bran oil, can relieve hot flashes.

Another area of women's health concerns that naturopathy has taken seriously is a growing preference for skin care and beauty products derived from natural sources rather than from chemical laboratories. Such products are often more beneficial to the skin and less likely to cause **rashes** or other allergic reactions.

Training and certification

Naturopathic medical students attend a four-year medical school and are educated in many of the same basic sciences as MDs, including anatomy and pathology. In the last two years, they also study such holistic therapies as nutrition, homeopathic medicine, botanical medicine, psychology, hydrotherapy, and counseling. The naturopathic curriculum places a strong emphasis on disease prevention and optimizing wellness.

After his or her education, a naturopath takes a national qualifying examination known as the Naturopathic Physicians Licensing Examination or NPLEX. A doctor should have graduated from a school that qualifies him or her to take these examinations. As of 2003, these schools include the National College of Naturopathic Medicine in Portland, Oregon; Bastyr University in Seattle, Washington; Southwest College of Naturopathic Medicine in Tempe, Arizona; Canadian College of Naturopathic Medicine in Toronto, Canada; and the University of Bridgeport College of Naturopathic Medicine in Bridgeport, Connecticut.

Some states license naturopathic physicians. As of late 2003, those states included Hawaii, Alaska, Washington, Oregon, Utah, Montana, Arizona, Connecticut, New Hampshire, Vermont, Maine, and Kansas, in addition to the territories of Puerto Rico and the Virgin Islands. Training via a correspondence school does not qualify a naturopath for licensure or to take the national qualifying examination.

Resources

BOOKS

Better Homes and Gardens. *Smart Choices in Alternative Medicine*. Meredith Books, 1999.

Burton Goldberg Group. *Alternative Medicine: The Definitive Guide*. Fife, WA: Future Medicine Publishing Inc., 1995.

Pelletier, Dr. Kenneth R. *The Best Alternative Medicine*. New York: Simon and Schuster, 2000.

PERIODICALS

Cramer, E. H., P. Jones, N. L. Keenan, and B. L. Thompson. "Is Naturopathy as Effective as Conventional Therapy for Treatment of Menopausal Symptoms?" *Journal of Alternatie and Complementary Medicine* 9 (August 2003): 529–538.

Engelhart, S., F. Saborowski, M. Krakau, et al. "Severe *Serratia liquefaciens* Sepsis Following Vitamin C Infusion Treatment by a Naturopathic Practitioner." *Journal of Clinical Microbiology* 41 (August 2003): 3986–3988.

Hudson, Tori. "Naturopathic Medicine, Integrative Medicine and Women's Health." *Townsend Letter for Doctors and Patients* (November 2001): 136.

Hudson, Tori, N.D. "Six Paths to Menopausal Wellness." *Herbs for Health* (Jan/Feb 2000): 47–50.

Kurtzweil, Paula. *An FDA Guide to Dietary Supplements*. FDA Consumer, 1998.

Lee, A. C., and K. J. Kemper. "Homeopathy and Naturopathy: Practice Characteristics and Pediatric Care." *Archives of Pediatric and Adolescent Medicine* 154, no. 1 (January 2000): 75–80.

Mills, E., R. Singh, M. Kawasaki, et al. "Emerging Issues Associated with HIV Patients Seeking Advice from Health Food Stores." *Canadian Journal of Public Health* 94 (September-October 2003): 363–366.

ORGANIZATIONS

American Association of Naturopathic Physicians. 601 Valley Street, Suite 105, Seattle, WA 98109. (206) 298-0126. http://www.naturopathic.org

Naturopathic Physicians Licensing Examination Board (NPLEX). P. O. Box 69657, Portland, OR 97201. (503) 250-9141. http://www.nabne.org/html/index2.html.

Barbara Boughton
Rebecca J. Frey, PhD

Nausea

Definition

Nausea is the sensation of having a queasy stomach or being about to vomit. **Vomiting**, or emesis, is the expelling of undigested food through the mouth.

Description

Nausea is a reaction to a number of causes that include overeating, infection, or irritation of the throat or stomach lining. Persistent or recurrent nausea and vomiting should be checked by a doctor.

A doctor should be called if nausea and vomiting occur:

- after eating rich or spoiled food or taking a new medication
- repeatedly or for 48 hours or longer
- following intense dizziness

It is important to see a doctor if nausea and vomiting are accompanied by:

- yellowing of the skin and whites of the eyes
- pain in the chest or lower abdomen
- trouble with swallowing or urination
- dehydration or extreme thirst
- drowsiness or confusion
- constant, severe abdominal pain
- a fruity breath odor

A doctor should be notified if vomiting is heavy and/or bloody; if the vomitus looks like coffee grounds or feces; or if the patient has been unable to keep food down for 24 hours.

An ambulance or emergency response number should be called immediately if:

- Diabetic shock is suspected.
- Nausea and vomiting continue after other symptoms of viral infection have subsided.
- The patient has a severe headache.
- The patient is sweating and having chest pain and trouble breathing.
- The patient is known or suspected to have swallowed a drug overdose or poisonous substance.
- The patient has a high body temperature, muscle cramps, and other signs of heat exhaustion or heat stroke.

- Nausea, vomiting, and breathing problems occur after exposure to a known allergen.

Causes and symptoms

Persistent, unexplained, or recurring nausea and vomiting can be symptoms of a variety of serious illnesses. It can be caused by simply overeating or drinking too much alcohol. It can be due to **stress**, certain medications, or illness. For example, people who are given morphine or other opioid medications for **pain** relief after surgery sometimes feel nauseated by the drug. Such poisonous substances as arsenic and other heavy metals cause nausea and vomiting. **Morning sickness** is a consequence of pregnancy-related hormone changes. **Motion sickness** can be induced by traveling in a vehicle, plane, or on a boat. Many patients experience nausea after eating spoiled food or foods to which they are allergic. Patients who suffer **migraine headache** often experience nausea. **Cancer** patients on chemotherapy are often nauseated. **Gallstones**, **gastroenteritis**, and stomach ulcer may cause nausea and vomiting. Such infectious illnesses as dengue **fever** and severe acute respiratory syndrome (SARS) may be accompanied by nausea and vomiting. These symptoms should be evaluated by a physician.

Diagnosis

Diagnosis is based on the severity, frequency, and duration of symptoms, and other factors that could indicate the presence of a serious illness.

Treatment

Getting a breath of fresh air or getting away from whatever is causing the nausea can solve the problem. Eating olives or crackers or sucking on a lemon can calm the stomach by absorbing acid and excess fluid. Coke syrup is another proven antiemetic remedy.

Vomiting relieves nausea immediately but can cause dehydration. Sipping clear juices, weak tea, and some sports drinks help replace lost fluid and minerals without irritating the stomach. Food should be reintroduced gradually, beginning with small amounts of dry, bland food like crackers and toast.

Biofeedback

Biofeedback uses **exercise** and deep **relaxation** to control nausea.

Acupuncture

Acupuncture is increasingly regarded as a useful adjunct to treating nausea. A growing body of literature shows that acupuncture is effective in treating nausea associated with **pregnancy**, surgery, and chemotherapy for cancer. The most effective acupuncture point for nausea appears to be PC-6.

A few patients, however, may experience temporary nausea as a side effect of acupuncture. It is not considered a serious side effect.

Acupressure

Acupressure (applying pressure to specific areas of the body) may be helpful in reducing nausea and vomiting and relaxes the gastrointestinal tract. Acupressure can be applied by wearing a special wristband or by applying firm pressure to the:

- back of the jawbone
- webbing between the thumb and index finger
- top of the foot
- inside of the wrist
- base of the rib cage

Nutritional therapy

- **Rehydration.** It is very important to replace fluid loss through prolonged vomiting. However, patients should take fluid in slowly to prevent shock to the body. Fruit juice or soup are even better than plain water because they also contain glucose and salt, which may also be deficient.
- **Avoid eating solids right away.** Patients should wait until the body has enough rests and the stomach has a chance to settle down before starting on solid foods.
- **Bland foods.** To avoid overworking the digestive system too soon, patients should resume eating with bland food such as toast or yogurt. In addition, they should not try to eat too much right away, as this also stresses out the digestive system.
- **Lactaid.** Lactaid helps prevent upset stomach in persons allergic to milk.

Herbal treatments

There are several herbal remedies that can help alleviate short bouts of nausea and vomiting.

- Chamomile (*Matricaria recutita*) or lemon balm (*Melissa officinalis*) tea may relieve symptoms.
- Ginger (*Zingiber officinale*), a very effective herbal remedy for nausea, can be drunk as tea or taken as candy or powered capsules. Ginger has been shown in several studies to relieve morning sickness associated with pregnancy.
- Peppermint tea is effective in alleviating nausea and vomiting associated with indigestion.

- Stomach tea, a combination of anise seed, fennel, peppermint and thyme, is a good herbal treatment for gas.
- Strong green tea can stop nausea especially if it is caused by eating spoiled foods.

Homeopathy

Depending on a patient's specific condition, a homeopathic practitioner may prescribe one of the following remedies: *Arsenicum album*, *Carbo vegetabilis*, *Ignatia*, homeopathic *ipecac*, and *Nux vomica*.

Aromatherapy

Peppermint or **lavender** oil when inhaled, calms the body and reduces nausea and vomiting.

Allopathic treatment

Meclizine (Bonine), a medication for motion sickness, also diminishes the feeling of queasiness in the stomach. Dimenhydrinate (Dramamine), another motion-sickness drug, is not effective on other types of nausea and may cause drowsiness.

Newer drugs that have been developed to treat postoperative or postchemotherapy nausea and vomiting include ondansetron (Zofran) and granisetron (Kytril). Another treatment that has been found to lower the risk of nausea after surgery is intravenous administration of supplemental fluid before the operation.

Prevention

Massage, **meditation**, **yoga**, and other relaxation techniques can help prevent stress-induced nausea. Antinausea medication taken before traveling can prevent motion sickness. Sitting in the front seat, focusing on the horizon, and traveling after dark can also minimize symptoms.

Food should be fresh, properly prepared, and eaten slowly. Overeating, tight-fitting clothes, and strenuous activity immediately after a meal should be avoided.

Resources

BOOKS

"Functional Vomiting," Section 3, Chapter 21 in *The Merck Manual of Diagnosis and Therapy*, edited by Mark H. Beers, MD, and Robert Berkow, MD. Whitehouse Station, NJ: Merck Research Laboratories, 2002.

Pelletier, Kenneth R., MD. *The Best Alternative Medicine*, Chapter 5, "Acupuncture: From the Yellow Emperor to Magnetic Resonance Imaging (MRI)." New York: Simon & Schuster, 2002.

Reader's Digest Guide to Medical Cures & Treatment: A Complete A to Z Sourcebook of Medical Treatment.

Neck pain

Definition

Neck pain is a nonspecific symptom of discomfort in the neck.

Description

Neck pain has a number of possible causes. Depending on the cause, neck pain may be experienced as limited to the neck itself (localized) or as radiating to the shoulders and upper arm. An individual may experience the pain as a dull ache, a sharp stabbing or burning sensation, or a feeling resembling a muscle cramp. Neck pain is often accompanied by stiffness or difficulty moving the neck.

Causes and symptoms

Possible causes of neck pain include:

- **Trauma.** Whiplash injuries from car accidents and fractures or sprains from rough contact sports or fights are examples of traumatic causes of neck pain.
- **Chronic strain on the muscles and tendons of the neck.** This stress is often related to the individual's occupation, as some jobs require workers to hold their neck and shoulders in one position for long periods. Computer programmers, dentists and dental hygienists, professional musicians (especially string and woodwind players), dancers, and long-distance truck drivers are especially vulnerable to this type of neck pain. In addition, teenagers who work are at higher risk of chronic neck pain than teenagers who participate in sports. Poor posture can also contribute to chronic strain on the neck.
- **Degenerative disorders that affect the neck and spine.** These include osteoarthritis, ankylosing spondylitis, and osteoporosis.
- A herniated disk in one of the cervical (neck) vertebrae. In a herniated disk, the disk projects outward between the vertebrae and can put pressure on a nerve.
- **Congenital abnormalities.** People who are born with abnormally shaped vertebrae or loose joints in the neck region may develop neck pain when the vertebrae begin to put pressure on the spinal cord.
- **Rheumatoid arthritis (RA).**
- **Fibromyalgia.**
- **Infectious diseases.** One of the earliest signs of mumps, meningitis, encephalitis, and poliomyelitis is stiffness and soreness in the neck.

Alternative Options and Home Remedies. Canada: The Reader's Digest's Association, 1996:310.

Zand, Janet, Allan N. Spreen, and James B. LaValle. "Nausea and Vomiting." In *Smart Medicine for Healthier Living: A Practical A-to-Z Reference to Natural and Conventional Treatments for Adults.* Garden City Park, NY: Avery Publishing Group, 1999: 437–439.

PERIODICALS

Ali, S. Z., A. Taguchi, B. Holtmann, and A. Kurz. "Effect of Supplemental Pre-Operative Fluid on Postoperative Nausea and Vomiting." *Anaesthesia* 58 (August 2003): 780–784.

Brunk, Doug. "Acupuncture Gains Favor as Adjunct (Controlling Headaches, Nausea, Dizziness)." *Pediatric News* 35 (December 2001): 1–2.

Cepeda, M. S., J. T. Farrar, M. Baumgarten, et al. "Side Effects of Opioids During Short-Term Administration: Effect of Age, Gender, and Race." *Clinical Pharmacology and Therapeutics* 74 (August 2003): 102–112.

Chung, A., L. Bui, and E. Mills. "Adverse Effects of Acupuncture. Which Are Clinically Significant?" *Canadian Family Physician* 49 (August 2003): 985–989.

O'Brien, C. M., G. Titley, and P. Whitehurst. "A Comparison of Cyclizine, Ondansetron and Placebo as Prophylaxis Against Postoperative Nausea and Vomiting in Children." *Anaesthesia* 58 (July 2003): 707–711.

Ratnaike, R. N. "Acute and Chronic Arsenic Toxicity." *Postgraduate Medical Journal* 79 (July 2003): 391–396.

Tan, M. "Granisetron: New Insights Into Its Use for the Treatment of Chemotherapy-Induced Nausea and Vomiting." *Expert Opinion in Pharmacotherapy* 4 (September 2003): 1563–1571.

Tiwari, A., S. Chan, A. Wong, et al. "Severe Acute Respiratory Syndrome (SARS) in Hong Kong: Patients' Experiences." *Nursing Outlook* 51 (September-October 2003): 212–219.

Treish, I., S. Shord, J. Valgus, et al. "Randomized Double-Blind Study of the Reliefband as an Adjunct to Standard Antiemetics in Patients Receiving Moderately-High to Highly Emetogenic Chemotherapy." *Supportive Care in Cancer* 11 (August 2003): 516–521.

Walling, Anne D. "Ginger Relieves Nausea and Vomiting During Pregnancy." *American Family Physician* 64 (November 15, 2001): 1745.

OTHER

"Nutrition Tips for Managing Nausea and Vomiting." *Mayo Clinic.* http://www.mayohealth.org/mayo/9709/htm/eating5.htm.

Mai Tran
Rebecca J. Frey, PhD

NDV *see* **Newcastle disease virus**

Nearsightedness *see* **Myopia**

Neck pain

• Cancer. Malignant tumors in the neck cause pain when they grow large enough to press on nerve endings and the spinal cord.

• Climatic factors. People whose jobs require them to work in drafty areas or outdoors in cold weather are at higher risk of developing neck pain.

Diagnosis

Diagnosis of neck pain is complicated not only by the number of possible causes but also by the fact that many patients suffer from two or more conditions at the same time. In most cases, the physician will begin by trying to determine if the neck pain is caused by a primary disorder in the neck and shoulder region or if the pain is the result of a systemic disease that is affecting the neck.

Patient history

Taking a careful patient medical and lifestyle history is particularly important in cases of neck pain because of the number of possible causes. A thorough history will include questions about the patient's occupation and sports or hobbies as well as a medical history.

Physical examination

The physician begins by touching, or palpating, the patient's neck and shoulder girdle. Because the underlying bones and muscles in the neck are close to the surface, an experienced examiner can feel swollen glands, tumorous swellings, muscle spasms, or abnormal protrusions between the vertebrae. The doctor then turns the patient's head gently from side to side to determine the neck's range of motion and whether movement worsens the pain. Examination of the inside of the patient's mouth and throat allows the doctor to check the salivary glands, which are swollen and inflamed if the patient has mumps.

Diagnostic imaging

An x ray of the neck may be ordered if the doctor suspects traumatic injury, osteoarthritis, osteoporosis, rheumatoid arthritis, a herniated disk, or congenital deformities. Chronic strain disorders of the neck do not always appear on a plain x ray. If cancer is suspected, the patient may be given a computed tomography (CT) scan of the head, neck, and chest, as well as a gallium scan and a bronchoscopy, laryngoscopy, and esophagoscopy. The patient's lungs and upper gastrointestinal tract are examined because most cancerous tumors in the neck are secondary tumors (metastases) from primary cancers located elsewhere in the body. The doctor may also order a CT scan before scheduling a lumbar puncture if the patient appears to have meningitis or another infection of the central nervous system.

Laboratory tests

The doctor may order a blood test to distinguish rheumatoid arthritis (RA) from systemic lupus erythematosus (SLE) or other inflammatory diseases. Abnormal values for the proteins in blood serum are often present in RA. In addition, a sample of the patient's joint fluid may be taken. Laboratory tests are most important, however, if the doctor suspects that neck pain is due to a central nervous system infection. Central nervous system infections are medical emergencies and require rapid treatment with intravenous antibiotics. Following a CT scan, a sample of the patient's spinal fluid is withdrawn through a lumbar puncture and cultured in order to identify the specific organism causing the infection.

Treatment

Most forms of alternative treatment for neck pain are directed at the milder forms of chronic pain caused by occupational or emotional stress. Many of them can be performed as self-help or self-treatment.

Lifestyle modification

Neck pain caused by chronic stress on the muscles of the neck can interfere significantly with overall quality of life as well as efficiency at work. Work-related neck pain may require a change in occupation or a modification of the equipment that the individual uses (e.g., an ergonomic chair for people who work long hours at the computer). People who have poor posture may benefit from various types of exercise or movement therapy. In some cases, psychotherapy may help to lower stress or relieve the painful feelings that are often associated with poor posture.

Acupressure and acupuncture

Acupressure and shiatsu are traditional Chinese and Japanese therapies that make use of pressure points (sometimes called acupoints) on the body to release muscular pain and tension. For most types of neck pain, the therapist makes use of acupoints on the neck and upper shoulders. Acupuncture as an alternative treatment for neck pain has become increasingly popular in the West since the early 1990s. While some studies indicate that acupuncture is effective in relieving pain in the neck and upper shoulders, other researchers as of 2008 were not convinced.

Chiropractic

Neck pain is a common reason for seeking chiro-practic treatment. A chiropractor treats neck pain by checking the cervical vertebrae for misalignment, which is called subluxation in chiropractic terminol-ogy. The misaligned vertebra is then moved back into proper position with manual pressure. A chiropractic adjustment is thought to restore normal functioning by reducing the stress on the joints, by lowering muscle tension resulting from subluxation, and by minimizing pressure on the spinal nerves. Some health insurance policies pay for chiropractic treatment.

Movement therapies

Both traditional **hatha yoga** and **breema**, a newer form of movement therapy, claim to treat neck pain by reducing or eliminating some of the underlying causes. Teachers of **yoga** maintain that the postures improve the flexibility of the spine and keep the disks between the vertebrae well nourished by spinal fluid. In breema, instructors individualize the exercises, so that persons with neck pain can be given a set of exercises for that specific problem. In addition, both yoga and breema emphasize the importance of cultivating healthy spiri-tual and emotional attitudes toward the body, thus lowering the level of psychological stress that often contributes to neck pain. Other systems that help to re-educate patients in body movement include **Feldenk-rais**, the **Alexander technique**, and **Hanna somatics.**

Reiki, reflexology, and polarity balancing

These methods of treatment rely on light or indirect contact with the affected area rather than on touching it with the techniques used in traditional massage. All three systems of treatment regard neck pain as a symp-tom of energy imbalance in the body. **Reiki** and **polarity therapy** practitioners seek to realign the energy flow by placing the hands lightly on or over parts of the body that are thought to redirect the energy. In **reflexology**, the feet are regarded as a map of the entire body. Neck pain would be treated by massaging the base of the large toes, which represent the neck area.

Traditional Chinese medicine

In **traditional Chinese medicine**, neck pain is treated by *Tui na* massage, followed by a herbal poul-tice on the neck; by suction cups, a traditional remedy for arthritis; or by skin scraping, a technique often used for ailments in the neck area. To perform **cup-ping**, the practitioner flames the inside of a glass suc-tion cup with a cotton ball dipped in alcohol and lighted. The heat from the fire reduces air pressure inside the cup, which is then pressed on the sore area and removed after 15 to 20 minutes. This treatment withdraws excess moisture from the tissues. In skin scraping, the skin on the back and sides of the neck is scraped with a coin dipped in salt water or by pinching a fold of skin, pulling sharply, and letting it fall back. These motions are performed rapidly until bright red stripes appear. Skin scraping is done to release excess heat and energy from the treated area.

Magnetic field therapy

Magnetic field therapy, which involves the appli-cation of a pulsed magnetic field to an injured area of the body, gained in popularity in the early 2000s as a treatment for chronic muscular and joint pain. It is thought that magnetic treatments relieve pain by increasing the flow of oxygenated blood to injured tissue. Some studies indicate that magnetic field ther-apy is useful in relieving chronic neck pain, particu-larly pain associated with whiplash injuries.

Allopathic treatment

Medications

Some forms of neck pain can be treated by med-ication. Osteoporosis is often treated with such compounds as alendronate (Fosamax) or etidronate (Didronel). These medications are intended to prevent further weakening of the bone. Pain caused by osteo-arthritis, **fibromyalgia**, rheumatoid arthritis, or **anky-losing spondylitis** is usually treated with aspirin or nonsteroidal anti-inflammatory drugs (NSAIDs, e.g., Advil, Motrin). Patients with RA may also be given injections of gold salts or methotrexate (MTX, Rheu-matrex). Pain from severe fibromyalgia may be treated with local anesthetics or muscle relaxants.

Appliances

Patients with neck pain caused by traumatic injury, chronic muscular strain, a herniated disk, some forms of osteoarthritis, or congenital deformity may need to have the neck temporarily kept from moving (immobilized) in order to heal. A cervical collar may be used in milder cases. Chronic or severe pain may require more extensive bracing or traction and a period of bed rest.

Surgery

Surgical treatment may be needed to replace dam-aged joints in severe cases of osteoarthritis or rheuma-toid arthritis. Herniated disks occasionally require surgery to fuse the vertebrae around the disk. Some patients with severe cases of ankylosing spondylitis may need to have the cervical spine stabilized by surgery. Most cancers of the neck are removed surgically after a course of radiation treatment.

KEY TERMS

Ankylosing spondylitis—A type of arthritis that causes gradual loss of flexibility in the spinal column. It occurs most commonly in males between the ages of 16 and 35 and may be initiated by a food allergy component, such as an allergy to wheat.

Bronchoscopy—A procedure in which a thin, flexible, lighted tube that is threaded through the airways to view the air passages in the lungs.

Cervical—Relating to the top part of the spine that is composed of the seven vertebrae of the neck and the disks that separate them.

Chiropractic—A method of treatment based on the interactions of the spine and the nervous system. Chiropractors adjust or manipulate segments of the patient's spinal column in order to relieve pain and increase the healthy flow of nerve energy.

Fibromyalgia—A chronic disorder causing pain in the bones and muscles along with severe fatigue.

Herniated—Characterized by an abnormal protrusion of a body part. In a herniated disk, the disk protrudes into the spinal canal between the vertebrae.

Nonsteroidal anti-inflammatory drugs (NSAIDs)—These compounds, which include aspirin, ibuprofen, and indomethacin, are first-choice drugs for treating pain associated with arthritis and autoimmune disorders.

Osteoporosis—A condition found in older individuals in which bones decrease in density and become fragile and more likely to break. It can be caused by lack of vitamin D and/or calcium in the diet.

Palpation—The examination of the body using the sense of touch.

Rheumatoid arthritis—A disease characterized by inflammation and degeneration of connective tissue in multiple joints at a young age.

Subluxation—A partial or incomplete dislocation of the bones that form a joint.

Systemic lupus erythematosus (SLE)—A chronic, inflammatory, autoimmune disorder in which the individual's immune system attacks, injures, and destroys the body's own organs and tissues. It may affect many organ systems, including the skin, joints, lungs, heart, and kidneys.

Prevention

Some potential causes of neck pain are difficult to prevent because they involve a genetic predisposition or component. These include ankylosing spondylitis, osteoarthritis, and RA. Others are easier to prevent by lifestyle choices. Attention to proper posture; the choice of office chairs and other furniture proportioned to the person's height and size; and exercise breaks from office work, study, or musical practice can help to lower the risk of neck pain from chronic muscular stress. Diet as well as exercise is a prominent factor in the prevention of osteoporosis. Observing safety guidelines and wearing protective equipment during contact sports can lower the risk of trauma to the neck. The use of certain types of shoulder harness while driving appears to lower the risk of whiplash injuries. Lastly, **meditation** and other spiritual practices are effective in lowering the level of emotional stress that often underlies chronic neck pain.

Expected results

The results of treatment for neck pain vary widely because of the number of possible causes. While mild arthritis and minor stress injuries in the neck respond well to treatment, cancers in the neck have low survival rates because they are often stage III or stage IV metastases of cancers elsewhere in the body.

Resources

BOOKS

Amir, Fred. *Rapid Recovery from Back and Neck Pain: A Nine-Step Recovery Plan*, 2nd ed. Santa Clara, CA: Health Advisory Group, 2002.

Bensky, Dan, et al. *Chinese Herbal Medicine: Materia Medica*, 3rd ed. Seattle, WA: Eastland Press, 2004.

Mayo Clinic Book of Alternative Medicine: The New Approach to Using the Best of Natural Therapies and Conventional Medicine. New York: Time Inc. Home Entertainment, 2007.

McKenzie, Robin. *Treat Your Own Neck*, 4th ed. Minneapolis, MN: Orthopedic Physical Therapy Products, 2006.

ORGANIZATIONS

Alternative Medicine Foundation, PO Box 60016, Potomac, MD, 20859, (301) 340-1960, http://www.amfoundation.org.

American Association of Oriental Medicine, PO Box 162340, Sacramento, CA, 95816, (866) 455-7999, (914) 443-4770, http://www.aaaomonline.org.

American Holistic Medical Association, PO Box 2016, Edmonds, WA, 98020, (425) 967-0737, http://www.holisticmedicine.org.

American Physical Therapy Association, 1111 North Fairfax Street, Alexandria, VA, 22314-1488, (800)

999-APTA (2782), (703) 684-APTA (2782), http://www.apta.org.

American Polarity Therapy Association, 122 N. Elm Street, Suite 512, Greensboro, NC, 27401, (336) 574-1121, http://www.polaritytherapy.org.

Touch for Health Kinesiology Association, PO Box 392, New Carlisle, OH, 45344-0392, (800) 466-8342, (937) 845-3404, http://www.tfhka.org.

Rebecca J. Frey, PhD
Tish Davidson, A.M.

Neem

Description

Neem is a compound that has a long history of use in both traditional Indian medicine and Ayurveda. Many of the popular herbal treatments in these two systems are still derived from it. Neem is a large evergreen tree, *Azadirachta indica*, in the mahogany family. It grows naturally in India and Sri Lanka, and has been successfully transplanted to other regions including West Africa, Indonesia, and Australia. The tree has small white flowers and produces a smooth, yellow-green fruit. All parts of the tree have medical uses. In India, neem is sometimes called "the village pharmacy." Over 100 pharmacologically active substances have been identified in this plant, and it has many traditional applications.

General use

Neem's wide variety of reported benefits include use in the treatment of **fever**, gastrointestinal disease, dermatologic (skin) disorders, immune dysfunction, respiratory disease, parasites, inflammatory conditions, and **infections** by some bacteria, fungi, and viruses. Some components have been shown to have antimalarial properties. The seeds contain an insecticidal substance that is EPA approved for use on non-food crops.

Some viral diseases have been treated by components of neem. It may inhibit the multiplication of viruses and prevent them from entering and infecting cells. Some of the diseases that have reportedly been relieved include colds, flu, and conditions caused by herpes, such as **chickenpox** and **shingles**.

Neem appears to be an appropriate treatment for numerous dermatologic indications. Its anti-inflammatory and **pain** relieving activity make it potentially useful against **psoriasis**, **eczema**, **acne**, **dermatitis**, and an assortment of fungal conditions. The neem leaf has been shown to have activity that suppresses the fungi that cause **athlete's foot**, ringworm, and *Candida*. Seed oil and aqueous leaf extracts have been used to treat **jock itch**, another fungal infection. The oil and leaf extract may be applied externally in the form of lotions and soaps. Leaf preparations may also be used internally for the **detoxification** properties. Poultices made from the leaf have antiseptic and astringent properties that treat **wounds** and **boils**.

Both internal and external parasites may be sensitive to the effects of neem. External parasites, such as lice and mites, are often treated in India with aqueous extracts of neem leaves. A medical research center in Nagercoil, India, found that a combination of neem and **turmeric** cured 97% of patients with **scabies** within 3–15 days of treatment. Teas are used against internal parasites, including intestinal **worms**. Perhaps one of the most interesting claims for neem is for the prevention and treatment of **malaria**. Leaf extracts are said to have the same effectiveness as quinine and chloroquine, the conventional medications that are used. Some studies show that even chloroquine-resistant **strains** of malaria are sensitive to neem, particularly a component called Irodin A. The recommended preventative measure is to chew and consume the leaves on a daily basis.

Twigs and leaves of the neem tree may be used for oral hygiene, and neem bark extracts used in toothpastes and mouthwashes are active against gingivitis. Ayurveda holds that neem has healthful properties for teeth and gum tissue.

Ayurvedic tradition holds that neem bark improves resistance to disease. It appears that certain carbohydrates contained in the bark do indeed stimulate the production of antibodies. One source recommends a cyclical use of neem to strengthen the immune system in order to lower the incidence of infections, particularly in people who have conditions that compromise the immune system.

Some studies show that neem can lower blood sugar levels. It has traditionally been used in Indian medicine for diabetes, and research with animals confirms this potential. Neem is an approved medication for the treatment of diabetes in India. Several forms of the supplement, including leaf extracts and teas, have been shown to have beneficial effects on reducing blood sugar.

There are several components of neem that may make it valuable in the treatment of both **osteoarthritis** and **rheumatoid arthritis**. It is a proven anti-inflammatory that decreases histamine and other

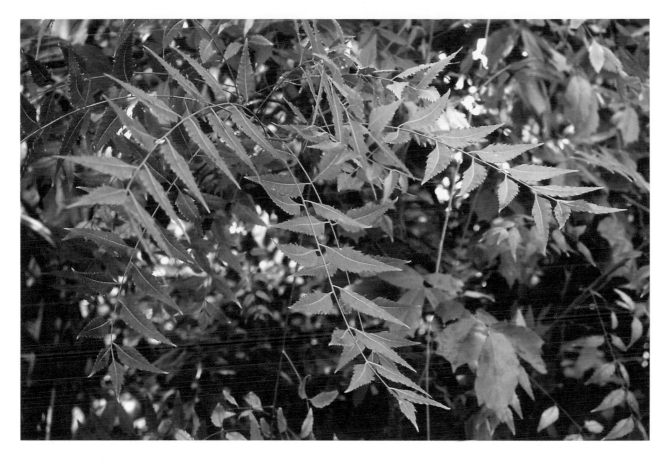

Neem plant. *(©PlantaPhile, Germany. Reproduced by permission.)*

mediators of inflammation in the body. Some of the important chemicals in neem that contribute to this effect are nimbidin, limonoids, and catechin. Warmed neem oil is also recommended for external use to reduce pain and inflammation in affected joints.

Neem has documented spermicidal properties when used intravaginally in women, and is sometimes used as a contraceptive. It is also being studied as a birth control measure for use by males.

Other claims for neem are extensive. They include treatment of high blood pressure, **cholesterol**, heart arrhythmia, kidney disorders, **indigestion**, **anxiety**, **epilepsy**, and many more. Some cancers may possibly be affected by the use of neem products. Consult a practitioner of Ayurveda or other expert in the use of botanicals for guidance in appropriate indications and products.

In addition to the treatment of human diseases and disorders, neem is being intensively studied as a natural insect repellent and pesticide. Studies in India and Pakistan have shown that it is an effective mosquito repellent. In 2002, the United States Department of Agriculture (USDA) reported that neem seed extract is toxic to the larvae of the Florida root weevil and other pests that attack citrus trees. As of 2000, 70 different patents had been granted for neem products intended for agricultural use.

Researchers in the textile industry are also finding uses for neem in the production of natural compounds for treating fabric. Neem seed hulls can be used to support the growth of fungi that produce an enzyme that will remove dye from cloth.

Preparations

There are many forms and routes of use for neem. Some of the preparations include seed oil, aqueous extracts of the leaf, powder from the leaf, smoke from burning dried leaves, and leaf pastes. Topically, neem oil and leaf extracts are incorporated into some soaps and lotions for the treatment of skin conditions. These act to relieve inflammation and kill some of the infectious causes of conditions including acne and many fungi. A decoction of the bark is used externally for **hemorrhoids**. Some bark extracts are also especially bactericidal.

KEY TERMS

Ayurveda—In Sanskrit, *Ayur,* means life, and *veda* means knowledge. Ayurveda is a system of holistic medicine from India that aims to bring the individual into harmony with nature. It provides guidance regarding food and lifestyle, so that healthy people can stay healthy and people with health challenges can improve their health.

Decoction—An herbal extract produced by mixing an herb in cold water, bringing the mixture to a boil, and letting it simmer to evaporate the excess water. The decoction is then strained and drank hot or cold. Decoctions are usually chosen over infusion when the botanical or herb in question is a root, seed, or berry.

Gingivitis—Inflammation of the gums in which the margins of the gums near the teeth are red, puffy, and bleeding. It is most often due to poor dental hygiene.

Scabies—A contagious parasitic skin disease caused by a tiny mite and characterized by intense itching.

Sequela (plural, sequelae)—An abnormal condition resulting from a previous disease or disorder.

The directions for use and application of products vary depending on the formulation. Refer to the label information or consult a health care provider.

Precautions

Due to a lack of sufficient study data and possible toxicity, it is inadvisable for children and pregnant or nursing women to use neem. Those who have impaired liver or kidney function should also use great caution. Large doses of seed or seed components may be toxic.

Traditional Ayurvedic practitioners advise against the use of neem if the patient suffers from obvious wasting or **fatigue**.

Side effects

The long history of the use of neem in India appears to show that there is a low incidence of side effects when used appropriately. Infants have suffered severe sequelae, and even death as a result of internal use of neem. Avoid using neem products on children.

Interactions

No clinically significant interactions between neem and other supplements or medications have been reported as of 2002.

Resources

BOOKS

Bratman, Steven, and David Kroll. *Natural Health Bible.* Roseville, Calif.: Prima Publishing, 1999.

Chevallier, Andrew. *The Encyclopedia of Medicinal Plants.* New York: DK Publishing, Inc., 1996.

Jellin, Jeff, Forrest Batz, and Kathy Hitchens. *Pharmacist's letter/Prescriber's Letter Natural Medicines Comprehensive Database.* Calif.: Therapeutic Research Faculty, 1999.

Pelletier, Kenneth R., MD. *The Best Alternative Medicine.* New York: Simon & Schuster, 2002.

PERIODICALS

Siddiqui, B. S., F. Afshan, S. Faizi, et al. "Two New Triterpenoids from *Azadirachta indica* and Their Insecticidal Activity." *Journal of Natural Products* 65 (August 2002): 1216-1218.

Verma, P., and D. Madamwar. "Production of Ligninolytic Enzymes for Dye Decolorization by Cocultivation of White-Rot Fungi *Pleurotus ostreatus* and *Phanerochaete chrysosporium* Under Solid-State Fermentation." *Applied Biochemistry and Biotechnology* 102-103 (July-December 2002): 109-118.

Weathersbee, A. A., 3rd, and Y. Q. Tang. "Effect of Neem Seed Extract on Feeding, Growth, Survival, and Reproduction of *Diaprepes abbreviatus* (Coleoptera: Curculionidae)." *Journal of Economic Entomology* 95 (August 2002): 661-667.

ORGANIZATIONS

The Ayurvedic Institute. 11311 Menaul NE, Albuquerque, NM 87112. (505) 291-9698. www.ayurveda.com.

National Institute of Ayurvedic Medicine. 584 Milltown Road, Brewster, NY 10509. (845) 278-8700. www.niam.com.

United States Department of Agriculture. Washington, DC 20250. www.usda.gov.

OTHER

Selvester, Joseph. "Neem: The Village Pharmacy." *The Original Neem Company.* http://www.askjoseph.com/ Ayurveda/villagepharmacy.htm. (1999).

Judith Turner
Rebecca J. Frey, PhD

Nerve pain *see* **Neuralgia**

Nettle

Description

Nettle is a member of the Urticaceae family, which includes as many as 500 species worldwide. Many species are tropical. The stinging nettle (*Urtica dioica*)

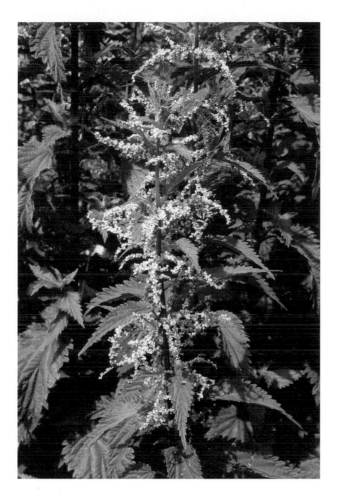

Nettle plant. *(©PlantaPhile, Germany. Reproduced by permission.)*

grows wild in nitrogen-rich soil on the edges of fields, stream banks, waste places, and close to stables and human habitations throughout the United States and Europe. This fibrous perennial is found throughout the world in temperate regions from Japan to the Andes Mountains. The plant seeds itself, and, in favorable conditions, nettle spreads freely from its tough, creeping yellow root. The hairy, erect, single stalks grow in dense clusters giving the plant a bushy look. The square stems produce heart-shaped, alternate leaves with pointed tips and deeply serrated edges. Leaves are dark green on the top and are a paler green and downy on the underside. The plant grows as tall as 4 ft (1.2 m). Leaves and stems are covered with needlelike hairs that pierce the skin on contact. The plant delivers a sharp sting and a lingering irritation caused by a combination of formic acid, serotonin, acetylcholine, and 5-hydroxytryptamine injected through the tiny needlelike hairs.

The common name nettle is taken from the Anglo-Saxon word *noedl* meaning "needle." Nettle's tiny green flowers grow in dangling clusters in the angles formed by the stalk and stem of the leaf. Flowers bloom from July to September. Each small fruit contains just one seed. Male and female flowers usually grow on separate plants of the stinging nettle, hence the species name *dioica*, meaning "separate," or "two houses." The genus name, *Urtica*, is taken from the Latin *uro*, "to burn." Small nettle (*U. urens*), an annual, usually has both male and female flowers on the same branched cluster. Its properties and uses are similar to those of the stinging nettle.

Older herbals cite the planet Mars with dominion over this common wayside plant. Nettle was certainly used in many battles. Roman nettle (*U. pilulifera*) is said to have been brought to Britain by Caesar's troops, who used the plant to flail themselves in an effort to keep warm in the cool, damp climate. Nettle's fibrous characteristics rival those of hemp and flax. Nettle fibers were woven into fabric for sails and ropes, and for German army uniforms as recently as World War I.

General use

Despite its piercing defense, the stinging nettle has long been valued as a medicinal and nutritional treasure. Nettle has astringent, expectorant, galactagogue (milk producing), tonic, anti-inflammatory, hemostatic, and diuretic properties. The plant is rich in chlorophyll, and a good source of **beta carotene**; vitamins A, C, and E; tannins; **iron**; **calcium**; phosphates; and various other minerals, especially **silica**. The active ingredients include water-soluble polysaccharides that stimulate the immune system, and large protein-sugar molecules known as lectins. The entire plant may be used in various medicinal preparations.

Nettle leaf is used in a simple infusion as a tonic decoction to cleanse the blood. Nettle can also be combined with **yellow dock** (*Rumex crispis*), **dandelion** (*Taraxacum officinale*), cleavers (*Galium aparine*), and **burdock root** (*Arctium lappa*). In folk medicine, the plant was used in a practice known as urtication. The fresh herb was thrashed across the skin to induce a stinging, burning sensation used to relieve the deeper **pain** of rheumatism. A leaf infusion, or a homeopathic tincture of nettle, may also be helpful as supportive therapy for rheumatism. With sufficient water intake, nettle acts as a diuretic and is helpful in treating arthritis and rheumatism. A team of German researchers has reported that the anti-inflammatory effect of nettle is related to its suppression of a type of cell that stimulates the inflammatory response.

An early twentieth-century herbalist reported that the juice of the fresh leaves and root (or the dried leaf when burned and inhaled) was useful to treat **asthma**. Nettle seeds, when ingested, were once thought to be beneficial in the treatment of **bites** from "mad dogs" or the stinging of "venomous creatures," according to Nicolas Culpeper, a seventeenth century doctor. Seeds were also used as an antidote to poisonous herbs such as nightshade (*Solanum dulcamara*) and henbane (*Hyoscyamus niger*), though no recent studies support this use.

Nettle is thought to be particularly helpful for treating urinary tract problems. An infusion of the leaves may be used for inflammatory diseases of the lower urinary tract. The infusion is thought to flush the system and to help expel kidney gravel. It has also been used internally to stop bleeding. An ointment preparation of the aerial parts, or a strong infusion, can be applied externally to relieve **hemorrhoids**. Nettle can increase and enrich the flow of milk in breast-feeding mothers.

Clinical studies have confirmed stinging nettle's benefit to men in reducing symptoms of benign prostatic hyperplasia (a noncancerous enlargement of the prostate gland). A concentrated root extract of nettle is sometimes combined with **saw palmetto** (*Serenoa repens*) and the bark of the pygeum evergreen tree (*Pygeum africanum*) to treat the early stages of the disease. The herbal combination helps to increase the urinary volume and maximize the rate of urine flow. German research suggests that active ingredients in the nettle root may reduce prostate swelling.

During allergy season, a tincture of the fresh herb, or an infusion as a tea, may reduce symptoms of **hay fever**, such as itchy eyes and **sneezing**. However, a study published in 2002 indicates that the antiallergic effects attributed to nettle require further study. Nettle's expectorant properties have been beneficial for coughs and have been used to expel phlegm from the lungs and stomach. The freshly gathered and cooked herb was used as a nutritive potherb in folk medicine to treat consumption. Nettle continues to be valued by wild-food foragers as an early spring potherb, rich in minerals. Nettle juice may be used as a vegetarian substitute for rennet to curdle milk when making cheese.

When boiled with equal parts vinegar and water, a decoction of the plant (particularly the root) is a beneficial and conditioning hair and scalp rinse useful in cases of **dandruff** and thinning hair. A nettle rinse won't restore hair to a bald head. However, it will lend a shine and enhance the color of the hair one does have. A small piece of cotton soaked in a nettle decoction and placed in the nostril can be used to stop a nosebleed. The root, when boiled, will produce a yellow dye, and the leaves produce a permanent, light green dye for wool.

Preparations

Numerous commercial preparations of the herb are available in the form of capsules, dried leaf for tea, homeopathic tinctures, or ointments. The medicinal potency of the herb will vary depending on the growing conditions and the manner and care with which the herb is harvested and prepared.

The fresh leaves and stems should be gathered from young plants on a dry day, just before the plant flowers. Caution should be used when harvesting to avoid the sting. Nettle's aerial parts may be used fresh or dried. To dry, the bunches are hung upside down out of direct sun in an airy room. The root is harvested in the fall when the plant has died back. It is washed thoroughly. Large roots may be chopped into slices while fresh and spread on a tray in a warm, sunny room for several days. Dried plant parts are stored in sealed containers in a dark place.

To make an infusion, 2 oz of fresh, finely chopped nettle leaves are combined with 2.5 cups of fresh, non-chlorinated water (2 tbsp of the dried herb may be used). This mixture is brought to a boil, removed from the heat, and covered. The tea is steeped for about 10 minutes. It is then strained and can be drunk warm or cold. The prepared tea can be stored for about two days in the refrigerator. Dosage for a general tonic is 3 or 4 cups per day. Ample fresh water should be drunk when using nettle as a diuretic tea.

To make a decoction, 2 oz of fresh or 1 tbsp of dried root is combined in a nonmetallic pan with 2.5 cups of water. The mixture is simmered for two minutes, then steeped for 10 minutes. The mixture is then strained.

To extract the juice, an abundance of nettle leaves and stems are gathered. A household food processor or juicer may be used to pulp the plant parts. The resulting pulp is then squeezed through a sieve. The juice is then sealed in dark glass containers and refrigerated.

To make an essential oil, the fresh nettle leaves and stems are packed in a large glass container. They are then covered completely with olive oil. A lid is placed on the container and the mixture is left on a sunny windowsill for two to three weeks. It is stirred daily. After this time period, the mixture is strained through cheesecloth and the oil is stored in a dark glass container.

To make an ointment, beeswax or petroleum jelly is melted in the top of a glass or ceramic double boiler. Finely chopped nettle leaf and stems are stirred in. The mixture is heated on low for about two hours. The mixture is strained through cheesecloth and, with gloved hands, the liquid is squeezed from the cloth. The liquid is then poured into clean, dark glass storage containers while still warm. The containers should be sealed with tight-fitting lids and stored away from direct sunlight.

Precautions

Gloves should always be worn when nettle is harvested to avoid the sharp sting. According to folk tradition, fresh yellow dock leaves may alleviate the burning when rubbed on nettle **stings**. When using stinging nettle preparations to irrigate and flush out the urinary tract, or as a treatment of kidney gravel, abundant fluid intake is required. Stinging nettle preparations are not to be used in the treatment of fluid retention brought on by reduced heart or kidney function. This plant should never be harvested after flowers appear because if harvested at this time, the plant can cause urinary tract damage.

Side effects

Aside from the distinctive sting when touching the fresh plant, there are few side effects from use of the herb in properly prepared therapeutic doses. Mild gastrointestinal distress may occasionally occur. Some people are allergic to nettle.

This plant should not be consumed raw because it can irritate mucous membranes. Leaves of the young plant can be safely consumed when cooked as a nutritional potherb. Boiling the young leaves and stems disarms the stinging hairs. Drying the herb also disarms the stinging hairs. The uncooked, mature nettles should not be eaten.

Interactions

Nettle appears to intensify the effects of nonsteroidal anti-inflammatory drugs, or NSAIDs, which are commonly given for arthritis and similar conditions. While this increased effect may be beneficial to patients with arthritis, they should nonetheless consult a healthcare provider before taking nettle.

Resources

BOOKS

The Alternative Advisor. Time/Life, 1999.

Lust, John. *The Herb Book*. New York: Bantam Books, 1994.

The PDR Family Guide to Natural Medicines And Healing Therapies. New York: Three Rivers Press, 1999.

PDR for Herbal Medicines. New Jersey: Medical Economics Company, 1998.

PERIODICALS

Broer, J., and B. Behnke. "Immunosuppressant Effect of IDS 30, a Stinging Nettle Leaf Extract, on Myeloid Dendritic Cells in Vitro." *Journal of Rheumatology* 29 (April 2002): 659-666.

Jaber, R. "Respiratory and Allergic Diseases: From Upper Respiratory Tract Infections to Asthma." *Primary Care* 29 (June 2002): 231-261.

Lowe, F. C., and E. Fagelman. "Phytotherapy in the Treatment of Benign Prostatic Hyperplasia." *Current Opinions in Urology* 12 (January 2002): 15-18.

Schulze-Tanzil, G., B. Behnke, S. Klingelhöfer, et al. "Effects of the Antirheumatic Remedy Hox Alpha–A New Stinging Nettle Leaf Extract–On Matrix Metalloproteinases in Human Chondrocytes in Vitro." *Histology and Histopathology* 17 (April 2002): 477-485.

Vahlensieck, W., Jr. "With Alpha Blockers, Finasteride and Nettle Root Against Benign Prostatic Hyperplasia. Which Patients Are Helped by Conservative Therapy?" [in German] *MMW-Fortschritte der Medizin* 144 (April 18, 2002): 33-36.

ORGANIZATIONS

American Botanical Council. 6200 Manor Road, Austin, TX 78714-4345. (512) 926-4900. www.herbalgram.org.

OTHER

"Nettle." *MotherNature.com*. http://www.mothernature.com/ency/Herb/Nettle.asp. (1998).

Clare Hanrahan
Rebecca J. Frey, PhD

Neural therapy

Definition

Neural therapy is a comprehensive healing system that focuses on the relief of chronic **pain** and long-term illness. These symptoms, practitioners say, can be stopped by injecting local anesthetics into scars, **acupuncture** points peripheral nerves, and glands. Other, less-invasive methods may also be used to correct "short circuits" and restore electrical conductivity in the body.

Origins

The earliest known use of neural therapy was in 1925, when two German doctors treated migraine headaches by injecting a local anesthetic (Novocain)

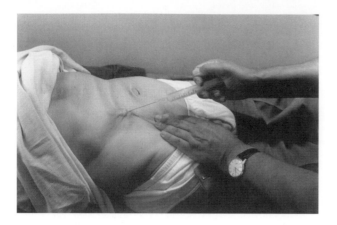

A patient is injected with a local anesthetic as part of neural therapy. *(Horacio Sormani / Photo Researchers, Inc.)*

into the veins. The injections immediately aborted not only the headaches but also a number of other symptoms (**dizziness**, **nausea**, a visual "flashing" sensation) also associated with migraine. In 1940, Dr. Ferdinand Huneke, a German physician, found that injecting procaine (Novocain) into an osteomyelitis scar on a patient's leg seemed to instantly cure chronic pain in her shoulder. Now called the lightning reaction or Huneke phenomenon, it showed that injuries in one part of the body may cause symptoms elsewhere in the body. Although it is still not fully understood, neural therapy has been widely practiced since the 1940s in both Europe and South America. More recently, some neural therapists have employed less-invasive procedures involving electricity, lasers, and other light sources.

Benefits

Neural therapy has been used in the treatment of hundreds of conditions. These include **depression**, hormonal imbalances, dizziness, **allergies**, **asthma**, skin diseases, **hemorrhoids**, ulcers, chronic bowel problems, prostrate and bladder problems, **headache** (including migraine), kidney disease, arthritis, back pain, as well as whiplash and other soft-tissue injuries.

Description

The most common procedures used by practitioners of neural therapy involve injections of procaine (Novocain), lidocaine, other local anesthetics, or saline solution into scars, glands, ganglia, peripheral nerves, acupuncture points, and other tissues. These injections are intended to correct abnormal electrical signaling caused by injuries, or to detoxify tissues or

enhance the effectiveness of drugs or nutrients. Other substances that may be injected include nutrients, isopathic dilutions of toxic substances, or diluted traditional medicines such as Benadryl or Demerol. It is argued that all scars cause problems and must be injected at least once. A typical course of treatment may involve between one and six sessions at a frequency of twice a week.

Precautions

Neural therapy involves invasive procedures that should be done only by properly licensed practitioners. It is not advisable for patients with allergies to local anesthetics. Anyone with serious illness should avoid using neural therapy as a sole method of treatment. In such cases, advice should also be sought from a medical practitioner. Neural therapy is thought, in some cases, to activate repressed psychological trauma. Patients may wish to consider whether their practitioner is competent to deal with the resurrection of these subconscious memories. Neural therapy is considered ineffective against **cancer** and metabolic disorders.

Side effects

When carried out by a competent, experienced therapist, neural therapy is considered generally free of adverse side effects. However, in one case reported in a German medical journal, serious internal bleeding resulted from an attempt to inject the adenoids. This indicates that life-threatening side effects are possible when neural therapists inject deeply into internal structures and organs, the article warned.

Research and general acceptance

Neural therapy has gained considerable acceptance among medical doctors and other practitioners in Germany, but is not widely known outside of Europe and South America. Its effectiveness as a pain-management tool is generally accepted, but there has been little scientific research into other claimed therapeutic benefits.

Training and certification

In Germany, neural therapy is available from many orthodox medical practitioners. Elsewhere in the world, a variety of medical doctors, osteopaths, dentists, naturopaths, chiropractors, and acupuncturists have undergone training in the discipline. The American Academy of Neural Therapy offers workshops, videos, and course manuals. Early in 2000, this group was moving toward board certification of neural therapists.

Resources

ORGANIZATIONS

American Academy of Neural Therapy. 410 East Denny Way, Suite 18, Seattle, WA, 98122. (206) 749-9967. http://www.Neuraltherapy.com.

David Helwig

Neuralgia

Definition

Neuralgia describes a variety of rare and painful conditions in which shooting, stabbing, burning, **pain**; electric-like shocks; or tingling, pins and needles, or numbness occur along the course of a nerve, usually in the head or neck.

Description

Neuralgia attacks tend to by cyclic, often coming and going without warning. They can last for minutes, hours, days, or longer, depending on the patient, and range from mild to debilitating. Often, no physical cause can be found, although some forms of neuralgia may be triggered when nerves are compressed by injuries, arteries, tumors, or, in rare cases, as the result of nerve damage from **multiple sclerosis**. Neuralgia is an uncommon condition, with trigeminal neuralgia occurring most often. Other types are occipital neuralgia, glossopharyngeal neuralgia, and postherpetic neuralgia. Most neuralgia patients are 50 or older, although younger patients can be affected as well.

Causes and symptoms

Most neuralgias appear suddenly, with no apparent physical basis for the pain, which can be severe. Other neuralgias may follow an injury, with pain, burning, tingling, or numbness in whatever part of the body the affected nerve supplies.

Trigeminal neuralgia (TN) also called *tic douloureux,* from the French for "painful spasm," is a disorder of the fifth cranial nerve, whose three branches supply the face. (There are 12 pairs of cranial nerves that supply the human head.) Most TN patients are 50 or older, with more women affected than men. Early attacks are short—one to two minutes long—but excruciating, with stabbing, shooting, pain on one side of the face. The location depends on which branch of the nerve is affected. At first, weeks or months separate incidents, but as the condition progresses the time between attacks shortens. Eventually, the area becomes hypersensitive, and painful bouts can even be triggered by eating, drinking, talking, cold, or even touching the face.

Glossopharyngeal is a relatively rare neuralgia, marked by recurring attacks of severe pain that occur for no apparent reason in the throat, ears, and neck. Glossopharyngeal neuralgia patients also tend to be middle-aged, but are more often male than female. The attacks can occur without warning, but, like other facial neuralgias, can also be triggered by **sneezing**, swallowing, talking, yawning, or clearing the throat.

Occipital neuralgia is caused by pain from one of the two occipital nerves that supply the back of the head. Unlike TN or glossopharyngeal neuralgia, occipital neuralgia may occur in conjunction with muscle tension or migraine headaches, with the spasms of nerve pain on top of nearly continual aching.

Although most neuralgias have no known cause, one type, postherpetic neuralgia (PHN) is only seen following an outbreak of **shingles**, a painful, blistering rash caused by the Herpes zoster virus, the same virus that causes chicken pox. Herpes zoster lives in nerve tissue, and never goes away, even after the initial outbreak of chicken pox has disappeared. Older people, especially those with weak immune systems, can suffer a relapse, with the rash appearing along the course of the nerve that is affected. This produces the searing pain of neuralgia, which can be made even worse by the touch of clothing, bedclothes, or another person. PHN and TN are the most common types of neuralgia.

Diagnosis

Physicians begin with a thorough examination, and often include a CT scan or MRI. These will sometimes uncover an artery or tumor that is compressing the nerve and creating the symptoms, but very often no obvious medical problem is found.

KEY TERMS

Desensitization—A treatment for phobias which involves exposing the phobic person to the feared situation. It is often used in conjunction with relaxation techniques. Also used to describe a technique of pain reduction in which the painful area is stimulated with whatever is causing the pain.

Dorsal root entry zone (DREZ)—A type of nerve surgery for postherpetic neuralgia that is occasionally used when the patient can get no other pain relief. The surgery destroys the area where damaged nerves join the central nervous system, thereby interfering with inappropriate pain messages from nerves to the brain.

Glossopharyngeal neuralgia—Sharp recurrent pain deep in the throat that extends to the area around the tonsils and possibly the ear. It is triggered by swallowing or chewing.

Occipital neuralgia—Pain on one side of the back of the head caused by entrapment or pinching of an occipital nerve.

Postherpetic neuralgia—Persistent pain that occurs as a complication of a herpes zoster infection. Although the pain can be treated, the response is variable.

Shingles—An disease caused by an infection with the *Herpes zoster* virus, the same virus that causes chickenpox. Symptoms of shingles include pain and blisters along one nerve, usually on the face, chest, stomach, or back.

Transcutaneous electrical nerve stimulation (TENS)—A technique used to control chronic pain. Electrodes placed over the painful area deliver a mild electrical impulse to nearby nerve pathways, thereby blocking transmission of pain signals to the brain.

Trigeminal neuralgia or tic douloureux—An affliction of the trigeminal or fifth cranial nerve. The condition is characterized by attacks of shooting, stabbing pain on one side of the face. These episodes are triggered by touching the affected area.

In addition, trigeminal neuralgia can be identified by several distinctive traits, many of which apply to other neuralgias as well:

- The patient has attacks of pain in the face that last less than two minutes.
- The pain follows the path of the trigeminal (or another) nerve.
- The pain is described as sudden, sharp, stabbing or burning, and severe.
- The pain may be triggered by certain activities.
- There are no symptoms between attacks.
- In many patients, TN can be positively diagnosed if the drug carbamazepine (Tegretol) diminishes the pain of an attack.

Glossopharyngeal neuralgia is identified in the same way as TN, that is, the patient complains of stabbing, spasmodic pain that follows the Glossopharyngeal nerve. A positive diagnosis is usually achieved if the pain stops when the nerve is blocked with a local anesthesia.

Occipital neuralgia is caused by pain from one of the two occipital nerves that supply the back of the head. Unlike TN or glossopharyngeal neuralgia, occipital neuralgia may occur in conjunction with muscle tension or migraine headaches, with the spasms of nerve pain on top of nearly continual aching. X rays and CT scans can help indicate if the nerve is compressed; numbing the nerve with anesthetics can pinpoint the cause.

Treatment

Trigeminal neuralgia was identified almost 2,000 years ago. Early treatments, like most medicine in those days, were mostly topical (applied to the skin) and ineffective. Today, the most effective treatments for neuralgia are allopathic, but alternative therapies may help support the patient's general well being and improve overall health.

Nutritional therapy

B-complex vitamins, taken orally or given by intramuscular injection, are important for a healthy nervous system, and may supplement medical treatment. A whole foods diet with adequate protein, carbohydrates, and fats that also includes yeast, liver, **wheat germ**, and foods that are high in B vitamins is important. **Essential fatty acids**, such as flax or **fish oil**, may also help reduce inflammation.

Herbal therapy

Capsaicin cream, made from capsicum, a substance found in hot peppers, has sometimes been helpful in desensitizing painful areas in postherpetic neuralgia. Capsaicin may diminish the amount of "substance P," a chemical used by nerves to send pain signals to the brain. **St. John's wort**, an antidepressant, may help the other forms of neuralgia, which are often treated allopathically with tricyclic antide-pressants (TCAs)

Acupuncture

Some patients found that **acupuncture** was help-ful in treating their neuralgia pain, especially that of postherpetic neuralgia. Others were unable to obtain relief from the procedure.

Chiropractic

Chiropractors can manipulate the jawbone, neck or spine to treat neuralgia pain. Like most alternative treatments for neuralgia, this is effective for some patients and not for others.

Homeopathy

Homeopathic treatment can also be tried. An experienced homeopathic practitioner will prescribe remedies to bolster the paitient's general health, tailor-ing remedies to the patient's overall personality profile as well as specific symptoms.

Other alternative therapies

The pain of neuralgia may also be relieved by **hydrotherapy** (hot shower or bath), deep massage, **reflexology** (massaging reflex points in the feet relat-ing affected painful areas in the body) or **yoga** exer-cises. In addition, **guided imagery**, **biofeedback** therapy, and hypnosis may be beneficial. Patients should also consider **t'ai chi**, **qigong**, and other **move-ment therapy**.

Patients may also be helped by transcutaneous electrical nerve stimulation (TENS), in which a weak electrical current applied to the skin interferes with the nerve's ability to send pain signals to the brain. Although somewhat controversial, initial results, espe-cially for postherpetic neuralgia, are promising.

Allopathic treatment

Once a diagnosis of neuralgia has been estab-lished, physicians prescribe drugs to alleviate the pain. The anticonvulsant drug carbamazepine (Tegre-tol) is often an effective treatment for TN, relieving or reducing the pain within a day or two. Unfortunately, it can also cause **dizziness**, drowsiness, **nausea**, and double vision, as well as other side effects. If Tegretol is not well tolerated, doctors can try another anitcon-vulsant, like gabapentin (Neurontin), antispasmodics like baclofen (Lioresal), or anti-anxiety drugs like clo-nazepam (Klonopin). These drugs are also frequently prescribed for other forms of neuralgia as well.

Injecting local anesthetics into the nerve can stop the pain for a few hours, and for some patients this is effective for a much longer time. Lidocaine cream may be somewhat helpful in treating PHN, probably by temporarily desensitizing nerves just under the skin. Lidocaine may also help atypical forms of TN. Alco-hol and glycerin injections that destroy part of the nerve (and thereby its ability to transmit pain) may also be an option.

One particularly unpleasant, but evidently suc-cessful, method of treating neuralgia seems to be desensitization. This means that if a patient is both-ered by the touch of clothing on the skin, the therapist may rub a towel briskly over the area for a few minutes. If the patient has trouble tolerating heat or cold, warm or cold water may be applied. Although initially quite painful, this method gradually dimin-ishes the frequency and intensity of the patient's pain, apparently by overwhelming (and eventually reduc-ing) the nerve's ability to send messages to the brain.

For PHN, the best treatment seems to be preven-tion. People with shingles should see a doctor as soon as the rash develops so they can receive treatment to ease the severity of the outbreak and minimize the risk of developing postherpetic neuralgia. It is not clear, however, whether treatment can prevent subsequent neuralgia. If PHN does develop, TCAs—especially amitriptyline—are often helpful. It's important to **stress**, though, that early attention to either a shingles outbreak or PHN episode will reduce the incidence and severity of future attacks. Some patients receive complete pain relief after treatment. Others are able only to reduce the pain (to greater or lesser degrees), while for a very few treatment is completely ineffec-tive. For these patients PHN becomes a lifelong, chronic condition; most cases, however, moderate on their own and disappear within five years. In 2002, clinical trials showed that gabapentin (Neurontin) was effective in treating patients with PHN with rela-tively low adverse effects.

As a last resort, surgery may bring relief for those neuralgia patients not helped by pharmaceuticals. Most procedures try to reduce the nerve's ability to send pain signals to the brain. One of the most prom-ising is dorsal root entry zone (DREZ) lesioning, which uses radio frequency to disrupt the nerves that are causing pain. Some studies showed that as many as 80% of DREZ patients were helped.

Expected results

Only a few neuralgia patients will not be helped by some combination of drugs and surgery. PHN, in particular, tends to fade away on its own, and only 2–3% of patients have pain that lasts a year or longer. For those unfortunate few, however, PHN can become a lifelong, debilitating condition.

Resources

BOOKS

Althoff, Susanne, Patricia N. Williams, Dianne Molvig, and Larry Schuster. *A Guide to Alternative Medicine*. Lincolnwood, IL: Publications International, Ltd., 1997.

Gottlieb, Bill, ed. "Sciatica." In *New Choices in Natural Healing: Over 1,800 of the Best Self-Help Remedies from the World of Alternative Medicine*. Emmaus, PA: Rodale Press, 1995.

Loeser, J. "Cranial Neuralgias." In *The Management of Pain*. 2nd ed. Philadelphia: Lea & Febiger, 1990.

"Neuralgia." In *The Hamlyn Encyclopedia of Complementary Medicine*. Great Britain: Reed International Books Limited, 1996.

PERIODICALS

Fields, H. "Treatment of Trigeminal Neuralgia." *The New England Journal of Medicine* 334 (April 1996): 1125–1126.

"Neurontin." *Formulary* 334 (July 2002): 335.

ORGANIZATIONS

American Chronic Pain Association. PO Box 850, Rocklin, CA 95677. (916) 632-0922.

National Chronic Pain Outreach. PO Box 274, Millboro, VA 24460. (540) 997-5004.

Trigeminal Neuralgia/Tic Douloureux Association. PO Box 340, Barnegat Light, NJ 08006. (609) 361-1014.

Amy Loerch Strumolo
Teresa G. Odle

Neurolinguisitic programming

Definition

Neurolinguistic programming (NLP) is aimed at enhancing the healing process by changing the conscious and subconscious beliefs of patients about themselves, their illnesses, and the world. These limiting beliefs are "reprogrammed" using a variety of techniques drawn from other disciplines including **hypnotherapy** and **psychotherapy**.

Origins

NLP was originally developed during the early 1970s by linguistics professor John Grinder and psychology and mathematics student Richard Bandler, both of the University of California at Santa Cruz.

Studying the well-known psychotherapist Virginia Satir, the hypnotherapist Milton Erickson, the anthropologist Gregory Bateson, and others whom they considered "charismatic superstars" in their fields, Grinder and Bandler identified psychological, linguistic and behavioral characteristics that they said contributed to the greatness of these individuals. On the other hand, they found that persons experiencing emotional difficulties could be similarly identified by posture, breathing pattern, choice of words, voice tone, eye movements, body language, and other characteristics.

Grinder and Bandler then focused on using these indicators to analyze and alter patterns of thought and behavior. After publishing their findings in two books in 1975, Grinder and Bandler parted company with themselves, with a number of other collaborators, and with the University of California, continuing their work on NLP outside the formal world of academia. As a result, NLP split into a number of competing schools.

Popularized by television "infomercial" personality Anthony Robbins and others, NLP was quickly adopted in management and self-improvement circles. During the 1990s, there was growing interest in NLP's healing potential.

Benefits

Neurolinguistic programming has been used to change the limiting beliefs of patients about their prospects of recovery from a wide variety of medical conditions including **Parkinson's disease**, **AIDS**, migraines, arthritis, and **cancer**. Practitioners claim to be able to cure most **phobias** in less than one hour, and to help in making lifestyle changes regarding **exercise**, diet, **smoking**, etc. NLP has also been used to treat **allergies**. In other fields, claimed benefits include improved relationships, communication, motivation, and business performance.

Description

In a health-care context, practitioners of neurolinguistic programming first seek to identify the negative attitudes and beliefs with which a client has been "programmed" since birth. This is accomplished by asking questions and observing physical responses such as changes in skin color, muscle tension, etc. Then, a wide variety of techniques is employed to "reprogram" limiting beliefs. For example, clients with chronic illness such as AIDS or cancer might be asked to displace the despair and loss of identity caused by the disease by visualizing themselves in vigorous health. Treatment by NLP practitioners is often of shorter duration than that of other alternative practitioners, but NLP self-help seminars and courses can be quite expensive.

For those who wish to try self-treatment with NLP, a wide variety of books, audio tapes, and videos are available.

Precautions

NLP is particularly popular in the self-improvement and career-development fields, and some trainers and practitioners have little experience in its use for healing. Practitioners should be specifically asked about this.

Because NLP is intended to enhance the healing process, it should not be used independently of other healing methods. In all cases of serious illness, a physician should be consulted.

Side effects

NLP is believed to be generally free of harmful side effects.

Research and general acceptance

Although some physicians and mental health practitioners employ principles of neurolinguistic programming, the field is generally considered outside of mainstream medical practice and academic thinking.

Training and certification

Since the originators of NLP parted company more than 20 years ago, a number of schools have been established to offer training and certification. Consumers should be aware that, in some cases, there has been considerable competition and even litigation among individuals and institutions involved in NLP. At the time of publication, there was no umbrella organization covering these institutions or offering uniform standards of training and certification.

Resources

ORGANIZATIONS

Association for NLP. PO Box 78, Stourbridge, UK DY8 2YP.

Australian Association of Professional Hypnotherapists and NLP Practitioners, Inc. PO BOX 1526, Southport, Gold Coast, Queensland 4215, Australia. http://www.members.tripod.com/~aaphan/index.html.

International NLP Trainers Association, Ltd. Coombe House, Mill Road, Fareham, Hampshire, UK PO16 0TN. (044) 01489 571171.

Society of Neuro-Linguistic Programming. PO Box 424, Hopatcong, NJ 07843. (201) 770-3600.

David Helwig

Niacin

Description

Niacin, also known as vitamin B_3 or nicotinic acid, is important for the normal function of many bodily processes. Like other B vitamins, it is water-soluble and plays a role in turning food into energy and in the metabolism of fats and carbohydrates. Niacin can also act as an antioxidant within cells, which means it can destroy cell-damaging free radicals. In conjunction with **riboflavin** and **pyridoxine**, it helps to keep the skin, intestinal tract, and nervous system

Recommended dietary allowance of niacin	
Age	**mg/day**
Children 0-6 mos.	2 (AI)
Children 7-12 mos.	4 (AI)
Children 1-3 yrs.	6
Children 4-8 yrs.	8
Children 9-13 yrs.	12
Boys 14-18 yrs.	16
Girls 14-18 yrs.	14
Men ≥ 19 yrs.	16
Women ≥ 19 yrs.	14
Pregnant women	18
Breastfeeding women	17
Foods that contain niacin	**mg**
Cereal, fortified, 1 cup	20-27
Tuna, light packed in water, 3 oz.	11.3
Chicken, light meat, 3 oz.	10.6
Salmon, 3 oz.	8.5
Cereal, unfortified, 1 cup	5-7
Turkey, light meat, 3 oz.	5.8
Beef, lean, 3 oz.	3.1
Pasta, enriched, 1 cup cooked	2.3
Bread, whole wheat, 1 slice	1.1
Asparagus, cooked, 1/2 cup	1
Carrots, raw, 1/2 cup	0.6
Coffee, brewed, 1 cup	0.5

AI = Adequate Intake
mcg = milligram

(Illustration by GGS Information Services. Cengage Learning, Gale)

functioning smoothly. The term *vitamin B₃* may also include the amide form of nicotinic acid, known as nicotinamide or niacinamide.

General use

The recommended daily allowance (RDA) of niacin for children from one to three years of age is 6 mg. It is 8 mg at four to eight years, and 12 mg at nine to 13 years. For males from age 14 to 18, the RDA is 16 mg; for females of that age range, 14 mg. Males 19 years and older require 16 mg, while females in that age range should have 14 mg per day. The RDA for pregnant females is 18 mg, and for lactating females, 17 mg. As of 2008, no RDA had been set for children under the age of one year, although an adequate intake (AI) is thought to be 2 mg for the first six months of life, and 4 mg for the next six months.

Niacin can be taken in very large doses to decrease blood **cholesterol** levels and reduce the risk of **heart attack**. Niacin is an important part of the treatment of familial hyperlipidemia, an inherited disorder characterized by high blood cholesterol levels and increased risk of heart disorders. The amount of niacin required is between 2 and 3 g per day. Although treatment with niacin is considered one of the best strategies for normalizing blood cholesterol levels, it should not be undertaken without professional medical advice and supervision. Niacin has been singled out as a dietary supplement for which people frequently exceed the upper limits of safe intake. One Canadian study found that 47% of adults who were taking dietary supplements were taking niacin above recommended levels.

Certain conditions preclude the use of high doses of niacin. These disorders include **gout**, diabetes, peptic ulcer, liver or kidney disease, and high blood pressure requiring medication. Even in the absence of these conditions, a patient on high doses of niacin should be closely monitored to be sure the therapy is both effective and without complications. A frequent, harmless but unpleasant side effect of this therapy is extreme flushing of the face and neck. An alternative form of nicotinic acid that does not cause flushing is **inositol** hexaniacinate. Slow-release niacin also causes less flushing, but it should not be taken as there is higher risk of liver inflammation.

There is some evidence that niacin used on a long-term basis can prevent the onset of juvenile diabetes in many susceptible children. Those who have been newly diagnosed with juvenile diabetes may also benefit by extending the time that the pancreas continues to produce a small amount of insulin. The advice of a healthcare provider should be sought for these uses.

Inositol hexaniacinate can be helpful for people suffering from intermittent claudication. This condition causes leg **pain** with **exercise** due to poor blood flow to the legs. Dilation of the blood vessels caused by the inositol hexaniacinate relieves this condition to some extent, allowing the patient to walk farther with less pain.

Other conditions that may be benefited by supplemental niacin include vertigo, **tinnitus**, **premenstrual syndrome** (PMS) headaches, and **osteoarthritis**. Raynaud's phenomenon reportedly may be improved by large doses of inositol hexaniacinate. A healthcare provider should be consulted for these uses. Niacin is not effective for the treatment of **schizophrenia**.

Preparations

Natural sources

Tuna is one of the best sources of niacin, but many other foods contain the vitamin. Most processed grain products are fortified with niacin, as well as other B vitamins. Although niacin is not destroyed by cooking, it does leach into water, so cooking with minimal liquid best preserves it. The amino acid tryptophan is widely found in foods high in protein, and about half of the tryptophan consumed is used to make niacin. Cottage cheese, milk, fowl, and tuna are some of the foods that are high in tryptophan.

Supplemental sources

Niacin can be purchased as an oral single vitamin product. A balanced B complex supplement is preferred over high doses of an individual vitamin unless there is a specific contraindication. Supplements should be stored in a cool, dry place, away from light, and out of the reach of children.

Deficiency

A serious deficiency of niacin causes a condition called pellagra. Once quite common in all countries, it has become rare outside areas in which poor **nutrition** is still the norm. Affected groups include refugees displaced by war as well as populations affected by such emergency situations as famine. The symptoms of pellagra include **dermatitis**, **dementia**, and **diarrhea**.

Milder deficiencies of niacin can cause similar, but less severe symptoms. Dermatitis, especially around the mouth, and other **rashes** may occur, along with **fatigue**, irritability, poor appetite, **indigestion**, diarrhea, **headache**, and possibly delirium.

Risk factors for deficiency

Severe niacin deficiency is uncommon in most parts of the world, but some people may need more than the RDA in order to maintain good health. Vegans, and other individuals who do not eat animal protein, should consider taking a balanced B vitamin supplement. Others who may need extra niacin and other B vitamins are people under high **stress**, including those experiencing chronic illnesses, liver disease, sprue, or poor nutritional status. People over 55 years old are more likely to have a poor dietary intake. Certain metabolic diseases also increase the requirement for niacin. Those who abuse nicotine, alcohol, or other drugs are very frequently deficient in B vitamins, but use of niacin with alcohol can cause seriously low blood pressure. A healthcare professional can determine if supplementation is appropriate.

Precautions

Niacin should not be taken by anyone with a B vitamin allergy, kidney or liver impairment, severe hypotension, unstable **angina**, arterial hemorrhage, or coronary artery disease. Supplemental niacin can exacerbate peptic ulcers. Diabetics should use caution as supplements of either niacin or niacinamide can alter medication requirements to control blood glucose. Supplements can raise uric acid levels and aggravate gout in people with this condition. Pregnant women should not take high doses of niacin, or any supplement, except on the advice of a healthcare provider.

Health care should be sought immediately if certain symptoms occur following niacin supplementation. These include abdominal pain, diarrhea, **nausea**, **vomiting**, yellowing of the skin, faintness, or headache. Such symptoms may indicate excessively low blood pressure or liver problems. Heart palpitations and elevated blood sugar are also potential effects.

Side effects

High doses of niacin can cause a harmless but unpleasant flushing sensation as well as darkening of the urine. The no-flush form can lessen this complication.

Interactions

Niacin supplements should not be taken by anyone on medication for high blood pressure, due to the vitamin's potential to reduce blood pressure. Isoniazid, a drug used to treat **tuberculosis**, inhibits the body's ability to make niacin from tryptophan. Extra niacin may be required. Supplements may also be needed by women taking oral contraceptives. Concomitant use of niacin with statin class drugs to lower cholesterol can cause myopathy. Cholestyramine and cholestipol, older medications to lower cholesterol, should be taken at a different time than niacin or they will reduce its absorption. Transdermal nicotine used with niacin is likely to cause flushing and **dizziness**. Carbamazepine, an anti-seizure medication, is more likely to cause toxicity in combination with niacin.

Resources

BOOKS

Elliot, Charlyn M. *Vitamin B: New Research*. Hauppauge, NY: Nova Science, 2008.

PERIODICALS

Birjmohun, R. S., et al. "Safety and Tolerability of Prolonged-release Nicotinic Acid in Statin-treated Patients." *Current Medical Research and Opinion* (July 2007): 1707–1713.

Ganji, Shobha H., et al. "Effect of Niacin on Lipoproteins and Atherosclerosis." *Future Lipidology* (October 2006): 549–557.

"Niacin ER Combinations Effective in Lipid Metabolism Disorders." *Inpharma* (November 17, 2007): 2.

Sanyal, Sanjukta, Richard H. Karas, and Jeffrey T. Kuvin. "Present-day Uses of Niacin: Effects on Lipid and Nonlipid Parameters." *Expert Opinion on Pharmacotherapy* (August 2007): 1711–1717.

KEY TERMS

Antioxidant—Any substance that reduces the damage caused by oxidation, such as the harm caused by free radicals.

Gout—A metabolic disorder characterized by sudden recurring attacks of arthritis caused by deposits of crystals that build up in the joints due to abnormally high uric acid blood levels. In gout, uric acid may be overproduced, underexcreted, or both.

Myopathy—Any abnormal condition or disease of muscle tissue, characterized by muscle weakness and wasting.

Pellagra—A condition caused by a dietary deficiency of niacin, one of the B vitamins. Symptoms include dementia, diarrhea, and dermatitis.

Sprue—A disorder in which the absorption of nutrients from the diet by the small intestine (malabsorption) is impaired, resulting in malnutrition. Two forms of sprue exist: tropical sprue, which occurs mainly in tropical regions; and celiac sprue, which occurs more widely and is due to sensitivity to wheat protein gluten.

Suryadevara, Ramya S., Richard H. Karas, and Jeffrey T. Kuvin. "Use of Extended-release Niacin in Clinical Practice." *Future Lipidology* (February 2008): 9–16.

ORGANIZATIONS

American Dietetic Association, 120 South Riverside Plaza, Suite 2000, Chicago, IL, 60606-6995, (800) 877-1600, www.eatright.org.

World Health Organization (WHO), Avenue Appia 20, 1211, Geneva, 27, Switzerland, +41 22 791-2111, www.who.int.

Judith Turner
Rebecca J. Frey, PhD
David Edward Newton, Ed.D.

Night blindness

Definition

Night blindness is the inability or reduced ability to see in dim light or darkness. It also refers to the condition in which the time it takes for the eyes to adapt to darkness is prolonged.

Description

Night blindness, also called nyctalopia, is a symptom of several different diseases or conditions. All of the possible causes of night blindness are associated with the way in which the eye receives light rays. Light travels through the cornea and lens and lands on the retina at the back of the eye. The retina is composed of photoreceptors. Photoreceptors are specialized nerve cells that receive light rays and convert them into electrical signals, which are then transmitted to the brain, creating an image.

There are two types of photoreceptors, rods and cones. There are three million cones and 100 million rods in each eye. The two different photoreceptors are similar in structure, however, rods have a larger outer segment than cones. The outer segments of photoreceptors contain light-sensitive photopigments which change shape whenever light rays strike them. Rods contain the photopigments retinal and rhodopsin, whereas cones contain retinal and three different opsins. Rhodopsin is only able to discriminate between different degrees of light intensity, whereas the opsins of cones distinguish between light wavelengths in the red, blue, and green ranges. Hence, rods see only black and white, but cones see colors. Also, rods enable the eyes to detect motion and provide peripheral vision.

Rods are responsible for vision in dim light, and cones are responsible for vision in bright light. The rods are spread throughout the retina, but the cones are only in the center of the retina. Vision in dim light or darkness is blurry because of the connections between the photoreceptors and the nerve cells which are linked to the brain. Each rod must share this connection to the brain with several other rods so the brain does not know exactly which rod produced the signal. Alternatively, vision in bright light is sharp because each cone has its own connection to the brain so the brain can determine exactly where on the retina the signal originated.

Another feature of rods is that they must adapt to darkness. This is best exemplified by walking into a dark movie theater. At first, one can see very little. With time, vision improves and one is able to discern objects. Ultimately, one can see moderately well. This dark adaptation process occurs because of the chemical nature of rhodopsin. Rhodopsin is decomposed in bright light making the rods nonfunctional. In darkness, rhodopsin is regenerated faster than it can be decomposed. Dark adaptation takes about 15–30 minutes and, when complete, increases light sensitivity by about 100,000 times.

Causes and symptoms

Several different conditions and diseases can cause night blindness.

These include:

- Cataracts. This condition is characterized by a cloudiness of the lens.
- Congenital night blindness. This is an inherited, stable disease in which persons suffer from night blindness. Recent advances in gene mapping have identified several mutations responsible for this form of night blindness.
- Liver conditions. Reduced night vision can be linked to poor liver functioning, due to a variety of conditions, which impairs vitamin A metabolism.
- Macular degeneration. Degeneration of the macula retinae, a specialized region of the retina, can cause night blindness.
- Retinitis pigmentosa. This is an inherited eye disease in which there is progressive deterioration of the photopigments of the photoreceptors, eventually resulting in blindness. The rods are destroyed early in the course of disease resulting in night blindness. Night blindness in children may be an early indicator of retinitis pigmentosa. Recent genetic studies have identified mutations related to retinitis pigmentosa on human chromosome 19.
- Vitamin A deficiency. Night blindness is commonly caused by a deficiency in vitamin A, in fact, it is one of the first indicators of vitamin A deficiency.
- Xerophthalmia. This condition is characterized by dryness of the conjunctiva (the membrane that covers the eyelids and exposed surface of the eye) and cornea, light sensitivity, and night blindness. It is caused by vitamin A deficiency. Xerophthalmia rarely occurs in countries with adequate supplies of milk products.
- Zinc deficiency. Zinc is a mineral that is necessary for vitamin A to improve vision.

Diagnosis

Night blindness can be diagnosed and treated by an ophthalmologist, a physician who specializes in eye disorders. Opticians can only dispense eye glasses but optometrists may be able to diagnose and treat vision problems.

Diagnosis begins with a detailed medical history regarding the night blindness. Questions include: severity of night blindness, when night blindness began, did it occur gradually or suddenly, etc. An eye examination is performed. A slit lamp examination, in which a narrow beam of intense light is used to examine the internal components of the eye, may also be performed. Additional testing may be performed based upon the results of these standard tests.

Treatment

Changes in vision should never be taken lightly. Because night blindness can be a symptom of a serious disease, an ophthalmologist should be consulted before a person embarks on self treatment.

Persons who experience night blindness should not drive during the evening or at night. Additional safety precautions should be taken. Alternative remedies may be effective at reducing night blindness, particularly when caused by a **vitamin A** deficiency.

Food remedies and supplements

Because night blindness can be caused by a vitamin A deficiency, supplementation with vitamin A, or eating foods rich in vitamin A, may help reduce symptoms. Vitamin A was found to slow the progression of retinitis pigmentosa. Foods rich in vitamin A include dairy products, egg yolks, fish liver oil, and liver. Pregnant women should consult a physician before taking vitamin A supplements because of the link between this vitamin and birth defects.

Vitamin A in humans is primarily obtained by conversion of beta-carotene, a pigment found in fruits and vegetables. Food sources for beta-carotene include apricots, asparagus, broccoli, brussel sprouts, cantaloupe, carrots, cherries, kale, lettuce, mango, mustard greens, papaya, peaches, pumpkin, red cabbage, seaweed, spinach, sweet potatoes, watermelon, winter squash, and yams.

Zinc is necessary to transport vitamin A from the liver to the retina, so zinc supplementation (up to 25 mg daily) may help improve night vision. Docosahexaenoic acid (DHA) helps to increase rhodopsin levels and lines the photoreceptor cells of the retina. DHA is converted from **omega-3 fatty acids**, both of which are found in certain fish oils. The suggested daily dose of DHA (from fish oils) is 500–1000 mg.

Herbal remedies

Herbals which may improve night vision include:

- bilberry (*Vaccinium myrtillus*)
- blueberry (*Vaccinium*) juice
- dandelion (*Taraxacum officinale*)
- eyebright (*Euphrasia officinalis*)
- matrimony vine (*Lycii fructus*, kou chi tza) berries
- passionflower (*Passiflora incarnata*)
- Queen Anne's lace (*Daucus carota sativas*)
- rose (*Rosa* species) flower eye wash
- yellow dock (*Rumex crispus*) leaves

Colored light therapy

One researcher found that some persons have reduced levels of photocurrent transmission (transmission of light signals from the eye to the brain) which can cause, among other things, night blindness. Colored **light therapy**, in which colored light stimulates the brain, can reduce night blindness caused by this photocurrent deficit. In colored light therapy, patients look at a device that cycles through 11 wave bands of color. Treatment involves 25–30 sessions over a period of four to six weeks.

Allopathic treatment

Night blindness caused by vitamin A deficiency will be treated with vitamin A supplements. Night vision devices are available which collect and magnify tiny amounts of light to help persons with night blindness see as well as they can during daylight.

Vitamin A supplementation may slow the progress of retinitis pigmentosa. There is no cure for retinitis pigmentosa or **macular degeneration**, but there are treatments, including laser surgery and the drug thalidomide, which slow down the growth of blood vessels. **Cataracts** require surgery.

Expected results

Vitamin A can effectively treat night blindness in persons who have a deficiency of this nutrient.

Prevention

Vitamin A may prevent night blindness and slow the progression of eye conditions, such as macular degeneration, which cause night blindness. Wearing sunglasses during the day can prevent eye damage.

Resources

PERIODICALS

Ramser, J., G. Wen, Y. Demirci, et al. "A Complete Gene Catalogue of Human Xp11.4 Harboring Disease Loci for Diabetes Mellitus Type I, Mental Retardation and Retinal Disturbances." *American Journal of Human Genetics* 69 (October 2001): 655.

Vithana, E. N., L. Abu-Safieh, M. J. Allen, et al. "A Human Homologue of Yeast Pre mRNA-Splicing Gene, PRP31, Underlies Autosomal Dominant Retinitis Pigmentosa on Chromosome 19q13.4 (RP11)." *American Journal of Human Genetics* 69 (October 2001): 229.

ORGANIZATIONS

The Foundation Fighting Blindness. 11435 Cronhill Drive, Owings Mills, MD 21117-2220. (888) 394-3937. info@blindness.org http://www.blindness.org.

OTHER

Haas, Elston M. "Vitamin A." *HealthWorld Online*. [cited October 2002]. http://www.healthy.net/hwlibrarybooks/haas/vitamins/avit.htm.

Belinda Rowland
Rebecca J. Frey, PhD

Non-Hodgkins lymphoma *see* **Malignant lymphoma**

Noni

Description

Noni, the common name for *Morinda citrifolia,* is a medicinal herbal substance derived from the noni tree, which is found in various areas of the South Pacific. Other names for the herb include morinda, Indian mulberry, nona, nonu, Polynesian bush fruit, Tahitian noni juice, and cheesefruit.

The noni tree is an evergreen shrub, up to 20 ft (6 m) tall, that grows in tropical areas of the South Pacific, including Australia, Malaysia, the West Indies, India, Vietnam, the Philippines, Taiwan, and Hawaii. Its branches and trunk are coarse, tough wood, and the leaves are glossy, oval, and dark green. Year-round, the tree yields a small fruit, which is cream-colored and about the size of a small potato. The noni fruit is noted for its bitter taste, unpleasant smell, and reportedly strong healing properties. Other parts of the plant also are used medicinally, including the leaves, bark, flowers, and roots.

Noni was first found in India, and migrating peoples may have carried it around regions in the Pacific. In Polynesia, the plant is considered a sacred healing herb with many uses. American soldiers stationed there during World War II were reportedly given noni as a health tonic. Other peoples of the South Pacific, including in Hawaii and Tahiti, use noni as a medicinal herb. Traditional uses of all parts of the plant for various conditions are numerous. Noni has been commercially grown for hundreds of years in the South Pacific region. The fruit is also a food source used by South Pacific peoples. The principal regions for commercial cultivation of noni are Hawaii, French Polynesia, and Tahiti.

Noni juice became an increasingly popular health drink during the 1990s, when a group of Hawaiians began internationally marketing the juice as an herbal remedy. Since then, many claims have been made

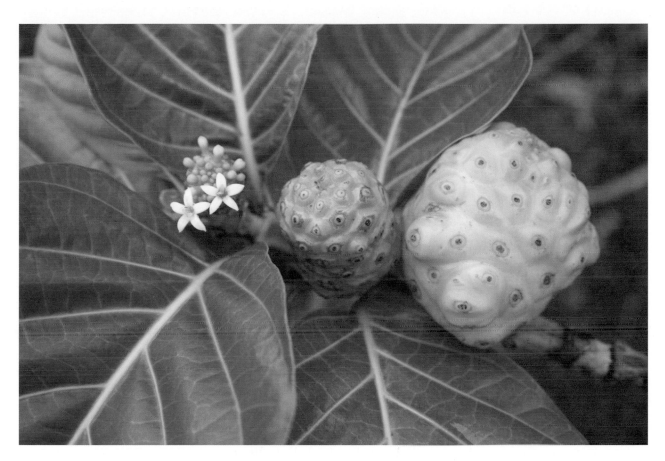

Noni (Morinda citrifolia) is a medicinal herbal substance derived from the noni tree, which is found in various areas of the South Pacific. *(inga spence / Alamy)*

about its healing powers, a few of which have been somewhat validated by controlled studies. However, there is a lack of research to conclusively back up the optimistic claims regarding the herb's healing powers, and most evidence of the herb's success exists in testimonial accounts.

General use

Traditionally, the fruit has been used for **aging**, diabetes, **halitosis**, **hemorrhoids**, tumors, **tuberculosis**, high blood pressure, and as a tonic for overall health and energy. The leaves have been ingested in remedies for arthritis, digestive problems, parasites, and dysentery (severe infection of the lower digestive tract characterized by acute **diarrhea** and dehydration). Topically, the leaves, fruit, and roots are used in poultices for arthritis and joint **pain**, headaches, for **burns** and lesions, poisonous **bites**, and to improve signs of aging.

Noni is used by some **cancer** patients for its anti-cancer and tumor-reducing possibilities. Some sufferers from immune-compromised diseases such as **AIDS**

and **chronic fatigue syndrome** use noni to boost immune system function. People with diabetes and **hypoglycemia** have reported that noni helps stabilize blood sugar levels in the body. People with arthritis, joint pain, and inflammatory conditions have used noni. It is also used as a sedative, painkiller, and sleeping aid. Noni juice is recommended to remove parasites, to cleanse the digestive tract and improve digestion, and to control weight. It is used as a general health tonic to improve energy and resistance and to slow the effects of aging. It is also used for **asthma**; digestive disorders including ulcers; **irritable bowel syndrome**; **constipation** and diarrhea; and **fibromyalgia**, a condition characterized by **fatigue** and chronic pain.

Scientific studies

A substance called ursolic acid found in the leaves of the noni plant has been shown to have anti-cancer properties in the body. A Japanese study found that noni fruit contains another substance (damnacanthal) that has some effectiveness against pre-cancerous cells. Some evidence points to noni's ability to increase immune system activity, due to substances found in the fruit (including a chemical called proxeronine). The leaves of the plant contain chemicals that may lower blood sugar levels, as well as reduce pain and inflammation. One study showed that laboratory mice with **lung cancer** had much longer survival times when given noni juice daily. A French study determined that the roots of the noni plant contain natural sedatives, while another study pointed to a compound that noni leaves may contain that is anti-malarial and antiparasitic in its effects. Finally, surveys of noni users have indicated testimonial success with the use of noni for cancer, strokes, diabetes, and as a general health and energy improver. Noni has been shown to contain vitamins, minerals, and **antioxidants**.

Preparations

Noni is available in several forms, including bottled juice from the fruit; essential oil; capsules containing dried fruit, leaves, roots, or combinations thereof; tablets; teas; and topical sprays. Organically grown sources of the supplement are recommended. Noni is best taken on an empty stomach, and can be taken daily. Between one quarter of an ounce and one ounce of the juice is a recommended daily dosage for adults. Up to ten ounces of the juice may be taken by those seeking therapeutic use of the herb and who are under the supervision of a health professional. Consumers should follow manufacturers' recommendations for capsules, tablets, and teas. In capsule form, it is estimated that 1,200 mg equals roughly one ounce of the juice.

Precautions

Although few allergic reactions to noni have been observed, consumers should ingest small amounts of the herb (one tablespoon of the juice) at first to test for adverse reactions. Noni should not be used by pregnant or nursing women, as there is insufficient evidence of its safety during **pregnancy** or for infants.

Side Effects

Reported side effects from the use of noni include **indigestion**; allergic reactions including **rashes**, swelling, and difficulty swallowing; diarrhea; and constipation.

Interactions

The use of noni with potassium-sparing drugs is not recommended, due to the high **potassium** content in the herb. It is recommended that noni not be taken with food, as stomach acid may render one of its active ingredients ineffective. Noni can cause discoloration of the urine and may interfere with diagnostic urine tests. Noni juice may increase the risk of hyperkalemia (higher than normal blood potassium levels) in people with kidney problems by elevating potassium levels in the body.

Resources

BOOKS

Elkins, Rita. *The Noni Revolution*. Woodland Publishing, 2002.
Solomon, Neil, M.D. *The Noni Phenomenon*. Direct Source Publishing, 1999.

OTHER

Cancer Research Center of Hawaii: The Noni Study. http://www.hawaii.edu/crch/CenStudyNoni.htm.
International Noni Certification Council (INCC). http://www.incc.org.

Douglas Dupler

Nosebleeds

Definition

A nosebleed is characterized by bleeding from the interior of the nasal cavity. It can be caused by heat, dry air, trauma to the nose, certain medications, or a medical condition.

Description

Anterior nosebleeds, or bleeding of the nose that comes from near the nose opening, are the most common nosebleeds in children. Children are twice as likely to experience nosebleeds as adults are. Bleeding that originates from deep within the nasal cavity is known as a posterior nosebleed, the type usually experienced by adults.

Causes and symptoms

The most common causes of nosebleeds are:

- Low humidity. Hot and dry climates can dry out the nasal cavities.
- Nasal trauma. Injuries to the nose can cause bleeding. Excessive nose picking can also injure the interior of the nose.
- Cold, allergies, and sinus infections. Excessive nose blowing and irritation to the mucous membrane can cause bleeding.

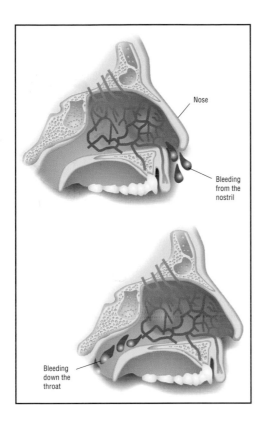

Two types of nosebleeds. *(Illustration by GGS Information Services, Inc. Cengage Learning, Gale)*

• Medications. Bleeding can be triggered by certain medications, particularly those with anticoagulant (or blood thinning) properties.

Nosebleeds can also be symptomatic of less common, but more serious, medical conditions. These include:

• nasal polyps
• high blood pressure
• blood clotting disorders (i.e., thrombocytopenia, liver disease)
• leukemia
• malaria

Diagnosis

A nosebleed is easily diagnosed by sight. Further examination of the nasal cavity may be necessary to determine the source of the bleeding, and a medical history should be taken if the cause of the nosebleed is not readily apparent.

Treatment

The first step in treating a nosebleed is to stop the bleeding. An individual experiencing a nosebleed

should lightly blow his or her nose, and then pinch both nostrils to encourage clotting of the blood flow. The nose should be pinched close for five to 10 minutes, or until bleeding has stopped. In most cases, this will resolve the nosebleed.

If pinching does not stop blood flow completely, an astringent can also be used to dry up the blood flow. A piece of cotton soaked in **witch hazel** (*Hamamelis virginiana*) can be inserted into the bleeding nostril(s) to tighten and seal the blood vessels. Sniffing a small pinch of powdered **yarrow** (*Achillea millefolium*) can also stop bleeding.

Allopathic treatment

Use of a spray decongestant is sometimes recommended to shrink blood vessels and stop bleeding. In severe cases where bleeding from the nose does not stop after 20 minutes, professional emergency care should be sought. Surgery to remove nasal polyps may be required in patients with this problem. In some cases of repeated, serious nosebleeds, cauterization of the blood vessels in the nasal passages is necessary.

Expected results

Most nosebleeds will resolve by themselves in 10–15 minutes. Nutritional and environmental measures can prevent further occurrences in many cases.

Prevention

The following precautions can prevent or lessen the frequency of nosebleeds:

• Vitamin C. An adequate supply of vitamin C is necessary to form collagen, the connective tissue that strengthens blood vessel walls.

• Humidify the air. Using a humidifier in the home and office can prevent nosebleeds caused by a dry environment.

• Vitamin E. Rubbing liquid vitamin E in the nose keeps the mucous membrane moist.

Resources

BOOKS

Hoffmann, David. *The Complete Illustrated Herbal.* New York: Barnes & Noble Books, 1999.

Paula Ford-Martin

Notoginseng root

Description

Notoginseng root is a frequently prescribed herb in Chinese medicine. The scientific names for the plant are *Panax notoginseng* and *Panax pseudoginseng*. The herb is also referred to as pseudoginseng, and in Chinese it is called Tien qi ginseng, San qi, three-seven root, and Mountain paint. Notoginseng belongs to the same scientific genus, *Panax*, as Asian ginseng. In Latin, the word *panax* means "cure-all," and the family of ginseng plants is one of the most famous and frequently used of all families of herbs.

Notoginseng grows naturally in China and Japan. The herb is a perennial with dark green, compound leaves and red clusters of berries. It is both cultivated and gathered from forests, with wild plants being the most expensive. The root of the plant is used medicinally, and tea is sometimes made from the leaves. At the top of the root is a section called the "age root," which has notches that indicate the age of the particular root. Chinese herbalists consider roots older than three years to be the most effective medicinally. Notoginseng root has a very bitter flavor.

Notoginseng root has been used in Chinese medicine for thousands of years. One of China's most famous herbalists once said that the root was "more valuable than gold." The herb is used as a general tonic, or a medicine to tone and strengthen the entire system. In particular, notoginseng is considered a blood and heart tonic. Chinese herbalists regard it as having a neutral to warm energy. In **traditional Chinese medicine**, notoginseng is believed to act on the heart and kidney meridians, which are the channels that contain the flow of qi (life energy) in the body. The herb was given the name "mountain paint" because herbalists sometimes recommend a liquid solution of it to reduce swelling and **boils** on the body.

General use

Notoginseng is used to treat external and internal bleeding, including **nosebleeds** as well as bloody stools and urine. Notoginseng has been used in the United States for some years to control postpartum bleeding in women and heavy bleeding associated with **menopause**. Some herbalists recommend notoginseng as an alternative to hormone replacement therapy.

Notoginseng is also used as a general tonic for the heart and circulatory system, and for such specific problems as coronary **heart disease** and high **cholesterol**. Chinese herbalists prescribe notoginseng to relieve the **pain** of **angina** pectoris, a condition that results in sharp pain in the chest region. Notoginseng is also used for painful **menstruation**, and for swelling and boils on the skin.

Research and general acceptance

Considerable research has been performed on notoginseng root in China and Japan over the years, but many of these findings have not been translated into English. Researchers from Western institutions have also taken a more recent interest in herbal treatments and have conducted their own notoginseng-related studies, many of which have been published since 2000.

From notoginseng, researchers have isolated chemicals called saponins and flavonoids, substances that are active biologically in the body. Some of the saponins in notoginseng are believed to provide the raw materials for the creation of important hormones that regulate energy levels and sexual function.

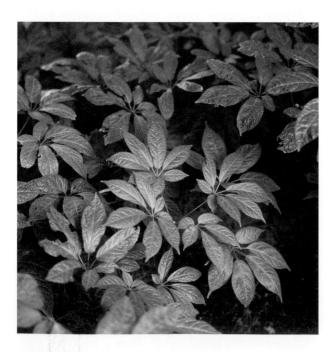

Notoginseng plant. *(© Arco Images / Alamy)*

Ginsenoside compounds are a group of saponins of special interest to biologists because they are found only among species in the Panax genus, and they are believed to be the primary source of these plants' pharmacological activity. Notoginseng has especially high concentrations of these compounds.

Notoginseng possesses anti-inflammatory properties, and research published in 2007 suggested that it may be helpful in treating arthritis, which is a chronic inflammatory condition that affects the joints. According to the study, notoginseng inhibits the secretion of a certain arthritis-related regulatory protein, known as a cytokine, and this contributes to notoginseng's anti-inflammatory effects.

In addition, notoginseng has been reported to stimulate the immune system. Other research has pointed to notoginseng's benefits for the heart and circulatory system, and the results of a preliminary study suggest that it may be useful in treating coma patients by decreasing pressure on brain tissue inside the skull.

Notoginseng also has been reported to have positive effects on the blood. It lowers low density lipoprotein (bad cholesterol), and is believed to help dissolve clots. At the same time, it is reputed to stop bleeding both internally and externally. Notoginseng root is one of the main herbs prescribed in Chinese medicine for traumatic injuries. In fact, the root has been distributed to members of armed forces in Asian countries to be used in case of traumatic injury and bleeding.

Possible newer uses for notoginseng root include treatment of HIV, or human immunodeficiency virus, infection. In 2002, researchers reported that they had isolated a compound known as a xylanase, which is a type of enzyme found in plant roots, from the roots of *Panax notoginseng*. According to their study, the new xylanase appeared to inhibit HIV-1 reverse transcriptase, which is an enzyme that allows HIV to integrate itself into the chromosomes inside a cell.

Researchers have also reported that an herbal product that combined extracts of **American ginseng**, *Panax quinquefolium*, and *Ginkgo biloba* showed promise as a treatment for **attention-deficit hyperactivity disorder**. They studied the treatment over a four-week span in three dozen children who were 3–17 years old and had been diagnosed with ADHD, and saw positive results.

Preparations

Notoginseng is available in Asian markets and some health food stores. It comes as dried root, powder, and in capsules. The root is sometimes steamed

and then powdered, which is believed to increase its healing effects for the blood. The powdered root can also be applied topically to **wounds** and swelling on the skin.

Notoginseng users sometimes decoct the dried root into a tea by briefly boiling and then simmering it for more than an hour. A daily dosage of the root by this method may be between 3–9 g. Some users instead stir 1–3 g of the powder into tea or juice as a daily serving. The dried root can be used in cooking as well. A common method of taking the herb in China is to prepare it with chicken or soups.

Precautions

Herbalists note that notoginseng root can usually be safely taken in normal doses, but advise that women avoid it during **pregnancy**. Some also recommend that persons who have heart or blood-vessel problems use caution when taking some notoginseng preparations.

Interactions

Notoginseng has been reported to interact with warfarin and heparin, which are medications to thin the blood, or anticoagulants; and with ticlopidine, a drug given to prevent blood platelets from clumping and to prolong bleeding time. Patients taking any of these medications may wish to avoid preparations containing notoginseng.

Resources

BOOKS

Fan Warner, J.W. *Manual of Chinese Herbal Medicine.* Boston: Shambhala, 2003.

Nutmeg

Lu, Henry C. *Chinese Natural Cures: Traditional Methods for Remedy and Prevention*. New York: Black Dog & Leventhal Publishers, 2006.

Teeguarden, Ron. *The Ancient Wisdom of the Chinese Tonic Herbs*. New York: Grand Central Publishing, 2000.

PERIODICALS

Frishman, William H., Stephen T. Sinatra, and Mohammed Moizuddin. " The use of herbs for treating cardiovascular disease." *Seminars in Integrative Medicine*. Volume 2, no. 1, March 2004: 23–25.

ORGANIZATIONS

American Herbalists Guild. 141 Nob Hill Road, Cheshire, CT 06410. (203) 272.6731. www.americanherbalists guild.com (accessed February 15, 2008).

Douglas Dupler
Rebecca J. Frey, Ph.D.
Leslie Mertz, Ph.D.

Nursing problems *see* **Breastfeeding problems**

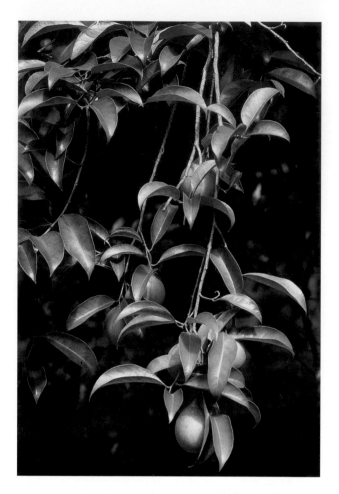

Nutmeg tree branch. *(©PlantaPhile, Germany. Reproduced by permission.)*

Nutmeg

Description

Nutmeg is known by many names, such *Myristica fragrans*, mace, magic, muscdier, muskatbaum, myristica, noz moscada, nuez moscada, and nux moschata. Nutmeg is most commonly used as a cooking spice, comes from the fruit of a 50 ft (15 m) tall tropical evergreen tree. This tree grows in Indonesia, New Guinea, and the West Indies. The bark is smooth and grayish brown with green young branches and leaves. The oblong, fleshy fruit, called the nutmeg apple, contains a nut from which nutmeg is made. The dried nut and essential oil are both used as medicine.

Nutmeg is used in both Western and Chinese herbal medicine. It is most popular as a spice in food and drinks, and is also used in cosmetics and soaps. In ancient Greece and Rome, where nutmeg was rare and expensive, people thought it stimulated the brain. The Arabs have used nutmeg since the seventh century.

General use

Nutmeg relaxes the muscles, sedates the body, and helps remove **gas** from the digestive track. It is most commonly used for stomach problems such as **indigestion**. It is also used for chronic nervous disorders, kidney disorders, and to prevent **nausea** and **vomiting**. In Chinese medicine, nutmeg is used to treat abdominal **pain**, **diarrhea**, inflammation, **impotence**, liver disease, and vomiting. In the Middle East, some cultures are said to use nutmeg in love potions as an aphrodisiac. The essential oil of nutmeg is used for rheumatic pain, toothaches, and bad breath. In Germany, it is used for problems related to the stomach and intestines, but this use is controversial. In **homeopathy**, nutmeg is used to treat **anxiety** or **depression**. Although nutmeg has been used to treat many ailments, it hasn't been proven to be useful or effective for any and it can be harmful. Nutmeg is used in medicines such as Vicks Vaporub, Agua del Carmen, Aluminum Free Indigestion, Incontinurina, Klosterfrau Magentoniuum, Melisana, and Nervospur.

Preparation

Nutmeg is made from the nut of the nutmeg apple. It is removed from the fruit and slowly dried. As an herbal medicine, nutmeg is commonly used in capsules (200 mg), powders, and essential oil. As a cooking

KEY TERMS

Anxiogenic—Tending to produce anxiety.

Homeopathy—A holistic system of treatment developed in the eighteenth century. It is based on the idea that substances that produce symptoms of sickness in healthy people will have a curative effect when given in very dilute quantities to sick people who exhibit those same symptoms. Homeopathic remedies are believed to stimulate the body's own healing processes.

Rheumatic—Refers to any of a variety of disorders marked by inflammation, deterioration, or metabolic damage of the body's connective tissues, especially the joints.

Trimyristin—A chemical found in nutmeg that causes anxiety.

spice, the nut is ground and cooked in food. The skin of the nuts is ground to produce another spice, called mace. Nutmeg butter, a mixture of fatty and essential oil, is made by chopping and steaming the nuts until they form a paste.

Some of the suggested doses of nutmeg can be harmful. For nausea, other stomach problems, and chronic diarrhea, one or two capsules or nutmeg kernel as a single dose or three to five drops of essential oil on a lump of sugar or on a teaspoon of honey is suggested. For diarrhea, 4-6 tbsp of powder could be taken every day. For a **toothache**, one or two drops of essential oil can be applied to the gum around the toothache to relieve pain; a visit to the dentist care is still necessary.

In Chinese medicine, 250–500 mg of nutmeg mixed with other herbs is recommended, once or twice a day. It can be taken in powder plain, capsules, pills, or infusion, and should be taken on an empty stomach. When used as a digestive stimulant in Chinese medicine, it is said to work best when ground and cooked in food.

Precautions

Nutmeg is not recommended for use as a medicine because it is too risky. An overdose of nutmeg is harmful and sometimes deadly. There are more effective treatments for all of the ailments that nutmeg could be used for.

Pregnant women should not use nutmeg because it can cause a miscarriage. Women who are breastfeeding should not use nutmeg either. Nutmeg should be used with caution in patients with psychiatric illnesses, as it can cause feelings of anxiety. Touching the nuts can cause an allergic skin reaction. In the home, nutmeg should be kept out of the reach of children and pets.

Side effects

There are no known side effects from using nutmeg properly. Too much nutmeg, however, can cause serious health problems and even death. Early symptoms of an overdose of nutmeg (one to three nuts) are thirst, nausea, and feelings of urgency. There may also be experiences of altered consciousness; this can range from mild to intensive hallucinations, and results in a stupor that lasts from two to three days. Sometimes shock and seizures occur. Immediate medical attention is necessary when someone has taken too much nutmeg.

Interactions

Recent studies of the anxiogenic, or anxiety-causing, effects of nutmeg indicate that it counteracts such tranquilizers as diazepam (Valium), ondansetron (Zofran), and buspirone (BuSpar). The specific substance in nutmeg that is responsible for this effect is a compound called trimyristin. There are, however, no known medical conditions that contraindicate the use of nutmeg in small quantities.

Resources

BOOKS

Fetrow, Charles W., and Jaun R. Avila. *Professional's Handbook of Complementary & Alternative Medicines.* Springhouse, 1999.

The PDR Family Guide to Natural Medicines & Healing Therapies. Three Rivers Press, 1999.

The PDR for Herbal Medicines. Medical Economics Company, 1998.

Reid, D. *A Handbook of Chinese Healing Herbs.* Shambhala, 1995.

PERIODICALS

Sonavane, G. S., et al. "Anxiogenic Activity of *Myristica fragrans* Seeds." *Pharmacology, Biochemistry and Behavior* 71 (January-February 2002): 239-244.

OTHER

"Semen Myristicae." China-med.net.http://www.china-med.net/research_center.html.

Lori De Milto
Rebecca J. Frey, PhD

Nutrition

Definition

Good nutrition can help prevent disease and promote health. There are six categories of nutrients that the body needs to acquire from food: protein, carbohydrates, fat, fibers, vitamins and minerals, and water.

Proteins

Protein supplies **amino acids** to build and maintain healthy body tissue. There are 20 amino acids considered essential because the body must have all of them in the right amounts to function properly. Twelve of these are manufactured in the body but the other eight amino acids must be provided by the diet. Foods from animal sources such as milk or eggs often contain all these essential amino acids while a variety of plant products must be taken together to provide all these necessary protein components.

Fat

Fat supplies energy and transports nutrients. There are two families of fatty acids considered essential for the body: the omega-3 and **omega-6 fatty acids. Essential fatty acids** are required by the body to function normally. They can be obtained from canola oil, **flaxseed** oil, cold-water fish, or **fish oil**, all of which contain **omega-3 fatty acids**, and primrose or **black currant seed oil**, which contain omega-6 fatty acids. The American diet often contains an excess of omega-6 fatty acids and insufficient amounts of omega-3 fats. Increased consumption of omega-3 oils is recommended to help reduce risk of cardiovascular diseases and **cancer** and alleviate symptoms of **rheumatoid arthritis**, **premenstrual syndrome**, **dermatitis**, and **inflammatory bowel disease**.

Carbohydrates

Carbohydrates are the body's main source of energy and should be a major part of total daily caloric intake. There are two types of carbohydrates: simple carbohydrates (such as sugar or honey) or complex carbohydrates (such as grains, beans, peas, or potatoes). Complex carbohydrates are preferred because these foods are more nutritious yet have fewer calories per gram compared to fat and cause fewer problems with overeating than fat or sugar. Complex carbohydrates also are preferred over simple carbohydrates for diabetics because they allow better blood glucose control.

Fiber

Fiber is the material that gives plant texture and support. Although it is primarily made up of carbohydrates, it does not have a lot of calories and usually is not broken down by the body for energy. Dietary fiber is found in plant foods such as fruits, vegetables, legumes, nuts, and whole grains.

There are two types of fiber: soluble and insoluble. Insoluble fiber, as the name implies, does not dissolve in water because it contains a high amount of cellulose. Insoluble fiber can be found in the bran of grains, the pulp of fruit and the skin of vegetables. Soluble fiber is the type of fiber that dissolves in water. It can be found in a variety of fruits and vegetables such as apples, oatmeal and oat bran, rye flour, and dried beans.

Although they share some common characteristics such as being partially digested in the stomach and intestines and have few calories, each type of fiber has its own specific health benefits. Insoluble fiber speeds up the transit of foods through the digestive system and adds bulk to the stools, therefore, it is the type of fiber that helps treat **constipation** or **diarrhea** and helps prevent colon cancer. On the other hand, only soluble fiber can lower blood **cholesterol** levels. This type of fiber works by attaching itself to the cholesterol so that it can be eliminated from the body, preventing cholesterol from re-circulating and being reabsorbed into the bloodstream.

Foods high in sugar

Chewing gum

Chocolate bar

Chocolate milk

Fruit yogurt

Jelly beans

Ice cream

Liqueurs

Peanut butter and jelly sandwich

Pork and beans

Soda

(Illustration by Corey Light. Cengage Learning, Gale)

Vitamins and minerals

Vitamins are organic substances present in food and required by the body in a minute amount for regulation of metabolism and maintenance of normal growth and functioning. The most commonly known vitamins are A, B_1 (**thiamine**), B_2 (**riboflavin**), B_3 (**niacin**), B_5 (**pantothenic acid**), B_6 (**pyridoxine**), B_7 (**biotin**), B_9 (**folic acid**), B_{12} (cobalamin), C (ascorbic acid), D, E, and K. The B and C vitamins are water-soluble, excess amounts of which are excreted in the urine. The A, D, E, and K vitamins are fat-soluble and will be stored in the body fat.

Minerals are vital to our existence because they are the building blocks that make up muscles, tissues, and bones. They also are important components of many life-supporting systems, such as hormones, oxygen transport, and enzyme systems.

There are two kinds of minerals: the major (or macro) minerals and the trace minerals. Major minerals are the minerals that the body needs in large amounts. The following minerals are classified as major: **calcium**, **phosphorus**, **magnesium**, **sodium**, **potassium**, **sulfur**, and chloride. They are needed to build muscles, blood, nerve cells, teeth, and bones. They also are essential electrolytes that the body requires to regulate blood volume and acid-base balance.

Unlike the major minerals, trace minerals are needed only in tiny amounts. Even though they can be found in the body in exceedingly small amounts, they are also very important to the human body. These minerals participate in most chemical reactions in the body. They also are needed to manufacture important hormones. The following are classified as trace minerals: **iron**, **zinc**, **iodine**, **copper**, **manganese**, fluoride, **chromium**, **selenium**, molybdenum, and **boron**.

Many vitamins (such as vitamins A, C, and E) and minerals (such as zinc, copper, selenium, or manganese) act as **antioxidants**. They protect the body against the damaging effects of free radicals. They scavenge or mop up these highly reactive radicals and change them into inactive, less harmful compounds. In so doing, these essential nutrients have been claimed to help prevent cancer and many degenerative diseases, such as premature **aging**, **heart disease**, autoimmune diseases, arthritis, **cataracts**, **Alzheimer's disease**, and **diabetes mellitus**.

Water

Water helps to regulate body temperature, transport nutrients to cells, and rid the body of waste materials.

Origins

Unlike plants, human beings cannot manufacture most of the nutrients they need to function. They must eat plants and/or other animals. Although nutritional therapy came to the forefront of the public's awareness in the late Twentieth century, the notion that food affects health is not new. John Harvey Kellogg was an early health food pioneer and an advocate of a **high-fiber diet**. An avowed vegetarian, he believed that meat products were particularly detrimental to the colon. In the 1870s, Kellogg founded the Battle Creek Sanitarium, where he developed a diet based on nut and vegetable products.

Benefits

Good nutrition helps individuals achieve general health and well-being. In addition, dietary modifications might be prescribed for a variety of complaints including **allergies**, **anemia**, arthritis, colds, **depression**, **fatigue**, gastrointestinal disorders, high or low blood pressure, **insomnia**, headaches, **obesity**, **pregnancy**, premenstrual syndrome (PMS), respiratory conditions, and **stress**.

Nutritional therapy also may be involved as a complement to the allopathic treatments of cancer, diabetes, and **Parkinson's disease**. Other specific dietary measures include the elimination of food additives for attention deficit hyperactivity disorder (ADHD), gluten-free **diets** for **schizophrenia**, and dairy-free diets for chronic respiratory diseases.

A high-fiber diet helps prevent or treat the following health conditions:

- High cholesterol levels. Fiber effectively lowers blood cholesterol levels. It appears that soluble fiber binds to cholesterol and moves it down the digestive tract so that it can be excreted from the body. This prevents the cholesterol from being reabsorbed into the bloodstream.
- Constipation. A high-fiber diet is the preferred non-drug treatment for constipation. Fiber in the diet adds more bulk to the stools, making them softer and shortening the time foods stay in the digestive tract.
- Hemorrhoids. Fiber in the diet adds more bulk and softens the stool, thus reducing painful hemorrhoidal symptoms.
- Diabetes. Soluble fiber in the diet slows down the rise of blood sugar levels following a meal and helps control diabetes.
- Obesity. Dietary fiber makes a person feel full faster.

• Cancer. Insoluble fiber in the diet speeds up the movement of the stools through the gastrointestinal tract. The faster food travels through the digestive tract, the less time there is for potential cancer-causing substances to work. Therefore, diets high in insoluble fiber help prevent the accumulation of toxic substances that cause cancer of the colon. New studies released in 2003 seemed to confirm these findings. Because fiber reduces fat absorption in the digestive tract, it also may prevent breast cancer.

A diet low in fat also promotes good health and prevents many diseases. Low-fat diets can help treat or control the following conditions:

• Obesity. High fat consumption often leads to excess caloric and fat intake, which increases body fat.

• Coronary artery disease. High consumption of saturated fats is associated with coronary artery disease.

• Diabetes. People who are overweight tend to develop or worsen existing diabetic conditions due to decreased insulin sensitivity.

• Breast cancer. A high dietary consumption of fat is associated with an increased risk of breast cancer.

Description

The four basic food groups, as outlined by the United States Department of Agriculture (USDA) are:

• dairy products (such as milk and cheese)

• meat and eggs (such as fish, poultry, pork, beef, and eggs)

• grains (such as bread, cereals, rice, and pasta)

• fruits and vegetables

The USDA recommendation for adults is that consumption of meat, eggs, and dairy products should not exceed 20% of total daily caloric intake. The rest (80%) should be devoted to vegetables, fruits, and grains. For children age two or older, 55% of their caloric intake should be in the form of carbohydrates, 30% from fat, and 15% from proteins. In addition, saturated fat intake should not exceed 10% of total caloric intake. This low-fat, high-fiber diet is believed to promote health and help prevent many diseases, including heart disease, obesity, and cancer.

Allergenic and highly processed foods should be avoided. Highly processed foods do not contain significant amounts of essential trace minerals. Furthermore, they contain lots of fat and sugar as well as preservatives, artificial sweeteners and other additives. High consumption of these foods causes buildup of these unwanted chemicals in the body and should be avoided. Food allergy causes a variety of symptoms including food cravings, weight gain, bloating, and water retention. It also may worsen chronic inflammatory conditions such as arthritis.

Preparations

An enormous body of research exists in the field of nutrition. Mainstream Western medical practitioners point to studies that show that a balanced diet, based on the USDA Food Guide Pyramid, provides all of the necessary nutrients. However, the USDA is working to revise the pyramid for the first time in a decade. Other pyramids are suggested by various research agencies, many of which emphasize different nutrition areas. A Harvard University researcher emphasizes whole grains and plant oils over meat, dairy and refined carbohydrates. Some nutritionists believe that the USDA will modify the Food Pyramid to reflect similar modifications. The basic pyramid will likely not change, but explanations about the types of fats, grains and carbohydrates that are best to choose are likely.

In the first revision of the Food Guide Pyramid in 2003, the USDA proposed new patterns about how much Americans eat. Calorie recommendations and vitamin intake will be based on a person's age, sex, and activity level. The complete revision was proposed for final publishing in the winter of 2005. As of early 2004, the Food Guide Pyramid recommends the following daily servings in six categories:

• Grains: Six or more servings

• Vegetables: Five servings

• Fruits: Two to four servings

• Meat: Two to three servings

• Dairy: Two to three servings

• Fats and oils: Use sparingly

A new food guide pyramid for various vegetarian diets has been released by the American Dietetic Association (ADA). The guide helps vegetarians obtain the vitamins and minerals they need from whole grains, vegetables, fruits, legumes, nuts and other protein-rich foods.

Precautions

Individuals should not change their diets without the advice of nutritional experts or health care professionals. Certain individuals, especially children, pregnant and lactating women, and chronically ill patients should only change their diets under professional supervision.

Side effects

It is best to obtain vitamins and minerals through food sources. Excessive intake of vitamins and minerals can cause serious physiological problems. 2001 guidelines to help nutritionists counsel cancer patients in use of complementary and alternative medicine reported that 73% of cancer patients used these therapies in addition to their allopathic treatment. Of those, only about 38% discussed the alternative therapies with their physicians. Patients using dietary supplements should document their use, discuss them with their doctor or nutritionist, and watch standard cautions like possible interactions with prescribed drugs, cumulative effects of several supplements containing the same vitamin or mineral, and to stop taking the supplements if adverse reactions occur.

The following is a list of possible side effects resulting from excessive doses of vitamins and minerals:

- vitamin A: Birth defects, irreversible bone and liver damage
- vitamin B_1: Deficiencies in B_2 and B_6
- vitamin B_6: Damage to the nervous system
- vitamin C: affects the absorption of copper; diarrhea
- vitamin D: Hypercalcemia (abnormally high concentration of calcium in the blood)
- phosphorus: affects the absorption of calcium
- zinc: affects absorption of copper and iron; suppression of the immune system

Research and general acceptance

Due to a large volume of scientific evidence demonstrating the benefits of the low-fat, high-fiber diet in disease prevention and treatment, this diet has been accepted and advocated by both complementary and allopathic practitioners.

Resources

BOOKS

Bruce, Debra Fulghum, and Harris H. McIlwain. *The Unofficial Guide to Alternative Medicine.* New York: Macmillan, 1998.

Casslieth, Barrie R. *The Alternative Medicine Handbook.* New York: W.W. Norton, 1998.

Credit, Larry P., Sharon G. Hartunian, and Margaret J. Nowak. *Your Guide to Complementary Medicine.* Garden City Park, New York: Avery Publishing Group, 1998.

U.S. Preventive Services Task Force Guidelines. "Counseling to Promote a Healthy Diet." *Guide to Clinical Preventive Services, 2nd edition.* http://epmcnet.columbia.edu/texts/gcps/gcps0006.html.

Winick, Myron. *The Fiber Prescription.* New York: Random House, Inc., 1992.

PERIODICALS

Halbert, Steven C. "Diet and Nutrition in Primary Care: From Antioxidants to Zinc." *Primary Care: Clinics in Office Practice* (December 1997): 825-843.

Mangels, Reed. "New Vegetarian Food Guide." *Vegetarian Journal* (July-August 2003): 12.

Shapiro, Alice C., et al. "Guidelines for Responsible Nutrition Counseling on Complementary and Alternative Medicine." *Nutrition Today* (November-December 2001): 291-297.

Sugarman, Carole. "USDA Proposes New Intake Patterns for Food Guide Pyramid." *Food Chemical News* (Sept. 15, 2003): 1.

Turner, Lisa. "Good 'n Plenty." *Vegetarian Times* (February 1999):48

"Two Studies Find High-fiber Diet Lowers Colon Cancer Risk." *Ca* (July-August 2003): 201.

VanBeusekom, Mary. "Converted Food Pyramid: the USDA Revises its Decade-old Food Guidelines." *MPLS-St. Paul Magazine* (August 2003): 60-64.

Vickers, Andrew, and Catherine Zollman. "Unconventional approaches to nutritional medicine." *British Medical Journal* (November 27, 1999): 1419.

ORGANIZATIONS

American Association of Nutritional Consultants, 810 S. Buffalo Street, Warsaw, IN 46580. (888) 828-2262.

American Dietetic Association. 216 W. Jackson Boulevard, Suite 800, Chicago, IL 60606-6995. (800) 366-1655. http://www.eatright.org/.

Teresa G. Odle

Nutritional supplements see **Orthomolecular medicine**

Nux vomica

Description

Nux vomica is the homeopathic remedy that is created from the seeds of the strychnos *Nux vomica* tree. Also known as poison nut or vomiting nut, this tree is an evergreen tree that is native to East India, Burma, Thailand, China, and Northern Australia.

The tree belongs to the *Loganiaceae* family and has small flowers and orange colored fruits that are the size of an apple or orange. Inside the fruit are five seeds surrounded by a jelly-like pulp. The ash gray seeds are round and measure 1 in (2.5 cm) in diameter and are

Nux vomica

Nux vomica affects the nervous system. When taken by a healthy person the remedy causes **muscle spasms and cramps**, and even convulsions. It affects all five senses and bodily reflexes and causes extreme sensitivity to light, touch, noise, and smells.

Nux vomica is one of the most frequently used homeopathic remedies, especially for acute conditions. Homeopaths prescribe this polychrest for hangovers, **back pain**, digestive problems, headaches, **allergies**, colds, flu, emotional **stress**, **constipation**, menstrual problems, and **hemorrhoids**.

General use

Medicinal use of the nut dates back to the middle of the sixteenth century, where it was written about extensively by Valerius Cordus. Germans used the nut as a treatment for **worms**, **rabies**, hysteria, rheumatism, **gout**, and as an antidote for the plague.

Strychnine produces a loss of appetite, hypersensitivity, **depression**, **anxiety**, and rigidity and stiffness of arms and legs. Toxic doses may cause convulsions and death. Some historians think that Alexander the Great died from drinking wine poisoned by strychnine.

Strychnine by itself is extremely poisonous taste. These alkaloids give the seeds their bitter brucine. The main alkaloids in the seeds are strychnine and central nervous stimulant. In larger doses, however, of urination. In the nineteenth century it was used as a appetite, aids digestion, and increases the frequency when given in small doses to humans it promotes

The main alkaloids in the seeds are strychnine and brucine. These alkaloids give the seeds their bitter taste. Strychnine by itself is extremely poisonous, but when given in small doses to humans it promotes appetite, aids digestion, and increases the frequency of urination. In the nineteenth century it was used as a central nervous stimulant. In larger doses, however,

.25 in (0.6 cm) thick. The seeds are coated with downy hairs that give them a satiny appearance.

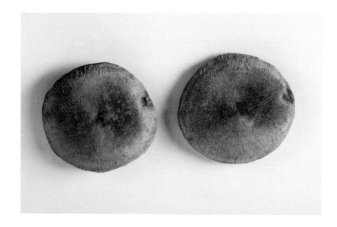

The main alkaloids in the seeds of nux vomica are strychnine and brucine. Strychnine by itself is extremely poisonous, but when given in small doses to humans it promotes appetite, aids digestion, and increases the frequency of urination. *(Bon Appetit / Alamy)*

The remedy is primarily indicated in ailments that are caused by abuse of narcotic drugs, alcohol, coffee, or tobacco, overindulgence in rich food and drink, and mental strain brought about by too much work. *Nux vomica* patients are typically thin and dark-complected workaholics who wear themselves down by working late, eating heavily, neglecting **exercise**, and overindulging in mood-altering foods such as coffee or alcohol. They are hurried and have an overactive mind, even at night, which is why they often suffer from **insomnia**. Their digestive systems are weakened by the rich, spicy, stimulating food and drink they crave and consume. As such, they suffer from **diarrhea**, constipation, hemorrhoids, digestive problems, and an overall weakened vitality. *Nux vomica* patients catch colds easily and are hypersensitive to light, touch, noise, smells, and the effect of medicines. They are also sensitive to the cold and dislike cold weather immensely. Patients may be tidy and fastidious.

Children who require *Nux vomica* are mischievous, stubborn, sensitive, and easily offended. They like to get their own way and become difficult if they do not.

Mentally, *Nux vomica* patients are irritable, impatient, jealous, suspicious, malicious, never satisfied or content, anxious, argumentative, critical, stubborn, and rude. They have a violent temper and are often suicidal. They also have a difficult time concentrating and their memory often fails them.

Physically they may suffer from **muscle spasms** and twitching of muscles, emaciation, **anemia**, internal muscle tension, numbness of the affected part, an ineffectual urge to urinate, cramping pains, and heat in the stomach, chest, uterus, head, face, and palms of

---

KEY TERMS

Gastritis—Inflammation of the lining of the stomach.

Placebo—An inactive substance with no pharmacological action that is administered to some patients in clinical trials to determine the relative effectiveness of another drug administered to a second group of patients.

Polychrest—A homeopathic remedy that is used in the treatment of many ailments.

Strychnine—A colorless, crystalline poison obtained from the seeds of *Nux vomica*.

Succussion—The act of shaking diluted homeopathic remedies as part of the process of potentization.

Nux vomica

the hands. The complaints are generally right-sided, especially in conditions of **tonsillitis**, hernias, and renal **colic**.

Symptoms are generally worse in the morning, at night (particularly after midnight or from 3:00 to 4:00 A.M.), in cold or open air, in dry weather, after eating, from cold food and drinks, from lying down or lying on the painful side, during the menstrual cycle, from mental strain, loss of sleep, and from use of alcohol, coffee, and tobacco. Symptoms are better with warmth, warm food and drinks, wet weather, and sleep.

Specific indications

The headaches indicative of *Nux vomica* are concentrated in the forehead (over the eyes) or back of the head. The pains are sharp, bursting pains and the scalp may feel sore and bruised. Constipation and other gastric symptoms are often present. This **headache** is typical of a **hangover** headache. It may be caused by alcohol, cold wind, damp weather, insomnia, mental strain, or overeating. The headache is aggravated by eating, cold air, moving the eyes, or shaking the head. Stillness and quiet relieves the headache, as does pressure, rising in the morning, or lying in bed at night.

The *Nux vomica* cold occurs as a result of exposure to cold, dry wind or from **indigestion**. Colds generally settle in the nose, throat, chest, and ears. Colds are accompanied by a hoarse voice, headache, **sore throat, sneezing, chills**, a tickling **cough, fever**, and bone pains. The voice sounds nasal from the stuffy nose, which is plugged in open air and at night. The nose emits a watery discharge during the day and in a warm room. The patient has a desire for cold water and the eyes are watery. Colds are better from fresh air and worse upon rising in the morning and after eating. The **earache** that accompanies the cold is made worse by swallowing. The ear is itchy and painful.

Flus and **hay fever** both exhibit the *Nux vomica* cold symptoms. The flu may be accompanied by an aching, sore sensation. The hay fever may last throughout the year.

The cough is a dry, tickling cough that comes about in violent fits. It is accompanied by headaches, a sore throat, and pain in the abdomen. Coughs are worse after midnight, from mental exertion, in cold air, and after eating. They are relieved by hot drinks and from fresh air.

Sore throat pains spread to the ears. The throat is raw and the patient may feel as though there is "a lump in his throat." The sore throat is worse from swallowing and cold air.

Fever is accompanied by chills, shivering, and an aching of the back, arms and legs. The fever begins early in the morning around 6:00 or 7:00 A.M. The fever is hot and dry and is often one-sided. The patient becomes chilled when he moves around in bed or when a limb becomes uncovered. He is thirsty and may perspire. The gastric symptoms typical of this remedy may occur with the fever.

Digestive complaints are brought about by overindulging in rich, spicy foods, alcohol, tobacco, or coffee. Disturbances include diarrhea, constipation, and abdominal pains and may be accompanied by **nausea**, vomiting, and indigestion. The patient feels bloated and full. The abdomen is painful and cramped and the patient may be doubled over. He may strain to urinate, defecate, or vomit. The pains are relieved by passing **gas** or passing a stool, from hot drinks, loose clothing, and warmth.

Menstrual difficulties occur throughout the cycle. The period is early, late, or too long. The menses may be heavy and clotted and accompanied by back pain and violent cramps that are aggravated by air or the cold and relieved by warmth and pressure.

Insomnia is caused by excitement, mental exertion, or the effects of alcohol. The patient is sleepy but as soon as her head hits the pillow she is awake. She often wakes up early in the morning, around 3:00 A.M., and cannot get back to sleep.

Recent research

Because *Nux vomica* is prescribed so frequently in homeopathic treatment, it has figured in several different areas of research into homeopathic remedies:

• Gastritis. Studies were done as early as 1966 comparing patients who received *Nux vomica* 4X for gastritis compared with a group that received a placebo. While one study showed that twice as many patients responded to the homeopathic remedy as responded to the placebo, other studies found no difference in the rate of response.

• Alcoholism. A study published in 2001 reported that *Nux vomica* reduced alcohol intake in rats that had been conditioned to crave alcohol. The rise in the number of animal studies using *Nux vomica*, however, has led to some debate among homeopaths regarding the morality of experimentation on animals.

• Abnormal psychology. The compilation of the Constitutional Type Questionnaire, or CTQ, as a homeopathic psychological research instrument has led to studies comparing its findings to those of mainstream psychological measures. One group of researchers reported that subjects who fit the *Nux*

Nux vomica

vomica profile on the CTQ scored high in neurotic traits as well as high in chemical intolerance.

Preparations

The seeds of the tree are ground until powdered then mixed with milk sugar. This solution is then diluted and succussed to create the final preparation.

Nux vomica is available at health food and drug stores in various potencies in the form of tinctures, tablets, and pellets.

Precautions

If symptoms do not improve after the recommended time period, a homeopath or healthcare practitioner should be consulted.

The recommended dose should not be exceeded, as the strychnine in *Nux vomica* is poisonous. People should be careful to use only preparations made by established manufacturers, as cases of accidental strychnine poisoning from non-homeopathic herbal preparations containing *Nux vomica* have been reported.

Side effects

There are no known side effects at recommended dosages, but individual aggravations may occur.

Interactions

When taking any homeopathic remedy, use of **peppermint** products, coffee, or alcohol should be avoided. These products may cause the remedy to be ineffective.

Resources

BOOKS

Cummings, M.D., Stephen, and Dana Ullman, M.P.H. *Everybody's Guide to Homeopathic Medicines.* New York, NY: Jeremy P. Tarcher/Putnam, 1997.

Kent, James Tyler. *Lectures on Materia Medica.* Delhi, India: B. Jain Publishers, 1996.

Pelletier, Kenneth R., MD. *The Best Alternative Medicine, Part I: Homeopathy.* New York: Simon & Schuster, 2002.

PERIODICALS

Bell, I. R., C. M. Baldwin, G. E. Schwartz, and J. R. Davidson. ''Homeopathic Constitutional Type Questionnaire Correlates of Conventional Psychological and Physical Health Scales: Individual Difference Characteristics of Young Adults.'' *Homeopathy* 91 (April 2002): 63-74.

Chan, T. Y. ''Herbal Medicine Causing Likely Strychnine Poisoning.'' *Human and Experimental Toxicology* 21 (August 2002): 467-468.

Sukul, N. C., S. Ghosh, S. P. Sinhababu, and A. Sukul. ''Strychnos *Nux-vomica* Extract and Its Ultra-High Dilution Reduce Voluntary Ethanol Intake in Rats.'' *Journal of Alternative and Complementary Medicine* 7 (April 2001): 187-193.

Thurneysen, A. ''*Nux vomica* and Animal Experiments.'' *Homeopathy* 91 (January 2002): 59.

ORGANIZATIONS

Foundation for Homeopathic Education and Research. 21 Kittredge St., Berkeley, CA 94704. (510) 649-8930.

International Foundation for Homeopathy. P. O. Box 7, Edmonds, WA 98020. (206) 776-4147.

National Center for Homeopathy. 801 N. Fairfax St., Suite 306, Alexandria, VA 22314. (703) 548-7790. www.homeopathic.org.

Jennifer Wurges
Rebecca J. Frey, PhD

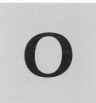

Oak

Description

Oak is the common name for many acorn-producing trees and shrubs that are members of the beech, or Fagaceae, family. Oak trees are classified as members of the genus *Quercus*, a Latin word said to be derived from a Celtic word meaning "fine tree." Worldwide there are more than 600 different species of oak. They thrive across the Northern Hemisphere in China, Japan, Europe, the British Isles, and in all of the continental United States except for Alaska. More than half of the 600 species are native to North America. Yet only about 60 varieties grow north of Mexico. In the forests of northern areas that have short summer growing seasons and long winters, such as Canada, northern Europe, and Siberia, varieties of oak are very scarce.

The oak family is a diverse group of trees and shrubs, influenced by climatic and environmental changes. Recent studies indicate that global warming contributes to oak dieback by speeding up the reproduction of beetles and fungi that attack oak trees. There are oaks that grow to heights of about 100 ft (30.5 m), while other types never grow larger than a small shrub. In warmer climates, oaks are evergreens, keep their leaves all year long, and are often used as ornamental trees in parks. In colder climates, they usually drop their leaves in autumn.

Many of these deciduous oaks have leaves that turn brilliant gold or scarlet in the autumn. In spring small, yellow green flowers appear. The male flowers hang in clusters called catkins and have profuse amounts of pollen. This oak pollen is carried by the wind to fertilize female flowers that produce acorns. Oak trees grow very slowly. In 80 years, it's estimated that one will grow to no more than 2 ft (0.6 m) in diameter. Oaks do not even produce acorns for their first 20 years, but they live a very long time. Average life expectancy for most oaks is between 200 and 400 years, and there are oak trees over 800 years old that are still alive.

Oaks are divided into two basic categories: white and red. The leaves of most of these are characteristically lobed, and depending upon the variety, can have anywhere from five to 11 lobes. Historically, the oak has been considered sacred by many civilizations. Abraham's Oak, the Oak of Mamre, is thought to be on the spot where the bible states Abraham pitched his tent. Legend states that anyone defacing this tree will lose their firstborn son. Both the ancient Greeks and Romans revered the oak, but its longest association has been with the British Isles. The Druids considered it to have both medicinal and mystical significance. For centuries, an oak sprig was inscribed on English coins. Legend states that King Arthur's round table was made from one gigantic slice of a very ancient oak tree. Oak has been used as a medicine since the ancient Greek and Roman times. The famous Roman doctor Galen first used oak leaves to heal **wounds**.

The American white oak, *Quercus alba*, and the English oak, *Quercus robur*, have bark with similar healing qualities. Oak bark contains saponins, tannins, calcium oxalate, starch, glycosides, oak-red, resin, pectin, levulin, and quercitol.

General use

Oak wood as timber is prized for its strength, elasticity, and durability. It is ideal for making furniture, barrels, railroad ties, and in the past, ships. Oak acorns are a source of food for wildlife and have been used as fodder for farm animals in the past. A flour made from ground acorns was also a part of the diet of Native Americans. The tannin in oak bark is used in leather preparation. Cork is made from the bark of some species that grow only in Spain and Portugal.

Recent advances in molecular genetics have shown that DNA from samples of oak can be isolated and analyzed. This type of analysis has a variety of potential applications in archaeology and forensic investigations.

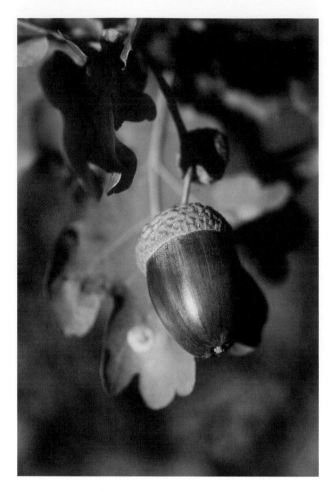

English Oak with acorn. (© ImageState / Alamy)

Oak used to make wine barrels has been found to increase the antioxidant activity of wines aged in the barrels as well as adding a distinctive aroma to the wine. The increase in antioxidant activity can be measured by a new technique known as electron paramagnetic resonance, or EPR.

Oak bark is used in medicine as a bowel astringent to treat **diarrhea** and as an anti-inflammatory gargle for soothing sore throats. It can be used topically for such skin inflammations as **dermatitis**, as an enema for hemorrhoids, or as a douche for vaginal **infections** and leukorrhea. A study in 1980 showed some evidence that oak bark may prevent kidney stone formation and act as a diuretic. A 1990 Russian study demonstrated that oak bark had antibacterial activity against *Staphylococcus*. One study in 1994 showed that oak bark could reduce serum cholesterol levels in animals.

Preparations

One teaspoonful of pulverized oak bark powder can be added to 1 cup of water, boiled, and then simmered at a reduced heat for 15 minutes to make an oak bark tea. This tea can be taken internally as an intestinal astringent up to three times per day. Oak bark is also available in both an extract and a tincture. For rinses, compresses, and gargles, 20 g of pulverized bark should be dissolved in 1 qt (1 L) of water, and prepared in the same manner as the tea. Oak bark is also available as snuff, tablets, and capsules.

Precautions

Oak bark should not be used externally over large areas of skin damage or used as a full bath. Oak bark for gargles, enemas, or douches should not be used for more than two weeks before consulting a doctor. A doctor should also be consulted for any episode of diarrhea that lasts longer than three days despite treatment with oak bark.

Side effects

No side effects have been reported when oak preparations are used at recommended dosage levels. Patients occasionally experience mild stomach upset or **constipation** if the dosage is exceeded.

Interactions

Oak bark preparations are believed to inhibit or reduce the absorption of such alkaline drugs as antacids. In addition, oak bark has been found to reduce the effectiveness of codeine and atropine.

Resources

BOOKS

Grieve, M., and C. F. Leyel. *A Modern Herbal: The Medical, Culinary, Cosmetic and Economic Properties, Cultivation and Folklore of Herbs, Grasses, Fungi, Shrubs and Trees With All of Their Modern Scientific Uses.* Barnes and Noble Publishing, 1992.

Hoffman, David, and Linda Quayle. *The Complete Illustrated Herbal: A Safe and Practical Guide to Making and Using Herbal Remedies.* Barnes and Noble Publishing, 1999.

PERIODICALS

Deguilloux, M. F., M. H. Pemonge, and R. J. Petit. "Novel Perspectives in Wood Certification and Forensics: Dry Wood as a Source of DNA." *Proceedings of the Royal Society of London, Series B, Biological Sciences* 269 (May 22, 2002): 1039-1046.

Diaz-Playa, E. M., J. R. Reyero, F. Pardo et al. "Influence of Oak Wood on the Aromatic Composition and Quality of Wines with Different Tannin Contents." *Journal of Agriculture and Food Chemistry* 50 (April 24, 2002): 2622-2626.

Kamata, N., N. Kamata, K. Esaki, et al. "Potential Impact of Global Warming on Deciduous Oak Dieback Caused by Ambrosia Fungus *Raffaelea sp.* Carried by Ambrosia Beetle *Platypus quercivorus* (Coleoptera: Platypodidae) in Japan." *Bulletin of Entomological Research* 92 (April 2002): 119-126.

Troup, G. J., and C. R. Hunter. "EPR, Free Radicals, Wine, and the Industry: Some Achievements." *Annual of the New York Academy of Science* (May 2002): 345-347.

ORGANIZATIONS

Herbal Advisor. http//www.AllHerb.com

OnHealth Herbal Index. "Oak Bark." http//www.OnHealth.com

Joan Schonbeck
Rebecca J. Frey, PhD

Oatstraw *see* **Wild oat**

Obesity

Definition

Obesity is an abnormal accumulation of body fat, usually 20% or more over an individual's ideal body weight. Obesity is associated with increased risk of illness, disability, and death.

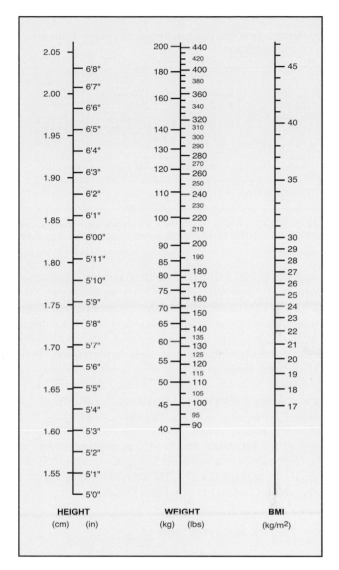

(Illustration by Argosy Inc. Cengage Learning, Gale)

The branch of medicine that deals with the study and treatment of obesity is known as bariatrics. As obesity has become a major health problem in the United States, bariatrics has become a separate medical and surgical specialty.

Description

Obesity traditionally has been defined as body weight at least 20% above the weight corresponding to the lowest death rate for individuals of a specific height, sex, and age (designated as the ideal weight). Twenty to forty percent over ideal weight is considered mildly obese; 40–100% over ideal weight is considered moderately obese; and 100% over ideal weight is considered severely, or morbidly, obese. According to some estimates, approximately 25% of the United

Percentage of healthy, overweight, and obese adults in the United States

Age ≥20 yrs.	Healthy weight BMI 18.5 to 24.9	Overweight BMI 25.0–29.9	Obese BMI 30 and above
All Adults	32.9%	34.1%	32.2%
Women	35.4%	28.6%	34.6%
Men	30.4%	39.7%	31.1%

SOURCE: National Institute of Diabetes and Digestive and Kidney Diseases, National Institutes of Health, U.S. Department of Health and Human Services

(Illustration by GGS Information Services. Cengage Learning, Gale)

States population can be considered obese, 4 million of whom are morbidly obese. Other studies state that over 50% of American adults are obese, based on body mass index (BMI) measurements. Excessive weight can result in many serious, and potentially deadly, health problems, including **hypertension**, Type II **diabetes mellitus** (non-insulin dependent diabetes), increased risk for coronary disease, increased unexplained **heart attack**, hyperlipidemia, **infertility**, and a higher prevalence of colon, prostate, endometrial, and possibly, **breast cancer**. Approximately 300,000 deaths a year are attributed to obesity, prompting leaders in public health, such as former Surgeon General C. Everett Koop to label obesity "the second leading cause of preventable deaths in the United States."

Causes and symptoms

The mechanism for excessive weight gain is clear—more calories are consumed than the body **burns**, and the excess calories are stored as fat (adipose) tissue. However, the exact cause is not as clear and likely arises from a complex combination of factors. Genetic factors significantly influence how the body regulates appetite and the rate at which it turns food into energy (metabolic rate). Studies of adoptees confirm this relationship. The majority of adoptees followed a pattern of weight gain that more closely resembled that of their birth parents than their adoptive parents. A genetic predisposition to weight gain, however, does not automatically mean that a person will be obese. Eating habits and patterns of physical activity also play a significant role in the amount of weight a person gains.

Some recent studies have indicated that the amount of fat in a person's diet may have a greater impact on weight than the number of calories the food contains. Carbohydrates like cereals, breads, fruits and vegetables, and protein (fish, lean meat, turkey breast,

KEY TERMS

Adipose tissue—Fat tissue.

Appetite suppressant— A drug that decreases feelings of hunger. Most work by increasing levels of serotonin or catecholamine, chemicals in the brain that control appetite.

Bariatrics—The branch of medicine that deals with the prevention and treatment of obesity and related disorders.

Ghrelin—A recently discovered peptide hormone secreted by cells in the lining of the stomach. Ghrelin is important in appetite regulation and maintaining the body's energy balance.

Hyperlipidemia—A condition characterized by abnormally high levels of lipids in blood plasma.

Hyperplastic obesity—Excessive weight gain in childhood, characterized by an increase in the number of new fat cells.

Hypertension—Abnormally high arterial blood pressure, which if left untreated can lead to heart disease and stroke.

Hypertrophic obesity—Excessive weight gain in adulthood, characterized by expansion of already existing fat cells.

Ideal weight—Weight corresponding to the lowest death rate for individuals of a specific height, gender, and age.

Leptin—A protein hormone that affects feeding behavior and hunger in humans. At present it is thought that obesity in humans may result in part from insensitivity to leptin.

skim milk) are converted to fuel almost as soon as they are consumed. Most fat calories are immediately stored in fat cells, which add to the body's weight and girth as they expand and multiply. There is continuing research on the theory that fat is metabolized as fuel and energy and that only excess carbohydrates are converted to stored fat. Current evidence shows that weight gain comes mostly from total calories consumed, rather than from the amount of carbohydrates. A study published in 2002 found that low-fat **diets** are no more effective in weight reduction programs than low-calorie diets. At any rate, a sedentary life-style, particularly prevalent in affluent societies like the United States, can contribute to weight gain. Psychological factors, such as **depression** and low self-esteem may, in some cases, also play a role in weight gain.

At what stage of life a person becomes obese can effect his or her ability to lose weight. In childhood, excess calories are converted into new fat cells (hyperplastic obesity), while excess calories consumed in adulthood only serve to expand existing fat cells (hypertrophic obesity). Since dieting and **exercise** can only reduce the size of fat cells, not eliminate them, persons who were obese as children can have great difficulty losing weight, since they may have up to five times as many fat cells as someone who became overweight as an adult.

Obesity can also be a side effect of certain disorders and conditions, including:

- Cushing's syndrome, a disorder involving the excessive release of the hormone cortisol
- hypothyroidism, a condition caused by an underactive thyroid gland
- neurologic disturbances, such as damage to the hypothalamus, a structure located deep within the brain that helps regulate appetite
- consumption of certain drugs, such as steroids, antipsychotic medications, or antidepressants

The major symptoms of obesity are excessive weight gain and the presence of large amounts of fatty tissue. Obesity can also give rise to several secondary conditions, including:

- arthritis and other orthopedic problems, such as lower back pain
- heartburn
- high cholesterol levels
- high blood pressure
- menstrual irregularities or cessation of menstruation (amenorhhea)
- shortness of breath that can be incapacitating
- skin disorders, arising from the bacterial breakdown of sweat and cellular material in thick folds of skin or from increased friction between folds

Diagnosis

Dignosis of obesity is made by observation and by comparing the patient's weight to ideal weight charts. Many doctors and obesity researchers refer to the body mass index (BMI), which uses a height-weight relationship to calculate an individual's ideal weight and personal risk of developing obesity-related health problems. Physicians may also obtain direct measurements of an individual's body fat content by using calipers to measure skin-fold thickness at the back of the upper arm and other sites. The most accurate means of measuring body fat content involves immersing a person in water and measuring relative displacement; however, this method is very impractical and is usually only used in scientific studies requiring very specific assessments. Women whose body fat exceeds 30% and men whose body fat exceeds 25% are generally considered obese.

Doctors may also note how a person carries excess weight on his or her body. Studies have shown that this factor may indicate whether or not an individual has a predisposition to develop certain diseases or conditions that may accompany obesity. "Apple-shaped" individuals who store most of their weight around the waist and abdomen are at greater risk for **cancer**, **heart disease**, **stroke**, and diabetes than "pear-shaped" people whose extra pounds settle primarily in their hips and thighs.

Treatment

Treatment of obesity depends primarily on the degree of a person's overweight and his or her overall health. However, to be successful, any treatment must affect life-long behavioral changes rather than short-term weight loss. "Yo-yo" dieting, in which weight is repeatedly lost and regained, has been shown to increase a person's likelihood of developing fatal health problems than if the weight had been lost gradually or not lost at all. Behavior-focused treatment should concentrate on:

- What a person eats and how much. This aspect may involve keeping a food diary and developing a better understanding of the nutritional value and fat content of foods. It may also involve changing grocery shopping habits (e.g. buying only what is on a prepared list and going only on a certain day), timing of meals (to prevent feelings of hunger, a person may plan frequent small meals), and actually slowing down the rate at which a person eats.
- How a person responds to food. This may involve understanding what psychological issues underlie a person's eating habits. For example, one person may binge eat when under stress, while another may always use food as a reward. In recognizing these psychological triggers, an individual can develop alternate coping mechanisms that do not focus on food.
- How people spend their time. Making activity and exercise an integral part of everyday life is a key to achieving and maintaining weight loss. Starting slowly and building endurance keeps individuals from becoming discouraged. Varying routines and trying new activities also keeps interest high.

For most who are mildly obese, these behavior modifications entail lifestyle changes they can make independently while being supervised by a family physician. Other mildly obese persons may seek the help of a commercial weight loss program (e.g. Weight Watchers). The effectiveness of these programs is difficult to assess, since programs vary widely, dropout rates are high, and few employ members of the medical community. However, programs that emphasize realistic goals, gradual progress, sensible eating, and exercise can be very helpful and are recommended by many doctors. Programs that promise instant weight loss or feature severely restricted diets are not effective and, in some cases, can be dangerous.

For individuals who are moderately obese, medically supervised behavior modification and weight loss are required. While doctors will put most moderately obese patients on a balanced low-calorie diet (1200–1500 calories a day), they may recommend that certain individuals follow a very low-calorie liquid protein diet (400–700 calories) for as long as three months. This therapy, however, should not be confused with commercial liquid-protein diets or commercial weight-loss shakes and drinks. Doctors tailor these diets to specific patients, monitor patients carefully, and use them for only a short period of time. In addition to reducing the amount and type of calories consumed by the patient, doctors will recommend professional therapists or psychiatrists who can help the individual effectively change his or her behavior in regard to eating.

The Chinese herb **ephedra** (*Ephedra sinica*, or ma huang), combined with exercise and a low-fat diet in physician-supervised weight-loss programs, can cause at least a temporary increase in weight loss. However, the large doses of ephedra required to achieve the desired result can also cause:

- anxiety
- heart arrhythmias
- heart attack
- high blood pressure
- insomnia
- irritability
- nervousness
- seizures
- strokes
- death

Ephedra should not be used by anyone with a history of diabetes, heart disease, or thyroid problems. It is not recommended for long-term use, and can cause serious medical or psychiatric problems if used too long. An article that appeared in the *Journal of the American Medical Association* in early 2003 advised against the use of ephedra.

Diuretic herbs, which increase urine production, can cause short-term weight loss but cannot help patients achieve lasting weight control. The body responds to heightened urine output by increasing thirst to replace lost fluids, and patients who use diuretics for an extended period of time eventually start retaining water again anyway. In moderate doses, **psyllium**, a mucilaginous herb available in bulk-forming laxatives like Metamucil, absorbs fluid and makes patients feel as if they have eaten enough. Red peppers and mustard help patients lose weight more quickly by accelerating the metabolic rate. They also make people more thirsty, so they crave water instead of food. Walnuts contain serotonin, the brain chemical that tells the body it has eaten enough. **Dandelion** (*Taraxacum officinale*) can raise metabolism and counter a desire for sugary foods.

The amino acid 5-hydroxytryptophan, or **5-HTP**, which is extracted from the seeds of the *Griffonia simplicifolia* plant, is thought to increase serotonin levels in the brain. Serotonin is a neurotransmitter, or brain chemical, that regulates mood and thus can be linked to mood-related eating behaviors. When physical and mental **stress** reduces serotonin levels in the body, 5-HTP may be helpful in regulating mood by boosting serotonin levels. Individuals should consult with their healthcare professional before taking 5-HTP, as the amino acid may interact with other medications and can have potentially serious side effects.

Acupressure and **acupuncture** can also suppress food cravings. Visualization and **meditation** can create and reinforce a positive self-image that enhances the patient's determination to lose weight. By improving physical strength, mental concentration, and emotional serenity, **yoga** can provide the same benefits. Also, patients who play soft, slow music during meals often find that they eat less food but enjoy it more.

Eating the correct ratio of protein, carbohydrates, and good-quality fats can help in weight loss via enhancement of metabolism. Support groups and self-help groups such as Overeaters Anonymous and TOPS (Taking Off Pounds Sensibly) that are informed about healthy, nutritious, and balanced diets can offer an individual the support he or she needs to maintain this type of eating regimen.

Allopathic treatment

For individuals who are severely obese, dietary changes and behavior modification may be accompanied by surgery to reduce or bypass portions of the stomach or small intestine. The risks of obesity surgery have declined in recent years, but it is still only performed on patients for whom other strategies have failed and whose obesity seriously threatens their health. Other surgical procedures are not recommended, including liposuction, a purely cosmetic procedure in which a suction device is used to remove fat from beneath the skin, and jaw wiring, which can damage gums and teeth and cause painful **muscle spasms**.

A newer approach to weight loss is the development of functional foods, which are food products that incorporate natural compounds shown to help in weight loss programs. These compounds include carbohydrates with a low glycemic index, which help to suppress appetite; **green tea** extract, which increases the body's energy expenditure; and **chromium**, which encourages the body to burn stored fat rather than lean muscle tissue. Functional food products are currently undergoing clinical testing.

Appetite suppressant drugs are sometimes prescribed to aid in weight loss. These drugs work by increasing levels of serotonin or catecholamine, which are brain chemicals that control moods and feelings of fullness. Appetite suppressants, though, are not considered truly effective, since most of the weight lost while taking them is usually regained after stopping. Also, suppressants containing amphetamines can be potentially abused by patients. While most of the immediate side effects of these drugs are harmless, the long-term effects in many cases, are unknown. Two drugs, dexfenfluramine hydrochloride (Redux) and fenfluramine (Pondimin) as well as a combination fenfluramine-phentermine (Fen/Phen) drug, were taken off the market when they were shown to cause potentially fatal heart defects. In 1999, the United States Food and Drug Administration (FDA) approved a new prescription weight loss drug, Orlistat. Unlike other anti-obesity drugs that act as appetite suppressants, Orlistat encourages weight loss by inhibiting the body's ability to absorb dietary fat. The drug can cause side effects of abdominal cramping, **gas**, and **diarrhea**.

Other weight-loss medications available with a doctor's prescription include:

- Sibutramine (Meridia)
- Diethylpropion (Tenuate, Tenuate Dospan)
- Mazindol (Mazanor, Sanorex)
- Phendimetrazine (Bontril, Prelu-2)
- Phentermine (Adipex-P, Fastin, Ionamin, Oby-Cap)

Phenylpropanolamine (Acutrim, Dextarim) is the only nonprescription weight-loss drug approved by the FDA. These over-the-counter diet aids can boost weight loss by 5%. Combined with diet and exercise

and used only with a doctor's approval, prescription anti-obesity medications enable some patients to lose 10% more weight than they otherwise would. Most patients regain lost weight after discontinuing use of either prescription medications or nonprescription weight-loss products.

Prescription medications or over-the-counter weight loss products can cause:

- constipation
- dry mouth
- headache
- irritability
- nausea
- nervousness
- sweating

None of the weight loss drugs should be used by patients taking monoamine oxidate inhibitors (MAO inhibitors).

Doctors sometimes prescribe fluoxetine (Prozac), an antidepressant that can increase weight loss by about 10%. Weight loss may be temporary and side effects of this medication include diarrhea, **fatigue**, **insomnia**, **nausea**, and thirst. Weight loss drugs currently being developed or tested include ones that can prevent fat absorption or digestion, reduce the desire for food and prompt the body to burn calories more quickly, and regulate the activity of substances that control eating habits and stimulate overeating.

Expected results

As many as 85% of dieters who do not exercise on a regular basis regain their lost weight within two years. In five years, the figure rises to 90%. Repeatedly losing and regaining weight (yo-yo dieting) encourages the body to store fat and may increase a patient's risk of developing heart disease. The primary factor in achieving and maintaining weight loss is a lifelong commitment to regular exercise and sensible eating habits.

Prevention

Obesity experts suggest that a key to preventing excess weight gain is monitoring fat consumption rather than counting calories, and the National **Cholesterol** Education Program maintains that only 30% of calories should be derived from fat. Only one-third of those calories should be contained in saturated fats (the kind of fat found in high concentrations in meat, poultry, and dairy products). Because most people eat more than they think they do, keeping a detailed food diary is a useful way to assess eating habits. Eating three balanced, moderate-portion meals a day—with the main meal at mid-day—is a more effective way to prevent obesity than **fasting** or crash diets. Exercise increases the metabolic rate by creating muscle, which burns more calories than fat. When regular exercise is combined with regular, healthful meals, calories continue to burn at an accelerated rate for several hours. Finally, encouraging healthful habits in children is a key to preventing childhood obesity and the health problems that follow in adulthood.

New directions in obesity treatment

The rapid rise in the incidence of obesity in the United States since 1990 has prompted researchers to look for new treatments. One approach involves the application of antidiabetes drugs to the treatment of obesity. Metformin (Glucophage), a drug that was approved by the Food and Dug Administration (FDA) in 1994 for the treatment of type 2 diabetes, shows promise in treating obesity associated with **insulin resistance**.

Another field of obesity research is the study of hormones, particularly leptin, which is produced by fat cells in the body, and ghrelin, which is secreted by cells in the lining of the stomach. Both hormones are known to affect appetite and the body's energy balance. Leptin is also related to reproductive function, while ghrelin stimulates the pituitary gland to release growth hormone. Further studies of these two hormones may lead to the development of new medications to control appetite and food intake.

A third approach to obesity treatment involves research into the social factors that encourage or reinforce weight gain in humans. Researchers are looking at such issues as the advertising and marketing of food products; media stereotypes of obesity; the development of eating disorders in adolescents and adults; and similar questions.

Resources

BOOKS

Ackerman, Norman. *5-HTP: The Natural Way to Overcome Depression, Obesity, and Insomnia.* New York: Bantam Books, 1999.

Flancbaum, Louis, MD, with Erica Manfred and Deborah Biskin. *The Doctor's Guide to Weight Loss Surgery.* West Hurley, NY: Fredonia Communications, 2001.

Harris, Dan R., ed. *Diet and Nutrition Sourcebook.* Detroit, MI: Omnigraphics, 1996.

"Nutritional Disorders: Obesity." Section 1, Chapter 5 in *The Merck Manual of Diagnosis and Therapy*, edited by Mark H. Beers, MD, and Robert Berkow, MD. Whitehouse Station, NJ: Merck Research Laboratories, 1999.

PERIODICALS

Aronne, L. J., and K. R. Segal. "Weight Gain in the Treatment of Mood Disorders." *Journal of Clinical Psychiatry* 64 (2003 Supplement 8): 22–29.

Bell, S. J., and G. K. Goodrick. "A Functional Food Product for the Management of Weight." *Critical Reviews in Food Science and Nutrition* 42 (March 2002): 163–178.

Brudnak, M. A. "Weight-Loss Drugs and Supplements: Are There Safer Alternatives?" *Medical Hypotheses* 58 (January 2002): 28–33.

Colquitt, J., A. Clegg, M. Sidhu, and P. Royle. "Surgery for Morbid Obesity." *Cochrane Database Systems Review* 2003: CD003641.

Espelund, U., T. K. Hansen, H. Orskov, and J. Frystyk. "Assessment of Ghrelin." *APMIS Supplementum* 109 (2003): 140–145.

Hundal, R. S., and S. E. Inzucchi. "Metformin: New Understandings, New Uses." *Drugs* 63 (2003): 1879–1894.

Pirozzo, S., C. Summerbell, C. Cameron, and P. Glasziou. "Advice on Low-Fat Diets for Obesity (Cochrane Review)." *Cochrane Database Systems Review* 2002: CD003640.

Schurgin, S., and R. D. Siegel. "Pharmacotherapy of Obesity: An Update." *Nutrition in Clinical Care* 6 (January-April 2003): 27–37.

Shekelle, P. G., M. L. Hardy, S. C. Morton, et al. "Efficacy and Safety of Ephedra and Ephedrine for Weight Loss and Athletic Performance: A Meta-Analysis." *Journal of the American Medical Association* 289 (March 26, 2003): 1537–1545.

Tataranni, P. A. "Treatment of Obesity: Should We Target the Individual or Society?" *Current Pharmaceutical Design* 9 (2003): 1151–1163.

Veniant, M. M., and C. P. LeBel. "Leptin: From Animals to Humans." *Current Pharmaceutical Design* 9 (2003): 811–818.

ORGANIZATIONS

American Dietetic Association. (800) 877-1600. www.eatright.org.

American Obesity Association (AOA). 1250 24th Street NW, Suite 300, Washington, DC 20037. (202) 776-7711 or (800) 98-OBESE. www.obesity.org.

American Society of Bariatric Physicians. 5453 East Evans Place, Denver, CO 80222-5234. (303) 770-2526. www.asbp.org.

American Society for Bariatric Surgery. 7328 West University Avenue, Suite F, Gainesville, FL 32607. (352) 331-4900. www.asbs.org.

North American Association for the Study of Obesity. 8630 Fenton St., Suite 412, Silver Spring, MD, 20910. (301) 563-6526. www.naaso.org.

Overeaters Anonymous. P.O. Box 44020, Rio Rancho, New Mexico, 87174-4020. (505) 891-2664. www.overeatersanonymous.org.

Weight-control Information Network (WIN). 1 WIN Way, Bethesda, MD 20892-3665. (202) 828-1025 or (877) 946-4627.

Paula Ford-Martin
Rebecca J. Frey, PhD

Obsessive-compulsive disorder

Definition

Obsessive-compulsive disorder (OCD) is a type of **anxiety** disorder characterized by distressing repetitive thoughts, impulses, or images that are intense, frightening, absurd, or unusual. These thoughts are followed by ritualized actions that are usually bizarre and irrational. These ritual actions, known as compulsions, help reduce anxiety caused by the individual's obsessive thoughts. Often described as the "disease of doubt," the sufferer usually knows the obsessive thoughts and compulsions are irrational but, on another level, fears they may be true.

Description

Almost one out of every 40 people will suffer from obsessive-compulsive disorder at some time in their lives. The condition is two to three times more common than either **schizophrenia** or manic **depression**, and strikes men and women of every ethnic group, age, and social level. Because the symptoms are so distressing, sufferers often hide their fears and rituals but cannot avoid acting on them. OCD sufferers are often unable to decide if their fears are realistic and need to be acted upon.

Most people with obsessive-compulsive disorder have both obsessions and compulsions, but occasionally a person will have just one or the other. The degree to which this condition can interfere with daily living also varies. Some people are barely bothered, while others find the obsessions and compulsions to be profoundly traumatic and spend a great deal of time each day in compulsive actions.

Obsessions are intrusive, irrational thoughts that keep popping up in a person's mind, such as, "My hands are dirty, I must wash them again." Typical obsessions include fears of dirt, germs, contamination, and violent or aggressive impulses. Other obsessions include feeling responsible for others' safety, or an irrational fear of hitting a pedestrian with a car. Additional obsessions

may involve intrusive sexual thoughts. The patient may fear acting out the strong sexual thoughts in a hostile way. People with obsessive-compulsive disorder may have an intense preoccupation with order and symmetry, or be unable to throw anything out.

Compulsions usually involve repetitive rituals such as excessive washing (especially handwashing or bathing), cleaning, checking and touching, counting, arranging, or hoarding. As the person performs these acts, he may feel temporarily better, but there is no long lasting sense of satisfaction or completion after the act is performed. Often, a person with obsessive-compulsive disorder believes that if the ritual isn't performed, something dreadful will happen. While these compulsions may temporarily ease **stress**, short-term comfort is purchased at a heavy price–time spent repeating compulsive actions and a long-term interference with life.

The difference between OCD and other compulsive behavior is that while people who have problems with gambling, overeating, or **substance abuse** may appear to be compulsive, these activities also provide pleasure to some degree. The compulsions of OCD, on the other hand, are never pleasurable.

KEY TERMS

Anxiety disorder—This is the experience of prolonged, excessive worry about circumstances in one's life. It disrupts daily life.

Cognitive-behavior therapy—A form of psychotherapy that seeks to modify behavior by manipulating the environment to change the patient's response.

Compulsion—A rigid behavior that is repeated over and over each day.

Obsession—A recurring, distressing idea, thought, or impulse that feels "foreign" or alien to the individual.

Scrupulosity—A spiritual disorder characterized by perfectionism and obsessive fears of God's punishment. Some patients with OCD also develop religious scrupulosity.

Selective serotonin reuptake inhibitors (SSRIs)—A class of antidepressants that work by blocking the reabsorption of serotonin in brain cells, raising the level of the chemical in the brain. SSRIs include Prozac, Zoloft, Luvex, and Paxil.

Serotonin—One of three major neurotransmitters found in the brain that is related to emotion, and is linked to the development of depression and obsessive-compulsive disorder.

OCD may be related to some other conditions, such as the continual urge to pull out body hair (trichotillomania); fear of having a serious disease (hypochondriasis), or preoccupation with imagined defects in personal appearance disorder (body dysmorphic disorder). Some people with OCD also have **Tourette syndrome**, a condition featuring tics and unwanted vocalizations (such as swearing). OCD is often linked with depression and other anxiety disorders.

Causes and symptoms

The tendency to develop obsessive-compulsive disorder appears to be inherited. In the summer of 2002, researchers at the University of Michigan identified a segment of human chromosome 9p as containing genes for susceptibility to OCD. Other chromosomes that may also be linked to OCD are 19q and 6p.

There are several theories behind the cause of OCD. Some experts believe that OCD is related to a chemical imbalance within the brain that causes a communication problem between the front part of the brain (frontal lobe) and deeper parts of the brain responsible for the repetitive behavior. Research has shown that the orbital cortex located on the underside of the brain's frontal lobe is overactive in OCD patients. This may be one reason for the feeling of alarm that pushes the patient into compulsive, repetitive actions. The higher-than-average rate of concurrent eating disorders in patients diagnosed with OCD has been attributed to the fact that hyperactivity in the orbital cortex is associated with both disorders. It is possible that people with OCD experience overactivity deep within the brain that causes the cells to get "stuck," much like a jammed transmission in a car damages the gears. This could lead to the development of rigid thinking and repetitive movements common to the disorder. The fact that drugs which boost the levels of serotonin (a brain chemical linked to emotion) in the brain can reduce OCD symptoms may indicate that to some degree OCD is related to brain serotonin levels.

Recently, scientists have identified an intriguing link between childhood episodes of **strep throat** and the development of OCD. It appears that in some vulnerable children, strep antibodies attack a certain part of the brain. Antibodies are cells that the body produces to fight specific diseases. That attack results in the development of excessive washing or germ **phobias**. A phobia is a strong but irrational fear. In this instance the phobia is fear of disease germs present on commonly handled objects. These symptoms would normally disappear over time, but some children who have repeated **infections** may develop full-blown OCD. Treatment with antibiotics has resulted in lessening of the OCD symptoms in some of these children.

If one person in a family has obsessive-compulsive disorder, there is a 25% chance that another immediate family member has the condition. It also appears that stress and psychological factors may worsen symptoms, which usually begin during adolescence or early adulthood.

Some studies indicate that the nature of parent-child interactions is an important factor in the development of OCD. Observers have often remarked that parents and children in OCD families can be differentiated from members of other types of families on the basis of behavior. One Australian study described the parents of children with OCD as "...less confident in their child's ability, less rewarding of independence, and less likely to use positive problem solving."

OCD has also sometimes been linked to religion, in that the symptoms of some persons diagnosed with OCD reflect religious beliefs or practices. Christian clergy have been trained since the Middle Ages to recognize a specific spiritual problem known as scrupulosity, in which a person is troubled by excessive fears of God's punishment or fears of having sinned and offended God. A new inventory for measuring scrupulosity in devout Jews as well as Protestants and Catholics has been tested at the University of Pennsylvania and appears to be a reliable instrument for evaluating OCD symptoms that take religious forms. Scrupulosity has been traditionally treated in both Judaism and Christianity by consultation with a rabbi, priest, or pastor who is able to correct the distorted beliefs that underlie the obsessions or compulsions. In some cases the clergyperson may also use an appropriate religious ritual in treating scrupulosity.

Diagnosis

People with obsessive-compulsive disorder feel ashamed of their problem and often try to hide their symptoms. They may avoid seeking treatment. Because they can be very good at keeping their problem from friends and family, many sufferers do not get the help they need until the behaviors are deeply ingrained habits and harder to change. As a result, the condition is often misdiagnosed or underdiagnosed. All too often, it can take more than a decade between the onset of symptoms and proper diagnosis and treatment.

While scientists seem to agree that OCD is related to a disruption in serotonin levels, there is no blood test for the condition. Instead, doctors diagnose OCD after evaluating a person's symptoms and history.

Treatment

Because OCD sometimes responds to selective serotonin reuptake inhibitors (SSRI) antidepressants, herbalists believe a **botanical medicine** called **St. John's wort** (*Hypericum perforatum*) might have some beneficial effect as well. Known popularly as "Nature's Prozac," St. John's wort is prescribed by herbalists for the treatment of anxiety and depression. They believe that this herb affects brain levels of serotonin in the same way that SSRI antidepressants do. Herbalists recommend a dose of 300 mg, three times per day. In about one out of 400 people, St. John's wort (like Prozac) may initially increase the level of anxiety. Homeopathic constitutional therapy can help rebalance the patient's mental, emotional, and physical well-being, allowing the behaviors of OCD to abate over time.

Other alternative treatments for OCD are intended to lower the patient's anxiety level; some are thought to diminish the compulsions themselves. Alternative recommendations include the following:

- Bach flower remedies: White chestnut, for obsessive thoughts and repetitive thinking.
- Traditional Chinese medicine: a mixture of bupleurum and dong quai, to strengthen the spleen and regulate the liver. In Chinese medicine, obsessive-compulsive disorder is due to liver stagnation and a weak spleen.
- Aromatherapy: a mixture of lavender, rosemary, and valerian for relaxation.
- Yoga: Yogis in India developed a special technique of yogic breathing specifically for OCD. The specific yogic technique for treating OCD requires blocking the right nostril with the tip of the thumb; slow deep inspiration through the left nostril; holding the breath; and slow complete expiration through the left nostril. This is followed by a long breath-holding out period.
- Schuessler tissue salts: for OCD, 10 tablets of *Ferrum phosphorica* 30X and 10 tablets of *Kali phosphorica* 200X, twice daily.
- Massage therapy: with special emphasis on loosening the muscles in the neck, back, and shoulders.

Cognitive-behavioral therapy (CBT) teaches patients how to confront their fears and obsessive thoughts by making the effort to endure or wait out the activities that usually cause anxiety without compulsively performing the calming rituals. Eventually their anxiety decreases. People who are able to alter their thought patterns in this way can lessen their preoccupation with the compulsive rituals. At the same time, the patient is encouraged to refocus attention elsewhere, such as on a hobby.

Allopathic treatment

Obsessive-compulsive disorder can be effectively treated by a combination of cognitive-behavioral therapy and medication that regulates the brain's serotonin levels. Drugs that are approved to treat obsessive-compulsive disorder include fluoxetine (Prozac), fluvoxamine (Luvox), paroxetine (Paxil), and sertraline (Zoloft), all SSRIs that affect the level of serotonin in the brain. Drugs should be taken for at least 12 weeks before deciding whether or not they are effective.

In a few severe cases where patients have not responded to medication or **behavioral therapy**, brain surgery may be attempted to relieve symptoms. Surgery can help up to a third of patients with the most severe form of OCD. The most common operation involves removing a section of the brain called the cingulate cortex. The serious side effects of this surgery for some patients include seizures, personality changes, and decreased ability to plan.

Expected results

Obsessive-compulsive disorder is a chronic disease that, if untreated, can last for decades, fluctuating from mild to severe and worsening with age. When treated by a combination of drugs and behavioral therapy, some patients go into complete remission. Unfortunately, not all patients have such a good response. About 20% of people cannot find relief with either drugs or behavioral therapy. Hospitalization may be required in some cases.

Resources

BOOKS

Dumont, Raeann. *The Sky is Falling: Understanding and Coping with Phobias, Panic and Obsessive-Compulsive Disorders*. New York: W.W. Norton & Co., 1996.

Pelletier, Kenneth R., MD. *The Best Alternative Medicine*, Part II, "CAM Therapies for Specific Conditions: Anxiety." New York: Simon & Schuster, 2002.

Schwartz, Jeffrey. *Brain Lock*. New York: HarperCollins, 1996.

Schwartz, Jeffrey. *Free Yourself from Obsessive-Compulsive Behavior: A Four-Step Self-Treatment Method to Change Your Brain Chemistry*. New York: HarperCollins, 1996.

Swedo, S.E., and H. L. Leonard. *It's Not All In Your Head*. New York: HarperCollins, 1996.

PERIODICALS

Abramowitz, J. S., J. D. Huppert, A. B. Cohen, et al. "Religious Obsessions and Compulsions in a Non-

Clinical Sample: The Penn Inventory of Scrupulosity (PIOS)." *Behaviour Research and Therapy* 40 (July 2002): 825-838.

Barrett, P., A. Shortt, and L. Healy. "Do Parent and Child Behaviours Differentiate Families Whose Children Have Obsessive-Compulsive Disorder from Other Clinic and Non-Clinic Families?" *Journal of Child Psychology and Psychiatry* 43 (July 2002): 597-607.

Hanna, G. L., J. Veenstra-Vanderweele, N. J. Cox, et al. "Genome-Wide Linkage Analysis of Families with Obsessive-Compulsive Disorder Ascertained through Pediatric Probands." *American Journal of Medical Genetics* 114 (July 8, 2002): 541-552.

Lin, H., C. B. Yeh, B. S. Peterson, et al. "Assessment of Symptom Exacerbations in a Longitudinal Study of Children with Tourette's Syndrome or Obsessive-Compulsive Disorder." *Journal of the American Academy of Child and Adolescent Psychiatry* 41 (September 2002): 1070-1077.

Pelchat, M. L. "Of Human Bondage: Food Craving, Obsession, Compulsion, and Addiction." *Integrative Physiological and Behavioral Science* 76 (July 2002): 347-352.

Sica, C., C. Novara, and E. Sanavio. "Religiousness and Obsessive-Compulsive Cognitions and Symptoms in an Italian Population." *Behaviour Research and Therapy* 40 (July 2002): 813-823.

Stein, D. J. "Obsessive-Compulsive Disorder." *Lancet* 360 (August 3, 2002): 397-405.

Talan, Jamie. "A Link to Strep, Behavior: The Infection May Trigger Obsessive-Compulsive Symptoms." *Newsday* (May 21, 1996): B31.

ORGANIZATIONS

American Academy of Child and Adolescent Psychiatry. 3615 Wisconsin Avenue, NW, Washington, DC 20016-3007. (202) 966-7300. Fax: (202) 966-2891. www.aacap.org.

American Psychiatric Association. 1400 K Street, NW. Washington, DC 20005. (202) 682-6220. www.psych.org.

Anxiety Disorders Association of America. 11900 Parklawn Dr., Ste. 100, Rockville, MD 20852. (301) 231-9350. http://adaa.org.

National Alliance for the Mentally Ill (NAMI). 200 N.Glebe Rd., #1015, Arlington, VA 22203-3728. (800) 950-NAMI. http://www.nami.org.

National Anxiety Foundation. 3135 Custer Dr., Lexington, KY 40517. (606) 272-7166. http://www.lexington-on-line.com/naf.html.

National Institutes of Mental Health (NIMH). Information Resources and Inquires Branch. 5600 Fishers Lane, Rm.7C-02, MSC 8030, Bethesda, MD 20892. (301) 443-4513. http://www.nimh.nih.gov.

Paula Ford-Martin
Rebecca J. Frey, PhD

OCD *see* **Obsessive-compulsive disorder**

Omega–3 fatty acids

Description

Omega-3 fatty acids are one of two groups of fatty acids—the omega-3s and the omega-6s—that are vital to human life. The omega-3 fatty acids get their name from the fact that the molecules of which they are made contain a double bond attached to the number 3 carbon atom, counting from the end of the molecule opposite the carboxyl group, the so-called omega end of the molecule. (This system of nomenclature is just the reverse of the one used by chemists.) The omega-3 fatty acids are called **essential fatty acids** (EFAs) because the body is unable to make them, but they are essential for normal growth and development. These fats must be supplied by diet. People living in industrialized western countries eat up to 30 times more omega-6 than omega-3 fatty acids, resulting in a relative deficiency of omega-3 fats. Omega-6 metabolic products (inflammatory prostaglandins, thromboxanes, and leukotrienes) are formed in excessive amounts causing allergic and inflammatory disorders

Sources of omega 3 fatty acids

Beans, navy or kidney

Canola oil

Fish, fatty
Albacore tuna
Anchovies
Herring
Lake trout
Mackerel
Salmon
Sardines

Flaxseed (ground) and flaxseed oil

Hemp seed/hemp nut (ground) and hemp oil

Olive oil

Soybeans and soybean oil

Tofu

Walnuts

Winter squash

(Illustration by Corey Light. Cengage Learning, Gale)

and making the body more prone to heart attacks, strokes, and **cancer**. Eating foods rich in omega-3 acids or taking **fish oil** supplements can restore the balance between the two fatty acids and can possibly reverse these disease processes.

General use

Heart disease and stroke

The American Heart Association (AHA) has endorsed omega-3 fatty acids as good for the heart. The omega-3 oils increase the concentrations of good **cholesterol** (high density lipoproteins, HDL) while decreasing the concentrations of bad cholesterol (low-density lipoproteins, LDL) and triglycerides. In addition, eating omega-3-rich food results in a moderate decrease in total cholesterol level. In one study of 38 women, **flaxseed** flour, which contains high amounts of omega-3 fatty acids, decreased total cholesterol level by 6.9% and LDL cholesterol by 14.7%. In addition, lipoprotein(a), which is associated with heart attacks in older women, decreased by almost 10%. Thus, omega-3 fatty acids are natural alternatives to estrogen in prevention of heart attacks in postmenopausal women.

Furthermore, omega-3 oils protect the heart by preventing **blood clots** or keeping other fats from injuring the arterial walls. They relax arteries and help to decrease constriction of arteries and thickening of blood.

Hundreds of studies have shown that **diets** rich in omega-3 fatty acids decrease risk of heart attacks, strokes, and abnormal heart rhythms. Eskimos, who eat a lot of cold-water fish, have low rates of heart attacks and strokes perhaps because they have thinner blood, high HDL to LDL cholesterol ratio, and less buildup of fatty deposits (plaques) in the arteries. A number of clinical trials have shown that regular consumption of fish or fish-oil supplements can prevent sudden deaths due to abnormal heart rhythms. In the Diet and Reinfarction Trial (DART) of 2,033 men who previously suffered a **heart attack**, men who ate two to three servings of fatty fish a week had their risk of sudden cardiac death lowered by 29% compared to those who had a low fat or high fiber diet. In the Physician's Health Study of 20,551 doctors, a 52% reduction in risk of heart attacks was observed in those who ate at least one fish meal per week compared with those who ate fish once a month or less.

Mild hypertension

Several studies have shown that eating 200 g of fatty fish or taking six to 10 capsules of fish oil daily will lower blood pressure (BP). Therefore, omega-3 can benefit patients with borderline high blood pressure. Omega-3 oils also effectively prevent **hypertension** in cardiac patients after transplantation.

Supplement for newborns and babies

Omega-3 fatty acids are essential for normal development of vision and brain function, especially in newborns and children. Very low birth weight preterm infants often have poor vision and motor skills, possibly because they receive less than one-third of the amount of omega-3 fatty acids outside the mother's womb that they would have received as a fetus. Human breast milk contains the appropriate amount of omega-3 and -6 fats and is believed best for babies. If mother's milk is unavailable, formulas with soybean oil that provide higher amounts of omega-3 fatty acids are more beneficial than those made from cow's milk. Even full-term babies benefit from the addition of essential fatty acids to cow-milk formulas. Studies have shown that babies given formulas supplemented with EFAs have better vision and score higher in skills and problem-solving tests compared to babies on formulas that do not contain additional EFAs.

Rheumatoid arthritis

Because omega-3 fatty acids inhibit the action of inflammatory prostaglandins and leukotrienes, they can help control arthritis symptoms. Significant reduction in the number of tender joints and morning stiffness, as well as an increase in grip strength, have been observed in patients taking fish oil capsules. Studies have shown that patients taking fish oil supplements for **rheumatoid arthritis** require fewer **pain** medications; some are able to discontinue their nonsteroidal anti-inflammatory treatment. Despite the beneficial effects of omega-3 fats, regular antirheumatic drugs and nonsteroidal anti-inflammatory medications most likely still are required to control this chronic condition.

Diabetes

Some studies in laboratories have indicated that omega-3 fatty acids in fish oils might prolong life in people with autoimmune disorders such as diabetes. One study looked at substituting fish oil for corn oil in diets and found a tendency to suppress immune system dysfunction and prolong life. As of 2008, more studies were required to prove the diet's benefits in humans.

Inflammatory bowel disease

High-dose fish-oil supplements have been shown to decrease abdominal cramping, **diarrhea**, and pain associated with **Crohn's disease**. In one study of 96 patients, patients who received 4.5 g of omega-3 fatty acids (15 fish oil capsules) required significantly less steroids to control symptoms. In another study of 78 Crohn's disease patients, 59% of patients who received nine fish oil capsules (2.7 g of omega-3 fatty acids) daily did not have any disease flare-ups for at least one year compared to 26% recurrence rate in patients who were not given fish oil. Omega-3 fatty acids also are effective in preventing reappearance of Crohn's disease after surgery to remove sections of diseased bowel. In a clinical trial involving 50 patients, patients who received 2.7 grams of omega-3 fats as fish oil cut their rate of disease reappearance in half compared to patients receiving placebo. However, the effectiveness of omega-3 oils varies depending on the type of omega-3 oils being used, length of use, and the patient's diet.

Asthma

Taking high dose omega-3 fatty acids can reduce inflammation of the airways and reduce **asthma** attacks. According to Donald Rudin, the author of *Omega-3 Oils*, allergic disorders such as asthma may be triggered by too much omega-6 and too little omega-3 fats in the body. Excessive amounts of omega-6 prostaglandins cause the body to produce antibodies that cause allergic reactions. Flaxseed or fish oil supplements can keep the omega-6 fats in check and decrease the inflammatory reactions associated with asthma.

Berger's disease (Immunoglobulin A (IgA) nephropathy)

Omega-3 fats may be effective in treating this autoimmune disease in which kidney function fails over time with few treatment options available. In a large, randomized study of 150 patients, those who received 3 g of omega-3 fatty acids daily for two years had significantly less reduction in renal function than those treated with placebo. Therefore, omega-3 fatty acids appear to have protective effects and may stabilize renal function in these patients.

Raynaud's disease

There have been few studies evaluating the effects of omega-3 fatty acids in treating Raynaud's disease; however, it appears that fish oil supplements may alleviate some blood clotting disorders.

Mental disorders

According to some studies, many common mental disorders, such as **depression**, **bipolar disorder** (manic-depression), attention-deficit hyperactive disorder (ADHD), **anxiety**, or **schizophrenia**, may be triggered by deficiencies of omega-3 fatty acids and/or B vitamins. The rates of depression are low in countries where people eat a lot of fish, while the rate of depression steadily rises in the United States as Americans eat increasingly more processed food and less fresh fish and vegetables containing omega-3 fats. In one study, 53% of bipolar patients on placebo (olive oil) became ill again within four months, while none of the patients who were given 9.6 g daily of omega-3 fatty acids (as fish oil) did. Supplements containing omega-3 fats also reportedly have been effective in children with ADHD precipitated by essential fatty acid deficiencies. Furthermore, a 25% decrease in schizophrenic symptoms was observed in patients receiving eicosapentanoic acid (EPA), one of the omega-3 fatty acids contained in fish oil.

A report in 2001 revealed that omega-3 fatty acids may have effects on stabilizing mood and relieving depression. As studies continued in the early 2000s, researchers found it more and more evident that omega-3 fatty acids can be effective for treating depression, though they remained uncertain about exactly how they work. A 2003 report linked depression to increased risk of sudden cardiac death.

Acquired immunodeficiency syndrome (AIDS)

In a small study of 20 **AIDS** patients, those who received fish oil supplements at dosage of 10 g of omega-3 fatty acids per day for 30 days gained more weight (2.4 kg) and significantly lowered their concentrations of tumor necrosis factor, which is believed to cause wasting in AIDS patients, compared to those who did not.

Cancer prevention

Omega-3 fatty acids inhibit tumor growth when injected into animals. Flaxseed oil, which is a plant source of omega-3 fatty acids, has been shown to prevent cancer of the breast, colon, and prostate. The **Mediterranean diet**, which is heart healthy, also can decrease risk of getting cancer. Omega-3 fats, it seems, strengthen the immune systems and inhibit the inflammation and blood circulation of the tumors.

Preparations

As of 2008, the U.S. Food and **Nutrition** Board had not issued recommended daily allowance (RDA) for omega-3 fatty acids. However, it has established adequate intake (IA) levels for some of the more common omega-3 fatty acids, including alpha linolenic acid (ALA), eicosapentaenoic acid (EPA), and docosahexaenoic acid (DHA). Those recommendations differ according to age and sex and for women who are pregnant or lactating. For men over the age of 14, the AI for ALA (the only omega-3 fatty acid for which an AI exists) is 1.6 grams per day; for women in the same age range, the AI for ALA is 1.1 grams per day.

The best way to achieve this dietary requirement is by eating fatty fish two or three times a week and/or eating vegetables and oils containing omega-3 fatty acids. Omega-3 fatty acids can be found naturally in the oil of cold-water fish, such as mackerel, salmon, sardines, anchovies, and tuna, or as extracted oils from plants, such as flaxseed, canola (rapeseed), or soybean. If fish oil supplement is preferred, then one to two capsules a day is sufficient. Each 1 g fish oil capsule typically contains 180 mg of EPA and 120 mg of DHA. **Vitamin E** is often contained in fish oil supplements to prevent spoilage and vitamin-E deficiency, which may occur with high dose fish-oil consumption. Patients should take supplements containing omega-3 fatty acids only under professional supervision to prevent an overdose, adverse reactions, or interactions with other medications. For treatment of diseases, flaxseed oil should be the first choice because it is the richest source of omega-3 fatty acids, relatively safe, and inexpensive.

Precautions

The safest and most effective way to get omega-3 fatty acids is through diets of at least three fish meals a week. Fish oil or flaxseed oil supplements should be taken only under a physician's supervision.

Although fish oils can be helpful in relieving arthritic symptoms, patients still may need anti-inflammatory medications to adequately control the disease.

Taking any medication during **pregnancy** is not recommended. Women who are pregnant or breast-feeding should talk to their doctor before taking fish oil supplements or any other medications.

Because of their blood thinning activity, aspirin, nonsteroidal anti-inflammatory drugs (NSAIDS), warfarin, or other anti-clotting medications should be used in conjunction with fish oil supplements only after consultation with a physician.

Side effects

Consuming excessive amounts of fish oil capsules can result in excessive bleeding, gastrointestinal distress, **anemia**, or strokes.

KEY TERMS

Essential fatty acid (EFA)—A fatty acid that the body requires but cannot make. It must be obtained from the diet. EFAs include omega-6 fatty acids found in primrose and safflower oils, and omega-3 fatty acids oils found in fatty fish and flaxseed, canola, soybean, and walnuts.

Prostaglandins—A group of hormone-like molecules that exert local effects on a variety of processes including fluid balance, blood flow, and gastrointestinal function. They may be responsible for the production of some types of pain and inflammation.

Interactions

Because of its blood-thinning activity, fish oil supplements may interact with aspirin, nonsteroidal anti-inflammatory drugs (NSAIDS), warfarin, or other anti-clotting medications to cause excessive bleeding.

Resources

BOOKS

Harris, Robert P. *Omega 3 Fatty Acids*. New York: Novinka Books, 2006.

Maisch, B., and R. Oelze, eds. *Cardiovascular Benefits of Omega-3 Polyunsaturated Fatty Acids*. Amsterdam: IOS Press, 2007.

Wexler, Barbara. *Fish Oil, Omega-3 and Essential Fatty Acids*. Chapmanville, WV: Woodland Press, 2007.

PERIODICALS

Freeman, M. P., et al. "Omega-3 Fatty Acids: Evidence Basis for Treatment and Future Research in Psychiatry." *Journal of Clinical Psychiatry* (December 2006): 1954–1967.

Harris, William S. "Omega-3 Fatty Acids and Cardiovascular Disease: A Case for Omega-3 Index as a New Risk Factor." *Pharmacological Research* (March 2007): 217–213.

MacLean, Catherine H, et al. "Effects of Omega-3 Fatty Acids on Cancer Risk: A Systematic Review." *Journal of the American Medical Association* (January 25, 2006): 403–415.

Opthof, T., and H. M. den Ruijter. "Omega-3 Polyunsaturated Fatty Acids (PUFAs or Fish Oils) and Atrial Fibrillation." *British Journal of Pharmacology* (December 2006): 258–260.

Surette, Marc E. "The Science behind Dietary Omega-3 Fatty Acids." *Canadian Medical Association Journal* (January 15, 2008): 177–180.

OTHER

"Essential Fatty Acids." Linus Pauling Institute, December 7, 2005. http://lpi.oregonstate.edu/infocenter/othernuts/omega3fa/. (February 19, 2008).

"Fish and Omega-3 Fatty Acids." American Heart Association. http://www.americanheart.org/presenter.jhtml?identifier=4632. (February 19, 2008).

"Omega-3 Fatty Acids." University of Maryland Medical Center, May 1, 20077. http://www.umm.edu/altmed/articles/omega-3-000316.htm. (February 19, 2008).

"Omega-3 Fatty Acids, Fish Oil, Alpha-linolenic Acid." MayoClinic.com, August 1, 2005. http://www.mayoclinic.com/health/fish-oil/NS_patient-fishoil. (February 19, 2008).

"Omega-3 Fatty Acids, Fish Oil, Alpha-linolenic Acid." MedlinePlus, November 1, 2006. http://www.nlm.nih.gov/medlineplus/druginfo/natural/patient-fishoil.html. (February 19, 2008).

ORGANIZATIONS

American Association of Naturopathic Physicians (AANP), 4435 Wisconsin Ave. NW, Suite 403, Washington, DC, 20016, (866) 538-2267, http://www.naturopathic.org.

DHA/EPA Omega-3 Institute, 150 Research Lane, Rm. 100, University of Guelph Research Park, Guelph, ON, Canada, N1G 4T2, http://www.dhaomega3.org/.

Teresa G. Odle
David Edward Newton, Ed.D.

Sources of Omega 6-Fatty Acids

- Baked goods
- Brazil nuts
- Cereals
- Corn oil
- Cottonseed oil
- Eggs
- Hemp oil
- Meats from grass-fed animals
- Pecans
- Pine nuts
- Pumpkin oil
- Safflower oil
- Sesame oil
- Soybean oil
- Sunflower oil
- Sunflower seeds
- Wheat germ oil
- Whole grains

(Illustration by GGS Information Services. Cengage Learning, Gale)

Omega-6 fatty acids

Description

Omega-6 fatty acids are one of two groups of **essential fatty acids** (EFAs) that are required in human **nutrition**. The other EFA is the omega-3 fatty acid group. The omega-6 fatty acids get their name from the fact that the molecules of which they are made contain a double bond attached to the number 6 carbon atom, counting from the end of the molecule opposite the carboxyl group, the so-called omega end of the molecule. (This system of nomenclature is just the reverse of the one used by chemists.) Omega-6 fatty acids include **linoleic acid** and its derivatives. Chemically, linoleic acid is *cis*, *cis*-9,12-octadecadienoic acid. The term *essential* means that these fatty acids must be consumed in the diet because humans cannot manufacture them from other dietary fats or nutrients, nor can they be stored in the body. They must be consumed daily to meet the body's requirements. They are macronutrients, required in amounts of grams per day (compared to micronutrients such as vitamins, which are required in milligrams per day). EFAs provide energy, are components of nerve cells and cellular membranes, and are converted to hormone-like substances known as prostaglandins.

In the body, prostaglandins and EFAs are necessary for normal physiology, including the following:

- producing steroids and synthesizing hormones
- regulating pressure in the eye, joints, and blood vessels
- mediating immune response
- regulating bodily secretions and their viscosity
- dilating or constricting blood vessels
- regulating collateral circulation
- directing endocrine hormones to their target cells
- regulating smooth muscles and autonomic reflexes
- being primary constituents of cell membranes
- regulating the rate of cell division
- maintaining the fluidity and rigidity of cellular membranes
- regulating the inflow and out-flux of substances into and out of cells
- transporting oxygen from red blood cells to the tissues
- maintaining proper kidney function and fluid balance
- keeping saturated fats mobile in the blood stream
- preventing blood cells from clumping together (conglomeration, which is the cause of atherosclerotic plaque and blood clots which can cause a stroke)
- mediating the release of inflammatory substances from cells that may trigger allergic conditions

- regulating nerve transmission and communication
- being the primary energy source for the heart muscle

Clinical trials have shown that EFAs protect against such conditions as **heart disease**; **cancer**; auto-immune diseases, including **rheumatoid arthritis** and **multiple sclerosis**; skin diseases, including **acne**, atopic **eczema**, and **psoriasis**; and may protect against **stroke**. The prevalence of heart disease in populations has been shown to be inversely proportional to the relative concentration of linoleic acid in the diet.

Both linoleic acid and its derivatives are obtained from plant and animal sources. Plant sources include unprocessed, unheated vegetable oils such as corn, sunflower seed, safflower, soy, sesame, and cottonseed oils. They are also found in plant materials such as evening primrose, black currant seeds, and gooseberry oils as well as in raw nuts and seeds, legumes, and leafy greens. Animal sources of omega-6 fatty acids (although in smaller amounts than in plants) are lean meats, organ meats, and breast milk.

Linoleic acid is an 18-carbon long polyunsaturated fatty acid containing two double bonds. Its first double bond occurs at the sixth carbon from the omega end, classifying it as omega-6 oil. As linoleic acid is absorbed and metabolized in the human body, it is converted into a derivative fatty acid, gamma linoleic acid (GLA), which is converted into di-homo-gamma linoleic acid (DGLA) and arachidonic acid (AA). The DGLA and AA are then converted into two types of prostaglandins by adding two carbon molecules and removing hydrogen molecules. There are three families of prostaglandins, PGE1, PGE2, and PGE3. DGLA is converted to PGE1, while AA is converted into PGE2. PGE3 is made by the conversion of **omega-3 fatty acids**. Both PGE1 and PGE3, anti-inflammatory agents, protect against coronary disease by keeping blood platelets slippery and flowing, thus preventing blood clotting. PGE2 has inflammatory effects and increases platelet stickiness and blood clotting. All three forms of prostaglandin must be present to ensure a functioning clotting system. There must be enough PGE2 to ensure healthy clotting, but enough PGE1 and PGE3 to protect against too much clotting, which can lead to hardening of the arteries, **heart attack**, and stroke. Likewise, PGE1 appears to act as a diuretic, whereas PGE2 aids in the retention of water and salts in the kidneys. PGE2 also is required for healthy brain and synapse functioning. The three types of prostaglandins serve as a system of checks and balances within the body.

However, if AA and its derivative, PGE2, are over-produced or imbalanced with PGE1 and PGE3, they can cause illness or disease. The over-consumption of land-based meats and the under-consumption of cold-water fish and unprocessed oils can lead to an over-production of inflammation-producing PGE2 and an under-production of anti-inflammatory agents PGE1 and PGE3. A healthy diet includes omega-6 fatty acids in a balance with omega-3 fatty acids. An optimal ratio is four parts omega-6 to one part omega-3. Ratios of healthy populations range from 2.5:1 in Inuit **diets** to 6:1 in other traditional diets.

Daily consumption of omega-6 fatty acids by many people may be excessive, due to the presence of omega-6 fatty acids in common cooking vegetable oils and processed foods. The ratio of omega-6 to omega-3 fatty acid consumption can reach 20:1. Achieve a more desirable ratio requires eliminating sources of omega-6 fatty acids, especially those hidden in processed foods, and increasing the amount of omega-3 fatty acids consumed through **fish oil** or **flaxseed** supplements. In addition, converting omega-6 fatty acids present in oils (such as corn, safflower, or soybean) to GLA requires that the oils be unprocessed and unheated and in the natural form (*cis* form). When oils undergo processing (heating and/or hydrogenation) to prolong shelf life or to form a solid at room temperature (e.g., shortening and margarine), the fatty acid structure is changed to the *trans* form, and the conversion process of omega-6 fatty acids to GLA may be inhibited.

General use

Most people receive sufficient amounts of omega-6 fatty acids in their diet. Deficiencies are rare and limited to people with severe malabsorption, short bowel syndrome, or extremely low-fat diets. For those who are unable to convert LA to GLA, dietary supplements containing GLA can be taken to increase the production of prostaglandins. Evening primrose, black currant, and **borage oil** all contain GLA. For individuals with diabetes, GLA supplementation can improve nerve function and help prevent diabetic nerve disease. Long-term exclusive or excessive use of flaxseed oil, which contains large amounts of omega-3 fatty acids, can result in omega-6 fatty acid deficiency and require the addition of oils containing omega-6 fatty acids to the diet.

Preparations

Omega-6 fatty acids may be consumed either as linoleic acid in oils that contain high levels of linoleic acid or in the converted form, GLA, in dietary supplements. Oils high in linoleic acid include soybean, peanut, corn, sunflower seed, cottonseed, soy, sesame,

KEY TERMS

Age-related macular degeneration (ARMD)— Degeneration of the macula (the central part of the retina where the rods and cones are most dense) that leads to loss of central vision in people over 60.

Atopic eczema—Inflammation of the skin caused by allergic reaction.

Multiple sclerosis (MS)—A progressive, autoimmune disease of the central nervous system characterized by damage to the myelin sheath that covers nerves. In most types, the disease, which causes progressive paralysis, is marked by periods of exacerbation and remission.

Omega-6 fatty acid—A fatty acid with its first double bond at the sixth carbon in its carbon chain.

and safflower. There is no official recommended daily dose for omega-6 fatty acids. The Food and Nutrition Board of the U.S. Department of Agriculture has, however, established recommended daily intakes of linoleic acid based on age and sex. Recommendations for pregnant and lactating women are also available. For males over the age of 19, the recommendation is for 17 grams per day; for females over the age of 19, the recommended intake is 11–12 grams per day, depending on age. Younger children, pregnant women, and women who are lactating generally need somewhat less linoleic acid than these levels.

For GLA supplementation, primrose oil, borage oil, and **black currant seed oil** are available in capsule form.

Precautions

Stress, alcohol consumption, and prescription medicines can interfere with the conversion of linoleic acid to its derivatives. Therefore, those with such conditions may benefit from the use of GLA supplementation to improve the production of prostaglandins. In addition, the use of unprocessed, unheated omega-6 oils in the cis form is recommended for improving prostaglandin production.

Side effects

Overconsumption of omega-6 oils in relation to consumption of omega-3 oils may lead to an overproduction of inflammation-producing prostaglandins (PGE2s) and a scarcity of anti-inflammatory prostaglandins (PGE1s and PGE2s), which may lead to a variety of health problems.

Linoleic acid appears to have at least one negative effect on the human body. It appears to increase a person's risk of developing age-related **macular degeneration** (ARMD), a disease of the eye that causes progressive loss of vision and eventual blindness.

Interactions

Nutrients essential for the use of omega-6 fatty acids in the body include **magnesium**, **selenium**, **zinc**, and vitamins A, carotene, B_3, B_6, C, and E.

Resources

BOOKS

Wexler, Barbara. *Fish Oil, Omega-3 and Essential Fatty Acids.* Chapmanville, WV: Woodland Press, 2007.

PERIODICALS

Conklin, S. M., et al. "High Omega-6 and Low Omega-3 Fatty Acids Are Associated with Depressive Symptoms and Neuroticism." *Psychosomatic Medicine* (November 2007): 932–934.

Kiecolt-Glaser J. K,, et al. "Depressive Symptoms, Omega-6; Omega-3 Fatty Acids, and Inflammation in Older Adults." *Psychosomatic Medicine* (April 2007): 217–214.

Lauretani, F., et al. "Omega-6 and Omega-3 Fatty Acids Predict Accelerated Decline of Peripheral Nerve Function in Older Persons." *European Journal of Neurology* (September 2007): 801–808.

Rashid, S., et al. "Topical Omega-3 and Omega-6 Fatty Acids for Treatment of Dry Eye." *Archives of Ophthalmology* (February 2008): 219–225.

Simopoulos, A. P. "Evolutionary Aspects of Diet, the Omega-6/Omega-3 Ratio and Genetic Variation: Nutritional Implications for Chronic Diseases." *Biomedicine and Pharmacotherapy* (August 2006): 502–507.

Judith Sims
Rebecca J. Frey, PhD
David Edward Newton, Ed.D.

Onion *see* **Allium cepa**

Ophiopogon

Description

Ophiopogon is a perennial herbaceous plant that is native to the Orient. Under the name *mai men dong*, its tuberous root is a highly prized and indispensable part of Chinese herbal medicine. In addition, this

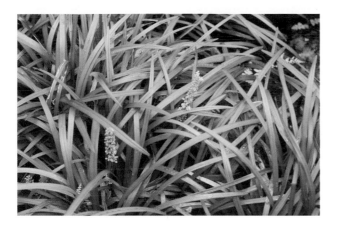

Ophiopogon. *(© Organica / Alamy)*

plant's graceful, grass-like leaves and tiny bell-shaped flowers have made it a popular landscaping ground cover. It is commonly known in the Western world as lily-turf or *Liriope spicata*, and is a member of the lily, or Liliaceac, family.

The tufted mounds that ophiopogon forms are usually about 1 ft (30cm) in height and diameter. On closer examination, the individual leaves of the plant resemble straps 0.25 in (0.6 cm) to almost 2 in (5 cm) in width and up to 16 in long (40.6 cm), depending upon the species. Ophiopogon leaves are evergreen and have a leathery appearance. *Ophiopogon japonicus* , the species most used in Oriental herbal medicine, has leaves with serrated edges. Subspecies of ophiopogon include several with a great variety of ornamental leaves, ranging from all-green to green with white, cream-colored or golden edges. The more decorative ophiopogon plants, such as *Liriope muscari* (blue lily-turf) or Christmas tree lily-turf, have larger **lavender**, blue-violet, or white bell-shaped flowers in clusters growing from upward-reaching spikes 4–6 in (approximately 10–15 cm) high. The flowers appear in mid-summer, and are followed by shining blackberry-like seeds that remain throughout the winter.

Ophiopogon grows best in warm climates, but is remarkably adaptable. There are species of this plant that grow and thrive in either full sun or full shade. Ophiopogon is able to tolerate a very wide variety of adverse conditions, including extreme heat, soil that is dry even to the point of drought, or high humidity. There are both erect and creeping types of ophiopogon. *Liriope spicata*, also known as *Ophiopogon japonicus*, is a creeping variety with fast spreading, slender tuberous roots that can prove to be quite invasive. It forms a rhizome with smaller fibrous roots growing outward; the tuber itself has a bittersweet taste.

Ophiopogon japonicus is also better able to tolerate cold than other varieties. All types of ophiopogon are propagated by division.

General use

Ophiopogon japonicus has long been used in Oriental herbal medicine. The earliest reference to its use is in the *Shennong Bencao Jing*, or *Herbal Classic of the Divine Plowman*. The oldest known edition of this classic was printed around A.D. 300. Ophiopogon is thought to be effective in clearing away what Chinese medical practitioners call "heat in the heart" and irritability. Ophiopogon is an antiseptic that is particularly useful in the healing of mouth sores. Its sedative qualities provide relief for **insomnia**, heart palpitations, **anxiety**, and restlessness. It is similar to the many chemical sedatives used in Western medicine in that it reduces muscle spasm.

Ophiopogon also moistens the mucous membranes of the body by stimulating the production of mucosal fluids. Moisturizing of the lungs reduces coughing. In the intestines, increasing the level of moisture improves elimination. Because of these qualities, ophiopogon is used in formulas to treat **constipation**, dry throat, and chronic dry bronchitis. Because ophiopogon has been shown to lower blood sugar and regenerates necessary cells in the pancreatic isles of Langerhans, it is also considered useful in treating the fluid imbalance caused by diabetes, as evidenced by excessive thirst and urination.

According to the United States Department of Agriculture phytochemical database developed at the Beltsville Agricultural Research Center in Maryland, the following varieties of ophiopogon all have medicinal uses:

- *Ophiopogon japonicus* is the species of this plant most commonly used in Oriental herbal medicine. It is useful in treating intestinal, kidney, and liver problems. It has been found to stimulate the production of milk in nursing mothers and to reduce inflammation. It has cough suppressing properties, and is used in treating nearly all lung-related illnesses, including bronchitis, whooping cough, tuberculosis, hemoptysis (coughing up blood), sore throat, laryngitis , and cough. A chemical present in the plant has shown effectiveness in the treatment of lung tumors. It is also used to treat fever, constipation, and stomach problems.

- *Ophiopogon ohwii* is used for its cough suppressant qualities. It is also an expectorant, a cardiac tonic, and an anti-inflammatory agent.

KEY TERMS

Aphrodisiac—A substance thought to stimulate erotic desire and enhance sexual performance. Aphrodisiacs are named for Aphrodite, the ancient Greek goddess of love.

Cardiac tonic—Any of a diverse group of remedies intended to relieve heart symptoms. Most tonics contain herbal extracts, vitamins, and minerals.

Diuretic—A group of medications that increase the amount of urine produced and relieve excess fluid buildup in body tissues. Diuretics may be used in treating high blood pressure, lung disease, premenstrual syndrome, and other conditions.

Galactogogue—A substance or medication that increases the flow of breast milk in nursing mothers.

Isles of Langerhans—Cellular masses of tissue in a space within the pancreas that secrete insulin.

Rhizome—The fleshy underground horizontal root of certain plants. Valerian preparations are made from dried rhizomes as well as from roots of the valerian plant.

Tuber—The thick, fleshy, underground stem of a plant.

- *Ophiopogon pendulus* has diuretic properties that are useful in reducing fluid retention in the body caused by either heart or kidney disease.
- *Ophiopogon spicatus* is considered an aphrodisiac, a treatment for digestive disturbance, and a galactogogue, or stimulator of lactation in nursing mothers.

Preparations

The slender, tuberous roots of ophiopogon are dug in summer, and the smaller, more fibrous roots are cut away. The rhizomes are dried in the sun, then pulverized and stored in a cool place in an airtight container. The usual daily dosage in Chinese herbal medicine is 4–10 g, when the plant is used in an infusion or decoction.

Precautions

It is important to remember that Chinese herbal medicine is based upon individual prescriptions developed for each patient and his or her unique symptoms. Chinese herbs should not be taken either individually or in combination formulas unless a practitioner of Chinese herbal medicine has been consulted.

It should also be remembered that coughing is a normal and helpful bodily reaction to irritation of the airway or lungs. It is designed to expel such harmful substances as excess phlegm or irritants from the lungs. **Cough** suppression can actually prevent or postpone recovery. It is persistent coughing that needs treatment. Moreover, a cough is merely a symptom of some other bodily illness, as are digestive problems. Therefore, ophiopogon preparations should not be taken for an extended period of time, and then only for dry, ticklish coughs. These preparations should only be used for temporary relief of symptoms. If the patient is bringing up a lot of phlegm, ophiopogon will make the cough worse. A physician should be consulted for persistent cough or gastrointestinal problems.

Side effects

Ophiopogon does not appear to produce serious side effects when used as directed.

Resources

BOOKS

Molony, David, and Ming Ming Pan Molony. *The American Association of Oriental Medicine's Complete Guide to Chinese Herbal Medicine.* New York: Berkley Publishing, 1999.

Phillips, Ellen, and C. Colston Burrell. *Rodale's Illustrated Encyclopedia of Perennials.* Emmaus, PA: Rodale Press, Inc., 1993.

OTHER

Michigan State University Extension Service. "*Ophiopogon Japonicus*—Dwarf Mondo Grass." http://www.msuo phiopogon.htm.

Joan Schonbeck

Opuntia *see* **Prickly pear cactus**
Oral herpes *see* **Cold sores**

Oregano essential oil

Description

Oregano (*origanum vulgare*)is a member of the Labiatae family (commonly referred to as the mint family). Its name is from the Greek word oreganos, which loosely translated means "joy of the mountains."

Native to Mediterranean regions, such as Greece and Crete, oregano is a perennial plant with an aromatic scent. With flowers that bloom from July to September, the plant is generally 2.5ft (75 cm) high

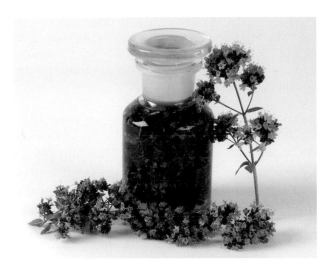

Oregano and oregano essential oil. (© *Arco Images / Alamy*)

and 2–3 ft (60–90 cm) wide. Its hairy, oval-shaped leaves are approximately 1.5 in (3.75 cm) in diameter and grow opposite of one another.

Oregano essential oil is produced from the oregano plant through the process of steam distillation. There are a variety of species referred to as oregano, but only a few qualify as high grade and are suitable for making oregano essential oil.

Oregano essential oil contains the following components:

- carvacrol (share 40–70%)
- gamma-terpinene (8–10%)
- p-cymene (5–10%)
- alpha-pinene
- myrcene
- thymol
- flavonoids
- caffeic acid derivatives

It should be noted that the *Physicians' Desk Reference for Herbal Medicines, Second Edition* also points out that there are various chemotypes with differing essential oil composition of thymol, linalool + terpinene-4-ol, linalool, caryophyllene + germacren D, or germacren D as chief components. However, those **strains**, especially ones high in thymol, are not suitable for preparing oregano essential oil intended for internal consumption. Some of these **essential oils** are toxic to the liver and kidney in very small quantities. However prudent, short term, topical use of these variants may be safe.

General use

Historically, Greek physicians used oregano essential oils for **wounds**, headaches, and venomous **bites** and even hemlock poisoning. It wasn't long before its medicinal benefits were used to treat lung conditions, **bronchitis**, sinusitis, and cold symptoms including **cough**. During the seventeenth century, it was heralded throughout Great Britain as an effective remedy for head colds. Used by physicians to induce **menstruation** as early as the nineteenth century, the benefits of using oregano essential oil have captured the interest of modern-day researchers.

Today, oregano essential oil has antiviral, antibacterial, antifungal, antiparasitic, and antiseptic properties. For external use, oregano essential oil is valued as a strong analgesic and antirheumatic agent. The diluted oil (usually 5 drops essential oil to 25 drops of carrier oil, like jojoba) can even be rubbed on a **toothache** to relieve **pain**. The oil is also believed to reduce the discomfort associated with insect bites. Its powerful antimicrobial properties are said to assist in the prevention of **infections** and to treat skin fungi such as **athlete's foot**. It has also been used to eliminate lice infestations and intestinal **worms**.

Oregano as a culinary spice became popular in the United States after World War II when the soldiers returned from Italy having developed a taste for pizza spiced with oregano. The problem is that medicinally speaking not all oregano is created equal. Growing conditions (soil, climate, rainfall, altitude) and harvesting and processing can produce variations in constituents and effects.

Having penned over ten books, Dr. Cass Ingram who is considered an expert on oregano essential oil, further explains the seriousness of mislabeled oregano oil in his book *The Cure is in the Cupboard*. He states that although many companies list products such as wild oregano or oil of oregano in their catalogues, "the problem is that the commercially available oil is almost exclusively **thyme** oil or marjoram oil," neither of which possesses the same medicinal properties as true oregano essential oil. Furthermore, Ingram states that thyme oil is usually made from a non-oregano plant, such as *Thymus capitus* from Spain, and even though it comes from an edible herb, thyme oil may be toxic. James A. Duke, Ph.D., a leading authority on healing herbs, agrees that thyme oil can be toxic; using it can lead to serious side effects and, in some cases, even cause death.

Therefore, it is critical when using oregano essential oil to be sure that its primary component is carvacrol and not thymol. As Ingram states, "true oregano grows only under specific soil and climate conditions and cannot be reproduced in your backyard." Oregano essential oil should be made only from high-grade oregano that grows wild in the mountains of the Mediterranean. Ingram provides seven key factors to consider when determining if the oil has been derived from a high-grade oregano plant. He suggests that it should be: 1) a wild spice, not farm-raised, 2) from a proven edible species of oregano, 3) a species high in carvacrol, 4) a type used in modern research at prestigious institutions such as Georgetown University, 5) extracted in a natural process (steam distilled), 6) free of all chemical residues, and 7) relatively low in thymol (less than 5%).

Provided that the oregano essential oil being used is authentic and high grade, there is a great deal of scientific evidence to support its medicinal properties. Indeed, several studies have shown that oregano essential oil can inhibit or destroy many strains of bacteria, fungi, and parasites.

One ambiguous study, published in the *Journal of Applied Microbiology* in 1999, compared 52 plant oils and extracts. Oregano essential oil was found to have significant antibacterial action against a wide number of bacteria including E coli, Staph, Salmonella enterica, and Klebsiella pneumonie, which is a **pneumonia** that frequently occurs in people with a weakened immune system. The following year, the *Journal of Applied Microbiology* published a study by Scottish researchers that showed oregano essential oil to be effective against 25 different bacteria. Other studies, such as the one done by researchers at the University of Tennessee in 2001, also showed oregano essential oil to have powerful antibacterial properties.

Research published in the *International Journal of Food Microbiology* in 1988 found oil of oregano to be an excellent antifungal, completely inhibiting the growth of the nine fungi tested. Since that time, numerous research studies have been published that repeatedly show the ability of oregano essential oil to kill yeast, including Candida albicans. In 2002, oregano essential oil was put to the test in an interesting study by researchers in Yugoslavia and the results were published in *Nahrung*. Among the 13 fungi tested were **food poisoning**, plant, animal, and human pathogenic species. Oregano essential oil high in carvacrol possessed the best and broadest antifungal properties.

A small clinical trial published in 2000 examined the effects of oregano oil in adults with intestinal parasites. Of the 14 adult participants, 11 tested positive for the intestinal parasite, Blastocystis hominis, which is known to cause **diarrhea**, anal **itching**, and weight loss. The 11 test-positive participants took 600 mg of emulsified oregano essential oil daily for six weeks. Eight were completely free of the parasite and the remaining three participants had a reduction in parasitic presence and symptoms.

Preparations

Oregano essential oil should never be used undiluted. Always dilute it in a suitable carrier oil, such as olive oil, almond oil, or v-6 mixing oil. As with any product used for medicinal purposes, it is important to read and follow the label instructions and warnings.

A skin patch test should be conducted prior to using oregano essential oil for the first time. To do this, place a small amount of diluted essential oil on the inside of your elbow and apply a bandage. Wait 24 hours to see if there is any negative reaction, such as redness or irritation, before proceeding with more extensive use

Because oregano essential oil is concentrated, a little bit goes a long way. At first, it may be wise to start out cautiously by using only 1 drop of oregano essential oil to 3 parts olive oil and massage into the affected area once or twice a day.

To topically treat **fungal infections** on the skin and nails, Dr. Jennifer Brett, a naturopathic physician and chair of the **botanical medicine** department at the University of Bridgeport College of **Naturopathic Medicine** in Connecticut suggests the following: Dilute 1 teaspoon oregano essential oil in 2 teaspoons olive oil and apply with a cotton swab to the affected area up to three times a day.

To treat bacterial and fungal infections in other parts of the body, 1 drop of oil may be placed in an 8-ounce glass of water or juice once or twice a day. One drop may also be placed under the tongue twice a day, but it should be mixed with 1 teaspoon of honey, maple syrup, or olive oil.

For use in the bath, mix 1 to 3 drops of diluted oregano essential oil with body gel or shampoo and add it to the bath water. As an antiseptic, the diluted oil can be used in cloths to wipe down kitchen and bathroom countertops.

Precautions

Do not use oregano essential oil, either topically or internally, while pregnant.

Nursing mothers should avoid applying the oil to their nipples, because it can be difficult to wash off and may be ingested inadvertently by their infants. During the weaning process, nursing mothers wishing to use a breast massage oil that contains oregano essential oil as a method to reduce milk production should do so with caution and be sure that all the oil is removed before breastfeeding. Because of safety issues regarding breast milk and infant care, nursing mothers should always obtain the approval of an obstetrician and/or pediatrician before using oregano essential oil either topically or internally.

Topically, oregano essential oil may be irritating to the skin, especially mucous membranes, and can cause burning. Therefore, it should always be suitably diluted, and according to Tisserand and Balacs, never applied topically to mucous membranes in concentrations greater than 1%. They also caution that people with damaged or very sensitive skin as well as children less than two years of age should not use the oil.

Special care should be taken when using oregano essential oil internally, because many of the commercially available products are erroneously labeled and are not made from high grade oregano. In fact, many contain dangerous levels of thymol. Some experts caution that oregano essential oil should never be taken internally, while others suggest that it is safe for internal use provided that it is suitably diluted and its source and contents are verified; it must be extracted from high grade oregano and meet seven strict requirements.

Internal use (swallowed or as a rectal suppository) should be highly restricted (ie, a few drops only of the pure essential oil per dose, and limiting duration of use to a few days to weeks) This is because essential oils represent highly concentrated extracts through distillation compared to the whole crude plant (essential oils have 100's of times more essential oil per drop due to purification, than does fresh or dried oregano herb) And although therapeutic in small, short term doses, these oils are toxic to liver, kidneys and the nervous system if taken in excess.

Always be sure to use true oregano essential oil (containing less than 5% thymol) and not thymol oil, which should never be taken internally and used topically only with extreme caution after being diluted in a suitable carrier oil.

People with any medical condition should use oregano essential oil only after consulting with a physician.

Side effects

The use of oregano essential oil can cause skin irritation, redness, and burning. If any of these negative side effects occur, discontinue use immediately.

When used either topically or internally to treat thrush, it has the potential to decrease a nursing mother's milk supply.

In low doses over a short period of time, oregano essential oil is considered generally safe. However, high doses may be toxic to the liver.

Interactions

In general, essential oils tend to be photosensitive. To avoid this interaction, stay away from direct sunlight or sun beds after applying oregano essential oil to prevent skin burn.

Do not apply oregano essential oil after perspiring; the combination of the oil and sweat could cause irritation.

Resources

BOOKS

Barnes J., L. A. Anderson, and J. D. Phillipson. *Herbal Medicines: A guide for Healthcare Professionals, second edition.* Pharmaceutical Press, 2002.

Brinker, F. *Herb Contraindications and Drug Interactions, second edition.* Eclectic Medical Publishers, 1998.

Duke, J. A. *Handbook of Medicinal Herbs.* CRC Press, 2001.

Fleming, T. (ed.). *Physicians' Desk Reference for Herbal Medicines.* Medical Economics Company, Inc., 2000.

Ingram, C. *The Cure is in the Cupboard.* Knowledge House, 1997.

Keville, K. *Herbs: An Illustrated Encyclopedia. A Complete Culinary, Cosmetic, Medicinal, and Ornamental Guide.* Friedman/Fairfax Publishers, 1999.

Rosengarten, F. *The Book of Spices.* Jove Books, 1973.

Tisserand, R. *Essential Oil Safety.* Churchill Livingston, 1995.

PERIODICALS

Dorman H. J., S. G. Deans. "Antimicrobial agents from plants: antibacterial activity of plant volatile oils." *Journal of Applied Microbiology* (February, 2000): 308-316.

Elgayyar M., F. A. Draughon, D. A. Golden, J. R. Mount. "Antimicrobial activity of essential oils from plants against selected pathogenic and saprophytic microorganisms." *Journal of Food Protection* (July, 2001): 1019–1024.

Force, M., W. S. Sparks, R. A. Ronzio. "Inhibition of enteric parasites by emulsified oil of oregano in vivo." *Phytotherapy Research* (May 2000): 213–214.

Hammer, K. A., C. F. Carson, T. V. Riley. "Antimicrobial activity of essential oils and other plant extracts." *Journal of Applied Microbiology* (June, 1999): 985–990.

Sokovic M., O. Tzakou, D. Pitarokili, M. Couladis. "Antifungal activities of selected aromatic plants growing wild in Greece." *Nahrung* (October, 2002): 317–320.

Lee Ann Paradise

Organic food

Definition

Organic foods are not specific foods, but are any foods that are grown and handled after harvesting in a particular way. In the United States, organic foods are crops that are raised without using synthetic pesticides, synthetic fertilizers, or sewage sludge fertilizer, and they have not been altered by genetic engineering. Organic animal products come from animals that have been fed 100% organic feed and raised without the use of growth hormones or antibiotics in an environment where they have access to the outdoors. Standards for organic foods vary from country to country. The requirements in Canada and Western Europe are similar to those in the United States. Many developing countries have no standards for certifying food as "organic."

Purpose

The organic food movement has the following goals:

- improve human health by decreasing the level of chemical toxins in food

- decrease the level of agricultural chemicals in the environment, especially in groundwater

- promote sustainable agriculture

- promote biodiversity

- promote genetic diversity among plants and animals by rejecting genetically modified organisms (GMOs)

- provide fresh, healthy, safe food at competitive prices

Pesticides in fruits and vegetables

Highest level	Lowest level
Peaches	Onions
Apples	Avocados
Sweet bell peppers	Corn, sweet, frozen
Celery	Pineapples
Nectarines	Mango
Strawberries	Peas, sweet, frozen
Cherries	Kiwi
Pears	Bananas
Grapes, imported	Cabbage
Spinach	Broccoli
Lettuce	Papaya
Potatoes	Blueberries

SOURCE: Developed by the Environmental Working Group

(Illustration by GGS Information Services. Cengage Learning, Gale)

Description

Organic farming is the oldest method of farming. Before the 1940s, what is today called organic farming was the standard method of raising crops and animals. World War II accelerated research into new chemicals that could be used either in fighting the war or as replacements for resources that were in short supply because of their usefulness to the military. After the war ended, many of the new technological discoveries were applied to civilian uses and synthetic fertilizers, new insecticides, and herbicides became available. Fertilizers increased the yield per acre and pesticides encouraged the development of single-crop mega-farms, resulting in the consolidation of agricultural land and the decline of the family farm.

Organic farming, although only a tiny part of American agriculture, originally offered a niche market for smaller, family-style farms. In the early 1980s this method of food production began to gain popularity, especially in California, Oregon, and Washington. The first commercial organic crops were vegetables that were usually sold locally at farmers' markets and health food stores.

By the late 1980s interest in organic food had reached a level of public awareness high enough that the United States Congress took action and passed the Organic Food Production Act of 1990. This act established the National Organic Standards Board (NOSB) under the United States Department of Agriculture (USDA). NOSB has developed regulations and enforcement procedures for the growing and handling of all agricultural products that are labeled "organic." These regulations went into effect on October 21, 2002.

Since the 1990s, the market for organic food has expanded from primarily fruits and vegetables to eggs, dairy products, meat, poultry, and commercially processed frozen and canned foods. In 2000, for the first time, more organic food was purchased in mainstream supermarkets than in specialty food outlets. By 2005, every state had some farmland that was certified organic, and some supermarket chains had begun selling their own brand-name organic foods. The demand for organic food is expected to continue to grow rapidly through at least 2010.

Organic certification is voluntary and applies to anyone who sells more than $5,000 worth of organic produce annually. (This exempts most small farmers who sell organic produce from their own farm stands). If a product carries the USDA Organic Seal indicating that it is "certified organic" it must meet the following conditions:

- The product must be raised or produced under an Organic Systems Plan that demonstrates and documents that the food meets the standards for growing, harvesting, transporting, processing, and selling an organic product.
- The producer and/or processor are subject to audits and evaluations by agents certified to enforce organic standards.
- The grower must have distinct boundaries between organic crops and non-organic crops to prevent accidental contamination with forbidden substances through wind drift or water runoff.
- No forbidden substances can have been applied to the land organic food is raised on for three years prior to organic certification.
- Seed should be organic, when available, and never genetically altered through bioengineering.
- Good soil, crop, and animal management practices must be followed to prevent contamination of groundwater, contamination of the product by living pathogens, heavy metals, or forbidden chemicals, and to reduce soil erosion and environmental pollution.

To meet these requirements, organic farmers use natural fertilizers such as composted manure to add nutrients to the soil. They control pests by crop rotation and interplanting. Interplanting is growing several different species of plants in an alternating pattern in the same field to slow the spread of disease. Pest control is also achieved by using natural insect predators, traps, and physical barriers. If these methods do not control pests, organic farmers may apply certain non-synthetic pesticides made from substances that occur naturally in plants. Weed control is achieved by mulching, hand or mechanical weeding, the use of cover crops, and selective burning.

Animals products that are USDA certified organic must come from animals that are fed only organic feed, are not given growth hormones, antibiotics, or other drugs for the purpose of preventing disease, and have access to the outdoors. This last requirement is rather vague, as regulations set neither a minimum amount of time the animal must spend outdoors nor any minimums concerning the amount of outdoor space available per animal.

Selecting organic food

The USDA allows three label statements to help consumers determine if a food is organic.

- Labels stating "100% organic" indicate that all of the ingredients in the product are certified organic. These items have the USDA Organic Seal on the label.
- Labels stating "organic" indicate that at least 95% of the ingredients are certified organic. These items also carry the USDA Organic Seal on the label.
- Labels stating "made with organic ingredients" indicate that at least 70% of the ingredients are certified organic. These items are not permitted to have the USDA Organic Seal on the label.
- Items that contain fewer than 70% organic ingredients are not permitted to use either the word "organic" or the USDA Organic Seal on the label.

Consumers may be bewildered by other words on food labels such as "natural" or "grass-fed" that may be confused with organic. Natural and organic are not interchangeable. "Natural" foods are minimally processed foods but, they are not necessarily grown or raised under the strict conditions of organic foods. "Grass-fed" indicates that the livestock were fed natural forage ("grass"), but not necessarily in open pasture or for their entire lives.

Debate continues about the exact requirements to label animal products "cage-free," "free-range," or "open pasture." Cage-free simply means the animals were not kept caged, but does not necessarily mean that they were raised outdoors or allowed to roam freely. There is no certification process for the designation "cage-free." Animals can spend as little as five minutes per day outdoors and still be considered "free-range." Animal rights organizations are working to clarify these designations and improve the conditions under which all animals, are raised.

Organic food and health

Certified organic food requires more labor to produce, which generally makes it more expensive than non-certified food. Some consumers buy organic food primarily because the way it is raised benefits the environment. Others believe absolutely in the health benefits of organic food. A larger group of consumers are uncertain if organic food offers enough health benefits to justify the additional cost.

Discussions of the health benefits of organic food can become quite heated and emotional. Advocates of buying organic foods firmly believe that they are preserving their health by preventing their bodies from becoming receptacles for poisonous chemicals that can cause **cancer**, **asthma**, and other chronic diseases. Non-organic food buyers take the position that the level pesticide and fertilizer residue in non-organic food is small and harmless. Neither side is likely to change the other's view. However, below are some conclusions from studies done comparing organic and non-organic foods.

- The food supply in the United States, whether organic or non-organic, is extremely safe.
- Fresh organic and non-organic produce are equally likely to become contaminated with pathogens such as *E. coli* that cause health concerns.
- Many, but not all, chemical contaminants can be removed from non-organic food by peeling or thorough washing in cool running water.
- Organic foods are not 100% pesticide and chemical free. However, their chemical load appears to be lower than that of non-organic foods.
- The nutrient value of identical organic and non-organic foods is the same.
- The long-term effect on humans of trace amounts of hormones, antibiotics, and drugs found in milk, meat, and other non-organic animal products is unclear.
- The long-term effect of genetically modified foods on both humans and the environment cannot yet be known.

Precautions

Individuals should be informed about food labeling requirements and read food labels carefully so that they can make informed decisions about their purchases.

Interactions

Organic food does not interact with drugs or other foods in a way that is different from non-organic foods.

Complications

No complications are expected from eating organic food.

Parental concerns

Chemicals found in foods may have a greater effect on the growth and development of younger children than older ones. Young children are rapidly growing while still developing their nervous system, immune system, and other organs. Chemicals may have a greater effect on these developing tissues than on adult tissues.

Resources

BOOKS

Fromartz, Samuel. *Organic, Inc.: Natural Foods and How They Grew*. Orlando, FL: Harcourt, 2006.

Goodman, Myra, with Linday Holland, and Pamela McKinstry, Pamela. *Food to Live By: The Earthbound Farm Organic Cookbook* New York: Workman Pub., 2006.

Lipson, Elaine. *The Organic Foods Sourcebook*. Chicago, IL: Contemporary Books, 2001.

Meyerowitz, Steve. *The Organic Food Guide: How to Shop Smarter and Eat Healthier* Guilford, CT: Globe Pequot Press, 2004.

OTHER

Barrett, Stephen. "'Organic' Foods: Certification Does Not Protect Consumers." Quackwatch, July 17, 2006. http://www.quackwatch.org/01Quackery Related Topics/organic.html.

Mayo Clinic Staff. "Organic Foods: Are They Safer? More Nutritious?" MayoClinic.com, December 26, 2006. http://www.mayoclinic.com/health/organic-food/NU00255.

National Organic Program. "Organic Food Standards &Labels: The Facts." United States Department of Agriculture, Agricultural Marketing Service, January 2007. http://www.ams.usda.gov/nop/Consumers/brochure.html

Nemours Foundation. "Organic and Other Environmentally Friendly Foods." March 2007. http://kidshealth.org/teen/food_fitness/nutrition/organics.html.

"Organic Foods in Relation to Nutrition and Health Key Facts." Medical News Today. July 11, 2004. http://www.medicalnewstoday.com/medicalnews.php?newsid=10587

Organic Trade Association. "Questions and Answers About Organic." 2003. http://www.ota.com/organic/faq.html

Pames, Robin B. "How Organic Food Works." How Stuff Works, undated, accessed April 26, 2007. http://home.howstuffworks.com/organic-food.htm

ORGANIZATIONS

National Organic Program, USDA-AMS-TM-NOP, ROOM 4008 s. Bldg, Ag Stop 0268, 1400 Independence Avenue, S.W., Room 1180, Washington, DC, 20250, (202)720-3252, http://www.ams.usda.gov/nop.

Organic Trade Association, PO Box 547, Greenfield, MA, 01302, (413) 774-7511, (413) 774-6432, http://www.ota.com.

Helen M. Davidson

Oriental Ginseng, *Panax ginseng see* **Ginseng, Korean**

Ornish diet

Definition

The Ornish diet was developed by Dean Ornish, M.D. Ornish was the first physician to demonstrate that **heart disease** can be reversed by natural methods, including specific dietary and lifestyle changes.

Origins

Dean Ornish, who was born in 1953, was a professor of clinical medicine at the University of California, San Francisco, and a practicing physician as of 2008. He received his Bachelor of Arts degree from the University of Texas, Austin, then attended Baylor College of Medicine and Harvard Medical School. He received further medical training at Massachusetts General Hospital. He is the founder and president of the Preventive Medicine Research Institute located in Sausalito, California.

While Ornish was a medical student he became interested in heart disease. In 1978 he began doing research on patients with coronary artery disease (a common form of heart disease). He created a diet that was very low in fat and completely vegetarian and studied its effects on the symptoms experienced by these patients. The patients also learned a variety of **stress** reduction techniques. He discovered that for many patients this diet caused a significant lessening of their symptoms. This was the beginning of his research on the effects of low fat, low or no-meat **diets** on weight loss, health, and heart disease.

It took Dr. Ornish several published studies before conventional medicine accepted his position that simple and inexpensive treatments, including diet, **exercise**, and stress reduction, could reverse heart disease. In a study begun in 1980, Ornish studied 48 people with severe heart disease. Half of them were assigned to a control group and were treated by conventional methods, while the other half participated for three weeks in Ornish's program of an ultra-low fat diet, **yoga**, **meditation**, social support groups, and no cigarettes. The diet that Ornish designed was similar to the regimen developed in the 1970s by Nathan Pritikin to combat heart disease, which continued to be used as of 2008 in several clinics. Both diets emphasize foods that are very low in fat and yet filling, including high-fiber grains and legumes (beans and peas).

Over the course of the study, Ornish's group experienced improvement in symptoms and significant drops in **cholesterol** and blood pressure. Dr. Ornish published the results in the prestigious *Journal of the American Medical Association*, and his study generated controversy. To convince his critics, Dr. Ornish set up a long-term controlled study. After one year, patients treated with Dr. Ornish's methods showed convincing results: 82% of them had significantly less blockage in their heart arteries and there was a drop of 91% in reported chest **pain**. After that study was published in the British medical journal *Lancet*, Dr. Ornish became internationally famous, and the Ornish diet was adopted by many heart disease patients.

Benefits

Because the Ornish diet includes almost only plant products, it is high in substances thought to promote health such as **antioxidants** and fiber, as well as low in substances that are harmful to the health such as fat and cholesterol. Following the diet's recommendation of light exercise can also be very beneficial. Walking 20 or 30 minutes a day instead of being completely sedentary has significant health benefits and may even reduce by half the chance of early death.

Although the Ornish diet is effective at causing weight loss and improved overall health, the most researched and discussed benefit of the program is the prevention and even reversal of heart disease. Dr. Ornish and colleagues have done extensive research showing that following a very strict, completely vegetarian form of his diet cannot only prevent heart disease from occurring or getting more severe, but it can actually cause a reverse of artery constriction allowing blood to flow to the heart better. Dr. Ornish also believes his diet may be effective at preventing or reversing other forms of disease such as **prostate cancer**.

Description

Heart disease develops when arteries that supply the heart with oxygen become narrowed due to the buildup of plaque on their walls. Plaque deposits are caused by cholesterol, a type of fat found in animal products and also made by the body from saturated fats in the diet. The narrowing of arteries is called **atherosclerosis**, a condition that develops over many years. When the coronary (heart) arteries become too blocked to supply the heart with enough oxygen, a **heart attack** occurs.

The first principle of the Ornish diet is to eliminate cholesterol, so all foods containing cholesterol and saturated fats are removed from the diet. Saturated fats are found in meat, dairy products, oils, nuts, seed, and avocados, which are all forbidden by the Ornish diet. Furthermore, the level of fat in the diet is reduced to only 10% of the total calories. This level is much lower than the diet recommended by the American Heart Association, which recommends up to 30% of calories from fat. The typical American diet consists of up to 50% fat. The Ornish diet is vegetarian, since cholesterol-containing meats are eliminated. The diet allows the use of egg whites and nonfat dairy products; technically it can be classified as a lacto-ovo-vegetarian diet.

Another feature of the Ornish diet is the ratios assigned to fat, protein, and carbohydrates, respectively. The typical American diet is 45% fat, 25% protein, and 30% carbohydrates, with nearly 500 mg of cholesterol per day. The Ornish diet is 10% fat, 20% protein, and 70% carbohydrates. The Ornish diet consists mainly of complex carbohydrates, commonly called starches. Complex carbohydrates are present in fruits, vegetables, grains, and beans. Simple carbohydrates include sugar, honey, and alcohol, which tend to be "empty calories," because they contain lots of calories but little fiber or nutrients. The Ornish diet restricts but does not eliminate simple carbohydrates. The Ornish diet also emphasizes high-fiber foods, which includes most complex carbohydrates. High-fiber diets have been shown to reduce cholesterol and have other beneficial effects.

The Ornish diet is slightly lower in protein than the American average, and lower protein intake has been shown by research to have potential health benefits for Americans. For those worried about the lack of protein in a vegetarian diet, the Ornish program teaches ways to ensure an adequate supply of complete proteins in the diet. Proteins are said to be complete when the body can fully utilize them. They can be obtained by combining grains with legumes (beans) or grains with nonfat dairy products. For instance, complete proteins in the Ornish diet are obtained by combining rice and beans, tofu and rice, pasta and beans, baked beans and wheat bread, or oatmeal with nonfat yogurt over the course of a day. Egg whites are another source of protein on the Ornish diet.

Another principle of the Ornish diet is that people are allowed to eat as much food as they wish, as long as the 10%-of-calories-from-fat rule is maintained, and as long as only approved foods are eaten. By allowing people to eat as much as they like, the Ornish diet reduces the risk of binge eating, to which many dieters resort when forced to restrict calories. Many diets have been shown to fail when calories are restricted.

To summarize, the Ornish diet excludes cholesterol and saturated fat, excluding all animal products (except egg whites and nonfat dairy products), nuts, seeds, avocados, chocolate, olives, and coconuts. Oils are eliminated except a small amount of canola oil for cooking, and oil that supplies omega-3 **essential fatty**

KEY TERMS

Atherosclerosis—A disease process whereby plaques of fatty substances are deposited inside arteries, reducing the inside diameter of the vessels and eventually causing damage to the tissues located beyond the site of the blockage.

Cholesterol—A steroid fat found in animal foods that is also produced in the human body from saturated fat. Cholesterol is used to form cell membranes and process hormones and vitamin D. High cholesterol levels contribute to the development of atherosclerosis.

Complete protein—A protein food that has all the essential amino acids the body requires to digest it.

Essential fatty acids—Fats that are essential to the diet because the body cannot make them. Omega-3 and omega-6 are the two major categories of essential fatty acids.

Plaque—A deposit, usually of fatty material, on the inside wall of a blood vessel. Also refers to a small, round demyelinated area that develops in the brain and spinal cord of an individual with multiple sclerosis.

Saturated fat—Fat that is usually solid at room temperature, found mainly in meat and dairy products but also in vegetable sources such as some nuts, seeds, and avocados.

acids. The Ornish diet also prohibits **caffeine** but allows a moderate intake of alcohol, sugar, and salt.

It should be noted that Ornish himself states that his diet alone is not sufficient for reversing heart disease but is only one part of an overall program that includes exercise, yoga, meditation, stress reduction, and lifestyle changes. In fact, Ornish calls some of his work "opening the heart" therapies because patients are encouraged to confront emotional aspects of their healing as well as physical concerns such as diet and high cholesterol.

Preparations

Anyone thinking of beginning a new diet should consult their physician. Requirements of calories, fat, and nutrients can differ significantly from person to person, depending on gender, age, weight, and many other factors such as the presence of any diseases or conditions. Pregnant or breastfeeding women should be especially cautious because deficiencies of vitamins or minerals can have a significant negative impact on a baby.

Patients with heart disease should be especially careful when beginning a diet. Although Dr. Ornish has published data about how his diet may be able to prevent or reverse heart disease, everyone reacts differently and no major dietary changes should be made without consulting a physician. The Ornish diet is not a replacement for cholesterol-lowering drugs or any other medications prescribed by a doctor and is not a replacement for medically recommended procedures. It is important to discuss all possible options with a physician and make all decisions based on professional recommendations.

Ornish states that one emphasis of his program is increasing the awareness of eating habits and the ingredients of food products. Those beginning the Ornish diet can prepare by becoming thoroughly familiar with the Ornish list of recommended and prohibited foods and by learning to read food labels and count calories. Another preparation dieters can make is determining their ideal weight for their particular height and body type. Daily calorie and fat allowances can then be derived from this ideal weight. Ornish has authored or co-authored several books that provide hundreds of recipes consistent with the diet.

Precautions

The Ornish diet is not a substitute for medical care of cardiovascular disease. Furthermore, the Ornish diet is designed to be used in conjunction with a holistic health program that includes exercise, yoga, meditation, lifestyle changes, and stress reduction. As with any diet program, research continued as of 2008 on its effectiveness. Critics of the program maintain that Dr. Ornish has not produced sufficient clinical research to support his claims; they also assert that a diet high in carbohydrates drives up insulin levels, increasing the risk of diseases such as diabetes. A 2003 study comparing low-fat diets to low-carbohydrate diets reported that obese patients lost more weight on the low-carbohydrate diet compared to a fat and calorie-restricted diet. They also appeared to have lower triglyceride levels and improved insulin sensitivity.

The Ornish diet is very low in fat and limits meat and animal product intake to little or none. Many important vitamins and minerals such as zinc and vitamin B-12 are acquired from these sources in a normal diet. Without these sources there is a significant possibility of deficiency. Also, because of the very low fat allowance of the diet there is some concern that people on this diet may not get enough vitamin E, which is found mainly in nuts and oil. These are too high in fat to be eaten regularly while on this diet. Dr. Ornish often recommends taking supplements while following his diet, and taking a complete multivitamin may help reduce the risk of a deficiency. Multivitamins and supplements, however, have their own risks, especially for pregnant or breast-feeding women and individuals with medical issues such as renal disease.

DEAN ORNISH (1953-)

Dr. Dean Ornish was born on July 16, 1953, in Dallas, TX. He attended Rice University and University of Texas at Austin, where he received his B.A. in 1975. He went on to graduate from Baylor College of Medicine in 1980 and completed his internship and residency at Massachusetts General Hospital and Harvard Medical School.

In 1989, Ornish began issuing data showing that the atherosclerotic patients he had been treating without drugs or invasive surgery had reduced the overall blockages in their arteries. That attention became international in 1990 with the issuance of the physician's best-selling book, Dr. Dean Ornish's Program for Reversing Heart Disease: The Only System Scientifically Proven to Reverse Heart Disease without Drugs or Surgery.

Ornish provides readers with information to help them make the comprehensive lifestyle changes he advocates. Among the alterations Ornish recommends is the incorporation of stress-management techniques such as meditation, imagery, breathing, and yoga exercises into their lives. Ornish also offers suggestions for healthier methods of coping with the emotional pain he believes everyone experiences in one form or another.

Although Ornish's lifestyle recommendations are similar to those advocated by most cardiologists, his prescription for health is much stricter. However, his research patients, all seriously ill at one time, have reduced their arterial blockages without the aid of pharmaceuticals or invasive surgical techniques.

Founder and president of the Preventive Medicine Research Institute of the University of California at San Francisco, Ornish believes there is a link between the causes of depression and heart disease and that bypasses and angioplasty only treat the symptoms, not the causes, of heart disease. Furthermore, he believes that having deeply intimate, loving relationships can be invaluable in preventing and treating heart disease.

Ornithosis see **Psittacosis**

Ortho-bionomy

Definition

Ortho-bionomy is a form of therapeutic bodywork, based on the principle that gentle and non-invasive body alignment has a positive influence on physical and emotional disorders.

Origins

Ortho-bionomy was developed in the 1970s by Dr. Arthur Lincoln Pauls, a British osteopathic physician who was also an accomplished martial artist. Pauls was influenced by the principles of **osteopathy** that state that the function of the body is related to its physical (skeletal) alignment; that proper circulation of the blood and lymph is crucial to health; and that the body contains built-in mechanisms that can be triggered to correct imbalances and diseases. Influenced also by Eastern philosophy, Dr. Pauls searched for a system of healing that was gentle, non-invasive, and that worked with the body's inherent wisdom, rather than using forceful methods to manipulate problems involving posture.

Dr. Pauls was guided toward his system of bodywork in the 1960s, when an American osteopath named Lawrence Jones published a paper on a phenomenon he called "Spontaneous Release Through Positioning." Jones claimed that **muscle spasms** and painful injuries can be treated by the gentle repositioning of the part of the body that was painful. For instance, if a person injures a knee, the muscles and tendons around that area tighten, sometimes to the point of **pain** and spasm. The tightening protects the knee from further injury. When the injury begins to heal, the muscles and tendons around the area retain the memory of the injury, and have changed in structure. This change affects the bones, joints, and overall alignment of the body. By gentle and comfortable repositioning of the area into its proper alignment, a therapist can prompt the muscles to self-correct, releasing tension and trauma while re-educating the body's memory of the injury, and speeding the healing process.

Dr. Pauls built upon this concept when developing Ortho-bionomy. Influenced by Eastern **martial arts**, Pauls built his idea on the premise that the physical body and the emotions are deeply connected. Pauls developed "Phased Reflex Techniques," which is based on the body healing itself in phases. In effect, there is a gradual release of the emotions and traumas that occur after physical injuries. Pauls also believed that reflex actions in the muscles play a key role in healing injuries, and that by utilizing knowledge of these reflexes the therapist can gently and effectively boost the body's ability to self-correct. These reflexes are contained in the proprioceptive nerves (nerves that are present in the muscles and tendons that provide feedback on the body's movement and alignment). These nerves are influenced by emotions, and they affect the movement of the body. Healing begins by re-educating these nerves toward correct alignment and movement. Emotions held inside are released. Pauls developed a detailed system of bodywork techniques based on these principles. For instance, he found that the greater the stored trauma around an

Resources

BOOKS

Ornish, Dean. *Dr. Dean Ornish's Program for Reversing Heart Disease.* New York: Random House, 2009.

Ornish, Dean. *The Spectrum: A Scientifically Proven Program to Feel Better, Live Longer, Lose Weight, and Gain Health.* New York: Ballantine Books, 2007.

PERIODICALS

Byrnes, Stephen. "Keeping Up with Nutritional Research." *Townsend Letter for Doctors and Patients* (July 2003): 119.

Danisinger, Michael L., et al. "Comparison of the Atkins, Ornish, Weight Watchers, and Zone Diets for Weight Loss and Heart Disease Risk Reduction." *Journal of the American Medical Association* 293 (January 5, 2005): 43–53.

Koertge, Jenny, et al. "Improvement in Medical Risk Factors and Quality of Life in Women and Men with Coronary Artery Disease in the Multicenter Lifestyle Demonstration Project." *American Journal of Cardiology* (June 1, 2003): 1316–1322.

"A Low-carbohydrate as Compared with a Low-fat Diet in Severe Obesity." *Journal of the American Academy of Physicians Assistants* (August 2003): 10–11.

OTHER

Ornish, Dean. "Dean Ornish, M.D., Lifestyle Program." *WebMD.* http://www.webmd.com/content/pages/9/3068_9408.htm (April 23, 2008).

ORGANIZATIONS

American Dietetic Association, 120 South Riverside Plaza, Suite 2000, Chicago, IL, 60606-6995, (800) 877-1600, http://www.eatright.org.

Douglas Dupler
Teresa G. Odle
Helen Davidson

Dr. Pauls termed his system Ortho-bionomy, which means, "the correct application of the laws of life." In the mid-1970s, he began teaching his system in the United States and Europe.

injury, the longer the therapist must reposition the area to provide a full release of healing potential.

Benefits

Ortho-bionomy is used to alleviate chronic pain associated with injuries, muscle and joint problems, and arthritis; reduce **stress**; increase circulation; enhance **relaxation**; and improve problems of posture or structural alignment. Its gentle technique is recommended for acute pain and rehabilitative injuries. Ortho-bionomy is incorporated into other healing treatments. For example, massage therapists may use this technique to relieve knotted muscles. Some of the techniques may be used to relieve cramps, back pain, sore muscles, and headaches.

Ortho-bionomy is safe for newborns, the elderly, and those in post-operative conditions. Athletes and dancers may improve performances with the therapy by increased balance and flexibility.

Description

A session with an Ortho-bionomy therapist is similar to other therapeutic massage sessions. The patient remains clothed. Emphasis is placed on comfort, and on a trusting and open relationship between patient and therapist. Open communication from the patient provides feedback and assists in the discovery and release of emotional issues. The therapist may use a range of hands-on techniques, including light touch, smooth movements, gentle pressure on reflex points, finding and working with points of tension and pain, gentle prolonged body-positioning for release, and re-education exercises. Therapeutic movements are done slowly and gently, so that they do not create additional stresses. Some therapists may employ non-physical touch, to work upon the energy field of the body, similar to the touch used in **reiki**. Generally, a series of treatments is recommended, as Ortho-bionomy is based on the idea that healing occurs in gradual phases. The goal of treatment is to ultimately increase the patient's awareness on the physical and emotional levels and—through this awareness—to promote re-education and elimination of unhealthy patterns.

Preparations

No special preparation is needed prior to Ortho-bionomy treatments.

Precautions

Consumers may check with a practitioner to determine the level of Ortho-bionomy training he or she has completed.

Side effects

There are no reported side effects of Ortho-bionomy. The therapy is gentle, painless, and non-invasive.

Research & general acceptance

Ortho-bionomy is done in countries around the world, indicating that it has grown in popularity since the early work of Dr. Pauls.

Training and certification

Ortho-bionomy is taught and practiced worldwide. Some **massage therapy** schools offer Ortho-bionomy as a specialty course in conjunction with general massage therapy. Ortho-bionomy is also done by other health practitioners including naturopathic and osteopathic physicians.

The Society of Ortho-bionomy International has developed two training programs for professionals, a basic practitioner program and a senior practitioner program. Both offer theoretical coursework and supervised hands-on training. Students choose individual advisors during their training. The Society's Web site has links to Ortho-bionomy practitioners in a number of states, as well as countries such as Australia and New Zealand.

Resources

BOOKS

Kain, Kathy L. *Ortho-Bionomy: A Practical Manual.* Berkeley, CA: North Atlantic, 1997.

Schultz, Louis R., Rosemary Feitis, and Diana Salles. *The Endless Web: Fascial Anatomy and Physical Reality.* Berkeley, CA: North Atlantic, 1996.

PERIODICALS

Tornick, Annie Woods. "Ortho-Bionomy: Dancing in the Still Point." *Massage Magazine* (March/April 2003): 114. http://www.massagemag.com.

KEY TERMS

Osteopathy—System of health care that emphasizes the musculoskeletal system.

Reiki—Form of therapeutic bodywork that strives to heal the body's energy field.

ORGANIZATIONS

Society for Ortho-Bionomy International. 5875 North Lincoln Avenue, Suite 225. Chicago, IL 60659. (800) 743-4890. http://www.ortho-bionomy.org. Publishes *Ortho-Bionomy News*.

Douglas Dupler

Orthomolecular medicine

Definition

Orthomolecular medicine is the prevention and treatment of disease by administering nutritional supplements. The patient's state of health, external or environmental factors and quality of diet are taken into account. The architect of orthomolecular medicine, Nobel Prize laureate Linus Pauling, coined the term in 1968. The aim of orthomolecular medicine is not merely to eliminate disease, but to aim for "optimum health."

Origins

Linus Carl Pauling was born in 1901 in Portland, Oregon. He published his first scientific paper at the age of 22. In 1925, he graduated summa cum laude from the California Institute of Technology with a Ph.D. in chemistry. He was to remain at this institute for the next 38 years.

Though by no means the first to investigate the properties of the nutrients contained in foods, or the first to consider the medical application of nutritional supplements, his contribution to our understanding of how nutrients work in our bodies and how supplements can affect our health, has not been matched, either before or since. It was not until 1966, after a long and distinguished career, that he changed direction in response to a letter from Irwin Stone and began to research the properties of micronutrients.

In 1970, Pauling published *Vitamin C and the Common Cold*, which established **vitamin C** as a favorite and effective remedy for colds and flu. In 1973, he founded the Institute of Orthomolecular Medicine, a non-profit research organization, with Arthur B. Robinson and Keene Dimick. The institute later became the Linus Pauling Institute of Science and Medicine. In the years that followed, Pauling published many research papers and books detailing his findings in the field of orthomolecular medicine until his death in 1994.

As a result of Pauling's research, orthomolecular medicine has become a specialized branch of alternative medicine, and its realm of application has widened to include not only **cancer** and other diseases, but many mental illnesses, including schizophrenia.

Benefits

In summarizing their philosophy, practitioners of orthomolecular medicine cite Hippocrates's watchword which was "First, do no harm." With their policy of rectifying **nutrition** first and then administering supplements in treating disease, they feel that they already have an advantage over allopathic methods such as chemotherapy, drug therapy, surgery and radiotherapy, which orthomolecular practitioners believe have potentially disastrous effects on the human organism. Despite the fact that when taken in "mega-doses" nutritional supplements have been known to cause harm, they can have a significantly lower potential for toxicity than allopathic drugs.

Orthomolecular practitioners recommend that patients improve their lifestyle and eating habits to consolidate benefits felt from the supplements themselves. Many of their "discoveries" have now become more or less common knowledge, for example the fact that a combination of vitamin C and **zinc** can speed the departure of a virus—particularly a cold—by many days.

Orthomolecular medicine can be of benefit to anyone for a wide range of illnesses and symptoms.

Some illnesses which have been treated with orthomolecular medicine are:

- depression, anxiety, and schizophrenia
- Raynaud's disease, heart problems, and atherosclerosis
- digestive disorders, irritable bowel syndrome, Crohn's disease, diverticulitis, obesity, and endometriosis
- chronic fatigue syndrome
- heavy metal toxicity and radiation sickness
- osteoarthritis and rheumatoid arthritis

KEY TERMS

Pellagra—A condition caused by a dietary deficiency of niacin, one of the B vitamins. The patient will have dementia, diarrhea and dermatitis.

Titration—Gradually adjusting dosage of a supplement until the desired result is obtained, but no unwanted side effects appear.

- infertility and other reproductive disorders
- high blood pressure
- asthma and other respiratory problems
- eczema and other skin disorders
- candidiasis
- cancer, AIDS, and other immune system problems
- neural tube defects in the fetus.

Description

The basic concept of orthomolecular medicine is that according to their genetic makeup, and other factors such as environment, stress levels, and levels of nutrition, individuals will have nutritional needs that are peculiar to themselves alone; no two people will be alike in this respect. Consequently, what will cause illness for one person, will produce good health in another.

Many degenerative diseases and even mental abnormalities are quite possibly the result of biochemical imbalances. Linus Pauling's research demonstrated that all illness and disease can be treated to some extent with nutritional supplements, such as vitamins, **amino acids**, trace minerals, electrolytes, and fatty acids.

Theoretically, fresh food that is of high quality should provide all the nutrients necessary for good health. However, the depletion of nutrients in soil result from over-use of pesticides and artificial fertilizers and intensive farming practices also means a gradual decline in the levels of nutrients in produce. Orthomolecular practitioners, therefore, recommend that laboratory tests should be conducted to assess nutritional status so that possible areas of insufficiency may be addressed with the use of supplements.

Orthomolecular psychiatric therapy

This is the treatment of diseases of the mind by providing optimum nutrients, thus enhancing the "chemistry of the brain." It has been found to be very effective in the treatment of mental illness, even schizophrenia.

For those in the allopathic medical profession who are sceptical, practitioners remind them that when nicotinic acid was introduced, it cured hundreds of thousands of pellagra patients of psychoses in addition to the physical symptoms of this disease. Vitamin C has been used successfully to treat some mental symptoms, in particular **depression**.

Many other micronutrients have been found to influence brain function, among them:

- thiamine
- pyridoxone

- folic acid
- tryptophan
- L(+)-glutamic acid
- cyanocobalamin

Preparations

Nutritional supplements are a growing business and can be obtained almost anywhere, even in the supermarket. It is advisable to obtain supplements from an establishment that specializes in this area, and to ensure that products are fresh and potent.

A reputable health store will have staff on hand to advise customers about what is suitable for them and how supplements should be taken.

Precautions

If taken incorrectly nutritional supplements can have a detrimental effect on the health. Some supplements can produce adverse effects when taken in combination with certain medications. Certain supplements also cause unwanted effects during **pregnancy**. Instructions should always be followed, and if in doubt, a nutritionally-oriented practitioner or a physician should be consulted. The U.S. Food and Drug Administration (FDA) has drawn up maximum and minimum recommended doses for the guidance of the public. However, orthomolecular practitioners point out that these levels are intended for normal healthy individuals and sometimes doses far in excess of the RDA (recommended daily allowance) are required to bring a sick person back to health.

In early 2002, the U.S. Pharmacopeial (USP) Convention announced that it would launch a voluntary dietary supplement verification program. Manufacturers of supplements can supply the USP with documentation that shows they have a quality standard system in place to address label accuracy, safety and efficacy of products. The USP then arranges for a quality audit to verify that good quality and safety practices are in place.

Patient should not try to prescribe their own supplements, but should instead consult a qualified practitioner for safer and more beneficial results. It should be noted that blood tests do not always give an accurate picture of nutritional status and most orthomolecular practitioners recommend titration of doses to suit the patient.

Side effects

Orthomolecular medicine, while generally harmless, can be dangerous if safe doses of nutritional supplements are not observed. Some supplements, notably the oil-based ones such as vitamins A, D, and E, can build up and cause undesirable consequences. Too much vitamin A, for example can cause very dry skin, among other things. Vitamin D can cause calcification of soft tissue if taken in excessive amounts, and all these items can cause liver damage if taken in excess.

Research and general acceptance

Since the beginning of this century, both nutrition and its "offshoot," orthomolecular medicine, have been extensively researched. Both the United States and British governments have special departments which determine safe doses of all supplements.

Orthomolecular medicine is possibly the branch of alternative therapies that has been the subject of most scientific research, and has certainly been validated by that research. Therefore, it is the one branch of alternative medicine that it is very difficult for allopathic medicine to call into question.

Linus Pauling was undoubtedly one of the most distinguished scientists of the twentieth century, and left over 400,000 research papers and other scientific documents to record his findings. Orthomolecular medicine research is based strongly on such other scientific fields as biochemistry, physiology, immunology, endocrinology, pharmacology, and toxicology.

Training and certification

Among those qualified to advise on treatment with nutritional supplements are board certified physicians, licensed nutritionists, and naturopaths. Although specialists in orthomolecular medicine tend to be highly qualified, it is advisable to check the credentials of any therapist or physician before consultation.

Resources

PERIODICALS

Levy, Sandra. "Watch for New Seals of Approval on Dietary Supplements."*Drug Topics*146 (January 7, 2002): 29.

"Tips for the Savvy Supplement User."*FDA Consumer*35, no. 2 (March - April, 2002): 17-25.

ORGANIZATIONS

American Holistic Medicine Association. http://www.holisticmedicine.org/index.html.

American Holistic Health Association. Dept. R P.O. Box 17400 Anaheim, CA 92817-7400. (714) 779-6152. ahha@healthy.net. http://www.healthy.net/pan/chg/ahha/rosen.html.

Center for Food Safety and Applied Nutrition, U.S. Department of Health and Human Services. 5100 Paint Branch Parkway, College Park, MD 20740 (888) SAFEFOOD. http://www.cfsan.fda.gov.

The Huxley Institute for Biosocial Research. American Academy of Orthomolecular Medicine. 900 North Federal Highway, Boca Raton, FL 33432 (800) 847-3802.

The Linus Pauling Institute. http://osu.orst.edu/dept/lpi/resagenda/timeline.html.

OTHER

"Holistic medicine." http://www.holisticmed.com/whatis.html.

National Center for Complementary and Alternative Medicine. http://nccam.nih.gov.

Orthomolecular medicine online. http://www.orthomed.org/.

Patricia Skinner
Teresa G. Odle

Osha

Description

Osha, whose botanical name is *Ligusticum porteri*, is a plant native to the western United States and Mexico. A member of the Umbelliferae family, osha has been used for centuries by Native Americans and Mexicans as a treatment for sore throats, fevers, and **influenza**. The plant belongs to the same family as **parsley** and dill, and it has the same long thin hollow stalk with large divided leaves. These leaves can reach heights of 2 ft (0.6 m). Osha's seeds and flowers are at the top of the plant and spread out in the form of an umbrella, whence its Latin family name. Osha flowers are white and the seeds have a sweet celery-like smell, as does the entire plant. The root is very hairy, brown on the outside and yellow on the inside. The plant has several other names: chuchupate, Indian parsley, Porter's lovage, mountain lovage, Colorado **cough** root. A plant related to osha, *Ligusticum wallichii*, is used in **traditional Chinese medicine**; most laboratory studies of osha have used this Chinese species.

General use

Osha root is a powerful antiviral and antibacterial agent, used for bronchial **infections** and sore throats. Taking a tincture or decoction of osha root, or chewing directly on the root, causes perspiration and enhances the body's immune function. Although osha has a bitter taste, its root has a numbing effect that soothes sore throats. Since it is also an expectorant, it is very useful for coughs and pharyngitis, and can also be used for very early stages of **tonsillitis**.

KEY TERMS

Decoction—An herbal extract produced by mixing an herb in cold water, bringing the mixture to a boil, and letting it simmer to evaporate the excess water. The decoction is then strained and drank hot or cold. Decoctions are usually chosen over infusion when the botanical or herb in question is a root, seed, or berry.

Expectorant—A drug that promotes the discharge of mucus from respiratory system.

Infusion—Introduction of a substance directly into a vein or tissue by gravity flow.

Tincture—A solution of alcohol and water containing plant matter. One available tincture of osha is 70% alcohol.

Osha root tea helps with gastrointestinal discomfort, in particular **indigestion** and stomach upset associated with **vomiting**. It can be used to increase appetite. Both osha root tincture and tea can be used topically on **cuts** and scrapes, as osha also has strong antibacterial qualities. Michael Moore, a contemporary American herbalist associated with the Southwest School of Herbal Medicine, states that osha can be used for head colds with dry cough; certain stages of pharyngitis; early stages of tonsillitis; coughs; influenza with persistent coughing; dry, hot fevers; and acute brochial **pneumonia**. Osha can be given together with **echinacea** for leukocytosis.

Preparations

Osha is available as whole or powdered dried roots. Dried osha root can be chewed directly. Michael Moore suggests taking a "walnut-sized root" every three to four hours. A cold infusion of osha, two to six ounces, can be taken as needed. Other products that contain osha come in different concentrations and should be mixed or diluted according to label instructions. If osha is used in tincture form, 20–60 drops can be taken up to five times a day. One part osha to two parts honey works well as a cough syrup, and is more appealing to children, who often dislike the plant's bitter taste.

Precautions

The most important precaution to take with osha is correct identification. The plant is often confused with hemlock parsley, which it closely resembles. Osha is also sometimes mistaken for poison hemlock, which can be fatal to humans if ingested. Osha has also been detected in the milk of lactating mothers, and should not be used by women who are pregnant or nursing.

Side effects

There are no known side effects with using osha other than allergy or hypersensitivity to it or to its plant family. High doses of osha taken over extended periods of time, however, may cause kidney or liver toxicity.

Interactions

No known adverse reactions have been reported with osha.

Resources

BOOKS

Moore, Michael. *Herbal Materia Medica*. Southwest School of Herbal Medicine, n.d.

Moore, Michael. *Herb/Medicine Contraindications*. Southwest School of Herbal Medicine, 1995.

Moore, Michael. *Medicinal Plants of the Mountain West*. Santa Fe, NM: Museum of New Mexico Press, 1979.

Moore, Michael. *Specific Indications for Herbs in General Use*. Southwest School of Herbal Medicine, 1994.

Katherine Y. Kim

Osteoarthritis

Definition

Osteoarthritis (OA), which is also known as osteoarthrosis or degenerative joint disease (DJD), is a progressive disorder of the joints caused by gradual loss of cartilage and resulting in the development of bony spurs and cysts at the margins of the joints. The name osteoarthritis comes from three Greek words meaning bone, joint, and inflammation.

Description

OA is one of the most common causes of disability due to limitations of joint movement, particularly in people over 50. It is estimated that 2% of the United States population under the age of 45 suffers from osteoarthritis; this figure rises to 30% of persons between 45 and 64, and 63–85% in those over 65. About 90% of the American population will have some features of OA in their weight-bearing joints by age 40. Men tend to develop OA at earlier ages than women.

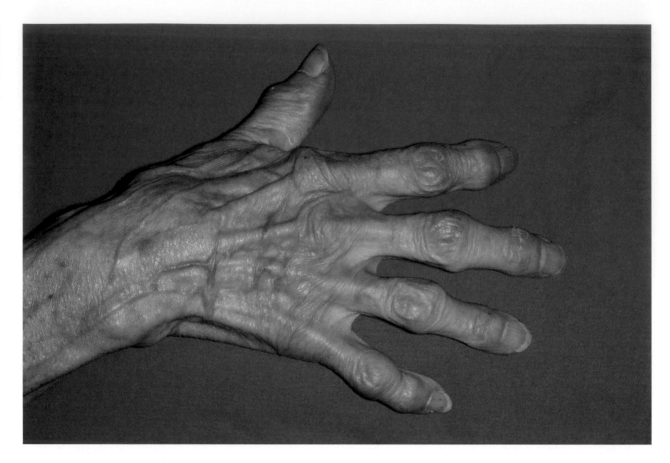

Osteoarthritis of the hand of a 78 year old woman. *(© Scott Camazine / Alamy)*

OA typically develops gradually over a period of years. Patients with OA may have joint **pain** on only one side of the body. It primarily affects the knees, hands, hips, feet, and spine.

Causes and symptoms

Osteoarthritis results from deterioration or loss of the cartilage that acts as a protective cushion between bones, particularly in weight-bearing joints such as the knees and hips. As the cartilage is worn away, the bone rubbing against bone forms spurs, areas of abnormal hardening, and fluid-filled pockets in the marrow known as subchondral cysts. As the disorder progresses, pain results from deformation of the bones and fluid accumulation in the joints. The pain is relieved by rest and made worse by moving the joint or placing weight on it. In early OA, the pain is minor and may take the form of mild stiffness in the morning. In the later stages of OA, chronic inflammation develops. The patient may experience pain even when the joint is not being used; and he or she may suffer permanent loss of the normal range of motion in that joint.

Until the late 1980s, OA was regarded as an inevitable part of **aging**, caused by simple "wear and tear" on the joints. This view has been replaced by recent research into cartilage formation. OA is now considered to be the end result of several different factors contributing to cartilage damage, and is classified as either primary or secondary.

Primary osteoarthritis

Primary OA results from abnormal stresses on weight-bearing joints or normal stresses operating on weakened joints. Primary OA most frequently affects the finger joints, the hips and knees, the cervical and lumbar spine, and the big toe. The enlargements of the finger joints that occur in OA are referred to as Heberden's and Bouchard's nodes. Some gene mutations appear to be associated with OA. **Obesity** also increases the pressure on the weight-bearing joints of the body. Finally, as the body ages, there is a reduction in the ability of cartilage to repair itself. In addition to these factors, some researchers have theorized that

Osteoarthritis

Risk Factors
  Age-related
  Overuse of joints
  Excessive weight

Physical Effects
  Affects joints
  Bony spurs
  Enlarged or malformed joints

Treatment Options
  Weight Management
  Non-steroidal anti-inflammatory drugs

Pain Management
  Support groups
  Exercise
  Joint splitting
  Physical therapy
  Passive exercise
  Joint replacement
  Heat and cold
  Message therapy
  Acupuncture
  Psychological approaches
    (relaxation, visualization)
  Tai Chi
  Low stress yoga

(Illustration by Corey Light. Cengage Learning, Gale)

primary OA may be triggered by enzyme disturbances, bone disease, or liver dysfunction.

Secondary osteoarthritis

Secondary OA results from chronic or sudden injury to a joint. It can occur in any joint. Secondary OA is associated with the following factors:

- trauma, including sports injuries
- repetitive stress injuries associated with certain occupations (like the performing arts, construction or assembly line work, computer keyboard operation, etc.)
- repeated episodes of gout or septic arthritis
- poor posture or bone alignment caused by developmental abnormalities
- metabolic disorders

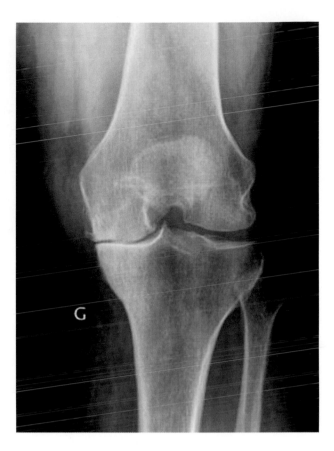

Colored x ray of the knee showing osteoarthritis. *(Phanie / Photo Researchers, Inc.)*

Diagnosis

History and physical examination

The two most important diagnostic clues in the patient's history are the pattern of joint involvement and the presence or absence of **fever**, rash, or other symptoms outside the joints. As part of the physical examination, the doctor will touch and move the patient's joint to evaluate swelling, limitations on the range of motion, pain on movement, and crepitus (a cracking or grinding sound heard during joint movement).

Diagnostic imaging

There is no laboratory test that is specific for osteoarthritis. Treatment is usually based on the results of diagnostic imaging. In patients with OA, x rays may indicate narrowed joint spaces, abnormal density of the bone, and the presence of subchondral cysts or **bone spurs**. The patient's symptoms, however, do not always correlate with x-ray findings. Magnetic resonance imaging (MRI) and computed tomography scans (CTscans) can be used to determine more precisely the location and extent of cartilage damage.

Treatment

Diet

Food intolerance can be a contributing factor in OA, although this is more significant in **rheumatoid arthritis**. Dietary suggestions that may be helpful for people with OA include emphasizing high-fiber, complex-carbohydrate foods, while minimizing fats. Plants in the Solanaceae family, such as tomatoes, peppers, eggplant, and potatoes, should be avoided, as should refined and processed foods. Citrus fruits should also be avoided, as they may promote swelling. Foods that are high in **bioflavonoids** (berries as well as red, orange, and purple fruits and vegetables) should be eaten often. Black cherry juice (2 glasses twice per day) has been found to be particularly effective for partial pain relief.

Nutritional supplements

In the past several years, a combination of **glucosamine** and **chondroitin** sulfate has been proposed as a dietary supplement that helps the body maintain and repair cartilage. Studies conducted in Europe have shown the effectiveness of this treatment but effects may not be evident until a month after initiating this treatment. These substances are nontoxic and do not require prescriptions. Other supplements that may be helpful in the treatment of OA include the antioxidant vitamins and minerals (vitamins A, C, E, **selenium**, and **zinc**) and the B vitamins, especially vitamins B_6 and B_5.

Naturopathy

Naturopathic treatment for OA includes **hydrotherapy**, **diathermy** (deep-heat therapy), nutritional supplements, and botanical preparations, including **yucca**, **devil's claw** (*Harpagophytum procumbens*), and **hawthorn** (*Crataegus laevigata*) berries.

Electromagnetic field therapy is believed to increase blood flow and oxygen exchange to enhance the body's natural healing processes. This treatment is not suggested for use over an open wound or in combination with transdermal drug delivery patches, or by those who are pregnant or have insulin pumps or pacemakers. Magnets may be worn within a shoe insole, anklet, bracelet, or back support.

Traditional Chinese medicine

Practitioners of **Traditional Chinese medicine** treat arthritis with suction cups, massage, **moxibustion** (warming an area of skin by burning a herbal wick a slight distance above the skin), the application of herbal poultices, and internal doses of Chinese herbal formulas.

Daily **acupressure** can also provide relief for stiff, achy joints. Massage of the achy joints with a blend of aromatic oils, especially **rosemary** and **chamomile** is beneficial. Periods of imagery are another suggested treatment—for 10-20 minutes twice daily—where the joint pain is pictured as transformed into a liquid that trickles from the body into the nearest body of water and eventually into the ocean waves.

Physical therapy

Patients with OA are encouraged to **exercise** as a way of keeping joint cartilage lubricated. Exercises that increase balance, flexibility, and range of motion are recommended for OA patients. These may include walking, swimming and other water exercises, **yoga** and other stretching exercises, or isometric exercises. Physical therapy may also include massage, moist hot packs, or soaking in a hot tub.

Allopathic treatment

Treatment of OA patients is tailored to the needs of each individual. Patients vary widely in the location of the joints involved, the rate of progression, the severity of symptoms, the degree of disability, and responses to specific forms of treatment. Most treatment programs include several forms of therapy.

Patient education and psychotherapy

Patient education is an important part of OA treatment because of the highly individual nature of the disorder and its potential impacts on the patient's life. Patients who are depressed because of changes in employment or recreation usually benefit from counseling. The patient's family should be involved in discussions of coping, household reorganization, and other aspects of the patient's disease and treatment regimen.

Medications

Patients with mild OA may be treated only with pain relievers such as acetaminophen (Tylenol) or propoxyphene (Darvon). Most patients with OA, however, are given nonsteroidal anti-inflammatory drugs, or NSAIDs. These include compounds such as ibuprofen (Motrin, Advil), ketoprofen (Orudis), and flurbiprofen (Ansaid). The NSAIDs have the advantage of relieving inflammation as well as pain. They also have potentially dangerous side effects, including stomach ulcers, sensitivity to sun exposure, kidney disturbances, and nervousness or **depression**.

Some OA patients are treated with corticosteroids injected directly into the joints to reduce inflammation and slow the development of Heberden's nodes. Injections should not be regarded as a first-choice treatment and should be given only two or three times a year. A series of hyaluronic acid injections into the affected joint may help to lubricate and protect cartilage.

Surgery

Surgical treatment of osteoarthritis may include the replacement of a damaged joint with an artificial part or appliance; surgical fusion of spinal bones; scraping or removal of damaged bone from the joint; or the removal of a piece of bone in order to realign the bone.

Protective measures

Depending on the location of the affected joint, patients with OA may be advised to use neck braces or collars, crutches, canes, hip braces, knee supports, bed boards, or elevated chair and toilet seats. They are also advised to avoid unnecessary knee bending, stair climbing, or lifting of heavy objects.

New treatments

Since 1997, several new methods of treatment for OA have been investigated. Although they are still being developed and tested, they appear to hold promise. They include:

- Disease-modifying drugs. These compounds may be useful in assisting the body to form new cartilage or improve its repair of existing cartilage.
- Gene therapy.
- Cartilage transplantation. This technique is presently used in Sweden.

Resources

BOOKS

"Bone, Joint, and Rheumatic Disorders: Osteoarthritis." In *The Merck Manual of Geriatrics,* edited by William B. Abrams, et al. Rahway, NJ: Merck Research Laboratories, 1995.

Hellman, David B. "Arthritis & Musculoskeletal Disorders." In *Current Medical Diagnosis & Treatment 1998,* edited by Lawrence M. Tierney, Jr., et al. Stamford, CT: Appleton & Lange, 1998.

"Musculoskeletal and Connective Tissue Disorders: Osteoarthritis (OA)." In *The Merck Manual of Diagnosis and Therapy,* edited by Robert Berkow, et al. Rahway, NJ: Merck Research Laboratories, 1992.

Neustadt, David H. "Osteoarthritis." In *Conn's Current Therapy,* edited by Robert E. Rakel. Philadelphia: W. B. Saunders Company, 1998.

"Osteoarthritis." In *Professional Guide to Diseases,* edited by Stanley Loeb, et al. Springhouse, PA: Springhouse Corporation, 1991.

Theodosakis, Jason, et al. *The Arthritis Cure.* New York: St. Martin's, 1997.

Kathleen D. Wright

Osteopathy

Definition

Osteopathy is a "whole person" philosophy of medicine, where doctors of osteopathic medicine (DOs) endorse an approach that treats the entire person, rather than a specific complaint. Attention is given to prevention, wellness, and helping the body to heal itself. Because the body is viewed as a single organism or unit, special focus is given to understanding body mechanics and the interrelationship of the body's organs and systems. A particular emphasis is placed on the musculoskeletal system. DOs may utilize physical manipulation of muscles and bones in conjunction with, or as an alternative to, conventional treatments, drug therapies, and surgery to provide complete health care.

Origins

Dr. Andrew Still developed the osteopathic approach to medicine. Still, whose father was a Methodist minister and physician, was himself a medical doctor who served as a Union surgeon during the Civil War. After the war, personal tragedy struck the Still household when three of his children died from spinal **meningitis**. This event angered and disillusioned him. He became dissatisfied with the state of medical knowledge and treatments available at that time. Consequently, he began an intense study of the human body to find underlying causes and cures for ailments.

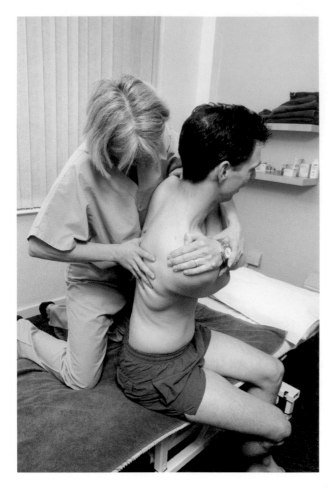

Upper spine examination. *(Paul Rapson / Photo Researchers, Inc.)*

Still gave great attention to anatomy. He recognized the importance of the musculoskeletal system, the body's ability for self-healing, and focused on prevention and the concept of "wellness." In an era when drug treatment was frequently dangerous and overused, and surgery often fatal, Still was able to develop alternative treatments. For example, by manipulating the ribs and spine, Still provided treatments for **pneumonia**. He gave attention to the lymphatic system (which filters foreign matter and removes excess fluids, proteins, and waste products from the tissues and transports them to the blood to be circulated and eliminated) and manipulating the fascia (connective tissue that is tough, but thin and elastic; it forms an uninterrupted three-dimensional network from head to foot, sheathing every muscle, bone, nerve, gland, organ, and blood vessel), allowing him to address a range of other ailments.

Still's sons learned his philosophies and techniques, but demand overwhelmed their ability to supply care. In 1892, Still founded the first college of osteopathic medicine, the American School of Osteopathy, in Kirksville, Missouri. When he died in 1917, there were more than 5,000 practicing osteopaths in the United States. Today, osteopaths are the fastest growing segment of the total population of physicians and surgeons in the United States. In 2002, there were more than 49,000 doctors of osteopathy. Osteopathy has spread outside of the United States and is now practiced in countries throughout the world.

Benefits

The osteopathic focus on prevention and wellness may help individuals to avoid illness by teaching healthy behaviors and encouraging health-promoting lifestyle changes. In addition to conventional treatments, drugs, and surgeries, DOs may offer manipulative therapies not available from their allopathic counterparts (MDs). Many people seek care from an osteopath for back or neck pains, joint pains, or injuries. However, DOs may use manipulative therapies to treat a variety of ailments and conditions including arthritis, **allergies**, **asthma**, **dizziness**, **carpal tunnel syndrome**, menstrual **pain**, migraine headaches, **sciatica**, sinusitis, **tinnitus** (ringing in the ears), and problems in the jaw joints. Manipulative therapies may be incorporated into the treatment plan to speed recovery from various conditions, such as **heart attack** or disc surgery, and to address pediatric concerns, such as otitis media (**ear infection**) and birth traumas. Various manipulative therapies may also be appropriate in alleviating discomforts associated with **pregnancy**, for example, back pain or digestive problems. Some osteopaths even feel that regular osteopathic treatments may help minimize the effects of **aging** on the spine and joints. Also, as noted by the American Osteopathic Association (AOA), the field of sports medicine has found particular benefit in osteopathic practitioners because of their emphasis on "the musculoskeletal system, manipulation, diet, **exercise**, and fitness. Many professional sports team physicians, Olympic physicians, and personal sports medicine physicians are DOs."

Description

Osteopathic medicine considers the human body to be a complex unit of interrelated parts, a unified organism. Organs and systems do not function independently and should not be treated as such. A disturbance in one part of the body affects the entire body. Illness is also impacted by many variables, such as emotions, **stress**, lifestyle, and environment. Therefore, illness must be addressed by taking a whole

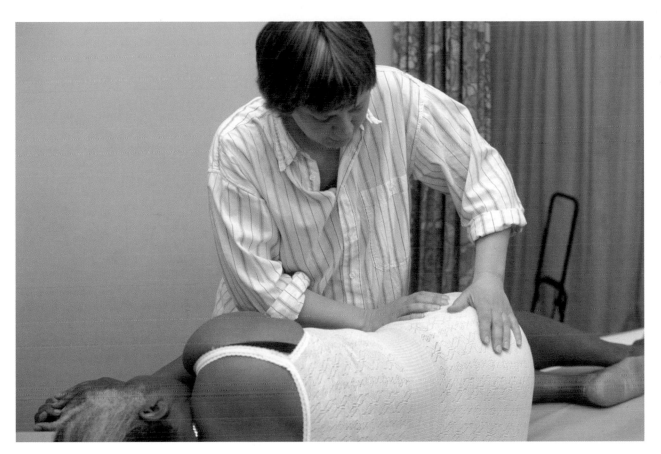

Elderly woman receiving osteopathy treatment. (© Sally and Richard Greenhill / Alamy)

person approach to treatment. Because the body is seen as self-regulating and self-healing, the osteopath gives special attention to illness prevention and helping the body maintain or re-establish wellness.

The nervous and circulatory systems play crucial roles in maintaining the functioning of the body's organs and systems; negative body-wide effects may occur when these two major systems are not functioning optimally. Relieving blocked blood flow or nerve impulses will help the body to heal itself by promoting blood flow through affected tissues. The blood supply will be better able to deliver vital nutrients and boost the immune system, the nerve supply to the area will be improved, and systemic balance can be restored.

The musculoskeletal system is key in this effort to achieve and maintain systemic balance and health. The musculoskeletal system is comprised of the bones, tendons, muscles, tissues, nerves, and spinal column. As the body's largest system, it encompasses over 60% of body mass and can suffer mechanical disorders or amplify illness processes anywhere in the body. Therefore, structural evaluation and attention to the musculoskeletal system is central to osteopathy.

In addition to conventional care such as drug therapies and surgery, osteopaths may use a variety of manipulative procedures to help the body systems function at peak levels. These techniques are commonly referred to as Osteopathic Manipulative Treatment (OMT). OMT is a form of noninvasive, "hands-on" care used for prevention, diagnosis, and treatment to reduce pain and restore motion, as well as help the body heal itself. OMT may be used to facilitate the movement of body fluids and normal tissue functioning, and release painful joints or dysfunctional areas. These therapies take different forms depending on patient needs.

In addition to easing the pain of physical disorders, OMT appears to be helpful in some psychiatric conditions as well. A recent study performed at the College of Osteopathic Medicine in Downers Grove, IL, found that OMT as an adjunct to **psychotherapy** alleviated the symptoms of **depression** in women, as measured by the Zung Depression Scale, a standard diagnostic instrument.

Manipulative procedures may be categorized and discussed in a variety of ways. According to the

American Association of Colleges of Osteopathic Medicine, the following groupings encompass some of the most commonly used procedures. Descriptions are compiled from the American Academy of Osteopathy, Leon Chaitow, N.D., DO, and others.

- Articulatory techniques. Procedures that move joints through their range of motion (articulating the joints) may be used to restore normal functioning.

- Counterstrain. This type of therapy is used to alleviate trigger points localized areas of hyperirritability in the muscles). The procedure involves first finding a body position that relieves the patient's pain. Through a process in which the patient and practitioner repeatedly use coordinated techniques of pushing (or compression), relaxing, and changing position, the trigger point is eased.

- Cranial treatment. Cranial treatments focus on the craniosacral system which consists of the brain, spinal cord, cerebrospinal fluid, dura (the membrane covering the brain and spinal cord), cranial bones, and the sacrum (triangular bone comprised of five fused vertebrae, and forming posterior section of the pelvis). Craniosacral release is a gentle technique that focuses on normalizing imbalances in the natural rhythms of this system. A light touch is used to detect and release restrictions in the system and encourage the body's own healing processes. Craniosacral therapies arose from the work of Dr. William Sutherland, a DO who developed and explored the concept that the bones of the skull allowed movement and could be manipulated to improve the system's rhythmic movements. Some DOs choose to specialize in cranial osteopathy. Craniosacral therapy is also practiced by a wide variety of health care professionals. As listed by the Upledger Institute, these practitioners include MDs, chiropractors, doctors of Oriental medicine, naturopaths, nurses, psychiatric specialists, psychologists, dentists, physical therapists, occupational therapists, acupuncturists, massage therapists, and other professional bodyworkers.

- Myofascial release treatment. Various direct or indirect treatments are applied to release fascia tissues.

- Lymphatic techniques. These techniques focus on improving lymphatic circulation, improving the ability of the lymphatic system to do its job of waste removal.

- Soft tissue techniques. Applied to tissue other than bone, these techniques use varying pressure and may stretch, roll, or knead, resulting in the relaxation or release of tissues.

- Thrust techniques. A quick, sharp thrust (which is often described as high velocity/low amplitude) to the area requiring treatment is used to force a correction, restoring normal joint function and movement. This is similar to chiropractic adjustment.

Precautions

DOs use the full range of conventional diagnostic techniques, drug therapies, treatments, and surgical interventions available to MDs. If deemed appropriate by the DO, OMT may be employed in addition to these conventional diagnoses, and treatments or may serve as an alternative to drug therapies. During the course of treatment, manipulative therapies may be interrupted or stopped if complications occur—for example, a rise in blood pressure. In some situations, the osteopath may determine that no further benefit will be gained from continuing manipulative treatment. Manipulation should not be applied in several medical conditions. As listed by Chris Belshaw, these conditions are mainly "acute **infections**; **fractures**; bone disease; **cancer**; gross structural deformities; such severe general medical conditions as gross high blood pressure or heart attack; vascular disease, for example, thrombosis; neurological conditions with nerve damage; spinal cord damage; and severe prolapse of an intervertebral disc." Additionally, as in any area of medicine, there is the possibility of mistaken diagnosis. Patients should always discuss all medical conditions, treatments, questions, and concerns with their physicians.

Side effects

Some patients, as noted by Belshaw, may experience mild headaches following neck treatments or discomfort after back manipulation. Some flushing and bruising may appear on those with sensitive skin. These reactions may last for several hours. Such symptoms may recur as treatment continues. Symptoms may return if treatment is stopped too soon.

Research and general acceptance

Research has shown the benefits of osteopathic care in a range of ailments and through improved recovery times. In addition to many of the conditions discussed above, the American Osteopathic Healthcare Association reports ongoing research on patient recovery times, length of hospital stays, chronic pain, **chlamydia** infection in women, reduction of deep vein thrombosis, and fall prevention for the elderly. Osteopathic colleges have increased their attention to biomedical research opportunities for students and those who desire to pursue research careers. The AOA Board of Research encourages and supports development of

ANDREW TAYLOR STILL (1828–1917)

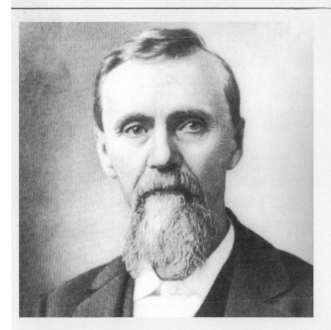

(Betmann/CORBIS. Reproduced by permission.)

Andrew Taylor Still, the father of osteopathy, was born on August 6, 1828, in Virginia to Abram and Martha Still. Growing up on the frontier lands of Tennessee and Missouri provided the impetus for his first studies of the musculoskeletal system. Skinning squirrels and deer, Still became familiar with the relationship between bones, muscles, nerves, and veins long before he picked up an anatomy book. He later studied medicine under his doctor-preacher father and served as a Union surgeon during the Civil War.

Following the war, his distrust of traditional medicine grew when three of his children died of cerebrospinal meningitis. Still decided that the medications of his day were useless and that there had to be another way.

Still studied the attributes of good health so he could understand disease. He saw the body as a complex machine that, when working properly, stayed free of disease. He turned to a drugless, manipulative therapy believing disease was caused by a failure of the human machinery to carry the fluids necessary to maintain health. He called his holistic approach osteopathy for the Greek words *osteon*, meaning bone, and *pathos*, to suffer.

Still gained a following working as an itinerant healer, and in October 1892, he opened the American School of Osteopathy in Kirksville, Missouri. Still welcomed women even as other medical schools denied them access.

As of 2000, there were 16 osteopathic medicine colleges in the United States and 35,000 practicing doctors of osteopathy. The Kirksville College of Osteopathic Medicine remains open.

scientific research in the osteopathic medical profession. The AOA has also conducted several campaigns to educate the public on osteopathy. In 2000, the AOA started a Women's Health Initiative, a three-year campaign to promote women's healthcare among osteopathic physicians and the public.

Training and certification

Training and certification for DOs exceed those of chiropractors and physical therapists, two groups to which their manipulative techniques are sometimes compared. **Chiropractic** training focuses on spinal manipulation only. Chiropractors typically have fewer years and types of required postgraduate training, and are more limited legally in their practice. DOs also have training and licensing well beyond that of physical therapists.

Osteopathic physicians, like their allopathic physician counterparts, are complete physicians. This means they are trained and licensed to prescribe medication and perform surgery, and qualified to render complete healthcare. DOs are fully licensed in all 50 states and the District of Columbia, to serve in the military medical corps, Veterans Administration, and Public Health Service, and are recognized by the American Medical Association as physicians. They hold the same practice rights as MDs, have passed the same or similar state licensing examinations, and practice in fully accredited hospitals. DOs can practice in all branches of medicine and surgery, and can specialize in any area, but the majority are primary care physicians.

As of spring 2002, the AOA lists 20 AOA-accredited colleges of osteopathic medicine. Training for DOs and MDs parallel in many ways. Osteopathic colleges, like medical schools, offer a basic, comprehensive four-year medical education. Added to this curriculum are the osteopathic philosophies and a holistic care emphasis on prevention and community care. In addition to stressing the interrelatedness of body organs and systems, students of osteopathy are taught to consider the whole person, including lifestyle, emotional factors, and environmental factors. Training also focuses on the musculoskeletal system and manual medicine. Manipulative therapies are taught for prevention, diagnosis, and treatment, and the osteopathic principle of helping the body toward good health.

After graduation from the four-year curriculum, DOs complete a one-year rotating internship, followed by several years in a residency program, if a specialty is desired. The areas covered during the internship period ensure that each DO is first trained as a primary care physician. Over half of all DOs are primary care physicians. Conversely, MDs are more likely to be specialists.

After the formal education process, the AOA requires members to earn continuing medical education (CME) credits every three years. To further enhance postgraduate medical education, the AOA has implemented the concept of Osteopathic Postdoctoral Training Institutions (OPTIs), which reflect the osteopathic emphasis on community care. These OPTIs are community-based consortia that include at least one hospital and college of osteopathic medicine. The intention of these is to promote institutional collaboration and enhance training opportunities that reflect the settings in which many osteopaths will practice. In early 2002, a new Osteopathic Research Center opened at the University of North Texas Health Science Center in Fort Worth. The new Research Center is the result of collaboration among the American Colleges of Osteopathic Medicine, the American Osteopathic Foundation, and the American Osteopathic Association.

Many aspects of traditional osteopathic philosophy, such as advice about diet and **smoking**, have entered mainstream medicine to the point that the lines between DOs and MDs are blurring. In addition, the dedication of osteopaths to **holistic medicine** and primary care has been a great benefit to rural areas of the United States that are often underserved by mainstream practitioners.

Resources

PERIODICALS

"Osteopathic Manipulative Treatment May Benefit Patients." *Health & Medicine Week* (October 8, 2001).

Patrick, Stephanie. "Fort Worth Chosen for Osteopathic Center." *Dallas Business Journal* 25 (October 26, 2001): 10.

Shepard, Scott. "Health Philosophies on Common Ground." *Cincinnati Business Courier* 18 (November 9, 2001): 38.

ORGANIZATIONS

American Association of Colleges of Osteopathic Medicine. 5550 Friendship Blvd., Suite 310, Chevy Chase, MD 20815-7231. (301) 968-4100. http://www.aacom.org.

American Osteopathic Association. 142 E. Ontario Chicago, IL 6061. (800) 621-1773. info@aoa-net.org. http://www.aoa-net.org.

The Upledger Institute, Inc. 11211 Prosperity Farms Road, D-325, Palm Beach Gardens, FL 33410-3487. Educational services: (800) 233-5880. Administration: (561) 622-4334. Fax: (561) 622&-4771. upledger@upledger.com. http://www.upledger.com.

OTHER

HealthWorld Online. "Osteopathy." [cited October 2002]. http://www.healthy.net/CLINIC/therapy/Osteo/Index.asp.

The Osteopathic Homepage. http://www.osteohome.com.

Kathy Stolley
Rebecca J. Frey, PhD

Osteoporosis

Definition

The word osteoporosis literally means porous bones. It occurs when bones lose an excessive amount of their protein and mineral content, particularly **calcium**. Over time, bone mass and, therefore, bone strength are decreased. As a result, the bones become fragile and break easily. Even a sneeze or a sudden movement may be enough to break a bone in someone with severe osteoporosis.

Description

Osteoporosis is a serious public health problem. Some 10 million people in the United States have osteoporosis and another 34 million have low bone mass, placing them at risk for osteoporosis. The disease is responsible for 1.5 million **fractures** (broken bones) annually. These fractures, which are often the first sign of the disease, can affect any bone, but the most common locations are the hip, spine, and wrist. Breaks in the hip and spine are of special concern because they almost always require hospitalization and major surgery and may lead to other serious consequences, including permanent disability and even death.

To understand osteoporosis, it is helpful to understand the basics of bone formation. Bone is living tissue that is constantly being renewed in a two-stage process (resorption and formation) that occurs throughout life. In the resorption stage, old bone is broken down and removed by cells called osteoclasts. In the formation stage, cells called osteoblasts build new bone to replace the old. During childhood

U.S. and FAO/WHO recommended amounts of calcium and vitamin D

Calcium

Age	Recommended dietary allowance, U.S.	FAO/WHO recommendations
Children 1-3 yrs.	500 (mg/day)	500 (mg/day)
Children 4-6 yrs.		600 (mg/day)
Children 4-8 yrs.	800 (mg/day)	
Children 7-9 yrs.		700 (mg/day)
Children 9-13 yrs.	900 (mg/day)	
Children 10-18 yrs.		1,300 (mg/day)
Adolescents 14-18 yrs.	1,300 (mg/day)	
Adults 19-50 yrs.	1,000 (mg/day)	
Adults 19-65 yrs.		1,000 (mg/day)
Adults > 50 yrs.	1,200 (mg/day)	
Adults ≥ 65 yrs.		1,300 (mg/day)
Postmenopausal women		1,300 (mg/day)

Vitamin D

Age	Adequate intake, U.S.		FAO/WHO recommendations	
Up to 50 yrs.	200 IU/day	5 mcg/day	200 IU/day	5 mcg/day
Adults 51-65 yrs.			400 IU/day	10 mcg/day
Adults 51-70 yrs.	400 IU/day	10 mcg/day		
Adults ≥ 65 yrs.			600 IU/day	15 mcg/day
Adults ≥ 71 yrs.	600 IU/day	15 mcg/day		

FAO/WHO = Food and Agriculture Organization and World Health Organization
IU = International Unit
mcg = microgram
mg = milligram

(Illustration by Corey Light. Cengage Learning, Gale)

and early adulthood, more bone is produced than removed, reaching its maximum mass and strength by the mid-30s. After that, bone is lost at a faster pace than it is formed, so the amount of bone in the skeleton begins to slowly decline. Most cases of osteoporosis occur as an acceleration of this normal **aging** process, which is referred to as primary osteoporosis. The condition can also be caused by other disease processes or prolonged use of certain medications that result in bone loss; if so, it is called secondary osteoporosis.

Osteoporosis occurs most often in older people, especially in women after **menopause**. It affects nearly half of all adults, men and women, over the age of 75. Women, however, are five times more likely than men to develop the disease. They have smaller, thinner bones than men to begin with, and they lose bone mass more rapidly after menopause (usually around age 50), when they stop producing a bone-protecting hormone called estrogen. In the five to seven years following menopause, women can lose about 20% of

their bone mass. By age 65 or 70, though, men and women lose bone mass at the same rate.

As an increasing number of men live longer, health professionals are increasingly aware that osteoporosis is an important health issue for men as well. In fact, men account for about 20% of all spinal fractures and up to 30% of all hip fractures due to osteoporosis.

Causes and symptoms

A number of factors increase the risk of developing osteoporosis. They include:

- Age. Osteoporosis is more likely as people grow older and their bones lose strength.

- Sex. Women are more likely to have osteoporosis because they start out with less bone. They also lose bone tissue more rapidly as they age. While women commonly lose 30 to 50% of their bone mass over their lifetimes, men lose only 20 to 33% of theirs.

Osteoporosis in the vertebrae

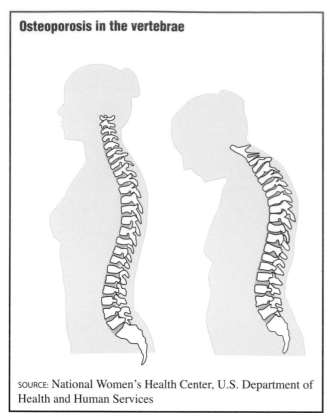

SOURCE: National Women's Health Center, U.S. Department of Health and Human Services

Osteoporosis is most common in the hips, wrist, and vertebrae (spine). The vertebrae are most important because these bones support the body to stand and sit upright. The vertebrae on the left is normal and the vertebrae on the right has been affected by osteoporosis. *(Illustration by GGS Information Services. Cengage Learning, Gale)*

- Race. Caucasian and Asian women are most at risk for the disease, but African American and Hispanic women can get it too.

- Body type. Women with small bones or thin frames are more liable to develop osteoporosis.

- Early menopause. Women who begin menopause early because of heredity, surgery, or lots of physical exercise may lose large amounts of bone tissue early in life. Such conditions as anorexia and bulimia may also lead to early menopause and osteoporosis.

- Lifestyle. People who smoke or drink too much or do not get enough exercise have an increased chance of getting osteoporosis.

- Medications. Certain prescription medications may speed up the loss of bone. These drugs include methotrexate, cimetidine, corticosteroids, and heparin.

- Diet. Adults who do not get enough calcium or protein may be more likely to have osteoporosis. People who constantly diet are more prone to the disease.

Osteoporosis is often called the silent disease because bone loss occurs without symptoms. People often do not know they have the disease until a bone breaks, frequently in a minor fall that would not typically cause a fracture. A common occurrence is compression fractures of the spine. These can happen even after a seemingly normal activity, such as bending or twisting to pick up a light object. The fractures can cause severe back **pain**, but sometimes they go unnoticed. Either way, the vertebrae collapse on themselves, and the person actually loses height. The hunchback appearance of many elderly women, sometimes called dowager's hump or widow's hump, is due to the effect of osteoporosis on the vertebrae.

Diagnosis

Certain types of doctors may have more training and experience than others in diagnosing and treating people with osteoporosis. These include a geriatrician, who specializes in treating the aged; an endocrinologist, who specializes in treating diseases of the body's endocrine system (glands and hormones); and an orthopedic surgeon, who treats fractures, such as those caused by osteoporosis.

Before making a diagnosis of osteoporosis, the doctor usually takes a complete medical history, conducts a physical examination, and orders x rays, as well as blood and urine tests, to rule out other diseases that cause loss of bone mass. The doctor may also recommend a bone density test, which is the only way to know for certain if osteoporosis is present. It can also show how far the disease has progressed.

Several diagnostic tools are available to measure the density of a bone. The ordinary x ray is one, though it is the least accurate for early detection of osteoporosis because it does not reveal bone loss until the disease is advanced and most of the damage has already been done. Two other tools that are more likely to catch osteoporosis at an early stage are computed tomography (CT) scans and machines called densitometers, which are designed specifically to measure bone density.

The CT scan, which takes a large number of x rays of the same spot from different angles, is an accurate test but uses higher levels of radiation than other methods. The most accurate and advanced of the densitometers uses a technique called DEXA (dual energy x ray absorptiometry). With the DEXA scan, a double x-ray beam takes pictures of the spine, hip, or entire body. It takes about 20 minutes, is painless, and exposes the patient to only a small amount of radiation—about 1/50 that of a chest x ray.

Medicare covers a test that measures bone resorption, an important measure for tracking a patient's response to osteoporosis therapy. The relatively inexpensive test measures a baseline amount then compares amounts from later tests to track progress. The test consists of simple urine collection.

People should talk to their doctors about their risk factors for osteoporosis and if and when to have a bone density test. Ideally, women should have bone density measured at menopause and periodically afterward, depending on the condition of their bones. Men should be tested starting at age 65. Men and women with additional risk factors, such as those who take certain medications, may need to be tested earlier.

Treatment

Alternative treatments for osteoporosis focus on maintaining or building strong bones. They include nutritional and herbal therapies and **homeopathy**.

Nutritional therapy

A healthful diet low in fats and animal products and containing whole grains, fresh fruits and vegetables, and calcium-rich foods (such as dairy products, dark-green leafy vegetables, sardines, salmon, and almonds), along with nutritional supplements (such as calcium, **magnesium**, and **vitamin D**) are important components of nutritional approaches to treating this disease.

Women should also eat more soy products such as tofu, soy burgers, other soy-based products, or miso. Soy beans contain a substance called isoflavones which have estrogen-like activity. Isoflavones may help to increase bone density, alleviate **hot flashes** and other menopausal symptoms, lower the risk of **cancer**, and even reduce the risk of heart attacks. Natural hormone therapy, such as the use of soy products, is a safer alternative to synthetic estrogenic hormones, which may increase the risk of **breast cancer**.

In addition, women should avoid foods that may accelerate bone loss. They should avoid having too much salt in their diet, not only because salt raises the blood pressure but also because it may contribute to osteoporosis. They should also cut down on coffee, caffeinated sodas, and alcohol. High consumption of these beverages, studies have shown, are associated with accelerated drop in bone density and increase risk of bone fracture in old age. Caffeinated sodas are especially bad for the bones because in addition to containing **caffeine**, they have high amounts of phosphoric acid. Phosphoric acid increases bone resorption, thus decreasing bone density.

Herbal supplements

Herbal supplements for osteoporosis emphasize such calcium-containing plants as **horsetail** (*Equisetum arvense*), oat straw (*Avena sativa*), **alfalfa** (*Medicago sativa*), **licorice** (*Glycyrrhiza glabra*), **marsh mallow** (*Althaea officinalis*), and sourdock (*Rumex crispus*). There are, however, few data from clinical trials to support the use of these herbs.

Homeopathy

Homeopathic remedies for osteoporosis focus on treatments believed to help the body absorb calcium. These remedies may include such substances as *Calcarea carbonica* (calcium carbonate) or *Silica* (flint). Again, there are few data other than isolated case reports regarding the effectiveness of these remedies.

Allopathic treatments

There are a number of good treatments for primary osteoporosis, most of them medications. For people with secondary osteoporosis, treatment may focus on curing the underlying disease.

Drugs

For most women who have gone through menopause, the best treatment for osteoporosis is hormone replacement therapy (HRT), also called estrogen replacement therapy. In addition to alleviating hot flashes, synthetic estrogens protect women against **heart disease** and they help to relieve and prevent osteoporosis. HRT increases a woman's supply of estrogen, which helps build new bone while preventing further bone loss.

The Women's Health Initiative (WHI), a large 15-year government-funded research study, concluded in a 2006 report that the drug Prempro (estrogen combined with progestin), which is used in hormone therapy, is associated with a modest increase in the risk of breast cancer, **stroke**, and **heart attack**. The WHI also demonstrated that in patients who had a hysterectomy, estrogen therapy alone was associated with an increase in the risk of stroke, but not of breast cancer or cardiovascular (heart) disease. A large study from the National Cancer Institute indicated that long-term use of estrogen therapy may be associated with an increased risk of **ovarian cancer**. Estrogen therapy is approved for treatment of menopausal symptoms but should be prescribed for the shortest period of time possible. When used solely for the prevention of postmenopausal osteoporosis, any estrogen/hormone therapy regimen should only be considered for women at significant risk of osteoporosis, and non-estrogen medications should be carefully considered first. The women in the WHI were participating in a follow-up phase of the study that was anticipated to last until 2010.

For people who cannot or decide not to take estrogen/hormone therapy, other medications can be good choices. These include a class of drugs called bisphosphonates, such as alendronate (Fosamax), risedronate (Actonel), and ibandronate (Boniva). Another bisphosphonate, zoledronic acid (Reclast), is approved to treat postmenopausal osteoporosis. Alendronate and another drug, calcitonin (Miacalein, Fortical), both stop bone loss, help build bone, and decrease fracture risk by as much as 50%. Both drugs attach to bone that has been targeted by bone-eating osteoclasts. They protect the bone from these cells. Osteoclasts help the body break down old bone tissue. Calcitonin is a hormone that has been used as an injection for many years. A subsequent version was on the market as a nasal spray in 2008. Side effects of these drugs are minimal, but calcitonin builds bone by only 1.5% a year. Fosamax has proven safe in very large multi-year studies and is as of 2008 indicated for treatment of osteoporosis in most men. Boniva is a pill that is taken once a month.

Another drug approved by the FDA to treat and prevent osteoporosis is raloxifene (Evista). It is from a class of drugs called estrogen agonists/antagonists, commonly called selective estrogen receptor modulators. Raloxifene appears to prevent bone loss in the spine, hips, and total body. It has been shown to benefit bone mass and turnover and can decrease the risk of vertebral fractures. Also approved for postmenopausal women and men with osteoporosis who have a high risk for fracture, is teriparatide (Forteo), an injectable form of human parathyroid hormone. Unlike other osteoporosis drugs, teriparatide works by stimulating new bone formation in the spine and hips.

Medications under study in the late 2000s include other biphosphonates that slow bone breakdown (such as alendronate), **sodium** fluoride, and vitamin D metabolites.

Surgery

Unfortunately, much of the treatment for osteoporosis is for fractures that result from advanced stages of the disease. For complicated fractures, such as broken hips, hospitalization and a surgical procedure are required. In hip replacement surgery, the broken hip is removed and replaced with a new hip made of plastic or a combination of metal and plastic. Despite often-successful surgeries, a large percentage of those who survive are unable to return to their previous level of activity, and many end up moving from self-care to a supervised living situation or nursing home. That is why prevention, getting early treatment, and taking steps to reduce bone loss are vital.

Expected results

There is no cure for osteoporosis, but it can be controlled. Most people who have osteoporosis fare well once they get treatment. The medicines available build bone, protect against bone loss, and halt the progress of this disease.

Prevention

Building strong bones, especially before the age of 35, and maintaining a healthy lifestyle are the best ways of preventing osteoporosis. To build as much bone mass as early as possible in life and to help slow the rate of bone loss later in life, individuals should do the following:

- Get calcium in foods: Experts recommend 500 to 1,300 milligrams (mg) of calcium per day for children, 1,300 mg for adolescents, 1,000 mg for ages 19 to 50, and 1,200 mg for people 51 and older. The dosage for pregnant or lactating women ages 14 to 18 is 1,300 mg daily and 1,000 mg for age 19 and older. Foods are the best source for this important mineral. Milk, cheese, and yogurt have the highest amounts. Other foods that are high in calcium are green leafy vegetables, tofu, shellfish, Brazil nuts, sardines, and almonds.

- Take calcium supplements: Many people, especially those who do not like or cannot eat dairy foods, do not get enough calcium in their diets and may need to take a calcium supplement. Supplements should be taken with meals and accompanied by six to eight glasses of water a day.

- Get vitamin D: Vitamin D helps the body absorb calcium. People can get vitamin D from sunshine with a quick (15–20 minute) walk each day or from foods such as liver, fish oil, and vitamin D fortified milk. During the winter months it may be necessary to take supplements. Four hundred mg daily is usually the recommended amount.

- Avoid smoking and alcohol: Smoking reduces bone mass, as does heavy drinking. To reduce risk, individuals ought not to smoke, and ought to limit alcoholic drinks to no more than two per day. An alcoholic drink is 1.5 oz of hard liquor, 12 oz of beer, or 5 oz of wine.

- Exercise regularly: Exercising regularly builds and strengthens bones. Weight-bearing exercises, in which bones and muscles work against gravity, are best.

KEY TERMS

Alendronate—A non-hormonal drug used to treat osteoporosis in postmenopausal women.

Anticonvulsants—Drugs used to prevent convulsions or seizures. They often are prescribed in the treatment of epilepsy.

Biphosphonates—Compounds (such as alendronate) that slow bone loss and increase bone density.

Calcitonin—A naturally occurring hormone made by the thyroid gland that can be used as a drug to treat osteoporosis and Paget's disease of the bone.

Estrogen—Female hormone produced mainly by the ovaries and released by the follicles as they mature. Responsible for female sexual characteristics, estrogen stimulates and triggers a response from at least 300 tissues. After menopause, the production of the hormone gradually decreases and eventually stops.

Glucocorticoids—A general class of adrenal cortical hormones that are mainly active in protecting against stress and in protein and carbohydrate metabolism. They are widely used in medicine as anti-inflammatories and immunosuppresives.

Osteoblasts—Cells in the body that build new bone tissue.

Osteoclasts—Cells that break down and remove old bone tissue.

Selective estrogen receptor modulator—A hormonal preparation that offers the beneficial effects of hormone replacement therapy (HRT) without the increased risk of breast and uterine cancer associated with HRT.

These include aerobics, dancing, jogging, stair climbing, tennis, walking, and lifting weights. People who have osteoporosis may want to attempt gentle exercise, such as walking, rather than jogging or fast-paced aerobics, which increase the chance of falling. Individuals ought to exercise three to four times per week for 20 to 30 minutes each time.

Resources

BOOKS

Bissinger, Margie. *Osteoporosis: An Exercise Guide.* Parsippany, NJ: Workfit Consultants, 2008.

Gueldner, Sarah H., et al. *Osteoporosis: Clinical Guidelines for Prevention, Diagnosis, and Management.* New York: Springer, 2007.

Nelson, Miriam E., and Sarah Wernick. *Strong Women, Strong Bones.* New York: Perigee Trade, 2006.

Pirello, Robert, and Bernardo A. Merizalde. *B.O.N.E.S : Beating Osteoporosis Naturally, Easily, Sensibly.* Philadelphia: Xlibris, 2006.

PERIODICALS

Arnst, Catherine. "Bones of Contention: Drugmakers Are Stoking Fears of Fracture Among Middle-Aged Women. But Experts Say the Risk Is Low." *Business Week* (February 11, 2008): 34.

Bates, Betsy. "Higher Vitamin D Doses Will Be Stressed in Fracture Guides." *Skin & Allergy News* (February 2008): 58.

Belt-Marchesi, June. "Osteoporosis in Men." *Clinical Reference Systems* (May 31, 2007): N/A.

Dean, Angela. "Get with the Strength: Complementary Therapies to Prevent & Treat Osteoporosis." *Pharmacy News* (November 22, 2007): 17.

Duck, Julie, and Carl T. Amodio. "Bone Health and Osteoporosis: Make No Bones About These Important Minerals." *Chiropractic Products* (January 2008): 26(2).

Hudson, Tori. "Phytoestrogen Intake Prevents Bone Loss." *Townsend Letter: The Examiner of Alternative Medicine* (February/March 2008): 141.

ORGANIZATIONS

Arthritis Foundation, PO Box 7669, Atlanta, GA, 30357-0669, (800) 283-7800, http://www.arthritis.org.

National Osteoporosis Foundation, 1232 Twenty-second St. NW, Washington, DC, 20036-4603, (800) 223-9994, http://www.nof.org.

Osteoporosis Canada, 1090 Don Mills Rd., Suite 301, Toronto, ON, M3C 3R6, Canada, (800) 463-6842, http://www.osteoporosis.ca.

Mai Tran
Ken R. Wells

Otitis media *see* **Ear infection**

Ovarian cancer

Definition

Ovarian **cancer** is a disease in which the cells in the ovaries become abnormal, start to grow uncontrollably, and form tumors. Ninety percent of all ovarian cancers develop in the cells that line the surface of the ovaries and are called epithelial cell tumors.

Description

The ovaries are a pair of almond-shaped organs that lie in the pelvis on either side of the uterus. The fallopian tubes connect the ovaries to the uterus. The

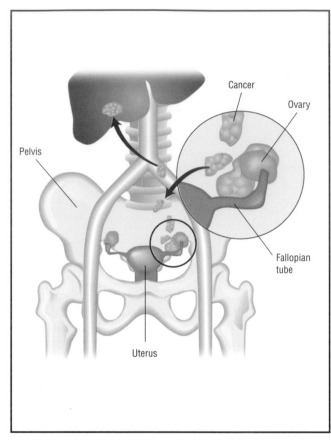

Pelvis

Cancer

Ovary

Fallopian
tube

Uterus

A close-up of a cancerous growth on the ovary. *(Illustration by GGS Information Services, Inc. Cengage Learning, Gale)*

ovaries produce and release usually one egg each month during the menstrual cycle. Along with the adrenal gland, the ovaries also produce the female hormones estrogen and progesterone, which regulate and maintain the secondary female sexual characteristics.

Ovarian cancer is the fifth most common cancer among women in the United States. It accounts for 4% of all cancers in women. However, the death rate due to this cancer is higher than that of any other cancer among women. About 1 in 70 women in the United States was anticipated to develop ovarian cancer, and 1 in 100 was anticipated to die from it. The National Cancer Institute (NCI) estimated that 21,650 new cases of ovarian cancer would be diagnosed in the United States in 2008, and that 15,520 women would die from the disease.

Ovarian cancer can develop at any age, but more than half the cases occur among women who are 65 years old or older. The incidence of the disease is highest among Native American women, followed by Caucasian, Vietnamese, Hispanic, and Hawaiian women. Only 50% of the women who are diagnosed with ovarian cancer survive five years after initial

diagnosis. This low survival rate is because at the time of initial diagnosis, the cancer is usually in an advanced stage. It is difficult to diagnose ovarian cancer early because often there are no warning symptoms, and the disease spreads relatively quickly. In addition, the ovaries are situated deep in the pelvis and small tumors cannot be detected easily during a routine physical examination.

Causes and symptoms

The actual cause of ovarian cancer is not known, but several factors are known to increase a woman's chances of developing the disease. These are called risk factors. The major risk factors for cancer in general are tobacco, alcohol, diet, sexual and reproductive behavior, infectious agents, family history, occupation, environment, and pollution. There are several risk factors particularly associated with ovarian cancer.

- Age. The incidence of the disease increases with age. Half of all cases are diagnosed after age 65.

- Race. The incidence of the disease is highest among Native American women and lowest among Korean and Chinese women.

- High-fat diet. When Asian women move to the more affluent Western countries and adopt a diet that is rich in fat, the incidence of ovarian cancer among them rises. Furthermore, ovarian cancer is highest in those countries with the highest consumption of dairy foods (Switzerland, Denmark, and Sweden) and lowest in those countries with the lowest dairy intake (Japan, South Korea, Singapore). Ovarian cancer is also linked to high socioeconomic status in women.

- Family history. Women who have even one close relative with the disease have a threefold increase in risk. In addition, if a woman has had breast cancer, she is at an increased risk for ovarian cancer.

- Early menstruation/late menopause. Menstruating early (before age 12) and experiencing menopause late seem to put women at a higher risk for ovarian cancer. It is believed that the longer a woman ovulates, the higher her risk of ovarian cancer (some researchers think exposure to estrogen during the monthly cycles is the cause). Since ovulation occurs only during the childbearing years, the longer she menstruates, the greater her risk. Pregnancy gives a break from ovulation and exposure to estrogen for nine months. Hence, multiple pregnancies actually appear to reduce the risk of ovarian cancer. Similarly, since oral contraceptives suppress ovulation and reduce exposure to estrogen, women who take birth control pills have a lower incidence of the disease.

- Fertility drugs. One study has shown that prolonged use of certain fertility drugs, such as clomiphene citrate, may increase a woman's risk of developing ovarian tumors.
- Talcum powder. Some studies have suggested that the use of talcum powder in the genital area may double a woman's risk of getting the cancer. The incidence of ovarian cancer is higher than normal among female workers exposed to asbestos. Since talc contains particles of asbestos, some researchers believe that is what accounts for the increased risk.

Ovarian cancer has no specific signs or symptoms in the early stages of the disease. There may be some vague, nonspecific symptoms that are often ignored. However, if any of the symptoms persist, it is essential to have them evaluated by a doctor immediately. Only a doctor can determine whether the symptoms are an indication of early ovarian cancer; however, the presence of two or more of the following symptoms is reason for concern. The patient may experience:

- pain or swelling in the abdomen
- bloating, and a general feeling of abdominal discomfort
- constipation, nausea, or vomiting
- loss of appetite, fatigue
- unexplained weight gain (generally due to an accumulation of fluid in the abdomen)
- vaginal bleeding in postmenopausal women.

Diagnosis

Patients with ovarian cancer were once thought to exhibit no symptoms in the early stage of the disease. But newer studies have shown that certain symptoms are more common in women with early stage ovarian cancer. These symptoms include bloating, pelvic or abdominal **pain**, difficulty eating or feeling full early, and urinary problems, such as frequency or urgency, according to the National Comprehensive Cancer Network. If ovarian cancer is suspected, the doctor typically begins the diagnosis by taking a complete medical history to assess all the risk factors. A thorough pelvic examination is conducted. Blood tests to determine the level of a particular blood protein, CA125, may be ordered. This protein is usually elevated in women with ovarian cancer. However, it is not a definitive test because the levels may also rise in other gynecologic conditions, such as **endometriosis** and ectopic **pregnancy**. Researchers have found another biological marker, a protein called prostasin that appears to be specific to ovarian cancer. While prostasin should not be used as the only blood test for ovarian cancer, assessment of prostasin levels together with CA125 levels improves the likelihood of early detection. Ultrasound is almost always used to check the size of the ovaries. Standard imaging techniques such as computed tomography scans (CT scans) and magnetic resonance imaging (MRI) may be used to determine the condition of the ovaries and if the disease has spread to other parts of the body. Ultrasonography, which uses ultrasound waves to produce images of the ovaries, is also used to diagnose ovarian cancer.

A noninvasive technique for early detection of ovarian cancer involves a genetically altered virus. Researchers at the University of Alabama engineered a **common cold** virus to infect ovarian cancer cells with a green fluorescent protein that reveals the cancer cells. The technique can also be used to monitor the effectiveness of therapy.

Other tests for the early detection of ovarian cancer were undergoing development as of 2008. One of the most promising is a blood test for asymptomatic early-stage ovarian cancer. The test, developed by researchers at Yale University, has shown a 99% accuracy rate in early trials. Further testing was underway as of early 2008, and if approved by the U.S. Food and Drug Administration (FDA), the test could be available in late 2008 or early 2009.

In order to determine if the tumor is benign or cancerous, surgery is necessary. If the tumor appears to be small from the imaging tests, then a procedure known as laparoscopy may be used. A tiny incision is made in the abdomen and a slender, hollow, lighted instrument is inserted through it. This device lets the doctor view the ovary more closely and to obtain a piece of tissue for microscopic examination. If the tumor appears large, a laparotomy is performed under general anesthesia. This procedure combines both diagnosis and treatment for ovarian cancer because the tumor is often completely removed at this time. A piece of the tissue that is removed will be examined under a microscope to determine whether the tumor was benign or malignant.

Surgery confirms the diagnosis, but ovarian cancer is often strongly suspected before surgery based on symptoms and ultrasound. The goal of surgery is to completely remove the cancer, but often this is not possible.

Diagnosis in alternative treatment uses mainstream diagnostic techniques and supplements them with thorough physical and psychological examinations. Considerations such as lifestyle, relationships, and emotional and psychological histories are used to complete an overall portrait of a patient's health in order to develop holistic strategies for healing.

Treatment

There are many alternative treatments available to help with ovarian cancer. Alternative treatments can be used in conjunction with, or separate from, surgery, chemotherapy, and radiation therapy. When used with conventional treatment, alternative treatments have been shown to decrease pain and side effects, aid in the recovery process, and improve the quality of life of cancer patients.

Alternative treatment of cancer is complicated, and there are many choices in therapies and alternative practitioners. Consumers should consult as many trained healthcare practitioners as possible when choosing alternative therapies. If consumers are willing to ask questions and thoroughly research their options, they can increase their chances of getting the best possible alternative support for the difficult task of treating cancer.

Alternative medicine generally views cancer as a holistic problem. That is, cancer represents a problem with the body's overall health and immunity. As such, treatment is holistic as well, striving to strengthen and heal the physical, mental, and emotional aspects of patients. Alternative cancer treatments may emphasize different basic approaches, which include traditional medicines, mind/body approaches, physical approaches, nutritional and dietary approaches, integrated approaches, and experimental programs.

Traditional medicines

Traditional Chinese medicine uses **acupuncture**, **acupressure** massage, herbal remedies, and movement therapies such as t'ai chi and **qigong** to treat cancer. Traditional Chinese herbal remedies have already contributed a significant number of anticancer drugs, and studies have shown their anticancer properties. Acupuncture has been shown to reduce some tumors, significantly reduce pain, and support and improve immune system activity.

Ayurvedic medicine uses **detoxification**, herbal remedies, massage, **exercise**, **yoga**, breathing techniques, and **meditation** as part of its cancer treatment. *Panchakarma* is an extensive detoxification and strengthening program that is recommended for cancer patients and those undergoing chemotherapy and radiation. **Panchakarma** uses **fasting**, special vegetarian **diets**, enemas, massage, herbal medicines, and other techniques to rid the body of excess toxins (believed to contribute to chronic diseases such as cancer) and to strengthen the immune system. Some Ayurvedic herbs may also have significant anticancer properties.

Naturopathy and **homeopathy** are traditional Western healing systems using herbal medicines and other techniques to strengthen the immune system and reduce the pain of cancer treatment. **Western herbalism** is also beginning to compile studies of many herbs that have potential anticancer and immune strengthening properties (such as **mistletoe**).

Mind/body approaches

Mind/body treatments seek to help patients with the mental and spiritual challenges posed by cancer and to mobilize the body's own defenses and immune system. Some of these therapies include **psychotherapy**, support groups, **guided imagery**, visualization techniques, meditation, **biofeedback**, hypnosis, breathing techniques, and yoga. Mind/body approaches work with the idea that the mind and emotions can profoundly influence the health of the body. These techniques help patients manage the **stress** and **anxiety** that accompany cancer. Mind/body techniques have also been shown to stimulate the immune system and to reduce the pain of symptoms and conventional treatments.

Physical approaches

Physical approaches to cancer include exercise; massage therapies; movement therapies, including yoga, t'ai chi, and qigong; breathing techniques; and **relaxation** techniques. These therapies strive to increase immune system response, promote relaxation and stress reduction, and reduce side effects (such as pain, **nausea**, **vomiting**, weakness, and physical immobility) of conventional treatments.

Nutritional and dietary approaches

Cancer patients have heightened needs for diets free of toxic chemicals and full of cancer-fighting nutrients. Diet and **nutrition** may improve both a cancer patient's chances for recovery and the patient's quality of life during treatment. In laboratory studies, vitamins such as A, C, and E, as well as compounds such as isothiocyanates and dithiolthiones found in broccoli, cauliflower, and cabbage, and beta-carotene found in carrots, tomatoes, and salad greens, have been shown to protect against cancer. The minerals **selenium** and **zinc** are also important nutrients in the ovarian cancer diet. Omega-3 **essential fatty acids** such as **flaxseed** oil or **evening primrose oil** are recommended as well.

Dietary approaches for ovarian cancer include **vegetarianism**, the raw food diet, and macrobiotics. Cancer diets generally emphasize raw and fresh fruits, vegetables, whole grains, beans, and peas. These diets also restrict or eliminate intake of fat, meat, dairy products, sugar, hydrogenated oils, processed foods, and foods with additives and artificial ingredients. **Caffeine** and alcohol are generally prohibited, and overeating is strongly discouraged.

Many herbs have been shown to have anticancer, immune enhancing, and symptom reducing properties. Some of the herbs used for ovarian problems include burdock, **mullein**, **yarrow**, vitex, **dandelion**, **black cohosh**, St. John's wort, red **raspberry**, nettles, and **Siberian ginseng**. Chinese herbs include **astragalus**, **ginger**, **dong quai**, cinnamon, rehmannia root, and scrophularia root. Patients should consult a competent herbalist or naturopathic doctor for individualized herbal support for ovarian cancer.

At least five plant extracts and 69 compounds isolated from plants have been shown to have antitumor activity against ovarian cancers. Recent additions to the list include triterpenes isolated from *Manihot esculenta*, a plant found in the Suriname rain forest, and from *Ligulariopsis shichuana*, a plant used in traditional Chinese medicine to bring down inflammation. **Green tea** consumption also improved the survival rate of women with epithelial ovarian cancer, a Chinese study reported in 2007. Green tea is high in polyphenols, which studies have shown to have powerful antioxidant and antitumor properties.

Integrated approaches

Keith Block, a conventional doctor and oncologist (cancer specialist), integrates many alternative practices into his cancer treatment center affiliated with the Chicago Medical School. His program seeks to provide individualized cancer treatment using both conventional therapies while integrating alternative healing techniques. Block advocates a special diet (based on vegetarianism and macrobiotics), exercise, psychological support, and herbal and nutritional supplements. Block's program has received acclaim for both treatment success and satisfaction of patients.

Experimental programs

Antineoplaston therapy was developed by Stanislaw Burzynski, a Polish doctor, who began practicing in Houston, Texas. Burzynski has isolated a chemical, deficient in those with cancer that he believes stops cancer growth, and his treatment has shown some promise.

Joseph Gold, the director of the Syracuse Cancer Research Institute, discovered that the chemical hydrazine sulfate has many positive effects in cancer patients, including stopping weight loss, shrinking tumors, and increasing survival rates.

The Livingston therapy was developed by the late Virginia Livingston, an American doctor. She asserted that cancer is caused by certain bacteria that she claimed are present in all tumors. She advocated a detoxification program and special diet that emphasized raw or lightly cooked, primarily vegetarian foods, with special vitamin and nutritional supplements.

The **Gerson therapy** has been the best known nutritional therapy for cancer. It is available in two clinics in California and Mexico. It consists of a basic vegetarian diet low in salt and fat, with high dosages of particular nutrients using raw fruit and vegetable juices. The Gerson therapy also requires patients to drink raw calf's liver juice, believed to aid the liver, and advocates frequent coffee enemas (thought to help the body evacuate toxins). There is no scientific evidence that supports the effectiveness of Gerson therapy.

Allopathic treatment

The cornerstone of allopathic treatment for ovarian cancer is surgery. The goal is to remove as much of the cancer as possible. Chemotherapy, which involves the use of powerful anticancer drugs to kill the cancer cells, is usually administered after the surgery to destroy any remaining cancer. As of 2008 some drugs to treat ovarian cancer were in the clinical trial stage, including monoclonal antibody treatment for advanced ovarian cancer. Radiation therapy is not routinely used for ovarian cancer.

The type of surgery depends on the extent of the disease. In most procedures, the ovaries, uterus, and fallopian tubes are completely removed. In rare cases, if the cancer is not very aggressive and the woman is young and has not had children, a more conservative approach may be adopted. Only one ovary may be removed, and, if possible, the fallopian tubes and the uterus may be left intact. Occasionally, in addition to the female reproductive organs, the appendix may also be removed. The liver and the intestine will be examined for signs of cancer and may be biopsied. Ovarian cancer spreads contiguously, which means that it moves to the organs that are next to it. In some cases, extensive surgery may be needed to remove as much of the cancer as possible.

If the patient's cancer is advanced, she may be treated with radiation therapy, chemotherapy, or both. Chemotherapy may be either systemic or intraperitoneal (IP), which means that the drugs are injected into the abdomen. The most common drug used is paclitaxel (Taxol), combined with either cisplatin or carboplatin. Cancers that do not respond to these combinations may be treated with topotecan (Hycamtin) or with a combination of paclitaxel and epirubicin (Ellence).

One drug treatment for ovarian cancer under development in 2008, enzastaurin, was undergoing clinical trial in combination with two existing drugs, docetaxel and prednisone, in several European countries. The clinical trials were expected to be completed in January 2010. The drug is also being tested in Europe to treat breast and colorectal cancers.

Expected results

Most often ovarian cancer is not diagnosed until it is in an advanced stage, making it the most deadly of the female reproductive cancers. More than 50% of the women who are diagnosed with the disease die within five years. If ovarian cancer is diagnosed while it is still localized to the ovary, more than 90% of the patients will survive five years or more. However, only 24% of all cancers are found at this early stage.

There are no clinical studies that show alternative medicine can cure cancer, but many treatments have been shown to help improve symptoms, control the pain and side effects of conventional treatments, speed healing, and increase the quality of life for cancer patients. Alternative therapies may be strongest as preventative measures, before major problems such as cancer occur in the body, and as supportive measures, used with allopathic medicine.

Prevention

There are ways to reduce one's risks of developing ovarian cancer. As of 2008, genetic tests were available that could help to determine whether a woman who has a family history of breast, endometrial, or ovarian cancer has inherited the mutated gene that predisposes her to these cancers. (However, this mutation affects only a few women.) If the woman tests positive for the mutation, then she may opt to have her ovaries removed (a procedure called an oophorectomy). Allopathic medicine often recommends removing the ovaries as prevention even when a clear genetic component is not found, and this procedure is called a prophylactic oophorectomy.

Having one or more children, preferably having the first before age 30, and breast-feeding may decrease a woman's risk of developing the disease. High-risk women are advised to undergo periodic screening with transvaginal ultrasound or a blood test for CA125 protein. The American Cancer Society recommends annual pelvic examinations for all women after age 40, in order to increase the chances of early detection of ovarian cancer.

Alternative medicine stresses preventative measures that avoid removing the ovaries, unless a clear genetic risk has been established. Some studies have shown that removal of the ovaries does not necessarily reduce the risk of cancer, and does not necessarily increase longevity rates in women.

Having sound physical and mental health can significantly reduce the chances of getting cancer of any type. The following guidelines are generally recommended by doctors, nutritionists, and alternative practitioners for cancer prevention and recovery.

- Do not smoke.
- Do not drink alcohol excessively.
- Exercise regularly, at least 20 minutes per day. It is better to exercise outdoors in the fresh air.
- Avoid exposure to radiation. This includes avoiding unnecessary x rays, not residing near sources of natural or man-made radiation, and avoiding occupational exposure to radiation.
- Avoid exposure to harmful chemicals, in food, the home, and the workplace.
- Maintain proper body weight and avoid obesity.
- Protect the skin from overexposure to sunlight. People should avoid direct exposure to sunlight between 11 a.m. and 3 p.m., and take other necessary precautions against sunburn.
- Eat a healthy diet. People should become educated on and practice dietary principles that reduce the risk of cancer. These principles include eating plenty of raw and fresh fruits, vegetables, beans, and whole grains. People should consume organically grown foods when possible, minimize overeating, reduced the intake of meat and dairy products, increase fiber, avoid processed and artificial foods. They should also avoid canned foods, including soft drinks; avoid sugar and refined starch products, such as white flour; reduce the intake of fat; avoid hydrogenated vegetable oils such as margarine and shortening; and drink filtered or spring water. A study of nearly 50,000 women, called the Women's Health Initiative, reported in 2008 that women who reduced their fat intake for at least four years had a 40% reduced risk of ovarian cancer compared to women who did not reduce their dietary intake of fat.
- Strive to maintain sound mental and emotional health. It is helpful to learn a technique such as yoga, t'ai chi, or meditation to reduce stress and promote relaxation. People should maintain healthy relationships and social support systems.

KEY TERMS

Computed tomography (CT) scan—A series of x rays that are put together by a computer in order to form detailed pictures of areas inside the body.

Ectopic pregnancy—A pregnancy that develops outside of the uterus, such as in the fallopian tube. Ectopic pregnancies often cause severe pain in the lower abdomen and are potentially life-threatening because of the massive blood loss that may occur as the developing embryo/fetus ruptures and damages the tissues in which it has implanted.

Endometriosis—A condition in which the tissue that normally lines the uterus (endometrium) grows in other areas of the body, causing pain, irregular bleeding, and frequently, infertility.

Magnetic resonance imaging (MRI)—An imaging technique that uses a large circular magnet and radio waves to generate signals from atoms in the body. These signals are used to construct detailed images of internal body structures and organs, including the brain.

Monoclonal antibody—A protein substance that is produced in the laboratory from a single clone of a B-cell, the type of cell of the immune system that makes antibodies. Monoclonal antibodies are used in cancer treatment.

Paclitaxel—A drug derived from the common yew tree (*Taxus baccata*) that is the mainstay of chemotherapy for ovarian cancer.

Prostasin—A blood protein that appears to be a reliable early indicator of ovarian cancer.

Transvaginal ultrasound—A technique for imaging the ovaries using sound waves generated by a probe inserted into the vagina. This diagnostic imaging procedure serves as the baseline for a hysterosonographic examination.

Resources

BOOKS

Alschuler, Lise N., and Karolyn A. Gazella. *Alternative Medicine Magazine's Definitive Guide to Cancer: An Integrative Approach to Prevention, Treatment, and Healing.* San Francisco: Celestial Arts, 2007.

Dizon, Don S. *100 Questions & Answers About Ovarian Cancer,* 2nd ed. Sudbury, MA: Jones and Bartlett, 2006.

Sheen, Barbara. *Diseases and Disorders—Ovarian Cancer.* Farmington Hills, MI: Lucent Books, 2005.

PERIODICALS

Hudson, Tori. "Green Tea Enhances Survival of Ovarian Cancer Patients." *Townsend Letter: The Examiner of Alternative Medicine* (August/September 2007): 161(2).

Jenkins, Rebecca. "New Hope for Early Ovarian Cancer Detection." *Australian Doctor* (February 22, 2008): 3.

Parch, Lorie A. "Silent No More: At Last There's Consensus About Symptoms that Could Allow Ovarian Cancer to be Detected at an Earlier, More Treatable Stage." *Town & Country* (November 2007): 146.

Pedersen, Amanda. "Higher Levels of HE4 May Be Sign of Ovarian Cancer, Study Reveals." *Diagnostics & Imaging Week* (December 20, 2007): 3.

Wendling, Patrice. "Serial Screening Combo May Flag Early Ovarian Cancer." *Internal Medicine News* (September 1, 2007): 25.

ORGANIZATIONS

American Cancer Society, 250 Williams St., Atlanta, GA, 30303, (800) 227-2345, http://www.cancer.org.

American Institute of Homeopathy, 801 N. Fairfax St., Suite 306, Alexandria, VA, 22314, (888) 445-9988, http://www.homeopathyusa.org.

British Association for Cancer Research, Institute of Cancer Research, McElwain Laboratories, Cotswold Road, Sutton, SM2 5NG, Great Britain, (44) 020-8722-4208, http://www.bacr.org.uk.

Canadian Cancer Society, 10 Alcorn Ave., Suite 200, Toronto, ON, M4V 3B1, Canada, (416) 961-7223, http://www.cancer.ca.

Women's Cancer Resource Center, 5741 Telegraph Ave., Oakland, CA, 94609, (888) 421-7900, http://www.wcrc.org.

Douglas Dupler
Ken R. Wells

Ovarian cysts

Definition

Ovarian cysts are fluid-filled sacs that form inside or on the surface of the ovaries, which are the female reproductive organs that lie in the lower abdomen. Ovarian cysts appear and disappear regularly as part of the normal menstrual cycle. The cysts can, however, become a medical problem if they remain in the ovaries, enlarge, and cause **pain** or other symptoms.

Description

Ovarian cysts develop as a normal part of a healthy menstrual cycle; mature ovaries very often have cysts in them. The cysts that appear during the regular activity of the ovaries are called functional cysts. There are two types of functional cysts, known as follicular cysts and luteal cysts respectively.

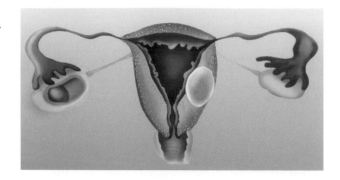

Ovarian cyst (on the left). *(VEM / Photo Researchers, Inc.)*

In the ovaries, immature eggs are stored in the follicles, which are tiny tube-like membranes. When **menstruation** begins in the early teens, women have nearly 400,000 follicles that store and produce eggs in the ovaries. During each menstrual cycle, an egg matures inside one of the follicles, and the follicle sac fills up with a liquid (*liquor folliculi*) that nourishes the growing egg. This swollen follicle is a follicular cyst. When the egg is released into the fallopian tube during ovulation, the follicle opens or ruptures and the fluid drains away. Sometimes there is pain associated with ovulation, known as *Mittelschmerz*, which is a German word that means middle pain. *Mittelschmerz* may last from a few minutes to several days. A small amount of bleeding may also accompany the normal release of an egg from the follicle.

After ovulation, another functional cyst forms on the ovary where the egg was released. This cyst is called the *corpus luteum*, or luteal cyst. The luteal cyst has the function of secreting progesterone, an important female hormone that regulates the reproductive cycle. If no **pregnancy** occurs, the luteal cyst should disappear with the continuation of the menstrual cycle.

Abnormalities in the menstrual cycle may cause cysts to remain and grow irregularly. Sometimes the follicles stay filled with liquid after the egg is released, or the egg does not get released in the proper way and the follicle continues to grow. These follicular cysts can reach 2 in (5 cm) or more in diameter, and may cause pain and pressure. They may rupture completely. Luteal cysts can also become abnormal. These cysts can grow quite large, to 3 in (8 cm) or more in diameter, and can cause sharp pain in the abdomen. Luteal cysts are often misdiagnosed as ectopic (tubal) pregnancies, particularly when they break open and cause bleeding and severe pain. Sometimes a cyst can bleed; it is then known as a *corpus hemorrhagicum*, meaning a body that bleeds. Bleeding often occurs when the cyst

KEY TERMS

Antiandrogen—A substance that blocks the action of androgens, the hormones responsible for male characteristics.

Dermoid tumor—A skin-like benign growth that may appear on the ovary and resemble a cyst.

Ectopic pregnancy—A pregnancy that develops outside of the mother's uterus, such as in the fallopian tube. Ectopic pregnancies often cause severe pain in the lower abdomen and are potentially life-threatening because of the massive blood loss that may occur as the developing embryo/fetus ruptures and damages the tissues in which it has implanted.

Functional cyst—A benign cyst that forms on the ovary and resolves on its own without treatment.

Hirsutism—An abnormal growth of hair on the face and other parts of the body caused by an excess of androgens. Also known as hypertrichosis.

McCune-Albright syndrome (MCAS)—A genetic syndrome characterized in girls by the development of ovarian cysts and puberty before the age of 8, together with abnormalities of bone structure and skin pigmentation.

Mittelschmerz—A German word for the pain that some women experience at ovulation.

Ovulation—The monthly process by which an ovarian follicle ruptures releasing a mature egg cell.

Polycystic ovarian syndrome (PCOS)—A condition in which the eggs are not released from the ovaries and instead form multiple cysts.

naturally breaks and begins to go away. When bleeding lasts for longer than several days and a large cyst remains, surgical intervention is sometimes called for. Surgery on the ovaries is usually performed through an instrument called a laparoscope. A laparoscope is a small device with a tiny camera.

Other types of cysts and growths may occur on the ovaries as well. Neoplastic (new growth) cysts may appear, which are benign (noncancerous) growths. These cysts occur when cells of the ovaries not related to ovulation begin to grow abnormally. Dermoid tumors are a type of benign growth that may occur on the ovaries and resemble cysts. Abnormal cysts may contain fluid or blood, and may be inside the ovary or next to it under the surface. Other cysts can be solid or contain cellular debris. All abnormal cysts require close watch by a doctor.

There is also a condition known as **polycystic ovary syndrome** (PCOS), in which the eggs and follicles are not released from the ovaries and instead form multiple cysts. **Obesity** is linked to this condition, as 50% of women with PCOS are also obese. Hormonal imbalances play a major role in this condition, including high levels of the hormone androgen and low levels of progesterone, the female hormone necessary for egg release. High levels of insulin, the hormone that regulates blood sugar, are often found in women with PCOS. PCOS is also characterized by irregular menstrual periods, **infertility**, and hirsutism (excessive hair growth on the body and face). Although PCOS was formerly thought to be an adult-onset condition, more recent research indicates that it begins in childhood, possibly even during fetal development.

In adolescent girls, ovarian cysts may be associated with a genetic disorder known as McCune-Albright syndrome, which is characterized by abnormal bone growth, discoloration of the skin, and early onset of puberty. The ovarian cysts are responsible for the early sexual maturation.

Causes and symptoms

The causes of nonfunctional ovarian cysts are not yet fully understood. Many factors are believed to play a role in the development of cysts, including a woman's general state of health, weight, diet, personal history, and lifestyle. The mind/body connection may also be a factor with cysts, as **stress** and **anxiety** may be prominent factors. Some alternative practitioners and psychotherapists believe that unexpressed creativity and repressed emotions like guilt and anger may be linked to problems in the ovaries. For PCOS, obesity, hormonal imbalances and high blood insulin levels are closely linked to the condition. For example, women with PCOS are five to ten times more likely to develop type 2 (adult-onset) diabetes than women in the general population.

PCOS is also known to run in families, which suggests that genetic factors contribute to its development. The specific gene or genes responsible for PCOS have not yet been identified; however, several groups of researchers in different countries have been investigating genetic variations associated with increased risk of type 2 diabetes in order to determine whether the same genetic variations may be involved in PCOS.

McCune-Albright syndrome is known to be associated with mutations in the GNAS1 gene. The mutation is sporadic, which means that it occurs during the child's development in the womb and that the syndrome is not inherited.

Some cysts can be asymptomatic (without symptoms), while others can cause swelling, aching, sharp pain, and bleeding. Pain from cysts may last from a few minutes to a few days. Other symptoms of cysts include late or missed periods, feelings of pressure or weight in the lower abdomen, and **constipation** and problems urinating due to internal pressure from cysts. Ruptured cysts can cause intense pain, and produce symptoms resembling those of appendicitis, infection or ectopic pregnancy. Medical attention should be sought at once for the following symptoms:

- sudden sharp pain in the lower abdomen
- persistent pain on the right side of the abdomen accompanied by sickness, fever, or vomiting
- abdominal pain along with vaginal discharge, fever, or swelling
- intermittant bursts of pain in the lower abdomen during intercourse, bowel movements, or exercise

Diagnosis

The majority of ovarian cysts in adults are found during routine pelvic examinations performed by doctors or gynecologists (specialists in women's sexual organs and health issues). An ultrasound test can be given to identify the location, size and probable type of cyst. Cysts less than 1.6 in (4 cm) in diameter are considered normal in premenopausal women. Doctors examine cysts closely to make certain they are not fibroid tumors or **cancer**. The cysts may be watched for a few months to allow them to go away or shrink on their own. For abnormal, painful or bleeding cysts, a biopsy may be performed. A biopsy is a procedure in which a small amount of tissue is surgically removed and examined to determine the exact type of growth. In alternative treatment, practitioners will closely consider lifestyle, diet, and emotional and psychological profiles in order to identify all the factors that may be playing a role in the development of cysts.

Ovarian cysts can be diagnosed in female fetuses by transabdominal ultrasound during the mother's pregnancy.

Treatment

Alternative treatment strives to reduce the possible causes and symptoms of cysts. Consumers should search for practitioners who have experience treating women's problems in general and ovarian cysts in particular. Because cysts may have many possible causes, ranging from hormone imbalances to emotional stress, a holistic approach to healing should include measures to balance and improve physical, emotional, and mental health. Preventive and supportive measures include dietary and nutritional changes, herbal supplementation, hot/cold compresses, daily **exercise**, and stress management through mind/body techniques. Treatments for existing cysts include such traditional healing systems as **traditional Chinese medicine**, Ayurveda, **homeopathy**, and **naturopathic medicine**.

Diet and nutrition

Dietary guidelines for treatment and prevention of cysts include:

- Eliminating caffeine and alcohol.
- Reducing intake of sugars, including honey and maple syrup, and refined starches such as white flour products.
- Increasing use of foods rich in vitamin A and carotenoids; good choices include carrots, tomatoes, and salad greens.
- Eating foods high in B vitamins such as whole grains.
- Including a dietary source of iodine such as seaweed for thyroid support.

Nutritional supplements include:

- Omega-3 essential fatty acids, such as flaxseed oil or evening primrose oil to promote hormonal balance. Essential fatty acids are also found in fatty fish like salmon and trout.
- Vitamins A, C, and E, and the minerals zinc and selenium. Zinc and selenium should be taken at different times. A good multivitamin and mineral supplement is also recommended.

Herbal therapies

Herbs that promote hormonal balance, steady blood sugar levels, and immune system strengthening are generally recommended. Herbs used to treat cysts include burdock, **mullein**, **yarrow**, vitex, **dandelion**, **black cohosh**, **St. John's wort**, red **raspberry**, nettles and **Siberian ginseng**. Chinese herbs include **astragalus**, **ginger**, **dong quai**, cinnamon, rehmannia root, and scrophularia root, although the specific formula that is given is tailored to the symptoms of the specific patient. A competent herbalist or naturopathic doctor should be consulted for herbal treatment of ovarian cysts.

Compresses

Compresses can be used to stimulate circulation and healing in the ovaries. A hot water bottle covered with a towel soaked in castor and **essential oils** can be applied to the lower abdomen near the ovaries.

Lavender, **rosemary**, and **chamomile** are recommended essential oils. A hot compress can also be made by heating in a warm oven a cloth soaked in castor and essential oils, which is then applied to the lower abdomen. Bags of ice covered with towels can be used alternately as cold treatments to increase local circulation.

Exercise and bodywork

Daily exercise for twenty minutes or more is recommended. Exercising outdoors in plenty of sunlight may help regulate hormones. **Yoga** includes exercises specifically designed to increase circulation and healing in the lower abdomen, and is an excellent stress-reduction technique as well.

Mind/body therapies

Mind/body therapies seek to heal the emotional and psychological components that may be contributing to cyst formation. Stress reduction can be achieved through yoga, **meditation**, **t'ai chi**, breathing techniques, progressive **relaxation**, and others. Visualization techniques, yoga, and **qigong** may help stimulate healing in the internal organs. Some practitioners have theorized that problems in the ovaries may be linked to certain emotional states. For instance, the ovaries are the organs that create life, and blocked creativity in women may contribute to their dysfunction. Furthermore, the ovaries are the specific female organs, and some healers have proposed that women who suffer abuse, low self-esteem, guilt and anger may be susceptible to ovarian problems. **Psychotherapy**, support groups, and other mind/body therapies seek to help women uncover and confront emotional issues.

Other systems

Traditional Chinese medicine utilizes **acupuncture**, **acupressure**, dietary and herbal remedies for ovarian cysts. **Ayurvedic medicine** uses herbal remedies, diet, exercise, yoga, massage, and **detoxification**. Homeopathic practitioners prescribe the remedies *Apis* for cysts on the right ovary and *Colocynthis* for cysts on the left ovary, as well as other remedies for hormone and immune system balance. Naturopathy tends to view ovarian cysts as associated with blood sugar problems, and uses herbal, dietary and other natural remedies to balance hormone and insulin levels.

Allopathic treatment

The treatment of ovarian cysts may vary according to the type of cyst and the patient's symptoms. Some cysts can be drained of fluid with the use of a fine needle, although this treatment has been shown to be no more effective in eliminating cysts than leaving them alone. Many cysts, particularly small ones, can be watched closely for several months to determine if they will go away on their own. Ultrasound is used to view cysts. A laparoscopy is a surgical procedure that may be used to correct bleeding cysts and other cyst conditions without removing the ovary, and allows doctors to view the ovaries. Doctors advise surgical removal for cysts that are larger than 4 in (10 cm) and for complex cysts. Complex cysts are solid or have additional growths inside them.

Most uncomplicated ovarian cysts in female infants resolve on their own shortly after delivery. Complicated cysts are treated by laparoscopy or laparotomy after the baby is born.

McCune-Albright syndrome is treated with testolactone (Teslac), an anti-estrogen drug that corrects the hormonal imbalance caused by the ovarian cysts.

Long-term management of PCOS has been complicated in the past by lack of a clear understanding of the causes of the disorder. Most commonly, hormonal therapy has been recommended, including estrogen and progesterone and such other hormone-regulating drugs as ganirelix (Antagon). Birth control pills have also been prescribed by doctors to regulate the menstrual cycle and to shrink functional cysts. In severe and painful cases, the ovaries have been removed by surgery.

More recent studies have shown that increasing sensitivity to insulin in women with PCOS leads to improvement in both the hormonal and metabolic symptoms of the disorder. This sensitivity is increased by either weight loss and exercise programs or by medications. Metformin (Glucophage), a drug originally developed to treat type 2 diabetes, has been shown to be effective in reducing the symptoms of hyperandrogenism as well as **insulin resistance** in women with PCOS.

Another strategy that is being tried with PCOS is administration of flutamide (Eulexin), a drug normally used to treat **prostate cancer** in men. Preliminary results indicate that the antiandrogenic effects of flutamide benefit patients with PCOS by increasing blood flow to the uterus and ovaries.

A surgical procedure known as ovarian wedge resection appears to improve fertility in women with PCOS who have not responded to drug treatments. In an ovarian wedge resection, the surgeon removes a portion of the polycystic ovary in order to induce ovulation.

Expected results

Neither type of functional ovarian cyst, follicular or luteal, has been shown to progress to cancer. When cysts do not go away on their own, they often can be removed without harming the ovaries. Some women have opted to live with large cysts instead of surgery without negative consequences. The chances for cysts recurring can vary. Some women never have cysts, others get them once or occasionally, while others see them appear and disappear almost constantly. Likewise, ovarian cysts can be painful and bothersome for some women, while other women experience no symptoms.

Resources

BOOKS

Blum, Jeanne. *Woman Heal Thyself: An Ancient Healing System for Contemporary Women.* New York: Tuttle, 1995.

Hobbs, Christopher, and Kathi Keville. *Women's Herbs, Women's Health.* Loveland, CO: Interweave Press, 1998.

Morgan, Peggy, and the Editors of Prevention Magazine. *The Female Body: An Owner's Manual.* Emmaus, PA: Rodale, 1996.

Northrup, Christiane, M.D. *Women's Bodies, Women's Wisdom.* New York: Bantam, 1994.

"Pelvic Pain." Section 18, Chapter 237 in *The Merck Manual of Diagnosis and Therapy*, edited by Mark H. Beers, MD, and Robert Berkow, MD. Whitehouse Station, NJ: Merck Research Laboratories, 1999.

"Physical Conditions in Adolescence." Section 19, Chapter 275 in *The Merck Manual of Diagnosis and Therapy*, edited by Mark H. Beers, MD, and Robert Berkow, MD. Whitehouse Station, NJ: Merck Research Laboratories, 1999.

"Pregnancy Complicated by Disease: Disorders Requiring Surgery." Section 18, Chapter 251 in *The Merck Manual of Diagnosis and Therapy*, edited by Mark H. Beers, MD, and Robert Berkow, MD. Whitehouse Station, NJ: Merck Research Laboratories, 1999.

PERIODICALS

Ajossa, S., S. Guerriero, A. M. Paoletti, et al. "The Antiandrogenic Effect of Flutamide Improves Uterine Perfusion in Women with Polycystic Ovary Syndrome." *Fertility and Sterility* 77 (June 2002): 1136–1140.

de Sanctis, C., R. Lala, P. Matarazzo, et al. "Pubertal Development in Patients with McCune-Albright Syndrome or Pseudohypoparathyroidism." *Journal of Pediatric Endocrinology and Metabolism* 16 (March 2003) (Suppl. 2): 293–296.

Ehrmann, D. A., P. E. Schwarz, M. Hara, et al. "Relationship of Calpain-10 Genotype to Phenotypic Features of Polycystic Ovary Syndrome." *Journal of Clinical Endocrinology and Metabolism* 87 (April 2002): 1669–1673.

Elkind-Hirsch, K. E., B. W. Webster, C. P. Brown, and M. W. Vernon. "Concurrent Ganirelix and Follitropin Beta Therapy is an Effective and Safe Regimen for Ovulation Induction in Women with Polycystic Ovary

Syndrome." *Fertility and Sterility* 79 (March 2003): 603–607.

Franks, S. "Adult Polycystic Ovary Syndrome Begins in Childhood." *Best Practice and Research: Clinical Endocrinology and Metabolism* 16 (June 2002): 263–272.

Kazerooni, T., and M. Dehghan-Kooshkghazi. "Effects of Metformin Therapy on Hyperandrogenism in Women with Polycystic Ovarian Syndrome." *Gynecological Endocrinology* 17 (February 2003): 51–56.

Legro, R. S. "Polycystic Ovary Syndrome. Long-Term Sequelae and Management." *Minerva ginecologica* 54 (April 2002): 97–114.

Marx, T. L., and A. E. Mehta. "Polycystic Ovary Syndrome: Pathogenesis and Treatment Over the Short and Long Term." *Cleveland Clinic Journal of Medicine* 70 (January 2003): 31–33, 36–41, 45.

Mittermayer, C., W. Blaicher, D. Grassauer, et al. "Fetal Ovarian Cysts: Development and Neonatal Outcome." *Ultraschall in der Medizin* 24 (February 2003): 21–26.

Ovalle, F., and R. Azziz. "Insulin Resistance, Polycystic Ovary Syndrome, and Type 2 Diabetes Mellitus." *Fertility and Sterility* 77 (June 2002): 1095–1105.

Vankova, M., J. Vrbikova, M. Hill, et al. "Association of Insulin Gene VNTR Polymorphism with Polycystic Ovary Syndrome." *Annual of the New York Academy of Sciences* 967 (June 2002): 558–565.

Yildirim, M., V. Noyan, M. Bulent Tiras, et al. "Ovarian Wedge Resection by Minilaparatomy in Infertile Patients with Polycystic Ovarian Syndrome: A New Technique." *European Journal of Obstetrics, Gynecology, and Reproductive Biology* 107 (March 26, 2003): 85–87.

ORGANIZATIONS

American College of Obstetricians and Gynecologists (ACOG). 409 12th Street, SW, P. O. Box 96920, Washington, DC 20090-6920. http://www.acog.org.

The Health Resource. 209 Katherine Drive. Conway, AR 72032. (501) 329-5272.

Herb Research Foundation. 1007 Pearl Street, Suite 200. Boulder, CO 80302.

Polycystic Ovarian Syndrome Association. P. O. Box 80517, Portland, OR 97280. (877) 775-PCOS. www.pcosupport.org.

Douglas Dupler
Rebecca J. Frey, PhD

Overweight *see* **Obesity**

Oxygen/ozone therapy

Definition

Oxygen/ozone therapy is a term that describes a number of different practices in which oxygen, ozone, or hydrogen peroxide are administered via **gas** or

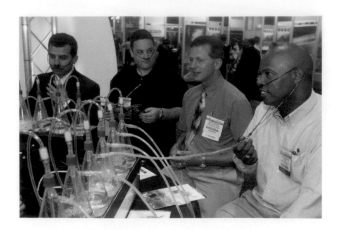

These men are receiving oxygen treatments at an oxygen bar. *(Jeff Greenberg / Alamy)*

water to kill disease microorganisms, improve cellular function, and promote the healing of damaged tissues. The rationale behind bio-oxidative therapies, as they are sometimes known, is the notion that as long as the body's needs for **antioxidants** are met, the use of certain oxidative substances will stimulate the movement of oxygen atoms from the bloodstream to the cells. With higher levels of oxygen in the tissues, bacteria and viruses are killed along with defective tissue cells. Healthy cells survive and multiply more rapidly. The result is a stronger immune system. The use of oxygen and/or ozone for therapeutic treatment is sometimes called hyperbaric, meaning high-pressure therapy.

Ozone itself is an allotrope (form) of oxygen, O_3, produced when ultraviolet light or an electric spark passes through air or oxygen. It is a toxic gas that creates free radicals, the opposite of what antioxidant vitamins do. Oxidation, however, is good when it occurs in harmful foreign organisms that have invaded the body. Ozone inactivates many disease bacteria and viruses.

Origins

The various forms of oxygen and ozone therapy have been in use since the late nineteenth century. The earliest recorded use of oxygen to treat a patient was by French surgeon J. A. Fontaine. who built a mobile operating device for the treatment in 1879. **Cancer** researchers first began using hyperbaric oxygen in the 1950s. The term hyperbaric means that the oxygen is given under pressure higher than normal air pressure. Recently, oxygen therapy has also been touted as a quick purification treatment for mass-market consumers. Oxygen bars can be found in airports and large cities, and provide pure oxygen in 20-minute sessions for less than $20. While proponents claim that breathing oxygen will purify the body, most medical doctors do not agree. What is more, oxygen can be harmful to people with severe lung diseases, and these people should never self-treat with oxygen.

Ozone has been used since 1856 to disinfect operating rooms in European hospitals and since 1860 to purify the water supplies of several large German cities. Ozone was not, however, used to treat patients until 1915, when the German doctor Albert Wolff began to use it to treat skin diseases with the gas. During World War I, the German Army used ozone to treat **wounds** and anaerobic **infections**. In the 1950s, several German physicians used ozone to treat cancer alongside mainstream therapeutic methods. According to some estimates, in the 2000s there were more than 15,000 ozone practitioners in Europe, although the number was much smaller in the United States. The European figure includes medical doctors as well as naturopaths and homeopaths.

Hydrogen peroxide is familiar to most people as an over-the-counter preparation that is easily available at supermarkets as well as pharmacies; it is used as an antiseptic for cleansing minor **cuts** and scrapes. It was first used as an intravenous infusion in 1920 by a British physician in India, T. H. Oliver, to treat a group of 25 Indian patients who were critically ill with **pneumonia**. Oliver's patients had a mortality rate of 48%, compared to the standard mortality rate of 80% for the disease. In the 1920s, an American physician William Koch experimented with hydrogen peroxide as a treatment for cancer. He left the United States after a legal battle with the Food and Drug Administration (FDA). In the early 1960s, researchers at Baylor University studied the effects of hydrogen peroxide in removing plaque from the arteries as well as its usefulness in treating cancer, but their findings were largely ignored.

Benefits

Oxygen and ozone therapies are thought to benefit patients in the following ways:

- Stimulating white blood cell production
- Killing viruses (ozone and hydrogen peroxide)
- Improving the delivery of oxygen from the blood stream to the tissues of the body
- Speeding up the breakdown of petrochemicals
- Increasing the production of interferon and tumor necrosis factor, thus helping the body to fight infections and cancers
- Increasing the efficiency of antioxidant enzymes

- Increasing the flexibility and efficiency of the membranes of red blood cells
- Speeding up the citric acid cycle, which in turn stimulates the body's basic metabolism

Description

Oxygen, ozone, and hydrogen peroxide are used therapeutically in a variety of different ways.

Hyperbaric oxygen therapy (HBO)

Hyperbaric oxygen therapy (HBO) involves putting the patient in a pressurized chamber in which he or she breathes pure oxygen for a period of 90 minutes to two hours. HBO may also be administered by using a tight-fitting mask, similar to the masks used for anesthesia. A nasal catheter may be used for small children.

Ozone therapy

Ozone therapy may be administered in a variety of ways:

- Intramuscular injection: A mixture of oxygen and ozone is injected into the muscles of the buttocks.
- Rectal insufflation: A mixture of oxygen and ozone is introduced into the rectum and absorbed through the intestines.
- Autohemotherapy: Between 10–15 mL of the patient's blood is removed, treated with a mixture of oxygen and ozone and reinjected into the patient.
- Intra-articular injection: Ozone-treated water is injected into the patient's joints to treat arthritis, rheumatism, and other joint diseases.
- Ozonated water: Ozone is bubbled through water that is used to clean wounds, burns, and skin infections, or to treat the mouth after dental surgery.
- Ozonated oil: Ozone is bubbled through olive or safflower oil, forming a cream that is used to treat fungal infections, insect bites, acne, and skin problems.
- Ozone bagging: Ozone and oxygen are pumped into an airtight bag that surrounds the area to be treated, allowing the body tissues to absorb the mixture.

Hydrogen peroxide

Hydrogen peroxide may be administered intravenously in a 0.03% solution. It is infused slowly into the patient's vein over a period of one to three hours. Treatments are given about once a week for chronic illness but may be given daily for such acute illnesses as pneumonia or **influenza**. A course of intravenous hydrogen peroxide therapy may range from one to 20 treatments, depending on the patient's condition and the type of illness being treated. Injections of 0.03% hydrogen peroxide have also been used to treat rheumatoid and **osteoarthritis**. The solution is injected directly into the inflamed joint.

Hydrogen peroxide is also used externally to treat stiff joints, **psoriasis**, and **fungal infections**. The patient soaks for a minimum of 20 minutes in a tub of warm water to which 1 pint of 35% food-grade hydrogen peroxide (a preparation used by the food industry as a disinfectant) has been added.

Preparations

Oxygen is usually delivered to the patient as a gas; ozone as a gas mixed with oxygen or bubbled through oil or water; and hydrogen peroxide as an 0.03% solution for intravenous injection or a 35% solution for external **hydrotherapy**.

Precautions

Patients interested in oxygen/ozone therapies must consult with a physician before receiving treatment. Hyperbaric oxygen treatment should not be given to patients with untreated pneumothorax, a condition in which air or gas is present in the cavity surrounding the lungs. Patients with a history of pneumothorax, chest surgery, **emphysema**, middle ear surgery, uncontrolled high fevers, upper respiratory infections, seizures, or disorders of the red blood cells are not suitable candidates for oxygen/ozone therapy. In addition, patients should be aware that oxygen should not be used near open flames since it greatly increases the rate of combustion.

Side effects

Typical side effects of oxygen or ozone therapy can include elevated blood pressure and ear pressure similar to that experienced while flying. Side effects may also include **headache**, numbness in the fingers, temporary changes in the lens of the eye, and seizures.

Research and general acceptance

Oxygen/ozone therapies are far more widely accepted in Europe than in the United States. In the 2000s, the most intensive research in these therapies was being conducted in the former Soviet Union and in Cuba. In the United States, the work of the Baylor researchers was not followed up. The National Center for Complementary and Alternative Medicine (NCCAM) of the National Institutes of Health sponsored four studies at the University of Pennsylvania on the use of hyperbaric oxygen in the treatment of four medical conditions.

KEY TERMS

Autohemotherapy—A form of ozone therapy in which a small quantity of the patient's blood is withdrawn, treated with a mixture of ozone and oxygen, and reinfused into the patient.

Hydrogen peroxide—A colorless, unstable compound of hydrogen and oxygen (H_2O_2). An aqueous solution of hydrogen peroxide is used as an antiseptic and bleaching agent.

Hyperbaric oxygen therapy (HBO)—A form of oxygen therapy in which the patient breathes oxygen in a pressurized chamber.

Ozone—A form of oxygen with three atoms in its molecule (O_3), produced by an electric spark or ultraviolet light passing through air or oxygen. Ozone is used therapeutically as a disinfectant and oxidative agent.

European research in ozone therapy has included studies in the oxygenation of resting muscles, the treatment of vascular disorders, and the relief of **pain** from herniated lumbar disks. Relatively little research on topics such as these was being conducted in the United States as of 2008.

Training and certification

In Europe, ozone therapies may be administered by licensed naturopaths and homeopaths as well as by medical doctors. In the United States and Canada, oxygen and ozone treatments are administered only by medical doctors.

Resources

BOOKS

Altman, Nathaniel. *The Oxygen Prescription: The Miracle of Oxidative Therapies.* Rochester, VT: Healing Arts Press, 2007.

Harch, Paul G., and Virginia McCullough. *The Oxygen Revolution: Hyperbaric Oxygen Therapy, The Groundbreaking New Treatment for Stroke, Alzheimer's, Parkinson's, Arthritis, Autism, Learning Disabilities and More.* Long Island City, NY: Hatherleigh Press, 2007.

Neuman, Tom S., and Stephen R. Thom. *Physiology and Medicine of Hyperbaric Oxygen Therapy.* St. Louis, MO: Saunders Elsevier, 2008.

PERIODICALS

Buettner, M. F., and D. Wolkenhauer. "Hyperbaric Oxygen Therapy in the Treatment of Open Fractures and Crush Injuries." *Emergency Medical Clinics of North America* (February 2007): 177–188.

Rockswold, S. B., G. L. Rockswold, and A. Defillo. "Hyperbaric Oxygen in Traumatic Brain Injury." *Neurological Research* (March 2007): 162–172.

Singhal, A. B. "A Review of Oxygen Therapy in Ischemic Stroke." *Neurological Research* (March 2007): 173–183.

Smerz, R. W. "Hyperbaric Oxygen Therapy: Caveat Doctor!" *Hawaii Medical Journal* (April 2005): 102–103.

OTHER

Neumeister, Michael. "Hyperbaric Oxygen Therapy." emedicine.com, July 21, 2005. http://www.emedicine.com/plastic/topic526.htm (February 19, 2008).

ORGANIZATIONS

American College of Hyperbaric Medicine, 9875 S. Franklin Dr., Suite 300, Franklin, WI, 53132, (414) 858-2240, http://www.hyperbaricmedicine.org/.

NIH National Center for Complementary and Alternative Medicine (NCCAM), NCCAM Clearinghouse. PO Box 7923, Gaithersburg, MD, 20898, (888) 644-6226, http://nccam.nih.gov.

Amy Cooper
Rebecca J. Frey, PhD
David Edward Newton, Ed.D.

P

Pain

Definition

Pain is an unpleasant feeling that is conveyed to the brain by sensory neurons. The discomfort signals actual or potential injury in the body. However, pain is more than a sensation or the physical awareness of pain; it also includes perception, the subjective interpretation of the discomfort. Perception gives information on the pain's location, intensity, and something about its nature. The various conscious and unconscious responses to both sensations and perception, including the emotional response, add further definition to the overall concept of pain.

Description

Pain arises from any number of situations. Injury is a major cause, but pain may also arise from a wide variety of illnesses. It may accompany a psychological condition, such as **depression**, or may even occur in the absence of a recognizable trigger.

Acute pain

Acute pain often results from ordinary tissue damage, such as a skin burn or broken bone. Acute pain can also be associated with headaches or **muscle cramps**. This type of pain usually goes away as the injury heals or the cause of the pain (stimulus) is removed.

To understand acute pain, it is necessary to understand the nerves that support it. Nerve cells, or neurons, perform many functions in the body. Although their general purpose, providing an interface between the brain and the body, remains constant, their capabilities vary widely. Certain types of neurons are capable of transmitting a pain signal to the brain.

As a group, these pain-sensing neurons are called nociceptors, and virtually every surface and organ of the body is wired with them. The central part of these cells is located in the spine, and they send threadlike projections to every part of the body. Nociceptors are classified according to the stimulus that prompts them to transmit a pain signal. Thermoreceptive nociceptors are stimulated by temperatures that are potentially tissue damaging. Mechanoreceptive nociceptors respond to a pressure stimulus that may cause injury. Polymodal nociceptors are the most sensitive and can respond to temperature and pressure. Polymodal nociceptors also respond to chemicals released by the cells in the area where the pain originates.

Nerve cell endings, or receptors, are at the front end of pain sensation. A stimulus at this part of the nociceptor unleashes a cascade of neurotransmitters (chemicals that transmit information within the nervous system) in the spine. Each neurotransmitter has a purpose. For example, substance P relays the pain message to nerves leading to the spinal cord and brain. These neurotransmitters may also stimulate nerves leading back to the site of the injury. This response prompts cells in the injured area to release chemicals that trigger an immune response and influence the intensity and duration of the pain.

Chronic and abnormal pain

Chronic pain refers to pain that persists after an acute injury heals, **cancer** pain, pain related to a persistent or degenerative disease, and long-term pain from an unidentifiable cause. It is estimated that one in three people in the United States experiences chronic pain at some point in their lives. Of these people, approximately 50 million are either partially or completely disabled.

Chronic pain may be caused by the body's response to acute pain. In the presence of continued stimulation of nociceptors, changes occur within the nervous system. Changes at the molecular level are dramatic and may include alterations in genetic transcription of neurotransmitters and receptors. These changes may also occur in the absence of an identifiable cause; one of the frustrating aspects of chronic pain is that the stimulus may be unknown. For example, the stimulus cannot be identified in as many as 85% of individuals suffering lower back pain.

Other types of abnormal pain include allodynia, hyperalgesia, and phantom limb pain. These types of pain often arise from some damage to the nervous system (neuropathic). Allodynia refers to a feeling of pain in response to a normally harmless stimulus. For example, some individuals who have suffered nerve damage as a result of viral infection experience unbearable pain from just the light weight of their clothing. Hyperalgesia is somewhat related to allodynia in that the response to a painful stimulus is extreme. In this case, a mild pain stimulus, such as a pin prick, causes a maximum pain response. Phantom limb pain occurs after a limb is amputated; although an individual may be missing the limb, the nervous system continues to perceive pain originating from the area.

Causes and symptoms

Pain is the most common symptom of injury and disease, and descriptions can range in intensity from a mere ache to unbearable agony. Nociceptors have the ability to convey information to the brain that indicates the location, nature, and intensity of the pain. For example, stepping on a nail sends an information-packed message to the brain: The foot has experienced a puncture wound that hurts a lot.

Pain perception also varies depending on the location of the pain. The kinds of stimuli that cause a pain response on the skin include pricking, cutting, crushing, burning, and freezing. These same stimuli would not generate much of a response in the intestine. Intestinal pain arises from stimuli such as swelling, inflammation, and distension.

Diagnosis

Pain is considered in conjunction with other symptoms and individual experiences. An observable injury, such as a broken bone, may be a clear indicator of the type of pain a person is suffering. Determining the specific cause of internal pain is more difficult. Other symptoms, such as **fever** or **nausea**, help narrow the possibilities. In some cases, such as lower back pain, a specific cause may not be identifiable. Diagnosis of the disease causing a specific pain is further complicated by the fact that pain can be referred to (felt at) a skin site that does not seem to be connected to the site of the pain's origin. For example, pain arising from fluid accumulating at the base of the lung may be felt in the shoulder.

Since pain is a subjective sensation, it may be very difficult to communicate its exact quality and intensity to other people. There are no diagnostic tests designed to determine the quality or intensity of an individual's pain. Therefore, a medical examination includes a lot of questions about where the pain is located, its intensity, and its nature. Questions seek to reveal what increases or relieves the pain, how long it has lasted, and whether there are any variations in it. An individual may be asked to use a pain scale to describe the pain. One such scale assigns a number to the pain intensity. For example, 0 may indicate no pain, and 10 may indicate the worst pain the person could imagine. Scales are modified for infants and children to accommodate their level of comprehension. Among the most painful non-trauma experiences are **childbirth** and **kidney stones**.

Treatment

Both physical and psychological aspects of pain can be dealt with through alternative treatment. Some of the most popular treatment options include herbal therapies, nutritional therapies, **homeopathy**, **acupressure** and **acupuncture**, massage, **chiropractic**, **guided imagery**, and **relaxation** techniques, such as **yoga**, hypnosis, and **meditation**. **Hydrotherapy** can also be beneficial for pain relief. A 2006 study reported that patients who received complimentary or alternative medical therapies before and after open heart surgery experienced less pain and tension during recovery than patients who received standard pain treatment. The therapies included music, massage, and guided imagery. The study of 104 men and women was conducted by the Minneapolis Heart Institute at Abbott Northwestern Hospital in Minneapolis.

Herbal therapies

Mild natural painkillers are used as herbal remedies for pain. They should only be used for mild to moderate chronic pain. However, unlike prescription drugs, they are not addictive and do not dull the senses. In addition, they can help heal the nervous system as well as relieve pain. The following herbal remedies have been known to provide pain relief:

- Capsaicin: found naturally in cayenne pepper. Its cream or gel form may be able to relieve some arthritic pain.
- Bromelain: reduce inflammation.
- Curcumin: reduces inflammation.
- Kava kava: helps relax the body.
- Pine-bark and grape-seed extracts: reduces inflammation.

- Pain-relief tea: is composed of white willow bark, chamomile, skullcap, valerian root, and licorice root. This herbal preparation may be effective in relieving normal aches and pain. However, persons with high blood pressure or those allergic to aspirin should avoid using this preparation.

Nutritional therapy

Diet and **nutrition** can play important roles in controlling chronic pain. Patients with chronic pain sometimes find relief just by eating healthy foods and by adding nutritional supplements with pain-killing properties. A diet high in fiber and complex carbohydrates is recommended. Because inflammation is often caused by allergic reactions, patients should eliminate allergic foods from their **diets**. They should also avoid foods high in fats or margarine, red meat, dairy products, shellfish, alcohol, and coffee. In addition, they may consider taking one of the following nutritional supplements: **flaxseed** oil, **bromelain**, **calcium** taken with **magnesium**, **vitamin C** taken with **bioflavonoids**, and **glucosamine**. Glucosamine sulfate is one of the best natural remedies available for arthritic pain, although studies show mixed results. Several studies have shown that it effectively reduces pain and improves joint movement in 80% of arthritic patients. It works by healing and regenerating new connective tissues damaged by the inflammatory process. It may also increase the level of endorphins, the body's natural painkillers, and reduces inflammation in most arthritic patients.

Researchers also have reported what thousands of people with arthritis have known for a long time—that cod liver oil eases the pain of arthritis. Several studies report that the **omega-3 fatty acids** in cod liver oil break down joint cartilage, slowing destruction of the joints and easing pain. This has been good news for arthritis sufferers who cannot tolerate the prescription drugs available for arthritis treatment. However, the Glucosamine/Chondroitin Arthritis Intervention Trial reported in 2006 that glucosamine and **chondroitin** did not reduce effectively pain in people with **osteoarthritis** of the knee. Nearly 1,600 patients with osteoarthritis of the knee took part in the study conducted at 16 centers across the United States. Not all of the news from the study was bad for the two-supplement combination. Study participants who reported moderate to severe pain, as opposed to mild pain, 79% reported significant pain reduction when taking glucosamine and chondroitin supplementation. The study lasted for six months and a majority of the participants said they suffered from mild osteoarthritis of the knee.

Homeopathy

Depending on a patient's specific condition, a homeopathic physician may prescribe one of the following medications for pain management:

- Arnica: for treatment of acute pain after an injury.

- Hypericum: for treatment of pain in nerves, fingers, or toes after injury or surgery.

- Ledum: for treatment of pain associated with black-and-blue bruises and puncture wounds.

In 2006, Miralus Healthcare began aggressively marketing its homeopathic **headache** formula HeadOn, which is applied topically to the forehead. In its now-famous television commercial, which many viewers deemed as annoying, an announcer quickly repeats three times the slogan, "HeadOn, apply directly to the forehead." It is not a coincidence that the ads are careful not to say that the product is for headache pain or can relieve headache pain. Making unsubstantiated medical claims is a violation of federal law. HeadOn is composed almost entirely of wax, with trace amounts of **potassium** bichromate (a chemical) and white bryony (a botanical) as active ingredients. As of early 2008, it came in six formulas: migraine relief, tension headache relief, headache relief, p.m. pain relief/sleep aid, sinus headache relief, and extra strength headache relief. The products cost about $8 to $10 and are primarily sold at discount pharmacies (Walgreens, CVS) and discount department store chains (Wal-Mart, Kmart). An article published in the September 2007 issue of *Consumer Reports* stated that HeadOn may "possibly" work "if users believe it will work." The article also stated that Miralus claimed clinical studies have been conducted on the product but refused to provide the magazine with details or copies of the studies. As of March 2008, there were no clinical studies posted on the Miralus Website (http://www.miralus.com). In 2006, the National Advertising Division (NAD) of the Council of Better Business Bureaus requested Miralus discontinue its ad claims regarding the performance and efficacy (effectiveness) of HeadOn due to insufficient evidence. In a written reply to NAD, Miralus disagreed with the conclusion but said it would consider the recommendation in developing future advertising. It did not provide NAD with any clinical studies of HeadOn. Miralus makes a number of other topical pain relief medications, including three formulations of RenewIn for joint care and ActivOn for arthritis pain. RenewIn and ActivOn retail for $12 to $15. As with HeadOn, Miralus does not claim RenewIn relieves pain, only that it provides "joint comfort."

Acupuncture

Acupuncture involves inserting needles at various points on the skin. These needles direct chi (life force) to organs or functions of the body. This therapy possibly works by triggering the release of endorphins, therefore dulling the perception of pain. Acupuncture can effectively reduce most chronic pain. However, it may require up to 10 sessions before results are noticeable. A 2002 study showed that acupuncture worked well for chronic **neck pain** and range of motion but that its long-term effects were limited. It is important that patients request disposable needles to prevent transmission of **AIDS**, **hepatitis**, and other infectious diseases.

Acupressure

There are some acupressure techniques that patients can train themselves to do to help relieve pain. Using thumbs or fingers to apply pressure at appropriate acupressure points in the body, a person can release muscular tension in the head, neck, or shoulder; calm the nervous system; and relieve painful symptoms. Like acupuncture, acupressure probably works by releasing endorphins.

Massage

Massage involves using physical manipulation techniques to make various parts of the body, such as muscles, connective tissues, and vertebrae, work together and function properly. This form of therapy may effectively reduce **stress** and physical pain.

Chiropractic

Chiropractors treat patients by manipulating joints and the spine. It is believed that pain, especially back pain, is caused by misalignment of the spine. This form of treatment is most effective in patients with persistent back pain and neck problems. It is also effective in some patients with acute, uncomplicated **low back pain**.

Relaxation therapy

Relaxation techniques include meditation, yoga, music, guided imagery, **biofeedback**, and **hypnotherapy**. When practiced regularly, these techniques have been shown to relax muscles and reduce tension and stress-related pain.

Lifestyle changes

Lifestyles can be changed to include a healthier diet and regular **exercise**. Regular exercise, aside from relieving stress, has been shown to increase endorphins.

Hydrotherapy

This form of therapy uses hot and cold compresses, whirlpools, saunas, and alternating cold/warm showers or body wraps to reduce the soreness of aching joints, inflamed muscles, chronic muscle **strains**, and backache. Some of these treatments can be done at home.

Allopathic treatment

There are many drugs aimed at preventing or treating pain. Nonopioid analgesics, narcotic analgesics, corticosteroids, anticonvulsant drugs, and tricyclic antidepressants work by blocking the production, release, or uptake of neurotransmitters. Nonopioid analgesics are used for treatment of minor pain. They include common over-the-counter medications such as aspirin, acetaminophen (Tylenol), and ibuprofen (Advil). Narcotic analgesics such as codeine, morphine, and methadone are used for more severe pain, such as cancer pain. These medications are available with a doctor's prescription. Initially developed to treat seizures and depression, some anticonvulsants and antidepressants also have pain-killing applications. Finally, corticosteroid injections directly into or near the nerve that is transmitting the pain signal are reserved for intractable (unrelenting) pain that is not treatable by other medications.

Drugs are not always effective in controlling pain. Surgical methods are used as a last resort if drugs and local anesthetics fail. Electrode implants are the least destructive surgical procedure. However, this method may not completely control pain and is not used frequently. Other surgical techniques involve destroying or severing the nerve, but the use of this technique is limited by side effects, including unpleasant numbness.

Expected results

Successful pain treatment is highly dependent on successful resolution of the pain's cause. Acute pain stops when an injury heals or when an underlying problem is treated successfully. Chronic pain and abnormal pain are more difficult to treat, and finding a successful resolution may take more time. Some pain is intractable and requires extreme measures for relief.

Prevention

Pain is generally preventable only to the degree that the cause of the pain is preventable; diseases and injuries are often unavoidable. However, increased pain, pain from surgery and other medical procedures, and continuing pain are preventable through drug treatments and alternative therapies.

KEY TERMS

Neuron—The fundamental nerve cell of the nervous system.

Neurotransmitters—Chemicals within the nervous system that transmit information from or between nerve cells.

Nociceptor—A nerve cell that is capable of sensing pain and transmitting a pain signal.

Referred pain—Pain that is experienced in one part of the body but originates in another organ or area. The pain is referred because the nerves that supply the damaged organ enter the spine in the same segment as the nerves that supply the area where the pain is felt.

Stimulus—Anything capable of eliciting a response in an organism or a part of that organism.

For many years, experts thought that arthritis patients should not exercise because it would damage their joints. However, a 2002 report stated that regular low-impact exercise such as water aerobics or riding a stationary bicycle can actually help arthritic patients prevent pain.

Resources

BOOKS

Berger, Phyllis. *The Journey to Pain Relief: A Hands-On Guide to Breakthroughs in Pain Treatment*. Alameda, CA: Hunter House, 2007.

Lewandowski, Michael J. *The Chronic Pain Care Workbook: A Self-Treatment Approach to Pain Relief Using the Behavioral Assessment of Pain Questionnaire*. Oakland, CA: New Harbinger, 2006.

Phillips, Maggie. *Reversing Chronic Pain: A 10-Point All-Natural Plan for Lasting Relief*. Berkeley, CA: North Atlantic Books, 2007.

Sadler, Jan. *Pain Relief Without Drugs: A Self-Help Guide for Chronic Pain and Trauma*. Rochester, VT: Healing Arts Press, 2007.

PERIODICALS

Archer, Shirley. "New Guidelines for Back Pain Including Yoga." *IDEA Fitness Journal* (January 2008): 89.

Archer, Shirley. "Qigong Helps Neck Pain." *IDEA Fitness Journal* (February 2008): 90.

Barrow, Karen. "The Right Pressure: Rolfing Eases Chronic Pain and Stress by Loosening the Connective Between Muscles and Bones." *Natural Health* (February 2008): 90(2).

Jackson, Emily, et al. "Does Therapeutic Touch Help Reduce Pain and Anxiety in Patients with Cancer?"
Clinical Journal of Oncology Nursing (February 2008): 113(8).

Menard, Martha Brown, and Cynthia Piltch. "Massage Soothes Chronic Pain." *Massage Therapy Journal* (Spring 2008): 153(3).

ORGANIZATIONS

American Chronic Pain Association, PO Box 850, Rocklin, CA, 95677-0850, (800) 533-3231, http://www.theacpa.org.

American Pain Society, 4700 W. Lake Ave., Glenview, IL, 60025, (847) 375-4715, http://www.ampainsoc.org/.

Canadian Pain Society. 701 Rossland Road East, Suite 373, Whitby, ON, L1N 9K3, Canada, (905) 668-9545, http://www.canadianpainsociety.ca.

Mai Tran
Ken R. Wells

Painful bladder syndrome *see* **Interstitial cystitis**

Paleolithic diet

Definition

The Paleolithic, or caveman, diet is a reversion to the foods eaten by humans prior to the advents of civilization, agriculture, and technology. Before those developments, the human diet during the Stone Age is thought to have consisted largely of lean red meat and vegetation. Modern-day adherents to Paleolithic **diets** add vigorous physical activity to mimic the Stone Age's hunter-gatherer lifestyle. In some cases, modern-day "Paleos" actually adopt such a lifestyle, hunting their own food in the natural environment.

Origins

The Paleolithic Period of human development, characterized by the use of chipped, stone tools, began about 2.5 million years ago. Whenever possible, Paleolithic peoples consumed large amounts of animal meat and offal, deriving 45-65% of their energy from animals. Among those aboriginal, hunter-gatherer societies in Australia, Africa, and South America that survived into the twentieth century, the rates of **cancer, rheumatoid arthritis, obesity**, diabetes, **osteoporosis, heart disease**, and other conditions were remarkably low until they switched to modern diets. In most other cultures, this switch to modern diets happened about 10,000 years ago, when it was discovered that many inedible plants could be rendered suitable for human consumption by cooking. This resulted in the introduction of grains, beans, and potatoes as foods, and later followed by sugar, milk, and milk products.

Benefits

Many nutritionists and scientists believe a Paleolithic diet and lifestyle might be an effective weapon against the adverse effects of modern affluence, reducing risk of heart disease, cancer, obesity, rheumatoid arthritis, and other conditions. Since this was the diet practiced during much of human evolution, advocates argue, it is the food that humans were designed to eat. Additionally, these advocates endorse the idea that milk (after weaning) and grains were never intended for human consumption.

Description

There is really no single Paleolithic diet. Hunter-gatherer cultures in different parts of the world ate widely differing diets, due to the availability in each locality. Stone Age diets also varied significantly depending on the season. Generally, however, such diets included much lean red meat from game, as well as eggs, fish, fruit, nuts, and vegetables. Excluded from most Paleolithic diets were grains (e.g., breads, pasta, cereals, corn), milk, refined sugars, beans, soy beans, or lentils. For twenty-first century adherents to Caveman diets, potatoes and peanuts are also forbidden. These diets are high in high-quality protein, fiber, vitamins, minerals, **iron**, mono-unsaturated fats, omega-3 fats, phytochemicals, and **antioxidants**. They are low in salt, saturated fats, enzyme inhibitors such as protease or amylase inhibitors, exorphins, and glycoalkaloids.

Precautions

Concerns have been expressed about the environmental effects of millions of people switching to diets heavy in red meats, requiring many agricultural operations to switch from growing crops to raising livestock. Sensitive wild areas could be ravaged in the search for insufficient quantities of Paleolithic foods. The global food supply is widely thought to be incapable of supporting widespread adoption of this diet. It is also believed that Stone Age peoples had access to a broader range of wild foods than are currently available, and modern-day "Paleos" should monitor their consumption to ensure a balanced diet. Some nutritionists caution against total dietary exclusion

---

of milk and milk products, arguing that low-fat dairy products can be useful to maintain sufficient levels of **calcium**.

Side effects

A balanced Paleolithic diet is thought to be generally free of harmful side effects, although anyone excluding milk and dairy products should be careful to maintain sufficient dietary levels of calcium to avoid problems such as osteoporosis, osteomalacia, rickets, and tetany.

Research and general acceptance

Many aspects of the Paleolithic diet have proven health benefits. There is absolutely no question that people who get plenty of **exercise** and eat lots of fruits and vegetables and avoid saturated fats tend to be healthier. Some experts are dubious, however, as to whether the benefits of the caveman diet extend into old age. They argue that diseases such as cancer, heart disease, and arthritis are found less frequently in hunter-gatherer societies because few members of those societies survive to an age at which those conditions become problems.

Training and certification

There is no organization dedicated specifically to training and certification of Paleolithic diet advisors, although a substantial number of scientists, physicians, and nutritionists are interested in the subject and can provide advice.

Resources

BOOKS

Audette, Raymond V. and Troy Gilchrist. *NeanderThin: Eat Like a Caveman to Achieve a Lean, Strong, Healthy Body*. New York: St. Martin's Press, 1999.

David Helwig

Palming *see* **Bates method**

Panax quinquefolius see **Ginseng, American**

Panchakarma

Definition

Panchakarma is the purification therapy used in **Ayurvedic medicine**. The word panchakarma means five actions, and refers to five procedures intended to intensively cleanse and restore balance to the body, mind, and emotions. Ayurvedic physicians use Panchakarma as a treatment for a wide variety of health conditions and as a preventative measure.

Origins

Ayurvedic medicine is the oldest healing system in the world, originating in the ancient civilizations of India some 3,000–5000 years ago. Ayurveda means knowledge of life in Sanskrit. Panchakarma is based on central concepts of Ayurveda, which state that disease is caused by the build-up of toxic substances in the body, and by imbalances in the body and mind.

Today, Ayurvedic medicine is used by millions of people, including at least half of the population of India. Ayurveda has become an increasingly accepted alternative medical treatment in America during the last couple of decades, aided by the efforts of Deepak Chopra, a conventionally trained M.D. who has written bestselling books based in part on Ayurvedic principles. Several Ayurvedic institutes and health clinics in America now perform panchakarma and conduct studies of its healing effects. A study in 2004 estimated that about three-quarters of a million Americans had used Ayurveda at least once, and 154,000 people had used it within the previous 12 months.

The ideas behind panchakarma have influenced other alternative treatments: Environmental medicine studies how the accumulation of environmental substances in the body may cause disease, and **detoxification** therapy relies upon cleansing the body as its central treatment.

Benefits

Panchakarma is used in Ayurvedic medicine to treat almost all diseases, particularly those that are chronic, metabolic, or stress-related in origin. Practitioners have used panchakarma to treat **allergies**, **asthma**, arthritis, **cancer**, **chronic fatigue syndrome**, **colitis**, high **cholesterol**, **depression**, diabetes, digestive disorders, **heart disease**, **hypertension**, immune problems, **infections**, inflammation, **insomnia**, nervous disorders, **obesity**, skin problems, and ulcers. Practitioners may use panchakarma alongside intensive conventional treatments, including chemotherapy and surgery, as a way to support healing and recovery. Panchakarma is limited in treating traumatic injuries, acute **pain**, and conditions requiring immediate surgery or invasive procedures.

Description

The first step of any Ayurvedic treatment is a thorough examination and diagnosis by an Ayurvedic practitioner, who determines the type and extent of panchakarma treatment required. According to Ayurvedic theory, physical and emotional traits are classified as three doshas—vata, kapha, and pitta. Each individual has all three doshas with one predominating. If an imbalance occurs, diseases or conditions appear. Panchakarma rebalances the doshas, bringing them back to equilibrium and returning the individual to good health. The physician may prescribe herbal remedies, and recommend that dietary and lifestyle changes be enacted before, during and after panchakarma.

Ayurvedic doctors believe that disease generally starts in the digestive tract. Poor **diets**, bad health habits, and other causes can lead to impaired digestion, and cause a toxic substance called *ama* to accumulate in the body. Ama interferes with normal functioning and the flow of energy, creating imbalances and disease. One goal of panchakarma is to cleanse the body of excess ama, and to restore the body's digestive power (*agni*).

A key part of panchakarma is *Shamana*, which is a collection of supportive therapies that include the preparation and post-therapy measures. The main treatment is called *shodhana* and refers to panchakarma's five main cleansing and elimination procedures. During preparation for panchakarma, oil therapy (termed *snehana* in Ayurveda) is the first treatment. Patients are given oil massages—*abhyanga* is full body massage and *shirodhaya* is forehead massage. They are fed dietary oils to lubricate the digestive tract, and are sometimes administered oil enemas. For stress-related and mental conditions, a special oil massage is given during which oil is steadily poured onto the patient's forehead. Practitioners may give oil therapy for up to a week before beginning the main treatment. Another preparation is sweating therapy (*swedana*). This employs saunas, steam rooms, heated clothing, herbal poultices, and **exercise**.

The five main methods of panchakarma are:

- therapeutic vomiting (*vamana*)
- purgation (*virechana*), which is the evacuation of the bowels
- medicated enema therapy (*niruha basti*)

- oil enema therapy (*anuvasana basti*)
- nasal cleansing (*nasya*).

Depending on an individual's health problem, one or more of these methods are used to cleanse the body and promote healing. Other Ayurvedic therapies may be used in conjunction with these methods.

Vamana uses herbal solutions or salt water to induce **vomiting**. This treatment is used for skin problems, asthma, diabetes, chronic sinus or lung infections, **epilepsy**, heart disease, and digestive disorders. Niruha basti uses special herbal solutions in a means to treat such conditions as skin diseases, liver problems, abdominal tumors, parasites, and chronic fevers. For therapeutic enemas, medicinal oils and herbal solutions are used to cleanse the lower bowels. Niruha and anuvasana basti are used to treat conditions such as **constipation**, arthritis, nervous disorders, colitis, headaches, muscle weakness, and lower back pain. During nasya, medicated oils or powders are administered into the nostrils to cleanse the sinuses. This therapy is used to treat conditions of the head, including mental disorders, headaches, and problems of the ear, nose, and throat.

After cleansing methods are performed, patients go through an important aftercare stage called *paschata karma*. Patients are advised to rest and avoid certain activities. In addition, they often receive attention from nurses and doctors. Psychological care and counseling may be part of the healing program, as panchakarma strives to cleanse the patient of emotional problems in addition to physical ones. Patients are also counseled about preventative practices. Dietary changes are carefully planned, and lifestyle considerations are examined and recommended. Exercise programs, such as **yoga**, and stress-management techniques, including **meditation**, may be introduced to patients during or after panchakarma, and herbal remedies may be prescribed as well.

Panchakarma treatment can vary in length from a couple of days to several weeks. Some clinics offer in-patient services, during which patients have medical supervision and are intensively treated around the clock with dietary therapy, exercise, yoga, meditation, massage, and other therapies. Most clinics offer out-patient services, during which panchakarma treatments may take two or more hours per day until completed. Some clinics provide housing arrangements for visiting patients.

Panchakarma treatment from Ayurvedic clinics typically cost $200–$400 per day, not including initial physician fees and herbal prescriptions. In addition, clinics with in-patient services are more expensive, and

KEY TERMS

Agni—Ayurvedic term for strength of digestion.

Meditation—A practice of concentrated focus upon a sound, object, visualization, the breath, movement, or attention itself in order to increase awareness of the present moment, reduce stress, promote relaxation, and enhance personal and spiritual growth.

Yoga—A method of joining the individual self with the divine, universal spirit, or cosmic consciousness. Physical and mental exercises are designed to help achieve this goal, also called self-transcendence or enlightenment. On the physical level, yoga postures, called asanas, are designed to tone, strengthen, and align the body. On the mental level, yoga uses breathing techniques (pranayama) and meditation (dyana) to quiet, clarify, and discipline the mind.

the costs vary with services. Insurance coverage of panchakarma varies, depending on the policy and whether the practitioner is a licensed physician.

Preparations

Patients should be thoroughly diagnosed and cared for by a qualified Ayurvedic practitioner. Patients should seek panchakarma treatment from reputable clinics with adequate staff and facilities.

Precautions

Certain panchakarma methods are not appropriate for specific health problems, and some should not be performed on children, pregnant women, and the elderly. Panchakarma treatments should only be administered by qualified and experienced practitioners.

Individuals should note that some Ayurvedic herbal products have been linked with unsafe levels of toxins. A 2004 study that appeared in *JAMA (the Journal of the American Medical Association)* cautioned that some Ayurvedic herbal medicine products may contain potentially harmful levels of heavy metals, including lead, mercury, and/or arsenic. Also in 2004, the Centers for Disease Control received a dozen reports of **lead poisoning** that was associated with the use of Ayurvedic products.

In addition, the National Center for Complementary and Alternative Medicine cautions that possible interactions may occur between certain Ayurvedic herbal products and other medications. For example, it notes that the extract of an Ayurvedic herb called **guggul** may enhance the activity of aspirin and possibly promote bleeding problems.

Side effects

During panchakarma, **fatigue**, malaise, headaches, congestion, general illness, and an increase in symptoms may occur as side effects. Also, because panchakarma seeks to release stored emotional problems from the patient, some people can experience mental disturbances and depression during treatment.

Research and general acceptance

The majority of the research surrounding Ayurveda has been conducted at research institutions in India, and its findings have mainly been published in Indian and European scientific journals. Much of the research in America is being supported by the Maharishi Ayur-Ved organization, which studies the Ayurvedic products it sells and its clinical practices, including panchakarma. Various studies have reported that panchakarma and/or Ayurvedic treatments have been successful in treating and in some cases, curing chronic illnesses such as asthma, **bronchitis**, hypertension, and diabetes. Other studies have shown that panchakarma can lower cholesterol and improve digestive disorders, and that Ayurvedic remedies can successfully treat diabetes, **acne**, and allergies. Proponents also claim that Ayurvedic treatments, including panchakarma, have been used successfully to support the healing process of patients undergoing chemotherapy.

As of 2007, however, the National Center for Complementary and Alternative Medicine cautions that most clinical trials of Ayurvedic approaches have been small, had problems with research designs, lacked appropriate control groups, or had other issues that affected how meaningful the results were.

Training and certification

In America, there is no standardized program for the certification of Ayurvedic practitioners. Many practitioners have primary degrees, either as MDs, homeopaths, or naturopathic physicians, with additional training in Ayurveda. Some institutions that provide training in Ayurvedic medicine include the following.

- The American Institute of Vedic Studies offers a program of Ayurvedic study.
- The Ayurvedic Institute offers training through classes and seminars, and performs panchakarma treatment. Its founder was Dr. Vasant Lad, one of the leading Ayurvedic practitioners in India and later America.
- Bastyr University of Natural Health Sciences offers training in Ayurvedic medicine.
- The Center for Mind-Body Medicine offers health services and professional training programs in Ayurveda. Dr. Deepak Chopra was one of its founders.
- The Rocky Mountain Institute of Yoga and Ayurveda offers a Panchakarma Practitioners Certification program that includes courses on Ayurvedic massage.

Resources

BOOKS

Godagama, Shantha. *Handbook of Ayurveda*. Berkeley: North Atlantic Books, 2004.

Krishan, Shubhra. *Essential Ayurveda: What It Is and What It Can Do for You*. Rockport, Novato, CA: New World Library, 2003.

Lad, Vasant. *Textbook of Ayurveda*. Albuquerque: Ayurvedic Press, 2001.

PERIODICALS

Saper, Robert B., Stefanos N. Kales, Janet Paquin, Michael J. Burns, David M. Eisenberg, Roger B. Davis, and Russell S. Phillips. "Heavy Metal Content of Ayurvedic Herbal Medicine Products" *JAMA*. Vol. 292, no. 23 (December 15, 2004): 2868-2873.

ORGANIZATIONS

American Institute of Vedic Studies. P.O. Box 8357, Santa Fe, NM 87504. (505) 983-9385. http://www.vedanet. com/ (accessed February 21, 2008).

Ayurvedic and Naturopathic Medical Clinic. 2115 112th Ave NE, Bellevue, WA 98004. (425) 453-8022. http:// www.ayurvedicscience.com/ (accessed February 21, 2008).

The Ayurvedic Institute. 11311 Menaul Blvd., Albuquerque, NM 87192.(505) 291-9698. http://www.ayurveda.com/ (accessed February 21, 2008).

Bastyr University. 14500 Juanita Dr. NE, Seattle, WA 98103. (206) 834-4100. http://www.bastyr.edu/ (accessed February 21, 2008).

Center for Mind-Body Medicine. 5225 Connecticut Ave, NW, Suite 414_Washington, DC 20015. (202) 966-7338. http://www.cmbm.org/ (accessed February 21, 2008).

Rocky Mountain Institute of Yoga and Ayurveda. P.O. Box 1091, Boulder, CO 80306. (303) 499-2910. http://www. rmiya.org/index.php/ (accessed February 21, 2008).

OTHER

Ayurveda Holistic Community. http://www.ayurvedahc. com (accessed February 21, 2008).

The Ayurvedic Institute. http://www.ayurveda.com (accessed February 21, 2008).

National Institute of Ayurvedic Medicine. http://www. niam.com (accessed February 21, 2008).

"What is Ayurvedic Medicine?" National Center for Alternative and Complementary Medicine, National Institutes of Health. http://nccam.nih.gov/health/ayurveda/ (accessed February 20, 2008).

Douglas Dupler
Leslie Mertz, Ph.D.

Pancreatic enzymes *see* **Digestive enzymes**

Pancreatitis

Definition

Pancreatitis is an inflammation of the pancreas, an organ that is important in digestion. Pancreatitis can be acute, beginning suddenly, usually with the patient recovering fully; or chronic, progressing slowly with permanent injury to the pancreas.

Description

The pancreas is located in the midline of the back of the abdomen, closely associated with the liver, stomach, and duodenum, the first part of the small intestine. The pancreas is considered a gland. A gland is an organ whose primary function is to produce chemicals that pass either into the main blood circulation (called an endocrine function), or pass into another organ (called an exocrine function). The pancreas is unusual because it has both endocrine and exocrine functions. Its endocrine function produces three hormones. Two of these hormones, insulin and glucagon, are central to the processing of sugars in the diet (carbohydrate metabolism or breakdown). The third hormone produced by the endocrine cells of the pancreas affects gastrointestinal functioning. This hormone is called vasoactive intestinal polypeptide (VIP). The pancreas's exocrine function produces a variety of **digestive enzymes** (trypsin, **chymotrypsin**, **lipase**, and amylase, among others). These enzymes are passed into the duodenum through a channel called the pancreatic duct. In the duodenum, the enzymes begin the process of breaking down a variety of food components, including, proteins, fats, and starches.

Acute pancreatitis occurs when the pancreas suddenly becomes inflamed but improves. Patients usually recover fully from the disease, and in almost 90% of cases, the symptoms disappear within about a week after treatment. The pancreas returns to its normal structure and functioning after healing from the illness. After an attack of acute pancreatitis, the tissue and cells of the pancreas typically return to normal. With chronic pancreatitis, damage to the pancreas occurs slowly over time. Symptoms may be persistent or sporadic, but the condition does not disappear and the pancreas is permanently impaired. Pancreatic tissue is damaged, and the tissue and cells function poorly.

Causes and symptoms

There are a number of causes of acute pancreatitis. The most common, however, are gallbladder disease and **alcoholism**. These two diseases are responsible for more than 80% of all hospitalizations for acute pancreatitis. Other factors in the development of pancreatitis include:

- certain drugs
- infections
- structural problems of the pancreatic duct and bile ducts (channels leading from the gallbladder to the duodenum)
- injury to the abdomen resulting in injury to the pancreas (including injuries occurring during surgery)
- abnormally high levels of circulating fats in the bloodstream
- malfunction of the parathyroid gland, with high blood levels of calcium
- complications from kidney transplants
- a hereditary tendency toward pancreatitis (recent advances in gene mapping have led to the discovery that a mutation in the gene responsible for cystic fibrosis is associated with a greatly increased risk of pancreatitis)

Pancreatitis caused by drugs accounts for about 5% of all cases. Some drugs that are definitely related to pancreatitis include:

- azathioprine, 6–mercaptopurine (Imuran)
- dideoxyinosine (Videx)
- estrogens (birth control pills)
- furosemide (Lasix)
- pentamidine (NebuPent)
- sulfonamides (Urobak, Azulfidine)
- tetracycline
- thiazide diuretics (Diuril, Enduron)
- valproic acid (Depakote)

Some drugs that are probably related to pancreatitis include:

- acetaminophen (Tylenol)
- angiotensin–converting enzyme (ACE) inhibitors (Capoten, Vasotec)
- erythromycin

KEY TERMS

Abscess—A localized collection of pus in the skin or other body tissue caused by infection.

Acute—Refers to a disease or symptom that has a sudden onset and lasts a relatively short period of time.

Autodigestion—A process in which pancreatic enzymes are activated prematurely and begin to digest the pancreas itself.

Chronic—Refers to a disease or condition that progresses slowly but persists or recurs over time.

Diabetes—A disease characterized by an inability to process sugars in the diet, due to a decrease in or total absence of insulin production.

Duodenum—The first of the three segments of the small intestine. The duodenum is about 10 in (25 cm) long and connects the stomach and the jejunum.

Endocrine—Refers to glands that secrete hormones circulated in the bloodstream or lymphatic system.

Enzyme—A protein that catalyzes a biochemical reaction without changing its own structure or function.

Exocrine—Refers to a system of organs that produces chemicals that go through a duct (or tube) to reach other organs or body surfaces whose functioning they affect.

Glands—Collections of tissue that produce chemicals needed for chemical reactions elsewhere in the body.

Necrosis—Localized tissue death due to disease or injury, such as a lack of oxygen supply to the tissues.

Pseudocyst—A fluid-filled space that may arise in the setting of pancreatitis.

Ranson's signs—A set of 11 signs used to evaluate the severity of a case of pancreatitis.

- methyldopa (Aldomet)
- metronidazole (Flagyl, Protostat)
- nitrofurantoin (Furadantin, Furan)
- nonsteroidal anti–inflammatory drugs (NSAIDs) (Aleve, Naprosyn, Motrin)
- salicylates (aspirin)

All of these causes of pancreatitis seem to have a similar mechanism in common. Under normal circumstances, many of the extremely potent enzymes produced by the pancreas are not active until they enter the duodenum, in which contact with certain other chemicals allows them to function. In pancreatitis, these enzymes become prematurely activated and actually begin their digestive functions within the pancreas. The pancreas, in essence, begins to digest itself. This process is known as autodigestion. A cycle of inflammation begins, including swelling and loss of function. Digestion of the blood vessels in the pancreas results in bleeding. Other active pancreatic chemicals cause the blood vessels to become leaky, and fluid begins to leak out of the normal circulation into the abdominal cavity. The activated enzymes also gain access to the bloodstream through the eroded blood vessels, and begin circulating throughout the body.

Pain is a major symptom of pancreatitis. The pain is usually quite intense and steady, located in the upper right hand corner of the abdomen, and often described as "piercing" or "boring." This pain is also often felt all the way through to the patient's back. The patient's breathing may become quite shallow because deeper breathing tends to cause more pain. Patients usually find some relief of pain by sitting up and bending forward; this postural relief is characteristic of pancreatic pain. **Nausea** and **vomiting**, and abdominal swelling are all common, as well. A patient will often have a slight **fever**, with an increased heart rate and low blood pressure.

Classic signs of shock may appear in more severely ill patients. Shock is a very serious syndrome that occurs when the volume (quantity) of fluid in the blood is very low. In shock, a patient's arms and legs become extremely cold, the blood pressure drops dangerously low, the heart rate is quite fast, and the patient may begin to experience changes in mental status.

In very severe cases of pancreatitis (called necrotizing pancreatitis) the pancreatic tissue begins to die and bleeding increases. Due to the bleeding into the abdomen, two distinctive signs may be noted in patients with necrotizing pancreatitis. Turner's sign is a reddish purple or greenish brown color in the flank area (the area between the ribs and the hip bone). Cullen's sign is the appearance of a bluish color around the navel.

Some of the complications of pancreatitis are due to shock. When shock occurs, all of the body's major organs are deprived of blood and the oxygen it carries, resulting in damage. Kidney, respiratory, and heart failure are serious risks of shock. The pancreatic enzymes that have begun circulating throughout the body (as well as various poisons created by the abnormal digestion of the pancreas by those enzymes) have severe effects on the major body systems. Any number of complications can occur, including damage to the heart, lungs, kidneys, lining of the gastrointestinal tract, liver, eyes, bones, and skin. As the pancreatic enzymes work on blood vessels surrounding the pancreas, and even blood vessels located at a distance, the risk of **blood clots** increases. These blood clots complicate the situation by blocking blood flow in the vessels. When blood flow is blocked, the supply of oxygen is decreased to various organs and the organ can be damaged.

The pancreas may develop additional problems, even after the pancreatitis decreases. When the entire organ becomes swollen and suffers extensive cell death (pancreatic necrosis), the pancreas becomes extremely susceptible to serious infection. A local collection of pus (called a pancreatic **abscess**) may develop several weeks after the illness subsides, and may result in increased fever and a return of pain. Another late complication of pancreatitis, occurring several weeks after the illness begins, is called a pancreatic pseudo-cyst. This occurs when dead pancreatic tissue, blood, white blood cells, enzymes, and fluid that has leaked from the circulatory system accumulates. In an attempt to enclose and organize this abnormal accumulation, a kind of wall forms from the dead tissue and the growing scar tissue in the area. Pseudocysts cause additional abdominal pain by putting pressure on and displacing pancreatic tissue, resulting in more pancreatic damage. Pseudocysts also press on other nearby structures in the gastrointestinal tract, causing more disruption of function. Pseudocysts are life-threatening when they become infected (abscess) and rupture. Simple rupture of a pseudocyst causes death 14% of the time. Rupture complicated by bleeding causes death 60% of the time.

As the pancreatic tissue is increasingly destroyed in chronic pancreatitis, many digestive functions become disturbed. The quantity of hormones and enzymes normally produced by the pancreas begins to seriously decrease. Decreases in the production of enzymes result in the inability to appropriately digest food. Fat digestion, in particular, is impaired. A patient's stools become greasy as fats are passed out of the body. The inability to digest and use proteins results in smaller muscles (wasting) and weakness. The inability to digest and use the nutrients in food leads to malnutrition and a generally weakened condition. As the disease progresses, permanent injury to the pancreas can lead to diabetes.

Diagnosis

Diagnosis of pancreatitis can be made very early in the disease by noting high levels of pancreatic enzymes circulating in the blood (amylase and lipase).

Later in the disease, and in chronic pancreatitis, these enzyme levels will no longer be elevated. Because of this fact, and because increased amylase and lipase can also occur in other diseases, the discovery of such elevations are helpful but not mandatory in the diagnosis of pancreatitis. Other abnormalities in the blood may also point to pancreatitis, including increased white blood cells (occurring with inflammation and/or infection), changes due to dehydration from fluid loss, and abnormalities in the blood concentration of **calcium**, **magnesium**, **sodium**, **potassium**, bicarbonate, and sugars.

X rays or ultrasound examination of the abdomen may reveal **gallstones**, perhaps responsible for blocking the pancreatic duct. The gastrointestinal tract will show signs of inactivity (ileus) due to the presence of pancreatitis. Chest x rays may reveal abnormalities due to air trapping from shallow breathing, or due to lung complications from the circulating pancreatic enzyme irritants. Computed tomography scans (CT scans) of the abdomen may reveal the inflammation and fluid accumulation of pancreatitis, and may also be useful when complications like an abscess or a pseudocyst are suspected.

In the case of chronic pancreatitis, a number of blood tests will reveal the loss of pancreatic function that occurs over time. Blood sugar (glucose) levels will rise, eventually reaching the levels present in diabetes. The levels of various pancreatic enzymes will fall, as the organ is increasingly destroyed and replaced by nonfunctioning scar tissue. Calcification of the pancreas can also be seen on x rays. Endoscopic retrograde cholangiopancreatography (ERCP) may be used to diagnose chronic pancreatitis in severe cases. In this procedure, the doctor uses a medical instrument fitted with a fiber-optic camera to inspect the pancreas. A magnified image of the area is shown on a television screen viewed by the doctor. Many endoscopes also allow the doctor to retrieve a small sample (biopsy) of pancreatic tissue to examine under a microscope. A contrast product may also be used for radiographic examination of the area.

Treatment

Pancreatitis is a serious condition that requires medical diagnosis and treatment. Alternative therapies should be used only to complement conventional treatment.

Nutritional therapy

Before taking nutritional supplements, patients should consult their doctors to make sure these supplements do not interfere with their overall treatment program. The following nutritional changes are recommended to help support pancreatic function and relieve pancreatitis symptoms:

- Follow a diabetic diet and avoid alcohol consumption.
- Limit intake of hydrogenated/saturated fats, sugar, and highly processed foods.
- Increase intake of yellow and orange fruits and dark-green vegetables, which are good sources of beta-carotene, whole foods, vitamin C, and other antioxidants.
- Take high-potency multivitamin/mineral supplements.
- Use chromium (300 mcg daily) supplements to help control blood sugar level and enhance insulin effectiveness.
- Take lipotrophic agents(which increase bile flow to and from the liver), such as vitamin B_6, vitamin B_{12}, folic acid, choline, betaine, and methionine.
- Take pancreatic enzymes at mealtime.

Other therapies

Other alternative treatments such as **acupuncture** or **relaxation** techniques can help patients cope with painful symptoms associated with pancreatitis. Reduce **stress** by **meditation**, **yoga**, **t'ai chi**, or other relaxation techniques. Stress can stimulate pancreatitis attacks.

Allopathic treatment

Treatment of acute pancreatitis involves quickly and sufficiently replacing lost fluids by giving the patient new fluids through a needle inserted in a vein (intravenous or IV fluids). Pain is treated with a variety of medications. In order to decrease pancreatic function (and decrease the discharge of more potentially harmful enzymes into the bloodstream), the patient is not allowed to eat. A thin, flexible tube (nasogastric tube) may be inserted through the patient's nose and down into his or her stomach. Oxygen may need to be administered by nasal prongs or by a mask.

Complications, such as **infections** that often occur in cases of necrotizing pancreatitis, abscesses, and pseudocysts, will require antibiotics administered intravenously. Severe necrotizing pancreatitis may require surgery to remove part of the dying pancreas. A pancreatic abscess can be drained by a needle inserted through the abdomen and into the collection of pus (percutaneous needle aspiration) or surgically removed, if necessary. Pancreatic pseudocysts may shrink on their own (in 25–40% of cases) or may continue to expand, requiring needle aspiration or surgery. When

diagnostic exams reveal the presence of gallstones, surgery may be necessary for their removal.

Because chronic pancreatitis often includes repeated flares of acute pancreatitis, the same kinds of basic treatment are necessary. Patients receive IV replacement fluids, receive pain medication, and are monitored for complications. Treatment of chronic pancreatitis caused by alcohol consumption requires that the patient stop drinking alcohol entirely. As chronic pancreatitis continues and insulin levels drop, a patient may require insulin injections in order to be able to process sugars in his or her diet. Pancreatic enzymes can be replaced with oral medicines, and patients sometimes have to take as many as eight pills with each meal. Drugs can be used to reduce the pain, but when narcotics are used for pain relief, there is danger of the patient becoming addicted.

Expected results

A number of systems have been developed to help determine the prognosis of an individual with pancreatitis. A very basic evaluation of a patient will allow some prediction to be made based on the presence of dying pancreatic tissue (necrosis) and bleeding. When necrosis and bleeding are present, as many as 50% of patients may die.

More elaborate systems have been created to help determine the prognosis of patients with pancreatitis. Ranson's signs, the most commonly used system, identifies 11 different signs that can be used to determine the severity of the disease. The first five categories are evaluated when the patient is admitted to the hospital:

- age over 55 years
- blood sugar level over 200 mg/Dl
- serum lactic dehydrogenase over 350 IU/L (increased with increased breakdown of blood, as would occur with internal bleeding, and with heart or liver damage)
- AST over 250 μ (a measure of liver function, as well as a gauge of damage to the heart, muscle, brain, and kidney)
- white blood count over 16,000 μL

The next six of Ranson's signs are reviewed 48 hours after admission to the hospital. These are:

- greater than 10% decrease in hematocrit (a measure of red blood cell volume)
- increase in BUN (blood urea nitrogen, an indicator of kidney function) greater than 5 mg/dL
- blood calcium less than 8 mg/dL

- PaO$_2$ (a measure of oxygen in the blood) less than 60 mm Hg
- base deficit greater than 4 mEg/L (a measure of change in the normal acidity of the blood)
- fluid sequestration greater than 6 L (an estimation of the quantity of fluid that has leaked out of the blood circulation and into other body spaces).

Once a doctor determines how many of Ranson's signs are present and gives the patient a score, the doctor can better predict the risk of death. The more signs present, the greater the chance of death. A patient with less than three positive Ranson's signs has a less than 5% chance of dying. A patient with three to four positive Ranson's signs has a 15–20% chance of dying.

The results of a CT scan can also be used to predict the severity of pancreatitis. Slight swelling of the pancreas indicates mild illness. Significant swelling, especially with evidence of destruction of the pancreas and/or fluid buildup in the abdominal cavity, indicates more severe illness. With severe illness, there is a worse prognosis.

Surgical treatment of pancreatitis is frequently followed by complications because of the leakage of pancreatic enzymes from the remaining portion of the organ. A team of French surgeons has reported that treating patients with somatostatin-14, a hormone that inhibits pancreatic secretion as well as pancreatic blood flow, appears to be effective in lowering the rate of complications from pancreatic surgery. In spite of recent advances in surgical technique, however, the mortality rate following surgery for pancreatitis is still 3%–10%.

Prevention

Alcoholism is essentially the only preventable cause of pancreatitis. Patients with chronic pancreatitis must stop drinking alcohol entirely. The drugs that cause or may cause pancreatitis should also be avoided.

Resources

BOOKS

Greenberger, Norton J., Phillip P. Toskes, and Kurt J. Isselbacher. "Acute and Chronic Pancreatitis." In *Harrison's Principles of Internal Medicine,* edited by Anthony S. Fauci, et al. New York: McGraw–Hill, 1998.
"Pancreatitis." In *Alternative Medicine: The Definitive Guide.* Tiburon, CA: Future Medicine Publishing, Inc., 1999.
"Pancreatitis." In *Reader's Digest Guide to Medical Cures & Treatments.* Canada: The Reader's Digest Association, Inc., 1997.

PERIODICALS

Amann, Stephen, et al. "Pancreatitis: Diagnostic and Therapeutic Interventions." *Patient Care* 31, no. 11 (June 15, 1997): 200+.
Goulliat, C., J. F. Gigot. "Pancreatic Surgical Complications— The Case for Prophylaxis." *Gut* 49 (December 2001): 32–39.
Le Marechal, C., O. Raguenes, I. Quere, et al. "Screening of Pancreatic Secretory Trypsin Inhibitor (PSTI) Mutations in Chronic Pancreatitis by DHPLC." *American Journal of Human Genetics* 69 (October 2001): 623.
Meissner, Judith E. "Caring for Patients with Pancreatitis." *Nursing* 27, no. 10 (October 1997): 50+.
"Mutations in the PSTI Gene Associated with Pancreatitis." *Gene Therapy Weekly* (December 27, 2001): 19.
Schlapman, Nancy. "Spotting Acute Pancreatitis." *RN* 64 (November 2001): 54.

ORGANIZATION

National Digestive Diseases Information Clearinghouse. 2 Information Way, Bethesda, MD 20892-3570. http://www.niddk.nih.gov.

Mai Tran
Rebecca J. Frey, PhD

Panic disorder

Definition

A panic attack is a sudden, intense experience of fear coupled with an overwhelming feeling of danger, accompanied by physical symptoms of **anxiety**, such as a pounding heart, sweating, and rapid breathing. A person with panic disorder may experience repeated panic attacks (at least several a month) and feel severe anxiety about having another attack.

Description

Each year, panic disorder affects one in every 63 Americans. While many people experience moments of anxiety, panic attacks are sudden and unprovoked, having little to do with real danger.

Panic disorder is a chronic, debilitating condition that can have a devastating impact on a person's family, work, and social life. Typically, the first attack strikes without warning. A person might be walking down the street, driving a car, or riding an escalator when suddenly panic strikes. Pounding heart, sweating palms, and an overwhelming feeling of impending doom are common features. While the attack may last only seconds or minutes, the experience can be profoundly disturbing. A person who has had one panic

KEY TERMS

Agoraphobia—Abnormal anxiety regarding public places or situations from which the person may wish to flee or in which he or she would be helpless in the event of a panic attack.

Aromatherapy—The therapeutic use of plant-derived, aromatic essential oils to promote physical and psychological well-being.

Benzodiazepines—A class of drugs that have a hypnotic and sedative action, used mainly as tranquilizers to control symptoms of anxiety or panic.

Cognitive-behavioral therapy—A type of psychotherapy in which people learn to recognize and change negative and self-defeating patterns of thinking and behavior.

Selective serotonin reuptake inhibitors (SSRIs)—A class of antidepressants that work by blocking the reabsorption of serotonin in the brain, thus raising the levels of serotonin. SSRIs include fluoxetine (Prozac), sertraline (Zoloft), and paroxetine (Paxil)

Tricyclic antidepressants—A class of antidepressants named for their three-ring structure that increase the levels of serotonin and other brain chemicals. They are used to treat depression and anxiety disorders, but have more side effects than the newer class of antidepressants called SSRIs.

attack typically worries that another one may occur at any time.

As the fear of future panic attacks deepens, the person begins to avoid situations in which panic occurred in the past. In severe cases of panic disorder, the victim refuses to leave the house for fear of having a panic attack. This fear of being in exposed places is often called agoraphobia.

People with untreated panic disorder may have problems getting to work or staying on the job. As the person's world narrows, untreated panic disorder can lead to **depression**, **substance abuse**, and in rare instances, suicide.

Causes and symptoms

Scientists aren't sure what causes panic disorder, but they know that a tendency to develop the condition can be inherited. In 2001, a team of geneticists pinpointed an abnormal duplication (known as DUP25) of a segment of human chromosome 15q as implicated in panic disorder. In addition to genetic

factors, some experts think that people with panic disorder may have a hypersensitive nervous system that unnecessarily responds to nonexistent threats. Research suggests that people with panic disorder may not be able to make proper use of their body's normal stress-reducing chemicals. And in some cases, panic disorder develops as a drug intolerance reaction to medications given to reduce high blood pressure.

People with panic disorder usually have their first panic attack in their 20s. Four or more of the following symptoms during panic attacks would indicate panic disorder if no medical, drug-related, neurologic, or other psychiatric disorder is found:

- pounding, skipping, or palpitating heartbeat
- shortness of breath or the sensation of smothering
- dizziness or lightheadedness
- nausea or stomach problems
- chest pains or pressure
- choking sensation or a "lump in the throat"
- chills or hot flashes
- sweating
- fear of dying
- feelings of unreality or being detached
- tingling or numbness
- shaking and trembling
- fear of losing control

A panic attack is often accompanied by the urge to escape, together with a feeling of impending doom. Others are convinced they are about to have a **heart attack**, suffocate, lose control, or "go crazy." Once people experience one panic attack, they tend to worry so much about having another attack that they avoid the place or situation associated with the original episode.

Diagnosis

Because its physical symptoms are easily confused with other conditions, panic disorder often goes undiagnosed. A thorough physical examination is needed to rule out a medical condition. Because the physical symptoms are so pronounced and frightening, panic attacks can be mistaken for a heart problem. Some people experiencing a panic attack go to an emergency room and endure batteries of tests until a diagnosis is made.

Once a medical condition is ruled out, a mental health professional is the best person to diagnose panic and panic disorder, taking into account not just the actual episodes, but how the patient feels about the attacks, and how they affect everyday life.

Treatment

One approach used in several medical centers focuses on teaching patients how to accept their fear instead of dreading it. In this method, the therapist repeatedly stimulates a person's body sensations (such as a pounding heartbeat) that can trigger fear. Eventually, the patient gets used to these sensations and learns not to be afraid of them. Patients who respond report almost complete absence of panic attacks.

Neurolinguistic programming and hypnotherapy can also be beneficial in treating panic attacks, since these techniques can help bring an awareness of the root cause of the attacks to the conscious mind.

Herbs known as *adaptogens* may also be prescribed by an herbalist or holistic healthcare provider to treat anxiety related to panic disorder. These herbs are thought to promote adaptability to **stress**, and include Siberian ginseng (*Eleutherococcus senticosus*), ginseng (*Panax ginseng*), wild yam (*Dioscorea villosa*), borage (*Borago officinalis*), licorice (*Glycyrrhiza glabra*), chamomile (*Chamaemelum nobile*), **milk thistle** (*Silybum marianum*), and nettles (*Urtica dioica*). Herbal preparations of **skullcap** (*Scutellaria lateriafolia*), **lemon balm** (*Melissa officinalis*), **passionflower** (*Passiflora incarnata*), and oats (*Avena sativa*) may also be recommended to ease the symptoms of panic disorder. Nutritional supplementation with B vitamins, magnesium, and antioxidant vitamins are also useful for relieving anxiety.

Chinese medicine regards anxiety as a disruption of *qi*, or energy flow, inside the patient's body. The practitioner of Chinese medicine chooses **acupuncture** and/or herbal therapy to rebalance the entire system. In acupuncture, the kidney meridian is associated with fear and may be out of balance. Reishi (*Ganoderma lucidum*), or ling-zhi is a medicinal mushroom prescribed in TCM to reduce anxiety and **insomnia**. It is available in extract form, but because reishi can interact with other prescription drugs and is not recommended in patients with certain medical conditions, individuals should consult their healthcare practitioner before taking the remedy. Other TCM herbal remedies for panic disorder include the **cordyceps** mushroom (also known as caterpillar fungus.) There are several herbal formulas, depending on the pattern of imbalance in an individual.

Meditation and mindfulness training can be beneficial to patients with **phobias** and panic disorder. **Hydrotherapy**, massage therapy, and **aromatherapy** are useful to some anxious patients because they can promote general **relaxation** of the nervous system. Popular aromatherapy prescriptions for anxiety relief include **essential oils** of lavender, ylang-ylang, and chamomile. Relaxation training, which is sometimes called anxiety management training, includes breathing exercises and similar techniques intended to help the patient prevent hyperventilation and relieve the muscle tension associated with the fight-or-flight reaction of anxiety. **Yoga**, aikido, **t'ai chi**, and dance therapy help patients work with the physical, as well as the emotional, tensions that either promote anxiety or are created by the anxiety.

Finally, patients can make certain lifestyle changes to help keep panic at bay, such as eliminating **caffeine** and alcohol, cocaine, amphetamines, and **marijuana**.

There are also homeopathic remedies that may be helpful by seeing a trained homeopathic practitioner.

It is important for patients who are using alternative treaments for panic disorder alongside allopathic medications or treatments to keep their health care provider informed about any herbal remedies they may be taking that could interact with prescription medications. A study done in 2001 found that Americans are more likely to seek alternative treatment for anxiety disorders than standard allopathic therapies, and that the percentage of alternative therapy users was the same in both sexes. In addition, the percentage was not affected by age, race, education, income, place of residence, marital status, or employment.

Allopathic treatment

Most patients with panic disorder respond best to a combination of cognitive-behavioral therapy and medication. Cognitive-behavioral therapy usually runs from 12–15 sessions. It teaches patients:

- How to identify and alter thought patterns so as not to misconstrue bodily sensations, events, or situations as catastrophic.
- How to prepare for the situations and physical symptoms that trigger a panic attack.
- How to identify and change unrealistic self-talk (such as "I'm going to die!") that can worsen a panic attack.
- How to calm down and learn breathing exercises to counteract the physical symptoms of panic.
- How to gradually confront the frightening situation step by step until it becomes less terrifying.
- How to "desensitize" themselves to their own physical sensations, such as rapid heart rate.

At the same time, many people find that medications can help reduce or prevent panic attacks by changing the way certain chemicals interact in the brain. People with panic disorder usually notice whether or not the drug is effective within two months, but most people take medication for at least six months to a year.

Several kinds of drugs can reduce or prevent panic attacks, including:

- Selective serotonin reuptake inhibitor (SSRI) antidepressants like paroxetine (Paxil) or fluoxetine (Prozac), some approved specifically for the treatment of panic.
- Tricyclic antidepressants such as clomipramine (Anafranil).
- Benzodiazepines such as alprazolam (Xanax) and clonazepam (Klonopin).
- A combination of sertraline, another SSRI, with clonazepam has been reported as especially effective in treating panic disorder.

Expected results

While there may be occasional periods of improvement, the episodes of panic rarely disappear on their own. Fortunately, panic disorder responds very well to treatment; panic attacks decrease in up to 90% of people after six to eight weeks of a combination of cognitive-behavioral therapy and medication.

Unfortunately, many people with panic disorder never get the help they need. If untreated, panic disorder can last for years and may become so severe that a normal life is impossible. Many people who struggle with untreated panic disorder and try to hide their symptoms end up losing their friends, family, and jobs.

Prevention

There is no way to prevent the initial onset of panic attacks. Antidepressant drugs or benzodiazepines can prevent future panic attacks, especially when combined with cognitive-behavioral therapy. There is some suggestion that avoiding stimulants (including caffeine, alcohol, or over-the-counter cold medicines) may help prevent attacks as well.

Resources

BOOKS

Bloomfield, Harold H. *Healing Anxiety with Herbs.* New York: Harper Collins, 1998.

Sheehan, Elaine. *Anxiety, Phobias and Panic Attacks: Your Questions Answered.* New York: Element, 1996.

Wilson, Robert R. *Don't Panic: Taking Control of Anxiety Attacks.* New York: HarperCollins, 1996.

PERIODICALS

"Alternative Treatment of Anxiety and Depression." *Harvard Mental Health Letter* 18 (October 2001): np.

Boschert, Sherry. "Drug Intolerance, Mood Disorders Linked in HT (Panic Attacks, Anxiety, Depression)." *Internal Medicine News* 34 (November 2001): 30.

Goddard, Andrew W. "Early Administration of Clonazepam with Sertraline for Panic Disorder." *Journal of the American Medical Association* 286 (October 24, 2001): 1955.

Gratacos, M., M. Nadal, R. Martin-Santos, et al. "Polymorphic Genomic Mutation on Human Chromosome 15 and Susceptibility to Anxiety Disorders (Panic Disorder and Social Phobia)." *American Journal of Human Genetics* 69 (October 2001): 177.

Katerndahl, David A. "Panic Attacks and Panic Disorder." *Journal of Family Practice* 43 (September 1996): 275- 283.

ORGANIZATIONS

Anxiety Disorders Association of America. 11900 Parklawn Dr., Ste. 100, Rockville, MD 20852. (301) 231-9350.

Anxiety Network Homepage. http://www.anxietynetwork.com.

National Institute of Mental Health, Anxiety Disorders Education Program. Rm 15C-05, 5600 Fishers Lane, Rockville, MD 20857. (800) 64-PANIC. www.nimh. nih.gov/anxiety.

Paula Ford-Martin
Rebecca J. Frey, PhD

Pantothenic acid

Description

Pantothenic acid, also known as vitamin B_5, is a member of the water-soluble B vitamin family. Every living organism needs pantothenic acid to survive. Humans do not make this vitamin and must obtain it from the food they eat. It is an essential ingredient of two substances, coenzyme A and acyl carrier protein, which are needed to metabolize carbohydrates and fats. The same coenzymes play a part in production of certain hormones, **vitamin D**, red blood cells, and the neurotransmitter acetylcholine. Pantothenic acid is necessary for proper growth and development. Studies of Mexican infants whose **diets** are deficient in micronutrients have shown that those who receive dietary supplements containing pantothenic acid do not show the growth retardation that appears in control groups.

General use

Pantothenic acid was discovered in 1936 and soon afterward was recognized as a vitamin essential to growth. Pantothenic acid is found in all living things. Its name is derived from the Greek word "pantos," which means "everywhere."

Pantothenic acid joins with another molecule to form coenzyme A (CoA). Coenzymes are small molecules that regulate enzyme reactions. CoA is involved in many essential metabolic reactions that produce energy and synthesize new molecules. Without pantothenic

Pantothenic acid

Recommended dietary allowance of pantothenic acid

Age	mg/day
Children 0-6 mos.	1.7
Children 7-12 mos.	1.8
Children 1-3 yrs.	2
Children 4-8 yrs.	3
Children 9-13 yrs.	4
Children 14-18 yrs.	5
Adults ≥ 19 yrs.	5
Pregnant women	6
Breastfeeding women	7

Foods that contain pantothenic acid	mg
Liver, beef, cooked, 3.5 oz.	5.3
Salmon, baked, 3.5 oz.	1.4
Yogurt, 8 oz.	1.35
Chicken, dark meat, cooked, 3.5 oz.	1.3
Chicken, light meat, cooked, 3.5 oz.	1.0
Milk, nonfat, 1 cup	0.80
Corn, cooked, 1/2 cup	0.72
Sweet potato, cooked, 1/2 cup	0.68
Lentils, cooked, 1/2 cup	0.64
Egg, 1 large, cooked	0.61
Broccoli, steamed, 1/2 cup	0.40
Tuna, canned, 3 oz.	0.18
Bread, whole wheat, 1 slice	0.16

mg = milligram

(Illustration by GGS Information Services. Cengage Learning, Gale)

nutrient needed to meet the health needs of 97–98% of the population. The Adequate Intake (AI) is an estimate set when there is not enough information to determine an RDA. The Tolerable Upper Intake Level (UL) is the average maximum amount that can be taken daily without risking negative side effects. The DRIs are calculated for children, adult men, adult women, pregnant women, and breastfeeding women.

The IOM has not set RDA values for pantothenic acid because of incomplete scientific information. Instead, it has set AI levels for all age groups. AI levels for pantothenic acid are measured by weight (milligrams or mg). No UL levels have been set for this vitamin because large doses of pantothenic acid do not appear to cause any side effects.

The following are the daily AIs of pantothenic acid for healthy individuals:

- children birth–6 months: 1.7 mg
- children 7–12 months: 1.8 mg
- children 1–3 years: 2 mg
- children 4–8 years: 3 mg
- children 9–13 years: 4 mg
- children 14–18 years: 5 mg
- adults age 19 and older: 5 mg
- pregnant women: 6 mg
- breastfeeding women: 7 mg

Pantothenic acid and pantethine are both available as supplements, and do appear to function somewhat differently. Pantethine can be used to lower serum **cholesterol** and triglycerides. It is more expensive and less effective than using **niacin** (vitamin B$_3$) for the same purpose, but does not have the potential side effects that niacin does. Generally a dose of 300 mg taken three times a day is recommended for this purpose. Pantethine may be a good cholesterol-lowering alternative for people with diabetes, who cannot take niacin due to the potential side effects on blood sugar regulation. Taking supplements of pantothenic acid does not affect cholesterol, as in this form it is immediately converted into coenzymes.

One very small study indicated that large daily doses of pantothenic acid (2 g of **calcium** pantothenate) were helpful to relieve symptoms of **rheumatoid arthritis**. Consult a healthcare provider regarding use of supplements for this purpose.

Panthenol is a derivative of pantothenic acid and is frequently an ingredient of shampoos and other hair care products. Experiments with rats have shown that a deficiency of pantothenic acid can cause hair to turn gray and fall out. Neither oral nor topical use of any

acid, there would be no CoA, and life would cease. Some of the activities that require CoA, and thus indirectly pantothenic acid, include:

- converting fats, carbohydrates, and proteins from food into energy that the body can use
- synthesizing heme, the molecule in red blood cells that picks up oxygen in the lung and carries it throughout the body
- synthesizing essential fatty acids, cholesterol, and steroid hormones needed to build new cells
- synthesizing acetylcholine, a neurotransmitter that carries electrical impulses between nerve cells
- stimulating chemical reactions in the liver that help rid the body of certain drugs and toxins (poisons).

The United States Institute of Medicine (IOM) of the National Academy of Sciences has developed values called Dietary Reference Intakes (DRIs) for vitamins and minerals. The DRIs consist of three sets of numbers. The Recommended Dietary Allowance (RDA) defines the average daily amount of the

form of pantothenic acid has been shown to prevent or treat gray hair or balding in humans. Some skin care products contain another form of pantothenic acid, called panthoderm, which may be helpful in treatment of minor skin injuries.

Other claims for pantothenic acid that remain unproven are that it improves immune function, decreases **allergies**, and acts as an anti-aging substance.

Preparations

Natural sources

Pantothenic acid is found small quantities in a wide variety of foods. Good sources include liver, kidney, fish, shellfish, egg yolk, broccoli, lentils, and mushrooms. Pantothenic acid is unstable. Much of it is lost during cooking, canning, freezing, and processing. Frozen meats and processed grains, for example, can lose up to half their pantothenic acid content.

The following list gives the approximate pantothenic acid content of some common foods.

- liver, beef, cooked, 3.5 ounces: 5.3 mg
- chicken, dark meat, cooked 3.5 ounces: 1.3 mg
- chicken, light meat, cooked 3.5 ounces: 1.0 mg
- salmon, baked, 3.5 ounces: 1.4 mg
- tuna, canned, 3 ounces: .18 mg
- egg, 1 large, cooked: .61 mg
- milk, nonfat, 1 cup: .80 mg
- yogurt, 8 ounces: 1.35 mg
- broccoli, steamed, 1/2 cup: .40 mg
- sweet potato, cooked 1/2 cup: .68 mg
- lentils, cooked, 1/2 cup: .64 mg
- corn, cooked 1/2 cup: .72
- bread, whole wheat, 1 slice: .16 mg

In order to get the most value out of the pantothenic acid contained in natural sources, use fresh foods whenever possible. Cook with minimal amounts of water since the water-soluble vitamin content may be leached out. Frozen foods lose some of their water-soluble vitamin content as they thaw. Processing can also destroy a significant amount of the vitamin content of foods. Pantothenic acid is fairly heat-stable, and is not broken down by cooking although it is destroyed by extremes of pH as may be created by adding such things as baking soda or vinegar.

Supplemental sources

Oral supplements of both pantothenic acid and pantethine are available. The latter is quite expensive, and less stable than other types. Calcium pantothenate

is one form of pantothenic acid made for oral use. Dexpanthenol is formulated for topical, intramuscular, or intravenous use. It is generally recommended that the B-vitamin family be taken in balanced amounts. Taking an excessive amount of an individual B-vitamin may have a detrimental effect on the absorption of others. As with all supplements, pantothenic acid should be stored in a cool, dry place, away from direct sunlight, and out of the reach of children. A dose of up to 500 mg is often recommended.

Deficiency

Pantothenic acid deficiency is so rare that it has only been seen in humans in severely malnourished prisoners of war in Asia after World War II and in research volunteers who were given a pantothenic-free diet. The main symptoms these groups experienced were burning, tingling, and numbness in the feet and **fatigue**. These symptoms disappeared when pantothenic acid was added to their diet.

It is possible for individuals to have low levels of pathothenic acid in conjunction with other B vitamins under certain conditions. This category may include people with severe nutritional deficiencies; and those with conditions affecting absorption, such as sprue or removal of portions of the gastrointestinal tract. People who chronically abuse alcohol or other drugs, and those under excessive amounts of **stress** including debilitating illnesses or recovery from **burns** or surgery are also at higher risk of general vitamin deficiency. The elderly are more susceptible both to poor nutritional status and decreased vitamin absorption. Use of tobacco is also detrimental to B vitamin absorption. Athletes who have a strenuous, daily physical regimen and people with physically active occupations may require larger than average amounts of pantothenic acid.

Precautions

People with hemophilia should not use dexpanthenol as it may prolong bleeding time. Anyone with a known or suspected obstruction of the gastrointestinal tract should also not use this product.

Side effects

Taken in very large doses, pantothenic acid may cause **diarrhea**. Topical use of dexpanthenol may cause a skin reaction.

Interactions

Using oral contraceptives may mildly increase the body's need for pantothenic acid. The effects of the medication levodopa may be decreased by supplemental pantothenic acid. This problem is not seen with combination carbidopa and levodopa products. These medications are often used to treat symptoms of **Parkinson's disease**. Anyone taking medication for this condition should consult a health care provider before taking nutritional supplements.

Resources

BOOKS

Berkson, Burt and Arthur J. Berkson. *Basic Health Publications User's Guide to the B-complex Vitamins*. Laguna Beach, CA: Basic Health Publications, 2006.

Bratman, Steven, and David Kroll. *Natural Health Bible*. Prima Publishing, 1999.

Feinstein, Alice. *Prevention's Healing with Vitamins*. Emmaus, PA: Rodale Press, 1996.

Griffith, H. Winter. *Vitamins, Herbs, Minerals & Supplements: The Complete Guide*. Arizona: Fisher Books, 1998.

Jellin, Jeff, Forrest Batz, and Kathy Hitchens. *Pharmacist's Letter/Prescriber's Letter Natural Medicines Comprehensive Database*. California: Therapeutic Research Faculty, 1999.

Lieberman, Shari and Nancy Bruning. *The Real Vitamin and Mineral Book: The Definitive Guide to Designing Your Personal Supplement Program*, 4th ed. New York: Avery, 2007.

Pressman, Alan H. and Sheila Buff. *The Complete Idiot's Guide to Vitamins and Minerals*, 3rd ed. Indianapolis, IN: Alpha Books, 2007.

PERIODICALS

Rivera, Juan A., Teresita Gonzalez-Cossio, Mario Flores, et al. "Multiple Micronutrient Supplementation Increases the Growth of Mexican Infants." *American Journal of Clinical Nutrition* 74 (November 2001): 657.

ORGANIZATIONS

Linus Pauling Institute, Oregon State University, 571 Weniger Hall, Corvallis, OR, 97331-6512, (541) 717-5075, (541) 737-5077, http://lpi.oregonstate.edu.

Judith Turner
Rebecca J. Frey, PhD
Helen Davidson

Parasitic infections

Definition

Parasites are organisms that live inside humans or other organisms who act as hosts. They are dependent on their hosts because they are unable to produce food or energy for themselves. Parasites are harmful to humans because they consume needed food, eat away body tissues and cells, and eliminate toxic waste, which makes people sick.

Because of sanitary living conditions in the United States, parasites do not cause widespread life-threatening **infections**. In other parts of the world, however, parasitic infections are epidemic. They kill and disable millions of people every year. Parasitic infection cases in the United States in the 2000s were on the rise, however, due to increased travel to and from underdeveloped countries. In addition, parasitic infections can cause severe infections in **AIDS** patients and other patients with weakened immune systems.

Because parasites can live inside the human body for years without making their presence known, they are more common than one might think. According to one study, approximately half of all Americans have at least one form of parasite. Their presence causes a variety of chronic diseases and conditions such as chronic **fatigue**, weakness, low energy levels, skin **rashes**, **pain**, **constipation**, and frequent colds and **influenza**.

Description

There are two types of parasites: large and small. Large parasites such as intestinal **worms** are easily seen with the naked eye. These are roundworms, flukes, and tapeworms. They usually lay their eggs on the intestinal walls. As they hatch, the young larvae feed on the food in the intestinal tract. Then they grow, reproduce, and start the cycle all over again. They sometimes dig through the digestive tract to get into the bloodstream, muscles, and other organs where they cause even more havoc. These types of parasites often cause malnutrition and **anemia** because they tend to rob the body of essential nutrients.

Small parasites—mostly protozoa and amoebae—are so tiny that they can only be seen with a microscope. These tiny parasites are even more dangerous to the body than the large ones. Although they usually stay in the intestines, they can migrate virtually anywhere in the body: into the bloodstream, muscles, and even vital organs such as the brain, the lungs, or the liver, where they do substantial damage.

Because parasites are everywhere, it is not difficult to become infected. People can become infested through the following ways:

- being bitten by insects
- walking barefoot
- eating raw or undercooked pork, beef, or fish
- eating contaminated raw fruits and vegetables
- eating foods prepared by infected handlers
- drinking contaminated water
- having contact with infected persons (including sexual contact, kissing, sharing drinks, shaking hands, or sharing toys)
- inhaling dust that contains parasitic eggs or cysts
- playing with or picking up pet litter contaminated with parasitic eggs or cysts

In 2002, the Centers for Disease Control (CDC) announced the first documented cases of transplant patients contracting a dangerous parasitic disease from infection with T. cruzi from organs harvested from a Central American donor. The infection caused Chagas disease, causing two of the three donor recipients to die. The CDC identified two additional cases of Chagas diseased in transplant patients. In one case, reported in 2006, the patient received a heart transplant in 2005 and showed symptoms of Chagas in January 2006. The patient was treated medically and recovered. However, he died several months later due to organ rejection. It was found that his donor lived in the United States but had traveled to a portion of Mexico infected with T. cruzi. Another case of Chagas disease was reported in February 2006, one month following a heart transplant. The patient's symptoms disappeared following treatment. He died several months later as a result of cardiac arrest. These represent the fourth and fifth reported cases of Chagas disease caused by T. cruzi. The fact that they occurred in Los Angeles prompted the CDC to encourage physicians in the area to suspect T. cruzi in transplant and transfusion patients, if appropriate symptoms are present.

Causes and symptoms

Risk factors for getting parasitic infections include:

- an immune system weakened by disease or long-term exposure to toxic chemicals or environmental pollution
- prolonged antibiotic use
- alcohol and/or drug abuse
- smoking
- emotional and/or physical stress
- diet high in fat and sugar and low in fiber
- food allergies
- malabsorption syndrome
- obesity

Causes

There are more than 100 types of human parasites. The following describe some of the most common species in the United States.

ARTHROPODS (INSECTS). In the United States, because of high sanitary standards and a temperate climate, parasitic insects do not flourish. Common bugs such as ticks, mites, fleas, lice, and bedbugs may cause intense **itching** in affected areas. They are a nuisance but generally not a major health risk. One exception is the deer tick, which is associated with the debilitating **Lyme disease**. Other parasites, spread by mosquitoes, cause more serious diseases such as western and eastern equine encephalitis, **malaria**, Dengue **fever**, and yellow fever.

INTESTINAL PARASITES. Some of the most common intestinal parasites are:

- Pinworms. This is the most common parasitic infection in the United States. The worm resides in the colon, yet it lays eggs outside the body, usually near the anus, a process that causes severe itching. The disease can be transmitted from one individual to another through dirty hands, clothing, bedclothes, and toys.
- Tapeworms. The two most common tapeworms are *Taenia solium* (pork tapeworm) and *Taenia saginata* (beef tapeworm). *Taenia solium* infestation is caused by eating undercooked pork while *Taenia saginata* (pork tapeworm) infestation is associated with consuming raw beef. Adult tapeworms may become quite big, some as long as 20 feet (6.1 m). Of the two, pork tapeworm is the more harmful. It often causes anemia and weight loss. More seriously, when adult pork tapeworm eggs, excreted in human feces, are ingested by other people (which can happen with poor hygiene and sanitation), the parasitic life cycle that occurs in pigs and cattle takes place in the human host. Once in the human digestive system, the tapeworm eggs, called proglottids, develop into an embryonic form of the parasite called onchospheres that burrow through the intestinal wall and into the bloodstream. From there they migrate into the muscles, eyes, and the brain, a condition called cysticercosis. Cysts in the brain often cause epileptic seizures.
- Protozoa (one-celled organisms) such as *Giardia lamblia, Entamoeba histolytica,* or *Cryptosporidium.* These organisms are some of the most common and infectious parasites in the world. They can be transmitted through contaminated food and water. They can also

be spread from one person to another. Protozoa may spread throughout the body, causing abscesses in the lungs, liver, heart, and brain. Cramps, watery diarrhea, abdominal pain, and serious weight loss are common symptoms of Giardia infection. *Entamoeba histolytica* can cause dysentery, a severe form of intestinal infection, as well as liver and lung damage. Cryptosporidia can cause severe diarrhea in AIDS or cancer patients who have weakened immune systems.

According to the Centers for Disease Control and Prevention (CDC), cases of *Cryptospordium* in the United States increased from 3,505 in 2003 to 8,269 cases in 2005. The largest portion of the increase was related to an outbreak in New York that was traced to use of a recreational water fountain. In 2003, 425 cases were linked to unpasteurized apple cider produced from contaminated apples.

CNS PARASITIC INFECTIONS. *Toxoplasma gondii* is the most common parasite that invades the central nervous system (CNS). Humans become infected with this organism by eating raw or undercooked meat or by handling infected cat litter, which can contain eggs. Pregnant women who are infected may miscarry or deliver stillborn babies. Infected babies are born with congenital toxoplasmosis and have symptoms that include eye inflammation, blindness, **jaundice**, seizures, abnormally small or large heads, and mental retardation. In people with weakened immune systems, such as AIDS patients, toxoplasmosis can affect the whole body, causing inflammation, convulsions, trembling, **headache**, confusion, paralysis in half of the body, or coma.

Symptoms

Parasitic infections are difficult to diagnose because many patients exhibit only vague symptoms or no symptoms at all. The following symptoms, however, may indicate parasitic infections:

- Diarrhea with foul-smelling stool that becomes worse in the later part of the day.
- Sudden changes in bowel habits (e.g. constipation that changes to soft and watery stool).
- Constant rumbling and gurgling in the stomach area unrelated to hunger or eating.
- Heartburn or chest pain.
- Flu-like symptoms such as coughing, fever, and nasal congestion.
- Nonspecific food allergies.
- Itching around the nose, ears, and anus, especially at night.
- Losing weight with constant hunger.

Other symptoms of parasitic infections include anemia, blood in the stool, bloating, **diarrhea**, **gas**, loss of appetite, intestinal obstruction, **nausea**, **vomiting**, sore mouth and gums, excessive nose picking, grinding teeth at night, chronic fatigue, headaches, muscle aches and pains, shortness of breath, skin rashes, **depression**, and **memory loss**.

Diagnosis

The following tests may be used to help doctors diagnose parasitic infections:

- *Ova and parasite (O & P) test.* Three to six stool samples are collected every one or two days to look for eggs and parasites.
- *Cellophane tape* (applied to the anal area). Ova (eggs) that stick to the tape prove pinworm infestation.
- *Endoscopy.* This procedure is used to obtain samples from the duodenum (the upper part of the small intestine), which are then analyzed for the presence of parasites.
- *Urine sample* and vaginal swab to detect *Trichomonas*, a parasite that causes vaginitis.
- *Blood tests.* High levels of eosinophils (a type of white blood cell) indicate infections. Antibodies against the parasites may also be detected. A study released in 2008 found that blood testing is often necessary to obtain a specific diagnosis. An increase in eosinophils, in particular, is associated with parasitic infections.
- *X ray, MRI, and CT scans.* X rays detect lesions in internal organs. Computed axial tomography (CT) scans and magnetic resonance imaging (MRI) are used to diagnose CNS parasitic infections.

Infected patients who are treated with anti-parasitic drugs or herbal remedies should be retested twice at the end of the treatment program; the two tests should be given one month apart.

Treatment

Alternative therapies for parasitic infections reduce parasitic infections by improving **nutrition** and strengthening the immune system through herbal therapy and **Ayurvedic medicine**. Some herbal remedies are directly anti-parasitic and actually eliminate the organisms that cause disease. Patients taking allopathic anti-parasitic remedies should consult their doctor before using any of these herbs. Care should be taken before giving them to children as they easily overdose.

Nutritional therapy

The following dietary changes may help prevent or treat parasitic infections:

- Eating a well-balanced diet with lots of fiber, vegetables, fruits, whole grains, nuts, and seeds. Fiber helps eliminate worms from the intestines; good nutrition improves immune function and protects the body against parasitic invasion.
- Limiting dairy foods, sugar, and fat. Parasites thrive on these foods.
- Avoiding raw or undercooked fish, pork, or beef.
- Take daily multivitamin/mineral supplements to prevent malnutrition and improve immune function.
- Supplementing the diet with probiotics such as *Lactobacillus acidophilus, Bifidobacteria,* and other beneficial intestinal bacteria that cultivate normal intestinal flora and suppress the spreading of parasites.

Herbal therapy

Herbal treatment should be given in combination with supportive dietary treatment and continued until the worms are completely eradicated. The following herbs are helpful in treating parasitic infestations:

- *Melaleuca alternifolia* (tea tree) oil. First discovered by Australian aborigines, tea tree oil has many uses, including treating intestinal parasites, lice, and ticks.
- *Artemisia annua* (wormwood herb) and citrus seed extract. These can be used together to help eliminate intestinal parasites such as *Giardia lamblia.*
- *Berberine-containing herbs.* Berberine is an antimicrobial alkaloid that can prevent parasites from attaching to the intestinal walls of human hosts. One study found that berberine was as effective against amoebal *Giardia lamblia* as metronidazole, the standard treatment. Herbs that contain berberine include goldenseal *(Hydrastis canadensis),* barberry *(Berberis vulgaris),* Oregon grape *(Berberis aquifolium),* and goldthread *(Coptis chinensis).*

Ayurvedic medicine

Momordica charantia (**bitter melon**) is a very safe remedy for pinworm infection. The melon is a vegetable shaped like a cucumber with a bitter taste. It can be found in most Oriental markets. It should be sliced thinly and eaten raw with other vegetables to reduce its bitter taste. Daily consumption of one to two bitter melons for seven to 10 days can eliminate pinworm infection. Patients may want to repeat the regimen after several months to prevent reinfection. Chinese herbal combinations also help treat parasitic infections by supporting the gastrointestinal system, stimulating immune response, and killing parasites.

Allopathic treatment

Insect infestations

Infestations with lice, ticks, fleas, or bedbugs can be controlled by insecticides and attention to hygiene and household or environmental contact.

Intestinal parasites

Treatment for intestinal parasites usually involves anti-parasitic drugs. Depending on the severity of the condition and the species involved, treatment may include one (or more) of the following drugs: albendazole, furazolidone, iodoquinol, mebendazole, metronidazole, niclosamide, paromomycin, pyrantel pamoate, pyrimethamine, quinacrine, sulfadiazine, or thiabendazole. Nitrazoxinide was approved in 2002 for treatment of *Cryptosporidium* in children ages 1 to 11 years. In 2004, the drug was approved for people older than age 11, including adults. The approval of this drug may have led to a rise in the number of reported cases.

To prevent reinfection and transmission of disease, thorough cleaning of hands, clothes, sheets, and toys is recommended. Treatments should involve all members of the family and repeated treatments may be necessary.

CNS parasitic infections

Babies or AIDS patients with toxoplasmosis are often given spiramycin or sulfadiazine plus pyrimethamine. Treatment may be continued indefinitely for AIDS patients to prevent recurrence.

Expected results

Though parasitic infections are difficult to diagnose, complete recovery from infestation can be achieved with appropriate herbal therapy or anti-parasitic drugs. Because reinfestation is common, multiple treatments may be necessary.

Prevention

The following measures can help prevent parasitic infections:

- Washing hands before eating and after using the restroom.
- Wearing gloves when gardening or working with soil or sand because soil can be contaminated with eggs or cysts of parasites.

KEY TERMS

Contaminated—Unclean or infected by contact with or the addition of something.

Eosinophil—A type of white blood cell that increases in number in response to certain medical conditions, such as allergy or parasitic infection.

Infest—To be parasitic in a host.

Intestines—Also called the bowels and divided into the large and small intestine. They extend from the stomach to the anus, where waste products exit the body. The small intestine is about 20 ft (6.1 m) long and the large intestine, about 5 ft (1.5 m) long.

Protozoa—Single-celled microorganisms belonging to the subkingdom Protozoa that are more complex than bacteria. About 30 protozoa cause diseases in humans.

- For pregnant women, avoiding handling of cat litter.

- Not allowing children to be licked by pets; not allowing children to kiss pets that are not dewormed regularly.

- Washing fresh vegetables carefully. Many people get *Entamoeba histolytica* by eating contaminated raw fruit and vegetables.

- Avoiding eating raw meat, which may contain *Giardia lamblia*.

- Wearing long-sleeved shirts, long pants, and boots when walking in the woods. In addition, spraying insect repellent on clothing to prevent tick bites.

Resources

PERIODICALS

"Chagas Disease after Organ Transplantation—Los Angeles, California, 2006." *MMWR Weekly.* 55, no. 29 (July 28, 2006): 798–800.

Page, Kathleen R., and Jonathan Zenilman. "Eosinophilia in a Patient from South America." *Journal of the American Medical Association* 299, no. 4 (January 30, 2008): 437-444.

OTHER

"General Information: Diagnosis of Parasitic Diseases." *Division of Parasitic Diseases: Public Information.* http://www.cdc.gov/ncidod/dpd/public/geninfo_diagnosis_diseases.htm. (February 28, 2008).

"Parasitic Infections." *The Merck Manual of Diagnosis and Therapy.* http://www.merck.com/pubs/mmanual/section13/chapter161/161a.htm. (February 28, 2008).

ORGANIZATIONS

AIDS Treatment Data Network, The NETWORK, 611 Broadway, Suite 613, New York, NY, 10012, (212) 260-8868, (800)734-7104, http://www.atdn.org/.

Centers for Disease Control and Prevention (CDC), International Traveler's Hotline: (404)332-4559, http://www.cdc.gov/travel/.

Mai Tran
Teresa G. Odle, PhD
Rhonda Cloos, RN

Parkinson's disease

Definition

Parkinson's disease (PD) is a motor system disorder caused by the chronic, progressive degeneration of neurons (nerve cells) in regions of the brain that control movement. PD causes a decline in the initiation, speed, and smoothness of movement. Over time it may come to affect many bodily functions.

Description

Parkinson's Disease (PD) was first described in 1817 by James Parkinson. It affects more than one million people in the United States, including some 500,000 people who have yet to be diagnosed. About 50,000 new cases are diagnosed each year. The average age of PD onset is 60. Symptoms of PD are seen in as many as 15% of those between the ages 65 and 74 and almost 30% of those between the ages of 75 and 84. Only 5 to 10% of PD cases occur before the age of 50. Young-onset PD occurs in those under age 40. A parent or sibling with PD increases one's risk of developing the disease.

PD results from the degeneration and death of neurons in the substantia nigra, movement control centers on each side of the brain. These cells secrete dopamine, a neurotransmitter that attaches to receptors on cell surfaces in another part of the brain—the corpus striatum—that controls muscle action. When dopamine levels fall, the neurons of the corpus striatum begin to misfire. It is estimated that dopamine-producing cells begin dying about 13 years before PD symptoms become evident. The symptoms of PD begin when about 60% of the dopamine-producing cells have died.

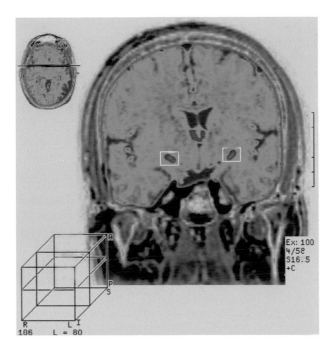

MRI image of Parkinson's Disease. *(James Cavallini / Photo Researchers, Inc.)*

Causes and symptoms

Causes

Although the cause of Parkinson's Disease (PD) is unknown, it appears to result from a combination of environmental and hereditary factors as well as oxidative damage and **aging**. Factors for PD may include:

- herbicide and pesticide exposure
- an as-yet-unidentified toxin or virus
- cellular damage from oxidation by free-radicals (atoms or molecules with an unpaired electron)
- loss of dopamine-secreting cells with age, particularly with accelerated aging
- fewer dopamine-secreting cells at birth

Symptoms

Early symptoms of PD often are quite subtle, developing on one or both sides of the body. The primary symptoms of PD are:

- tremors (shaking) while at rest. The classic PD tremor is the rubbing of the thumb and forefinger at a frequency of about three rubs per second. Tremors may spread to the hands, arms, legs, feet, jaw, and face. The tremors increase with stress. However, many people with PD do not experience tremors.
- slow movement (bradykinesia) or freezing during movement (akinesia).

- stiffness or rigidity of the limbs and trunk
- poor balance leading to frequent falls

Other early symptoms of PD include:

- short, shuffling steps
- stooped posture
- masking (reduction) of facial expression and infrequent blinking
- slow or rapid, soft, monotonic (without inflection) speech
- other speech changes
- insomnia, restlessness, and nightmares
- depression
- emotional changes, including fear, irritability, and insecurity
- incontinence
- constipation
- small, illegible handwriting
- frequent, dramatic swings in mobility and moods

Later-stage PD symptoms may include:

- frozen muscles that prevent the initiation of movement
- oily or very dry skin
- sweating
- digestive tract shutdown causing difficulties in swallowing, digesting, and elimination
- auditory and/or visual hallucinations
- progressive deterioration of intellectual function
- dementia, affecting 30 to 40% of those with late-stage PD
- loss of contact with reality (psychosis)

Medications for PD can also cause some of these symptoms.

Diagnosis

There is no definitive test for PD. Diagnosis is based on a careful medical history and complete neurological examination.

In addition to PD, anything that damages the substantia nigra can cause Parkinson's-like symptoms, called parkinsonism. Possible causes of parkinsonism include:

- infection
- nausea
- trauma
- stroke
- exposure to manganese or other toxins
- medications for psychiatric disorders, such as haloperidol (Haldol) or chlorpromazine (thorazine)

- a chemical called MPTP, present as an impurity in some illegal drugs
- epilepsy
- Alzheimer's disease
- other neurodegenerative diseases that sometimes are referred to as Parkinson's plus or parkinsonism plus syndromes

Brain scans, blood tests, lumbar puncture, or x rays may be used to rule out causes of parkinsonism other than PD.

Treatment

There is no cure for Parkinson's disease. In a study released in 2007, gene therapy showed promise. Study participants were given either low, medium, or high doses of a gene involved in the production of dopamine. The gene was injected directly into the brain cells of the participants. Three months following the injection, researchers found improvements that were similar to those previously seen after surgical intervention, such as deep brain stimulation. No side effects were noted; however, scientists believe that more research is needed.

Many factors can help relieve PD symptoms, at least temporarily:

- maintaining general health
- regular, moderate, muscle-building exercise
- frequent rest
- smaller, more frequent, meals to accommodate gastrointestinal slowdowns
- physical, occupational, and/or speech therapies
- encouragement and emotional support

Fatigue, **anxiety**, and **depression** can aggravate PD symptoms significantly.

Therapies that may relieve muscle tightness in PD include:

- acupuncture
- massage
- yoga
- Feldenkrais
- t'ai chi
- qigong
- meditation

A physical therapist can design an appropriate **exercise** program and suggest strategies and techniques for improving balance and stimulating movement during slowdowns or freezing.

Supplementation therapies for PD include:

- amino acids

- essential fatty acids, including omega-3 and omega-6 fatty acids, fish oil, and flax oil
- antioxidants, including carotenoids (dark green and orange fruits and vegetables) and other bioflavonoids (antioxidants derived from foods)
- vitamins A, B, C, and E
- selenium and zinc
- calcium and magnesium
- coenzyme Q_{10} (CoQ_{10}).

For more than 4,000 years, practitioners of Ayurveda—traditional Indian medicine—have prescribed mucuna seeds (*Mucuna pruriens*) to treat Parkinson's disease. Mucuna contains a natural form of levodopa.

Allopathic treatment

Drugs

The pharmacological treatment of Parkinson's disease is very complex. Although many drugs may relieve at least some symptoms of PD, their effectiveness varies with the patient and the progression of the disease. Side effects may preclude the use of the most effective dose or require another drug to counteract them.

A study released in 2007 found that a blood pressure medication known as israpidine forced the neurons of mice to use dopamine in a more youthful manner of generating electrical impulses. Researchers hoped that further investigation would show a link to slowing the progression of PD.

LEVODOPA. Levodopa (L-dopa, L-3,4-dihydroxyphenylalanine) has been the standard treatment for PD since the 1960s and remains one of the best drugs for treating symptoms, particularly tremors and movement problems. Levodopa (Laradopa) is a naturally occurring derivative of dopamine that is converted into dopamine in the brain. However, unlike dopamine, levodopa can reach the brain from the bloodstream. Levodopa treatment may begin at the onset of PD symptoms or when the symptoms begin to interfere with daily life. At least 75% of patients are helped to some degree by levodopa, and the drug enables many people with PD to live relatively normal lives for a number of years. Levodopa normally is prescribed only in combination with other drugs.

Side effects of levodopa include:

- nausea and vomiting
- low blood pressure, particularly when standing up, resulting in dizziness and fainting
- dyskinesias (abnormal movements, including twisting and tics) in at least 50% of patients
- agitation
- hallucinations

These effects usually lessen after several weeks on levodopa.

After five or more years on levodopa, many patients develop the following:

- motor fluctuations, including "peak-dose" dyskinesias when the drug is at its highest level in the brain
- on-off phenomena—significant changes in response as the drug levels fluctuate
- unpredictable responses to the drug

The levodopa dosage is usually increased when these changes occur. However, dyskinesias may increase with increasing dosages.

Levodopa is an amino acid that is absorbed from the digestive system by the same transporters that carry **amino acids** from dietary proteins. Therefore some healthcare practitioners may limit or redistribute protein intake to improve levodopa adsorption into the bloodstream.

ENZYME INHIBITORS. Since levodopa and dopamine are amino acids, they can be broken down by the same enzyme systems that break down other amino acids. Therefore, the two most commonly prescribed forms of levodopa are an amino-acid-decarboxylase (AADC) inhibitor: carbidopa (in Sinemet) or benzascride (in Madopar). These drugs enable more levodopa to enter the brain and may reduce some side effects. Controlled-release formulations (Sinemet CR) can prolong the interval between doses. Carbidopa also prevents vitamin B_6 (pyridoxin) from interfering with levodopa.

Catechol-O-methyltransferase (COMT) also breaks down levodopa. The COMT inhibitor entacapone (Comtan) prolongs the effects of levodopa and may moderate its fluctuations. Stalevo contains levodopa, carbidopa, and entacapone. Although the COMT inhibitor tolcapone (Tasmar) reduces the average required dosage of levodopa by 25%, as of 2008 it was no longer commonly used because of severe side effects and possible liver damage and failure.

Selegiline (deprenyl) inhibits monoamine oxidase B (MAO-B), which metabolizes dopamine in the brain. Selegiline can delay levodopa treatment for an average of nine months and also is used in combination with levodopa (Eldepryl) in early-stage PD. Common side effects include dyskinesias, **dry mouth**, and mood swings.

DOPAMINE AGONISTS. Dopamine agonists (DAs) are drugs that activate dopamine receptors, mimicking the effects of dopamine. In younger adults with early-stage PD, DAs appear to be more effective than levodopa. More often, DAs are used in conjunction with Sinemet to prolong the action of levodopa and reduce levodopa-induced dyskinesias. Although they are expensive, DAs may postpone or prevent the need for expensive neurosurgery at later stages of PD.

DAs include the following:

- bromocriptine (Parlodel)
- pergolide (Permax)
- pramipexole (Mirapex)
- ropinirole (Requip)

Side effects of DAs are similar to those of levodopa, including drowsiness and confusion. DAs may cause dyskinesias in at least 50% of patients. Pergolide has been associated with a type of **heart disease**.

ANTICHOLINERGIC DRUGS. The neurotransmitters dopamine and acetylcholine balance one another's effects in the brain. Anticholinergics help maintain this balance when dopamine levels fall. Although they may control tremors in early-stage PD, their side effects—including dry mouth, urine retention, severe **constipation**, blurred vision, confusion, **memory loss**, and hallucinations—are usually too severe for older patients or those with **dementia**. Anticholinergics rarely work for very long. Trihexyphenidyl (Artane) and benztropine (Cogentin) are the most common anticholinergics for PD.

OTHER DRUGS. Other common PD medications include:

- Diphenhydramine (Benadryl), an antihistamine, and antidepressants such as amitryptiline (Elavil), have similar effects as anticholinergics and may be appropriate for older patients.
- Amantadine (Symmetrel) is an antiviral drug used in later-stage PD, particularly to treat tremors and levodopa-induced dyskinesias. Its effects include increased dopamine release and blocking of glutamate, an amino acid that destroys neurons. Side effects include swollen ankles and purple mottling of the skin.
- Clozapine (Clozaril) is particularly effective for psychiatric symptoms of late-stage PD, including psychosis and hallucinations.

Although drug therapies can relieve most symptoms of early-stage PD, as the disease advances, drug responses begin to fluctuate and their overall effectiveness decreases.

Surgery

Surgery may be used to help manage severe or debilitating PD symptoms when drug treatments fail.

Pallidotomy uses an electrical current to destroy a small amount of brain tissue in the globus pallidus,

KEY TERMS

Acetylcholine—A major neurotransmitter that balances the effects of dopamine in the brain.

Akinesia—Inability to move.

Allopathic—The practice of medicine that combats disease with remedies that produce effects different from those produced by the disease.

Amino acid decarboxylate (AADC) inhibitors—Drugs, such as carbidopa and benserazide, that block the enzyme AADC, which breaks down levodopa in the blood.

Antioxidants—Nutrients in food that help maintain health by slowing the destructive aging process of cell molecules and improving immune responses.

Ayurveda—India's traditional health system.

Bioflavonoids—A group of chemical compounds naturally found in certain fruits, vegetables, teas, wines, nuts, seeds, and roots. Not considered vitamins, they function nutritionally as antioxidants to prevent cell destruction.

Bradykinesia—Slow movement.

Catechol-O-methyltransferase (COMT) inhibitors—Drugs, such as entacapone and tolcapone, that block COMT, an enzyme that breaks down levodopa in the blood.

Corpus striatum—Regions on each side of the brain that transmit signals for movement in response to dopamine from the substantia nigra.

Dopamine—A brain neurotransmitter that sends signals that help to control movement.

Dopamine agonist (DA)—A drug that binds to dopamine receptors on cell surfaces and mimics the effects of dopamine.

Dyskinesia—An abnormal involuntary movement or tic.

Feldenkrais—An educational method dedicated to improved movement and enhanced functioning originated by Moshe Feldenkrais (1904–1984), an engineer, physicist, and Judo expert.

Globus pallidus—Areas on each side of the brain that transmit signals controlling movement.

Levodopa—A naturally occurring amino acid that is converted to dopamine in the brain; the primary treatment for Parkinson's disease.

Monoamine oxidase (MAO-B) inhibitors—Drugs such as selegiline that inhibit the enzyme MAO-B that breaks down dopamine in the brain.

Neurotransmitter—A chemical that helps to transmit signals between two nerves or between a nerve and a muscle.

Pallidotomy—Surgery that destroys a small amount of tissue in the globus pallidus, which is over-stimulated by the corpus striatum in PD. The surgery can improve tremors, rigidity, and bradykinesia.

Parkinsonism—A disease or condition with symptoms similar to those of Parkinson's disease.

Substantia nigra—Movement control centers of the brain containing dopamine-producing cells.

T'ai chi—An ancient Chinese martial art consisting of slow, rhythmic movements to relieve stress, anxiety, and depression, and provide cardiovascular, respiratory, and pain relief benefits. Qigong is a form of T'ai chi.

Thalamotomy—Surgery that destroys a small amount of tissue in the thalamus to control PD tremors.

Thalamus—An important relay center for sensory signals in the cerebral cortex of the brain.

which is over-stimulated by the corpus striatum in PD. Pallidotomy may relieve tremors and slow, rigid movements, and decrease dyskinesia caused by drug therapy, by interfering with the neural pathway between the globus pallidus and the thalamus (a major transmission center in the brain). The benefits often do not last and the surgery may cause slurred speech, disabling weakness, and vision problems, particularly with a double pallidotomy (surgery on both sides of the brain).

Thalamotomy reduces hand and arm tremors by destroying small amounts of tissue in the thalamus.

Because a double thalamotomy leaves patients extremely weak and with slurred speech, it usually is performed on only one side of the brain, relieving tremors on the opposite side of the body.

With deep brain stimulation (DBS), a device similar to a heart pacemaker sends signals to fine electrodes implanted in the subthalamic nuclei or the globus pallidus (Activa Therapy). The electrical pulses appear to interrupt signals from the thalamus that are involved in tremors. DBS restores a balance between excitatory (tending to excite) and inhibitory (interfering or retarding) signals in brain signal transmission centers, thereby decreasing or abolishing dyskinesias without slowing normal movement. Patients use a magnetic device to adjust stimulation in one or both halves of the brain, as the response dictates. DBS usually results in a significant improvement in some motor symptoms, including tremors and peak-dose dyskinesias and improves motor function and mobility. It also enables patients to take higher doses of levodopa. The best candidates for DBS are persons who have been afflicted with PD for 10 to 20 years and who have wearing-off motor fluctuations, periods of extreme slowness in movement, and twisting motions caused by medications. Risks may be as minor as drowsiness or **headache** or as serious as hemorrhage, **stroke**, or infection.

The implantation of fetal cells to replace the dopamine-producing cells of the substantia nigra appears to benefit only patients under age 60. It can have serious side effects and about 15% of patients later develop severe dyskinesia due to dopamine-overproduction.

The use of stem cells derived from embryos discarded by **infertility** clinics is a potentially useful treatment for PD. However, it remains morally and ethically controversial, and as of 2008, the treatment was linked to law-making decisions and opinions.

Prognosis

There is no way to predict the course of PD. Many people live active, productive lives for 12 to 15 years. However, in others the disease progresses rapidly. Regardless of treatment, PD symptoms worsen with time and become less responsive to drug therapy. Most people with PD experience some additional problem every year. A small number of patients eventually become completely incapacitated. Although PD is not fatal, its effects can lead to fatal accidents or illnesses.

Prevention

There are no clear risk factors or preventions for PD. Central body **obesity** may increase the risk. Some studies have found that coffee drinking or hormone replacement therapy (HRT) in postmenopausal women may decrease the risk of PD. However, heavy coffee drinking in combination with HRT appears to increase the risk of Parkinson's disease.

Resources

BOOKS

Christensen, Jackie Hunt. *The First Year—Parkinson's Disease: An Essential Guide for the Newly Diagnosed.* New York: Marlowe, 2005.
Ford, Blair. *Deep Brain Stimulation for Parkinson's Disease.* New York: Parkinson's Disease Foundation, 2005.

Weiner, William J. *Parkinson's Disease: A Complete Guide for Patients and Families (A Johns Hopkins Press Health Book)*. Baltimore, MD: Johns Hopkins University Press, 2007.

PERIODICALS

Bean, Bruce P. "Neurophysiology: Stressful Pacemaking." *Nature* 60, no. 447 (June 28, 2007): 1059–1060.

OTHER

Gardner, Amanda. "First Gene Therapy Trial Effective Against Parkinson's." *Healthfinder.gov* (2007). http://www.healthfinder.gov/news/newsstory.asp?docID= 605764. (February 18, 2008).

ORGANIZATIONS

American Parkinson Disease Association, Inc, 1250 Hylan Blvd., Suite 4B, Staten Island, NY, 10305, (800) 223-2732, http://www.apdaparkinson.com.
Michael J. Fox Foundation for Parkinson's Research, Grand Central Station, PO Box 4777, New York, NY, 10163, (800) 708-7644, http://www.michaeljfox.org.
National Parkinson Foundation, 1501 NW Ninth Ave./Bob Hope Rd., Miami, FL, 33136-1494, (800) 327-4545, http://www.parkinson.org.
Parkinson Alliance, PO Box 308, Kingston, NJ, 08528-0308, (800) 579-8440, http://www.parkinsonalliance.net.
Parkinson's Action Network, 1000 Vermont Ave. NW, Washington, DC, 20005, (800) 850-4725 , (202) 842-4101, http://parkinsonsaction.org.
Parkinson's Disease Foundation, 710 West 168th Street, New York, NY, 10032-9982, (800) 457-6676 , (212) 923-4778, http://www.parkinsons-foundation.org.

Paula Ford-Martin
Margaret Alic, PhD
Rhonda Cloos, RN

Parotitis *see* **Mumps**
Parrot fever *see* **Psittacosis**

Parsley

Description

Parsley (*Petroselinum crispum* and *P. sativum*) is a member of the Apiaceae family of plants. Relatives of this common culinary herb include the garden vegetables carrot, parsnip, and celery. Parsley belongs to the same family as poison hemlock (*Conium maculatum L.*), a deadly narcotic herb. Parsley is native to the Mediterranean area but is now naturalized and cultivated throughout the world. Nicolas Culpeper, the seventeenth-century English herbalist and astrologer, placed parsley under the dominion of the planet Mercury. Common names for

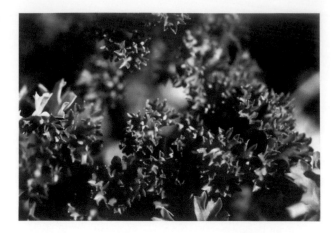

Fresh parsley. *(Photo by Kelly Quin. Reproduced by permission.)*

this herb include parsley breakstone, garden parsley, rock parsley, persely, and petersylinge. A variety known as Hamburg parsley (*P. crispum, "Tuberosum"*), first cultivated in Holland, has a root as much as six times as large as garden parsley.

In ancient times parsley was dedicated to Persephone, the wife of Hades and goddess of the underworld. Parsley is slow to germinate. Folk legend explains this characteristic with the myth that parsley must first visit Hades seven times before it may freely germinate and flourish on the earth. It was also believed that the herb would flourish only in gardens where a strong woman presides over the household. Parsley was used as a ceremonial herb in ancient Greek and Roman cultures. The herb was sprinkled on corpses to cover the stench, and planted on the graves of loved ones. Roman gladiators ate parsley before facing foes in the arena. Victorious Greek athletes were crowned with parsley. In the Middle Ages this lovely herb was known as merry parsley and was credited with lethal powers. It was believed that one could bring certain death to an adversary by pulling a parsley root from the earth while calling out the enemy's name.

Parsley is a self-seeding biennial that thrives in rich, moist soil in full sun or partial shade. It grows from a single spindle-shaped taproot producing smooth, many-branched and juicy stems. The bright green leaves are feather-like in appearance, tri-pinnate and finely divided. Some varieties are flat-leafed, others are more compact and curly. Diminutive five-petaled flowers are yellow-green and borne in dense, flat-topped clusters. They bloom in midsummer. The gray-brown seeds are tiny, ribbed and ovate (egg-shaped). Parsley can grow as much as 3 ft (1 m) tall

in its second year as the flower-bearing stems become nearly leafless and reach for the sun.

General use

Parsley's taproot, leaves, and seeds are used medicinally. The leaf is used extensively as a culinary herb and garnish. Parsley's volatile oil, particularly the oil from the seed, contains the chemicals apiole, also known as parsley camphor, and myristicin in varying quantities depending on the variety of parsley. These constituents are diuretic, and also act as uterine stimulants. The diuretic effect of parsley appears to be related to increased retention of **potassium** in the small intestine.

Internal uses

In folk tradition, parsley has been used to promote **menstruation**, facilitate **childbirth**, and increase female libido. Its emmenagogic properties can bring on delayed menstruation. Parsley juice also inhibits the secretion of histamine; it is useful in treating **hives** and relieving other allergy symptoms. A decoction of parsley root can help eliminate bloating and reduce weight by eliminating excess water gain. Parsley has also been used traditionally as a liver tonic and as a means of breaking up **kidney stones**. The German Commission E, an advisory panel on herbal medicines, has approved parsley for use in the prevention and treatment of kidney stones. The saponin content of parsley may help relieve coughs. Parsley root is laxative and its carminative action can relieve flatulence and **colic**. Parsley is rich in vitamins and minerals, including A and C, as well as **calcium**, thiamin, **riboflavin**, **niacin**, **zinc**, potassium, and **iron**. The **boron** and fluorine in parsley give strength to the bones. Parsley's high chlorophyll content makes this beneficial herb a natural as a tasty breath freshener.

More recently, the natural deodorizing activity of parsley has been put to use by the food industry. More particularly, parsley can be added to processed foods containing onions or **garlic** in order to minimize the odors associated with these vegetables.

External uses

The freshly gathered leaves of parsley have been used as a poultice to relieve breast tenderness in lactating women. Parsley poultices may also soothe tired, irritated eyes, and speed the healing of **bruises**. The juice will relieve the itch and sting of insect **bites**, and serves well as a mosquito repellent. A juice-soaked gauze pad can be applied to relieve **earache** or **toothache**, or used as a face wash to lighten freckles. The

KEY TERMS

Abortifacient—An agent that induces abortion.

Biennial—A plant that takes two years to complete its life cycle. It produces fruit and flowers only in the second year.

Carminative—A substance or preparation that relieves digestive gas.

Diuretic—A medication or substance that increases urine output.

Emmenagogue—A type of medication that brings on or increases a woman's menstrual flow.

Infusion—The most potent type of extraction of a herb into water. Infusions are steeped for a longer period of time than teas.

Photosensitivity—An abnormal reaction to light exposure caused by a disorder or resulting from the use of certain drugs.

Pinnate—Having leaflets arranged on each side of a common stalk. Parsley has a tripinnate leaf.

Saponin—A compound found in parsley, soapwort, and other plants, that forms a stable foam when added to water. Saponin is used commercially in beverages.

Tincture—An alcoholic solution of a chemical or drug.

powdered seeds, sprinkled on the hair and massaged into the scalp for three days, are a folk remedy said to stimulate hair growth. Parsley has also been used as a hair rinse in efforts to eradicate head lice.

Preparations

The root and seed of parsley should be harvested in the fall from plants in the second year of growth. The leaves can be harvested throughout the growing season. It is important not to confuse wild parsley with the herb *Aethusa cynapium*, also known as "fool's parsley." It would be a toxic mistake.

After harvesting, remove parsley leaves from the stems and place them in a single layer on a drying tray out of direct sunlight in an airy room. When the herb is thoroughly dry, store it in tightly sealed, clearly labeled dark glass containers.

Decoction: Many of parsley's medicinal properties are concentrated in the root and are best extracted by decoction. Add about 1 tsp of thinly-sliced fresh or dried parsley root to 8 oz of cold water in a glass or ceramic pot. Bring to a boil; reduce heat and simmer for about ten minutes and infuse for an additional ten minutes. Drink up to three cups daily.

Infusion: Place 2 oz of fresh parsley leaves or root in a warmed glass container. Bring 2.5 cups of fresh nonchlorinated water to the boiling point and add it to the herbs. Cover and infuse the tea for about ten minutes, then strain. Drink the herb after the infusion cools. The prepared tea can be kept for about two days in the refrigerator. Parsley tea may be enjoyed by the cupful up to three times a day.

Tincture: Combine 4 oz of finely-cut fresh or powdered dry herb with 1 pt of brandy, gin, or vodka in a glass container. There should be enough alcohol to cover the plant parts and have a 50/50 ratio of alcohol to water. Place the mixture away from light for about two weeks, shaking several times each day. Strain and store in a tightly capped dark glass bottle. A standard dose is 1/2–1 tsp of the tincture up to three times a day

Juice: Large amounts of organic fresh parsley are needed for juicing. An electric home juicer or food processor may be used. Squeeze any pulp through a sieve to extract all the juice. Prepare parsley juice fresh as needed, and store in clearly labeled glass containers. Keep refrigerated.

Precautions

A chemical found in the oil-rich seeds of parsley has abortifacient properties. For this reason, women should not use parsley during **pregnancy** or lactation. Parsley irritates the epithelial tissues of the kidney, increasing blood flow and filtration rate; therefore persons with kidney disease should not take this herb internally without consultation with a qualified herbalist or physician. According to the *PDR for Herbal Medicine*, the daily dose of parsley in medicinal preparations is 2.1 oz (6 g). Parsley's volatile oil is toxic in high doses, and overdose can lead to poisonings.

Side effects

Parsley contains furocoumarins– compounds that can cause photosensitivity in fair-skinned persons exposed to sunlight after "intensive skin contact" with the freshly harvested herb. Parsley may also cause allergy in sensitive persons.

Interactions

No interactions have been reported between parsley and standard allopathic medications.

Resources

BOOKS

Coon, Nelson. *An American Herbal: Using Plants For Healing.* Emmaus, PA: Rodale Press, 1979.

Duke, James A., Ph.D. *The Green Pharmacy.* Emmaus, PA: Rodale Press, 1997.

Foster, Steven, and James A. Duke. *Peterson Field Guides, Eastern/Central Medicinal Plants.* Boston and New York: Houghton Mifflin Company, 1990.

Hoffmann, David. *The New Holistic Herbal,* 2nd ed. Boston: Element, 1986.

Hutchens, Alma R. *A Handbook of Native American Herbs.* Boston: Shambhala Publications, Inc., 1992.

PDR for Herbal Medicines. Montvale, NJ: Medical Economics Company, 1998.

Tyler, Varro E., Ph.D. *Herbs of Choice.* New York: Pharmaceutical Products Press, The Haworth Press, Inc., 1994.

Weiss, Gaea, and Shandor Weiss. *Growing & Using the Healing Herbs.* New York: Wings Books, 1992.

PERIODICALS

Kreydiyyeh, S. I., and J. Usta. "Diuretic Effect and Mechanism of Action of Parsley." *Journal of Ethnopharmacology* 79 (March 2002): 353-357.

Negishi, O., T. Negishi, and T. Ozawa. "Effects of Food Materials on Removal of Allium-specific Volatile Sulfur Compounds." *Journal of Agriculture and Food Chemistry* 50 (June 19, 2002): 3856-3861.

ORGANIZATIONS

United States Department of Agriculture. Washington, DC 20250. www.usda.gov.

Clare Hanrahan
Rebecca J. Frey, PhD

Partridge berry *see* **Squawvine**
Pasque flower *see* **Pulsatilla**

Passionflower

Description

Passionflower (*Passiflora incarnata*) is a creeping perennial vine with white, purple-tinged flowers and orange berries that grows to a height of up to 30 ft (9 m). First used by Native Americans and the Aztecs of Mexico as a sedative, passionflower has been a popular folk remedy for centuries in Europe and North America. Other names for passionflower include maypop, granadilla, passion vine, and apricot vine. The herb, which is generally used today to alleviate **anxiety** and **insomnia**, received its curious name from the Spanish conquistadors who overran Mexico and Peru in the sixteenth century. In the flowers of the vine, they saw various symbols of the Passion of Christ, which in Christian tradition refers to the period of time between the Last Supper and Christ's death. In the Spaniard's elaborate analogy, the corona in the center of the flower was thought to resemble the crown of thorns worn by Jesus during the crucifixion. The flower's tendrils symbolized whips, the five stamens represented Christ's **wounds**, the total number of petals corresponded to the 10 faithful apostles (Peter and Judas did not make the cut), and so on.

While there are over 400 species belonging to the genus *Passiflora*, the variety used for medicinal purposes is called *incarnata*, which can be translated "embodied." The plant is obtained primarily from the southern United States, India, and the West Indies, though passionflower also grows in Mexico as well as Central and South America. Only the parts of the plant that grow above the ground are used as a drug, in fresh and dried form.

Some investigations of passionflower have been conducted in humans; in addition, animal and other studies suggest that the herb has sedative, anxiolytic, and antispasmodic properties. The German Commission E, considered an authoritative source of information on alternative remedies, reported that passionflower appears to reduce restlessness in animals. In a 1988 study involving rats that was published in a German journal of pharmacology, passionflower was shown to prolong sleep, reduce motor activity, and protect the rodents from convulsions. Despite findings such as these, researchers have been unable to identify the herb's active ingredients. Attention has focused on flavonoids (medicinal passionflower contains up to 2.5% of these chemicals); maltol; and harmala alkaloids such as harman, harmine, harmaline, and harmalol. (The Germans attempted to use harmine as a truth serum during World War II because of the chemical's reputation for inducing a euphoria-like state.) Some researchers speculate that it is the interaction, or synergy, of several chemicals in passionflower that is responsible for the herb's therapeutic effects.

General use

Although it has not been approved by the Food and Drug Administration (FDA), passionflower is mainly used in the United States and Europe to relieve anxiety, restlessness, and insomnia. It is also recommended for the relief of **nausea** caused by nervousness or anxiety. The herb appears to work, at least in part, by mildly depressing the central nervous system and preventing **muscle spasms**. In its capacity as a sedative and sleep aid, passionflower has been endorsed by

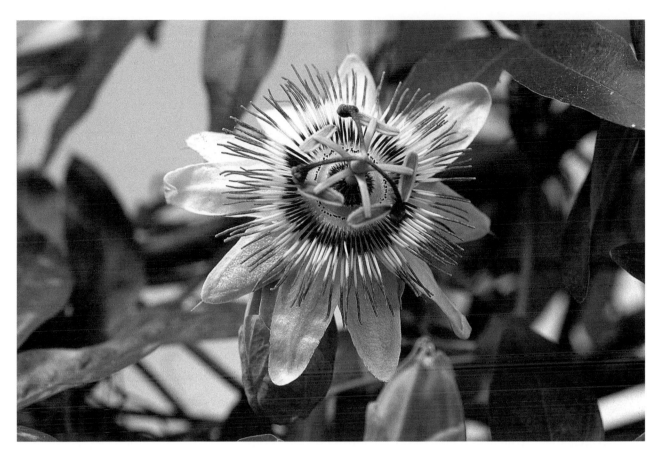

Passionflower blossom. *(©PlantaPhile, Germany. Reproduced by permission.)*

several important European research organizations. For over 15 years, passionflower has been approved by Commission E for the treatment of nervous unrest. The European Scientific Cooperative on Phytotherapy has approved the herb for use in people who experience tension, restlessness, and insomnia associated with irritability. Passionflower is listed in many national pharmacopoeiae as a drug plant.

Passionflower is often used in combination with other sedative plants. In the United Kingdom, it is an ingredient in several dozen over-the-counter (OTC) sedatives. In Germany, the herb is used as an ingredient in sedative preparations that also include **valerian** and **lemon balm**. The standardized sedative tea formula approved by Commission E contains 30% passionflower, 40% valerian root, and 30% lemon balm. Passionflower is also used in Germany in a special sedative tea for children. The ingredients of this tea typically include 30% passionflower, 30% lemon balm, 30% **lavender** flower, and 10% **St. John's wort**. In combination with **hawthorn**, passionflower is also used to alleviate digestive spasms associated with **gastritis** and **colitis**.

In the past, passionflower was approved by the FDA as an ingredient in OTC sleep aids and sedative products. This approval was revoked in 1978 during a review by the agency, but not because the reviewers found passionflower to be unsafe or ineffective. Drug manufacturers were responsible for submitting information about the safety and effectiveness of OTC medications under review by the FDA. No companies submitted data for passionflower, so the herb was denied approval because it had no sponsors.

Throughout its history, passionflower has been used to treat a variety of medical problems in addition to those mentioned above. These include **epilepsy**, **diarrhea**, **neuralgia**, **asthma**, **whooping cough**, seizures, painful **menstruation**, and **hemorrhoids** (when used externally). Some herbalists also recommend passionflower as a treatment for **Parkinson's disease**, based on their belief that the harmine and harmaline in the herb may help to counteract the effects of the disorder. As of 2000, these additional uses for passionflower are considered speculative.

In 2002, a team of American researchers published a report finding that passionflower shows promise as a chemopreventive for **cancer**. The scientists found that passionflower extract inhibits an early antigen of Epstein-Barr virus, which suggests that it may also inhibit the growth of cancerous tumors.

Preparations

Recommended dosages of passionflower generally range from 4–8 g of herb a day. While it is typically used in preparations containing other sedative ingredients, it may also be used alone. Passionflower tea can be prepared by steeping 1 teaspoonful of the herb in 150 ml of simmering water. The mixture should be strained after about 10 minutes. Dosage is usually two or three cups of tea a day, taken during the day and a half-hour before going to bed. The liquid extract preparation is usually taken three times a day in doses of 0.5–1.0 ml. Dosage for the tincture is 0.5–2.0 ml three times a day. Tablets containing passionflower are available in the United Kingdom. Persons who use a combination product containing passionflower should follow the package directions for use.

Precautions

Passionflower is not known to be harmful when taken in recommended dosages, though there are some precautions to consider. The herb contains two potentially dangerous alkaloids called harman and harmaline. In large amounts, these chemicals may stimulate the tissue of the uterus. However, most authorities believe that the amounts of harman and harmaline contained in medicinal passionflower are too small to have an adverse effect when the herb is used in normal amounts. Caution should also be exercised when combining passionflower with certain medications (see below).

While self-care measures such as passionflower may be effective in relieving anxiety or insomnia, these problems may be a symptom of a more serious psychological disorder that requires consultation with a mental health professional. Nighttime sleep aids should not be used for longer than two weeks without seeking medical advice. Due to lack of sufficient medical study, passionflower should be used with caution in children, women who are pregnant or breast-feeding, and people with liver or kidney disease.

Side effects

When taken in recommended dosages, passionflower has not been associated with any significant or bothersome side effects.

Interactions

Passionflower has the potential to interact adversely with certain medications. The harman and harmaline in passionflower may increase the effects of prescription antidepressants called monoamine oxidase inhibitors (MAOIs), which are generally used to treat **depression**, panic attacks, and eating disorders. Passionflower may also increase the effects of OTC sedatives as well as those sold by prescription.

Resources

BOOKS

Gruenwald, Joerg. *PDR for Herbal Medicines.* New Jersey: Medical Economics, 1998.

Newall, Carol A. *Herbal Medicines: A Guide for Health Care Professionals.* London: Pharmaceutical Products Press, 1996.

Sifton, David W. *PDR Family Guide to Natural Medicines and Healing Therapies.* New York: Three Rivers Press, 1999.

Tyler, Varro E. *Herbs of Choice.* New York: Pharmaceutical Products Press, 1994.

PERIODICALS

Kapadia, G. J., M. A. Azuine, H. Tokuda, et al. "Inhibitory Effect of Herbal Remedies on 12-o-Tetradecanoylphorbol-13-Acetate-Promoted Epstein-Barr Virus Early Antigen Activation." *Pharmacological Research* 45 (March 2002): 213-222.

ORGANIZATIONS

American Botanical Council. P.O. Box 144345. Austin, TX 78714-4345. http://www.herbalgram.org.

Herb Research Foundation. 1007 Pearl Street. Suite 200. Boulder, CO 80302. http://www.herbs.org.

OTHER

Discovery Health. http://www.discoveryhealth.com.
OnHealth. http://www.onhealth.com.

Greg Annussek
Rebecca J. Frey, PhD

Past life therapy

Definition

Past life therapy is a therapy in which an individual is regressed to past lives in order to heal and resolve ailments and situations from the current life.

Origins

Past life therapy is based on the ancient belief of reincarnation. The foundation of Hindu philosophy, reincarnation dates back thousands of years. It is the notion that the soul is eternal and incarnates again and again, retaining all the knowledge of events that occur during each lifetime.

Karma is an important component of reincarnation. It is a Sanskrit word meaning action. The basis of karma is that every action has a reaction: cause and effect. Each lifetime is lived in order to resolve unwholesome actions in previous lifetimes. The circumstances of each life are determined by the growth and progress achieved in a past life. According to this theory, a person's actions in one lifetime determine the conditions, situations, relationships, environment, and opportunities of the next life.

The actions carried out in one lifetime are often carried through to the next life. For instance, someone who committed a murder in a previous life may encounter a lifetime in which he will have to deal with anger and violence. Although "past lives" began as a religious concept, since the 1960s it has been used in the therapeutic community to help people reframe current issues in their lives that are blocking their health and well-being. Whether or not there are past-life experiences and memories is debatable and ultimately unprovable. They may be metaphors of the mind. Even so, they can serve as useful processes for bringing understanding and resolution to present conflicts.

Benefits

Past life therapy is reported to have a myriad of benefits. Memories revealed from a past life allow individuals to alter their perspectives on their current lives. This therapy helps people to understand who they are, learn how past life events have affected present life circumstances, and to offer insight into hidden conflicts so that repeating patterns may be stopped.

Awareness created through regression therapy allows mental, physical, and emotional release. Patients may let go of deep-seated emotions, fears, and guilt that often result in the relief of such problems as chronic **pain**,

alcoholism, jealousy, arthritis, claustrophobia, agoraphobia, migraine headaches, weight problems, **insomnia**, obsessive/compulsive behaviors, chemical dependencies, **depression**, and sexual dysfunctions. The release of fear and other painful emotions strengthens will and self-esteem and fosters forgiveness towards others and towards the self.

Throughout their lives individuals may have felt negativity towards certain persons or places. They may be averse to particular foods, be prone to illness or disease, or have recurring dreams. This may be the result of a past life connection. By becoming aware of the roots of these conditions the negativity is released and healing often occurs.

Description

Past lives may be accessed through regression therapy, hypnosis, **guided imagery**, dreams, craniosacral therapy and other types of bodywork, spontaneous regressions, automatic writing, **meditation**, or contact with one's higher self. Dealing with one's higher self is achieved through meditation and hypnosis and is based on the belief that the soul retains information of past lives and uses this to set the destiny of the current life. Contacting the higher self is said to help change one's destiny. The therapy is usually performed on an individual basis.

Past life therapy is usually undertaken to reach the source of problems or conflicts in the current life. The purpose of a regression session is to release guilt, fears, and other emotions tied to past events in order to make appropriate decisions in the present lifetime and gain an understanding of present relationships.

One common method of exploring past lives is through hypnosis. During a hypnotic regression, the patient is relaxed into a light trance state in which he or she is often completely aware of the surroundings. In order to achieve this state, the therapist may lead the patient through a guided fantasy. The patient may begin to intuit an awareness of a scene or see moving pictures as in a movie or on television. The patient may see or hear words describing a scene and feel emotions relating to that scene. The therapist acts as a coach, encouraging the patient to explain what she is seeing and feeling until the scene has stopped.

BRIAN WEISS (1944-)

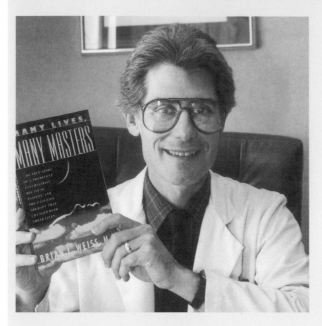

(AP/Wide World Photos. Reproduced by permission.)

Brian L. Weiss graduated from Columbia University and Yale Medical School, where he received his degree in medicine with a specialty in psychiatry. He is Chairman Emeritus of Psychiatry at the Mount Sinai Medical Center in Miami and a former professor of psychiatry at the University of Miami School of Medicine. He is an advocate of the clinical applications of regression or past life therapy in treating phobias, addictions, depression, and psychosomatic disorders. Weiss uses hypnosis to access patients' memories of their childhood and past lives. His interest began when a woman he had hypnotized said she had communicated with his dead infant son through spirits called the Masters. The woman claimed to have lived at least 86 previous lives.

He conducts lectures around the world and is a frequent guest on radio and television talk shows. Weiss is author of several books, including *Many Lives, Many Masters* (1988), *Through Time Into Healing* (1993), *Only Love is Real: A Story of Soulmates Reunited* (1995), and *Messages from the Masters* (2000). He is founder of the Weiss Institute and maintains a practice at 6701 SW 72nd St, Miami, FL.

In the past life regression, the patient may recognize people from her current life. According to the karmic theory, souls who are closely related in one life will meet in another. Often people who bond together in this lifetime, such as family, lovers, or friends, have also been together in previous lives. The significance of meeting again is to resolve karmic issues from other lives in order to promote growth and healing.

Past lives generally are not experienced in a sequential fashion. This is due to the karmic understanding that past lives are revealed at a time when the individual will benefit most by the lesson learned through the review.

Research and general acceptance

Much research has been conducted on past life therapy. One of the proponents of the past life movement, Dr. Brian Weiss, has written several books detailing the experiences he has encountered while performing past life regressions.

Dr. Ian Stevenson, professor of psychiatry at the University of Virginia, has conducted research on children who consciously recall their past lives. One of his cases involved a girl from India named Shanti Devi. When she was very young, Shanti began to talk about a husband and children. She gave the address of

her "former" home and the identity of her husband. When she was nine, Shanti was taken to the house, where she retrieved some jewelry she had buried in the garden in her former life.

Past life therapy is not generally accepted by most Western medical practitioners. Although the idea of discovering past lives through hypnosis became popularized in the 1970s, it is now under criticism by modern psychologists. Many contend that patients under hypnosis are directed to remember past lives by the suggestions of hypnotherapists, and subsequently fabricate false memories of past lives.

Training and certification

Past life therapy may be performed by trained psychologists, persons trained in **hypnotherapy** or regression techniques, or psychics or mediums. The techniques used for past life regressions are the same techniques used for age regression therapy.

Resources

BOOKS

Andrews, Ted. *How to Uncover Your Past Lives*. Minnesota: Llewellyn Publications, 1997.

Avery, Jeanne. *Past Lives, Present Loves*. Signet, 1999.

Eason, Cassandra. *Discover Your Past Lives*. England: Foulsham, 1996.

ORGANIZATIONS

Association for Past Life Research and Therapies, Inc., P.O. Box 20151 Riverside, CA 92516. http://www.pastlifehealing.com/.

Jennifer Wurges

Pau d'arco

Description

Pau d'arco (pronounced pow-darko) is a large tree that grows in the Amazon rain forest and in tropical areas of South America. The botanical names for the species most commonly used are *Tabebuia heptaphylla* and *Tabebuia impetiginosa*. The tree is called taheebo or lapacho in South America. The inner bark of pau d'arco is used as an herbal medicine, most notably in the treatment of **cancer** and **infections**.

The pau d'arco tree grows up to 150 ft (45 m) tall and 10 ft (3 m) in diameter, and is prized for its lumber. The wood is extremely hard, and makes fine furniture. The tree produces large purple flowers, making it popular for landscaping and decoration. The bark of the tree has been used medicinally by native South American peoples for centuries. Rainforest medicine men scrape the inner bark and brew a tea from it. The tea has been used to treat conditions as varied as **malaria**, infections, **fever**, arthritis, skin problems, **syphilis**, **AIDS**, and cancer. Pau d'arco has long been a common herbal remedy for Europeans who moved to South America as well, and is sometimes drunk there as a refreshing tea. The tea has a cool, bitter flavor.

Pau d'arco became known to the mainstream medical community during the 1960s. At that time, a doctor named Theodore Meyer learned of the herb from a rainforest tribe, and used it to treat patients suffering from **leukemia** (cancer of the blood). He reported that the herb completely cured five cases of advanced cancer. Then, a hospital in South America used a tea made from the herb to treat cancer patients, and reported that pau d'arco reduced **pain** and cured tumors in some patients. These stories made it to the press, and pau d'arco was touted around the world as a miracle cancer cure.

Pau d'arco caught the attention of American researchers and drug companies, and scientific studies on it were performed. Scientists isolated an active

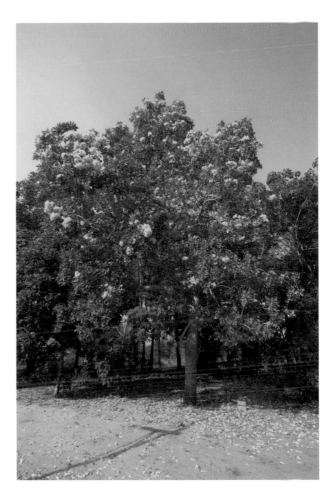

The inner bark of pau d'arco is used as an herbal medicine, most notably in the treatment of cancer and infections.
(Genevieve Vallee / Alamy)

chemical found in the bark, and termed it lapachol. Several studies showed that lapachol was effective against cancerous tumors in rats, giving it promise as a cancer cure. In 1974, however, the National Cancer Institute concluded that the amounts of lapachol required for beneficial effects against cancer in humans would result in toxic side effects, and stopped researching pau d'arco as a cancer treatment.

Although research in general did not support the huge claims made for pau d'arco, it continued to generate stories of miraculous cancer cures and other successes treating infections and chronic conditions. Some researchers have theorized that other ingredients in the bark besides lapachol may have therapeutic effects; and it has been shown that the use of the whole herb does not create the side effects that extracted lapachol causes. Researchers have isolated over 20 active chemicals in pau d'arco. Research, mainly on laboratory animals, has shown pau d'arco to have anti-microbial and anti-viral properties, helping to destroy bacteria, fungi, parasites and viruses by increasing the supply of oxygen to cells. It has demonstrated effectiveness against yeast infections, malaria, **tuberculosis**, strep, and dysentery. Pau d'arco has also been shown to influence the activity of the immune system. In small dosages, it increases immune system activity and in large doses suppresses some immune responses such as inflammation. Its anti-inflammatory actions have given pau d'arco promise as a remedy for **allergies**, arthritis, skin problems, ulcers and other inflammatory conditions.

General use

Pau d'arco is used frequently in the herbal treatment of cancer and infections, including candidiasis and other yeast infections. Pau d'arco is also used for allergies, arthritis, diabetes, flu, lupus, parasites, skin diseases, and ulcers.

Preparations

Pau d'arco is available in health food stores in capsules, tinctures, and as dried bark. The recommended dosage is 1-2 capsules or 1-2 droppersful of tincture taken one to four times per day, depending on the condition and patient.

Tea can be made from the bark by adding 1 tbsp of bark for every 3 cups of water. The tea should be boiled for 20 minutes or longer in a non-aluminum pot. One cup of tea can be taken three or four times daily for acute conditions. One-half cup three or four times daily is recommended for other conditions.

Precautions

Pregnant and lactating women should not use pau d'arco, as its effects during **pregnancy** have not been sufficiently researched. Pau d'arco has been shown to have blood-thinning actions in some people, and may cause **anemia** (shortage of red blood cells) when used over long periods. For this reason, pau d'arco should not be used before surgery or by patients with anemia or bleeding problems.

Another precaution consumers should take is assuring that the product they purchase is produced by a reputable manufacturer. Pau d'arco is a valuable resource in South America, and there has been a history of fraudulent products being exported. Some of these products have caused uncomfortable side effects that do not occur with real pau d'arco. In Canada in 1987, a chemical analysis of 12 commercial products revealed that only one contained the active ingredient lapachol, and that was in minute amounts. Some manufacturers have begun to offer products with standardized quantities of active ingredients to assure quality. The pau d'arco imported from Argentina is generally considered to be the highest quality bark.

Side effects

Possible side effects from ingesting too much pau d'arco include **nausea**, **vomiting**, **diarrhea**, **dizziness**, and stomach cramps. Long-term usage has been reported to cause anemia.

Interactions

Pau d'arco products should be avoided by those taking anticoagulant (blood thinning) medication.

Resources

BOOKS

Jones, Kenneth. *Pau d'Arco: Immune Power From the Rain Forest*. Rochester, VT: Healing Arts Press, 1995.

Taylor, Leslie. *Herbal Secrets of the Rainforest*. Rocklin, CA: Prima, 1998.

PERIODICALS

HerbalGram (a quarterly journal of the American Botanical Council and Herb Research Foundation). P.O. Box 144345, Austin, TX 78714-4345. (800) 373-7105.

Douglas Dupler

Pediculosis *see* **Lice infestation**

Pelvic inflammatory disease

Definition

Pelvic inflammatory disease (PID) is a term used to describe any infection in the lower female reproductive tract that spreads upward to the upper female

Pelvic inflammatory disease (PID) risk factors

Age: the rate of infection in women drops as they get older. Risk is highest for sexually active women under 25 years of age.

Ethnicity: the rate of infection is higher in nonwhite groups.

Socioeconomic status: the rate of infection is higher in women of lower socioeconomic status.

IUD: the rate of infection is higher with the use of IUDs, and frequent douching.

Barrier contraception: consistent use of barrier contraceptives protects against PID, although they may not protect against other STDs, such as HPV.

Lifestyle: the rate of infection is higher in women who abuse drugs and alcohol, have had intercourse for the first time at an early age, and have had a higher number of sexual partners.

STDs: the rate of infection is higher in women who have had sexually transmitted diseases.

(Illustration by Corey Light. Cengage Learning, Gale)

reproductive tract. The lower female genital tract consists of the vagina and the cervix. The upper female genital tract consists of the body of the uterus, the fallopian or uterine tubes, and the ovaries.

Description

PID is the most common and the most serious consequence of infection with sexually transmitted diseases (STD) in women. Over one million cases of PID are diagnosed annually in the United States, and it is the most common cause for hospitalization of reproductive-age women. Sexually active women aged 15–25 are at highest risk for developing PID. The disease can also occur, although less frequently, in women having monogamous sexual relationships. The most serious consequences of PID are increased risk of infertility and ectopic **pregnancy**.

To understand PID, it is helpful to understand the basics of inflammation. Inflammation is the body's response to disease-causing (pathogenic) microorganisms. The affected body part may swell due to accumulation of fluid in the tissue or may become reddened due to an excessive accumulation of blood. A discharge (pus) may be produced that consists of white blood cells and dead tissue. Following inflammation, scar tissue may form by the proliferation of scar-forming cells (fibrosis). Adhesions of fibrous tissue form and cause organs or parts of organs to stick together.

PID may be used synonymously with the following terms:

- salpingitis (inflammation of the fallopian tubes)
- endometritis (inflammation of the inside lining of the body of the uterus)
- tubo-ovarian abscesses (abscesses in the tubes and ovaries)
- pelvic peritonitis (inflammation inside of the abdominal cavity surrounding the female reproductive organs)

Causes and symptoms

A number of factors affect the risk of developing PID. They include:

- Age. The incidence of PID is very high in younger women and decreases as a woman ages.
- Race. The incidence of PID is 8–10 times higher in nonwhites than in whites.
- Socioeconomic status. The higher incidence of PID in women of lower socioeconomic status is due in part to a woman's lack of education and awareness of health and disease, and due in part to barriers to her accessibility to medical care.
- Use and method of contraception. Induced abortion, use of an IUD, nonuse of such barrier contraceptives as condoms, and frequent douching are all associated with a higher risk of developing PID.
- Lifestyle. Such high-risk behaviors as drug and alcohol abuse; early age at first intercourse; a high number of sexual partners; and smoking all are associated with a higher risk of developing PID.

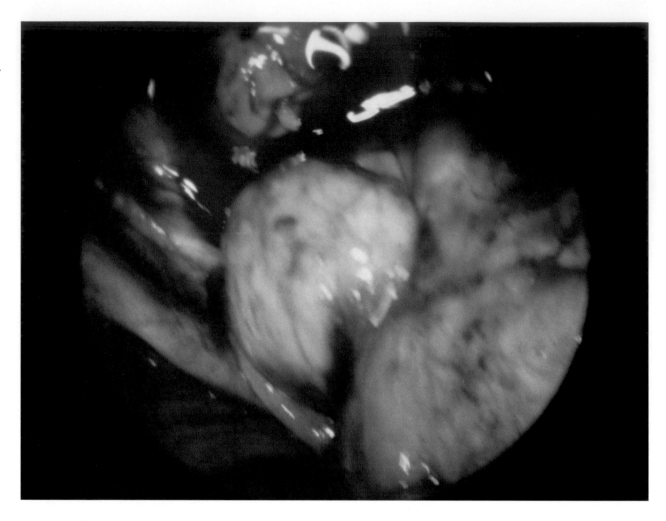

Laparoscopic view of pelvic inflammatory disease. *(Custom Medical Stock Photo. Reproduced by permission.)*

- Specific sexual practices. Intercourse during the menses and frequent intercourse may offer more opportunities for the admission of pathogenic organisms to the inside of the uterus.
- The presence of a sexually transmitted disease. Sixty to seventy-five percent of PID cases are associated with STDs. A prior episode of PID increases the chances of developing subsequent infections.

The two major organisms that cause STDs are *Neisseria gonorrhoeae* and *Chlamydia trachomatis*. The main symptom of *N. gonorrheae* infection (**gonorrhea**) is a vaginal discharge of mucus and pus. Sometimes bacteria from the colon normally in the vaginal cavity may travel upward to infect the upper female genital organs, facilitated by the infection with gonorrhea. **Infections** with *C. trachomatis* and other nongonoccal organisms are more likely to have mild or no symptoms.

Although PID is unusual in women who are not sexually active, disease organisms other than the gonococcus and *C. trachomatis* can occasionally gain entrance to the upper female reproductive tract and cause PID. Cases have been reported from Canada, Norway, and South America of PID caused by pinworms, pneumococci, and *Entamoeba histolytica*, a pathogenic amoeba.

Normally the cervix produces mucus that acts as a barrier to prevent disease-causing microorganisms, called pathogens, from entering the uterus and moving upward to the tubes and ovaries. This barrier may be breached in two ways. A sexually transmitted pathogen, usually a single organism, invades the lining cells, alters them, and gains entry. Another way for organisms to gain entry happens when trauma or alteration to the cervix occurs. **Childbirth**, spontaneous or induced abortion, or use of an intrauterine contraceptive device (IUD) are all conditions that may alter or weaken the normal lining cells, making them susceptible to infection, usually by several organisms.

KEY TERMS

Adhesion—The joining or sticking together of parts of an organ that are not normally joined together.

C-reactive protein (CRP)—A protein present in blood serum in various abnormal states, like inflammation.

Ectopic—Located away from normal position; ectopic pregnancy results in the attachment and growth of the fertilized egg outside of the uterus, a life-threatening condition.

Endometriosis—The presence and growth of functioning endometrial tissue in places other than the uterus; often results in severe pain and infertility.

Erythrocyte sedimentation rate (ESR)—The rate at which red blood cells settle out in a tube of unclotted blood, expressed in millimeters per hour; elevated sedimentation rates indicate the presence of inflammation.

Fibrosis—The formation of fibrous, or scar, tissue which may follow inflammation and destruction of normal tissue.

Hysterectomy—Surgical removal of the uterus.

Laparoscope—A thin flexible tube with a light on the end which is used to examine the inside of the abdomen; the tube is inserted into the abdomen by way of a small incision just below the navel.

Ligase chain reaction—A laboratory technique for detecting sexually transmitted disease organisms in urine by rapidly copying and recopying the organism's DNA, thus making the presence of infection easier to detect.

During **menstruation**, the cervix widens and may allow pathogens entry into the uterine cavity.

Recent evidence suggests that bacterial vaginosis (BV), a bacterial infection of the vagina, may be associated with PID. BV results from the imbalance of normal organisms in the vagina— by douching, for example. While the balance is altered, conditions then favor the overgrowth of anaerobic bacteria that thrive in the absence of free oxygen. A copious discharge is usually present. Should some trauma occur in the presence of anaerobic bacteria, such as menses, abortion, intercourse, or childbirth, these organisms may gain entrance to the upper genital organs.

The most common symptom of PID is pelvic pain. However, many women with PID have symptoms so mild that they may be unaware that they are infected.

In acute salpingitis, a common form of PID, swelling of the fallopian tubes may cause tenderness on physical examination. Fever may be present. Abscesses may develop in the tubes, ovaries, or in the surrounding pelvic cavity. Infectious discharge may leak into the peritoneal cavity and cause peritonitis; or abscesses may rupture, causing a life-threatening surgical emergency.

Chronic salpingitis may follow an acute attack. Subsequent to inflammation, scarring and resulting adhesions may result in chronic **pain** and irregular menses. Due to blockage of the tubes by scar tissue, women with chronic salpingitis suffer a high risk of having an ectopic pregnancy. An ectopic pregnancy develops when a fertilized ovum is unable to travel down the fallopian tube to the uterus and implants itself in the tube, on the ovary, or in the peritoneal cavity. This condition can also be a life-threatening surgical emergency.

IUDs

The use of intrauterine devices, or IUDs, has been strongly associated with the development of PID. Bacteria may be introduced to the uterine cavity while the IUD is being inserted or may travel up the tail of the IUD from the cervix into the uterus. Surrounding uterine tissue may show areas of inflammation, increasing its susceptibility to pathogens.

Some researchers, however, maintain that the connection between IUDs and PID has been exaggerated and that further research is necessary.

Susceptibility to STDs

Susceptibility to STDs involves many factors, some of which are not known. The ability of the organism to produce disease and the circumstances that place the organism in the right place at a time when a trauma or alteration to the lining cells has occurred are factors. The woman's own immune response also helps to determine whether infection occurs.

Diagnosis

If PID is suspected, the physician will take a complete medical history and perform an internal pelvic examination. Other diseases that may cause pelvic pain, such as appendicitis and **endometriosis**, must be ruled out. If pelvic examination reveals tenderness or pain in that region, or tenderness on movement of the cervix, these are good physical signs that PID is present.

Specific diagnosis of PID is difficult to make because the upper pelvic organs are hard to reach for samplings. The physician may take samples directly from the cervix to identify the organisms that may be responsible for infection. Two blood tests may help to establish the existence of an inflammatory process. A positive C-reactive protein (CRP) and an elevated erythrocyte sedimentation rate (ESR) indicate the presence of inflammation. The physician may take fluid from the cavity surrounding the ovaries called the *cul de sac*; this fluid may be examined directly for bacteria or may be used for culture. Diagnosis of PID may also be done using a laparoscope, but laparoscopy is expensive, and it is an invasive procedure that carries some risk for the patient.

A newer diagnostic technique that has dramatically improved the accuracy of laboratory testing for PID and other STDs is the ligase chain reaction (LCR) technique. The LCR technique detects DNA from *N. gonorrhoeae* and *C. trachomatis* in a patient's urine sample. LCR technology is less invasive as well as more accurate.

Treatment

Alternative therapy should be complementary to antibiotic therapy. Because of the potentially serious nature of this disease, a patient should first consult an allopathic physician to start antibiotic treatment for infections. Traditional medicine is better equipped to quickly eradicate the infection, while alternative treatments can help the body fight the disease and relieve painful symptoms associated with PID. Some of the alternative treatments include **diets**, nutritional supplements, herbal remedies, **homeopathy**, **acupressure**, and **acupuncture**.

General recommendations

- Bed rest. Patients need to rest and reduce physical activity to help the body recuperate faster.
- Avoid sexual activity. Both patient and her partner should be treated for PID infections. They should also avoid sexual activity until their infections are completely eradicated.
- Healthy diet. Diet should include a variety of fresh fruits and vegetables. These foods contain high amount of phytonutrients and essential vitamins that help keep the body strong and stimulate the immune system to fight infections.

Nutritional supplements

The following nutritional supplements may be helpful:

- Daily vitamin and mineral supplements. These supplements can ensure that the body receives all the essential nutrients for normal body function. They also help keep the body strong to fight diseases including PID.
- Vitamin C. High-dose vitamin C (1–2 g) boost the immune function and help the body fight infection better.

Herbal treatment

The following herbal remedies may be helpful:

- Castor oil packs. Patients can make warm packs by pouring castor oil on a clean piece of cloth wrapped in layers and warming it before placing on the lower part of their abdomen for up to 20 minutes. It is recommended that patients repeat this therapy every day for up to seven days.
- *Echinacea* spp., goldenseals and *Calendula officinalis*. These herbs are believed to have antimicrobial activity and may be taken to augment the action of prescribed antibiotics.
- Grapefruit seed extract. This herb has been used to fight a variety of infections including bacterial, viral, fungal, parasitic, and worm infections.
- Blue cohosh (*Caulophyllum thalictroides*) and false unicorn root (*Chamaelirium luteum*). These remedies are recommended as tonics for the general well-being of the female genital tract.

Homeopathy

A homeopathic practitioner may prescribe a patient-specific remedy to help reduce some of the symptoms associated with PID. Herbs that are used in PID patients include **Apis** mellifica, **Arsenicum album**, **Belladonna**, Colocynthis, Magnesia phosphorica, and Mercurius vivus.

Acupressure

Acupressure (applying pressure on specific pressure points) can increase blood flow to the pelvic region, reduce pain, and promote general health.

Acupuncture

Acupuncture involves inserting needles at various points on the skin of the body. These needles are like antennae that direct qi (life force) to organs or functions of the body. This treatment may help with pain and also strengthen immunity. It is important that patients request disposable needles to prevent transmission of **AIDS**, hepatitis, and other infectious diseases.

Allopathic treatment

If acute salpingitis is suspected, treatment with antibiotics should begin immediately. The patient is usually treated with at least two broad-spectrum antibiotics that can kill both *N. gonorrhoeae* and *C. trachomatis* plus other types of bacteria that may have the potential to cause infection. Hospitalization may be required to ensure compliance. Treatment for chronic PID may involve hysterectomy. Early treatment of suspected PID is essential because some **strains** of *N. gonorrhoeae* are showing increasing resistance to standard antibiotics as of 2002.

If a woman is diagnosed with PID, she should see that her sexual partner is also treated to prevent the possibility of reinfection.

Expected results

PID can be cured if the initial infection is treated immediately. If infection is not recognized, as frequently happens, the process of tissue destruction and scarring that results from inflammation of the tubes results in irreversible changes in the tube structure that cannot be restored to normal. Subsequent bouts of PID increase a woman's risk of complications. Thirty to forty percent of female **infertility** cases are due to acute salpingitis.

With modern antibiotic therapy, death from PID is almost nonexistent. In rare instances, death may occur from the rupture of tubo-ovarian abscesses and the resulting infection in the abdominal cavity. One recent study has linked infertility, a consequence of PID, with a higher risk of **ovarian cancer**.

Prevention

The prevention of PID is a direct result of the prevention and prompt recognition and treatment of STDs or of any suspected infection involving the female genital tract. The main symptom of infection is an abnormal discharge. To distinguish an abnormal discharge from the mild fluctuations of normal discharge associated with the menstrual cycle takes vigilance and self-awareness. Sexually active women must be able to detect symptoms of lower genital tract disease. Frank dialogue regarding sexual history, risks for PID, and treatment options is necessary with a physician. Also, open discussions with sexual partners regarding symptoms and possible infection is imperative.

Lifestyle changes should focus on preventing the transfer of organisms when the body's delicate lining cells are unprotected or compromised. Barrier contraceptives, such as condoms, diaphragms, and cervical caps, should be used. Women in monogamous relationships should use barrier contraceptives during menses and take their physician's advice regarding intercourse following abortion, childbirth, or biopsy procedures.

Resources

BOOKS

Buhner, Stephen Harrod. *Herbal Antibiotics: Natural Alternatives for Treatment of Drug-Resistant Bacteria*. Pownal, VT: Schoolhouse Road, 1999.

Kurman, Robert J., ed. *Blaustein's Pathology of the Female Genital Tract*. New York: Springer-Verlag, 1994.

Landers, D.V., and R. L. Sweet, eds. *Pelvic Inflammatory Disease*. New York: Springer, 1997.

The PDR Family Guide to Natural Medicine and Herbal Therapies: The Most Comprehensive Book of Its Kind. New York, NY: Three Rivers Press, 1999.

Zand, Janet, Allan N. Spreen and James B. LaValle. "Pelvic Inflammatory Disease." In *Smart Medicine for Healthier Living: A Practical A-to-Z Reference to Natural and Conventional Treatments for Adults*. Garden City Park, NY: Avery Publishing Group,1999: 467-469.

PERIODICALS

Bucher, A., and F. Muller. "Spectrum of Abdominal and Pelvic Infections Caused by Pneumococci in Previously Healthy Adult Women." *European Journal of Clinical Microbiology and Infectious Diseases* 21 (June 2002): 474-477.

Calore, E. E., N. M. Calore, and M. J. Cavaliere. "Salpingitis Due to *Entamoeba histolytica*." *Brazilian Journal of Infectious Diseases* 6 (April 2002): 97-99.

Centers for Disease Control and Prevention. "Sexually Transmitted Diseases Treatment Guidelines 2002." *Morbidity and Mortality Weekly Report* 51 (May 10, 2002)(RR-6): 1-78.

Espey, E., and T. Ogburn. "Perpetuating Negative Attitudes About the Intrauterine Device: Textbooks Lag Behind the Evidence." *Contraception* 65 (June 2002): 389-395.

Kissin, D. M., S. Holman, H. L. Minkoff, et al. "Epidemiology and Natural History of Ligase Chain Reaction Detected Chlamydial and Gonococcal Infections." *Sexually Transmitted Infections* 78 (June 2002): 208-209.

Tandan, T., et al. "Pelvic Inflammatory Disease Associated with *Enterobius vermicularis*." *Archives of Diseases of Childhood* 86 (June 2002): 439-440.

ORGANIZATIONS

American College of Obstetricians and Gynecologists (ACOG). 409 12th St., S.W., PO Box 96920, Washington, D.C. 20090-6920. www.acog.org.

Centers for Disease Control and Prevention (CDC). 1600 Clifton Road, Atlanta, GA 30333. (404) 639-3311. www.cdc.gov.

Mai Tran
Rebecca J. Frey, PhD

Pennyroyal

Description

Pennyroyal (*Hedeoma pulegioides*), known as American pennyroyal, and *Mentha pulegium*, known as English or European pennyroyal, are both members of the Lamiaceae or mint family. These two beneficial herbs, though classified in different genera, have similar chemical constituents and medicinal properties.

American pennyroyal is also known as mock pennyroyal, mosquito plant, fleabane, tickweed, stinking balm, and hedeoma. This aromatic American native thrives in limestone-rich soil, in fields, and in sunny patches of open woodlands throughout North America. American pennyroyal was used extensively by Native Americans to treat a variety of ailments from **headache** and stomach distress to **itching**, watery eyes, and fevers. For external use, the leaves were crushed and applied to the skin to repel mosquitoes and other insects. American pennyroyal came to be called squawmint and squaw balm because of its traditional use by native women to promote menstrual flow. Women in some Native American tribes reportedly drank hot pennyroyal tea regularly as a method of contraception. Pennyroyal was listed as a medicinal drug in official publications from 1831–1931. It was included in the *U.S. Pharmacopoeia* as an abortifacient (an agent that induces abortion) until 1931.

American pennyroyal is an annual mint with small, oval leaves arranged opposite each other on a square stem. Leaves are entire and may be sparsely-toothed or smooth on the margins. The erect stems grow to 1 ft (31 cm) high from a many-branched root system. The tiny blue-violet flowers grow in whorls from the leaf axils on the top half of the stems. The fragrant herb blossoms in midsummer. The entire plant exudes a strong, acrid aroma and has a mint flavor. The scent is offensive to fleas, chiggers, mosquitoes, and other irritating insects.

European pennyroyal, also known as English pennyroyal, is a perennial mint native to Europe and Asia. The herb has naturalized throughout North America since its introduction to the continent by early European colonists. European pennyroyal was mentioned in Greek literature as early as 421 B.C. in the plays of Aristophanes where it was noted for its use as an abortifacient. In the first century A.D. the herbalist and physician Pliny wrote of pennyroyal's action to repel fleas. The specific name for the herb is from the Latin word *pulex*, meaning flea. European pennyroyal thrives in moist areas along stream banks, around ponds, in irrigated fields, and in boggy grasslands. This growing habit is reflected in some of European pennyroyal's other common names, including run-by-the-ground, lurk-in-the-ditch, and pudding grass.

European pennyroyal can be distinguished from the American native pennyroyal not only by its preferred habitat, but also, with careful observation, by its appearance. European or English pennyroyal hugs the ground where it grows, with only the flower stalk rising to a height of about 1 ft (31 cm). The oval leaves are opposite along the square stem, but are smaller than those of the American pennyroyal, measuring about 0.5 in (1.3 cm) long. The tiny, tubular blossoms each have four stamens in the European herb, and bear only two stamens in the American native.

General use

Pennyroyal has been used traditionally as a stimulating tea to relieve digestive disorders, gall bladder disorders, **gout**, **nausea**, and nervous conditions. Pennyroyal leaf, prepared as a hot infusion, will promote perspiration. Some herbalists suggest the additional treatment of a hot footbath while drinking the herbal infusion as a remedy at the onset of colds and flu. Pennyroyal may relieve headache, bring down **fever**, and quiet coughs. It has also been used to treat **bronchitis** and sinusitis. As a carminative (gas-reliever),

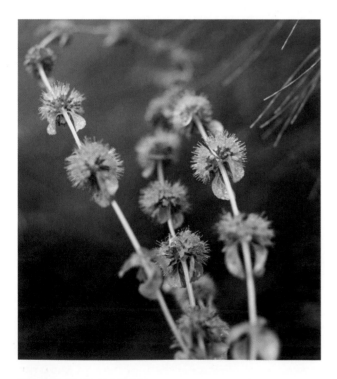

Pennyroyal. (© dk / Alamy)

KEY TERMS

Abortifacient—A drug or other substance that causes abortion.

Emmenagogue—A herbal remedy or medication that brings on a woman's menstrual period.

Hepatotoxic—Poisonous to the liver.

Pulegone—The toxic chemical found in pennyroyal oil.

pennyroyal is considered an effective remedy for flatulence, a virtue it shares with other mints. The herbal infusion has also been used traditionally to treat suppressed **menstruation**.

By far the most controversial and dangerous use of pennyroyal is as an abortifacient. Its emmenagogic properties stimulate uterine contraction and promote menstrual flow. The essential oil has been used for centuries to induce abortion. This use of the essential oil of pennyroyal is extremely risky, and has sometimes been lethal to both the mother and the fetus. The U.S. Food and Drug Administration reported on a 1998 fatal case of pennyroyal overdose in a self-induced abortion. Both pennyroyals contain as much as 85% of the toxic phytochemical pulegone in the essential oil.

Pennyroyal is also considered potentially dangerous because of its hepatotoxicity, or ability to harm the liver. Of four cases of pennyroyal poisoning reported in San Francisco in 1996, one patient died from liver damage. As of late 2001, researchers are studying the pathways of pulegone metabolism in the human body in order to determine the degree of toxicity more precisely.

The best use for this potent herb is an external application as an insect repellent to deter mosquitoes, fleas, chiggers, and other pests. It is also soothing as a skin wash to relieve itching and rash. Pet collars, woven from the freshly gathered stems and leaves, will deter fleas, and bunches of the herb, hanging to dry, will also keep pests at bay. Many commercial products contain the oil of pennyroyal in insect-repellent preparations. Other chemical constituents in pennyroyal include tannins, such as rosmaric acid, and flavonoids, including diosmin and **hesperidin**.

Preparations

The essential oil of pennyroyal and the fresh or dried leaves and stems are medicinally active. Gather fresh leaves in the summer, on a dry and sunny day when the herb is in blossom. Hang bundles of the herb to dry in a light, airy room out of direct sunlight. When the herb is thoroughly dry, strip the leaves from the stems and store in tightly sealed, clearly labeled, dark-glass containers.

Infusion: Place 2 oz of fresh, or 1 oz of dried, pennyroyal leaves in a warmed glass container. Bring 2.5 cups of fresh, nonchlorinated water to a boil and add it to the herbs. Do not boil the tea. Cover and infuse the tea for about 10 minutes. Strain. The prepared tea will store for about two days in the refrigerator. This infusion may be used externally as a soothing skin wash. According to some herbalists, pennyroyal leaf infusion may also be safely consumed as a medicinal tea, taking up to two cups throughout the day. Others, however, including the *PDR For Herbal Medicines*, recommend that pennyroyal not be ingested due to its hepatotoxicity. Other non-toxic herbs, such as **peppermint** (*Mentha piperita*) and **spearmint** (*Mentha spicata*) may be used to remedy many of the same conditions that pennyroyal treats without the toxic risk.

Precautions

Pregnant women should never ingest pennyroyal, particularly the oil, nor should they apply the oil externally as it may be absorbed through the skin. Pennyroyal essential oil contains as much as 85% of the ketone pulegone, an extremely toxic phytochemical. Overdose of the essential oil has been reported to cause severe liver damage, coma, and death. Quantities as small as 0.5 tsp of the essential oil have caused extremely toxic reactions. The effective abortifacient dosage is dangerously close to the lethal dose. Women have died when attempting to induce abortion by ingesting pennyroyal oil. American pennyroyal contains twice as much of the toxic volatile oil as European pennyroyal. The *PDR For Herbal Medicines* recommends that the drug not be used because of its hepatotoxicity, although with proper dosage and administration of the foliage drug, poisoning is not likely.

Side effects

Contact dermatitis is possible when using crushed leaf or the undiluted oil extract on the skin to repel insects.

Interactions

None reported.

Resources

BOOKS

Duke, James A. *The Green Pharmacy*. Emmaus, PA: Rodale Press, 1997.

Foster, Steven, and James A. Duke. *Peterson Field Guides, Eastern/Central Medicinal Plants*. Boston-New York: Houghton Mifflin Company, 1990.

Medical Economics Company. *PDR for Herbal Medicines*. Montvale, NJ: Medical Economics Company, 1998.

Tyler, Varro E. *The Honest Herbal*. New York: Pharmaceutical Products Press, 1993.

Weiss, Gaea, and Shandor Weiss. *Growing & Using The Healing Herbs*. New York: Wings Books, 1992.

PERIODICALS

Anderson, Ilene B., Walter H. Mullen, et al. "Pennyroyal Toxicity: Measurement of Toxic Metabolite Levels in Two Cases and Review of the Literature." *Annals of Internal Medicine* 124 (April 1996): 726–734.

Chen, L. J., et al. "Metabolism of (R)-(+)-pulegone in F344 Rats." *Drug Metabolism and Disposal* 29 (December 2001): 1567–77.

U.S. Food and Drug Administration, Center for Food Safety and Applied Nutrition, Office of Special Nutritionals. *FDA/CFSAN Report, October 20, 1998*.

OTHER

"Herbal Abortifacients." *Westside Crisis Pregnancy Center*. [cited January 2033]. http://w-cpc.org/abortion/herbal.html.

"Pennyroyal." *Viable Herbal Solutions*. [cited January 2003]. http://www.viable-herbal.com/herbdesc3/1pennyro.htm.

Clare Hanrahan
Rebecca J. Frey, PhD

Peony *see* **White peony root**

Peppermint

Description

Peppermint (*Mentha piperita*) is an aromatic perennial plant that grows to a height of about 3 ft (1 m). It has light purple flowers and green leaves with serrated edges. Peppermint belongs to the Lamiaceae family and grows throughout North America, Asia, and Europe. There are more than 25 species of true mint grown throughout the world.

The plant is harvested when the oil content is highest. When ready for harvest, it is always collected in the morning, before noon sun reduces the leaf essential oil content. This generally takes place shortly before the plant blooms, which occurs in the summer (July through August) or during dry, sunny weather. The United States is responsible for producing 75% of the world's supply of peppermint.

History

Peppermint is a natural hybrid of water mint (*Mentha aquatica*) and **spearmint** (*Mentha spicata*) and was first cultivated in England in the late seventeenth century. The herb has been used as a remedy for **indigestion** since Ancient Egyptian times. In fact, dried peppermint leaves were found in Egyptian pyramids dating back to 1000 B.C. The ancient Greeks and Romans valued it as a stomach soother. During the eighteenth century, peppermint became popular in Western Europe as a folk remedy for **nausea**, **vomiting**, **morning sickness**, respiratory **infections**, and menstrual disorders. Peppermint was first listed in the *London Pharmacopoeia in 1721*. In modern times it appears in the *British Herbal Pharmacopoeia* as a remedy for intestinal **colic**, **gas**, colds, morning sickness, and **menstruation pain**.

Properties

Peppermint is a cooling, relaxing herb that contains properties that help ease inflamed tissues, calm **muscle spasms** or cramps, and inhibit bacteria and microorganisms. It also has pain-relieving and infection-preventing qualities.

The medicinal parts of peppermint are derived from the whole plant, and include a volatile oil, flavonoids, phenolic acids, and triterpenes. The plant is primarily cultivated for its oil, which is extracted from the leaves of the flowering plant.

The essential oil contains the principal active ingredients of the plant: menthol, menthone, and menthyl acetate. Menthyl acetate is responsible for peppermint's minty aroma and flavor. Menthol, peppermint's main active ingredient, is found in the leaves and flowering tops of the plant. It provides the cool sensation of the herb.

The menthol content of peppermint oil determines the quality of its essential oil. This varies depending upon climate, habitat, and where the peppermint is grown. For instance, American peppermint oil contains 50–78% menthol, while English peppermint oil has a menthol content of 60–70%. Japanese peppermint oil contains 85% menthol. Peppermint and its oils help with intestinal function.

Peppermint also contains vitamins A and C, **magnesium**, **potassium**, **inositol**, **niacin**, **copper**, **iodine**, silicon, **iron**, and **sulfur**.

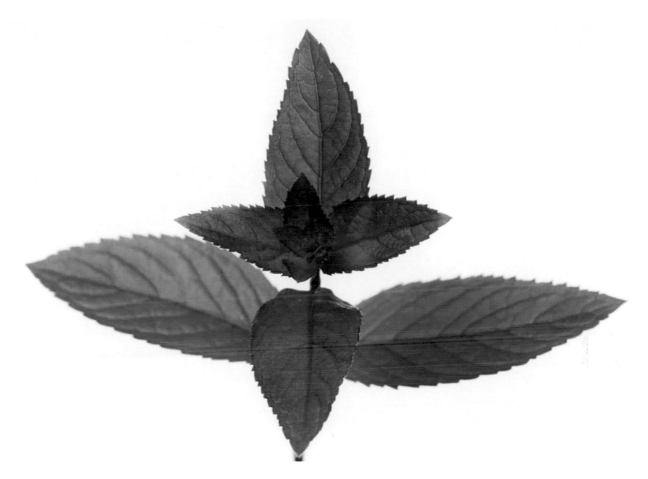

Peppermint. *(© Arco Images / Alamy)*

General use

Peppermint is one of the most popular flavoring agents. Many products contain peppermint, including chewing gum, mints and candies, ice cream and other sweets, tobacco, toothpaste, mouthwash, **cough** drops, teas, alcoholic liqueurs, and digestive aids. It is also used to scent soaps, perfumes, detergents, lipsticks and other cosmetics, and is an ingredient in many over-the-counter medications. Therapeutically, peppermint is used to treat many ailments of the skin, circulatory system, respiratory system, digestive system, immune system, and nervous system.

Peppermint and headaches

Peppermint's pain-relieving effects on headaches have been known for many years. The first documented report to link peppermint and **headache** relief was published in 1879. A more recent study took place in Germany in 1996. In this double-blind study, researchers found that an ethanol solution containing 10% peppermint oil was as effective in relieving headache pain as 1,000 mg of acetaminophen. In another study, 32 people with headaches massaged peppermint oil on their temples. The results showed that the peppermint oil significantly relieved their pain.

When applied to the skin, peppermint reduces sensitivity and relieves pain. Rubbed on the temples, across the forehead, and behind the neck, peppermint oil helps to ease digestive-related headaches and migraines by generating a cooling effect on the skin and relaxing cranial muscles.

Peppermint as a digestive aid

Peppermint is employed in the treatment of various digestive ailments, such as **irritable bowel syndrome**, **Crohn's disease**, **diverticulitis**, liver and gallbladder complaints, loss of appetite, spastic colon, **diarrhea**, gas, bloating, colic, cramps, and **heartburn**. The infused herb tea of peppermint or a few drops of its essential oil stimulate the flow of digestive juices and the production

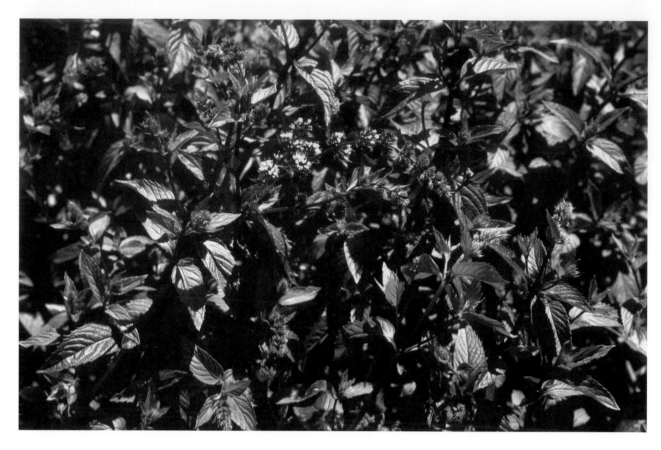

Peppermint. *((c) Photo Researchers, Inc. Reproduced by permission.)*

of bile, a substance that helps to digest fats. This eases indigestion, relieves gas, reduces colon spasms, and eases **motion sickness** and nausea. When peppermint is taken after a meal, its effects will reduce gas and help the digestion of food by reducing the amount of time the food is in the stomach. This is one reason after-dinner mints are so popular.

The compounds of the essential oil have antispasmodic properties that reduce spasms of the colon and intestinal tract and relax the stomach muscles. Peppermint has a soothing effect on the lining and muscles of the colon, which helps to relieve diarrhea and spastic colon.

Menthol acts to stimulate the stomach lining. Its cooling properties soothe the stomach and ease stomach pain. Peppermint oil is popular in the treatment of motion and sea sickness and nausea associated with **pregnancy**. It acts as an anesthetic to the stomach wall and eases vomiting and nausea. An account on the effects of peppermint on nausea appeared in the September 1997 issue of the *Journal of Advanced Nursing*, in which gynecological patients were given peppermint oil to counter post-operative nausea. The patients reported less nausea and required fewer drugs to treat the nausea.

A German health commission, German Commission E, has endorsed peppermint tea as a treatment for indigestion. Clinical trials in Denmark and Britain in the 1990s confirmed peppermint's actions as a therapeutic treatment for irritable bowel syndrome. In 1996, a German study was performed to research the therapeutic benefits of peppermint essential oil on irritable bowel syndrome. Subjects with irritable bowel syndrome were given enteric-coated capsules containing peppermint and caraway oils. Results showed that the pain symptoms, which ranged from moderate to severe, improved in 89.5% of the group.

Peppermint and respiratory ailments

Peppermint is an expectorant and decongestant. It is used to help treat many respiratory ailments including **asthma**, **bronchitis**, sinusitis, and coughs.

Peppermint is an element of many cough preparations, not only for its pleasant flavor, but also because it contains compounds that help ease coughs. Constituents of peppermint increase the production of saliva, causing frequent swallowing and suppressing the cough reflex.

German Commission E has officially recognized peppermint's ability to reduce inflammation of nasal passageways. When menthol vapors are inhaled, nasal passageways are opened to provide temporary relief of nasal and sinus congestion.

Peppermint essential oil is an ingredient in many commercial chest and cold rubs. These are popularly rubbed onto the chest to ease congestion.

A tea made from the leaves can stimulate the immune system and relieve the congestion of colds, flus, and upper respiratory infections.

Other conditions

Peppermint is an effective relaxant and can be helpful in treating nervous **insomnia**, **stress**, **anxiety**, and restlessness.

Many over-the-counter balms and liniments contain peppermint essential oil. These are applied externally to relieve muscle pain, arthritis, **itching**, and **fungal infections**.

Peppermint induces sweating and can help bring down fevers. It is said that it contains **antioxidants** that help prevent **cancer** and **heart disease**. The essential oil is a powerful antiseptic and is useful in treating bad breath and sore throats. It is also beneficial in preventing tooth decay and **gum disease**.

A plant with potent antiviral properties, peppermint can help fight viruses that cause ailments such as **influenza**, herpes, yeast infections, and **mumps**. Peppermint is also used as an **earache** remedy, to dissolve **gallstones**, to ease muscle tightness, and to ease menstrual cramps.

A 2002 report announced that peppermint also helped participants in a study run faster, do more pushups, and show greater grip strength than those who were not exposed to peppermint scent. Although researchers concluded the effect may have been psychological, a result of peppermint's effect on mood and increased motivation, it still resulted in measurable performance improvement.

Preparations

Peppermint is available as a tincture, tea, essential oil, oil capsules, and tablets. The fresh and dried leaves may be purchased in bulk.

Tablets and capsules are often coated so the oil's therapeutic properties are released in the intestine and not in the stomach. These enteric-coated pills are used in the treatment of irritable bowel syndrome, diverticulitis, and other chronic digestive ailments. Peppermint oil capsules are effective in treating lower intestinal disorders:

- Irritable bowel syndrome: 1–2 capsules three times daily between meals.
- Gallstones: 1–2 capsules three times daily between meals.

Peppermint tea

Peppermint tea may be used to relieve migraine headaches, minor colds, digestive ailments, and morning sickness, as well as many other conditions. Taken after a meal, the tea acts to settle the stomach and improve digestion. To prepare the tea, pour one cup of boiling water over 1–2 tsp of dried peppermint leaves, cover, and steep for 10 minutes. Strain the mixture before drinking.

DOSAGE. For relief of migraine pressure, drink 1–2 cups of cool tea daily.

For digestive disorders, drink one cup of tea with meals.

For cough relief, drink 3–4 cups of cool tea throughout the day, taking frequent sips (every 15–30 minutes).

For morning sickness, women may drink a tea that has been diluted.

Aromatherapy and peppermint

The essential oil of peppermint is a pale yellow or greenish liquid that is made by distilling the flowering herb. When inhaled, the oil can reduce **fever**, relieve nausea and vomiting, improve digestion, and soothe the respiratory system. Various studies have been performed on the oil's ability to improve the sense of taste and smell and improve concentration and mental acuity when inhaled.

The oil blends well with other **essential oils** such as benzoin, **rosemary**, **lavender**, marjoram, lemon, **eucalyptus**, and other mints. Essential oils are available at many health food stores or through a qualified aromatherapist.

Peppermint essential oil can be used in several ways: inhaled, rubbed on **reflexology** points on the bottom of the feet, diffused into the air, or as a therapeutic bath. Below are some applications for the use of peppermint essential oil:

- Steam inhalation for congestion relief: A few drops of the essential oil of peppermint are placed in a large bowl of hot water. The person should cover his or her head with a towel, lean over the bowl, and inhale the steam.
- Motion sickness: A few drops of essential oil should be places on a tissue and inhaled.
- Headaches: A few drops can be placed on a cool, wet towel and used as a compress on the forehead. Or, massaged into the neck, back, temples, and/or forehead.
- Digestion: Several drops of diluted oil massaged on the stomach or the pure oil rubbed onto the bottoms of the feet.
- Breath freshener: Several drops placed on the tongue.
- Therapeutic bath: Several drops of diluted oil placed into a tepid bath to relieve stomach complaints, nasal congestion, headache, or menstrual cramps. If essential oil is not available, a bath can be made by adding to the water a cloth bag filled with several handfuls of dried or fresh peppermint leaves.

As with any essential oil, caution should be taken when using it. Essential oils are highly concentrated and should be diluted with a vegetable oil prior to external use to prevent adverse reactions, as some people are allergic to peppermint or its essential oil. The oil may cause a skin reaction if the dosage is excessive. Avoid contact with the eyes.

Precautions

Extreme caution should be used when administering to children under five years of age as the menthol can cause a choking reaction in young children.

Peppermint oil should not be applied to the faces of infants or small children.

The essential oil of peppermint should not be ingested unless under professional supervision.

Pure menthol or pure peppermint should not be ingested. Pure peppermint may cause an irregular heartbeat. Pure menthol is poisonous and fatal in doses as small as 1 tsp.

Pregnant women with a history of miscarriage should use peppermint with caution. Large amounts of peppermint may trigger a miscarriage. Additional caution should be practiced by women who are breast-feeding their infants.

Side effects

If the essential oil is not used properly it can cause **dermatitis** and other allergic reactions.

Rare reactions to enteric-coated capsules may occur. These reactions include skin rash, heartburn, slow heart rate, and muscle tremors.

Large internal doses of peppermint essential oil may result in kidney damage.

Interactions

Peppermint should not be used in conjunction with homeopathic treatment.

Resources

BOOKS

Foster, Steven, and Varro E. Tyler, Ph.D. *Tyler's Honest Herbal.* The Haworth Herbal Press, 1999.

PERIODICALS

Moxey, Beth. "A Peppermint Twist: New Research Shows that a Whiff of Peppermint May Improve Your Running (Health and Fitness)." *Runner's World* (January 2002): 21.

"Peppermint Oil and Tea Best for Nose and Stomach, Not Lungs." *Environmental Nutrition* (January 1997):7.

Siegel–Maier, Karyn. "Peppermint: More Than Just Another Pretty Flavor." *Better Nutrition* (February 1998): 24.

Jennifer Wurges
Teresa G. Odle

Periodontal disease *see* **Gum disease**

Peripheral neuropathy

Description

Peripheral neuropathy, sometimes called peripheral neuritis, is damage to the nerves that connect peripheral (outlying) portions of the body (especially the hands, arms, legs, and feet) to the central nervous system. It may involve only one peripheral nerve (mononeuropathy) or several nerves (polyneuropathy).

Description

Similar to electrical wiring in a house, the body has a highly complex network of nerves made up of bundles of neurons, axons, and dendrites. This network originates in the brain and extends down through the spinal cord. These nerves branch off at junctures along this pathway to connect each portion of the body to the brain and spinal cord, the central nervous system. Nerves relay necessary information to and from every area, notifying the brain of sensations and external conditions. The brain, in turn, sends messages back to those areas. With peripheral neuropathy, damage has occurred to the nerves that connect peripheral portions of the body, and the patient feels **pain** or numbness.

Peripheral neuropathy is not usually considered a disease. It is more often thought of as a symptom of other diseases or conditions, or results from damage caused by the introduction of toxic substances. There are an estimated two million Americans who suffer from peripheral neuropathy. It becomes more common as people age, and the majority of its victims are 65 years old or older.

Causes and symptoms

The symptoms of peripheral neuropathy depend upon which type of nerve fiber is affected. Sensory nerve fiber damage is more likely to generate various sensations, while motor nerve fiber is more apt to result in weakening and wasting of muscle tissue in the affected area. It is a condition that develops quite gradually, usually over a period of months or even years. A tingling, prickly sensation in the toes and/or feet is commonly the first sign that is noticed, or there may be numbness in this area. Typically this feeling progresses to the lower legs, fingers, hands, arms, and then the trunk of the body in severe cases. As the situation worsens, the tingling sensation feels more like burning or severe discomfort followed by sharp, almost electric shock-like jabs of pain. These sensations may begin in the toes and feet, and then progress to other affected areas. Later symptoms often include increasing muscle weakness, poor coordination, numbness, and lack of feeling. **Urinary incontinence**, **diarrhea**, **constipation**, **impotence**, and postural hypotension (dramatic drops in blood pressure when a person stands) causing **dizziness** or dangerous falls are other potential negative effects, especially in the elderly.

Peripheral nerves are extended and delicate, easily damaged by a variety of things. Diabetes, **alcoholism**, diseases of the autoimmune system such as rheumatoid arthritis and lupus, and exposure to health damaging substances can cause peripheral neuropathy. Chronic liver and kidney disease, thyroid gland imbalances, bacterial or viral **infections**, and **cancer** can also cause the damage. Many of the strong anticancer drugs used and certain vitamin deficiencies can also lead to this condition. Repetitive mechanical actions that put pressure on a particular nerve, like the wrist in carpal-tunnel syndrome, or even inherited abnormalities in the body can cause peripheral neuropathy. However, in many cases no one single reason for this condition can be found.

Guillain-Barre syndrome, also called acute polyneuritis or ascending paralysis, is the only form of peripheral neuropathy that develops differently. It is a rare and very serious form that is believed to be caused by an autoimmune reaction to infection. Its primary difference from other types of peripheral neuropathy is the terrific rapidity of its onset.

A few rare forms of peripheral neuropathy are inherited. The best known inherited peripheral neuropathy is called Charcot-Marie-Tooth syndrome, or CMT. More than 20 different genes and loci on human chromosomes are now known to be associated with CMT.

Diagnosis

Because peripheral neuropathy can be caused by a variety of factors, outcomes vary depending upon the reason for the nerve damage. Some causes, such as vitamin or metabolic deficiencies, can be reversed if caught early; other causes may not be reversible. Because of these factors, early diagnosis is very important. A neurologist (a doctor who specializes in the nervous system) can diagnose the disorder, try to determine the cause, and assess the extent of the damage. Sensations of pain, temperature, and touch in various parts of the body are tested by observing the person's ability to respond to a stimulus. If areas of either hypersensitivity or loss of sensation are found, the boundaries of that feeling are mapped by further testing.

An electromyogram (EMG) tests the electrical activity occurring in muscles and can be used in the diagnostic process. X rays, blood tests, and muscle biopsies are common tests used in determining the cause of peripheral neuropathy. For example, blood tests that show elevated blood sugar would indicate diabetes, or elevated liver function tests or thyroid levels could indicate liver or thyroid disease.

Treatment

Treating the underlying cause of the peripheral neuropathy is the key to reversing this condition. For example, diabetics who closely follow their diabetic diet and keep their blood sugar in good control stand the best chance of recovering. Nutritional deficiencies often related to alcoholism may indicate that the person needs to stop drinking and requires vitamin supplements. Changes in lifestyle or treatment of the disease condition causing the neuropathy is a highly important facet of reversing, arresting, or simply reducing the symptoms of this uncomfortable condition.

Several simple self-care actions can also relieve symptoms. They include:

- That shoes and stockings should never be tight, but rather loose cotton socks and shoes with good support and padding should be worn. Good foot care includes daily or twice daily foot soaks in tepid to cool water for 15 minutes followed by application of a moistening cream.
- Keeping heavy bed covers off of feet at night either by turning back the covers or using a bed cradle.
- Improving circulation and stimulating regeneration of nerves by frequently massaging the affected areas and walking as much as possible. Hydrotherapy with whirlpool baths may also be used to improve circulation.
- Reducing the intake of caffeine and nicotine, both of which may increase pain.
- Lowering the stress level as much as possible, including taking steps to treat the depression and/or insomnia that often accompany peripheral neuropathy. This may include relaxation therapies or herbal remedies.

Herbal remedies used for peripheral neuropathy include gingko, **St. John's wort**, vervain, oats, and gotu kola. Nutritional supplements that may provide relief and are thought to help repair nerve fibers include supplemental **carnitine**, gamma-linolenic acid, alpha-lipoic acid, **magnesium**, **chromium**, **choline**, **inositol**, vitamins B_6 and B_{12}, **niacin**, **thiamine**, **biotin**, and **folic acid**. Additional therapies thought to provide relief include **detoxification** and **fasting**, used to cleanse the system and eliminate poisons that may cause nerve damage.

Control of symptoms is a significant part of the treatment. Pain relief is usually the highest priority. Bodywork such as massage and movement therapies like **t'ai chi** and **qigong** may provide relief. **Acupuncture** can also be used to promote general health and provide some symptomatic relief. **Meditation** or **yoga** may help with **relaxation** and pain control.

Another alternative approach to peripheral neuropathy is the **Feldenkrais** method, which works on improving the patient's sense of balance, and thus helps to prevent falls.

Allopathic treatment

It may take months for the symptoms to subside. Milder pain can be treated with over-the-counter pain medications, including Tylenol or aspirin, while more severe episodes of pain may require pain relievers such as nonsteroidal anti-inflammatory drugs (NSAIDs) like ibuprofen or naproxen, or narcotics such as codeine,

Demerol, or morphine. Sometimes tricyclic antidepressants such as Elavil, Tofranil, or Norpramin are used both for pain relief and the depression that may accompany chronic pain. Anticonvulsant medications such as Tegretol, Neurontin, or Dilantin are effective against electric-like, jabbing pain. Less frequently used drugs include heart and blood pressure drugs such as Mexitil and clonidine, which may alleviate burning sensations.

The acute onset and potentially serious symptoms that can develop in Guillain-Barre syndrome, including nerve and muscle damage affecting swallowing and breathing, make this the type of peripheral neuropathy most likely to require in-patient hospital treatment. The person suffering from this syndrome must be carefully monitored, may require intubation in order to breathe, and may even have blood plasma removed in order to reduce the number of antibodies in the blood.

Expected results

Full recovery from peripheral neuropathy is possible if the nerves are not damaged beyond repair. The outcome is dependent upon the extent of damage. Research is now being conducted that may lead to the manufacture of substances similar to the naturally produced chemicals in the body that stimulate repair of small nerve fibers.

The majority of people suffering from Guillain-Barre syndrome recover completely, often without even receiving medical treatment, but some will develop residual, permanent weakness in the affected area or have further episodes.

Prevention

The best way to prevent peripheral neuropathy is to treat the underlying disease or eliminate the toxic substance that may cause the symptoms.

Resources

BOOKS

Thomas, Clayton L., ed. *Taber's Cyclopedic Medical Dictionary*. F. A. Davis Co., 1997.

PERIODICALS

Kauffman, T. "Balance Falls Assessment: Low Tech to High Tech, Peripheral Neuropathy, and Alternative Considerations." *The Gerontologist* (October 15, 2001): 264.

Palau, F., A. Cuesta, L. Pedrola, et al. "Mutations in the Ganglioside-Induced Differentiation-Associated Protein 1 (GDAP1) Gene Cause Axonal Charcot-Marie-Tooth Disease." *American Journal of Human Genetics* 69 (October 2001): 196.

ORGANIZATIONS

MayoClinic.com. http://www.mayoclinic.com.

Joan Schonbeck
Rebecca J. Frey, PhD

Periwinkle

Description

An herbal remedy with a rich history in folk medicine, periwinkle is the common name for a pair of perennial flowering shrubs belonging to the dogbane (Apocynaceae) family. The herb has been used for centuries to treat a variety of ailments and was a favorite ingredient of magical charms in the Middle Ages. The purple-flowered plant was called sorcerer's violet by superstitious Europeans and was renowned for its

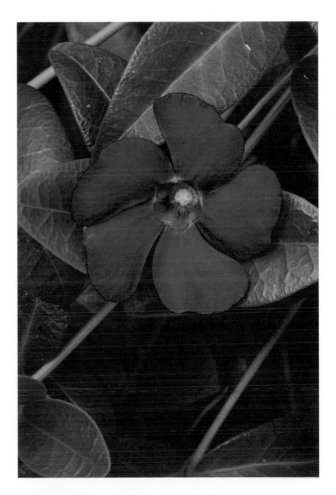

Periwinkle flower. *(©PlantaPhile, Germany. Reproduced by permission.)*

power to dispel evil spirits. There are two main varieties: lesser periwinkle (*Vinca minor*), which is also called common periwinkle, and greater periwinkle (*Vinca major*). Lesser periwinkle originated in Spain, France, and other areas of Europe but can now be found growing in many parts of the world, while greater periwinkle is native to southern Europe. While not widely recommended for medicinal purposes today, periwinkle is sometimes used to improve brain circulation and alleviate heavy menstrual periods. Only the aboveground parts of the plant are used as a drug.

It is important to distinguish lesser and greater periwinkle from a close relative called Madagascar periwinkle. The Latin name for this herb is *Catharanthus roseus*, but it was formerly classified as *Vinca rosea*, and is still called by that name in some of the herbal literature. Another member of the dogbane family, this plant originated on the island of Madagascar but now grows in the southern United States and many other temperate regions of the world. Madagascar periwinkle has been used for centuries to treat a variety of medical problems, from diabetes and eye **infections** to sore throats and tumors. Modern research has indicated that Madagascar periwinkle contains dozens of alkaloids, some of which may have the ability to lower blood sugar levels and stop bleeding. Two of these alkaloids, vincristine and vinblastine, are recognized by Western medicine as potent anticancer agents. (A shaman in Madagascar who used the plants to treat tumors and **cancer** gave Western scientists the lead.) They are used to make important prescription drugs. Madagascar periwinkle is not widely recommended as a dietary supplement because some of the alkaloids in the plant can cause serious and potentially dangerous side effects.

General use

While not approved by the Food and Drug Administration (FDA), periwinkle has been reported to have a number of beneficial effects. Unfortunately, there is scarcely any scientific evidence to support these claims. Both forms of the herb have been used as an astringent for centuries and may be useful in alleviating excessive bleeding during **menstruation**, according to some herbalists. Lesser periwinkle is generally recommended for improving circulation, particularly in the brain. Greater periwinkle has been used to combat nervousness or **anxiety** and help reduce high blood pressure. Periwinkle is also reputed to be effective in treating diabetes, perhaps by stimulating the pancreas.

While they do not recommend periwinkle for a wide variety of ailments, some practitioners of alternative

medicine claim that the herb is useful in treating certain conditions. Periwinkle has been used as an effective astringent that can be used orally or topically. It is mainly used to treat excessive menstrual bleeding but may also be a helpful choice in cases of **colitis**, **diarrhea**, bleeding gums, **nosebleeds**, sore throats, and mouth ulcers.

Perhaps the most intriguing dietary supplement derived from periwinkle is vinpocetine, which is made from an alkaloid chemical in lesser periwinkle called vincamine. While vinpocetine is not what most people would consider a natural remedy, since it is produced via chemical manipulation in the laboratory, it is sold in the United States as a dietary supplement. Several studies of vinpocetine suggest that it may improve brain function and memory, particularly in people affected by diseases that decrease mental capacity such as **Alzheimer's disease** or **dementia**. In a double-blind, placebo-controlled trial published in the *Journal of the American Geriatrics Society* in 1987, vinpocetine appeared to improve the condition of several dozen elderly patients who suffered from mental impairment due to **aging**. Researchers found that the 42 patients who took vinpocetine for three months performed better on several tests of mental functioning than those in the placebo group. In the study, no significant side effects were associated with vinpocetine.

Exactly how vinpocetine works is unknown. According to one theory, vinpocetine may protect brain cells from damage caused by oxygen deprivation. The apparent effectiveness of vinpocetine, which is made partly from a chemical contained in lesser periwinkle, may help to explain the herb's traditional reputation as a brain booster. It is important to remember, however, that periwinkle itself has not been proven to have the same effects as vinpocetine.

Preparations

The optimum daily dosage of periwinkle has not been established with any certainty. Readers who wish to use this herb should follow the package directions for proper usage or consult a doctor experienced in the use of alternative remedies.

The dosage of vinpocetine is generally 30 mg a day, divided into three equal doses. Taking vinpocetine with food may enhance its effectiveness by increasing the amount of drug absorbed.

Precautions

Periwinkle is not known to be harmful when taken in recommended dosages, though it is important to remember that the long-term effects of taking the herb (in any amount) have not been investigated. Periwinkle should not be used by people with low blood pressure or **constipation**. Due to lack of sufficient medical study, periwinkle should be used with caution in children, women who are pregnant or breastfeeding, and people with liver or kidney disease.

Taking too much periwinkle can cause a potentially dangerous drop in blood pressure (symptoms include **dizziness** and fainting). In case of overdose, seek emergency care.

Vinpocetine should not be combined with certain medications or dietary supplements (see below).

Side effects

Periwinkle may cause flushing and gastrointestinal problems.

When taken in recommended dosages, vinpocetine is not associated with any bothersome or significant side effects.

Interactions

Periwinkle is not known to interact adversely with any drugs or dietary supplements. Periwinkle may be combined with cranesbill and agrimony. It may also be used in conjunction with beth root for menstrual problems.

Vinpocetine should not be combined with agents that thin the blood, except under medical supervision. These include drugs such as warfarin (Coumadin) and aspirin as well as dietary supplements like ginkgo, **vitamin E** in high dosages, and **garlic**.

Resources

BOOKS

Crellin, John K. and Jane Philpott. *A Reference Guide to Medicinal Plants: Herbal Medicine Past and Present.* Durham, NC: Duke University Press, 1997.

ORGANIZATIONS

American Botanical Council. PO Box 144345. Austin, TX 78714-4345.

OTHER

Discovery Health. http://www.discoveryhealth.com.

Greg Annussek

Pertusis *see* **Whooping cough**

Pet therapy

Definition

Animal-assisted therapy (AAT), also known as pet therapy, utilizes trained animals and handlers to achieve specific physical, social, cognitive, and emotional goals with patients.

Origins

The enjoyment of animals as companions dates back many centuries, perhaps even to prehistoric times. The first known therapeutic use of animals started in Gheel, Belgium in the ninth century. In this town, learning to care for farm animals has long been an important part of an assisted living program designed for people with disabilities.

Some of the earliest uses of animal-assisted healing in the United States were for psychiatric patients. The presence of the therapy animals produced a beneficial effect on both children and adults with mental health issues. It is only in the last few decades that AAT has been more formally applied in a variety of therapeutic settings, including schools and prisons, as well as hospitals, hospices, nursing homes, and outpatient care programs.

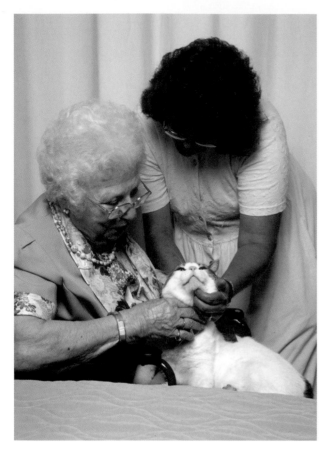

Pet therapy used to engage senior woman in an assisted living facility. *(© Mira / Alamy)*

Benefits

Studies have shown that physical contact with a pet can lower high blood pressure, and improve survival rates for **heart attack** victims. There is also evidence that petting an animal can cause endorphins to be released. Endorphins are chemicals in the body that suppress the **pain** response. These are benefits that can be enjoyed from pet ownership, as well as from visiting therapeutic animals.

Many skills can be learned or improved with the assistance of a therapy animal. Patient rehabilitation can be encouraged by such activities as walking or running with a dog, or throwing objects for the animal to retrieve. Fine motor skills may be developed by petting, grooming, or feeding the animal. Patient communication is encouraged by the response of the animal to either verbal or physical commands. Activities such as writing or talking about the therapy animals or past pets also develop cognitive skills and communication. Creative inclusion of an animal in the life or

therapy of a patient can make a major difference in the patient's comfort, progress, and recovery.

Description

The way in which AAT is undertaken depends on the needs and abilities of the individual patient. Dogs are the most common visiting therapy animals, but cats, horses, birds, rabbits, and other domestic pets can be used as long as they are appropriately screened and trained.

For patients who are confined, small animals can be brought to the bed if the patient is willing and is not allergic to the animal. A therapeutic plan may include a simple interaction aimed at improving communication and small motor skills, or a demonstration with educational content to engage the patient cognitively.

If the patient is able to walk or move around, more options are available. Patients can walk small animals outside, or learn how to care for farm animals. Both of these activities develop confidence and motor abilities. Horseback riding has recently gained great therapeutic popularity. It offers an opportunity to work on balance, trunk control, and other skills. Many patients who walk with difficulty, or not at all, get great emotional benefit from interacting with and controlling a large animal.

One advantage of having volunteers provide this service is that cost and insurance are not at issue.

Precautions

AAT does not involve just any pet interacting with a patient. Standards for the training of the volunteers and their animals are crucial in order to promote a safe, positive experience for the patient. Trained volunteers will understand how to work with other medical professionals to set goals for the patient and keep records of progress. Animals that have been appropriately trained are well socialized to people, other animals, and medical equipment. They are not distracted by the food and odors that may be present in the therapy environment and will not chew inappropriate objects or mark territory.

Animals participating in AAT should be covered by some form of liability insurance.

Research and general acceptance

The research evidence supporting the efficacy of AAT is slim, although the anecdotal support is vast. Although it may not be given much credence by medical personnel as a therapy with the potential to assist the progress of the patients, some institutions do at least allow it as something that will uplift the patients or distract them from their discomforts.

Training and certification

AAT is carried out by volunteers who are trained to provide therapy along with their animals. There are a growing number of groups that will provide screening and certification. These include Delta Society, Therapy Dogs Inc., Therapy Dogs International, and St. John Ambulance Therapy Dogs in Canada. Each program has somewhat different qualifications. The Pet Partners Program sponsored by Delta is exemplary. Animals receive a veterinary screening, an aptitude test to evaluate socialization, and a skills test of training and behavior. The owner also receives training hours and agrees to a code of ethics in order to join Pet Partners.

Resources

BOOKS

Burch, Mary. *Volunteering With Your Pet.* New York: Howell Book House, 1996.

ORGANIZATIONS

Delta Society. http://www.deltasociety.org/.

Judith Turner

Pharyngitis *see* **Sore throat**

Phlebitis

Definition

Thrombophlebitis is the inflammation of a vein, with **blood clots** forming inside the vein at the site of inflammation. Thrombophlebitis is also known as phlebitis, phlebothrombosis, and venous thrombosis.

Description

There are two aspects of thrombophlebitis, inflammation of a vein and blood clot formation. If the inflammation component is minor, the disease is usually called venous thrombosis or phlebothrombosis. Thrombophlebitis can occur in both deep veins and superficial veins, but most often occurs in the superficial veins of the extremities (legs and arms). Most cases occur in the legs. When thrombophlebitis occurs in a superficial vein, one that is near the surface of the skin and is visible to the eye, the disease is called superficial thrombophlebitis. Any form of injury to a blood vessel can result in thrombophlebitis. In the case of superficial thrombophlebitis, the blood clot usually attaches firmly to the wall of the affected blood vein. Since superficial veins do not have muscles that massage the veins and help the blood to circulate, blood clots in superficial veins tend to remain where they form and seldom break loose. When thrombophlebitis occurs in a deep vein, a vein that runs deep within muscle tissue, it is called deep venous thrombosis. Deep venous thrombosis presents the threat of producing blood clots that will break loose to form emboli. Emboli are clumps of cells that are carried by the circulation to other tissues where they can lodge and block the blood supply. Emboli typically come to rest in the lungs and cause tissue damage that can sometimes be serious or fatal.

Causes and symptoms

The main symptoms of phlebitis are tenderness and **pain** in the area of the affected vein. Redness and/or swelling may also be seen. In the case of deep venous thrombosis, there is more swelling than is caused by superficial thrombophlebitis, and the patient may experience muscle stiffness in the affected area. There are many causes of thrombophlebitis. The main causes can be grouped into three categories: injury to veins, increased blood clotting, and blood stasis. When blood veins are damaged, collagen in the vein wall is exposed. Platelets respond to collagen by initiating the clotting process. Damage to a vein can occur as a consequence of in-dwelling catheters, trauma, infection, Buerger's disease, or the injection of irritating substances. Increased tendency of the blood to clot can be caused by malignant tumors, genetic disorders, high-fat **diets**, and oral contraceptives. Stasis, in which the blood clots due to decreased blood flow in an area, can happen following surgery, as a consequence of **varicose veins**, as a complication of postpartum states, and following prolonged bed rest. In the case of prolonged bed rest, blood clots form because of inactivity, allowing blood to move sluggishly and stagnate (collect) in the veins. Stasis can lead to blood clots. These clots (also called emboli) are sometimes released when the patient stands up and

KEY TERMS

Emboli, embolus—Emboli is the plural form of embolus. Embolus refers to any mass of air, blood clot, or foreign body that travels through the bloodstream and is capable of lodging in smaller blood vessels where it can obstruct the blood flow to that vessel.

Embolism—The obstruction of a blood vessel by a blot clot.

Phlebitis—Inflammation of a vein.

Stasis—Stagnation in the flow of blood or any body fluid.

Thrombus—A blood clot that forms within a blood vessel or the heart.

resumes activity. Emboli can present a problem if they lodge in vital organs. In the case of postpartum patients, a **fever** developing four to 10 days after delivery may indicate thrombophlebitis. It is also known that thrombophlebitis in some patients involves hereditary factors, including mutations of genes that control the amount of clotting factors in the blood.

Questions have been raised in recent years as to whether frequent long-distance air travel increases the risk of thrombophlebitis in airline pilots and passengers. As of 2001, studies of the effects of long-distance flights on blood circulation in human test subjects have yielded conflicting results.

Diagnosis

In superficial thrombophlebitis, the location of the clot can sometimes be seen by the unaided eye. Blood clots are hard and can usually be detected by a physician using palpation (massage). Deep venous thrombosis requires specialized diagnostic instruments to detect the blood clot. Among the instruments a physician may use are ultrasound and x ray, coupled with dye injection (venogram).

Treatment

While patients have to rely on conventional medicine to resolve major blood clots in the veins, alternative therapies help prevent future blood clots and bring relief from pain due to superficial thrombophlebitis.

Physical therapy

Physical therapy helps prevent blood clots in patients who are temporary bed-ridden after a major surgery or accidents. Physical therapists help patients exercise their arms and legs while they are restricted in bed, use massage to stimulate muscles, and encourage them to regain their mobility as soon as possible.

Nutritional therapy

The following dietary changes may help prevent phlebitis and further vein damage:

- Limit fat intake. Saturated and hydrogenated fats are associated with increased risk of thrombosis and poor blood circulation.
- Eat a heart-healthy, high-fiber diet with emphasis on fruits, vegetables, grains, beans, nuts and seeds, and fish.
- Eat lots of garlic, ginger, onions, and hot pepper. These spices have blood-thinning activity and prevent clot formation.
- Increase consumption of cherries, blueberries, and blackberries. They contain chemicals called proanthocyanidins and anthocyanidins that help improve vein function and keep veins healthy.
- Take nutritional supplements. Supplements that help prevent blood clots and keep veins healthy include B-complex vitamins, especially folic acid (2,500 mg/day), vitamin B_6 (25 mg/day) and vitamin B_{12} (2 mcg/day); vitamin C (500 - 3,000 mg/day) and vitamin E (800 - 1,200 IU).

Herbal therapy

Several herbs help keep veins healthy and strong and/or prevent blood clots. They include:

- Butcher's broom (*Ruscus aculeatus*)
- Gingko biloba
- Gotu Kola (*Centella asiatica*)
- Horse chestnut (*Aesculus hippocastanum*)
- Bromelain (a natural enzyme found in pineapple that inhibits clot formation, therefore preventing thrombophlebitis)

Allopathic treatment

Superficial thrombophlebitis usually resolves without treatment. Application of heat or anti-inflammatory drugs (aspirin or ibuprofen) can help relieve the pain. It can take from several days to several weeks for the clot to resolve and the symptoms to completely disappear. Rarely, anticoagulant drugs may be administered.

Deep venous thrombosis is a serious condition. To prevent pulmonary embolism, anticoagulant drugs are given and the patient's limbs are elevated. The primary objective in treating deep venous thrombosis (DVT) is prevention of a pulmonary embolism. The patient usually is hospitalized during initial treatment. The prescribed anticoagulant drugs limit the ability of blood clots to grow and new clots to form. Sometimes, a drug that dissolves blood clots is administered. Recent advances in drug treatment of DVT include the use of low molecular weight heparin (LMWH), which is safer for use in pregnant women and also allows more patients with DVT to be treated on an outpatient basis.

Surgery may be used to treat DVT if the affected vein is likely to present a long term threat of producing blood clots that will release emboli. The affected veins are either removed or tied off to prevent the release of the blood clots. Tying off superficial blood veins is an outpatient procedure that can be performed with local anesthesia. The patient is capable of immediately resuming normal activities.

Expected results

Superficial thrombophlebitis seldom progresses to a serious medical complication, although non-lethal embolisms may be produced. Deep venous thrombosis may lead to embolism, especially pulmonary embolism. This is a serious consequence of deep venous thrombosis, and is sometimes fatal.

Prevention

To prevent phlebitis, people should eat a high-fiber, heart-healthy diet and engage in regular physical exercises such as walking, bicycling, or running. If temporarily bedridden, they should stretch their arms and legs frequently and try to become mobile as soon as possible.

Resources

BOOKS

Alexander, R.W., R. C. Schlant, and V. Fuster, eds. *The Heart,* 9th edition. New York: McGraw-Hill, 1998.

Berkow, Robert, ed. *Merck Manual of Medical Information.* Whitehouse Station, NJ: Merck Research Laboratories, 1997.

Larsen, D.E., ed. *Mayo Clinic Family Health Book* New York: William Morrow and Company, Inc., 1996.

Murray, Michael T., and Joseph Pizzorno. "Varicose Veins." In *Encyclopedia of Natural Medicine, revised 2nd ed.* Rocklin, CA: Prima Publishing, 1998.

"Phlebitis." In *Prevention's Healing with Vitamins: The Most Effective Vitamin and Mineral Treatment for Everyday Health Problems and Serious Disease-From Allergies and Arthritis to Water Retention and Wrinkles.* Emmaus, PA: Rodale Press, Inc., 1996.

"Phlebitis/Venous Thrombosis." In *Reader's Digest Guide to Medical Cures & Treatments: A Complete A-to-Z Sourcebook of Medical Treatments, Alternative Options, and Home Remedies.* Canada: Reader's Digest Association, Inc., 1996.

PERIODICALS

Egermayer, Paul. "The 'economy class syndrome': Problems with the assessment of risk factors for venous thromboembolism." *Chest* 120 (October 2001): 1047-1048.

Evans, A. D. B., and R. V. Johnston. "Venous Thromboembolic Disease in Pilots." *Lancet* 358 (November 17, 2001): 1734.

Ulutin, T. A., J. Altinisik, H. O. Ates, et al. "Screening of Factor V Leiden (G1691A), Prothrombin G20210A and Protein C Mutations in Thrombosis Patients." *American Journal of Human Genetics* 69 (October 2001): 430.

Zoler, Mitchel L., and Winnie Anne Imperio. "Drug Update: Outpatient Treatment of Deep Vein Thrombosis." *Internal Medicine News* 34 (December 1, 2001): 24.

Mai Tran
Rebecca J. Frey, PhD

Phobias

Definition

A phobia is an intense but unrealistic fear that can interfere with the ability to socialize, work, or go about everyday life, brought on by an object, event or situation.

Description

Just about everyone is afraid of something—an upcoming job interview or being alone outside after dark. But about 18% of all Americans are tormented by irrational fears that interfere with their daily lives. They aren't crazy—they know full well their fears are unreasonable—but they can't control the fear. These people suffer from phobias.

Phobias belong to a large group of mental problems known as **anxiety** disorders that include **obsessive-compulsive disorder** (OCD), **panic disorder**, and **post-traumatic stress disorder**. Phobias themselves can be divided into three specific types:

- specific phobias
- social phobia
- agoraphobia

Specific phobias

As its name suggests, a specific phobia is the fear of a particular situation or object, including anything

KEY TERMS

Agoraphobia—A phobia characterized by intense fear of open or public places with no way to leave or escape easily if panic develops.

Benzodiazepine—A class of drugs that have a hypnotic and sedative action, used mainly as tranquilizers to control symptoms of anxiety.

Beta blockers—A group of drugs usually prescribed to treat heart conditions, but are also used to reduce the physical symptoms of anxiety and phobias, such as sweating and palpitations.

Monoamine oxidase inhibitors (MAO inhibitors)—A class of antidepressants used to treat social phobia.

Neuroimaging—The use of x ray studies and magnetic resonance imaging (MRIs) to detect abnormalities or trace pathways of nerve activity in the central nervous system.

Selective serotonin reuptake inhibitors (SSRIs)—A class of antidepressants that work by blocking the reabsorption of serotonin in the brain, raising the levels of serotonin. SSRIs include Prozac, Zoloft, and Paxil.

Serotonin—One of three major types of neurotransmitters found in the brain that is linked to emotions.

Specific phobia—An intense but irrational fear of a specific place, object, or animal. Common specific phobias include fear of spiders, snakes, or dogs; fear of flying or highway driving; fear of blood; and fear of elevators and other closed spaces.

from airplane travel to dentists. Found in one out of every 10 Americans, specific phobias seem to run in families and are roughly twice as likely to appear in women. If the person doesn't often encounter the feared object, the phobia doesn't cause much harm. However, if the feared object or situation is common, it can seriously disrupt everyday life. Common examples of specific phobias, which can begin at any age, include fear of snakes, flying, dogs, escalators, elevators, high places, disease, or open spaces.

Social phobia

People with social phobia have deep fears of being watched or judged by others and being embarrassed in public. This may extend to a general fear of social situations—or be more specific, such as a fear of giving speeches or of performing (stage fright). More rarely, people with social phobia may have trouble using a public restroom, eating in a restaurant, or signing their name in front of others.

Social phobia is not the same as shyness. Shy people may feel uncomfortable with others, but they don't experience severe anxiety, they don't worry excessively about social situations beforehand, and they don't avoid events that make them feel self-conscious. On the other hand, people with social phobia may not be shy—they may feel perfectly comfortable with people except in specific situations. Social phobias may be only mildly irritating, or they may significantly interfere with daily life. It is not unusual for people with social phobia to turn down job offers or avoid relationships because of their fears.

Agoraphobia

Agoraphobia is the intense fear of feeling trapped and having a panic attack in a public place. It usually begins between ages 15 and 35, and affects three times as many women as men—about 3% of the population.

An episode of spontaneous panic is usually the initial trigger for the development of agoraphobia. After an initial panic attack, the person becomes afraid of experiencing a second one. Sufferers literally fear the fear, and worry incessantly about when and where the next attack may occur. As they begin to avoid the places or situations in which the panic attack occurred, their fear generalizes. Eventually the person completely avoids public places. In severe cases, people with agoraphobia can no longer leave their homes for fear of experiencing a panic attack.

Causes and symptoms

Experts don't really know why phobias develop, although research suggests they may arise from a complex interaction between heredity and environment. Some hypersensitive people have unique chemical reactions in the brain that cause them to respond much more strongly to **stress**. These people also may be especially sensitive to **caffeine**, which triggers certain brain chemical responses.

Advances in neuroimaging have also led researchers to identify certain parts of the brain and specific neural pathways that are associated with phobias. One part of the brain that is currently being studied is the amygdala, an almond-shaped body of nerve cells involved in normal fear conditioning. Another area of the brain that appears to be linked to phobias is the posterior cerebellum.

While experts believe the tendency to develop phobias runs in families and may be hereditary, a specific stressful event usually triggers the development of a specific phobia or agoraphobia. For example, someone predisposed to develop phobias who experiences severe turbulence during a flight might go on to develop a phobia about flying.

Social phobia typically appears in childhood or adolescence, sometimes following an upsetting or humiliating experience. Certain vulnerable children who have had unpleasant social experiences (such as being rejected) or who have poor social skills may develop social phobias. The condition also may be related to low self-esteem, unassertive personality, and feelings of inferiority.

A person with agoraphobia may have a panic attack at any time for no apparent reason. While the attack may last only a minute or so, the person remembers the feelings of panic so strongly that the possibility of another attack becomes terrifying. For this reason, people with agoraphobia avoid places where they might not be able to escape if a panic attack occurs.

While the specific trigger may differ, the symptoms of different phobias are remarkably similar (e.g., feelings of terror and impending doom, rapid heartbeat and breathing, sweaty palms, and other features of a panic attack). Patients may experience severe anxiety symptoms in anticipating a phobic trigger. For example, someone who is afraid to fly may begin having episodes of pounding heart and sweating palms at the mere thought of getting on a plane in two weeks.

Diagnosis

A mental health professional can diagnose phobias after a detailed interview and discussion of both mental and physical symptoms. Social phobia is often associated with other anxiety disorders, **depression**, or **substance abuse**.

Treatment

People who have a specific phobia that is easy to avoid (such as snakes) and that doesn't interfere with their lives may not need to seek treatment. In all types of phobias, symptoms may be eased by lifestyle changes, such as:

- eliminating caffeine
- cutting down on alcohol
- eating a good diet
- getting plenty of exercise
- reducing stress

Meditation and mindfulness training can be beneficial to patients with phobias and panic disorder. **Hydrotherapy**, **massage therapy**, and **aromatherapy** are useful to some anxious patients because they can promote general **relaxation** of the nervous system. Relaxation training, which is sometimes called anxiety management training, includes breathing exercises and similar techniques intended to help the patient prevent hyperventilation and relieve the muscle tension associated with the fight-or-flight reaction of anxiety. **Yoga**, aikido, **t'ai chi**, and **dance therapy** help patients work with the physical, as well as the emotional, tensions that either promote or are created by anxiety.

Herbs known as adaptogens may be prescribed to treat the anxiety related to phobias. These herbs are thought to promote adaptability to stress, and include **Siberian ginseng** (*Eleutherococcus senticosus*), and ginseng (*Panax ginseng*). Adrenal modulators such as **licorice** (*Glycyrrhiza glabra*) and borage (*Borago officinalis*), nervine herbs such as **chamomile** (*Chamaemelum nobile*) and **skullcap** (*Scutellaria lateriafolia*), and antioxidal herbs like **milk thistle** (*Silybum marianum*) are also beneficial. Tonics of skullcap and oats (*Avena sativa*) may also be recommended to ease anxiety.

Allopathic treatment

When phobias interfere with a person's daily life, a combination of **psychotherapy** and medication can be quite effective. Medication can block the feelings of panic, and when combined with cognitive-behavioral therapy, can be quite effective in reducing specific phobias and agoraphobia.

Cognitive-behavioral therapy adds a cognitive approach to more traditional **behavioral therapy**. It teaches patients how to change their thoughts, behavior, and attitudes, while providing techniques to lessen anxiety, such as deep breathing, muscle relaxation, and refocusing.

One cognitive-behavioral therapy is desensitization (also known as exposure therapy), in which people are gradually exposed to the frightening object or event until they become used to it and their physical symptoms decrease. For example, someone who is afraid of snakes might first be shown a photo of a snake. Once the person can look at a photo without anxiety, he might then be shown a video of a snake. Each step is repeated until the symptoms of fear (such as pounding heart and sweating palms) disappear. Eventually, the person might reach the point where he can actually touch a live snake. Three-fourths of patients are significantly improved with this type of treatment.

Another more dramatic cognitive-behavioral approach is called flooding, which exposes the person immediately to the feared object or situation. The person remains in the situation until the anxiety lessens.

Several drugs are used to treat specific phobias by controlling symptoms and helping to prevent panic attacks. These include anti-anxiety drugs (benzodiazepines) such as alprazolam (Xanax) or diazepam (Valium). Blood pressure medications called beta blockers, such as propranolol (Inderal) and atenolol (Tenormin), appear to work well in the treatment of circumscribed social phobia, when anxiety gets in the way of performance, such as public speaking. These drugs reduce overstimulation, thereby controlling the physical symptoms of anxiety.

In addition, some antidepressants may be effective when used together with cognitive-behavioral therapy. These include the monoamine oxidase inhibitors (MAO inhibitors) phenelzine (Nardil) and tranylcypromine (Parnate), as well as selective serotonin reuptake inhibitors (SSRIs) like fluoxetine (Prozac), paroxetine (Paxil), sertraline (Zoloft), and fluvoxamine (Luvox).

A medication that shows promise as a treatment for social phobia is valproic acid (Depakene or Depakote), which is usually prescribed to treat seizures or to prevent migraine headaches. Researchers conducting a twelve-week trial with 17 patients found that about half the patients experienced a significant improvement in their social anxiety symptoms while taking the medication. Further studies are underway.

Treating agoraphobia is more difficult than other phobias because there are often so many fears involved, such as open spaces, traffic, elevators, and escalators. Treatment includes cognitive-behavioral therapy with antidepressants or anti-anxiety drugs. Paxil and Zoloft are used to treat panic disorders with or without agoraphobia.

Expected results

Phobias are among the most treatable mental health problems; depending on the severity of the condition and the type of phobia, most properly treated patients can go on to lead normal lives. Research suggests that once a person overcomes the phobia, the problem may not return for many years—if at all.

Untreated phobias are another matter. Only about 20% of specific phobias will go away without treatment, and agoraphobia will get worse with time if untreated. Social phobias tend to be chronic, and without treatment, will not likely go away. Moreover, untreated phobias can lead to other problems, including depression, **alcoholism**, and feelings of shame and low self-esteem.

A group of researchers in Boston reported in 2003 that phobic anxiety appears to be a risk factor for **Parkinson's disease** (PD) in males, although it is not yet known whether phobias cause PD or simply share an underlying biological cause.

While most specific phobias appear in childhood and subsequently fade away, those that remain in adulthood often need to be treated. Unfortunately, most people never get the help they need; only about 25% of people with phobias ever seek help to deal with their condition.

Prevention

There is no known way to prevent the development of phobias. Medication and cognitive-behavioral therapy may help prevent the recurrence of symptoms once they have been diagnosed. Early detection and treatments may decrease severity.

Resources

BOOKS

American Psychiatric Association. *Diagnostic and Statistical Manual of Mental Disorders*, 4th edition, text revision. Washington, DC: American Psychiatric Association, 2000.

Bloomfield, Harold H. *Healing Anxiety with Herbs.* New York: Harper Collins, 1998.

Peurifoy, Reneau Z. *Anxiety, Phobias and Panic: A Step by Step Program for Regaining Control of Your Life.* New York: Warner Books, 1996.

"Phobic Disorders." Section 15, Chapter 187 in *The Merck Manual of Diagnosis and Therapy*, edited by Mark H. Beers, MD, and Robert Berkow, MD. Whitehouse Station, NJ: Merck Research Laboratories, 2002.

Schneier, Franklin, and Lawrence Welkowitz. *The Hidden Face of Shyness: Understanding and Overcoming Social Anxiety.* New York: Avon Books, 1996.

Stern, Richard. *Mastering Phobias: Cases, Causes and Cures.* New York: Penguin USA, 1996.

PERIODICALS

Kinrys, G., M. H. Pollack, N. M. Simon, et al. "Valproic Acid for the Treatment of Social Anxiety Disorder." *International Clinical Psychopharmacology* 18 (May 2003): 169–172.

Modica, Peter. "Social phobia may run in the family." *American Journal of Psychiatry* 155 (1998): 90-97.

Ploghaus, A., L. Becerra, C. Borras, and D. Borsook. "Neural Circuitry Underlying Pain Modulation:

Expectation, Hypnosis, Placebo." *Trends in Cognitive Science* 7 (May 2003): 197–200.

Rauch, S. L., L. M. Shin, and C. I. Wright. "Neuroimaging Studies of Amygdala Function in Anxiety Disorders." *Annals of the New York Academy of Sciences* 985 (April 2003): 389–410.

Weisskopf, M. G., H. Chen, M. A. Schwarzschild, et al. "Prospective Study of Phobic Anxiety and Risk of Parkinson's Disease." *Movement Disorders* 18 (June 2003): 646–651.

ORGANIZATIONS

Agoraphobics Building Independent Lives. 1418 Lorraine Ave., Richmond, VA 23227.

Agoraphobics In Motion. 605 W. 11 Mile Rd., Royal Oak, MI 48067.

American Psychiatric Association (APA). 1400 K Street, NW, Washington, DC 20005. (888) 357-7924. http://www.psych.org.

Anxiety Disorders Association of America. 11900 Parklawn Dr., Ste. 100, Rockville, MD 20852. (301) 231-9350.

National Anxiety Foundation. 3135 Custer Dr., Lexington, KY 40517. (606) 272-7166. http://www.lexington-on-line.com/naf.html.

National Institute of Mental Health (NIMH) Office of Communications. 6001 Executive Boulevard, Room 8184, MSC 9663, Bethesda, MD 20892-9663. (866) 615-NIMH or (301) 443-4513. http://www.nimh.nih.gov.

OTHER

Anxiety Network Homepage. http://www.anxietynetwork.com.

National Institute of Mental Health (NIMH). *Anxiety Disorders*. NIH Publication No. 02-3879. Bethesda, MD: NIMH, 2002.

Paula Ford-Martin
Rebecca J. Frey, PhD

❚ Phosphorus

Description

Phosphorus (chemical symbol P) is a chemical element discovered by the German alchemist Hennig Brand in 1669. It plays an essential part in multiple biochemical reactions for both plants and animals and is essential to all life. Phosphorus is found in living things and in soil and rock, mostly as chemical compounds known as phosphates. Rock and soil phosphorus are mined extensively throughout the world, but especially in the People's Republic of China and the United States.

Elemental phosphorus exists in a number of allotropic forms, primarily white, red, and black phosphorus.

Allotropes are forms of an element with differing physical and chemical properties. White (also called yellow or common) phosphorus is a wax-like substance formed by heating phosphorus until it vaporizes and the condensate solidifies. One of this form's characteristics has given the English language the adjective *phosphorescent*, from white phosphorus's tendency to glow in the dark when exposed to air.

White phosphorus is highly toxic, causes **burns** if it comes in contact with skin, and is so combustible that it has to be stored underwater for safety. Red phosphorus is a rust-colored powder created by heating white phosphorus and exposing it to sunlight. It is not as combustible as the white form. Black phosphorus is made by heating white phosphorus under extremely high pressure until it resembles graphite.

In plants, phosphorus is necessary for photosynthesis to take place. In the human body, phosphorus works in tandem with another element, **calcium**, in much the same way that two other electrolyte components, **sodium** and **potassium**, do. Though phosphorus is found in every cell of the human body and accounts for 1% of the body's total weight, its primary function is working in conjunction with calcium to form teeth and bones.

Eighty-five percent of the phosphorus found in the body is located in these structures. In a delicately balanced chemical reaction, parathyroid hormone (PTH), alcitonin, and 25-dihydroxy **vitamin D** regulate the absorption of both calcium and phosphorus from the intestinal tract, thus making it available for the production of bones and teeth. If an excessive amount of phosphorus is absorbed, the phosphorus combines with all available calcium and prevents the calcium's efficient use in making and maintaining bones and teeth.

PTH balances the proportions of calcium and phosphorus in the body by increasing the release of calcium and phosphate from bone and the loss of phosphorus via the kidneys while limiting the excretion of calcium. PTH also increases the activity of the 25-Dihydroxy v25-Dihydroxy vitamin D, which, in contrast, increases the absorption of both phosphorus and calcium from the intestinal tract.

General use

Compounds of phosphorus are used to make fertilizers, detergents, and water softeners. They are also used in the manufacture of steel, plastics, insecticides, medical drugs, and animal feeds. Phosphorus is used in the manufacture of safety matches and pesticides, including rat poison.

Phosphorus found in the blood stream and in soft tissue has a highly significant role to play in a variety of body functions. Working with vitamin B, phosphorus is involved in the metabolism of fats and carbohydrates, in both the repair of damaged cells and tissues and the routine maintenance of healthy ones. Phosphorus is necessary for the regularity of the heartbeat and aids in the contraction of all other muscles throughout the body. Phosphorus is needed for the functioning of the kidneys and plays a part in the conduction of impulses along the network that makes up the nervous system.

Preparations

According to the American Dietetic Association, phosphorus intake in the United States is generally above what is needed and in the 1990s and 2000s actually increased. Therefore, under normal circumstances with normal food intake, there is seldom if ever a need to supplement intake of phosphorus. Persons suffering from eating disorders such as anorexia and bulimia can be deficient in phosphorus intake as well as other nutrients. As the best source of phosphorus is in protein foods such as meat, eggs, and milk products. Some vegetarians may also need to evaluate their intake of this element. Excess consumption of processed foods, inadequate intake of whole foods, and fertilizers and pesticides are some of the causes for excess phosphorus.

Beside high-protein foods, phosphorus is also found in decreasing quantities in wholegrain breads and cereals, especially unprocessed ones, and in minute amounts in fruits and vegetables. The phosphorus present in wholegrain breads and cereals, however, exists as a substance called *phytin*. Phytin combines with calcium to create a salt that the human body is incapable of absorbing, thus making grains that are unprocessed and not enriched a negligible source of phosphorus. But both commercially prepared cereals and breads may provide this element as they are frequently enriched with it. Phosphates can also be taken by mouth as a tablet.

Precautions

White phosphorus is poisonous. Red phosphorus is not. As noted, white phosphorus is a highly toxic, flammable substance capable of burning the skin on contact, and of igniting at room temperature. It should be handled with extreme care. Accidental phosphorus poisoning can happen from both fertilizers and pesticides. Humans rarely come into contact with elemental phosphorus, so these precautions apply primarily to

KEY TERMS

Anorexia nervosa—A serious and sometimes fatal eating disorder characterized by intense fear of being fat and severe weight loss. It primarily affects teenage and young adult females. Sufferers have a distorted body image wherein they see themselves as fat even when they are at normal weight or even emaciated.

Bulimia—An eating disorder characterized by bouts of gross overeating usually followed by self-induced vomiting.

Calcitonin—A hormone produced by the thyroid gland that controls the calcium level in the blood by slowing the rate that calcium is lost from bone.

Deciliter—A fluid measurement that is equal to one-tenth of a liter, or 100 cubic centimeters (27 fluid drams or teaspoonfuls).

Diabetic ketoacidosis—A potentially serious condition in which ketones become present in the blood stream because of the metabolism of fats *burned* in lieu of carbohydrates that would normally be used, which occurs because there is insufficient insulin available to cause carbohydrates to be used as fuel.

Electrolyte—Substances that split into ions, or electrically charged particles, within the body to regulate many important bodily processes. Examples of electrolytes are sodium, potassium, hydrogen, magnesium, calcium, bicarbonate, phosphates, and chlorides.

Multiple endocrine neoplasia—Tumor formation characterized by a progressive, abnormal multiplication of cells that are not necessarily malignant in any of the glands that secrete chemicals directly into the blood stream, such as the thyroid gland, adrenal glands, or ovaries.

Osteomalacia—Softening, weakening, and removal of the minerals from bone in adults caused by vitamin D deficiency.

Osteoporosis—Loss of formative protein tissue from bone, causing it to become brittle and easily fractured; considered a normal part of aging, but with hormonal causes that make it much more common in women than men.

Sarcoidosis—A rare disease of unknown cause as of 2008 that occurs mostly in young adults. Inflammation occurs in the lymph nodes and other tissues throughout the body, usually including the lungs, liver, skin, and eyes.

workers in the phosphorus industry. Phosphates sometimes are leached into water systems through sewage and can drastically alter the chemical makeup of lakes and rivers. In sufficient quantities, they can lead to the death of nearly all forms of aquatic life.

A normal blood serum level of phosphorus is 2.4–4.1 mg per deciliter of blood. An abnormal serum phosphorus level should be evaluated by a physician.

Phosphorus levels higher than normal can indicate a diet that includes an excessive phosphorus intake, inadequate intake of calcium, or lack of PTH (parathyroid hormone) in the system. It can be related to bone metastasis associated with **cancer**, liver or kidney disease, or *sarcoidosis*.

Serum phosphorus levels that are below normal can be related to insufficient phosphorus or vitamin D in one's diet leading to rickets in children and osteomalacia in adults. Disorders of the parathyroid gland, causing it to secrete excessive quantities of PTH, or of the pancreas, causing it to secrete too much insulin, also affect blood levels of phosphorus. Diabetic ketoacidosis or too much calcium are other possible causes. Multiple endocrine neoplasia (MEN) is yet another condition that often is associated with lower than normal levels of phosphorus.

Side effects

Phosphorus preparations taken to supplement low phosphorus levels in the body can cause **diarrhea**.

Interactions

Antacids can decrease the absorption of phosphorus. Laxatives and enemas that contain the chemical compound sodium phosphate and excessive intake of vitamin D can increase phosphorus levels in the body. Administration of intravenous glucose solutions will cause phosphorus to combine with the glucose that is being absorbed by the cells.

Resources

BOOKS

Berdanier, Carolyn D., and Janos Zempleni. *Advanced Nutrition: Macronutrients, Micronutrients, and Metabolism.* Boca Raton, FL: CRC Press, 2008.
Panel on Macronutrients. *Dietary Reference Intakes for Energy, Carbohydrate, Fiber, Fat, Fatty Acids, Cholesterol, Protein, and Amino Acids (Macronutrients).* Washington, DC: National Academies Press, 2005.
Shils, Maurice E., et al., eds. *Modern Nutrition in Health and Disease,* 10th ed. Philadelphia: Lippincott Williams & Wilkins, 2005.

PERIODICALS

Karp, H., et al. "Acute Effects of Different Phosphorus Sources on Calcium and Bone Metabolism in Young Women: A Whole-Foods Approach." *Calcified Tissue International* (April 2007): 251–258.
Rigo, Jacques, et al. "Enteral Calcium, Phosphate and Vitamin D Requirements and Bone Mineralization in Preterm Infants." *Acta Pædiatrica* (July 2007): 969–974.

OTHER

"Phosphorus." Linus Pauling Institute, August 2007. http://lpi.oregonstate.edu/infocenter/minerals/phosphorus/. (February 19, 2008).
"Nutrition Fact Sheet: Phosphorus." Northwesternutrition, July 2007. http://www.feinberg.northwestern.edu/nutrition/factsheets/phosphorus.html. (February 19, 2008).

Joan Schonbeck
David Edward Newton, Ed.D.

Phytolacca

Definition

Phytolacca is a genus of plants belonging to the family Phytolaccaceae, commonly known as the pokeweeds. That common name is also used for members of the genus Phytolacca. Some well known members of the genus include "P. americana", native to North America; "P. dioica" (South America); "P. decadra" (North America); "P. heteropetala" (Mexico), "P. icosandra (South America); and "P. octandra(New Zealand). Members of the Phytolacca genus are also known by a number of common names, including American nightshade, **cancer** root, cocum, inkberry, ombú, pigeon berry, poke, pokebush, pokeberry, pokeroot, polk salad, polk sallet, red ink plant, red nightshade, red weed, scoke, and shang–lu .

Description

Pokeweed is a perennial plant that adjusts readily to a variety of growing conditions. It prefers open areas, such as recently cleared spaces, open meadows, or pastureland. It is anchored by large, fleshy, bulbous root that sends out a single erect stem each year that may grow to a height of 10 feet (3 meters). One of the most robust examples of the plants grows on the South American pampas, where it attains the height and appears of a small tree. The stem is green at first, but turns red or purple later in the season as flowers appear. Leaves are alternate, pointed, and crinkly. White flowers, which form at the terminus of pendulous stems, eventually change into round deep purple berries filled with a beautiful purple juice. American botanist Edmond Preston first noted in 1884 that leaves of the pokeweed emit a faint and continuous fluorescent light in the dark at the end of its growing season in fall.

Pokeweed contains a number of organic compounds toxic to mammals, including phytolaccine (an alkaloid), phytolaccatoxin (a resin), and phytolaccigenin (a saponin). Alkaloids are nitrogen–containing organic compounds with physiological effects on animals. Saponins are glycosides, sugar–like substances. Resins are semi–solid materials commonly produced by plants. Most animals avoid pokeweed, apparently because of its noxious taste. Small children are sometimes attracted to the colorful berries and may become ill if they eat the plant. The toxins in pokeweed act as an emetic, producing **nausea** and **vomiting** within a few hours of being ingested. Without treatment, symptoms because worse and may include convulsions, spasms, paralysis of the respiratory system, and death. Interestingly, birds appear to be immune to the toxic effects of the pokeweed plant. Scientists hypothesize that the plant seeds, which contain toxins, pass through a bird's digestive system unchanged, thus avoiding any harmful effects on the animals. This hypothesis helps explain the fact that pokeweed plants often grow in isolated areas where no parent plant has been able to drop seeds. The volunteer plants in such cases arise out of seeds that have passed through a bird's digestive system.

Uses

Physicians and public health authorities have long advised against the human consumption of phytolacca, pointing out the serious risk of poisoning. Nonetheless, pokeweed products have had a long history as foods and herbal remedies. In the American south, for example, the plant is often prepared by boiling it three times over (to remove toxic components) and then served as poke salad, pokeberry juice, or in combination with other juices and jellies.

The plant's appeal, in spite of its toxic risks, lies in a number of supposed therapeutic uses to which it can be put. It is taken either orally, as a tonic or infusion, or topically, by rubbing on the skin or other injured or diseased area. Proponents of it say that pokeweed is

- alterative (gradually improving one's overall health)
- anodyne (relieving pain and discomfort)
- anti–inflammatory
- cathartic (capable of relieving constipation)
- emetic (capable of inducing nausea and vomiting)

- expectorant (an agent that stimulates the expulsion of mucus from the lungs and throat)
- hypnotic (capable of inducing sleep)
- narcotic (capable of inducing deep sleep or unconsciousness)
- purgative (stimulating movement of the bowels)

Some specific conditions for which phytolacca has been recommended include **bronchitis**, catarrh (inflammation of the mucous membranes), chronic **eczema**, diphtheria, dysentery, glandular **fever**, immune disorders, **influenza**, **mumps**, **psoriasis**, rheumatism, **sore throat**, **sprains**, swollen glands, tender nipples and sore breasts, tinea capitis (**fungal infections** of the scalp), **tonsillitis**, and ulcers of the leg. On its website review of the medicinal uses of phytolacca in 2008, the Memorial Sloan–Kettering Cancer Center concluded that "[n]o study supports the use of pokeweed for any proposed claim."

In spite of that general observation, some researchers believe that phytolacca or one or more of its components may be effective in treating certain diseases, especially cancer and viral **infections**, such as autoimmundeficiency syndrome (**AIDS**). Since the late 1990s, for example, researchers have been exploring the use of pokeweed antiviral protein (PAP) as treatment for certain types of cancers and viral infections. The compound has been effective in killing viruses and cancer cells in vitro and in experimental animals. At this point, however, there is not enough evidence to assess the safety and efficacy of PAP for use with humans. Research also continues on the use of another product obtained from phytolacca called PAPF–s as an antifungal agent. So far, laboratory results are promising, but no human studies have been completed.

Side Effects

Some homeopathic practitioners claim that there are no side effects associated with the use of phytolacca preparations. Medical sources, however, report that a number of adverse effects have been reported during the use of the product. These effects include chest **pain**, difficulty in breathing, **hives**, itchy or swollen skin, nausea, vomiting, stomach cramps, **diarrhea**, muscular weakness, hypotension, and irregular heart beat. As indicated above, the product is also toxic if taken in sufficient amounts.

Interactions

Relatively little research has been conducted on possible interactions of phytolacca with drugs and other herbs. Some hypothesized interactions are the following:

KEY TERMS

Alkaloid—A nitrogen–containing plant product that has pharmacological effects on animals.

Alterative—Having the tendency to improve one's general health gradually over time.

Anodyne—A substance that reduces pain and discomfort

Cathartic—Capable of reducing or relieving constipation.

Emetic—Having a tendency to induce nausea and vomiting

Expectorant—A substance that loosens phlegm in the lungs and throat, leading to its expulsion by coughing and spitting

Hypnotic—Capable of inducing sleep.

Narcotic—Capable of inducing deep sleep or unconsciousness.

Purgative—Having a tendency to stimulate movement of the bowels.

Resin—A gummy, semi–solid material produced by many kinds of plants.

Saponin—Soapy–like substances found in many plants with a chemical structure related to that of the simple sugar glucose.

- an increase in the action of anticoagulants
- inhibition, in general, of the action of drugs because of the increase in transit time through the gastrointestinal system
- an increase in the action of antidepressants
- a reduction in the efficacy of phytolacca with the use of chlorophenylalanine, cyproheptadine HCl, and phenobarbital
- an increase in the antibiotic activity of echinacea
- a reduction in pokeroot's efficacy if milk is used in tea concoctions

Resources

BOOKS

Bensky, Dan, Steven Clavey, and Erich Stoger. *Chinese Herbal Medicine: Materia Medica, 3rd edition.* Vista, Calif.: Eastland Press, 2004.

Gruenwald, Joerg. *PDR for Herbal Medicines.* London: Thomson PDR, 2004.

PERIODICALS

Park, Sand–Wok, et al. "Isolation and Characterization of a Novel Ribosome–inactivating Protein from Root Cultures of Pokeweed and Its Mechanism of Secretion from Roots." *Plant Physiology* (September 2002): 164–178.

Zhao, Y., et al. "A Pokeweed Antiviral Protein Gene in Roots of Phytolacca Americana." *Acta Virologica* (October 2004): 131–132.

OTHER

Alternative Nature Online Herbal. "Pokeweed." http://www.altnature.com/gallery/pokeweed.htm (February 27, 2008).

Henriette's Herbal Homepage. "Phytolacca." http://www.henriettesherbal.com/eclectic/kings/phytolacca.html (February 27, 2008).

Plants for a Future. "Phytolacca americana – L. Pokeweed" http://www.pfaf.org/database/plants.php?Phytolacca + americana (February 27, 2008).

David Edward Newton, Ed.D.

PID *see* **Pelvic inflammatory disease**

Pilates

Definition

Pilates or Physical Mind method, is a series of non-impact exercises designed by Joseph Pilates to develop strength, flexibility, balance, and inner awareness.

Origins

Joseph Pilates (pronounced pie-LAH-tes), the founder of the Pilates method (also simply referred to as "the method") was born in Germany in 1880. As a frail child with rickets, **asthma**, and **rheumatic fever**, he was determined to become stronger. He dedicated himself to building both his body and his mind through practices which included **yoga**, zen, and ancient Roman and Greek exercises. His conditioning regime worked and he became an accomplished gymnast, skier, boxer, and diver.

While interned in England during World War I for being a German citizen, Pilates became a nurse. During this time, he designed a unique system of hooking springs and straps to a hospital bed in order to help his disabled and immobilized patients regain strength and movement. It was through these experiments that he recognized the importance of training the core abdominal and back muscles to stabilize the torso and allow the entire body to move freely. This experimentation provided the foundation for his style of conditioning and the specialized **exercise** equipment associated with the Pilates method.

KEY TERMS

Yoga—A system of physical, mental, and breathing exercises developed in India.

Zen—A form of meditation that emphasizes direct experience.

Pilates emigrated to the United States in 1926 after the German government invited him to use his conditioning methods to train the army. That same year he opened the first Pilates studio in New York City. Over the years, dancers, actors, and athletes flocked to his studio to heal, condition, and align their bodies.

Joseph Pilates died at age 87 in a fire at his studio. Although his strength enabled him to escape the flames by hanging from the rafters for over an hour, he died from smoke inhalation. He believed that ideal fitness is "the attainment and maintenance of a uniformly developed body with a sound mind fully capable of naturally, easily, and satisfactorily preforming our many and varied daily tasks with spontaneous zest and pleasure."

Benefits

Pilates is a form of strength and flexibility training that can be done by someone at any level of fitness. The exercises can also be adapted for people who have limited movement or who use wheel chairs. It is an engaging exercise program that people want to do. Pilates promotes a feeling of physical and mental well-being and also develops inner physical awareness. Since this method strengthens and lengthens the muscles without creating bulk, it is particularly beneficial for dancers and actors. Pilates is also helpful in preventing and rehabilitating from injuries, improving posture, and increasing flexibility, circulation, and balance. Pregnant women who do these exercises can develop body alignment, improve concentration, and develop body shape and tone after **pregnancy**. According to Joseph Pilates, "You will feel better in 10 sessions, look better in 20 sessions and have a completely new body in 30 sessions."

Although Pilates is often associated with dancers, athletes, and younger people in general who are interested in improving their physical strength and flexibility, a simplified version of some Pilates exercises is also being used as of 2003 to lower the risk of hospital-related deconditioning in older adults. A Canadian study of hospitalized patients over the age of 70 found that those who were given a set of Pilates exercises that could be performed in bed recovered more rapidly than a control group given a set of passive range-of-motion exercises.

Description

During the initial meeting, an instructor will analyze the client's posture and movement and design a specific training program. Once the program has been created, the sessions usually follow a basic pattern. A session generally begins with mat work and passive and active stretching. In passive stretching, the instructor moves and presses the client's body to stretch and elongate the muscles. During the active stretching period, the client preforms the stretches while the instructor watches their form and breathing. These exercises warm up the muscles in preparation for the machine work. The machines help the client to maintain the correct positioning required for each exercise.

There are over 500 exercises that were developed by Joseph Pilates. "Classical" exercises, according to the Pilates Studio in New York involve several principles. These include concentration, centering, flowing movement, and breath. Some instructors teach only the classical exercises originally taught by Joseph Pilates. Others design new exercises that are variations upon these classical forms in order to make the exercises more accessible for a specific person.

There are two primary exercise machines used for Pilates, the Universal Reformer and the Cadillac, and several smaller pieces of equipment. The Reformer resembles a single bed frame and is equipped with a carriage that slides back and forth and adjustable springs that are used to regulate tension and resistance. Cables, bars, straps, and pulleys allow the exercises to be done from a variety of positions. Instructors usually work with their clients on the machines for 20-45 minutes. During this time, they are observing and giving feedback about alignment, breathing, and precision of movement. The exercises are done slowly and carefully so that the movements are smooth and flowing. This requires focused concentration and muscle control. The session ends with light stretching and a cool-down period.

Once the basics are learned from an instructor, from either one-on-one lessons or in a class, it is possible to train at home using videos. Exercise equipment for use at home is also available and many exercises can be performed on a mat.

A private session costs between $45–$75, depending on the part of the country one is in. This method is not specifically covered by insurance although it may be covered when the instructor is a licensed physical therapist.

Precautions

The Pilates method is not a substitute for good physical therapy, although it has been increasingly used and recommended by physical therapists since the mid-1980s. People with chronic injuries are advised to see a physician.

Research and general acceptance

As of early 2004, several physical therapists and gerontologists have done research studies on the Pilates method, although much more work needs to be done in this area. The appeal of the Pilates method to a wide population, coupled with a new interest in it on the part of rehabilitation therapists, suggests that further studies may soon be underway. Dancers and actors originally embraced the Pilates method as a form of strength training that did not create muscle bulk. Professional and amateur athletes also use these exercises to prevent reinjury. Sedentary people find Pilates to be a gentle, non-impact approach to conditioning. Pilates equipment and classes can be found in hospitals, health clubs, spas, and gyms.

Training and certification

There are two main centers for training and certification. The Pilates Studio in New York City certifies teachers in the "classical" exercises of "The Pilates Method." The teacher training program of The Pilates Studio involves seminar training and 600 apprenticeship hours. Perspective teachers need a strong background in Pilates. There is an extensive application and examination process. Classes are available throughout the United States and in 20 international locations.

The PhysicalMind Institute in Santa Fe, New Mexico, offers a 275-hour basic certification program in "The Method." Prerequisites include a 15-hour course, knowledge of functional anatomy, and 10 hours of private sessions. After completing an apprenticeship, students must pass a written and practical final exam. Advanced training is also offered. Students at this center receive training in the original exercises of Joseph Pilates, as well as the concepts of body mechanics. Understanding the concepts behind the exercises enables teachers to create appropriate variations for their clients. Classes are available throughout the United States and Canada.

Resources

BOOKS

Knaster, Mirka. *Discovering the Body's Wisdom*. New York: Bantam Books, 1996.

Pilates, Joseph H., et al. *The Complete Writings of Joseph Pilates: Return to Life Through Contrology and Your Health*. New York: Bantam Doubleday, 2000.

Robinson, Lynne, et al. *Body Control: Using the Techniques Developed by Joseph Pilates*. Trans-Atlantic Publications, 1998.

Siler, Brooke. *The Pilates Body: The Ultimate At-Home Guide to Strengthening, Lengthening and Toning Your Body-Without Machines*. New York: Bantam Doubleday, 2000.

PERIODICALS

Anderson, Brent D. "Pushing for Pilates." *Rehab Management* 14 (June-July 2001): 23–25.

Argo, Carol. "The Pilates Method for a Balanced Body." *American Fitness* (March/April 1999):52-54.

Blum, C. L. "Chiropractic and Pilates Therapy for the Treatment of Adult Scoliosis." *Journal of Manipulative and Physiological Therapeutics* 25 (May 2002): E3.

Chang, Yahlin. "Grace Under Pressure." *Newsweek* (February 28, 2000).

Coleman-Brown, L., and V. Haley-Kanigel. "Movement with Meaning." *Rehab Management* 16 (July 2003): 28–32.

Mallery, L. H., E. A. MacDonald, C. L. Hubley-Kozey, et al. "The Feasibility of Performing Resistance Exercise with Acutely Ill Hospitalized Older Adults." *BMC Geriatrics* 3 (October 7, 2003): 3.

ORGANIZATIONS

PhysicalMind Institute. 1807 Second Street, Suite 15/16, Santa Fe, New Mexico 87505. (505) 988-1990 or (800) 505-1990. Fax: (505) 988-2837. themethod@trail.com. http:\\www.the-method.com.

The Pilates Studio. 2121 Broadway, Suite 201, New York, New York, 10023-1786. (800)474-5283 or (888) 474-5283 or (212)875-0189. Fax: (212) 769-2368. http:\\www.pilates-studio.com.

Linda Chrisman
Rebecca J. Frey, PhD

Piles *see* **Hemorrhoids**

Pinched nerve

Definition

A pinched nerve is caused by some anatomical structure putting pressure on a nerve and impairing its function. This problem may occur in many different

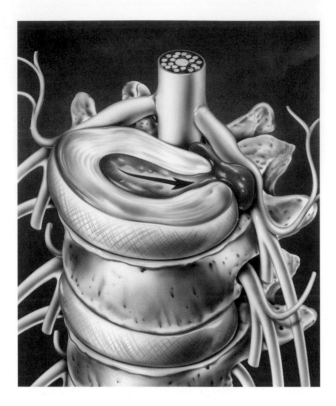

Illustration of an intervertebral disc that has ruptured, leading to the internal jelly-like material putting pressure on a nerve. *(John Bavosi / Photo Researchers, Inc.)*

areas of the body. The most common places are those in which a nerve must travel through a small space. Examples include the region where the nerve roots exit the spine called the intervertebral foramen, and the carpal tunnel at the wrist, where a nerve must travel through a tunnel created by the wrist bones and ligaments.

Description

A pinched nerve may go by several different names. It may be called nerve compression, entrapment, or impingement. Many problems involving pinched nerves will be called syndromes. Examples include **carpal tunnel syndrome**, thoracic outlet syndrome, and piriformis syndrome. If the nerve is pinched right near its root where it attaches to the spinal cord it is often called a radiculopathy.

The nerves that exit the spine and go down the upper limb and lower limb are gathered together in groups. Each group of nerves is called a plexus. In the neck region the nerves that leave the neck and go down the upper arm make up the brachial plexus. In the low back region, the nerves that go down the leg may come from the lumbar plexus or the sacral plexus. If a nerve is pinched where it is part of a plexus, it may be called a

plexopathy. If the nerve is pinched farther along its length after it has left the plexus it is called a neuropathy.

A nerve is responsible for carrying two different types of signals. It carries sensory information, such as sensations of heat, pressure, texture, **pain**, or body position back to the spinal cord where that information will eventually be transmitted directly to the brain. These sensory signals that travel through the nerves are called afferent signals. A nerve also carries motor signals from the brain and spinal cord that tell the muscles when and how much to contract in order to create movement in the body. These motor signals that go from the brain and spinal cord out to the muscles are called efferent signals. When a nerve is pinched it may cause dysfunction with either the sensory (afferent) or motor (efferent) signals.

Causes and symptoms

A pinched nerve may occur from a direct blow. Most people are familiar with this sensation when they bang their elbow on a hard surface and get a sharp pain or prickling sensation down the arm. The symptoms of this kind of pinched nerve are usually very short-lived and are not a significant problem unless the force of the impact was severe.

What is much more common is the sensation of small amounts of pressure on the nerve from such adjacent structures as bones, muscles, tendons, and ligaments. This pressure most often occurs when the nerve has to travel through a small space between these structures. The nerve may get compressed with a small amount of pressure for a long period of time. It is the long time period of pressure on the nerve that causes the most damage. In many cases these long periods of pressure are related to the person's job. Occupations in which a person must hold the wrist, forearm or shoulder in one position for long periods of time and/or perform repetitive movements have a high rate of workers with pinched nerve syndromes. Dental hygienists, keyboard instrumentalists, violinists, data entry workers, assembly line and construction workers, and professional athletes are examples of workers at risk for pinched nerve syndromes.

When pressure is placed on the nerve a person may feel a variety of different symptoms. Paresthesia (the sensation of pins and needles) is often felt first. The sensations of paresthesia are usually felt anywhere along the nerve from the site of compression toward the far end of the extremity. Symptoms may also go from the site of compression toward the spinal cord, but it is not as common. In addition to paresthesia sensations, a person with a pinched nerve may also feel sharp, shooting pain, or pain that feels like an

KEY TERMS

Afferent—Sensory signals that go from the sensory cells at the periphery of the body back to the brain and spinal cord.

Chiropractic—A method of treatment based on adjustment or manipulation of the segments of the spinal column.

Cupping—A procedure in traditional Chinese medicine in which heated air is trapped underneath a specially shaped glass cup that is placed over the skin and then rubbed along the skin. The heated air trapped in the cup creates a suction effect on the skin. Sometimes cups are used with a vacuum pump instead of heating.

Efferent—Motor signals that go from brain and spinal cord out to the muscles of the body.

Neuropathy—Compression of a peripheral nerve somewhere along its length.

Paresthesia—The sensation of pins and needles or tingling that is often the result of nerve compression.

Plexopathy—Compression of a nerve where it is part of a bundle of nerves called a plexus.

Radiculopathy—Compression of a nerve root at the point where it exits the spinal cord.

Transcutaneous electrical nerve stimulation (TENS)—A form of treatment for chronic pain in which a self-operated portable device is used to send electrical impulses through electrodes placed on the skin over the affected area. The pain is relieved because the electrical impulses interrupt the transmission of pain signals traveling along the nerve.

electrical shock going down the extremity. All of these symptoms are from impairment of the afferent (sensory) nerve signal transmission. The sensation is not necessarily near the area where the pressure is occurring.

Motor (efferent) signals can also be impaired from nerve compression. This will most likely show up as muscle weakness or problems with coordination. For example, people with carpal tunnel syndrome will frequently report losing grip strength. This is because the nerve has been compressed and signals are not getting through to the muscles of the hand that produce the grip.

Diagnosis

Most pinched nerve conditions can be diagnosed with physical examination. The practitioner will take a thorough history, including an occupational history, and investigate the nature of the signs and symptoms to see if they indicate the likelihood of nerve compression. A number of physical examination tests may also be performed to see if nerve compression is aggravated with specific movements or pressure in certain areas. In addition to physical examination and information from the patient's history, nerve conduction tests may be run to see if the nerves are transmitting signals at the proper rate. If a nerve compression problem exists, there will be a slowing in the velocity of signal transmission in that nerve and it will likely be detected by the nerve conduction velocity test.

As of 2003, diagnostic imaging is being increasingly used to aid in the diagnosis of nerve entrapment and compression syndromes. Recent refinements in ultrasound and magnetic resonance imaging (MRI) provide doctors with detailed pictures of the anatomy of peripheral nerves and the changes that take place in them with compression syndromes.

Treatment

Alternative therapy practitioners who specialize in such manual therapy methods as **chiropractic**, **osteopathy**, or **massage therapy** will look closely at the mechanical factors in the region of pain to identify what is pinching the nerve. If it is determined that the nerve is being compressed by some structure like a muscle that is pressing on the nerve, then therapy will be aimed at reducing tightness in that muscle so that it no longer presses on the nerve. This will generally be done through a variety of soft tissue therapy methods. In some instances there are other postural or mechanical distortions that may lead to nerve compression, and those will be addressed through manual therapy or various movement retraining methods.

Treatment will also focus on changing mechanical factors that may have led to nerve compression. For example, in carpal tunnel syndrome it is often some repetitive use activity that has led to the problem. If that activity can be altered so there is not an accumulation of **stress** on the soft tissues, it is likely that the symptoms of the nerve compression will be resolved. However, nerve compression symptoms may be slow to fully resolve even after the primary cause of the compression has been addressed.

Acupuncture can be quite helpful in treating pinched nerves since it has been shown to be a very effective method for producing pain relief. The primary goals of an acupuncture treatment will be both to reduce pain sensations and to get proper energy moving along the pathways that have been impaired.

Needles will be inserted in areas that will help encourage proper neurological flow through the involved area. Acupuncture with electrical stimulation of the needles may also be used for treating pinched nerves.

In addition to acupuncture, other approaches from **traditional Chinese medicine** may be used. Both topical and oral herbal preparations may be used to help restore proper function and address any underlying causes of the pinched nerve symptoms. **Cupping** may be used to help free soft tissue restrictions that may be compressing the nerve structures in the area.

Allopathic treatment

Traditional allopathic treatment for pinched nerves will also focus on the site of nerve compression and try to manage the symptoms first through conservative therapy. Oral medications may be given to relieve pain or reduce any inflammation that may be contributing to the nerve compression. Physical therapy may be used to help address any mechanical factors that may be contributing to the nerve compression. Physical therapy approaches are likely to include stretching, joint mobilization, soft tissue treatments, or such other modalities as ultrasound to address the causative factors of the nerve compression. Splinting is an additional conservative approach to nerve compression syndromes.

Depending on where the nerve compression is located, surgical treatment may sometimes be necessary. Surgery is often performed for such common nerve compression problems as carpal tunnel syndrome and thoracic outlet syndrome. Most of these surgical procedures will be aimed at relieving pressure on the affected nerve.

Some newer allopathic treatments that are used to relieve the pain of pinched nerve syndromes include low-level laser therapy (LLLT) and transcutaneous electrical nerve stimulation (TENS). In LLLT, a continuous-wave red-beam laser is aimed at acupuncture points on the affected area. In TENS, the affected nerve is stimulated with high-frequency electrical signals, which disrupt the transmission of pain impulses along the nerve so that the pain is no longer felt. Both these approaches give good results in treating pinched nerve syndromes, as they are non-invasive and painless.

In some cases in which the pinched nerve is related to the patient's job, a change of occupation may be necessary.

Expected results

Most problems with pinched nerves will be resolved as soon the pressure on them is released. If the symptoms have been present for a long time, the relief of the condition may not be immediate. The longer the pressure has been applied, the longer it is likely to take for the symptoms to be resolved.

Prevention

Most pinched nerve conditions can be avoided with proper body mechanics. Repetitive motions of the upper extremity are notorious for causing pinched nerves in several places, and it is wise to make sure a person is conditioned for the level of activity he or she is engaging in so as to prevent this from occurring. The individual should also be careful of activities that might put pressure on nerves for long periods. For example, nerves can be compressed in the shoulder region from the wearing of heavy backpacks or handbags for long periods.

Resources

BOOKS

Beinfield, H. *Between Heaven & Earth: A guide to Chinese Medicine* New York: Ballantine, 1991.

Butler, D. *Mobilisation of the Nervous System.* London: Churchill Livingstone, 1999.

Dawson, D., M. Hallet, and A. Wilbourn. *Entrapment Neuropathies.* Philadelphia: Lippincott-Raven, 1999.

Hammer, W. *Functional Soft Tissue Examination and Treatment by Manual Methods, Second Ed.* Gaithersburg, MD: Aspen, 1999.

Maciocia, G. *Foundations of Chinese Medicine.* London: Churchill Livingstone, 1989.

Stux, G. *Basics of Acupuncture.* New York: Springer-Verlag, 1991.

PERIODICALS

Anton, D., J. Rosecrance, L. Merlino, and T. Cook. "Prevalence of Musculoskeletal Symptoms and Carpal Tunnel Syndrome Among Dental Hygienists." *American Journal of Industrial Medicine* 42 (September 2002): 248-257.

Becker, J., D. B. Nora, I. Gomes, et al. "An Evaluation of Gender, Obesity, Age and Diabetes Mellitus as Risk Factors for Carpal Tunnel Syndrome." *Clinical Neurophysiology* 113 (September 2002): 1429-1434.

Gerritsen, A. A., H. C. de Vet, R. J. Scholten, et al. "Splinting vs Surgery in the Treatment of Carpal Tunnel Syndrome: A Randomized Controlled Trial." *Journal of the American Medical Association* 288 (September 11, 2002): 1245-1251.

Naeser, M. A., K. A. Hahn, B. E. Lieberman, and K. F. Branco. "Carpal Tunnel Syndrome Pain Treated with Low-Level Laser and Microamperes Transcutaneous Electric Nerve Stimulation: A Controlled Study."

Archives of Physical Medicine and Rehabilitation 83 (July 2002): 978-988.

Nathan, P. A., K. D. Meadows, and J. A. Istvan. "Predictors of Carpal Tunnel Syndrome: An 11-Year Study of Industrial Workers." *Journal of Hand Surgery* 27 (July 2002): 644-651.

Roquelaure, Y., J. Mariel, S. Fanello, et al. "Active Epidemiological Surveillance of Musculoskeletal Disorders in a Shoe Factory." *Occupational and Environmental Medicine* 59 (July 2002): 452-458.

Spratt, J. D., A. J. Stanley, A. J. Grainger, et al. "The Role of Diagnostic Radiology in Compressive and Entrapment Neuropathies." *European Radiology* 12 (September 2002): 2352-2364.

Werner, R. A., and M. Andary. "Carpal Tunnel Syndrome: Pathophysiology and Clinical Neurophysiology." *Clinical Neurophysiology* 113 (September 2002): 1373-1381.

ORGANIZATIONS

American Academy of Medical Acupuncture (AAMA). 4929 Wilshire Blvd., Suite 428, Los Angeles, CA 90010. (323) 937-5514. www.medicalacupuncture.org.

American College of Occupational and Environmental Medicine (ACOEM). 1114 North Arlington Heights Road, Arlington Heights, IL 60004. (847) 818-1800. www.acoem.org.

American Physical Therapy Association (APTA). 1111 North Fairfax Street, Alexandria, VA 22314. (703)684-APTA or (800) 999-2782. www.apta.org.

Centers for Disease Control and Prevention, National Institute for Occupational Safety and Health (NIOSH). (800) 35-NIOSH. Fax: (513) 533-8573. www.cdc.gov/niosh.

Whitney Lowe
Rebecca J. Frey, PhD

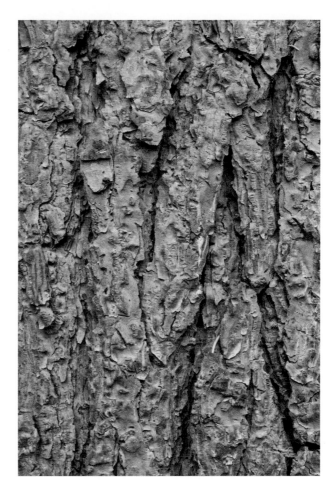

Pine bark extract is a new nutritional supplement used for its antioxidant properties, which are believed to be effective for a wide range of healing and preventative purposes. (© *Andrew Darrington / Alamy*)

Pine bark extract

Description

Pine bark extract is made from the bark of a European coastal pine tree called the Landes or maritime pine, whose scientific name is *Pinus maritima*. The maritime pine is a member of the Pineaceae family. Pine bark extract is a new nutritional supplement used for its antioxidant properties, which are believed to be effective for a wide range of healing and preventative purposes. Pine bark extract has been patented by a French researcher under the name Pycnogenol (pronounced pick-nah-jen-all).

Pine bark extract has a 450-year-old legend surrounding it. There is a written account of an event that happened in 1534, when a French ship led by explorer Jacques Cartier became stranded in ice near Quebec, Canada. Cartier's crew became severely sick from scurvy, which used to be a fatal disease caused by a lack of **vitamin C** in the diet. Cartier's crew was saved when a Quebec Indian instructed them to drink a brew made from pine bark and needles. Four centuries later, a French researcher named Jacques Masquelier discovered the reason for the effectiveness of this remedy. A substance found in pine bark acts as an antioxidant in the body, and greatly increases the effectiveness of the vitamin C found in the pine needles.

During the 1950s, Masquelier had heard the story of Cartier when he was in Canada performing research. He was investigating a group of substances called flavonols, which he originally found in peanut skins. Flavonols and **bioflavonoids** are substances in fruits and vegetables that give them their color. Masquelier found that these substances have beneficial effects in the body, particularly in improving circulation and repairing tissue. He later found that an abundant source of these substances was the bark of pine trees that grew on the coasts of southern France. Pine bark was also the most efficient source of the substance, because it took only warm water and pressure to extract the substance from trees that were considered a waste product. Masquelier called his pine bark extract Pycnogenol, and continued his research on pine bark extract and bioflavonoids for decades. In 1987, the United States awarded him a patent. Only Masquelier's pine bark extract can legally claim to have antioxidant properties.

Antioxidants play a key role of repairing and protecting cells in the body. They help protect against free radicals, which are damaging byproducts of metabolism and exposure to environmental pollutants. Free radical damage is believed to contribute to **aging**, as well as too severe conditions including **heart disease** and **cancer**. Common antioxidants are vitamins A, C, E, and the mineral **selenium**. Researchers have termed the group of antioxidants found in pine bark extract oligomeric proanthocyanidins, or OPCs for short. OPCs (also referred to as PCOs) are some of the most powerful antioxidants available.

OPCs are found in many common foods. In fact, OPCs are at the center of what has been called the French paradox. The French paradox has to do with the fact that the French eat as much **cholesterol** as Americans, yet have a significantly reduced incidence of heart disease. Researchers have theorized that one reason for this paradox is the French consumption of red wine with meals. Red wine is rich in bioflavonoids, including OPCs, which have been shown to protect blood vessels from cholesterol. Another OPC supplement on the market besides pine bark extract is **grape seed extract**, which is the cheapest and most widely used source of OPCs.

Much research has been conducted on OPCs and on pine bark extract. In France, pine bark extract and OPCs have been rigorously tested for safety and effectiveness, and pine bark extract is a registered drug. Pine bark extract has been shown to contain a powerful antioxidant that helps protect cells from free radical damage and increases the effectiveness of vitamin C. Pine bark extract has been shown to help lower cholesterol, and to decrease the risk and severity of **atherosclerosis**, or damage to the arteries. It has been demonstrated to help strengthen and repair tissues made of collagen, a protein that builds blood vessels, skin, and connective tissue. The OPCs in pine bark extract have also been shown to help reduce swelling and inflammation in the body.

General use

Pine bark extract is used to reduce the risk and severity of heart disease, strokes, high cholesterol, and circulation problems. It is used in the nutritional treatment of **varicose veins** and **edema**, which is swelling in the body due to fluid retention and leakage of blood vessels. Arthritis and inflammation have also been improved in studies using pine bark extract, as well as the uncomfortable symptoms of PMS and **menopause**. The OPCs in pine bark extract are recommended for various eye conditions that are caused by blood vessel damage, such as diabetic **retinopathy** and **macular degeneration**. Pine bark extract is recommended to improve the health and smoothness of the skin, including damage caused by overexposure to sunlight. Pine bark extract is a supplement used for anti-aging and preventive care as well.

Preparations

Pine bark extract is available in health food stores as powder and capsules. For prevention and general health, a daily dosage of 50 mg (1–2 capsules) is recommended. For treatment of health conditions, the dosage may be increased to 300 mg or more, depending on the advice of a physician and the specific condition. Pine bark extract can be taken either with or between meals.

Precautions

While pine bark extract is used in the nutritional treatment of many conditions, it is not meant to replace proper medical supervision.

Side effects

Pine bark extract has been extensively tested for safety, and no dangerous side effects have been observed with its use.

Interactions

The effectiveness of pine bark extract may be increased with the use of other antioxidants, including vitamins A, C, E, and the mineral selenium. **Diets** rich in foods that contain antioxidants and bioflavonoids, such as fresh fruits and vegetables, may also contribute to its effectiveness.

Resources

BOOKS

Kilham, Chris. *OPC: The Miracle Antioxidant*. New Canaan, CT: Keats, 1997.

Passwater, Richard, PhD. *The New Superantioxidant Plus*. New Canaan, CT: Keats, 1992.

Douglas Dupler

KEY TERMS

Adjuvant—A substance or medication used together with a vaccine or other drug to assist the effect of the main ingredient.

Antiemetic—A medication or preparation given to stop vomiting.

Chi—The Chinese name for "life force."

Decoction—An extract of a herb obtained by boiling the herb in water or alcohol.

Expectorant—A drug given to help bring up mucus or phlegm from the respiratory tract.

Goiter—Swelling of the thyroid gland caused by under or over production of thyroxine.

Materia medica—The branch of medical science concerned with the study of drugs or herbs.

Rhizome—A horizontal underground stem that sends up shoots from its upper surface.

Scrofula—Tuberculosis of the lymphatic glands.

Pinellia

Description

Pinellia (*Araceae pinellia ternatae*) is a member of the Aroid family. Originating from China and Japan, it is a small plant that is popular for ornamental use and known in Asia as "green dragon." Pinellia is a small plant, growing only to a height of 6–12 in (15–30 cm) high. It has black shiny stems, and glossy arrowhead-shaped leaves that are highlighted by a silver stripe along the veins. It produces purple tongue-like flowers in late summer.

General use

Athough not widely used in Western herbal medicine, pinellia is particularly useful for chest complaints. It relieves coughs and **cuts** through mucus, being especially good for sinus congestion and nasal discharge. It is also recommended for **asthma**, emphysema, and any form of **wheezing**, which makes it valuable as not many herbs are suited to the treatment of these particular ailments. It is more widely used in Oriental medicine than in Western natural therapies, however, and it is often an ingredient of herbal mixtures in both Western and Chinese herbal medicine.

Pinellia in Chinese herbalism

Known as "ban xia" or "wu bing shao" to the Chinese, Pinellia is widely used in a variety of combinations in Chinese herbal medicine. They consider that its properties are "pungent, warm, and toxic," and it is considered a treatment for the areas of the Chinese concepts of Spleen, Stomach, and Lung. Remedies are generally prepared from the roots and stems of the plant and are used to treat digestive and respiratory problems.

Pinellia is most useful for chest complaints, in which it is used in conjunction with **magnolia** bark or perilla leaf—both common ingredients of Chinese remedies. It is especially useful when dealing with phlegm and congestion, which are both cold in nature. Pinellia is also used in combination with other herbal ingredients for the treatment of **nausea** and **vomiting**. It is considered an antiemetic (nausea suppressant). Depending on the patient's body type, it may be used with fresh **ginger**, bamboo shavings, loquat leaf, perilla stem, or amomum fruit. It may also be used with ginseng or jujube.

Chinese herbalists also recommend pinellia for the treatment of swollen glands, and certain cases of goiter, for which it is used in conjunction with seaweed and fritillary bulb. It is recommended for sinus problems in which there is **pain** and a feeling of fullness across the sinus area.

Pinellia is also used for coughing and asthma. In addition, the Chinese use it for the treatment of scrofula and subcutaneous cysts.

Pinellia also appears to have antidepressant effects. It is the primary ingredient in Banxia Houpu decoction, a traditional Chinese formula that has been used for centuries to treat **depression**. A recent chemical analysis of this decoction showed that its antidepressant activity is close to that of fluoxetine (Prozac).

A new use for pinellia is its role as an adjuvant (substance given to assist the effectiveness of a vaccine or medication) to a nasal vaccine for **influenza**. Researchers isolated a compound called pinellic acid from pinellia, and found that an oral preparation of it measurably increased the effectiveness of a nasal vaccine against influenza without any harmful side effects.

Preparations

The parts of the plant used, particularly in Chinese herbalism, are generally the rhizomes, or tubers. These should be dug during late summer, early autumn. The bark and fibrous roots are then removed and the rhizomes should be dried in sunlight. The raw herbs are toxic and must be prepared bydrying them and then frying them in ginger and vinegar to make them usable. The preparation is called *fa ba xia* and is available in health food stores.

Dosage may be in the form of readily prepared pills, again especially in the case of Chinese herbalism, or in the form of a syrup, in which case the recommended dosage should be followed. The dried rhizome may be taken in doses of 5–10 grams.

Precautions

Pinellia is best used as an expectorant for congestive chest conditions. Another remedy should be used for dry coughs accompanied by chills, due to its drying and warming properties. Pinellia should not be used by pregnant women, those suffering from blood disorders, particularly if there is bleeding, **fever** or conditions which cause heat in the body. Pinellia is used to treat **morning sickness**, but only under the strict supervision of an experienced herbalist.

A general precaution to observe when using any Chinese patent medicine is to purchase only well-known brands recommended by a practitioner of **traditional Chinese medicine**. Cases have been reported of incorrect labeling, contamination with heavy metals, and substitution of Western pharmaceuticals for the Chinese ingredients. Any of these occurrences can present a serious health hazard.

Side effects

Pinellia is registered as a toxic herb in the United States and should be used with caution. The Chinese Materia Medica also acknowledges that it has toxic potential. Never use the herb in its raw form or exceed the recommended doses of herbal mixtures containing pinellia.

Pinellia has been reported to trigger asthmatic attacks in people who have been sensitized to it.

Interactions

Pinellia should not be taken in conjunction with aconite, as it may increase the toxic properties of this substance.

Resources

BOOKS

Reid, Daniel. *Chinese Herbal Medicine*. Boston, MA: Shambhala, 1996.

PERIODICALS

Lee, S. K., H. K. Cho, S. H. Cho, et al. "Occupational Asthma and Rhinitis Caused by Multiple Herbal Agents in a Pharmacist." *Annals of Allergy, Asthma and Immunology* 86 (April 2001): 469-474.

Luo, L., J. Nong Wang, L. D. Kong, et al. "Antidepressant Effects of Banxia Houpu Decoction, a Traditional Chinese Medicinal Empirical Formula." *Journal of Ethnopharmacology* 73 (November 2000): 277-281.

Nagai, T., H. Kiyohara, K. Munakata, et al. "Pinellic Acid from the Tuber of *Pinellia ternata Breitenbach* as an Effective Oral Adjuvant for Nasal Influenza Vaccine." *International Immunopharmacology* 2 (July 2002): 1183-193.

ORGANIZATIONS

American Association of Oriental Medicine. 5530 Wisconsin Avenue, Suite 1210, Chevy Chase, MD 20815. (301) 941-1064. www.aaom.org.

Institute of Traditional Medicine. 2017 SE Hawthorne Blvd., Portland, OR 97214. (503) 233-4907. www.itmonline.org.

OTHER

"A Healing Place." www.healingplace.com/formulas/pinellia.html.

"Herbal Medicine" In: Holistic-Online.com. www.holisticonline.com/w_herbal_medicine.html.

Patricia Skinner
Rebecca J. Frey, PhD

Pink eye *see* **Conjunctivitis**

Piper methysticum see **Kava kava**

Pityriasis rosea

Definition

Pityriasis rosea is a skin disease of uncertain origin characterized by lesions bordered by collar-like areas that tend to peel off in tiny scales. Pityriasis comes from the Greek word for bran, *pityron*, because the flakes of skin shed from the lesions resemble small pieces of wheat bran. Rosea comes from a Latin word that means "rose-colored" or "pink."

Description

Pityriasis rosea is a common benign skin disease, or exanthem, that was first described by a French physician named Camille Gibert in 1860. It is classified as a papulosquamous disorder, which means that its lesions are marked by small raised areas (papules) as well as scaly areas. Pityriasis rosea begins in 60%–90% of patients with a pinkish-brown or salmon-colored herald patch—sometimes called a mother patch—on the chest, back, or neck. The herald patch is a small spot when it first appears, but enlarges over a period of several days to form a circular or oval-shaped area between 3/4-in and 2-1/2 in in diameter. The herald patch develops a scaly border known as a collarette, and is often misdiagnosed in its early stages as **eczema** or ringworm.

The herald patch is followed within 5–10 days by a series of similar but smaller oval-shaped patches that appear on the patient's chest, back, and legs, although the general eruption may appear as rapidly as a few hours after the herald patch or as long as three months later. The general rash lasts for about six weeks. The smaller patches range between 1/8 in and 1/2 in in diameter, and are sometimes described as resembling cigarette paper. Lesions on the trunk and abdomen are commonly distributed along the midline of the body in a pattern resembling the outline of a Christmas tree. The lesions of the general eruption are found most commonly on the chest, back, and upper arms, but are sometimes limited to such smaller areas of the body as the armpits, groin, palms of the hands, or feet. Between 9% and 16% of patients develop ulcers or plaques inside the mouth. It is relatively unusual, however, for patches to appear on the face. A small minority of patients may have the herald patch as the only sign of pityriasis rosea.

Pityriasis rosea is a common skin disorder, accounting for 3% of visits to dermatologists in the United States and Canada. The overall prevalence of the disease in the general North American population is thought to be about 0.13% in males and 0.14% in females. It is rare in infants and the elderly; most cases are diagnosed in persons between the ages of 10 and 35. Pityriasis rosea tends to cluster in families, which is

one reason why some researchers have been investigating various viruses as possible causes; however, it is not known to spread by casual contact. The disease affects all races and ethnic groups equally.

Pityriasis rosea may occur at any time of year but is most common in temperate climates in the spring and fall.

Causes and symptoms

Causes

The cause of pityriasis rosea is debated as of early 2004. Various researchers have reported isolating a mycoplasma (a type of gram-negative bacterium), a picornavirus, and human herpesviruses 6 and 7 from skin samples of patients diagnosed with the disease, but these findings are not yet considered definitive. Certain medications, including diphtheria vaccines, barbiturates, gold, bismuth compounds, captopril (Capoten), metronidazole (Flagyl), isotretinoin (Accutane), clonidine (Catapres), omeprazole (Prilosec), penicillamine (Cuprimine or Depen), and terbinafine (Lamisil) have been reported to cause skin **rashes** that resemble the lesions of pityriasis rosea. High levels of emotional **stress** appear to increase the severity of the skin lesions in some patients.

Symptoms

The most common symptom associated with the lesions of pityriasis rosea is pruritus or **itching**, which affects about 75% of patients, with 25% reporting severe itching. Many patients find that athletic activity or hot weather makes the itching worse. In addition to pruritus, some patients have prodromal symptoms, which are warning symptoms that occur before the herald patch appears. Prodromal symptoms of pityriasis rosea may include **fever**, loss of appetite, **nausea**, **headache**, joint pains, and swelling of the lymph nodes. Lymph node swelling is more common among African Americans diagnosed with the disease than among Caucasian or Asian Americans.

Diagnosis

The diagnosis of pityriasis rosea is usually made through taking a patient history—with particular attention to prescription medications—and a skin biopsy ordered by a dermatologist. Although there is no blood test for pityriasis rosea itself, most primary care physicians will order a rapid plasma reagin (RPR) or Venereal Disease Research Laboratory (VDRL) blood test to screen for **syphilis**. The reason for this precaution is that the lesions of pityriasis rosea resemble the skin rash associated with secondary syphilis. The skin biopsy is done to distinguish between pityriasis rosea and such other skin diseases as lichen planus, **psoriasis**, ringworm, **Kaposi's sarcoma**, and seborrheic **dermatitis**.

Treatment

Pityriasis rosea is a self-limiting disease, which means that it goes away on its own even without alternative or allopathic treatment. Both mainstream physicians and naturopaths, however, recommend adding a cup of oatmeal or baking soda to a tub of warm (not hot) water to minimize itching. In addition, patients whose lesions increase in size or number due to emotional stress may be helped by **hydrotherapy**, **aromatherapy**, **meditation**, or other therapies intended to reduce stress. **Massage therapy**, however, is contraindicated because the disease usually affects large areas of skin.

Homeopathic practitioners suggest the following remedies for pityriasis rosea, to be taken in 6C potency four times daily for 7 days:

- *Arsenicum.* Recommended for patients whose rash is accompanied by anxiety, restlessness, and thirst.
- *Radium bromide.* For patients whose lesions are fiery red in color, burning, and painful.

- *Natrum muriaticum.* For patients whose lesions have a red appearance under thin white scales, or whose pruritus is made worse by warmth or exercise.

In addition, a homeopathic remedy known as *Urtica urens* is available in cream or ointment form for direct application to affected areas.

Allopathic treatment

Allopathic treatment of pityriasis rosea is directed toward symptom relief, as the cause of the disease is still uncertain. To relieve the itching, the doctor may prescribe calamine lotion, **zinc** oxide ointment, oral antihistamine medications, or topical ointments containing corticosteroids or a combination of phenol and 25% menthol. Some physicians prescribe creams containing pramoxine, a local anesthetic. Steroid medications taken by mouth are not recommended unless the pruritus is extremely severe; although these drugs relieve itching, they may also prolong the course of the disease or make the lesions worse.

Some patients are benefited by exposure to sunlight or by treatment with ultraviolet light; however, there is some risk that the skin lesions will develop hyperpigmentation (become darker than the surrounding skin) after ultraviolet treatment. Hyperpigmentation is most likely to occur in African American patients.

There is no need to keep children with pityriasis rosea from attending school, as the disease is not considered contagious.

Expected results

The prognosis for patients with pityriasis rosea is excellent. The disease does not cause long-term health problems, is not dangerous even during **pregnancy**, and usually clears completely in 6–8 weeks. A few patients have lesions that last as long as 3–4 months, but fewer than 3% of patients experience recurrences.

Prevention

As the cause of pityriasis rosea is still debated as of 2004, there are no known preventive measures.

Resources

BOOKS

"Pityriasis Rosea." Section 10, Chapter 117 in *The Merck Manual of Diagnosis and Therapy*, edited by Mark H. Beers, MD, and Robert Berkow, MD. Whitehouse Station, NJ: Merck Research Laboratories, 2002.

PERIODICALS

Allen, Robert A. MD, and Robert A. Schwartz, MD, MPH. "Pityriasis Rosea." *eMedicine*, 11 November 2002. http://www.emedicine.com/derm/topic335.htm.

Scott, L. A., and M. S. Stone. "Viral Exanthems." *Dermatology Online Journal* 9 (August 2003): 4.

Stulberg, J. L., and J. Wolfrey. "Pityriasis Rosea." *American Family Physician* 69 (January 1, 2004): 87–91.

Watanabe, T., T. Kawamura, S. E. Jacob, et al. "Pityriasis Rosea Is Associated with Systemic Active Infection with Both Human Herpesvirus-7 and Human Herpesvirus-6." *Journal of Investigative Dermatology* 119 (October 2002): 793–797.

ORGANIZATIONS

American Academy of Dermatology. P. O. Box 4014, Schaumburg, IL 60168-4014. (847) 330-0230. Fax: (847) 330-0050. http://www.aad.org.

OTHER

American Academy of Dermatology (AAD). *Pityriasis Rosea*. Schaumburg, IL: AAD, 2003.

Rebecca Frey, PhD

Placebo effect

Definition

A placebo effect occurs when a treatment or medication with no therapeutic value (a placebo) is administered to a patient and the patient's symptoms improve. The patient believes and expects that the treatment is going to work; therefore, it does. The placebo effect is also a factor to some degree in clinically effective therapies and explains why some patients respond better than do others to treatment despite similar symptoms and illnesses.

Origins

The word placebo is from the Latin "I shall please." Throughout most of medical history, the placebo effect was the principal treatment physicians offered their patients; for example, reassurance, attention, and belief in treatment would mobilize patients' internal powers to fight their illnesses. This effect is apparent in indigenous cultures using shamanistic healing, which places healing power in objects and rituals. In fact, placebos are sometimes called sham treatments.

Placebos were used throughout the nineteenth century in blind assessments of medical treatments. These blind assessments were created to test controversial medical treatments of the time (e.g., mesmerism and **homeopathy**) and involved using a blindfold on or withholding information from patients so they were unaware of the exact nature of the treatment being studied. For example, in blind assessments of homeopathy conducted in 1834 in France, homeopathic remedies were replaced with an inert placebo substance without the patient's knowledge. These blind assessments were the forerunners to modern double-blind randomized controlled trials used in drug development and in the study of other therapeutic techniques.

According to some medical historians, from the early 1800s through as late as World War II, placebos (usually in the form of sugar pills or saline injections) were regularly prescribed for up to 80% of patients. Doctors used placebos to appease patients when no effective treatment for their symptoms was available or prescribed placebos to patients they perceived as difficult.

The first documented American clinical study using placebos was conducted in the late 1920s. In 1937 scientists at Cornell University Medical School published a study on an **angina** drug that used placebo and blind assessment techniques. They found that the patients who were given a placebo instead of the angina drug experienced an improvement of symptoms. This was the first published account in the United States that discussed the possible therapeutic value of the placebo effect.

Benefits

The placebo effect is usually positive by its nature because it indicates that a patient believes in the therapy and that the therapy has some sort of a beneficial effect. The placebo effect has been documented in a wide variety of diseases and disorders. Certain conditions such as headaches, arthritis, and **hot flashes** are especially responsive to placebos, as are some individuals.

Description

Every available medical treatment is subject to the placebo effect. If patients believe the therapy will benefit them, it usually will to some degree. Even if the placebo does not improve the symptoms directly, the peace of mind patients may feel after taking a treatment they believe will help them is often enough to encourage a sense of improved well-being. For this reason, controlled, scientific studies are so crucial to determining the actual clinical efficacy of medications and therapies.

The person prescribing the placebo treatment may also have an impact on the effect it has on the patient. For example, the doctor's enthusiasm about a new treatment may heighten its placebo effect for the patient. In addition, if a healthcare provider is perceived as a trusted, well-respected figure by the patient, the patient may experience benefits from any treatments the provider prescribes.

Placebos are often used in scientific trials of new medications and treatments to determine their efficacy. A randomly selected group of study subjects known as the control group is given placebo medication (usually a sugar or water-based substance) or treatment while the rest of the subjects are administered the actual therapy. The patients do not know which group they are in during the study, and the researchers and study authors do not know which subjects are in which group (hence the term double-blind). This system helps researchers to determine if new treatments work because they are clinically effective or because the subjects believe they will work.

Some authorities have estimated that the average placebo effect is 33%, though it can range lower and higher. Therefore, to demonstrate that a treatment, procedure, or medication is effective, a trial has to show that it does significantly better than the placebo given to a control group. For example, a study of single-remedy homeopathy was conducted with a group of 487 patients with an influenza-like syndrome. Patients treated with a single, non-individualized remedy were 70% more likely to have recovered within 48 hours than those receiving the placebo. Mathematical analysis allows a researcher to determine whether this effect is statistically significant or not.

Preparations

Placebos have therapeutic value only if the patient believes they will work. If the healthcare provider elicits trust and respect and engenders comfort, the patient is likely to find the prescribed treatments beneficial, whether they are clinically effective or unproven.

The use of a placebo in scientific studies requires informed consent of the entire population of subjects. The study subjects must know that they have a 50/50 chance of receiving a placebo treatment instead of the treatment under investigation.

Precautions

Using placebos with patients presents ethical issues if the healthcare provider knows there is no therapeutic value to the treatment and other available treatments could possibly benefit the patient. For patients with progressive or life-threatening illnesses, taking a medication or therapy with no clinical value other than its placebo effect can be harmful if it causes them to ignore proven treatments that could improve their condition.

Some clinical trials of surgical procedures require the placebo or control subjects to undergo what is essentially unnecessary surgery, involving incisions and other invasive procedures while the final therapeutic portion of the procedure is withheld (the placebo). Although as of 2008 this is standard scientific procedure recommended by the U.S. Food and Drug Administration (FDA) for the approval of new medical procedures and devices, it is also commonly accepted knowledge that unnecessary surgery is never beneficial to a patient and can result in serious complications such as infection, hemorrhaging, and possible death.

Side effects

The placebo effect can have a negative influence also, a nocebo. If a placebo is given that patients believe to be harmful to their health in some way, the patients may develop symptoms appropriate to this belief. A toxic or negative placebo suggests the great degree to which attitudes and expectations can affect one's state of health or course of an illness. People who believe they have been cursed or are the victim of voodoo have been known to die.

Research and general acceptance

The placebo effect is a well-known phenomenon in the scientific community, and clinical trials and other scientific studies are built around it. Ethical concerns can arise when there is a risk that patients are not getting the potentially life-saving treatments they need. In some cases, the placebo effect is enough to compensate for this lack. For example, a study published in the *Archives of General Psychiatry* found that in 45 controlled trials of antidepressants, subjects in the control group experienced a significant positive therapeutic effect with the placebo only. In cases of treatments involving potentially fatal diseases such as **cancer** and **AIDS**, the ethical implications of placebo use may not be as clear-cut.

Surgical placebo procedures, which are a relatively new type of clinical study, are not as universally accepted as placebo drug trials. A heated debate in the medical community concerns the value of such studies. However, the use of placebo surgery for controlled clinical trials is endorsed by the National Institutes of Health, the medical research arm of the U.S. Department of Health and Human Services.

KEY TERMS

Double-blind randomized controlled trial—A study that uses two groups of subjects. One group (the experimental group) receives the treatment being tested, while the other group (the control group) receives a placebo. Double-blind means that neither the subjects nor the researchers know which subjects are in which group.

Homeopathy—A practice of medicine based on the theory that certain substances that produce a specific symptom will cure those same symptoms if administered in small, extremely diluted doses.

Resources

BOOKS

Jopling, David. *Talking Cures and Placebo Effects.* New York: Oxford University Press, 2008.

Kradin, Richard. *The Placebo Response and the Power of Unconscious Healing.* New York: Routledge Press, 2008.

Thompson, W. Grant. *The Placebo Effect and Health: Combining Science and Compassionate Care.* Amherst, NY: Prometheus Books, 2005.

PERIODICALS

Hrobjartsson, Asbjorn, and Peter C. Gotzsche. "Is the Placebo Powerless? Update of a Systematic Review with 52 New Randomized Trials Comparing Placebo with No Treatment." *Journal of Internal Medicine* (April 2005): 91–100.

Hunter, Philip. "A Question of Faith. Exploiting the Placebo Effect Depends on Both the Susceptibility of the Patient to Suggestion and the Ability of the Doctor to Instill Trust." *EMBO Reports* (February 2007): 125–128.

Paterson, Charlotte, and Paul Dieppe. "Characteristic and Incidental (Placebo) Effects in Complex Interventions such as Acupuncture." *BMJ* (May 21, 2005): 1202–1205.

Sartorius, Norman. "Praised Be Placebo, May Its Glory Shine." *Croatian Medical Journal* (February 2006): 189–190.

Paula Ford-Martin
David Edward Newton, Ed.D.

Plantain

Description

Plantain, *Plantago major*, was considered to be one of the nine sacred herbs by the ancient Saxon people, and has been celebrated in Anglo-Saxon

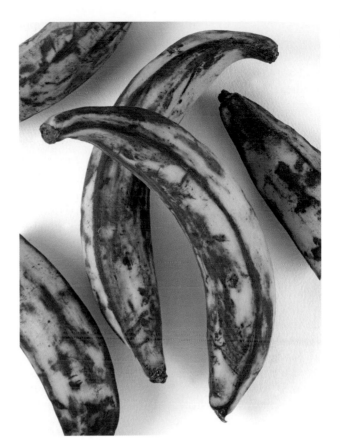

Plantains. *(© foodfolio / Alamy)*

poetry as the "mother of herbs." There are more than 200 species of plantain and nearly as many recorded uses for this humble herb. Plantain is native to northern and central Asia and Europe. Early colonists brought plantain to North America as one of their favored healing remedies. Native Americans called this persistent herb "white man's foot" as it is often found growing along well-trodden foot paths. The Latin generic name means "sole of the foot." The indigenous Americas adopted many of the traditional European uses for this beneficial herb. They also used the plant to draw out the poison of rattlesnake bite, to soothe rheumatic **pain**, as a poultice to treat battle **wounds**, and as an eyewash. They used the fresh young leaves and seeds in their diet.

Plantain is a member of the Plantaginaceae family. Some of the familiar species, naturalized throughout North America, are: *Plantago major*, commonly known as common plantain, dooryard plantain, broad-leaved plantain, greater plantain, round-leafed plantain, way bread, devil's shoestring, bird seed, snakeweed, and white man's foot; *Plantago media L.*, known as hoary plantain; and *Plantago lanceolata L.*, also known as English plantain, lance-leaf plantain, buckhorn, chimney-sweeps, headsman, ribgrass, ribwort, ripplegrass, hen plant, snake plantain, fire weed, and soldier's herb. Two species of plantain, valued medicinally primarily for the seed, are *Plantago psyllium L.* and *Plantago indica*, also known as flea seed and plantago. The dried, ripe seeds of these species, generally called **psyllium**, is high in mucilage and is widely used as a bulk-forming laxative.

Plantain is a hardy and prolific perennial found in fields, lawns, roadsides, footpaths, and marginal areas throughout the temperate regions of the world. It thrives even in poor, compacted soil. The sturdy leaves and flower stalks grow in a basal rosette directly from the mass of light-brown rootlets. Depending on the species, the leaves are broadly ovate or narrow and lance-like. The dark-green leaves have distinct, parallel ribs along their length and are slightly bitter to the taste. The yellow-green stamens and the rust-colored sepals of the tiny flowers encircle the wand-like spikes at the end of each stalk. Plantain's flower spikes resemble tiny cattail spikes. The yellow-green stamens are more prominent in *P. lanceolata L.*, encircling the flower spike like a delicate wreath. The tapered flower spikes in this species are longer than those of *P. major* stretching up well beyond the height of the basal leaves. Plantain flowers from June through September. Blossoms are followed by flea-size, light-brown seeds. The plant may reach to 2 ft (0.6 m) in height, and self-seeds freely.

General use

The leaves and seeds of plantain are most often used medicinally. The fresh leaves, crushed and applied to wounds, sores, insect **bites**, bee and wasp **stings**, **eczema**, and sunburn are healing to tissue because of the high allantoin content. Plantain is an ancient remedy used widely for relieving coughs, **bronchitis** , **tuberculosis**, **sore throat**, **laryngitis**, urinary **infections**, and digestive problems. The infusion has been used as a blood purifying tonic, a mild expectorant, and a diuretic. The juice from crushed leaves may also stem the flow of blood from **cuts**, and soothe the itch of poison ivy or the sting of **nettle** (*Urtica dioica*). The root of the herb has been used to relieve **toothache**. The juice may relieve **earache**. A decoction of plantain has been used in douche preparations to relieve leucorrhea, and the juice or infusion can ease the pain of ulcers and inflammation of the intestines. All plantains contain high amounts of mucilage and tannin, and have similar medicinal properties. Plantain is high in minerals and vitamins C and K.

Plantain is used throughout the world. It is an effective treatment for chronic **colitis**, acute **gastritis**, enteritis, and enterocolitis according to the Russian Ministry of Health. The German Commission E, an advisory panel on herbal medicines for that country, lists plantain as a safe and effective herb with demulcent, astringent and antibacterial properties. A poultice (salve prepared from the leaf) or an infusion used as a skin wash, have been shown to reduce pain, **itching**, and bleeding from **hemorrhoids**. Studies in Italy and Russia have confirmed plantain's usefulness as a weight-loss remedy. In Chinese medicine plantain is considered a remedy for male **impotence**. The species *P. major* and *P. lanceolata* contain mucilage, the iridoid glycosides cubin and catapol, flavonoids, tannins, and **silica**.

Plantain seeds, particularly those of the species *P. psyllium* and *P. ovata* soaked in water and ingested, are widely used as a gentle and safe bulk laxative and antidiarrheal. Plantago seeds from these two species are listed in *The United States Pharmacopoeia XXII* as an official laxative herb. Psyllium is found in numerous commercial laxative preparations. Psyllium seed has also been proven beneficial in reducing high levels of blood **cholesterol**. Psyllium seeds contain a high mucilage content in addition to other phytochemicals including monoterpene alkaloids, glycosides, sugars, triterpenes, fixed oil, fatty acids, and tannins. The entire plant may be used with an alum mordant to dye wool a bronze-gold color. A newer use of plantain starch is in the manufacture of pharmaceuticals; like corn starch, plantain starch can be used as an inert ingredient to mix with drugs in order to form tablets containing consistent measured doses of the drugs.

Preparations

Harvest plantain leaves throughout the spring and summer, before the herb is in full blossom. Fresh young leaves may be eaten in salads or cooked as a potherb. The juice of fresh, bruised leaves has an antibacterial effect. However this property is lost when the herb is infused with boiling water. Harvest seeds when they can be easily removed from the flower spikes. Dry the leaves quickly to avoid discoloration and store in clearly labeled, dark glass containers.

Leaf infusion: Place 2–4 tbsp of fresh plantain leaf, half if dried, in a warmed glass container. Bring 2-1/2 c of fresh, non-chlorinated water to the boiling point, add it to the herbs. Cover. Steep five to seven minutes. No need to decoct plantain leaves. Drink warm or cold throughout the day, up to three cups per day. The prepared tea will store for about two days in the refrigerator in a sealed jar.

Tincture: Combine 4 oz of finely-cut, fresh plantain leaf, or 2 oz dry, powdered herb with one pint of brandy, gin, or vodka, in a glass container. Cover and store the mixture away from light for about two weeks, shaking several times each day. Strain and store in a tightly capped, clearly labeled, dark glass bottle. A standard dose is 10–30 drops of the tincture in water, up to three times a day.

Precautions

Pregnant women should not use plantain, particularly the laxative psyllium preparations. Nursing mothers should consult a qualified herbalist before using psyllium or treating young children with the herb. Avoid inhaling psyllium seed powder as it may induce **asthma** attacks. Ingesting seeds without first soaking them in water may cause gastrointestinal problems. It is critical to drink large amounts of water when using psyllium, as the seeds absorb water in the intestine.

Persons who are interested in using herbal preparations as dietary supplements or to treat minor health conditions should note that the United States Food and Drug Administration (FDA) does not subject herbal preparations to the same set of regulations applied to prescription drugs. It is up to the manufacturer to make sure that a dietary supplement is safe before it is marketed. The FDA's role is that of post-marketing surveillance. Since the mid-1990s, there have been reports of herbal products that were mislabeled. In 1997, a young woman with a heart condition purchased a product that was labeled as "plantain" and experienced an abnormally rapid heartbeat. It turned out that the product was contaminated with **digitalis**, a powerful heart stimulant derived from **foxglove**. It is best to purchase herbs or herbal preparations only from established and reliable manufacturers. Questions about the safety of a specific product or reports of adverse reactions to a herbal product should be sent to the FDA's Center for Food Safety and Applied **Nutrition**, listed under Resources below.

Side effects

Psyllium seed and plantain may cause allergic reactions in sensitive persons.

Interactions

Plantain has been reported to decrease the absorption of digoxin (a heart medication) and lithium from the intestine. Its **Vitamin K** content may interfere with blood-thinning medications (anticoagulants). Plantain should not be taken together with prescription diuretics as it increases the risk of **potassium** loss from the bloodstream (hypokalemia). Persons taking any of these prescription medications should consult a physician before taking plantain as a dietary supplement.

Resources

BOOKS

Culpeper, Nicholas. *Culpeper's Complete Herbal & English Physician*. IL: Meyerbooks, 1990.

Duke, James A., Ph.D. *The Green Pharmacy*. PA: Rodale Press, 1997.

Elias, Jason, and Shelagh Ryan Masline. *The A to Z Guide to Healing Herbal Remedies*. Lynn Sonberg Book Associates, 1996.

PDR for Herbal Medicines. New Jersey: Medical Economics Company, 1998.

Pelletier, Kenneth R., MD. *The Best Alternative Medicine, Part I: Western Herbal Medicine*. New York: Simon & Schuster, 2002.

Tyler, Varro E., Ph.D. *Herbs of Choice, The Therapeutic Use of Phytomedicinals*. New York: Pharmaceutical Products Press, 1994.

PERIODICALS

Alebiowu, G., and O. A. Itiola. "Compressional Characteristics of Native and Pregelatinized Forms of Sorghum, Plantain, and Corn Starches and the Mechanical Properties of Their Tablets." *Drug Development and Industrial Pharmacy* 28 (July 2002): 663-672.

ORGANIZATIONS

American Botanical Council. 6200 Manor Road, Austin, TX 78714-4345. (512) 926-4900. www.herbal gram.org.

Herb Research Foundation. 1007 Pearl St., Suite 200, Boulder, CO 80302. (303) 449-2265. www.herbs.org.

United States Food and Drug Administration (FDA), Center for Food Safety and Applied Nutrition. 5100 Paint Branch Parkway, College Park, MD 20740. (888) SAFEFOOD. www.cfsan.fda.gov.

Clare Hanrahan
Rebecca J. Frey, PhD

Pleurisy

Definition

Pleurisy is an inflammation of the membrane that surrounds and protects the lungs (the pleura). Inflammation occurs when an infection or damaging agent irritates the pleural surface. Sharp chest pains are the primary symptom of pleurisy.

Description

Pleurisy, also called pleuritis, is a condition that generally stems from an existing respiratory infection, disease, or injury. In people who have otherwise good health, respiratory **infections** or **pneumonia** are the main causes of pleurisy. This condition used to be more common, but with the advent of antibiotics and modern disease therapies, pleurisy has become less prevalent.

The pleura is a double-layered structure made up of an inner membrane, which surrounds the lungs, and an outer membrane, which lines the chest cavity. The pleural membranes are very thin, close together, and have a fluid coating in the narrow space between them. This liquid acts as a lubricant, so that when the lungs inflate and deflate during breathing, the pleural surfaces can easily glide over one another.

Pleurisy occurs when the pleural surfaces rub against one another, due to irritation and inflammation. Infection within the pleural space is the most common irritant, although the abnormal presence of air, blood, or cells can also initiate pleurisy. These disturbances all act to displace the normal pleural fluid, which forces the membranes to rub, rather than glide, against one another. This rubbing irritates nerve endings in the outer membrane and causes **pain**.

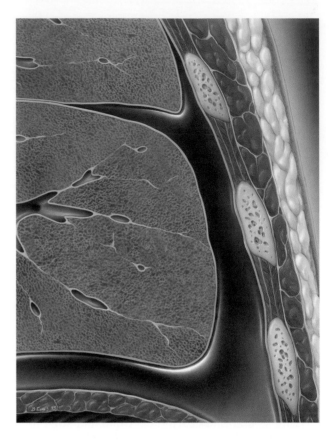

Pleural effusion, the oozing of fluid from the blood or lymph into a pleural cavity, the space between the two layers of the pleura. *(Brian Evans / Photo Researchers, Inc.)*

Pleurisy also causes a chest noise that ranges from a faint squeak to a loud creak. This characteristic sound is called a "friction rub."

Pleurisy cases are classified either as having pleural effusion or as being "dry." Pleural effusion is more common and refers to an accumulation of fluid within the pleural space; dry pleurisy is inflammation without fluid build-up. Less pain occurs with pleural effusion because the fluid forces the membrane surfaces apart. However, pleural effusion causes additional complications because it places pressure on the lungs. This leads to respiratory distress and possible lung collapse.

Causes and symptoms

A variety of conditions can give rise to pleurisy. The following represent the most common sources of pleural inflammation:

- infections, including pneumonia, tuberculosis, and other bacterial or viral respiratory infections
- immune disorders, including systemic lupus erythematosus, rheumatoid arthritis, and sarcoidosis

KEY TERMS

Effusion—The accumulation of fluid within a cavity, such as the pleural space.

Empyema—An infection that causes pus to accumulate in the pleural space which may cause a tear in the pleural membrane and allow the infection to spread to other areas in the body.

Inflammation—An accumulation of fluid and cells within tissue that is often caused by infection and the resultant immune response.

Pneumonia—A condition caused by bacterial or viral infection that is characterized by inflammation of the lungs and fluid within the air passages.

Referred pain—The presence of pain in an area other than where it originates. In some pleurisy cases, referred pain occurs in the neck, shoulder, or abdomen.

- diseases, including cancer, pancreatitis, liver cirrhosis, and heart or kidney failure

- injury, from a rib fracture, collapsed lung, esophagus rupture, blood clot, or material such as asbestos

- drug reactions, from certain drugs used to treat tuberculosis (isoniazid), cancer (methotrexate, procarbazine), or the immune disorders mentioned above (hydralazine, procainamide, phenytoin, quinidine).

The hallmark symptom of pleurisy is sudden, intense chest pain that is usually located over the area of inflammation. Although the pain can be constant, it is usually most severe when the lungs move during breathing, coughing, **sneezing**, or even talking. The pain is usually described as shooting or stabbing, but in minor cases it resembles a mild cramp. When pleurisy occurs in certain locations, such as near the diaphragm, the pain may be felt in other areas such as the neck, shoulder, or abdomen (referred pain). Another indication of pleurisy is that holding one's breath or exerting pressure against the chest causes pain relief.

Pleurisy is also characterized by certain respiratory symptoms. In response to the pain, pleurisy patients commonly have a rapid, shallow breathing pattern. Pleural effusion can also cause shortness of breath, as excess fluid makes expanding the lungs difficult. If severe breathing difficulties persist, patients may experience a blue-colored complexion (cyanosis).

Diagnosis

The distinctive pain of pleurisy is normally the first clue physicians use for diagnosis. Doctors usually feel the chest to find the site of inflammation. A stethoscope is used to listen for abnormal chest sounds (such as the friction rub) as the patient breathes. Sometimes, a friction rub is masked by the presence of pleural effusion and further examination is needed for an accurate diagnosis.

To diagnose the illness that is causing pleurisy, doctors must evaluate the patient's history, additional symptoms, and laboratory test results. A chest x ray may also be taken to look for signs of accumulated fluid and other abnormalities. Computed tomography (CT) scan and ultrasound scans are more powerful diagnostic tools used to visualize the chest cavity.

The most helpful information in diagnosing the cause of pleurisy is a fluid analysis. Once the doctor knows the precise location of fluid accumulation, a sample is removed using a procedure called thoracentesis. In this technique, a fine needle is inserted into the chest to reach the pleural space and extract fluid. Several laboratory tests are performed to analyze the chemical components of the fluid and determine whether bacteria or viruses are present. Pleurisy associated with **rheumatoid arthritis** produces a distinctive pattern of tissue cells in the pleural fluid. Cancerous growths also shed cells into the tissue fluid. While most cases of pleurisy associated with **cancer** are secondary developments from a primary tumor, in some instances the pleurisy is the first indication of a malignancy.

In certain instances a biopsy of the pleura may be needed for microscopic analysis. A sample of pleural tissue can be obtained several ways: with a biopsy needle, by making a small incision in the chest wall, or by using a thoracoscope (a video-assisted instrument for viewing the pleural space and collecting samples).

Treatment

Alternative treatments can be used in conjunction with conventional treatment to help heal pleurisy. **Acupuncture** and botanical medicines are alternative approaches for alleviating pleural pain and breathing problems.

Herbal remedies

Poultices (crushed herbs applied directly to the skin) of respiratory herbs can assist in the healing process. An herbal remedy commonly recommended is pleurisy root (*Asclepias tuberosa*), so named because of its use by early American settlers who learned of this medicinal plant from Native Americans. Pleurisy root helps to ease pain, inflammation, and breathing difficulties brought on by pleurisy. This herb is often used in conjunction with **mullein** (*Verbascum thapsus*) or elecampane (*Inula helenium*), which serve as expectorants to clear excess mucus from the lungs. Other respiratory herbs that are used in the treatment of pleurisy include **boneset** (*Eupatorium perfoliatum*), **catnip** (*Nepata cataria*), and **feverfew** (*Chrysanthemum parthenium*).

Herbs thought to combat infection, such as **echinacea** (*Echinacea* species), are also included in herbal pleurisy remedies. Antiviral herbs, such as *Lomatium dissectum* and *Ligusticum porteri*, can be used if the pleurisy is of viral origin.

Chinese medicine

Traditional Chinese treatments are chosen based upon the specific symptoms of the patient. The treatment principles are to harmonize the collaterals, regulate the qi, and possibly to treat stagnation of phlegm and blood. Acupuncture, ear acupuncture, and herbal remedies are used to treat chest pains. The herb **ephedra** (*Ephedra sinica*) opens air passages and alleviates respiratory difficulties in pleurisy patients. One pill of Xue Fu Zhu Yu Wan (Blood Mansion Eliminating Stasis Pill) can be taken twice daily to treat stabbing chest pain. The basic herbal formula, to which additional herbs are added for specific symptoms, is:

- Chuan Lian Zi (*Fructus meliae toosendan*), 10 g
- Jiang Xiang (*Ligum dalbergiae odoriferae*), 3 g
- Jie Geng (*Radix platycodi*), 5 g
- Xiang Fu (*Rhizoma cyperi*), 10 g
- Xuan Fu Hua (*Flos inulae*), 6 g
- Yan Hu Suo (*Rhizoma corydalis*), 10 g
- Yu Jin (*Tuber curcumae*), 10 g
- Zhi Ke (*Fructus aurantii*) 5 g

Other remedies

Other alternative remedies for pleurisy include:

- Aromatherapy. Essential oils can be effective when used as massage oils or inhaled with steaming water. Rosemary relieves pain. Peppermint relieves pain and decreases inflammation. Eucalyptus eliminates infection.
- Diet. Dietary recommendations include eating fresh fruits and vegetables, and adequate protein. The patient should ingest omega–3 fatty acids, which are fats with anti-inflammatory activity found in salmon, mackerel, herring, and flaxseed oil.

- Homeopathy. Homeopathic treatment, chosen by a trained practitioner based on the pattern of symptoms experienced by the patient, can be effective in resolving pleurisy.
- Hydrotherapy. Contrast hydrotherapy applied to the chest and back, along with compresses (cloths soaked in an herbal solution), can assist in the healing process.
- Supplements. Taking certain nutritional supplements, especially large doses of vitamin C, may also provide health benefits to persons with pleurisy.

Allopathic treatment

The pain of pleurisy is usually treated with analgesic and anti-inflammatory drugs, such as acetaminophen, ibuprofen, and indomethacin. Sometimes, a painful **cough** will be controlled with codeine-based cough syrups. However, as the pain eases, a person with pleurisy should try to breathe deeply and cough to clear congestion, otherwise pneumonia may occur.

The treatment used to cure pleurisy is determined by the underlying cause. Pleurisy from a bacterial infection is treated with antibiotics. Specific therapies designed for more chronic illnesses can often cause pleurisy to subside. In some cases, excess fluid must be removed by thoracentesis or a chest tube. If left untreated, a more serious infection, called empyema, may develop.

Expected results

Prompt diagnosis, followed by appropriate treatment, ensures a good recovery for most pleurisy patients. Generally speaking, the prognosis for pleurisy is linked to the seriousness of its cause.

Prevention

Preventing pleurisy is often a matter of providing early medical attention to conditions that can cause pleural inflammation. Maintaining a healthy lifestyle and avoiding exposure to harmful substances (for example, asbestos) are more general preventative measures.

Resources

BOOKS

The Burton Goldberg Group. *Alternative Medicine: The Definitive Guide*. Fife, WA: Future Medicine Publishing, 1999.

Light, Richard W. "Disorders of the Pleura, Mediastinum, and Diaphragm." In *Harrison's Principles of Internal Medicine*. 14th ed., edited by Anthony S. Fauci, et al. New York: McGraw-Hill, 1998.

Light, Richard W. *Pleural Diseases*. Baltimore, MD: Williams and Wilkins, 1995.

Stauffer, John L. "Lung: Pleural Diseases." In *Current Medical Diagnosis and Treatment 1998*. edited by Lawrence M. Tierney, Jr., et al. Stamford, CT: Appleton and Lange, 1998.

Ying, Zhou Zhong, and Jin Hui De. "Chest Pain." *Clinical Manual of Chinese Herbal Medicine and Acupuncture*. New York: Churchill Livingston, 1997.

PERIODICALS

Brechot, J. M., T. Molina, and P. Jacoulet. "Secondary Tumoral Pleurisy." [Article in French] *Presse Med* 31 (March 30, 2002): 556-561.

Chow, C. W., and S. C. Chang. "Pleuritis as a Presenting Manifestation of Rheumatoid Arthritis: Diagnostic Clues in Pleural Fluid Cytology." *American Journal of Medical Science* 323 (March 2002): 158-161.

ORGANIZATIONS

American Lung Association. 1740 Broadway, New York, NY 10019-4374. (800) 586-4872. http://www.lungusa.org.

National Heart, Lung, and Blood Institute. Information Center. PO Box 30105, Bethesda, MD 20824-0105. (301) 496-4236. http://www.nhlbi.nih.gov.

Belinda Rowland
Rebecca J. Frey, PhD

PMS *see* **Premenstrual syndrome**

Pneumonia

Definition

Pneumonia is an infection of the lung that can be caused by nearly any class of organism known to cause human **infections**. These include bacteria, amoebae, viruses, fungi, and parasites.

Description

Anatomy of the lung

To better understand pneumonia, it is important to understand the basic anatomic features of the respiratory system. The human respiratory system begins at the nose and mouth, where air is breathed in (inspired) and out (expired). The air tube extending from the nose is called the nasopharynx. The tube carrying air breathed in through the mouth is called the oropharynx. The nasopharynx and the oropharynx merge into the larynx. The oropharynx also carries swallowed substances, including food, water, and salivary secretion that must pass into the esophagus and then into the stomach. The larynx is protected by a trap door called the epiglottis, which prevents substances that have been swallowed, as well as substances that have been regurgitated (thrown up), from heading down into the larynx toward the lungs.

A useful method of picturing the respiratory system is to imagine an upside-down tree. The larynx flows into the trachea, which is the tree trunk, and thus the broadest part of the respiratory tree. The trachea divides into two tree limbs, the right and left bronchi. Each one of these branches off into multiple smaller bronchi, which course through the tissue of the lung. Each bronchus divides into tubes of smaller and smaller diameter, finally ending in the terminal bronchioles. The air sacs of the lung, in which oxygen-carbon dioxide exchange actually takes place, are clustered at the ends of the bronchioles like the leaves of a tree. They are called alveoli.

The tissue of the lung that serves only a supportive role for the bronchi, bronchioles, and alveoli is called the lung parenchyma.

Function of the respiratory system

The main function of the respiratory system is to provide oxygen, the most important energy source, for the body's cells. Inspired air (the air taken in when a person breathes) contains oxygen and travels down the respiratory tree to the alveoli. The oxygen moves out of the alveoli and is sent into circulation throughout the body as part of the red blood cells. The oxygen in the inspired air is exchanged within the alveoli for the waste product of human metabolism, carbon dioxide. The air people breathe out contains carbon dioxide. This **gas** leaves the alveoli during expiration. To restate this exchange of gases simply, humans breathe in oxygen, and they breathe out carbon dioxide.

Respiratory system defenses

The healthy human lung is sterile. There are normally no resident bacteria or viruses (unlike the upper respiratory system and parts of the gastrointestinal system, where bacteria dwell even in a healthy state). There are multiple safeguards along the path of the respiratory system. These are designed to keep serious, pathogenic organisms from invading and leading to infection.

The first line of defense includes the hair in the nostrils, which serves as a filter for larger particles. The epiglottis is a trap door of sorts, designed to prevent food and other swallowed substances from entering the larynx and then trachea. **Sneezing** and coughing, both provoked by the presence of irritants within the respiratory system, help to clear such irritants from the respiratory tract.

Mucus produced by the respiratory system also serves to trap dust and infectious organisms. Tiny hair-like projections (cilia) from cells lining the respiratory tract beat constantly. They move debris trapped by mucus upwards and out of the respiratory tract. This mechanism of protection is referred to as the mucociliary escalator.

Cells lining the respiratory tract produce several types of immune substances that protect against various organisms. Other cells (called macrophages) along the respiratory tract actually ingest and kill invading organisms.

The organisms that cause pneumonia, then, are usually carefully kept from entering the lungs by these host defenses. However, when an individual encounters a large number of organisms at once, the usual defenses may be overwhelmed. Infection may happen either by inhaling contaminated air droplets or by aspiration of organisms inhabiting the upper airways.

Demographics

In the United States, pneumonia, in combination with **influenza**, is the eighth most common disease leading to death. An estimated 2.3 million Americans develop pneumonia each year, and about 58,500 die from it, according to 2004 statistics published by the Centers for Disease Control and Prevention (CDC). In developing countries, pneumonia ties with **diarrhea** as the most common cause of death.

Pneumonia is the most common fatal infection acquired by already hospitalized patients. Even in nonfatal cases, pneumonia is a significant economic burden on the healthcare system. One study estimates that people in the U.S. workforce who develop pneumonia cost employers five times as much in health care as the average worker.

Causes and symptoms

Causes

The list of organisms that can cause pneumonia is very large and includes nearly every class of infectious organism: viruses, bacteria, bacteria-like organisms, fungi, and parasites (including certain **worms**). Different organisms are more frequently encountered by different age groups. Further, other characteristics of individuals may place them at greater risk for infection by particular types of organisms:

- Viruses cause the majority of pneumonia cases in young children (especially respiratory syncytial virus, parainfluenza and influenza viruses, and adenovirus).
- Adults are more frequently infected with bacteria (such as *Streptococcus pneumoniae, Haemophilus influenzae,* and *Staphylococcus aureus*).
- Pneumonia in older children and young adults is often caused by the bacteria-like *Mycoplasma pneumoniae* (the cause of what is often referred to as "walking" pneumonia).
- *Pneumocystis carinii* is an extremely important cause of pneumonia in patients with immune problems, such as patients being treated for cancer with chemotherapy or patients with AIDS. Classically considered a parasite, it appears to be more related to fungi.
- People who have reason to come into contact with bird droppings, such as poultry workers, are at risk for pneumonia caused by the organism *Chlamydia psittaci.*
- A very large, serious outbreak of pneumonia occurred in 1976, when many people attending an American Legion convention were infected by a previously unknown organism. Subsequently named *Legionella pneumophila,* it causes what is was later called "Legionnaire's disease." The organism was traced to air conditioning units in the convention's hotel.

CONDITIONS PREDISPOSING TO PNEUMONIA. In addition to exposure to sufficient quantities of causative organisms, certain conditions may make an individual more likely to become ill with pneumonia. Certainly, the lack of normal anatomical structure could result in an increased risk of pneumonia. For example, there are certain inherited defects of cilia which result in less effective protection. Cigarette smoke, inhaled directly by a smoker or secondhand by an innocent bystander, interferes significantly with ciliary function, as well as inhibiting macrophage function.

Stroke, seizures, alcohol, and various drugs interfere with the function of the epiglottis. A weak epiglottis leads to a leaky seal on the trap door, with possible contamination by swallowed substances and/or regurgitated stomach contents. Alcohol and drugs also interfere with the normal **cough** reflex. This interference further decreases the chance of clearing unwanted debris from the respiratory tract.

Viruses may interfere with ciliary function, allowing themselves or other microorganism invaders (such as bacteria) access to the lower respiratory tract. One of the most important viruses is HIV (Human Immunodeficiency Virus), the causative virus in **AIDS** (acquired immunodeficiency syndrome). Between the 1980s and early 2000s this virus resulted in a huge increase in the incidence of pneumonia. Because AIDS results in a general decreased effectiveness of many aspects of the host's immune system, a person with AIDS is susceptible to all kinds of pneumonia, which includes some previously rare parasitic types that would be unable to cause illness in an individual with a normal immune system.

The elderly have an increased risk of developing pneumonia due to a less effective mucociliary escalator, as well as immune system changes that occur naturally with the **aging** process.

Various chronic conditions predispose a person to infection with pneumonia. These include **asthma**, cystic fibrosis, and neuromuscular diseases that may interfere with the seal of the epiglottis. Esophageal disorders may result in stomach contents passing upwards into the esophagus, which increases the risk of aspiration into the lungs of those stomach contents with their resident bacteria. Diabetes, **sickle cell anemia**, lymphoma, **leukemia**, and **emphysema** also predispose a person to pneumonia.

Genetic factors appear to be involved in susceptibility to pneumonia. Certain changes in DNA appear to affect some patients' risk of developing such complications of pneumonia as septic shock.

Pneumonia is also one of the most frequent infectious complications of all types of surgery. Many drugs used during and after surgery may increase the risk of aspiration, impair the cough reflex, and cause patients to underfill their lungs with air. **Pain** after surgery also discourages patients from breathing deeply enough and from coughing effectively.

Radiation treatment for **breast cancer** increases the risk of pneumonia in some patients by weakening lung tissue.

In addition, the use of mechanical ventilators to assist patients in breathing after surgery increases their risk of developing pneumonia. This condition, now referred to as ventilator-associated pneumonia, has a mortality exceeding 50%.

Symptoms

Pneumonia is suspected in any patient who has **fever**, cough, chest pain, shortness of breath, and increased respirations (number of breaths per minute). Fever with a shaking chill is even more suspicious. Many patients cough up clumps of sputum, commonly known as spit. These secretions are produced in the alveoli during an infection or other inflammatory condition. They may appear streaked with pus or blood. Severe pneumonia results in the signs of oxygen deprivation, which includes blue appearance of the nail beds or lips (cyanosis).

The invading organism causes symptoms, in part, by provoking an overly strong immune response in the lungs. In other words, the immune system that should help fight off infections, kicks into such high gear, that it damages the lung tissue and makes it more susceptible to infection. The small blood vessels in the lungs (capillaries) become leaky, and protein-rich fluid seeps into the alveoli, which results in less functional area for oxygen-carbon dioxide exchange. The patient becomes relatively oxygen deprived, while retaining potentially damaging carbon dioxide. The patient breathes faster and faster, in an effort to bring in more oxygen and blow off more carbon dioxide.

Mucus production is increased, and the leaky capillaries may tinge the mucus with blood. Mucus plugs actually further decrease the efficiency of gas exchange in the lung. The alveoli fill further with fluid and debris from the large number of white blood cells being produced to fight the infection.

Consolidation, a feature of bacterial pneumonia, occurs when the alveoli, which are normally hollow air spaces within the lung, instead become solid, due to quantities of fluid and debris.

Viral pneumonia and mycoplasma pneumonia do not result in consolidation. These types of pneumonia primarily infect the walls of the alveoli and the parenchyma of the lung.

Severe acute respiratory syndrome (SARS)

Severe acute respiratory syndrome (SARS) is a contagious and potentially fatal disease that first appeared in the form of a multi-country outbreak in early February 2003 in Asia, North America, and Europe. The CDC later worked with the World Health Organization (WHO) to investigate the cause(s) of SARS and to develop guidelines for infection control. SARS was described as an atypical pneumonia of unknown etiology and the disease agent was identified as a previously unknown coronavirus.

Early symptoms of SARS include a high fever with **chills**, **headache**, **muscle cramps**, and weakness. This early phase is followed by respiratory symptoms, usually a dry cough and painful or difficult breathing. About 10 to 20% of patients require mechanical ventilation due to insufficient blood oxygen levels. The median incubation period of SARS is four to five days. The primary mode of transmission is direct mucus membrane (eyes, nose, and mouth) contact with infectious respiratory droplets. If the patient is isolated and receives prompt treatment within the first five days after the onset of symptoms, the risk of infecting other people is greatly reduced, particularly if the SARS-designated care facility adheres to strict airborne precautions, according to the WHO. Treatments include antibiotics known to be effective against bacterial pneumonia; ribavirin and other antiviral drugs; and steroids. The mortality of SARS is estimated at 7 to 9%.

Diagnosis

For the most part, diagnosis of pneumonia is based on the patient's report of symptoms, combined with examination of the chest. Listening with a stethoscope reveals abnormal sounds, and tapping on the patient's back (which should yield a resonant sound due to air filling the alveoli) may instead yield a dull thump if the alveoli are filled with fluid and debris.

Laboratory diagnosis can be made of some types of bacterial pneumonia by staining sputum with special chemicals and looking at it under a microscope. Identification of the specific type of bacteria may require culturing the sputum (using the sputum sample to grow greater numbers of the bacteria in a lab dish.).

X-ray examination of the chest may reveal certain abnormal changes associated with pneumonia. Localized shadows obscuring areas of the lung may indicate a bacterial pneumonia, while streaky or patchy appearing changes in the x-ray picture may indicate viral or mycoplasma pneumonia. These changes on x ray, however, are known to lag behind the patient's actual symptoms.

Treatment

Pneumonia is a potentially serious condition that requires prompt medical attention. Patients should contact their doctors for immediate diagnosis and treatment. Alternative treatment such as nutritional support, however, can help alleviate some of the symptoms associated with pneumonia and boost the body's immune function.

Diet and nutrition

The following nutritional changes are recommended:

- Avoid all potentially allergenic foods and determine allergenic foods with an elimination diet.
- Reduce intake of sugar and processed foods.
- Get plenty of rest.
- Get plenty of fluids to prevent dehydration and help loosen phlegm.

- Consume nutritional supplements such as vitamins C, bioflavonoids, vitamin A, beta-carotene, and zinc.

Herbal treatment

Over-the-counter herbal preparations such as glycerol guaiacolate can help clear the lungs of phlegm and speed up the recovery process. Antimicrobial herbs, such as **goldenseal** (*Hydrastis canadenis*) and Chinese herbs, which stimulate the immune system, may be taken for treatment.

Other treatment

Other treatments include **yoga**, help with breathing, movement, and **relaxation**. Also recommended are **meditation** and the use of **guided imagery**. Individuals can contact local practitioners to enroll in such therapies.

Allopathic treatment

Prior to the discovery of penicillin antibiotics, bacterial pneumonia was almost always fatal. In the late 2000s, antibiotics, especially given early in the course of the disease, are very effective against bacterial causes of pneumonia. Erythromycin and tetracycline improve recovery time for symptoms of mycoplasma pneumonia. They do not, however, eradicate the organisms. Amantadine and acyclovir may be helpful against certain types of viral pneumonia.

Another antibiotic linezolid (Zyvox) was being used to treat penicillin-resistant organisms that cause pneumonia in the late 2000s. Linezolid is the first of a line of antibiotics known as oxazolidinones. Another drug known as ertapenem (Invanz) was reported to be effective in treating bacterial pneumonia.

Expected results

Rate of recovery varies according to the type of organism causing the infection. Recovery following pneumonia with *Mycoplasma pneumoniae* is nearly 100%. *Staphylococcus pneumoniae* has a death rate of 30 to 40%. Similarly, infections with a number of gram negative bacteria (such as those in the gastrointestinal tract which can cause infection following aspiration) have a high death rate of 25 to 50%. *Streptococcus pneumoniae,* the most common organism causing pneumonia, produces a death rate of about 5%. More complications occur in very young or very old individuals who have multiple areas of the lung infected simultaneously. Individuals with other chronic illnesses (including **cirrhosis** of the liver, congestive heart failure, individuals without a functioning spleen, and individuals who have other diseases that

KEY TERMS

Alveoli—The little air sacs clustered at the ends of the bronchioles, in which oxygen-carbon dioxide exchange takes place.

Aspiration—An action during which solids or liquids that should be swallowed into the stomach are instead breathed into the respiratory system.

Cilia—Hair-like projections from certain types of cells.

Consolidation—A condition in which lung tissue becomes firm and solid rather than elastic and air-filled because it has accumulated fluids and tissue debris.

Coronavirus—One of a family of RNA-containing viruses known to cause severe respiratory illnesses. In March 2003, a previously unknown coronavirus was identified as the causative agent of severe acute respiratory syndrome (SARS).

Cyanosis—A bluish tinge to the skin that can occur when the blood oxygen level drops too low.

Parenchyma—The supportive tissue surrounding a particular structure. An example is that tissue that surrounds and supports the actually functional lung tissue.

Sputum—Material produced within the alveoli in response to an infectious or inflammatory process.

result in a weakened immune system) experience complications. Patients with immune disorders, various types of **cancer**, transplant patients, and AIDS patients also experience complications.

Prevention

Because many types of bacterial pneumonia occur in patients who are first infected with the influenza virus, yearly vaccination against influenza can decrease the risk of pneumonia for the elderly and people with chronic diseases such as asthma, cystic fibrosis, diabetes, kidney disease, and cancer.

Maintaining a healthy diet that includes whole foods and **vitamin C** and B-complex vitamins aids in prevention. Also helpful in terms of both good health and prevention of pneumonia is developing a regular **exercise** regimen, as well as reducing **stress**.

A specific vaccine against *Streptococcus pneumoniae* is very protective and should also be administered to patients with chronic illnesses.

Patients who have decreased immune resistance are at higher risk for infection with *Pneumocystis carinii*. They are frequently put on a regular drug regimen of Trimethoprim sulfa and/or inhaled pentamidine to avoid Pneumocystis pneumonia.

Resources

BOOKS

Mandell, Gerald L., John E. Bennett, and Raphael Dolin. "Clinical Evaluation and Therapy for Pneumonia." In *Principles and Practice of Infectious Diseases,* 6th ed. Philadelphia: Churchill Livingstone/Elsevier, 2005.

Pizzorno, Joseph E., Michael T. Murray, and Herb Joiner-Bey. "Bronchitis and Pneumonia." In *The Clinician's Handbook of Natural Medicine,* 2nd ed. Philadelphia: Churchill Livingstone/Elsevier, 2007.

PERIODICALS

Minino, A. M., Melonie P. Heron, Sherry L. Murphy, and Kenneth D. Kochanek. "Deaths: Final Data for 2004." *National Vital Statistics Reports,* National Centers for Health Statistics, Centers for Disease Control and Prevention, 55, no. 19 (August 21, 2007): 1–120.

Ruffell, A., and L. Adamcova. "Ventilator-Associated Pneumonia: Prevention Is Better than Cure." *Nursing in Critical Care* 13, no. 1 (January/February 2008): 44–53.

ORGANIZATIONS

American Lung Association, 61 Broadway, 6th Floor, New York, NY, 10006, (800) 548-8252, (212) 315 8700, http://www.lungusa.org.

Centers for Disease Control and Prevention, 1600 Clifton Rd., NE, Atlanta, GA, 30333, (800) 311-3435, (404) 498-1515, http://www.cdc.gov.

Global Alliance Against Chronic Respiratory Diseases (GARD), World Health Organization, Department of Chronic Diseases and Health Promotion, 20, Avenue Appia, CH-1211 27, Geneva, Switzerland, http://www.who.int/respiratory/gard/en/.

National Heart, Lung, and Blood Institute Information Center, PO Box 30105, Bethesda, MD, 20824-0105, (301) 592-8573, http://www.nhlbi.nih.gov.

Mai Tran
Rebecca J. Frey, PhD
Angela M. Costello

Poison ivy and poison oak *see* **Contact dermatitis**

Poison oak (plant) *see* **Rhus toxicodendron**

Pokeweeds *see* **Phytolacca**

Polarity therapy

Definition

Polarity therapy is a holistic, energy-based system that includes bodywork, diet, **exercise**, and lifestyle counseling for the purpose of restoring and maintaining proper energy flows throughout the body. The underlying concept of polarity therapy is that all energy within the human body is based in electromagnetic force and that disease results from improperly dissipated energy.

Origins

Austrian-American chiropractor, osteopath, and naturopath Randolph Stone (1888–1981) developed polarity therapy as an integration of Eastern and Western principles and techniques of healing. Stone discovered the ancient principles of the Ayurvedic philosophy in the course of his travels during a sojourn in India. On a life-long quest to learn the fundamentals of human vitality, he also studied **reflexology** and **traditional Chinese medicine**.

Stone became committed to the principles of **Ayurvedic medicine**, which he interpreted in conjunction with his scientific and medical knowledge to define polarity therapy. According to the philosophy of Ayurved, which is based in a set of principles called the tridosha—the energy of the human body is centered in five organs or regions (the brain; the cardiopulmonary [heart and lungs] region, the diaphragm, the smaller intestine, and the larger intestine). One of five airs or energy forms controls each respective region: prana in the brain, vyana in the heart and lungs, udana in the diaphragm, samana in the smaller intestine, and apana in the larger intestine. The five airs control all directional motion in the body, with each air in command of a different type of movement. Stone established further that the prana, centered in the brain, ultimately controlled the combined forces of the body. Any impediment or restriction to the flow of prana in turn affects the health of the entire body. The prana force is nurtured through the flow of food and air into the body as well as through our interactions with other living beings and through the intake of the five sensory organs.

Stone devoted much of his life to defining an elaborately detailed cause and effect relationship between the human anatomy and illness, based in the energy flow of the prana. He further attributed electromagnetic energy as the basis of the energy forces. He used the medical symbol of the Caduceus to define the patterns of the flow and described the energy movement in detail in charts of the human body. Polarity therapy is based in charted energy flows. The primary energy pattern is defined in a spiral motion that radiates from the umbilicus and defines the original energy flow of the fetus in the womb.

Benefits

Polarity therapy unblocks and recharges the flow of life energy and realigns unbalanced energy as a means of eliminating disease. Patients learn to release tension by addressing the source of the **stress** and by maintaining a healthy demeanor accordingly.

This treatment may be effective to promote health and healing to anyone willing to embrace the appropriate lifestyle. Polarity therapy is reportedly effective for anyone who has been exposed to toxic poisons. Likewise HIV-positive individuals may find comfort in polarity therapy. Additionally this is an appropriate therapy for relieving general stress, back **pain**, stomach cramps, and other recurring maladies and conditions.

Description

After determining the exact source of a patient's energy imbalance, the therapist begins the first of a series of bodywork sessions designed to rechannel and release the patient's misdirected prana. This therapy, akin to massage, is based in energetic pressure and involves circulating motions. In performing the regimen, the therapist pays strict attention to the pressure exerted at each location—even to which finger is used to apply pressure at any given point of the patient's anatomy. This technique, which comprises the central regimen or focal point of polarity therapy is very gentle and is unique to polarity therapy. It typically involves subtle rocking movements and cranial holds to stimulate body energy. Although firm, deep pushing touches are employed in conjunction with the massage technique, the polarity therapist never exerts a particularly forceful contact.

To support the bodywork, the therapist often prescribes a diet for the patient, to encourage cleansing and eliminate waste. The precepts of polarity therapy take into consideration specific interactions between different foods and the human energy fields.

Likewise, a series of exercises is frequently prescribed. These exercises, called polarity **yoga** include squats, stretches, rhythmic movements, deep breathing, and expression of sounds. They can be both energizing

Apana—life sustaining energy centered in the larger intestine; the fifth of the five airs of Ayurvedic philosophy; the life force governing expulsion activity.

Ayurveda—(Sanskrit, *Ayur,* life, and *veda,* knowledge) is translated as "knowledge of life" or "science of longevity." It became established as the traditional Hindu system of medicine.

Caduceus— the ancient and universal symbol of medicine consisting of the winged staff of Mercury and two intertwining serpents.

Prana—life sustaining energy centered in the human brain; the first of the five airs of Ayurvedic philosophy; the life force governing inspiration and the conscious intellect.

Primary energy pattern—a spiral motion that radiates from the umbilicus; the energy pattern associated with a child in the womb.

QV—quantum vacuum, a theory coined by physicists, which defines the interactions of energy that combine to form reality.

Reflexology—Belief that reflex areas in the feet correspond to every part of the body, including organs and glands, and that stimulating the correct reflex area can affect the body part.

Samana—life sustaining energy of the smaller intestine; the fourth of the five airs of Ayurvedic philosophy; the life force governing side-to-side motion.

Tridosha—the combination of three basic principles of energy, or biological humor, that comprise life, according to Ayurvedic philosophy.

Udana—life sustaining energy of the diaphragm, the third of the five airs of Ayurvedic philosophy, the life force governing upward motion.

Vyana—life sustaining energy of the heart and lungs; the second of the five airs of Ayurvedic philosophy; the life force governing circular motion.

and relaxing. Counseling may be included whenever appropriate as a part of a patient's highly individual therapy regimen to promote balance.

Preparations

Therapists take a comprehensive case history from every patient prior to beginning treatment. This preliminary verbal examination often monopolizes the first therapy session. Depending upon circumstances a therapist might have a need to assess the patient's physical structural balance through observation and physical examination.

Precautions

Polarity therapy is safe for virtually anyone, even the elderly and the most frail patients, because of the intrinsic gentleness of the **massage therapy**.

Side effects

Highly emotional releases of energy (laughter, tears, or a combination of both) are associated with this therapy.

Research and general acceptance

This is a complementary therapy of holistic, spiritually based treatment, which may be used in conjunction with a medical approach. Polarity therapy is practiced worldwide, but the majority of practitioners are based in the United States. Modern physicists employ concepts similar to Stone's basic theories of polarity in defining the quantum vacuum (QV) as a foundation of all reality. Still, by 2000, this holistic regimen had not achieved the widespread acceptance anticipated by Stone before his death in 1981.

When St. Paul Fire and Marine insurers offered a liability insurance package to therapy providers, the company recognized polarity therapy as an alternative medical treatment along with **acupuncture**, **biofeedback**, **homeopathy**, reflexology, and others.

Training and certification

The American Polarity Therapy Association (APTA) sanctions two levels of training. The Associate Polarity Practitioner (APP) is the preliminary level, based on a minimum level of excellence in this field. Registered Polarity Practitioner (RPP) is bestowed upon the graduates of an approved training curriculum. Post-graduate and specialty training is available in a variety of fields, and APTA certifies practitioners accordingly.

RANDOLF STONE (1890-1981)

Randolf Stone was born Rudolph Bautsch in 1890 in Austria. He immigrated with his family to the United States in 1898. As he grew, Stone started studying many medical practices and soon was experienced in the healing arts of naturopathy, osteopathy, and chiropractic. He changed his name to Randolf Stone in the 1920s.

Stone's quest for knowledge continued to grow. He soon turned to the study of physics, including quantum physics and the study of energy fields, in search of a more effective healing art. In pursuit of greater knowledge in these areas, he traveled throughout the United States. Additionally he returned to Europe and traveled to India to investigate the esoteric arts of different cultures.

Through his travels, Stone grew to believe in energy fields that surround people. When these fields are weak or disrupted, it results in sickness and disease. Stone developed polarity therapy. This is the manipulation of these human energy fields through nutrition, touch, and environmental factors. Stone based his theories of polarity therapy extensively on the precepts that he learned throughout the course of his travels, most fundamentally on the Ayurveda system of five energies that he learned in India. He also drew from his knowledge of chiropractic, naturopathy, and osteopathy medical treatments.

In 1947, Stone published his first book, *Energy,* discussing his views on the energy fields. He followed up this work with six other books, all expanding on polarity therapy. His writing, *The Physical Anatomy of Man,* became the foundation for all healing arts in the United States.

Resources

BOOKS

Stone, Randolph. *Polarity Therapy—The Complete Collected Works.* Reno, CRCS Publications, 1986.

PERIODICALS

Modern Medicine (August 1, 1999): 15.

ORGANIZATIONS

American Polarity Therapy Association. P.O. Box 19858, Boulder Colorado 80308. (303) 545-2080. Fax: (303) 545-2161.

Trans-Hyperboreau Institute of Science. P.O. Box 2344 Sausalito, California 94966. (415) 331-0230. (800) 485-8095. Fax: (415) 331-0231.

OTHER

Young, Phil. "Prana." http://www.eclipse.co.uk/masterworks/Polarity/PolarityArticles.htm. (16 June 2000).

Gloria Cooksey

Polycystic ovary syndrome

Definition

Polycystic Ovary Syndrome (PCOS) is a collection of hormonal and metabolic imbalances marked by virilization, anovulation and polycystic ovaries.

Description

The condition known as PCOS was first defined by Drs. Stein and Leventhal in 1935, who observed that female patients with multiple **ovarian cysts** often had other distinct physical symptoms including excessive male-pattern hair growth, menstrual cycle disturbances leading to **infertility**, and **obesity**. In 2004, the American Society of Reproductive Medicine and European Society of Human Reproduction and Embryology redefined diagnostic criteria to include two out of three of the following: anovulation, hyperandrogenism, and polycystic ovaries.

Demographics

PCOS is the most common hormonal disorder of premenopausal women, affecting 5-7% of women of childbearing age. Symptoms typically begin to occur shortly after the onset of menses, however the syndrome may remain undiagnosed until later in life. There can be many different clinical presentations that fall under the category of PCOS. It has been suggested that PCOS may actually have several subcategories based on the variety of symptoms. The most common symptoms are excessive hair growth, menstrual irregularities and obesity. It is estimated that 95% of women with this collection of symptoms have PCOS.

Causes and Symptoms

The cause of PCOS is not fully understood. Several different mechanisms have been identified as contributing to PCOS: dysfunction of the central nervous system, ovarian disorders, and **insulin resistance**. Additionally, there appears to be a genetic component.

The central nervous system regulates autonomic processes of the body, and is in communication with the endocrine system via the hypothalamus. The hypothalamus is responsible for regulating aspects of the autonomic nervous system and communicating with the pituitary gland via neuroendocrine agents. The hypothalamic hormone regulating reproduction, Gonadotropin-releasing hormone (GnRH), influences the pituitary gland to secrete follicle-stimulating hormone (FSH) and leutinizing hormone (LH). In PCOS, GnRH secretion is disrupted, resulting in elevated LH. The effect of LH on the ovary is to increase androgen production.

Alteration of ovarian function is another component of PCOS. Typically, there is a failure of the follicle to fully mature and ovulate. As a result, the ovaries may be quite enlarged by multiple unreleased follicles, now fluid-filled follicular cysts. Androgen production by the ovaries is enhanced, including testosterone and dehydroepiandrosterone (**DHEA**).

Metabolic alterations involving insulin likely play a role in PCOS. Between 40-80% of women with PCOS experience some degree of insulin resistance or dysglycemia, and about 40% will go on to develop Type II diabetes. Insulin resistance is the decreased sensitivity of insulin receptors of skeletal muscle. Decreased sensitivity to insulin leads to a need for more insulin to be released, resulting in chronically elevated levels of both insulin and glucose. Dysglycemia is certainly present in the general population and is not unique to PCOS, but there is a correlation between the two for many women. It has been proposed that the insulin resistance of PCOS is qualitatively different from that which occurs independently, and involves a problem with the signaling pathway of insulin. Insulin interferes with ovulation and the normal menstrual cycle.

In addition to the local effects of excess insulin, there are many systemic effects. About 40-60% of women with anovulatory menstrual cycles and PCOS are obese. The weight distribution tends to be abdominal, with an increased waist-to-hip ratio. This abdominal obesity is known to contribute to elevated risk of diabetes, **hypertension**, hyperlipidemia, and cardiovascular disease. Obesity further contributes to the abnormal hormone profile in women with PCOS by promoting estrogen conversion in adipose tissue.

Obesity is also linked with a decrease in sex-hormone-binding globulin (SHBG), a transport protein that binds to and carries estrogen and testosterone, which in their unbound form are metabolically active. The effect of estrogen on the ovary is to stimulate androgen production and increase ovarian receptors to LH, amplifying the androgen effect. Elevated testosterone produced by the ovary and unbound from SHBG is responsible for the symptoms of virilization that often occur with PCOS. These symptoms include excess hair growth, loss of hair from the head, and **acne**.

Testosterone is normally produced in small amounts by the ovaries and adrenal glands, as are weaker androgens **androstenedione**, dehydroepiandrosterone (DHEA) and dehydroepiandrosterone sulfate (DHEA-S). These can be converted to the highly active hormone dihydroxytestosterone (DHT) by the enzyme 5-a-reductase. Testosterone acts on receptors on hair follicles to promote hair growth, also known as hirsutism, on the chest, back, abdomen and face.

Hirsutism doesn't necessarily correlate with testosterone levels measured in the blood, as androgens may be elevated enough to cause hair growth and still be within normal limits on testing. The number of androgen receptors in the hair follicle determines the degree of hirsutism, and this has great genetic and ethnic variation.

Other skin changes may occur as part of the polycystic ovary syndrome. Acne is a fairly common symptom and presents as a result of an increase in circulating androgens. Skin discoloration at the neck and under the breasts, called *acanthosis nigricans*, is a unique symptom that is caused by elevated insulin. Skin tags, thickening of the skin (*hyperkeratosis*) and **infections** of hair follicles called *hydradenitis suppurativa* are also caused by hyperinsulinemia and may occur in PCOS.

Diagnosis

PCOS is considered a diagnosis of exclusion, made after a full workup to rule out other endocrine disorders. The first part of evaluation is a clinical assessment of medical history, family history and a physical examination. Signs and symptoms looked for on the physical exam include:

- hair loss on head
- facial hair growth: cheeks, chin, upper lip, sideburns
- acne
- thyroid enlargement
- skin discoloration
- skin tags
- body hair on chest, back, abdomen, between umbilicus and pubic area, thighs
- enlarged or tender ovaries
- weight, body mass index (BMI), waist-hip ratio

Next, the physician will order laboratory evaluation and ultrasound of the pelvis. A diagnosis of PCOS can be made if the patient has clinical symptoms, laboratory abnormalities or multiple cysts on ultrasound. Often a woman will have all of these, but all two of the three must be present to make a diagnosis.

There are numerous laboratory tests that may be helpful for the diagnosis and management of PCOS. Many of these tests evaluate hormone levels:

- thyroid-stimulating hormone (TSH)
- prolactin
- LH and FSH
- testosterone, androstenedione, DHEA
- estrogen
- SHBG

Further tests to evaluate glucose regulation are indicated and include **fasting** glucose, insulin, and hemoglobin A1C (HgbA1C). HgbA1C measures glycosylated hemoglobin, a marker of the effects of prolonged elevated glucose. A glucose tolerance test (GTT) could also be performed, in which a series of serum samples are drawn after the patient consumes a standardized bolus of glucose. Fasting glucose and HgbA1C may be used to monitor treatment of insulin resistance.

Women with PCOS are at increased risk of cardiovascular disease, a problem associated with dysglycemia. Additional screening tests may be ordered:

- Lipid panel - includes total cholesterol, high-density and low-density lipoproteins (HDL and LDL), and triglycerides
- Homocysteine - a predictor of coronary, cerebral and peripheral vascular disease associated with vitamin B12 or folate deficiency
- C-Reactive protein (CRP) - a marker of inflammation and an independent risk factor for cardiovascular disease

Treatment

Conventional treatment for PCOS typically centers around drug therapy for dysglycemia. The most widely used drug is metformin (Glucophage), a non-sulfonylurea which increases cell receptor response to insulin, decreases intestinal absorption of glucose, and decreases production of glucose by the liver. Several studies have evidenced that metformin both decreases hyperinsulinemia and promotes ovulation in women with anovulatory cycles. It may also help with weight loss in overweight patients with PCOS.

Another pharmaceutical strategy for treating PCOS is suppressing ovarian function with oral contraceptive pills (OCPs). Treatment with OCPs will often initiate regular menses in women with **amenorrhea** or

oligomenorrhea. The birth control pill decreases androgen levels, regulates menses and protects against uterine hyperplasia. However, there is conflicting evidence regarding the effect of OCPs on metabolic issues, some studies suggesting that oral contraceptive use promotes dysglycemia and leads to frank diabetes. Another obvious disadvantage of the oral contraceptive pill in PCOS is the problem of infertility.

Conventional treatment with PCOS seeking fertility is often metformin, clomifene, or a combination of the two. Clomifene (Clomid) acts on the ovaries to induce ovulation, and increases the rate of ovulation with use of metformin alone from 46% to 76%.

Women struggling with the often disruptive symptoms of PCOS may be seeking treatment for the virilizing effects of testosterone. One such treatment is spironolactone, a diuretic drug with antiandrogenic effects.

Nutrition/dietetic concerns

Of primary importance are lifestyle factors that can be modified to improve overall health and manage hyperinsulinemia. A high fiber diet rich in complex carbohydrates such as whole grains and vegetables, and avoidant of refined carbohydrates like pasta, breads, pastries and sweets, is crucial for glucose regulation. Developing dietary habits of eating small, frequent meals and snacks will help regulate glucose and insulin. Lean proteins consumed with every meal and snack make for slow-burning sources of fuel. Lastly, decreasing overall calorie consumption may be part of a holistic nutritional plan if weight loss is a goal of treatment. In overweight women, a loss of 10% body weight will reduce insulin resistance and often the weight loss alone can restore ovulation.

Regular **exercise** also reduces insulin resistance and promotes weight loss. Exercising five to seven days per week for thirty minutes is optimal. Walking or other movement after meals is another way to utilize excess circulating glucose, as active skeletal muscle is not dependent on insulin for its uptake.

Therapy

There are many complementary and alternative treatments for PCOS, often using similar strategies as pharmaceutical therapy to address insulin resistance, anovulation, infertility and hyperandrogenism. The goals of natural remedies for PCOS are to:

- increase insulin sensitivity, lower blood glucose and insulin levels
- induce ovulation and restore fertility

KEY TERMS

Adipose—Fat tissue, which can act as an endocrine organ by converting androgens to estrogen via the enzyme aromatase.

Adrenal glands—Composed of an outer cortex and inner medulla, the adrenal glands sit above both kidneys. The adrenal cortex produces several hormones including cortisol, DHEA, estrogen and progesterone, and aldosterone.

Amenorrhea—The absence of menses in women of childbearing age in the absence of pregnancy.

Androgen—Precursors to male hormones testosterone and androsterone.

Dysglycemia—Disrupted glucose regulation resulting in periods of hypoglycemia, hyperglycemia, elevated insulin and insulin resistance.

Hirsutism— Male-pattern growth of increased coarse hair in females.

Insulin—A protein produced by the pancreas, insulin regulates glucose uptake for use by cells.

Oligomenorrhea—Irregular, infrequent menses.

Virilization—Male sexual characteristics such as deepening voice, male-pattern hair growth and balding in women.

- lower estrogen and adrogens by increasing SHBG

- inhibit 5-alpha reductase to reduce conversion of androgens to dihydrotestosterone

Several nutrients are important cofactors needed for glucose metabolism. **Chromium**, often referred to as "glucose-tolerance factor," has been shown in several studies to lower blood glucose, insulin and Hgb A1C. Additionally, the botanical agents **fenugreek**, momordica, **gymnema** and cinnamon are used for lowering glucose and insulin.

The hyperandrogenism of PCOS can be improved by increasing SHBG and by inhibiting 5-a-reductase from converting androgens to dihydrotestosterone. **Saw palmetto** has traditionally been used in men with benign prostatic hypertrophy (BPH), and is anti-androgenic through its inhibition of 5-a-reductase. **Green tea**, soy and flax seeds have been found to increase SHBG, also acting to inhibit testosterone activity.

Menstrual irregularities including amenorrhea and anovulation often improve with management of insulin. Further treatments for hormone regulation include **acupuncture** and **botanical medicine**. Acupuncture has been shown to improve fertility when used in conjunction with conventional therapies. Western botanicals that may be helpful in PCOS include **black cohosh**, which may decrease elevated levels of LH.

Prognosis

The hormonal and metabolic imbalances of PCOS can usually be well managed with diet, exercise and medical or natural therapies.

Prevention

Because PCOS has an unclear etiology and includes a genetic component, it is difficult to determine how to prevent its onset. Maintaining a healthy weight and eating a nutritious diet low in refined carbohydrates are crucial in managing PCOS, and may help prevent some symptoms from developing.

Resources

BOOKS

Gordon J., Speroff L. *Handbook for Clinical Gynecologic Endocrinology and Infertility*. Lippincott. 2002.

Thatcher, S. *Polycystic Ovary Syndrome: The Hidden Epidemic*.Perspectives Press. 2000.

PERIODICALS

Diamante-Kandarakis E, JP Baillargeon, MJ Iuorno, DJ Jakubowicz, JE Nestler. A Modern Medical Quandary: Polycystic Ovary Syndrome, Insulin Resistance, and Oral Contraceptive Pills. *Journal of Clinical Endocrinology and Metabolism*. 2003. 88(5):1927-1932.

Dunaif A et al. Insulin Resistance and the Polycystic Ovary Syndrome: Mechanism and Implications for Pathogenesis. *Endocrine Reviews*.1997. 18(6):774-800.

Eagelson CA, AB Bellows, M Hu, MB Gingrich, JC Marshall. Obese Patients with Polycystic Ovary Syndrome: Evidence that Metformin Does Not Restore Sensitivity of the Gonadotropin-Releasing Hormone Pulse Generator to Inhibition by Ovarian Steroids. *Journal of Clinical Endocrinology and Metabolism*. 2003. 88(11):5158-5162.

Ehrmann DA, MK Cavaghan, J Imperial, J Sturgis, RL Rosenfeld, KS Polonsky. Effects of Metformin on Insulin Secretion, Insulin Action and Ovarian Steroidogenesis in Women with Polycystic Ovary Syndrome. *Journal of Clinical Endocrinology and Metabolism*. 1997. 82(2):524-530.

Fagelman E, FC Lowe. Saw Palmetto Berry as a Tretment for BPH. *Reviews in Urology*. 2001 Summer 3(3):134-8.

Fleming R, ZE Hopkinson, MA Wallace, IA Greer, N Sattar. Ovarian Function and Metabolic Factors in Women with Oligomenorrhea Treated with Metformin in a Randomized Double Blind Placebo-Controlled Trial. *Journal of Clinical Endocrinology and Metabolism*. 2002. 87(2):569-574.

Godsland IF, C Walton, C Felton, A Proudler, A Patel, V Wynn. Insulin Resistance, Secretion and Metabolism in Users of Oral Contraceptives. *Journal of Clinical Endocrinology and Metabolism.* 1992. 72(1):64.

Korythowski MT, M Mokan, MH Horwitz, SL Berga, Metabolic Effects of Oral Contraceptives in Women with PCOS. *Journal Clinical Endocrinology and Metabolism.* 1995. 80(11):3327.

Martin J, ZQ Wang, XH Zhang, D Wachtel, J volaufova, DE Matthews, WT Cefalu. Chromium Picolinate Supplementation Attenuates Body Weight Gain and Increases Insulin Sensitivity in Subjects with Type 2 Diabetes. *Diabetes Care.* 2006 August 29(8):1826-32.

Persaud SJ, H Al-Majed, A Raman, PM Jones. *Gymnema sylvestre* Stimulates Insulin Release In Vitro by Increased Membrane Permeability. *Journal of Endocrinology.* 1999. (63):207-212.

Rotterdam ESHRE/ASRM-Sponsored PCOS Consensus Workshop Group. Revised 2003 Consensus on Diagnostic Criteria and Long-Term Health Risks. *Fertility and Sterility.* 2004. 81:19-25.

Diana Christoff Quinn, ND

Polygonum *see* **Fo ti**

Postpartum depression

Definition

Postpartum **depression** is a mood disorder that begins after **childbirth** and usually lasts at least six weeks.

Description

Postpartum depression, or PPD, affects approximately 15% of all childbearing women. The onset of postpartum depression tends to be gradual and may persist for many months or develop into a second bout following a subsequent **pregnancy**. Mild to moderate cases are sometimes unrecognized by women themselves. Many women feel ashamed and may conceal their difficulties. This is a serious problem that disrupts women's lives and can have effects on the baby, other children, partners, and other relationships. Levels of depression for fathers can also increase significantly.

Postpartum depression is often divided into two types: early onset and late onset. Early-onset PPD most often seems like the "blues," a mild brief experience during the first days or weeks after birth. During the first week after the birth, up to 80% of mothers experience the "baby blues." This period is usually a time of extra sensitivity; symptoms include tearfulness, irritability, **anxiety**, and mood changes, which tend to peak between three to five days after childbirth. The symptoms normally disappear within two weeks without requiring specific treatment apart from understanding, support, skills, and practice. In short, some depression, **fatigue**, and anxiety may fall within the "normal" range of reactions to giving birth.

Late-onset PPD appears several weeks after birth. It involves slowly growing feelings of sadness, depression, lack of energy, chronic fatigue, inability to sleep, change in appetite, significant weight loss or gain, and difficulty caring for the baby.

Causes and symptoms

Experts cannot always say what causes postpartum depression. Most likely, it is caused by a combination of factors that vary from person to person. Some researchers think that women are vulnerable to depression at all major turning points in their reproductive cycle, childbirth being only one of these markers. Factors before the baby's birth that are associated with a higher risk of PPD include severe **vomiting** (hyperemesis), premature labor contractions, and psychiatric disorders in the mother. In addition, new mothers commonly experience some degree of depression during the first weeks after birth. Pregnancy and birth are accompanied by sudden hormonal changes that affect emotions. Additionally, the 24-hour responsibility for a newborn infant represents a major psychological and lifestyle adjustment for most mothers, even after the first child. These physical and emotional stresses are usually accompanied by inadequate rest until the baby's routine stabilizes, so fatigue and depression are not unusual.

In addition to hormonal changes and disrupted sleep, certain cultural expectations appear to place women from those cultures at increased risk of postpartum depression. For example, women who bear daughters in societies with a strong preference for sons (such as Communist China) are at increased risk of postpartum depression. In other cultures, a strained relationship with the husband's family is a risk factor. In Western countries, domestic violence is associated with a higher rate of PPD.

Experiences of PPD vary considerably but usually include several symptoms.

Feelings:

- persistent low mood
- inadequacy, failure, hopelessness, helplessness

- exhaustion, emptiness, sadness, tearfulness
- guilt, shame, worthlessness
- confusion, anxiety, and panic
- fear for the baby and of the baby
- fear of being alone or going out

Behaviors:

- lack of interest or pleasure in usual activities
- insomnia or excessive sleep, nightmares
- not eating or overeating
- decreased energy and motivation
- withdrawal from social contact
- poor self-care
- inability to cope with routine tasks

Thoughts:

- inability to think clearly and make decisions
- lack of concentration and poor memory
- running away from everything
- fear of being rejected by the partner
- worry about harm or death to partner or baby
- ideas about suicide

Some symptoms may not indicate a severe problem. However, persistent low mood or loss of interest or pleasure in activities, along with four other symptoms occurring together for a period of at least two weeks, indicate clinical depression and require adequate treatment.

There are several important risk factors for postpartum depression, including the following:

- stress
- lack of sleep
- poor nutrition
- lack of support from one's partner, family, or friends
- family history of depression
- labor/delivery complications for mother or baby
- premature or postmature delivery
- problems with the baby's health
- separation of mother and baby
- a difficult baby (temperament, feeding, sleeping problems)
- pre-existing neurosis or psychosis

Diagnosis

Diagnosis of postpartum depression can be made through a clinical interview with the patient to assess symptoms.

Treatment

Postpartum depression can be effectively alleviated through counseling and support groups, so that the mother does not feel she is alone in her feelings. **Acupuncture**, **traditional Chinese medicine**, **yoga**, **meditation**, and herbs can all help the mother suffering from postpartum depression return to a state of balance.

Recommended herbal remedies to ease depressive episodes may include **damiana** (*Turnera diffusa*), ginseng (*Panax ginseng*), lady's slipper (*Cypripedium calceolus*), **lavender** (*Lavandula angustifolia*), oats (*Avena sativa*), **rosemary** (*Rosmarinus officinalis*), **skullcap** (*Scutellaria laterifolia*), St. John's wort (*Hypericum perforatum*), and vervain (*Verbena officinalis*). Women who are breastfeeding or are suffering from a chronic medical condition should consult a healthcare professional before taking any herbal remedies.

Some strategies that may help new mothers cope with the **stress** of becoming a parent include:

- Valuing her role as a mother and trusting her own judgment.
- Making each day as simple as possible.
- Avoiding extra pressures or unnecessary tasks.
- Trying to involve her partner more in the care of the baby from the beginning.
- Discussing with her partner how both can share the household chores and responsibilities.
- Scheduling frequent outings, such as walks and short visits with friends.
- Sharing her feelings with her partner or a friend who is a good listener.
- Talking with other mothers to help keep problems in perspective.
- Trying to sleep or rest when the baby is sleeping.
- Taking care of her health and well being.

Allopathic treatment

Several treatment options exist, including medication, **psychotherapy**, counseling, and group treatment and support strategies, depending on the woman's needs. One effective treatment combines antidepressant medication and psychotherapy. These types of medication are often effective when used for three to four weeks. Any medication use must be carefully considered if the woman is breastfeeding, but with some medications, continuing breastfeeding is safe. There are many classes of antidepression medications. Two of the most commonly prescribed for PPD are selective serotonin reuptake inhibitors (SSRIs) such as citalopram (Celexa), escitalopram (Lexapro), fluoxetine (Prozac), paroxetine (Paxil, Pexeva), and sertraline (Zoloft), and tricyclids, such as amitriptyline (Elavil), desipramine (Norpramin), imipramine (Tofranil), and nortriptyline (Aventyl, Pamelor). Nevertheless, medication alone is never sufficient and should always be accompanied by counseling or other support services. Also, many women with postpartum depression feel isolated. It is important for these women to know that they are not alone in their feelings. There are various postpartum depression support groups available in local communities, often sponsored by non-profit organizations or hospitals. Also, support information is available by calling the PPD helpline. Women can find a local support group by calling the Kristin Brooks Hope Center helpline at (800) 442-4673. For women who have thoughts of suicide, it is imperative to immediately call the toll-free 24-hour suicide hotline at (800) 784-2433.

Expected results

When a woman has supportive friends and family, mild postpartum depression usually disappears quickly. If depression becomes severe, a mother cannot care for herself and the baby, and in rare cases, hospitalization may be necessary. However, medication, counseling, and support from others usually work to cure even severe depression in three to six months.

Prevention

Exercise, including yoga, can help enhance a new mother's emotional wellbeing. New mothers should also try to cultivate good sleeping habits and learn to rest when they feel physically or emotionally tired. It is important for a woman to learn to recognize her own warning signs of fatigue and respond to them by taking a break.

Resources

BOOKS

Poulin, Sandra. *The Mother-to-Mother Postpartum Depression Support Book*. New York: Berkley Trade, 2006.

Shields, Brooke. *Down Came the Rain: My Journey Through Postpartum Depression*. New York: Hyperion Books, 2006.

Venis, Joyce A., and Suzanne McCloskey. *Postpartum Depression Demystified: An Essential Guide for Understanding the Most Common Complication After Childbirth*. New York: Marlowe, 2007.

PERIODICALS

Gaby, Alan R. "Fish Oil for Postpartum Depression." *Townsend Letter: The Examiner of Alternative Medicine* (October 2006): 40.

Hung, Chich-Hsiu. "The Hung Postpartum Stress Scale." *Journal of Nursing Scholarship* (Spring 2007): 71(4).

Klotter, Jule. "Exercise and Postpartum Depression." *Townsend Letter: The Examiner of Alternative Medicine* (October 2007): 42(2).

McGinnis, Marianne. "Baby Blues? Get Help Early." *Prevention* (January 2006): 107.

Ramashwar, S. "In China, Women Who Give Birth to Girls Face an Increased Risk of Postpartum Depression." *International Family Planning Perspectives* (December 2007): 191(2).

ORGANIZATIONS

Kristin Brooks Hope Center, 615 Seventh St. NE, Washington, DC, 20002, (202) 536-3200, (800) 442-4673, http:www//hopeline.com.

National Institute of Mental Health, 6001 Executive Blvd., Room 8184, MSC 9663, Bethesda, MD, 20892, (866) 615-6464, http://www.nimh.nih.gov.

Postpartum Support International, PO Box 60931, Santa Barbara, CA, 93160, (805) 967-7636, (800) 944-4773, http://www.postpartum.net.

Paula Ford-Martin
Ken R. Wells

Post-traumatic stress disorder

Definition

Post-traumatic **stress** disorder (PTSD) is a debilitating psychological condition triggered by a traumatic event, such as rape, war, a terrorist act, sudden or violent death of a loved one, natural disaster, or catastrophic accident. It is marked by recurring memories or thoughts of the event, "blunting" of emotions, increased arousal, and sometimes severe personality changes.

Description

Officially termed post-traumatic stress disorder since 1980, descriptions of post-traumatic stress were

Common characteristics that increase the risk of developing PTSD

Female

Middle-aged (40 to 60 years old)

No experience coping with traumatic events

Ethnic minority

Lower socioeconomic status

Children in the home

Having family members with PTSD

Pre-existing psychiatric condition

Primary exposure to the trauma

Living in traumatized community

Lacking a good support system (close family and friends)

(Illustration by Corey Light. Cengage Learning, Gale)

documented as early as the Civil War and in nineteenth century train crash victims. In the period between World War I and II, a condition known as "shell shock" or "battle fatigue" was recognized. Initially, it was thought that shrapnel entered the brain during battle explosions and caused small brain hemorrhages. When symptoms occurred in war veterans who had not been exposed to explosions, it was then often viewed as a character flaw.

In the 1970s, during and after the Vietnam War, post-traumatic stress received more serious research and documentation. In 1989, the National Center for Post-traumatic Stress Disorder was established in the U.S. Department of Veterans Affairs. Another benchmark was its addition to the third edition of the Diagnostic and Statistical Manual of Mental Disorders (DSM-III) published by the American Psychiatric Association. In the past 20 years, those who have been diagnosed with PTSD have been rape victims, victims of violent crimes, and survivors of natural disasters, terrorist attacks, and random shootings in schools and the workplace.

Although people of all ages, cultures, and socioeconomic backgrounds can develop PTSD if exposed to a life-threatening event, statistics gathered from past events indicate that the risk of PTSD increases in order of the following factors:

- female gender
- middle-aged (40 to 60 years old)
- little or no experience coping with traumatic events
- ethnic minority
- lower socioeconomic status
- children in the home
- women with spouses exhibiting PTSD symptoms
- pre-existing psychiatric conditions
- primary exposure to the event including injury, life-threatening situation, and loss
- living in a traumatized community

For example, over a third of the survivors of the 1995 Murrah Federal Building bombing in Oklahoma City developed PTSD and over half showed signs of **anxiety**, **depression**, and alcohol abuse. More than a year later, Oklahomans in general had an increased use of alcohol and tobacco products, as well as PTSD symptoms.

Children are also susceptible to PTSD and their risk is increased exponentially as their exposure to the event increases. Children experiencing abuse, the death of a parent, or those located in a community suffering a traumatic event can develop PTSD. Two years after the Oklahoma City bombing, 16% of children in a 100-mile radius of Oklahoma City with no direct exposure to the bombing had increased symptoms of PTSD. Weak parental response to the event, having a parent suffering from PTSD, and increased exposure to the event via the media all increase the possibility of the child developing PTSD symptoms.

Causes and symptoms

Specific causes for the onset of post-traumatic stress disorder are not clearly defined, although experts suspect it may be influenced both by the severity of the event, by the person's personality and genetic make-up, and by whether or not the event was expected. First response emergency personnel and those directly involved in the event or families who have lost loved ones in the event are most like to experience PTSD.

People exposed to mass destruction or death, toxic contamination, the sudden or violent death of a loved one, or the loss of home or community, are also at high risk for PTSD. Victims of human-caused trauma have a higher incidence of PTSD than those of natural disasters. Among rape and Holocaust survivors, the rate of PTSD is 50%.

A sampling of the types of traumatic events and the percentage of those exposed to them who develop PTSD includes:

- natural disaster, 4–5%
- mass shooting, 28%
- plane crash into hotel, 29%
- bombing, 34%

For men, events most likely to trigger PTSD are rape, combat exposure, childhood neglect, and childhood physical abuse. For women, these events are rape, sexual molestation, physical attack, threat with a weapon, and childhood physical abuse.

A related condition, Acute Stress Disorder (ASD), which occurs two days to four weeks after a traumatic event, is thought to be an indicator of the occurrence of PTSD. This is especially true if the following factors are present:

- lack of emotional and social support
- the presence of other stressors such as fatigue, cold, hunger, fear, uncertainty, and loss
- continued difficulties at the scene of the event
- lack of information about the event
- lack of self-determination
- treatment given in an authoritarian or impersonal manner
- lack of follow-up

PTSD symptoms are distinct and prolonged stress reactions that naturally occur during a highly stressful event. Common symptoms are:

- hyperalertness
- fear and anxiety
- nightmares and flashbacks
- sight, sound, and smell recollection
- avoidance of recall situations
- anger and irritability
- guilt
- depression
- increased substance abuse
- negative world view
- decreased sexual activity

Symptoms usually begin within three months of the trauma, although sometimes PTSD does not develop until years after the initial trauma occurred. Once the symptoms begin, they may fade away again within six months. Others suffer with the symptoms for far longer and in some cases, the problem may become chronic.

Among the most troubling symptoms of PTSD are flashbacks, which can be triggered by sounds, smells, feelings, or images. During a flashback, the person relives the traumatic event and may completely lose touch with reality, suffering through the trauma for minutes or hours at a time, believing that the traumatizing event is actually happening all over again.

Research conducted in the late 20th century suggests that PTSD sufferers undergo neurological and physiological changes stemming from altered brain activity. A decrease in size of the hippocampus (one of two seahorse-shaped parts of the brain generally believed by scientists to pay an essential role in formation of new memories) may affect the processing and integration of memory while abnormal activation of the amygdala (almond-shaped parts of the brain believed to have strong connections to mental and physical reactions) may be tied to fear response. This altered brain activity can lead to hyper-arousal of the sympathetic nervous system, increased sensitivity of the startle reflex, and sleep abnormalities.

The hormone levels of PTSD patients may also show abnormalities: for example, high levels of thyroid, epinephrine, and natural opiates coupled with low levels of cortisol. Blunted, or depressed, responses to a trauma may be the result of the body's increased production of opiates (narcotic-like hormones that induce mental lethargy), which masks the emotional **pain**.

People with post traumatic stress disorder are also like to suffer from other psychiatric disorders. Eighty-eight percent of men and 79% of women with PTSD meet the diagnostic criteria for other disorders. Physical ailments such as headaches, gastrointestinal ailments, immune system weaknesses, **dizziness**, chest pain, and general body discomfort are also common in PTSD sufferers.

Diagnosis

Consultation with a mental health professional for diagnosis and a plan of treatment is always advised. Many of the responses to trauma, such as shock, terror, irritability, blame, guilt, grief, sadness, emotional numbing, and feelings of helplessness, are natural reactions. For most people, resilience is an overriding factor and trauma effects diminish within six to sixteen months. It is when these responses continue or become debilitating that PTSD is often diagnosed. The third edition of the Diagnostic and Statistical Manual of Mental Disorders (DSM-III) outlined three forms of the disorder:

- Acute: onset within six months of the event and lasting less than six months
- Chronic: symptoms lasting six months or more
- Delayed: onset at least six months after the event

As outlined in DSM-IV, the exposure to a traumatic stressor means that an individual experienced, witnessed or was confronted by an event or events involving death or threat of death, serious injury or the threat of bodily harm to oneself or others. The individual's response must involve intense fear, helplessness, or horror. A two-pronged approach to evaluation is considered the best way to make a valid diagnosis because it can gauge under-reporting or over-reporting of symptoms. The two primary forms are structured interviews and self-report questionnaires. Spouses, partners and other family members may be interviewed. Because the evaluation may involve subtle reminders of the trauma in order to gauge a patient's reactions, individuals should ask for a full description of the evaluation process beforehand. Asking what results can be expected from the evaluation is also advised.

A number of structured interview forms have been devised to facilitate the diagnosis of post traumatic stress disorder:

- The Clinician Administered PTSD Scale (CAPS) developed by the National Center for PTSD
- The Structured Clinical Interview for DSM (SCID)
- Anxiety Disorders Interview Schedule-Revised (ADIS)
- PTSD-Interview
- Structured Interview for PTSD (SI-PTSD)
- PTSD Symptom Scale Interview (PSS-I)

Self-reporting checklists provide scores to represent the level of stress experienced. Some of the most commonly used checklists are:

- The PTSD Checklist (PCL), which has one list for civilians and one for military personnel and veterans
- Impact of Event Scale-Revised (IES-R)
- Keane PTSD Scale of the MMPI-2
- The Mississippi Scale for Combat Related PTSD and the Mississippi Scale for Civilians
- The Post Traumatic Diagnostic Scale (PDS)
- The Penn Inventory for Post-Traumatic Stress
- Los Angeles Symptom Checklist (LASC)

Treatment

A definitive treatment does not yet exist for PTSD nor is there a known cure. However, a number of therapies such as cognitive-behavior therapy, group therapy, and exposure therapy are showing promise. Cognitive-behavioral therapy focuses on changing specific actions and thoughts with the help of **relaxation** training and breathing techniques. In exposure therapy, the person relives the traumatic event repeatedly in a controlled environment and then works through the trauma.

A treatment technique known as eye movement desensitization and reprocessing (EMDR) has been employed with some success to treat PTSD. EMDR involves desensitizing the patient to his or her traumatic memories by associating a series of eye movements with both negative and positive events and emotions. The specific eye movements associated with the negative memories are thought to help the brain process the event and come to terms with the trauma. EDMR should only be performed by a healthcare practitioner, usually a clinical psychologist, certified in the technique.

Relaxation training, which is sometimes called anxiety management training, includes breathing exercises and similar techniques intended to help the patient prevent hyperventilation and relieve the muscle tension associated with the fight-or-flight reaction of anxiety. **Yoga**, aikido, t'ai chi, and **dance therapy** help patients work with the physical as well as the emotional tensions that either promote anxiety or are created by the anxiety.

Other alternative or complementary therapies are based on physiological and/or energetic understanding of how the trauma is imprinted in the body. These therapies affect a release of stored emotions and resolution of them by working with the body rather than merely talking through the experience. One example of such a therapy is Somatic Experiencing (SE), developed by Dr. Peter Levine. SE is a short-term, biological, body-oriented approach to PTSD or other trauma. This approach heals by emphasizing physiological and emotional responses, without re-traumatizing the person, without placing the person on medication, and without the long hours of conventional therapy.

When used in conjunction with therapies that address the underlying cause of PTSD, relaxation therapies such as **hydrotherapy**, **massage therapy**, and **aromatherapy** are useful to some patients in easing PTSD symptoms. **Essential oils** of lavender, chamomile, neroli, sweet marjoram, and ylang-ylang are commonly recommended by aromatherapists for stress relief and anxietyreduction.

Research into the prevention of PTSD is also undergoing intensive research. The National Mental Health Association provides RAPID grants that allow researchers to visit disaster scenes to study acute effects and the effectiveness of early intervention. Rapid disaster relief and positive community response appear to be key. Not identifying individual survivors as "victims" also seems to help. Debriefing survivors as quickly as possible after the event can stem the development of PTSD symptoms.

Allopathic treatment

As of mid-2004, allopathic (medical practice that combats disease with remedies to produce effects different from those produced by the disease) treatment consists of a combination of medication along with supportive and cognitive-behavioral therapies. Effective medications include anxiety-reducing medications and antidepressants, especially the selective serotonin reuptake inhibitors (SSRIs) such as fluoxetine (Prozac) and sertraline (Zoloft). In 2001, the U.S. Food and Drug Administration (FDA) approved Zoloft as a long-term treatment for PTSD. In a controlled study, Zoloft was effective in safely improving symptoms of PTSD over a period of 28 weeks and reducing the risk of relapse. Sleep problems can be lessened by brief treatment with an anti-anxiety drug such as a benzodiazepine like alprazolam (Xanax). However, long-tem use of these drugs can lead to disturbing side effects, such as increased anger. The new research into the biological changes manifested in PTSD patients is leading to additional research on drugs used to monitor hormone levels and brain activity.

Expected results

With appropriate medication, emotional support, and counseling, most people show significant improvement. Behavior therapies can help reduce negative thought patterns and self talk. The patient typically moves back and forth through three recovery phases:

- Phase One, Safety: the elimination and/or management of dangerous behaviors and/or relationships. Becoming less fearful of thoughts, feelings, and dissociative (separated from the main stream of consciousness) episodes
- Phase Two: resolution of traumatic memory processing. Developing a narrative account of the trauma without becoming re-traumatized
- Phase Three: personality re-integration and rehabilitation

Successful treatment depends in part on whether or not the trauma was unexpected, the severity of the trauma, if the trauma was chronic (such as for victims of sexual abuse), and the person's inherent personality and genetic makeup. However, prolonged exposure to severe trauma such as experienced by victims of prolonged physical or sexual abuse and survivors of the Holocaust may cause permanent psychological scars.

Resources

BOOKS

Knaster, Mirka. *Discovering the Body's Wisdom: A Guide to Exploring Bodyways.* New York: Bantam Books, 1996.

Shapiro, Francine, Ph.D., and Margot Silk Forrest. *The Breakthrough Therapy for Overcoming Anxiety, Stress, and Trauma.* New York: Basic Books, 1997.

PERIODICALS

DiGiovanni, C. "Domestic Terrorism with Chemical or Biological Agents: Psychiatric Aspects." *American Journal of Psychiatry–* (1999): 15001505.

Kessler, R., et al. "Post-traumatic Stress Disorder in the National Comorbidity Survey." *Archives of General Psychiatry–* (1996): 10481060.

North, C., S. Nixon, S. Hariat, S. Mallonee et al. "Psychiatric Disorders Among Survivors of the Oklahoma City Bombing." *Journal of the American Medical Association–* (1999): 755762.

Pfefferbaum, B., R. Gurwitch, N. McDonald et al. "Post-traumatic Stress Among Children After the Death of a Friend or Acquaintance in a Terrorist Bombing." *Psychiatric Services–*(2000): 386388.

"Sertraline HCl Approved for Long-Term Use." *Women's Health Weekly* (September 20, 2001).

Sloan, M. "Response to Media Coverage of Terrorism." *Journal of Conflict Resolution–* (2000): 508522.

Smith, D, E., Christiansen, R. Vincent, and N. Hann. "Population Effects of the Bombing of Oklahoma City." *Journal of Oklahoma State Medical Association–* (1999): 193198.

ORGANIZATIONS

American Psychiatric Association. 1000 Wilson Blvd., Ste. 1825, Arlington, VA 22209-3901. (703) 907-7300. http://www.psych.org.

Anxiety Disorders Association of America. 8730 Georgia Ave., Ste. 600, Silver Spring, MD 20910. (240) 485-1001. http://www.adaa.org.

Freedom From Fear. 308 Seaview Ave., Staten Island, NY 10305. (718) 351-1717. http://www.freedomfrom fear.com.

International Society for Traumatic Stress Studies, 60 Revere Dr., Ste. 500, Northbrook, IL 60062. (847) 480-9028. http://www.istss.org.

National Anxiety Foundation. 3135 Custer Dr., Lexington, KY 40517. (606) 272-7166. http://www.lexington-on-line.com.

National Institute of Mental Health. 6001 Executive Blvd, Rm. 8184, MSC 9663, Bethesda, MD 20892. (866) 615-6464. http://www.nimh.nih.org.

National Mental Health Association. 2001 N. Beauregard St., 12th floor, Alexandria, VA 22311. (800) 969-NMHA. http://www.nmha.org.

OTHER

"Effects of Traumatic Stress in a Disaster Situation." *National Center for PTSD*. [cited May 2, 2004]. http://www.ncptsd. org/facts/disasters/fs_effects_disaster.htmlgt;.

"How is PTSD Measured?" National Center for PTSD. [cited May 2, 2004]. http://www.ncptsd.org/facts/treatment/ fs/ lay/assess.htmlgt;.

Mary McNulty

Potassium

Description

Potassium is one of the electrolytes essential to the smooth running of the human body; in fact, just about all bodily functions depend on it to some extent. It is also one of the most abundant minerals in the body, constituting 70% of the positive ions inside cells; the rest are a mixture of **sodium**, **magnesium**, **calcium**, **arginine**, and others. Potassium is distributed to the cells by a process of passive diffusion and is regulated by an enzyme called adenosinetriphosphatase together with the level of sodium concentration inside the cell. Potassium and sodium are antagonistic, which means that an imbalance of one will automatically cause an imbalance of the other; normally potassium should predominate inside the cell.

General use

Potassium is necessary for normal cell respiration. A deficiency can cause decreased levels of oxygen, which will reduce the efficiency of cell function. Adequate supplies of potassium are also required to regulate heartbeat, facilitate normal muscle contraction, regulate the transfer of nutrients to cells, and regulate kidney function and stomach juice secretion, among other functions. One of the most important uses of potassium in the body is in the process of nerve transmission, as it is a cofactor catalyst for the activation of several enzyme systems, but since only minute amounts are required for these processes, deficiency in this respect is unlikely.

Potassium is thought to be therapeutically useful in many ways, including assisting in the treatment of **alcoholism** and **acne**, alleviating **allergies**, promoting the healing of **burns**, and preventing high blood pressure. It can also help with such problems as congestive heart failure, **chronic fatigue syndrome**, or **kidney stones**. People suffering from any of the above conditions should consider increasing their intake of potassium after talking to a professional.

Symptoms of potassium deficiency

A deficiency of potassium in the blood is referred to as hypokalemia and manifests itself in many ways. Among the most serious symptoms are arthritis, high blood pressure, **heart disease**, **stroke**, **cancer**, and even **infertility**, as potassium constitutes a vital element of seminal fluid.

Potassium deficiency will increase acid levels in the body, lowering the natural pH, which will have far reaching effects. Lack of potassium can also aggravate problems caused by lack of protein. If potassium levels are down, the liver cannot operate normally, particularly regarding transformation of glucose to glycogen. A healthy liver should have about twice as much potassium as sodium.

Potassium deficiency can cause problems with the formation of connective tissue and can render normally strong body tissue vulnerable to all kinds of problems. The collagen of a healthy person is approximately as strong as steel, and the strength of bone tissue can be likened to that of cast **iron**. Lack of potassium may create a susceptibility to **fractures**, skin lesions that do not heal, or other connective tissue problems. So important is potassium for the protection of collagen that many natural health gurus claim that along with other vital nutrients, it constitutes an essential element of protection against premature **aging**. In the 1920s, German physician Max Gerson became the first person ever to cure lupus lesions with a diet entirely raw fruit and vegetables designed to reduce abnormally high sodium levels and raise potassium levels to normal.

Potassium is essential to the efficient processing of foods in the body; without it they cannot be broken down into the proper compounds. This condition can lead to rheumatism, and is one reason why adequate potassium prevents rheumatism.

Potassium requirements

In the past potassium was more plentiful in the diet than salt, but gradually, the situation has been reversed. The widespread lack of potassium in modern **diets** is largely due to modern processing and high levels of salt added to most processed foods. Cooking and processing remove potassium, and added salt further robs the body of vital potassium. This departure from traditional cooking of fresh homegrown fruit and vegetables is likely the cause of many health problems faced by modern society.

Who needs potassium supplements?

Those who may need to take potassium supplements include women who take oral contraceptives, abusers of alcohol or drugs, smokers, athletes, workers whose job involves physical exertion, patients who have had their gastrointestinal tract surgically removed, anyone suffering from any degree of malabsorption syndrome, and vegetarians. People who have eating disorders, especially bulimia and anorexia, are particularly at risk of damage due to low potassium levels. Also, individuals who have been ill, anyone who has undergone surgery, and those who are taking cortisone or **digitalis** preparations, and those suffering from high levels of **stress** will probably have low potassium levels.

The U.S. Food and Drug Administration (FDA) has established a Daily Reference Value (recommended daily intake) of potassium as 3,500 mg. The actual average daily intake of potassium for Americans ranges significantly from a low of about 1,200 mg/day to as high as 4,000 mg/day. However, in general, nutritionists recommend reducing salt intake and ensuring adequate supply by increasing the amount of fresh fruit and vegetables in the diet.

If individuals feel that they may be suffering from a potassium deficiency but would like to make sure before taking supplements, there are a variety of laboratory tests that can be conducted. These include serum-potassium determinations (although these may be unreliable unless levels are very low), serum creatinine, electrocardiograms, serum-pH determinations, whole blood, sublingual cell smears, and red blood cell potassium level determinations.

Preparations

The best sources of potassium are fresh natural foods. Supplements may have side effects and large doses must be taken to approach the levels of potassium that can be obtained from food; the average tablet contains about 90 mg, for example, and a medium banana contains 500 mg. Vegetables containing the highest levels of potassium are generally those containing the lowest levels of starch. Seaweed has amazingly high potassium content, containing roughly ten times as much as leafy vegetables, but it also contains a large amount of mineral salt. Green coconut milk is another good source of potassium.

Plentiful sources of potassium

There is a great variety of natural foods that are an excellent source of potassium. These include avocados; bananas; chard; citrus fruits; juices such as grapefruit, tomato, and orange; dried lentils; green leafy vegetables; milk; molasses; nuts such as almonds, brazils, cashews, peanuts, pecans, and walnuts; parsnips; dried peaches; potatoes; raisins; sardines; spinach; and wholegrain cereals.

Cooking

Boiling food in water is a sure way to lose the potassium in it, unless it is to make soup. Baking and broiling are ways in which food can be cooked while at the same time preserving the potassium content; indeed, these methods preserve all the nutrients apart from **vitamin C** and some of the B vitamins, which are destroyed by heat. Broiling also oxidizes **essential fatty acids**. Stir-frying is also a good way of preserving nutrients. It is important to vary the intake of potassium rich foods in order to ensure adequate intake of other nutrients and to avoid the possibility of toxicity, as some vegetables contain elements that are toxic if they are eaten in large amounts (oxalic acid in rhubarb, for example). It is important to note that freezing also depletes potassium levels in foods.

RECIPE FOR POTASSIUM BROTH. Many variations of potassium broth can be found, and most natural health practitioners recommend one version or another, but the main constituents are the following vegetables, generally any vegetable of choice can be added to this base.

Ingredients

- 2 lb potatoes
- 1 lb carrots
- 1/2 lb peas
- bones for stock, or a vegetable bouillon cube
- 4 oz cracked wheat or pearl barley

First, in a stainless steel pan, boil the stock bones, if they are used. After about one hour, add the remaining ingredients and continue to simmer in plenty of water for about another hour. It is preferable to use the potatoes and carrots well scrubbed, but with their skins on, as this retains valuable nutrients. Keep any unused soup in the refrigerator.

Potassium supplements

Potassium supplements come in either tablet or liquid form, and anything over 390 mg requires a prescription in the United States. Enteric-coated tablets have been known to cause ulcers, as they do not dissolve until they reach the intestines and may prove too concentrated for the undefended intestinal wall. To be on the safe side, supplements should be taken with a glass of juice. Slow-release enteric-coated supplements are available, which decrease the danger of ulcers. Potassium gluconate is the ideal supplement, as it more closely resembles the potassium found in plants. Small divided doses should be taken, as opposed to one large dose, when treating a potassium deficiency. Athletic drinks are an electrolyte replacement and as such contain potassium. Potassium supplements should be kept in a cool, dry place, out of direct light. They should not be frozen and should not be kept in the bathroom medicine cabinet as heat and moisture may reduce their effectiveness.

Precautions

In general, the multitude of nutrients that humans require in order to stay healthy are synergistic, which means they are interdependent. If one is depleted, it is highly likely others will be deficient. Many nutrients, for example, require the presence of either calcium or vitamin C for efficient use by the body, and if individuals have a deficiency of any of the B vitamins, they almost certainly will have a deficiency in the B vitamins in general, as these occur together in nature. Given the factor of synergy, it is very unwise to take large amounts of any one nutrient without making sure that the full spectrum of nutrients is plentifully available for the body to use, which can best be achieved by making sure that a large proportion of the daily diet consists of raw fruit and vegetables, whole grains, and unroasted nuts.

Of all the essential nutrients that are commonly taken as supplements, potassium is perhaps the most dangerous. Only 14 grams of potassium can cause death under certain circumstances, particularly when intake is low at other times. When potassium intake is restricted, somehow the mechanism for utilizing it is altered, so that large amounts cannot be processed.

Just the right amount of potassium is essential. Too much or too little can cause **muscle spasms and cramps** if a calcium deficiency also exists. Thus, it is important to ensure adequate intake of calcium and **vitamin D**, which will promote the uptake of calcium in the body.

Many sufferers of degenerative diseases such as **tuberculosis**, cancer, and arthritis, suffer from high serum potassium levels. This is not because they have too much serum, but because the disease affects body functions in such a way that it throws off this valuable nutrient instead of using it. In such cases, natural sources of potassium, such as fresh fruit or vegetable juice, can be more effective than supplements.

Potassium and heart disease

Potassium has been recommended for the treatment of heart disease since the 1930s, but some heart disease that is due to malnutrition does not respond to potassium. Indeed, because of the impaired ability of the body to take up potassium, it can be dangerous. Most heart disease patients of the Western world, however, can benefit from an increase in potassium levels.

Potassium and arthritis

Some individuals who begin to eat a well-balanced selection of fresh vegetables and fruits and eliminate a large proportion of processed, denatured foods begin to feel amazingly well very quickly, as the potassium/sodium balance in the body is restored. Tiredness and other symptoms, such as arthritis, are soon replaced with renewed energy and vigor, and the body is able to replenish itself and finds new strength. However, potassium is only partially successful at treating **osteoarthritis**.

Side effects

Those who are taking potassium-sparing diuretics, such as spironolactone, triamterene, or amiloride should not take potassium supplements. Anyone allergic to potassium supplements or those who have kidney disease should not take them either. Those suffering from Addison's disease, heart disease, intestinal blockage, stomach ulcers, those using medication for heart disease, or taking diuretics, or who are above the age of 55, should consult a doctor before taking potassium supplements. There are no contradictions for pregnant or breast feeding women, although they should not take mega-doses.

ECG and kidney function tests can be affected by potassium supplementation. A doctor should be informed if one is taking potassium supplements. However, supplementation will not affect blood tests, unless they are to measure serum-potassium levels.

Symptoms of potassium overdose

Overdose symptoms of potassium include listlessness, mental confusion, tingling of limbs, weakness, pallid complexion, low blood pressure, and an irregular or fast heartbeat. These symptoms can progress to a drop in blood pressure, convulsion, coma, and eventually cardiac arrest, and can also be triggered by any kind of shock to the system. If any of the above symptoms occur, or in cases of bloody stool (may appear black and tarry), or difficulty in breathing or **nausea**, medical help should be sought immediately.

High serum-potassium is the major problem with shock and is the major cause of death in cases of shock or injury. This is a life-threatening situation, and self treatment is not appropriate.

If such an emergency occurs and medical help is not available, a glass of water containing half a teaspoon of salt, a quarter of a teaspoon of bicarbonate soda and a little honey will help. Potassium supplements should be taken with extreme care in cases of dehydration, as this can be fatal. Adequate liquids, particularly juice, should always accompany the supplement.

Interactions

Care should be taken when taking potassium supplements in conjunction with diuretics. A practitioner should be consulted. A doctor should be informed when a patient is taking potassium supplements. In addition, the following are known to react with potassium:

- Amilorid: causes a dangerous rise in blood potassium
- Atropine: increases the possibility of intestinal ulcers, which may be caused by potassium supplements
- Belladonna: increases possibility of intestinal ulcers
- Calcium: increases likelihood of heartbeat irregularities
- Captopril: increases likelihood of potassium overdose
- Digitalis preparations: may cause irregular heartbeat
- Enalapril: increases chance of overdose
- Laxatives: may decrease effectiveness of potassium (due to the fact that they leach potassium from the body)
- Spironolactone: increases blood potassium
- Triamterene: increases blood potassium
- Vitamin B_{12}: slow release supplements may decrease the absorption of vitamin B_{12}, increasing requirements

Resources

BOOKS

Duyff, Roberta Larson. *American Dietetic Association Complete Food and Nutrition Guide*, 3rd ed. New York: Wiley, 2006.

Haas, Elson M., and Buck Levin. *Staying Healthy with Nutrition*. Berkeley, CA: Celestial Arts, 2006.

Hark, Lisa, and Darwin Deen. *Nutrition for Life*. Harlow, Essex, UK: DK Adult, 2005.

PERIODICALS

Ferrara, L. A., et al. "Fast Food Versus Slow Food and Hypertension Control." *Current Hypertension Reviews* (February 2008): 30–35.

Geleijnse, Johanna M., et al. "Sodium and Potassium Intake and Risk of Cardiovascular Events and All-cause Mortality: The Rotterdam Study." *European Journal of Epidemiology* (November 2007): 763–770.

Lin, Shih-Hua, and Mitchell Halperin. "Hypokalemia: A Practical Approach to Diagnosis and Its Genetic Basis." *Current Medicinal Chemistry* (June 2007): 1551–1565.

Schaefer, Timothy J., and Robert W. Wolford. "Disorders of Potassium." *Emergency Medical Clinics of North America* (August 2005): 723–747.

OTHER

"Potassium in Diet." *New York Times,* Health Guide, March 2, 2007. http://health.nytimes.com/health/guides/nutrition/potassium-in-diet/overview.html. (February 20, 2008).

Patricia Skinner
David Edward Newton, Ed.D.

Pranic healing

Definition

Pranic healing encompasses a broad array of therapeutic approaches, both ancient and modern, based on the notion that illnesses of body or mind involve an imbalance and/or blockage in the flow of vital life energy. In ancient India, this energy was known as *prana*, as it still is in the contemporary practice of yoga and **Ayurvedic medicine**. Traditional Chinese medicine uses the term *qi* to describe this vital energy. Pranic healing seeks, by widely varying means, to strengthen and equalize the pranic flow. And, as the number of alternative therapies has mushroomed during the last several decades, the concept of prana/qi has become almost a common denominator among approaches that may otherwise seem wildly diverse.

Origins

The belief in a fundamental life force flowing through the human body (and, by extension, through all living things) is an ancient one, common to many healing systems worldwide. More recently, many Western therapies have incorporated a similar concept.

Prana

The concept of prana evolved thousands of years ago in India, apparently in connection with esoteric religious practices. A central concept in both yoga and Ayurveda (an ancient healing system), it is discussed in the earliest written sources for these disciplines—the *Yoga Sutras* of Patanjali and the ancient Hindu scriptures known as *vedas*.

Qi

As with prana, the origins of the concept of qi are lost in the distant past. **Acupuncture**, which uses needles inserted at specific points to stimulate the flow of qi, has been practiced extensively in China for thousands of years. Archaeologists have unearthed stone acupuncture needles dated to around 3000 B.C. The *Nei Jing* (or *Classic of Internal Medicine*), the oldest known text that discusses the theoretical basis of traditional Chinese medicine, is believed to have been written roughly 2,000 years ago. In addition to acupuncture, one type of Chinese massage is known as qi healing or healing with external qi.

Benefits

Because it is a general conceptual approach rather than a specific healing modality, pranic healing cannot be said to provide a specific list of benefits; although pranayama, or yogic breathing, is said to directly benefit the respiratory system. Some practitioners might argue that dealing with imbalances at such a fundamental level, rather than treating symptoms at a superficial level, benefits the patient by getting to the root of the problem and avoiding the risk of merely masking it by treating symptoms. Pranic healing also makes a good fit with the concept of wellness, as opposed to

the mere absence of disease, that underlies many alternative therapies.

Description

The diverse array of therapies loosely described as pranic healing may be grouped under several subheads, depending on both their origins and the nature of the healing techniques they employ.

Traditional healing systems

Both Ayurveda and **traditional Chinese medicine** are ancient medicinal systems that view health and disease in terms of blockage and flow of vital energy. Both use various diagnostic techniques, herbs/diet, and other treatments (notably acupuncture, therapeutic **exercise**, and massage, in the case of TCM) to stimulate and balance energy flow.

Pranayama

Practitioners of pranayama, or yogic breathing, believe that prana is moving when the human breath, which is a manifestation of universal prana, is flowing freely. When the body's energy is blocked, this stagnation can lead to illness and disease. Because Ayurvedic medicine considers prana a kind of nutrient that one can take in through the breath, breathing exercises play an important role in health promotion in Ayurveda. Pranayama soothes the nervous system, induces **relaxation**, regulates respiration, and balances the hemispheres of the brain. The major technique of pranayama is alternate nostril breathing.

Bodywork

Over the last century or so, more especially in recent decades, a number of alternative therapies have emerged that manipulate the body and/or noninvasively stimulate specific points to promote wellness, achieve healing, and strengthen the vital force. Among the many such modalities are reflexology, **polarity therapy**, breema, and **reiki**.

Nonphysical approaches

The many different schools of meditation generally involve some combination of breathing, chanting, special postures, and mental exercises to produce enhanced or altered states of being. The focus of different **meditation** techniques can range from simple relaxation to mainstream religious devotion to esoteric spiritual evolution.

Exercise systems

Various ancient systems—including **yoga**, qigong and t'ai chi—represent a blending of exercise, therapeutic benefits, and spiritual path. To the extent that these disciplines are viewed as healing modalities, they can be said to represent forms of pranic healing. Qigong, for example, literally means "energy cultivation." In each case, specific postures and/or movements—practiced daily, often in combination with breathing exercises—are said to encourage optimal energy flow.

Preparations

Preparations for the various types of pranic healing range from wearing comfortable non-binding clothing for bodywork to fasting and spiritual preparation for certain forms of meditation. Students of yoga are advised not to eat a full meal for two to three hours prior to a yoga class because some of the postures are uncomfortable on a full stomach.

Precautions

Despite the widespread adoption of the concept of prana by contemporary alternative therapies, it is not accepted in Western scientific circles. Although controlled studies have confirmed specific therapeutic benefits for both yoga and acupuncture—which, in different ways, are based on the idea of pranic healing—there is as yet no generally accepted scientific evidence for the theories that underlie these systems. Because so many different techniques and practitioners are said to employ some form of pranic healing, it can be difficult even to determine what, exactly, is meant by their respective uses of this terminology. And there is always the risk that a focus on maximizing pranic flow might interfere with more mainstream attempts to address tangible physiological problems.

Given the variety of practices and techniques that can be classified under pranic healing, persons who are interested in a specific form should find out beforehand what level of physical exercise is involved (if any) and what belief system (if any) underlies the practice. Some forms of bodywork may be too strenuous for people with heart disease, fragile bones, or other major health problems. In addition, some forms of pranic healing may produce physical or psychological phenomena that can startle those not expecting them. For example, a type of yoga known as kundalini yoga works with energy stored at the base of the spine that is activated by exercises. Some people who have experienced the movement of kundalini energy found it unsettling because they had not been prepared for it. It may be helpful to seek out an experienced guide or mentor who has practiced a specific form of pranic healing long enough to be aware of possible reactions.

Side effects

The side effects of pranic healing can range from headaches and muscular soreness or stiffness after bodywork sessions to edginess or nervousness resulting from energies released by meditation. These side effects are usually mild and disappear after further practice.

Research and general acceptance

Some forms of pranic healing, including yoga, Ayurveda, and traditional Chinese medicine, have been intensively studied. The Office of Alternative Medicine of the National Institutes of Health (NIH) funds research into various forms of pranic healing, including mind/body interventions. The NIH's National Center for Complementary and Alternative Medicine (NCCAM) maintains a clearinghouse of information about alternative therapies and clinical trials of their effectiveness.

Training and certification

The training and certification of practitioners of prana healing ranges from the equivalent of medical school and government licensing for practitioners of traditional Chinese medicine to various forms of certification conferred by other professions or groups. **Breema** and reiki have formal degrees or certification programs. The Shalem Institute in Washington, DC, has a program for training spiritual directors in the mainstream Christian churches. There are various yoga institutes in the United States that provide courses of instruction for teachers of yoga.

Resources

BOOKS

Cassileth, Barrie R. *The Alternative Medicine Handbook.* New York: W.W. Norton & Company, 1998.

Gach, Michael Reed, with Carolyn Marco. *Acu-Yoga: Self Help Techniques to Relieve Tension.* Tokyo and New York: Japan Publications, Inc., 1998.

Stein, Diane. *Essential Reiki: A Complete Guide to an Ancient Healing Art,* Chapter VI, "Opening the Kundalini." Freedom, CA: The Crossing Press, Inc., 1995.

Svoboda, Robert, and Arnie Lade. *Tao and Dharma: Chinese Medicine and Ayurveda.* Twin Lakes, WI: Lotus Press, 1995.

Woodham, Anne, and Dr. David Peters. *DK Encyclopedia of Healing Therapies.* New York: DK Publishing, 1997.

ORGANIZATIONS

American Foundation of Traditional Chinese Medicine (AFTCM). 505 Beach Street. San Francisco, CA 94133. (415) 776-0502. Fax: (415) 392-7003. aftcm@earthlink.net.

National Center for Complementary and Alternative Medicine (NCCAM) Clearinghouse. P. O. Box 8218. Silver Spring, MD 20907-8218. TTY/TDY: (888) 644-6226.

Shalem Institute for Spiritual Formation. Mount Saint Alban. Washington, DC 20016.

Peter Gregutt

Praniyama *see* **Breath therapy**

Prayer and spirituality

Definition

Prayer is an act of communication with God or the Absolute. The spiritual beliefs of the person praying influence how the Absolute is perceived. For some, the Absolute is known as the Great Goddess. Others experience the Absolute as God, Allah, the Tao, the Universal Mind, Brahma, the Void, or a myriad of other forms. Spiritual, or faith, healing is the relief of illness through some type of religious belief system held by the sick person or by someone praying for them.

Origins

Prayer in one form or another is a spiritual practice found in nearly every culture. The use of prayer for healing is a vital principle of Christianity, Judaism, and Islam. Even in a non-theistic religion such as Buddhism, prayer is important in healing. In the traditional medicine of Mexico, **curanderismo**, health is perceived as a gift from God. Disease is seen as a punishment for sins and God's help is necessary for a cure. Patients may pray or make a spiritual pilgrimage as part of their medical treatment.

Spiritual healing in the West dates back to Biblical times, when some of the Hebrew prophets and Jesus used the power of prayer to heal the sick and injured. In the Jewish and Christian religions, praying for healing and medical miracles has been common for 3,000 years. The Christian tradition of faith healing formally developed out of a first-century prayer ritual for healing. Among contemporary Christians belonging to liturgical churches (Roman Catholics, Eastern Orthodox, Episcopalians, and Lutherans), spiritual healing is related to the sacraments of the Eucharist and anointing the sick, especially in churches, shrines, or sites where miracles have taken place. In the United States, numerous spiritual healing or faith healing groups and movements have appeared since the early 1800s, such as the Emmanuel movement and the John Alexander Dowie movement.

Christian Science, a movement that grew out of the Association formed by Mary Baker Eddy in 1876, holds faith healing at the core of its principles. Christian Scientists believe that death and illness are illusions. Eddy claimed that the end result of knowledge gained through Christian Science is the power to heal. Eddy's beliefs stemmed from her claims that she was cured of various illnesses in 1862 through massage, positive reinforcement, and mental healing. In 1875, she published *Science and Health*, the founding text of Christian Science.

People have always prayed, especially when sick or facing death. Still, despite the scientific evidence pointing to the effectiveness of prayer, it is not generally accepted as a treatment method by the Western medical community. Hippocrates, the father of modern medicine, believed that the mind and body were separate, and this point of view is the foundation of modern Western medicine.

Beginning in the seventeenth century, with the philosophy of René Descartes, the West has increasingly focused on a material view of the world. In medicine this has meant that an almost exclusive concentration on the physical aspects of disease. The contribution of emotions, thoughts, relationships, and spirituality to disease and health were either ignored or discounted. Only since the 1960s has there been an increase in interest about the effectiveness of prayer, **meditation**, and other mind-body approaches to health and healing.

Benefits

Perhaps the two most obvious benefits of faith healing is that the cost is minimal or zero, and that it involves no medications or medical devices. The medical, scientific, and religious communities almost unanimously agree that the human mind has a tremendous amount of untapped potential, including the power to heal physical and emotional ailments. A person's faith has a strong influence over his or her sense of well-being, ability to fight disease, and desire to get well, according to many researchers.

Prayer and other spiritual approaches can be particularly beneficial for people with stress-related disorders. Dr. Herbert Benson reports that meditative prayer can ease **anxiety**, mild **depression**, **substance abuse**, ulcers, **pain**, **nausea**, tension and migraine headaches, **infertility**, **premenstrual syndrome** (PMS), **insomnia**, and high blood pressure.

Prayer also plays an important role in helping people cope with difficult circumstances such as chronic illness and death. Prayer offers new meaning, purpose, hope, and a sense of guidance or control. These perceptions may help instill a fighting spirit, which has been reported to be an important factor in healing. Prayer can enrich the quality of one's life and also bring a feeling of peace and acceptance at the time of death. In addition, being part of a religious community can benefit patients by counteracting the social isolation that many sick people experience. Visits from friends or their spiritual leader are reminders that they are still part of a faith community and the larger human community.

More recently, researchers have recognized that prayer and spiritual practice are often related to people's connections with other creatures. Although the strength of the bond between humans and animals was first discussed in the context of people's grieving for dead pets, the human-animal connection and its role in spirituality is now being studied in its own right.

Description

Spiritual healing can involve a person praying alone by themselves for healing, one person praying for the healing of another person, or a group of persons praying for an ill person. It can involve formal ritual and the administration of the sacraments. Many Roman Catholic, Episcopal, and Lutheran congregations in the United States hold special Eucharists for healing; people can come for their own healing or in behalf of someone else.

Another common type of prayer is meditative prayer, which involves quieting the mind and focusing on an object, sound, movement, visualization, or simply the breath. Eastern types of meditative prayer may involve the repetition of a sound or phrase (mantra) or repeating the name of the Divine (japa). In India, there is a tradition of sacred temple dance as a form of meditative prayer. Western types of meditative prayer

may focus on quieting the mind and opening the heart to listen to God, often repeating prayer-like mantras. Dr. Herbert Benson has studied the effects of meditative prayer and found many significant health benefits.

Many healers also use prayer as a form of spiritual healing. Healing utilizing prayer can be done at a distance or through the laying on of hands. Spiritual healing is often not distinguished from psychic and energy healing, although some researchers do make a distinction. A spiritual healer is primarily concerned with a way of being, while other types of healers are concerned with the sick person's body and try to heal the physical symptoms of the disease. A spiritual healer allows an infinite consciousness, intelligence, and love (known as God, or nonlocal mind) to express itself through the healer. Other types of healers direct their energy outward and concentrate on replenishing or changing the energy flow of the patient. Energy healers do this by using their hands or fingers. Examples of subtle energy healing include **reiki**, **therapeutic touch**, **qigong**, and **pranic healing**. Psychic healers are able to relieve symptoms from a distance with their minds.

Preparations

People can pray at any time at any place. There is no advance preparation needed. However, most of the major religious traditions have developed certain patterns or practices associated with prayer, such as the use of rosaries, prayer books, or prayer shawls, that are meaningful to members of those traditions and help them to focus their attention when they pray. There are many clergy and spiritual leaders in the major faith traditions in the United States who can explain the various practices associated with prayer and why they can be helpful preparation for praying.

Precautions

Prayer and spirituality are not a substitute for other medical care. It is a complementary practice. Patients with serious illnesses should not choose prayer over other medical therapies and delay seeking necessary treatment.

There is also potential for harm in prayer and spiritual practices. Studies have shown that the growth of microorganisms can be retarded or inhibited depending upon the intention of the healer. There is also evidence of negative prayer in many different cultures.

Side effects

There are no known side effects of positive prayer, although negative energy focused on an individual has been shown to produce negative results.

Research and general acceptance

A 1996 Gallup poll showed that nine out of 10 Americans pray and 75% pray every day. The most common prayers were for family well-being (98%), prayers of thanks (94%), prayers for strength or guidance (92%), and prayers for forgiveness (92%). Eighty-two percent of Americans prayed for health and healing. Prayer is one of the most common complementary practices to standard medical treatment.

As of 1993, one American researcher had compiled a list of over 130 English-language clinical studies that have documented the effectiveness of faith and prayer in healing. For example, a 1987 study at the University of California Medical School in San Francisco involving 393 patients with heart problems were divided into two groups. One group had people pray for them at a distance (intercessory prayer), and the other group did not. The prayed-for group had fewer deaths, medical interventions, and complications than the control (not prayed-for) group. Dr. Larry Dossey, who was co-chair of the Panel on Mind/Body Interventions in the Office of Alternative Medicine at the National Institutes of Health in 2000, has written several books on laboratory studies of prayer and the historical reluctance of the mainstream scientific community to examine the connections between prayer and healing.

A number of studies, also at Duke University, have shown that the combination of active involvement in a religious community and frequent prayer has powerful effects on blood pressure and **smoking**.

Over the past three decades approximately 200 studies have examined the ability of prayer to affect human beings, animals, plants, and even microorganisms. Evidence so far shows that there is no one best way to pray.

Acceptance of prayer and spiritual healing among medical professionals varies. Some feel quite strongly that medicine and spiritual practice should not be mixed and that doctors and nurses should refer patients to religious professionals for spiritual needs. Surveys have shown, however, that as of 2002 a majority (about 76%) of physicians and nurses in the United States feel comfortable praying with patients if asked to do so, and 96% would discuss spiritual or religious matters with patients confronting a life-threatening illness or end-of-life issues.

Some researchers have attempted in recent years to develop scales for measuring spiritual experiences, in order to have some basis for comparing findings from different studies. Two such measures are the Daily Spiritual Experience Scale (DSES), a 16-item questionnaire; and the Ironson-Woods Spirituality-Religion (SR) Index, which measures four factors—faith in God, sense of peace, religious behavior, and compassionate view of others. The Ironson-Woods Index has been used to study the effects of spirituality and religious practice on the long-term survival of **AIDS** patients.

Training and certification

Clergy and pastoral counselors in the mainstream religious bodies in the United States receive extensive training in the spiritual and mental health needs of patients. The American Association of Pastoral Counselors (AAPC) is a professional organization that certifies Christian clergy who have undergone advanced training in **psychotherapy** as well as theology. The AAPC supports about 100 counseling centers across the United States as well as certifying clergy who serve in hospital chaplaincies or mental health clinics. The corresponding certification body for Jewish rabbis and pastoral counselors is the National Association of Jewish Chaplains.

Spiritual healers in less structured traditions may be certified through a school of energy healing, recognized within a particular religious group for their healing aptitude, or initiated into healing by another means. Native American healers have formed the Indigenous Traditional Healing Council to provide certification for healers as well as to protect the integrity of Native American healing rituals. Many other healers develop their healing gifts on their own. Any caring person can develop a certain amount of healing ability through meditation, prayer, study with other experienced healers, and practice. There are many self-help books on prayer and meditation, but personal guidance is usually helpful to learn the subtleties of any approach to healing. Churches and other religious centers usually offer spiritual direction through prayer, meditation, or study.

Resources

BOOKS

Benor, Daniel J. "Spiritual Healing." *Essentials of Complementary and Alternative Medicine.* Edited by Wayne Jonas and Jeffrey Levin. New York, NY: Lippincott Williams & Wilkins, 1999.

Benson, Herbert, M.D. *Timeless Healing: The Power and Biology of Belief.* New York, NY: Fireside, 1997.

Dossey, Larry, M.D. *Healing Words: The Power of Prayer and the Practice of Medicine.* New York, NY: HarperCollins, 1993.

Koenig, H.G., and M. McConnell. *The Healing Power of Faith.* New York, NY: Simon & Schuster, 1999.

Koenig, Harold G. "Spiritual Healing." *Clinician's Complete Reference to Complementary and Alternative Medicine.* Edited by Donald Novey. St. Louis, Missouri: Mosby, 2000.

Targ, Russel, and Jane Katra. *Miracles of Mind: Exploring Nonlocal Consciousness and Spiritual Healing.* Novato, CA: New World Library, 1998.

PERIODICALS

Ironson, G., G. F. Solomon, E. G. Balbin, et al. "The Ironson-Woods Spirituality/Religiousness Index Is Associated with Long Survival, Health Behaviors, Less Distress, and Low Cortisol in People with HIV/AIDS." *Annals of Behavioral Medicine* 24 (Winter 2002): 34-48.

Lawrence, R. J. "The Witches' Brew of Spirituality and Medicine." *Annals of Behavioral Medicine* 24 (Winter 2002): 74-76.

Lliff, S. A. "An Additional "R": Remembering the Animals." *Institute for Laboratory Animal Research Journal* 43 (2002): 38-47.

Siegel, B., A. J. Tenenbaum, A. Jamanka, et al. "Faculty and Resident Attitudes About Spirituality and Religion in the Provision of Pediatric Health Care." *Ambulatory Pediatrics* 2 (January-February 2002): 5-10.

Tricycle: The Buddhist Review (Spring 2000): 66–81.

Underwood, L. G., and J. A. Teresi. "The Daily Spiritual Experience Scale: Development, Theoretical Description, Reliability, Exploratory Factor Analysis, and Preliminary Construct Validity Using Health-Related Data." *Annals of Behavioral Medicine* 24 (Winter 2002): 22-33.

ORGANIZATIONS

American Association of Pastoral Counselors. 9504–A Lee Highway, Fairfax, VA 22031-2303. (703)385–6967. www.aapc.org. info@aapc.org.

Indigenous Traditional Healing Council. P. O. Box 646, Tempe, AZ 85280. (602) 209-4759.www.azitlan.org/sweatlodge/council/htm..

National Association of Jewish Chaplains. 901 Route 10, Whippany, NJ 07981-1156. (973) 736-9193.www.najc.org.

Linda Chrisman
Ken R. Wells
Rebecca J. Frey, PhD

Pregnancy

Definition

Pregnancy is the period from conception to birth. After an egg is fertilized by a sperm and implanted in the lining of the uterus, it develops into an embryo, and later into a fetus. Pregnancy usually lasts 40 weeks, beginning from the first day of the woman's

Recommended weight gain for pregnant women

If you are:	You should gain:
Underweight	About 27 to 40 pounds
Normal weight	About 25 to 35 pounds
Overweight	About 15 to 25 pounds
Obese	About 15 pounds or less

SOURCE: National Institute of Diabetes and Digestive and Kidney Diseases, National Institutes of Health, U.S. Department of Health and Human Services

General weight-gain recommendations for women who are expecting only one baby. *(Illustration by GGS Information Services. Cengage Learning, Gale)*

last menstrual period. The condition is divided into trimesters, each lasting three months.

Description

Pregnancy is a state in which a woman carries a fertilized egg inside her body as it develops into a fetus and prepares to be born.

First month

At the end of the first month, the embryo is about 1/3 in long (.85 cm), and its head, trunk, and the beginnings of arms and legs have started to develop. The embryo gets nutrients and eliminates waste through the umbilical cord and placenta. By the end of the first month, the liver and digestive system begin to develop, and the heart starts to beat.

Second month

In this month, the heart starts to pump and the nervous system (including the brain and spinal cord) begins to develop. The 1 in (2.5 cm) long fetus has a complete cartilage skeleton, which is replaced by bone cells by month's end. Arms, legs, and all of the major organs begin to appear. Facial features begin to form.

Third month

By now, the fetus has grown to 4 in (10 cm) and weighs a little more than 1 oz (28 g). Now the major blood vessels and the roof of the mouth are almost completed. The face starts to take on a more recognizably human appearance. Fingers and toes appear. All the major organs are forming; the kidneys are now functional, and the four chambers of the heart are complete.

Fourth month

The fetus begins to kick and swallow, although most women still cannot feel fetal movement at this time. Now 4 oz (112 g) in weight, the fetus can hear and urinate and has established sleep-wake cycles. All organs are now fully formed, although they continue to grow for the next five months. The fetus has skin, eyebrows, and hair.

Fifth month

Now weighing up to 1 lb (454 g) and measuring 8 to 12 in (20–30 cm), the fetus experiences rapid growth as its internal organs continue to grow. At this point, the mother may feel fetal movement, and she can hear the heartbeat with a stethoscope.

Sixth month

Even though its lungs are not fully developed, some fetuses born during this month can survive with intensive care. Weighing 1 to 1.5 lbs (454–681 g), the fetus is red, wrinkly, and covered all over its body with fine hair. The fetus grows very rapidly during this month as its organs continue to develop.

Seventh month

There is a better chance that a fetus born during this month will survive. The fetus continues to grow rapidly and may weigh as much as 3 lbs (1.3 kg). Now the fetus can suck its thumb and look around its watery environment with open eyes.

Eighth month

Growth slows as the fetus begins to take up most of the space inside the uterus. Now weighing between 4 and 5 lbs (1.8–2.3 kg) and measuring 16 to 18 in (40–45 cm) in length, the fetus may at this time prepare for delivery next month by moving into the head-down position.

Ninth month

Adding 0.5 lb (227 g) each week as the due date approaches, the fetus drops lower into the mother's abdomen and prepares for the onset of labor, which may begin any time between the 37th and 42nd week of pregnancy. Most healthy babies weigh 6 to 9 lbs (2.7–4 kg) at birth and will be about 20 in (50 cm) long.

Causes and symptoms

Pregnancy is caused by a sperm fertilizing an egg. The first sign of pregnancy is usually a missed menstrual period, although some women bleed in the beginning. A woman's breasts swell and may become tender as the mammary glands prepare for eventual breastfeeding. Nipples begin to enlarge and the veins over the surface of the breasts become more noticeable.

Nausea and **vomiting** are common symptoms during the first three months of pregnancy. Since these symptoms are usually worse in the morning, this condition is known as **morning sickness**. Many women also feel extremely tired during the early weeks or pregnancy. Frequent urination is common, and there may be a creamy white discharge from the vagina. Some women crave certain foods, and an extreme sensitivity to odors may worsen the nausea. Maternal weight begins to increase.

In the second trimester (13–28 weeks) a woman begins to look noticeably pregnant and the enlarged uterus is easy to feel. The nipples get bigger and darker, the skin of Caucasians may darken, and some women may feel flushed and warm. Appetite may increase. By the twenty-second week, most women have felt the fetus move. During the second trimester, nausea and vomiting often diminish or disappear, and the pregnant woman often feels better and more energetic than in early pregnancy. Heart rate increases as does the volume of blood in the body.

By the third trimester (29–40 weeks), many women begin to experience a range of symptoms. Stretch marks (striae) may develop on the abdomen, breasts and thighs, and a dark line may appear from the navel to pubic hair. A thin fluid may be expressed from the nipples. Many women feel hot, sweat easily, and often find it hard to get comfortable. Kicks from an active fetus may cause sharp pains, and lower backaches are common. More rest is needed as the woman copes with the added **stress** of extra weight. Braxton Hicks contractions may get stronger.

At about the thirty-sixth week in a first pregnancy (later in repeat pregnancies), the fetus's head drops down low into the pelvis. This shift may relieve pressure on the upper abdomen and the lungs, allowing a woman to breathe more easily. The fetus's new position, however, places more pressure on the bladder.

The average woman gains 28 lb (12.7 kg) during pregnancy, 70% of it during the last 20 weeks. An average healthy full-term baby at birth weighs 7.5 lbs (3.4 kg), and the placenta and fluid together weigh another 3 lbs (1.3 kg). The remaining weight that a woman gains during pregnancy is mostly due to water retention and fat stores.

In addition to the typical symptoms of pregnancy, some women experience other problems that may be annoying but usually disappear after delivery. **Constipation** may develop as a result of food passing more slowly through the intestine. **Hemorrhoids** and **heartburn** are fairly common during late pregnancy. Gums may become more sensitive and bleed more easily. Eyes may dry out, making contact lenses feel painful. Pica (a craving to eat substances other than food) may occur. Swollen ankles and **varicose veins** may be a problem in the second half of pregnancy, and chloasma (light brown spots) may appear on the face.

While the preceding symptoms are considered normal, there are some symptoms that may indicate more dangerous underlying problems. A pregnant woman experiencing any of the following should contact her doctor immediately:

- abdominal pain
- rupture of the amniotic sac or leaking of fluid from the vagina
- bleeding from the vagina
- no fetal movement for 24 hours (after the fifth month)
- continuous headaches
- marked sudden swelling of eyelids, hands, or face during the last three months
- dim or blurry vision during the last three months
- persistent vomiting

Diagnosis

Many women first discover they are pregnant after a positive home pregnancy test. Pregnancy urine tests check for the presence of human chorionic gonadotropin (hCG), which is produced by a placenta. Home tests can detect pregnancy as early as the first day of the missed menstrual period.

Home pregnancy tests are more than 97% accurate if the result is positive, and about 80% accurate if the result is negative. If the result is negative and there is no menstrual period within another week, the pregnancy test should be repeated. While home pregnancy tests are reliable, they are less accurate than a pregnancy test evaluated by a laboratory. For this reason, a woman may want to have a second pregnancy test conducted at her doctor's office to be sure of the accuracy of the result.

Blood tests to determine pregnancy are usually used only when a very early diagnosis of pregnancy is needed. This more expensive test, which also looks for hCG, can produce a result within nine to twelve days after conception.

Once pregnancy has been confirmed, there are a range of screening tests that can be done to screen for birth defects, which affect about 3% of unborn children. Two tests are recommended for all pregnant women: alpha-fetoprotein (AFP) and the triple marker test.

Other tests are recommended for women at higher risk for having a child with a birth defect. These groups include women over age 35 who have another child or a close relative with a birth defect or who have been exposed to certain drugs or high levels of radiation. Women with any of these risk factors may want to consider amniocentesis, chorionic villus sampling (CVS) or ultrasound.

Other prenatal tests

Other prenatal tests that are routinely performed include:

- pap test
- gestational diabetes screening test at 24–28 weeks
- tests for sexually transmitted diseases
- urinalysis
- blood tests for anemia or blood type
- screening for immunity to various diseases, such as German measles

Treatment

Alternative medicine offers a variety of treatments for conditions ranging from morning sickness to stretch marks. Before starting any treatment, a pregnant woman should consult with her doctor or healthcare practitioner. Note that except for **ginger**, the effectiveness of these herbs has not been proven to the satisfaction of conventional medical practitioners.

Prenatal care is vitally important for the health of the fetus. A pregnant woman should eat a balanced, nutritious diet of frequent small meals. Many physicians prescribe pregnancy vitamins, including **folic acid** and **iron** supplementation during pregnancy.

Herbal remedies

Numerous herbs are believed to remedy a range of conditions experienced by pregnant women. Many remedies can be taken as herbal teas, and packaged tea bags are sold at health food stores. The following herbs are recommended for pregnant women:

- Red raspberry leaf tea (*Rubus idaeus*) is regarded as an all-purpose remedy. It is said to be a good source of iron, to tone the uterus, protect against miscarriage, and prevent infection, cramps, and anemia. Furthermore, red raspberry is believed to aid the birth process by stimulating contractions. The herb also is believed to prevent excessive bleeding during labor and afterwards.

- For morning sickness, several forms of ginger (*Zingiber officinale*) provide relief. A cup of ginger tea, ginger capsules, ginger ale, or ginger cookies can ease the queasiness.
- Lemon balm (*Melissa officinalis*) can be taken for nausea. It also aids digestion.
- Wild yam (*Dioscorea villosa*) and burdock root (*Arctium luppa*) are effective against morning sickness. Wild yam can be taken for pregnancy pain and cramping. The herb is taken to reduce the risk of miscarriage. Burdock root aids with water retention; it also protects against infant jaundice.
- Peppermint (*Mentha piperita*) can be taken after the first trimester to combat nausea. It helps with digestion, provides stomach relief, and serves as a body strengthener.
- Echinacea (various species) boosts the immune system to fight colds, flu, and infection.
- Chamomile (*Matricaria recutita*) provides soothing relaxation and can be used to help with sleep. It also helps with digestive problems and bowel difficulties.
- Yellow dock (*Rumex crispus*) thwarts infant jaundice. The herb helps with iron absorption.
- Bilberry (*Vaccinium myrtillus*) serves as a diuretic for bloating; it also strengthens vein and capillary support.
- Nettles (*Urtuca dioica*) and oat straw (*Avena sativa*) are sources of calcium. In addition, nettles and dandelion reportedly prevent high blood pressure and water retention. Nettles contain vitamin K and help to prevent excessive bleeding. Nettles can also be taken to avoid hemorrhoids and to enhance kidney function.
- Blue cohosh (*Caulophyllium thalictroides*) is taken during the last weeks of pregnancy to induce labor contractions and ease spasmodic pains.
- Lobelia (*Lobelia inflata*) works to relax the mother during delivery. The herb also aids with delivery of the placenta.

HERBS TO AVOID. Some herbs can cause complications to mother or fetus and should not be taken during pregnancy. Uterine contractions can be caused by **angelica** (*Angelica archangelica, A. atropurpurea*), lovage (*Levisticum vulgaris*), **mistletoe** (*Viscum album*), **mugwort** (*Artemesia vulgaris*), tansy (*Tanacetum vulgare*), wild ginger (*Asarum europaeum*), and **wormwood**

(*Artemisia absinthium*). Other herbs to be avoided include cinchona (*Chinchona pubescens*), **eucalyptus** oil (*Eucalyptus globulus*), **juniper** (*Juniperus communis*), ma huang (**ephedra**) (*Ephedria sinica*), male fern (*Dryopteris filix-mas*), **pennyroyal** (*Mentha pulegium*), poke root (*Phytolacca americana*), rue (*Ruta graveolens*), shepherd's purse *Capsella bursa-pastoris*), and **yarrow** (*Achillea millefolium*).

Aromatherapy

Aromatherapy involves the use of **essential oils** as remedies. The application of combined oils to the skin is said to counteract stretch marks. An aromatherapist can recommend specific oil combinations.

Traditional Chinese medicine and acupuncture

In addition to using herbs for **infertility** problems, **traditional Chinese medicine** recommends herbal formulas for such problems associated with pregnancy as morning sickness, threatened miscarriage, and **postpartum depression**. One well-known formula, recommended to be taken three to six months before attempting conception, is called the Rock on Tai Mountain decoction. The formula is intended to build up both the woman's qi, or life energy, and her blood. In traditional Chinese medicine, it is thought that the mother's blood nourishes, the qi protects, and the qi in the kidneys holds the fetus.

Chinese practitioners use **acupuncture** to assist conception by clearing the stagnation of qi in the liver; to prevent miscarriage by conserving qi in the kidney; and to induce labor.

Traditional Chinese medicine recommends abstinence from intercourse during pregnancy in order to allow the placenta to develop normally and to prevent harm caused by sexual excess to the various organs and substances in the mother's body.

Hydrotherapy

Although pregnant women should avoid saunas and hot tubs, other forms of **hydrotherapy** can provide relief. To ease nausea, a warm compress is placed between the chest and abdomen 30 minutes before eating. The compress is a cloth soaked in hot water and wrung out. A foot bath can soothe swollen feet.

Homeopathy

Morning sickness can be treated by several homeopathic remedies. If a homeopathic remedy is a decimal potency, it is indicated by an "x". This indicates the number of times that one part of a remedy was diluted in nine parts of a diluent. Distilled water is the preferred diluent.

Ipecacuanha 30x is recommended if the woman feels worse lying down, has **diarrhea**, and is salivating heavily. If morning sickness is accompanied by queasiness about eating, *Colchicum autumnale* 6x is recommended. **Nux vomica** 6x is the remedy when a woman vomits in the morning, but her condition improves after eating. *Phosphorus* 6x is taken when a woman vomits after drinking water. For nausea only, *Natrum phosporicum* 6x may provide relief.

Each remedy is taken every 15 minutes until the feeling of nausea lessens. However, no more than four doses should be taken in one day unless specified by a homeopath.

Flower remedies

Flower remedies are liquid concentrates made by soaking flowers in spring water. Also known as flower essences, 38 remedies were developed by homeopathic physician Edward Bach during the 1930s. Walnut, a Bach remedy for difficulty in adjusting to change, may be helpful to pregnant women. A thirty-ninth combination formula, the **rescue remedy**, is taken to relieve stress. A pregnant woman should, however, check with her doctor before beginning flower therapy. Flower essences, which contain alcohol, are taken in water and usually sipped.

Relaxation techniques

Relaxation techniques can be used to cope with such conditions as stress or morning sickness. Helpful techniques include **meditation**, deep breathing, and listening to relaxation tapes. Another useful technique is **guided imagery**. The mother does some deep breathing and then visualizes a positive image or affirmation.

Bodywork

Massaging sore areas of the body during pregnancy can reduce aches and stress. Another form of bodywork is the **Alexander technique**, developed by actor Frederick Matthias Alexander during the 1800s. An Alexander technique practitioner can show a woman how to release muscle tension, with emphasis on the neck. The technique focuses on posture and movement. It is said to reduce stress and relieve **pain** in such areas as the back.

Allopathic treatment

No medication (not even nonprescription drugs, herbal, or homeopathic remedices) should be taken except under medical supervision, since certain substances can pass from the mother through the placenta and into the developing fetus. Some drugs have been proven harmful to a fetus, but all drugs should be considered suspect and taken only with medical supervision. Drugs taken during the first three months of a pregnancy may interfere with the normal formation of the fetus's organs, leading to birth defects. Drugs taken later on in pregnancy may slow the fetus's growth rate, or they may damage specific fetal tissue (such as the developing teeth).

To have the best chance of having a healthy baby, a pregnant woman should avoid:

- smoking
- alcohol
- street drugs
- large amounts of caffeine
- artificial sweeteners.

Expected results

Pregnancy is a natural condition that usually causes little discomfort provided the woman takes care of herself and gets adequate prenatal care. **Childbirth** education classes for the woman and her partner help prepare the couple for labor and delivery.

Prevention

There are many ways to avoid pregnancy. A woman has a choice of many methods of contraception that will prevent pregnancy, including (in order of least to most effective):

- spermicide alone
- natural (rhythm) method
- diaphragm or cap alone
- condom alone
- diaphragm with spermicide
- condom with spermicide
- intrauterine device (IUD)
- contraceptive pill
- sterilization (either a man or woman)
- avoiding intercourse

KEY TERMS

Alpha-fetoprotein—A substance produced by a fetus's liver that can be found in the amniotic fluid and in the mother's blood. Abnormally high levels of this substance suggest there may be defects in the fetal neural tube, a structure that will include the brain and spinal cord when completely developed. Abnormally low levels suggest the possibility of Down syndrome.

Braxton Hicks contractions—Short, fairly painless uterine contractions during pregnancy that may be mistaken for labor pains. They allow the uterus to grow and help circulate blood through the uterine blood vessels.

Chloasma—A skin discoloration common during pregnancy, also known as the mask of pregnancy or melasma, with which blotches of pale brown skin appear on the face. The blotches may appear in the forehead, cheeks, and nose, and may merge into one dark mask. It usually fades gradually after pregnancy, but it may become permanent or recur with subsequent pregnancies.

Embryo—The result of fertilization of an egg by a sperm during the first eight weeks of development following conception. For the rest of pregnancy, the embryo is called a fetus.

Fetus—A developing unborn infant from the end of the eighth week after fertilization until birth.

Human chorionic gonadotropin (hCG)—A hormone produced by the placenta during pregnancy.

Placenta—The organ that develops in the uterus during pregnancy that links the blood supplies of the mother and fetus.

Rhythm method—The oldest method of contraception with a very high failure rate, in which partners refrain from having sex during ovulation. Ovulation is predicted on the basis of a woman's previous menstrual cycle.

Resources

BOOKS

Chevallier, Andrew. *Herbal Remedies.* New York: DK Publishing, 2007.

Dolan, Deirdre, and Alexandra Zissu. *The Complete Organic Pregnancy.* New York: Collins, 2006.

Mayo Clinic Book of Alternative Medicine: The New Approach to Using the Best of Natural Therapies and Conventional Medicine. New York: Time Inc. Home Entertainment, 2007.

Murkoff, Heidi, and Sharon Mazel. *What to Expect When You're Expecting,* 4th ed. New York: Workman, 2008.

Raffelock, Dean, and Robert Roundtree. *A Natural Guide to Pregnancy and Postpartum Health.* New York: Avery, 2002.

Romm, Aviva J. *The Natural Pregnancy Book: Herbs, Nutrition and Other Holistic Choices.* Berkeley, CA: Celestial Arts, 2003.

ORGANIZATIONS

Alternative Medicine Foundation, PO Box 60016, Potomac, MD, 20859, (301) 340-1960, http://www.amfoundation.org.

American Holistic Medical Association, PO Box 2016, Edmonds, WA, 98020, (425) 967-0737, http://www.holisticmedicin.org.

Association of Women's Health, Obstetric, and Neonatal Nurses, 2000 L St. NW, Suite 740, Washington, DC, 20036, (800) 673-8499 , (202) 261-2400, Toll free in Canada (800) 245-0231, http://www.awhonn.org.

National Women's Health Network, 514 Tenth Street NW, Suite 400, Washington, DC, 20004, (202) 628-7814, http://www.nwhn.org.

Liz Swain
Tish Davidson, A.M.

Pregnancy massage

Definition

Pregnancy massage is the prenatal use of **massage therapy** to support the physiologic, structural, and emotional well-being of both mother and fetus. Various forms of massage therapy, including Swedish, deep tissue, neuromuscular, movement, and Oriental-based therapies, may be applied throughout pregnancy as well as during labor and the postpartum period.

Origins

Cultural and anthropological studies indicate that massage and movement during the childbearing experience were and continue to be a prominent part of many cultures' health care. Indian Ayurvedic medical manuals detail therapists' instructions for rubbing specially formulated oils into pregnant patients' stretched abdominal skin. Traditional sculptures depict Eskimo fathers supporting and lovingly stroking their laboring wives' backs. In certain Irish hospitals laboring women are held and touched by a doula (labor assistant) or midwife through most of their notably short, uncomplicated labors. For billions of women, over thousand of years, midwives' highly developed hands-on skills

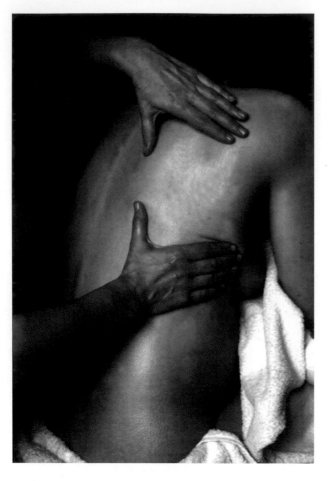

Pregnancy massage increases blood flow, relaxes muscles, reduces water retention, and makes the skin more supple. It is particularly useful in relieving the back pain of late pregnancy. *((c) Photo Researchers, Inc. Reproduced by permission.)*

have provided loving support and eased childbearing discomforts. As massage therapy resumes its place within Western healthcare methods, pregnancy massage is becoming one of its fastest growing specialized applications.

Benefits

Profound physiologic, functional, emotional, relational, and lifestyle changes occur during gestation and labor, often creating high **stress** levels. Too much stress can negatively affect maternal and infant health, resulting in reduced uterine blood supply and higher incidence of miscarriage, prematurity, and other complications. Massage therapy can help a woman approach her due date with less **anxiety** as well as less physical discomfort. Even apart from easing specific aches, massage can act as an overall tonic and increase the expectant mother's body awareness.

Massage therapy can address the various physical challenges of pregnancy: **edema**; foot, leg, or hand discomforts; and **pain** in the lower back, pelvis, or hips. **Swedish massage** may facilitate gestation by supporting cardiac function, placental and mammary development, and increasing cellular respiration. It can also reduce edema and high blood pressure as well as contribute to sympathetic nervous system sedation. Deep tissue, trigger point, and both active and passive movements alleviate stress on weight-bearing joints, muscles, and fascial tissues to reduce neck and back pain caused by poor posture and strain on the uterine ligaments. During labor, women whose partners use basic massage strokes on their backs and legs have shorter, less complicated labors. After the baby's birth, massage therapy can gently facilitate the body's return to its pre-pregnancy state, alleviate pain, foster a renewed sense of body and self, and help maintain flexibility despite the physical stresses of infant care. For post-Caesarean mothers, specific therapeutic techniques can also reduce scar tissue formation and facilitate the healing of the incision and related soft tissue areas.

Description

When nestled with pillows or other specialty cushions into a side-lying or semi-reclining position, most women are more comfortable for the 30–60 minutes of a typical massage session. A pregnant woman can expect to enjoy many of the same techniques, draping, and professional demeanor offered all massage therapy clients. The lower back, hips, and neck benefit from sensitively applied deep tissue, neuromuscular, and **movement therapy**. Edema in the legs and arms may be relieved with the gliding and kneading strokes of Swedish or **lymphatic drainage** massage. Pregnant women should expect a thorough health and prenatal intake interview with their therapists. Cost, procedures, and insurance coverage are similar to those for other massage client populations.

Preparations

In addition to the preparations listed in the massage therapy entry, some expectant women will be asked to secure a release from their maternity healthcare provider, especially those with complications or high risk factors.

Precautions

In addition to those listed in the massage therapy entry, the following other precautions are prudent:

- The abdomen should be touched only superficially with a flat, gentle hand.
- Any pressure applied to the inner leg should also be superficial.
- Women who must be on bed rest for any complication are at higher risk of blood clots forming in their legs; therefore, most massage of the legs should be avoided.
- Massage is safest when a woman is either lying on the side or propped semi-sitting at a 45–70 degree angle rather than lying on her back or belly.
- Because there are many other specific body areas and types of techniques that must be avoided or modified according to an individual woman's health condition, advanced specialized training of the therapist and consultation with her physician or midwife are highly recommended. It is better to avoid massage if the woman has vaginal bleeding, abdominal pain, or diarrhea.

Side effects

There are no known side effects to receiving appropriate prenatal massage therapy.

Research and general acceptance

Current research on the benefits of touch is providing a contemporary basis for its reintroduction into maternity care. Scientists have found that rats restricted from cutaneous self-stimulation had poorly developed placentas and 50% less mammary gland development. Their litters were often ill, stillborn, or died shortly after birth due to poor mothering skills. Women who are nauseated and/or **vomiting** prenatally experienced a decrease in these discomforts when they applied finger pressure to a specific **acupuncture** point (**acupressure**) on their forearm several times each day. Pregnant women massaged twice weekly for five weeks experienced less anxiety, leg, and back pain. When compared with control groups who practiced **relaxation** exercises only, the women who had had massage reported better sleep and improved moods, and their labors had fewer complications, including fewer premature births. Studies

show that when women receive nurturing touch during later pregnancy, they touch their babies more frequently and lovingly. During labor the presence of a doula, a woman providing physical and emotional support, including extensive touching and massage, reduces the length of labor and number of complications, interventions, medications, and Caesarean sections.

Training and certification

Some massage therapy schools include comprehensive courses in pregnancy massage therapy. More often, however, therapists receive only introductory guidance in maternity applications during their 500–1000 hours of basic training and then pursue specialization certification in pre- and perinatal massage therapy. Several nationwide programs offer such advanced training in 24–34 hour workshop programs.

Resources

BOOKS

Curties, Debra. *Breast Massage.* Moncton, New Brunswick, Canada: Curties-Overzet Publications Inc., 1999.

Goldsmith, Judith. *Childbirth Wisdom.* New York: Congdon and Weed, 1984.

Klaus, Marshall H., M.D., John H. Kennell, M.D., and Phyllis H. Klaus, M.Ed. *Mothering the Mother.* New York: Addison-Wesley Publishing Company, 1993.

Osborne-Sheets, Carole. *Pre- and Perinatal Massage Therapy: A Comprehensive Practitioners' Guide to Pregnancy, Labor, and Postpartum.* San Diego: Body Therapy Associates, 1998.

Rich, Laurie. *When Pregnancy Isn't Perfect.* New York: Dutton, 1991.

Samuels, Mike, and Nancy Samuels. *The New Well Pregnancy Book.* New York: Fireside, 1996.

Yates, John, PhD. *A Physician's Guide to Therapeutic Massage: Its Physiological Effects and Their Application to Treatment.* Vancouver, BC: Massage Therapists' Association of British Columbia, 1999.

ORGANIZATIONS

National Association of Pregnancy Massage Therapy. (888) 451-4945.

Carole Osborne-Sheets

Premenstrual syndrome

Definition

Premenstrual syndrome (PMS) refers to over 150 symptoms that occur between ovulation and the onset of **menstruation**. The symptoms include both physical

Symptoms of PMS

Physical	Emotional/behavioral
Weight gain	Moodiness/irritability
Fluid retention	Anxiety or tension
Breast tenderness	Depression
Headaches and body aches	Panic attacks
Acne	Suicidal thoughts
Hot flashes	Crying fits
Nausea	Aggressiveness
Cold sores and herpes outbreaks	Social withdrawal
Constipation or diarrhea	
Food cravings/Appetite changes	
Insomnia	
Fatigue	

(Illustration by Corey Light. Cengage Learning, Gale)

ones, such as breast tenderness, back **pain**, abdominal cramps, **headache**, and changes in appetite; behavioral symptoms such as clumsiness, poor concentration, and sleep problems; and psychological symptoms of **anxiety**, irritability, **depression**, and unrest. Severe forms of this syndrome are referred to as premenstrual dysphoric disorder (PMDD). These symptoms may be related to hormonal imbalances and emotional disorders.

Description

Between 40 and 75% of all menstruating women experience symptoms that occur before or during menstruation. PMS encompasses a wide range of symptoms, some as minor as appetite change or others so severe that they may interfere with daily life. Some women experience an increase in their sexual libido (sex drive). Only 3 to 7% of women experience the much more severe premenstrual dysphoric disorder (PMDD). These symptoms can last 4 to 10 days and can have a substantial impact on a woman.

The reason some women get severe PMS whereas others get little or none of the symptoms is not understood. PMS symptoms usually begin at puberty and last until **menopause**. Women more sensitive to hormonal change may experience PMS more than others. **Stress** also contributes and the relief of tension often lessens the other symptoms as well. Overall, however, it is difficult to predict who is most at risk for PMS.

Causes and symptoms

Because PMS is restricted to the second half of a woman's menstrual cycle, after ovulation, it is thought that hormones play a role. During a woman's monthly menstrual cycle, which lasts from 24 to 35 days, hormone levels change. The hormone estrogen gradually rises during the first half of a woman's cycle, the pre-ovulatory phase, and falls dramatically at ovulation. After ovulation, the post-ovulatory phase, progesterone levels gradually increase until menstruation occurs. Both estrogen and progesterone are secreted by the ovaries, which are responsible for producing the eggs. The main role of these hormones is to cause thickening of the lining of the uterus (endometrium).

However, estrogen and progesterone also affect other parts of the body, including the brain. In the brain and nervous system, estrogen can affect the levels of neurotransmitters, such as serotonin. Serotonin has long been known to have an effect on emotions and eating behavior. It is thought that when estrogen levels go down during the post-ovulatory phase of the menstrual cycle, decreases in serotonin levels follow. Whether these changes in estrogen, progesterone, and serotonin are responsible for the emotional aspects of PMS is not known with certainty. However, most researchers agree that the chemical transmission of signals in the brain and nervous system is in some way related to PMS. This position is supported by the fact that the times following **childbirth** and menopause are also associated with both depression and low estrogen levels.

Nutritional deficiencies, food **allergies**, and **hypoglycemia** (low blood sugar) have been linked with PMS. A diet deficient in **essential fatty acids**, **zinc**, **magnesium**, and vitamin B_6 may affect estrogen and progesterone production and their balance in the body.

Over 150 symptoms for PMS have been identified. These include physical, behavioral, and emotional aspects that range from mild to severe. The physical symptoms include bloating, headaches, food cravings, abdominal cramps, headaches, tension, **fatigue, acne**, muscle aches, and breast tenderness. Behavioral symptoms may include

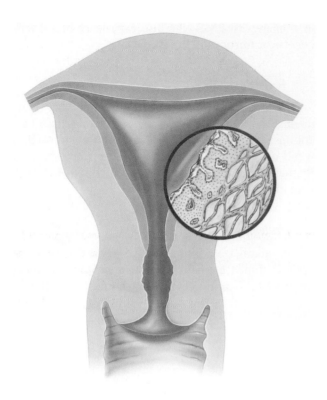

Conceptual illustration of menstrual pain. *(© PHOTOTAKE Inc. / Alamy)*

insomnia, lack of concentration, and clumsiness. Emotional aspects include mood swings, irritability, and depression.

Diagnosis

The best way to diagnose PMS is to review a detailed diary of a woman's symptoms for several months. PMS is diagnosed by the presence of physical, psychological, and behavioral symptoms that are cyclic and occur in association with the premenstrual period of time. PMDD, which is far less common, was officially recognized as a disease in 1987. Its diagnosis depends on the presence of at least five symptoms related to mood that disappear within a few days of menstruation. These symptoms must interfere with normal functions and activities of the individual.

Treatment

There are many natural treatments for PMS and PMDD depending on the symptoms and their severity. **Hypnotherapy**, spiritual healing, **color therapy**, **reflexology**, **Ayurvedic medicine**, **traditional Chinese medicine**, **acupuncture**, **acupressure**, **aromatherapy**, herbal treatment, Naturopathic treatment, and **homeopathy** are all used to treat PMS.

Vitamins and minerals

Some women find relief with the use of vitamin and mineral supplements. Magnesium can reduce the fluid retention that causes bloating, whereas **calcium** may decrease both irritability and bloating. Magnesium and calcium also help relax smooth muscles, which may reduce cramping. Some studies indicate that calcium supplements can reduce premenstrual complaints by nearly half. **Vitamin E** reduces breast tenderness, nervous tension, fatigue, and insomnia. Vitamin B_6 decreases fluid retention, fatigue, irritability, and mood swings. Vitamin B_5 supports the adrenal glands and may help reduce fatigue.

Phytoestrogens and natural progesterone

The Mexican wild yam, *Dioscorea villosa*, contains a substance that may be converted to progesterone in the body. Because this substance is readily absorbed through the skin, it can be found as an ingredient in many skin creams. (Some products also have natural progesterone added to them.) Some herbalists believe that these products can have a progesterone-like effect on the body and decrease some of the symptoms of PMS.

The most important way to alter hormone levels may be by eating more phytoestrogens. These plant-derived compounds have an effect similar to estrogen in the body. One of the richest sources of phytoestrogens is soy products, such as tofu and soy milk. Additionally, many supplements contain **black cohosh** (*Cimicifuga racemosa*) or **dong quai** (*Angelica sinensis*), which are herbs high in phytoestrogens. **Red clover** (*Trifolium pratense*), **alfalfa** (*Medicago sativa*), **licorice** (*Glycyrrhiza glabra*), **hops** (*Humulus lupulus*), and legumes are also high in phytoestrogens. Increasing the consumption of phytoestrogens is also associated with decreased risks of **osteoporosis**, **cancer**, and **heart disease**.

Herbal treatment

Herbal treatment has been used to treat many symptoms of PMS. Herbs to alleviate cramps include **angelica** root, **cramp bark**, **kava kava**, red **raspberry**, **black haw**, and **rosemary**. Black cohosh, **peppermint**, strawberry leaf, and **valerian** root have been used to decrease mood swings. **Dandelion**, couch grass, and **hawthorn** are effective diuretic herbs used to reduce bloating and swelling. **Burdock root** and red clover are liver cleansing herbs that can be useful in eliminating excess estrogen from the system. Herbs to balance hormones include **blessed thistle**, dong quai, false unicorn root, **fennel** seed, sarsaparilla root, and squaw vine. **Feverfew** may be effective for migraine headaches.

Many herbs may be beneficial as a natural antidepressant. St. John's wort (*Hypericum perforatum*) has been shown in scientific trials to be an effective antidepressant. As with the standard antidepressants, however, it must be taken continuously and does not show an effect until used for four to six weeks. A preliminary study conducted at the University of Exeter in England indicated that St. John's wort may also be an effective treatment for the moods associated with PMS. For two menstrual cycles, each woman in the study took one 300 milligram tablet of St. John's wort daily and maintained a diary in which each woman rated her symptoms on a scale of zero to four. Of the 19 women who completed the study, symptom ratings improved by about 50%. Scores on tests of anxiety and depression also dropped significantly after the first month on St. John's wort. There are also herbs, such as **skullcap** (*Scutellaria lateriflora*) and kava kava (*Piper methysticum*), that can relieve the anxiety and irritability that often accompany depression. An advantage of these herbs is that they can be taken when symptoms occur rather than continually.

Chaste-berry tree (*Vitex agnus-castus*) in addition to helping rebalance estrogen and progesterone in the body also may relieve the anxiety and depression associated with PMS. It is also used to treat menstrual irregularities, painful menstruation, and breast pain in women with PMS. Two surveys of its effectiveness were done on 1,542 women who took a liquid extract (42 drops daily) for spans up to 16 years. The patients' doctors rated its effectiveness as very good, good, or satisfactory in 92% of cases. An article on the surveys was published in the February 2000 issue of *Let's Live* magazine.

Another natural PMS remedy is **evening primrose oil** (EPO) *Oenothera biennis*. EPO is derived from the plant's seeds and is valued for its oil-containing essential fatty acids. These include **linoleic acid** and **gamma-linoleic acid** (GLA). Women with PMS have been shown to have impaired conversion of linoleic acid to GLA. Because a deficiency of GLA might be a factor in PMS and because evening primrose oil contains significant amounts of GLA, researchers have studied EPO as a potential way to reduce PMS symptoms. In several double blind studies, EPO was found to be beneficial, whereas in other studies it was no more effective than a placebo. The studies were done in the 1980s and 1990s. Despite these conflicting results, many homeopathic health practitioners recommend EPO. The usual recommended dose is 3 to 4 grams per day. EPO seems to work best when used over several menstrual cycles and may be more helpful in women with PMS who also experience breast tenderness or **fibrocystic breast disease**.

Aromatherapy

Aromatherapy oils can be a useful adjunct treatment for PMS. **Lavender** oil reduces headaches, cramps, and painful breasts. **Chamomile** and sandalwood oils may be used to relieve stress and tension. Premenstrual fatigue may be remedied by geranium, bergamot, and rosemary oils.

Homeopathy

A number of homeopathic remedies may be applied in the treatment of PMS, depending upon the individual's symptoms. Natrum muriaticum may be the appropriate remedy when irritability, lack of self-confidence, depression, anxiety, and headaches are present. **Sepia** may be given when PMS is accompanied by stress, weepiness, and to calm nerves. Symptoms of indifference, panic attacks, anger, tension, **hair loss**, sugar cravings, and a reduced sex drive may indicate that Kali carbonicum may be the appropriate remedy.

Allopathic treatment

Allopathic treatments available include over-the-counter anti-inflammatory drugs such as ibuprofen or acetominophen, antidepressant drugs, hormone treatment, or (only in extreme cases) surgery to remove the ovaries. Anti-inflammatory drugs are useful in reducing headaches, muscle aches, and cramping. One recommendation is to begin taking the anti-inflammatory one to two days before the onset of cramps. Doing so will block the cramp-causing hormones, prostaglandins, and may prevent any **nausea**, **vomiting**, and **diarrhea** associated with PMS. Hormone treatment usually involves oral contraceptives. This treatment is used to prevent ovulation and the changes in hormones that accompany ovulation. Some studies, however, indicate that hormone treatment has little effect over placebo. In 2006, the U.S. Food and Drug Administration (FDA) approved Sarafem for the treatment of premenstrual dysphoric disorder (PMDD), a severe form of PMS. As of April 2008, it was the only prescription medication indicated for the treatment of this condition. Sarafem, however, is not a new drug. It is actually a new brand name for the antidepressant fluoxetine (Prozac), which has had some very serious allegations leveled against it. Opponents of the drug claim that it is a trigger for violent and/or suicidal behavior in certain susceptible individuals.

Antidepressants

Besides Prozac, other antidepressants prescribed for PMS include sertraline (Zoloft) and paroxetine (Paxil). They are termed selective serotonin reuptake inhibitors (SSRIs) and act by indirectly increasing the brain serotonin levels, thus stabilizing emotions. Some doctors prescribe antidepressant treatment for PMS throughout the cycle, while others direct patients to take the drug only during the latter half of the cycle. Antidepressants should be avoided by women wanting to become pregnant. Side effects of sertraline were found to include nausea, diarrhea, and decreased libido.

Expected results

The prognosis for women with both PMS and PMDD is good. Most women experience relief from symptoms when treated.

Prevention

Women who have PMS typically have very poor **diets**. Maintaining a good diet, one low in sugars, salt, fats, alcohol, and **caffeine**, and high in phytoestrogens and complex carbohydrates, may prevent some of the symptoms of PMS. Consumption of more complex carbohydrates may relieve PMS symptoms since carbohydrates drop serotonin levels as they raise insulin levels. For instance, two cups of cereal or a cup of pasta has enough carbohydrate to effectively increase serotonin levels. Carbohydrates also provide steady levels of blood sugar and act to stabilize one's mood. One recommendation is to eat 100 calories of complex carbohydrates every three hours beginning one week before menstruation. Complex carbohydrates include whole wheat bread and pasta, brown rice, and whole grain foods. Caution should be taken due to the fact that a high carbohydrate diet causes water retention, which in turn is a symptom of PMS. Also, excess caffeine consumption has been associated with breast tenderness and fibrocystic breasts. Because of the potential that PMS is caused by estrogen dominance, one might also consider steps that eliminate or reduce the consumption of xenoestrogens (estrogenic compounds from the hormones and pesticides in the food supply). A vegetarian diet or consumption of organically grown meats, eggs, fruits, vegetables, and dairy products are two ways one might reduce xenoestrogen exposure.

Women should try to **exercise** three times a week, keep in generally good health, and maintain a positive self image. Because PMS is often associated with stress, avoidance of stress or developing better means

KEY TERMS

Antidepressant—A drug used to control depression.

Estrogen—A female hormone important in the menstrual cycle.

Neurotransmitter—A chemical messenger used to transmit an impulse from one nerve to the next.

Phytoestrogens—Compounds found in plants that can mimic the effects of estrogen in the body.

Progesterone—A female hormone important in the menstrual cycle.

Serotonin—A neurotransmitter important in regulating mood.

to deal with stress can be important. Chronic stress has two very important effects on the body related to PMS: it increases cortisol, a hormone produced by the adrenal glands, that keeps women going through times of stress and it increase production of prolactin. Cortisol competes for progesterone receptor sites. If it is chronically elevated, women end up with the symptoms of progesterone deficiency, even though their bodies may be producing enough for their needs. Further, cortisol can stimulate feelings of irritability, anger and rage, familiar symptoms for women with PMS. Stress reduction techniques such as **biofeedback** training, exercise, time management skills, **yoga**, and **meditation** may all be useful to women who are chronically stressed.

Resources

BOOKS

Glenville, Marilyn. *Overcoming PMS the Natural Way.* London: Piatkus Books, 2006.

Jones, Andrew. *The All-Natural Cure to Your PMS.* Akron, OH: 48 Hour Books, 2007.

O'Brien, P., M. Shaun, et al. *The Premenstrual Disorders: PMS and PMDD.* New York: Informa Healthcare, 2007.

Scalis, Dagmara. *Everything Health Guide to PMS: The Essential Guide to Reducing Discomfort, Minimizing Symptoms, and Feeling Your Best.* Cincinnati, OH: Adams Media, 2007.

PERIODICALS

Crain, Esther. "The PMS Diet: What You Consume Pre-period Can Control Annoying Symptoms." *Cosmopolitan* (October 2007): 224.

Graham, Janis. "Hormone Help: It's Not Just About Birth Control Anymore. New Methods Can Help Manage Heavy Periods, Killer Cramps, PMS, Even Hot Flashes." *Good Housekeeping* (June 2007): 43(4).

Guthrie, Catherine. "Herbs for Hormones: Tame PMS, Hot Flashes, and Even Hormone-Related Depression with Herbs and Supplements." *Natural Health* (March 2008): 91(3).

Kane, Emily A. "Marvel at Milk Thistle's Many Uses: This Ancient Medicine Has a Range of Modern Uses. Treating Liver Disease, Resolving Skin Conditions and Alleviating PMS Symptoms Are Just a Few." *Better Nutrition* (June 2007): 24.

Parch, Lorie. "The Nine Best Herbs for Women: The Latest Research on What Really Works to Prevent PMS, Hot Flashes, Migraines, Heart Disease, and More." *Natural Health* (September 2006): 74(6).

Perkins, Melissa. "Banish PMS Forever! Cramps, Bloating, Mood Swings—Yeah, Periods Can Suck. But with These Expert Tips, You Can Beat Even the Ickiest PMS Symptoms and Make It Through the Month." *Girl's Life* (February/March 2007): 50(2).

ORGANIZATIONS

American Institute of Homeopathy, 801 N. Fairfax St., Suite 306, Alexandria, VA, 22314, (888) 445-9988, http://www.homeopathyusa.org.

Australian Homeopathic Association, 6 Cavan Ave., Renown Park, SA 5008, Australia, (61) 8-8346-3961, http://www.homeopathyoz.org.

European Institute of Women's Health, 33 Pearse St., Dublin, 2, Ireland, 353-1-671-5691, http://www.eurohealth.ie.

Homeopathic Medical Council of Canada, 3910 Bathurst St., Suite 202, Toronto, ON, M3H 3N8, Canada, (416) 638-4622, http://www.hmcc.ca.

Office of Women's Health. U.S. Department of Health and Human Services, 200 Independence Ave. SW, Room 712E, Washington, DC, 20201, (800) 994-9662, http://www.womenshealth.gov.

Jennifer Wurges
Ken R. Wells

Prickly heat

Definition

Prickly heat is a common disorder of the sweat glands characterized by a red, **itching**, prickling rash following exposure to high environmental temperatures.

Description

Prickly heat is also known as heat rash, sweat retention syndrome, and miliaria rubra. This disorder occurs during the summer months or year-round in hot, humid climates, and is caused by blockage of the sweat glands. The skin contains two types of glands: one produces oil and the other produces sweat. The sweat glands are coil-shaped and extend deep into the skin. Blockage can occur at several different depths, producing four distinct skin rashes:

- Miliaria crystallina. This is the most superficial blockage and affects only the thin upper layer of skin, the epidermis. Sweat that cannot escape to the surface forms little blisters. A bad sunburn as it just starts to blister can look exactly like miliaria crystallina.

- Miliaria rubra. Blockage at a deeper layer causes sweat to seep into the living layers of skin, causing irritation and itching.

- Miliaria pustulosais. A complication of miliaria rubra in which the sweat is infected with pyogenic (pus-producing) bacteria and contains pus.

- Miliaria profunda. The deepest of all blockages causes dry skin and possibly goose bumps.

These four types of heat rash can cause complications because they prevent sweat from cooling the body, as normally occurs when the sweat evaporates from the skin surface. Sweating is the most important human cooling mechanism available in hot environments. If it does not work effectively, the body can rapidly become overheated, with severe and potentially fatal consequences.

Causes and symptoms

The best evidence to date suggests that bacteria form the plugs in the sweat glands. These bacteria are probably normal inhabitants of the skin, and why they suddenly interfere with the free flow of sweat is not understood.

Heat rash appears suddenly and has a hot, itching, prickling sensation. Infants are more likely to get miliaria rubra than adults. Obese persons are also more susceptible to heat rash. All the sweat retention **rashes** are also more likely to occur in hot, humid weather.

Failure to secrete sweat can cause the body to overheat. Before the patient suffers heat **stroke**, there will be a period of heat exhaustion symptoms (**dizziness**, thirst, weakness) when the body is still effectively maintaining its normal temperature. Then the patient's temperature rises, often rapidly, to 104 or 105° F (40° C) and beyond. Heat stroke is an emergency that requires immediate and rapid cooling. The best method of treatment is immersion in ice water.

Diagnosis

Prickly heat can be diagnosed and treated by a dermatologist (skin disease specialist). The symptoms of a rash and dry skin in hot weather are usually sufficient to diagnose these conditions.

KEY TERMS

Ambient—Surrounding.

Antipruritic—A type of medication applied to the skin to stop itching.

Pyogenic—Capable of generating pus. Streptococci, staphylococci, and bowel bacteria are the primary pyogenic organisms.

Syndrome—A collection of abnormalities that occur together often enough to suggest that they have a common cause.

Treatment

Naturopaths maintain that **essential fatty acids** can speed the clearing of the rash. The patient should eat fish rich in fatty acids (salmon, mackerel, or herring). Other sources include dark green leafy vegetables and **flaxseed** oil.

The homeopathic remedy for prickly heat is a dose of *apis* in 30c potency, taken when the itching or prickling sensation begins. *Apis* may be taken every 2 hours for up to 10 days.

An alkaline bath is the **hydrotherapy** treatment for prickly heat. The patient should soak for 30–60 minutes in a tub filled with lukewarm water containing 1 cup of baking soda.

Herbal treatments to relieve itching include sprinkling arrow root powder over the rash or rubbing a slice of fresh daikon radish or raw potato over the rash. A sponge bath with **ginger** will increase circulation. Fresh grated ginger is steeped in boiling-hot water, cooled, and then sponged over the rash. For widespread itching the patient can take cool baths with corn starch and/or oatmeal.

Chinese herbal medicines are used internally for widespread prickly heat or externally for small areas of rash. The medicines Zhi Yang Po Fen (Relieve Itching Powder), Jie Du Cha Ji (Resolve Toxin Smearing Liquid), and Qing Dai San Cha Ji (Natural Indigo Powder Smearing Liquid) can be applied to the rash. Fresh lotus leaf with a decoction of Jin Yin Hua (*Flos lonicerae*) can be taken as a tea. A decoction of the following herbs can be taken by mouth:

- Qing Hao (*Herba artemisiae annuae*): 5g
- Bo He (*Herba menthae*): 5 g
- Jin Yin Hua (*Flos lonicerae*): 10 g
- Dan Zhu Ye (*Herba lophatheri*): 10 g
- Lu Dou Yi (*Pericarpium phaseoli munginis*): 10 g
- Ju Hua (*Flos chrysanthemi*): 5 g
- fresh lotus leaf: one piece

Allopathic treatment

Heat rash may be treated with topical antipruritics (itch relievers) containing calamine, **aloe**, menthol, camphor, **eucalyptus** oil, and similar ingredients. Dermatologists can peel off the upper layers of skin using a special ultraviolet light. This treatment will remove the plugs and restore sweating, but is not necessary in most cases.

Expected results

With cooler temperatures, the rash disappears in a day, but the skin may not recover its ability to sweat for two weeks (the time needed to replace the top layers of skin with new growth from below).

Prevention

Because the body cannot cool itself adequately without sweating, careful monitoring for symptoms of heat exhaustion is important, especially in infants or the elderly. If the symptoms of heat exhaustion do appear, the person should move into the shade or take a cool bath or shower. Clinical studies have found that application of topical antiseptics like hexachlorophene almost completely prevented these rashes. General measures to prevent prickly heat include:

- wearing loose-fitting clothing
- removing sweat-soaked clothing
- taking a cool shower or bath after sweating
- limiting outdoor activities to the mornings and evenings during hot weather
- staying in an air-conditioned environment during hot weather.

Resources

BOOKS

Berger, Timothy G. "Skin and Appendages." In *Current Medical Diagnosis and Treatment*, edited by Lawrence M. Tierney, Jr., et al. Stamford, CT: Appleton & Lange, 1996.

"Sweat Retention Syndrome." In *Dermatology in General Medicine*, edited by Thomas B. Fitzpatrick et al. New York: McGraw-Hill, 1993.

Ying, Zhou Zhong, and Jin Hui De. "Prickly Heat and Summer Dermatitis." *Clinical Manual of Chinese Herbal Medicine and Acupuncture*. New York: Churchill Livingston, 1997.

Belinda Rowland

Prickly pear cactus

Description

A member of the Cactaceae (or cactus) family, prickly pear cactus, also known as nopal, grows in the United States, Mexico, and South America. It also flourishes in Africa, Australia, and the Mediterranean.

Although prickly pear cactus can tolerate a wide range of temperature and moisture levels, it grows best in sunny, desert-like conditions. Over a dozen species of prickly pear cactus belong to the *Opuntia* genus, but all of them have flat, fleshy, green-colored pads that look like large leaves and are oval to round in shape. With a tendency to grow quickly and at odd angles, the pads are actually the stems of the plant. It is in the pads that the moisture is stored. In general, the pads range from 4 in (10 cm) to 18 in (46 cm) in length. Larger pads have been known to grow as wide as 9 in (23 cm) or

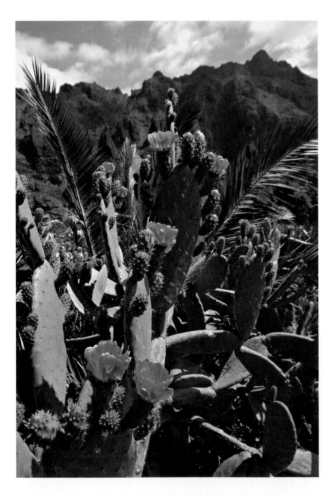

Prickly pear cactus. *(© Chris Howes/Wild Places Photography / Alamy)*

more. The height of a prickly pear cactus can vary and be anywhere from less than a foot to 7 ft (2.1 m) tall.

Like most cactus plants, the prickly pear cactus has long, sharp spines that protrude from the pads. In addition, harder-to-see tiny spines, called glochids, can be found at the base of the more predominant spines. Disguised in fuzzy-looking patches, the glochids appear harmless. However, they come off the pad easily and once they've gotten into a person's skin, they can be difficult to remove and cause irritation for days.

The pads and fruit of the prickly pear cactus are edible. The fruit can be peeled and eaten raw. However, many experts suggest that the fruit is best when it is made into candy, jelly, juice, or wine. It is also available dried or in extract form.

From early spring to summer, the cactus blossoms and sets fruit, which line the edges of the pads. Anytime thereafter, until late fall, the fruit ripens and is ready to be picked. The fruit should be harvested only when ripe and, according to Savio, "Those that are best for eating fresh ripen from September to November." Once picked, the fruit has a brief shelf life—typically under a week.

Most often, the flowers of the prickly pear cactus are red, yellow, or purple with each flower yielding one fruit. On average, the fruit grows to be about 2.5 in (7 cm) long and is cylindrical in shape. Although the fruit's flesh can be found in many different colors, such as white, green, yellow, red, or purple, most people in the United States are familiar with the reddish-purple or dark red variety; whereas in Mexico, the white-skinned varieties are most common.

In a 1998 paper presented in Santiago, Chile, at the International Symposium on Cactus Pear and Nopalitos Processing and Uses, Armida Rodriguez-Felix and Monica A. Villegas-Ochoa reported that the chemical composition of prickly pear cactus pads is not unlike most vegetables. High in **amino acids** (building blocks of proteins and highly bioactive, generally), prickly pear cactus is said to be high in fiber, B vitamins, **magnesium**, and **iron**. Rodriguez-Felix and Villegas-Ochoa listed the following ingredients as well:

- water
- carbohydrates
- protein
- fat
- minerals
- vitamin C
- beta carotene

General use

Prickly pear cactus has been used for healing purposes and as food for centuries. Loaded with protein and vitamins, the cactus, also known as nopal, has been used to treat diabetes, stomach problems, **cuts** and **bruises**, **sunburn**, windburn, **constipation**, and cold symptoms. Folk remedies abound, such as the one that involves heating the pads and placing them on a cold sufferer's chest to relieve congestion.

In an article published in *The Hindu*, India's national newspaper, Ms. Margarita Barney de Cruz, president of the Group to Promote Education and Sustainable Development, was quoted as having said that nopal was even used in the sixteenth to eighteenth centuries for painting churches and convents. Apparently, according to Barney de Cruz, this practice originated in rural Mexico when it was discovered that prickly pear cactus could be used to make a highly effective waterproof paint for homes.

Rural residents, especially farmers, in Mexico and elsewhere have utilized the prickly pear cactus for years as an effective way to mark property lines, as well as a protective barrier against predators, both animal and human. In central Africa, the juice from the pads has long been considered an effective mosquito repellent.

An important part of the Mexican culture for centuries, prickly pear cactus is still being used there for medicinal and nutritional purposes. In *Worldwide Gourmet*, edited by Michele Serre, prickly pear cactus reportedly is one of the most important food crops collected by the native population and is widely eaten as both a fruit and vegetable. In northern Mexico, the pads are often fed to dairy cows in order to add a unique and sweet flavor to their milk. Not only is this feed inexpensive, but also the resulting dairy product is highly prized among local consumers.

Today, prickly pear cactus is still being used as a remedy for many of the same problems it was used for in the past. For example, it is still commonly used topically to treat cuts, insect **bites**, sunburn, and windburn. Over the past three decades, some interesting studies have been conducted on the healing properties of prickly pear cactus, with a primary research focus on its effectiveness in lowering blood sugar levels. Wholehealthmd.com reported that animal studies done in the 1990s indicate that extracts of the prickly pear at doses lower than traditionally used can reduce blood sugar levels. This is promising for the possible development of easy-to-use extracts that may some day be effective for use in treating diabetes in humans. With regard to the cactus pads themselves, not the extract, some interesting studies have indicated that the cooked pads do help reduce sugar levels, thereby validating traditional medicinal usage. According to the experts at wholehealthmd.com, one theory of the mechanism of blood sugar lowering is that the high fiber from the pad's gooey pectin absorbs sugar in the body, and then enables the body to very slowly release sugar through the course of the day.

Two 1988 studies, one published in *Diabetes Care* and the other in the *Archives of Investigative Medicine*, conducted by Frat-Munari and colleagues indicated that consuming 100 to 500 grams of cooked pads was beneficial in treating humans with diabetes. Results confirmed a drop of between 8 to 31% of blood glucose readings. The Frati-Munari studies involved three groups on three separate "treatments." One group took nopal, one group took a water placebo, the third took zucchini squash. The water group experienced no change in serum glucose levels, whereas a slight increase of serum glucose concentrations was measured in the zucchini squash group. Those taking nopal displayed improvements in elevated blood sugar.

In a similar study published by the *Texas Journal of Rural Health* in 1998, Keith Rayburn, M.D., and colleagues had an interestingly different outcome. In the study by Rayburn et al, although blood sugar readings also fell after consumption, the water ingestion group showed a declining glucose concentration, whereas in the studies by Frati-Munari that was not the case. Dr. Rayburn and colleagues compared their study to two studies with similar findings (one by Chen et al conducted in 1988 and another by Gannon et al conducted in 1989) and made three important assessments. One explanation for the different findings might have to do with the water control group. It may have had a declining glucose reading because its members were allowed to drink as much water as they liked, which could have had a blood-sugar-lowering effect. Secondly, although the use of nopal in folk culture is not limited to one species, Rayburn and colleagues did point out that the nopal used in their study differed from the nopal used in the 1988 studies by Frati-Munari and colleagues. In fact, Rayburn and his colleagues specifically stated, "We cannot rule out the possibility that *O. streptacantha* might have more activity than other species." Finally, and perhaps most importantly, Rayburn and colleagues concluded, "Despite lacking an acute hypoglycemic effect in our subjects, it is possible that nopal has other important metabolic effects, such as lowering lipids or increasing insulin sensitivity, as suggested by Frati-Munari et al [in two studies published in 1991]."

In a literature review published in 2002 by the *Journal of American Pharmacists Association,* Drs. Shapiro and Gong investigated the uses of several products and conclude that based on the evidence, several natural products in common use can lower blood glucose in patients with diabetes.

Interesting research continues to be conducted to validate or discover new ways in which prickly pear cactus can be used medicinally. For example, in a 1998 study published in *Archives of Pharmaceutical Research* by Dr. E. H. Park and colleagues, it was suggested that prickly pear cactus pads could be used to reduce inflammation and help relieve stomach problems. Some evidence also exists that prickly pear cactus could be effective in reducing **cholesterol** levels, but more research needs to be conducted.

Preparations

Gloves should be worn when the pads and fruit are removed from the cactus. Even those varieties regarded as "spineless" have glochids, so beware. To avoid getting punctured by the spines, use a long, sharp knife to cut and tongs to lift the pads and fruit away from the plant. Place the cuttings in a bowl or basket with handles. Novices should continue to wear gloves until all the spines are removed. To remove the spines, simply scrape them off with a blunt knife, while holding the pad at its base. Another way to remove the spines is to burn them off by passing the pad over an open flame, but this should be done with great care and suitable utensils such as tongs with heat resistant handles. Many experts recommend cutting off the edges or peeling them entirely. Most experts agree that the young, bright green pads are the most tender and the best ones for culinary purposes.

If the pads are small, they can be sautéed in a covered pan with some olive oil and vegetables, such as mushrooms, peppers, onions, or tomatoes. The ingredients should be simmered over low heat until the pad is very tender. Some people also prefer to add ground

pepper and herbs such as cilantro, basil, or **rosemary**. The nopales can also be sautéed until cooked. The pads can also be sliced thin to resemble green beans. As Savio states, "They can be eaten raw in salads, boiled and fried like eggplant, pickled with spices, or cooked with shellfish, pork, chilies, tomatoes, eggs, coriander, **garlic**, and onions." In an article published by *Wilderness Way,* Christopher Nyerges suggests that the cut slices be boiled in water, drained, and then boiled again to reduce the sliminess. The slices can then be seasoned with butter and garlic powder prior to serving them. Once dried, the peeled and sliced pads are known as leather britches, according to Nyerges. Much like string beans, the leather britches add texture and fiber to stews and soups.

Omelets containing prickly pear cactus are common in the southwestern United States. When a young cactus pad is cooked in a skillet for use in an omelet, its bright green color will change to "a dull green-almost tan-as it cooks," Nyerges explained.

An interesting suggestion regarding "the importance of a penny" can be found in the *Worldwide Gourmet.* In an article on prickly pear cactus, the reader is encouraged "to rub a **copper** penny with baking soda and lemon, heat it on the grill until it turns red, and then put it in the water used to cook the nopal. This allows the water to reach its boiling point more quickly and also neutralizes the viscous substance found in the cactus."

Often tasting similar to watermelon, the fruit can be eaten raw and is delicious chilled. It is filled with little seeds, which account for its grainy texture. The seeds are edible, too, but some people prefer to remove them. In the Native American culture, it is customary to dry and grind the seeds for later use in flour.

According to Nyerges, making juice is simple. Just "press the peeled fruit through a colander to remove the seeds and add an equal amount of water to the sweet, pulpy mass." When chilled, it's a refreshing summer beverage.

For soft, shiny hair, cut a peeled cactus pad into 10 small pieces. Put them in a blender with two cups of water. Turn the blender on low for a few seconds, just enough to get the cactus juices into the water but not so long that the mixture turns to mush. Then strain the pieces out, leaving only the juicy water. The juicy water can then be used as a hair massage, which should be thoroughly rinsed out after one minute. If the mixture is allowed to thicken, it can still be used, although it will take more time to rinse out.

For minor cuts, the juice from the pads has been used traditionally much like **aloe** vera. Savio suggests to "simply cut off a portion of a [peeled] pad, crush it, and squeeze the juice into the cut; the sap will soothe the wound." When an equal measure of prickly pear cactus and water are mixed, the juice can be somewhat jelly-like, making it an ideal salve for windburn.

Recommended dosages vary, but most experts agree that eating 100 to 500 grams of the prickly pear cactus daily is reasonable, provided that there are no contraindications for doing so. For those that prefer juice, 2 to 4 ounces a day are suggested. If in doubt, consult with a physician or registered dietician for an individual assessment.

Precautions

Even Opuntia cacti, regarded as spineless, have glochids, so beware.

Consuming prickly pear cactus is not recommended while pregnant or breast-feeding. In addition, it has not been established whether it is safe for young children or anyone with severe liver or kidney disease to consume nopal.

In general, prickly pear cactus is considered safe in food form, which has been consumed for centuries by native peoples. However, less is known about the extract form, which should be taken only after consulting a physician.

People taking drugs for diabetes should not consume nopal without first consulting with a physician, since insulin or diabetes medication dosage may be affected.

Because water causes dried nopal to swell, oral doses of dried nopal should be taken with at least 8 ounces of water to avoid potentially dangerous blockages of the esophagus or intestines.

Side effects

Adverse side effects such as mild bloating, **diarrhea**, **headache**, and **nausea** have been reported after consuming nopal.

The experts at wholehealthmd.com caution that it is possible to be allergic to prickly pear cactus, although it isn't common. Signs of an allergic reaction are those typically associated with other food **allergies**. They include skin rash, **hives**, swelling, chest **pain**, breathing problems such as tightness in the chest or throat, and digestive symptoms such as diarrhea or constipation. If any of these reactions occur, one should contact a physician immediately.

Although rare, **contact dermatitis** has been reported from touching the nopal plant or applying it to broken skin. People with sensitive skin should consult a physician before using nopal as a topical ointment. More common is skin irritation caused by coming in contact with the plant's spines during the collection and cleaning process, which is why gloves should be worn, especially during the collection process.

Interactions

Because some studies have shown that consuming nopal may cause lower blood sugar by increasing the body's ability to absorb insulin, people taking drugs for diabetes, such as Actos, Avandia, Glyset, and Prandin, to name a few, should consult with their physician before adding nopal to their **diets**.

In order to avoid **hypoglycemia**, which is blood sugar that is too low, nopal should not be used in conjunction with other blood sugar medication and herbs such as **bitter melon**, **chromium**, **kudzu**, panax ginseng, or high amounts of **ginger** without the guidance of a health professional. Symptoms of hypoglycemia include shakiness, confusion, distorted speech, and loss of muscle control. Hypoglycemia is potentially an emergency and even deadly problem, and requires immediate intervention (offering fruit juice or professional health care management).

In theory, because dried nopal becomes gel-like when combined with water, taking it within two hours of other medications (or even after meals) could alter the way food and medications are absorbed in the body. Always consult with a physician or pharmacist before adding dried nopal (or any form of nopal) to your health care regime. Be sure to make a complete list of any other herbal product being taken, as well as any prescribed or over-the-counter medicine, so that an informed decision can be made.

Resources

PERIODICALS

Chen, Y. D., C. Y. Jeng, C. B. Hollenbeck, M. S. Wu, and G. M. Reaven. "Relationship between plasma glucose and insulin concentration, glucose production, and glucose disposal in normal subjects and patients with non-insulin dependent diabetes." *Journal of Clinical Investigation.* (1988): 21–25.

Frati-Munari, A. C., B. E. Gordillo, P. Altamirano, and C. R. Ariza. "Hypoglycemic effects of *Opuntia streptacantha* Lemaire in NIDDM." *Diabetes Care.* (1988): 63–66.

Frati-Munari, A. C., J. L. Q. Lazaro, P. Altamirano Bustamante, M. Banales Ham, S. Islas-Andrade, and C. R. Ariza-Andraca. "The effect of different doses of prickly pear cactus (*Opuntia streptacantha* Lemaire) on the glucose tolerance test in healthy individuals." *Archives of Investigative Medicine.* (1988): 143–148.

Frati-Munari, A. C., B. E. Gordillo, P. Altamirano, C. R. Ariza, R. Cortes-Franco, A. Chavez-Negrete, and S. Islas-Andrade. "Influence of nopal intake upon fasting glycemia in type 2 diabetics and healthy subjects." *Archives of Investigative Medicine*. (1991): 51–56.

Frati-Munari, A. C., N. X. Diaz, P. Altamirano, C.R. Ariza, and R. Lopez-Ledesma. "The effect of two sequential doses of *Opuntia streptacantha* upon glycemia." *Archives of Investigative Medicine* (1991): 431–436.

Gannon, M. C., F. Q. Nuttall, S. A. Neil, and E. R. Seaquest. "Effects of dose ingested glucose on serum metabolite and hormone responses in type 2 diabetic subjects." *Diabetes Care* (1989): 544–552.

Park, E. H., J. H. Kahng, E. A. Paek. "Studies on the pharmacological action of cactus: identification of its anti-inflammatory effect." *Archives of Pharmaceutical Research*. (1998): 30–34.

Rayburn, K., R. Martinez, M. Escobedo, F. Wright, and M. Farias. "Glycemic effects of various species of nopal (*Opuntia sp.*) in type 2 diabetes mellitus." *Texas Journal of Rural Health*. (1998): 68–74.

Shapiro, K., and W. C. Gong. "Natural products used for diabetes." *Journal of American Pharmacists Association*. (2002): 217–226.

OTHER

Nyerges, C. "Prickly pear cactus." *Wilderness Way* [cited June 14, 2004]. http://www.wwmag.net/pricklycactus.htm.

"Prickly pear." Wholehealthmd.com [cited June 14, 2004]. http://www.wholehealthmd.com.

"Prickly pear and barbary fig." *The Worldwide Gourmet* [cited June 14, 2004]. http://gourmet.sympatico.ca/vegetables/south/nopal.htm.

"Prickly pear cactus crop with multiple uses." *The Hindu* [cited June 14, 2004]. http://www.hindu.com.

Rodriguez-Felix, A., and M. A. Villegas-Ochoa. "Postharvest handling of cactus leaves (nopalitos)." Paper presented at the *International Symposium of Cactus Pear and Nopalitos Processing and Uses*. Santiago, Chile (September 24-26, 1998).

Savio, Yvonne. *Prickly pear cactus*. Brochure. Small Farm Center, University of California. July 1989 [cited June 14, 2004]. http://www.sfc.ucdavis.edu/pubs/brochures/pricklypear.html.

Lee Ann Paradise

Prince's pine

Description

Prince's pine, the evergreen shrub *Chimaphila umbellate,* is closely related to the wintergreens and is sometimes confused with striped **wintergreen** (*C. maculata*). Other names for prince's pine are pipsissewa (the most common alternate name), king's curse, ground holly, love in winter, rheumatism weed, butter weed, winter green, and pyrola umbellata.

Prince's pine grows in deep or moderate shade and requires moist, well-drained soil. It is most often found growing under conifers (pines, firs) and along mountain streams to an altitude of about 7,700 ft (2,500 m). The plant is widely distributed in the northern hemisphere and can be found in northern Europe, Siberia, Canada, Alaska, and across most of the continental United States, except for a region stretching from Florida to Texas and north through Nebraska. Prince's pine is on the endangered species list in the state of Illinois, is a threatened species in Iowa and Ohio, and is listed as vulnerable in New York. In Germany it is a protected species.

Prince's pine grows slowly, reaching a mature height of 8–10 inches (10–25 cm). The leaves, shiny dark green on top and lighter green underneath, are 2 to 3 inches (5–8 cm) long and about .5 inches (1.2 cm) wide and tapered at both ends. The leaves remain green all year. Scented light purple to cream-colored flowers develop in July and August. The leaves are used in healing. In some cultures, the yellow rhizome (root-like part) is also ground and used medicinally.

General use

Prince's pine is used as a food additive as well as a healing herb. An extract of the leaves is used to flavor root beer and candy. In Mexico, prince's pine is used to flavor an alcoholic drink made from fermented sprouted corn. The plant is also used in the perfume industry because of its pleasant scent.

Prince's pine is thought to have diuretic, astringent, antibacterial, and tonic properties. A chemical analysis of the herb shows that, among other compounds, it contains hydroquinones, which are known to have antibacterial actions, and tannins, which are known astringents.

Historically, many different Native American tribes used prince's pine to treat urinary problems and to regulate **menstruation**. The herb was also used to induce sweating and treat fevers. Some Native American tribes made a tea of the ground rhizome and used it for treating **tuberculosis** and other lung **infections**. Other traditional uses are treatment of **gonorrhea** (a sexually transmitted disease), stomach **cancer**, and rheumatism. Externally the leaves were used to treat skin diseases.

Modern herbalists mainly use prince's pine to treat urinary tract infections and as a general tonic. Prince's pine is thought to have many of the same actions as uva-ursi (*Acrtostaphylos uva-ursi*), although less intense. In 1999, a United States patent was filed for an herbal treatment for **chronic fatigue syndrome** that has prince's pine as one of its four ingredients. Prince's pine, under the name pipsissewa, was included in the *United States Pharmacopoeia* from 1820 to 1916.

Prince's pine is also used in homeopathic medicine. Homeopathic medicine operates on the principle that "like heals like," which means that a disease can be cured by treating the person with substances that produce the same symptoms as the disease, while also working in conjunction with the homeopathic law of infinitesimals. In opposition to traditional medicine, the law of infinitesimals states that the *lower* a dose of curative, the more effective it is. To achieve a low dose, the curative is diluted many, many times until only a tiny amount remains in a huge amount of the diluting liquid. In homeopathic medicine, prince's pine is used to treat disorders of the urinary tract, female reproductive system, and male prostate.

Preparations

The leaves of prince's pine are usually harvested from wild-growing plants in the summer when the plant is in flower. They are dried for future use but lose much of their fragrance when dried. Leaves are crushed or ground and prepared as a decoction, fluid extract, or syrup. Dosage varies depending on the preparation and condition being treated. Fresh leaves are often crushed and put directly on the skin to treat skin diseases, although an extract of prince's pine can also be used externally.

Precautions

No studies have been done on the safety of prince's pine, so pregnant and breastfeeding women would do well to avoid using this herb.

Side effects

No side effects from the internal use of prince's pine have been reported. Given that this herb is also used as a food additive, it is highly likely to be safe when used internally in moderate quantities. Fresh leaves placed directly on the skin can cause **blisters** in some sensitive individuals.

Interactions

No studies have been done on interactions between prince's pine and other herbs or traditional pharmaceuticals. Individuals who regularly take dietary supplements, herbs, or pharmaceutical drugs

---

KEY TERMS

Astringent—A substance that reduces secretions, dries and shrinks tissue, and helps control bleeding.

Decoction—A preparation made by boiling an herb, then straining the solid material out. The liquid is then taken internally as a drink.

Diuretic—A substance that removes water from the body by increasing urine production.

---

should discuss the use of prince's pine with their healthcare provider before beginning treatment.

Resources

BOOKS

PDR for Herbal Medicines, 4th ed. Montvale, NJ: Thompson Healthcare, 2007.

PERIODICALS

Moerman, D.E "An Analysis of the Food Plants and Drug Plants of Native North America." *Journal of Ethnorharmacology* 52 (1996): 1-22.

ORGANIZATIONS

Alternative Medicine Foundation, PO Box 60016, Potomac, MD, 20859, (301) 340-1960, http://www.amfoundation.org.

American Holistic Medical Association, PO Box 2016, Edmonds, WA, 98020, 425-967-0737, http://www.holisticmedicine.org.

American Institute of Homeopathy, 801 N. Fairfax St., Suite 306, Alexandria, VA, 22314, (888) 445-9988, http://homeopathyusa.org.

Tish Davidson, A. M.

Pritikin diet

Definition

The Pritikin diet is a heart-healthy high-carbohydrate, low-fat, moderate-exercise lifestyle diet developed in the 1960s. It promotes eating whole grains, vegetables, and fruit instead of animal protein, eggs, processed grains, and sugar.

Origins

Nathan Pritikin, the originator of the Pritikin Diet, was diagnosed with **heart disease** at the age of 42. In the late 1950s when Pritikin was diagnosed, about 40% of calories in the average American diet came from fats. Pritikin was given little medical guidance on how lifestyle changes might slow his heart disease. Although educated as an engineer, Pritikin worked to devise his own heart-healthy diet. He spent the next 20 years researching diet and **nutrition**, experimenting with a variety of **diets**, such as eating only meats or only lentils. He recorded the information and his reactions to the various diets along with blood and other medical tests. He finally concluded that a program combining moderate **exercise** with a diet low in fat and high in fiber was most beneficial, and credits it with reversing his own heart disease. Based on his experience, he opened the Pritikin Longevity Center in Florida in 1975. Here people could come and immerse themselves for one or more weeks in the Pritikin Eating Plan.

In 1976, he opened the Pritikin Longevity Center in Santa Barbara, California, which moved a few years later to Santa Monica, California. Pritikin detailed his program of diet and exercise in his 1979 book, *The Pritikin Program for Diet and Exercise*, which quickly became a bestseller. He and his son, Robert Pritikin, have published eight additional books on diet and exercise. Robert Pritikin took over management of the longevity center following the death of his father in 1985.

Pritikin's diet came to national attention when Pritikin and Florida cardiologist David Lehr appeared in the CBS program "60 Minutes" in 1977. The Pritikin Diet soon became the most popular diet of the 1970s. The Pritikin Program took on new credibility in 1984 when the National Institutes of Health published its landmark lipid study that said lowering **cholesterol** reduced the risk of heart disease. Since that time, many research studies have been done to evaluate the effectiveness of the Pritikin Plan, the results of which have been published in mainstream, refereed medical journals. More than 75,000 people have experience the Plan at what is now the upscale Pritikin Longevity Center & Spa at the Turnberry Isle Yacht Club in Aventura, Florida. Millions of others have bought Pritikin's books and tried the Plan.

Benefits

The consensus among health professionals is that a diet low in fat and high in fiber can help prevent a wide range of medical problems. It also provides significant health benefits to people who already have many different health conditions. Additionally, it can also be effective in weight loss and ideal weight maintenance.

Pritikin Diet emphasizes the following specific health benefits:

- lowered total cholesterol and LDL or "bad" cholesterol
- lowered blood pressure, so that people with high blood pressure may no longer need pressure-lowering drugs
- better control of insulin levels, so that people with type 2 diabetes can often control their disease through diet and without drugs
- decrease in the circulating levels of compounds that increases the risk of heart disease and blood vessel damage
- a substantially reduced risk of heart disease, hypertension, type 2 diabetes, and breast, colon, and prostate cancers.
- lifetime freedom from obesity and all of its associated health risks and lifestyle-limiting conditions

Description

The Pritikin diet is basically the opposite of another popular program, the **Atkins diet**. While the Atkins regimen is high in fat and protein and low in carbohydrates, the Pritikin program is low in fat and protein and high in whole-grain natural complex carbohydrates. Pritikin believed the reason a large number of Americans are overweight is because they do not eat enough complex carbohydrates, such as whole-grain corn, rice, and wheat.

The Pritikin diet is based on a wide variety of foods, including fruits, vegetables, beans, and low-fat dairy products. There are four levels to the Pritikin diet, each based on calories. Individuals pick the level they want based on how overweight they are, how much weight they want to lose, and how quickly they want to. In his book, "The Pritikin Permanent Weight-Loss Manual," Pritikin lists two weeks of sample menus for each level. The book also contains information on a free-form version of the diet, in which the dieter selects any food that has low calorie density.

The Pritikin Plan is based on eating a particular number of servings of each group of foods as follows:

- at least five 1/2-cup servings of whole grains such as wheat, oats, and brown rice or starchy vegetables such as potatoes, and dried beans and peas. Refined grain products (white flour, regular pasta, white rice) are limited to two servings daily, with complete elimination of refined grain products considered optimal.
- at least four 1-cup servings of raw vegetables or 1/2-cup servings of cooked vegetables. Dark green, leafy, and orange or yellow vegetables are preferred.

- at least three servings of fruit, one of which can be fruit juice.
- two servings of calcium-rich foods such as nonfat milk, nonfat yogurt or fortified and enriched soymilk.
- no more than one 3.5 ounce cooked serving of animal protein. Fish and shellfish are preferred. Lean poultry should optimally be limited to once a week and lean beef to once a month. This diet is easily adapted to vegetarians by replacing animal protein with protein from soy products, beans, or lentils.
- no more than one caffeinated drink daily. Instead drink water, low-sodium vegetable juices, grain-based coffee substitutes (e.g. Postum) or caffeine-free teas.
- no more than four alcoholic drinks per week for women and no more than seven for men, with red wine preferred over beer or distilled spirits.
- no more than seven egg whites per week
- no more than 2 ounces (about 1/4 cup) of nuts daily

Other foods such as unsaturated oils, refined sweeteners (e.g. concentrated fruit juice, corn syrup), high-sodium condiments (e.g. soy sauce), and artificial sweeteners (e.g. Splenda) are "caution" foods. They are not recommended, but if they are used, the Plan gives guidance in how to limit them to reasonable amounts. Animal fats, processed meat, dairy products not made with non-fat milk, egg yolks, salty snacks, cakes, cookies, fried foods and similar high-calorie choices are forbidden.

An important component of the Pritikin program is exercise. Pritikin encourages many types of exercise routines, but aerobic exercises like walking, jogging, swimming, and indoor machines that simulate these activities are recommended for optimum weight loss. The suggested routine should include 5-10 minutes of warm-up, 20-30 minutes of workout, and 5-10 minutes of cool-down.

Unlike the Atkins diet, the Pritikin program can be easily followed by vegetarians, including vegans.

Preparations

No advance preparation is required for the diet.

Precautions

As with any diet, overweight individuals and those with serious medical conditions such as heart disease or diabetes who are contemplating the Pritikin diet should first check with their doctor or health care practitioner. Individuals taking certain prescription drugs may find the need for these drugs will decrease and should be monitored by their physician during and following the weight loss period.

Side effects

The Pritikin diet is not believed to cause any adverse side effects.

Research and general acceptance

Unlike many diets, the Pritikin Plan has the respect of much of the medical community and has a thirty-year history of delivering on most of its health promises. Supporters of the diet point to many studies done by both Longevity Center doctors and outside investigators and published in highly respected journals such as the *Journal of the American Medical Association* and the *New England Journal of Medicine*. People do lose weight and keep it off, along with decreasing the risk of heart disease when following the plan.

Dietitians and nutritionists also like the fact that the diet teaches people how to eat well using ordinary foods rather than special pre-packaged foods. This keeps the cost of following the Plan low, especially since the Plan calls for dieters to eat only small quantities of meat. In addition, the Plan is designed to provide a balance of vitamins and minerals from food and does not rely on dietary supplements.

The biggest criticism of the Pritikin Plan is that it requires rigorous self-discipline to stay on for a lifetime. People who do well on the Pritikin Plan tend to be highly motivated and zealous about following the diet. Many healthcare professionals feel long-term success for most people is more likely to occur if the dieter follows a well-balanced but less rigorous diet.

Some nutritionists also take issue with whether the low fat component of the diet allows people to get enough beneficial fats such as **omega-3 fatty acids** and whether absorption of the fat-soluble vitamins A, D, E, and K is impaired. To date these criticisms have not been supported by research findings. However, critics were handed more ammunition by a long-term study of 49,000 American women ages 50–79 that found that a low-fat diet had no effect on the risk of developing heart disease or **cancer**. The study was published in February 2006 in the *Journal of the American Medical Association*. The findings are controversial, and go against much current medical thinking. This study will certainly stimulate additional research on low-fat diets.

Training and certification

The diet can be followed by nearly anyone and requires no special training or certification.

Resources

BOOKS

Pritikin, Nathan. *The Pritikin Permanent Weight Loss Manual*. New York: Grosset & Dunlap. 1981.

Pritikin, Nathan. *Pritikin Program for Diet and Exercise*. New York: Bantam Books. 1987.

Pritikin, Robert. *The Pritikin Principle: The Calorie Density Solution*. New York: Time Life. 2000.

Pritikin, Robert. *The New Pritikin Program: The Easy and Delicious Way to Shed Fat, Lower Your Cholesterol, and Stay Fit*. New York: Pocket Books. 1991.

Pritikin, Robert. *The Pritikin Weight Loss Breakthrough: Five Easy Steps to Outsmart Your Fat Instinct*. New York: Signet. 1999.

Scales, Mary Josephine. *Diets in a Nutshell: A Definitive Guide on Diets from A to Z*. Clifton, VA: Apex Publishers, 2005.

PERIODICALS

Pritikin, Robert. "Go Out and Eat Thin! 32 Slimming Tricks from the Newest Pritikin Diet Program." *Redbook* (Jan. 1990): 74.

ORGANIZATIONS

American Dietetic Association, 120 South Riverside Plaza, Suite 2000, Chicago, Illinois, 60606-6995, (800) 877-1600, http://www.eatright.org.

The Pritikin Longevity Center, 19735 Turnberry Way, Aventura, FL, 33180, (305) 935-7131, (800) 327-4914, (305) 935-7371, http://www.pritikin.com.

Ken R. Wells

Proanthocyanidin *see* **Grape seed extract**

Probiotics

Definition

Probiotics, as defined by the Food and Agricultural Organization of the United Nations (FAO), are "live microorganisms administered in adequate amounts which confer a beneficial health effect on the host." The microorganisms referred to in this definition are non-pathogenic bacteria (small, single celled organisms which do not promote or cause disease), and one yeast, *Saccharomyces*. They are considered "friendly germs," due to benefits to the colon and the immune system. The word probiotic is a compound of a Latin and a Greek word; it means "favorable to life." Probiotics is also sometimes used to refer to a form of nutritional therapy based on eating probiotic foods and dietary supplements. Although probiotic supplements have also been used with farm animals, most are produced for human consumption in the form of dairy products containing two types of microbes—lactobacilli and bifidobacteria. As with the extended use of **royal jelly**, probiotics are now also being used in face creams and similar cosmetic products.

A new category called prebiotics now also appears in the literature. Prebiotics refer mainly to certain foods, and occasionally to certain food products, that support probiotic microorganism viability, enhancing their survivability. Included among prebiotics are foods such as Jerusalem and regular artichokes, oats, leeks, onions and whole grain breads or cereals. Examples of prebiotic food products are the **Fructooligosaccharides** (fructo-oligo-saccharides, or fruit derived, digestion resistant sugars) (FOS), also in honey, and the galactooligosaccharides (galacto-oligo-saccharides), sugars in galactose-containing foods like goats milk.

Origins

Although the term probiotics is relatively recent, as are science-based investigations, the use of probiotic-containing fermented foods in many cultures of the world predates the advent of refrigeration. The applied notion of improving health by supplementing the natural microflora of the human intestines with additional bacteria taken by mouth goes back to the late nineteenth century. At that time, some physicians attributed sickness and the **aging** process to a build up of waste products (or, putrefaction) in the colon (the lower part of the large intestine that empties into the rectum), and toxic materials leaking from the colon into the bloodstream. The process of leakage—

now referred to as gut permeability or leaky gut syndrome— and the poisoning that resulted from it, were called autointoxication. The autointoxication theory assumed that dietary changes aimed at reducing toxic decomposition in the colon would be beneficial to health. Some observers knew about the use of lactic acid bacteria in sausage-making to ferment the meat and protect it from spoilage. Because these bacteria are harmless to humans, it was thought that adding them to the diet by eating fermented foods would reduce the amount of toxins produced in the colon. The Lactobacilli group of bacteria, some of which are found in yogurt, was the first identified probiotic. In the 1920s and 1930s, many doctors recommended **acidophilus** milk, which contains the lactobaccili bacterium called *Lactobacillus acidophilus,* for the treatment of **constipation** and **diarrhea**. This treatment was effective for many patients.

The next phase in the development of probiotics came in the 1950s, when medical researchers began to study *L. acidophilus* as a possible answer to some of the digestive side effects of taking antibiotics. It was known that antibiotic medications upset the natural balance of the intestinal microflora by killing of the beneficial as well as the pathogenic bacteria. The researchers thought that taking oral preparations of *L. acidophilus* might offset the side effects of the antibiotics.

One of the chief difficulties in benefiting from probiotic supplementation has been assuring survivability of the bacteria as it passes through the acidity of the stomach and the digestive processes of the small intestine and successfully colonizing in the colon. Recently, a new probiotic with exceptional survivability and colonization characteristics, as demonstrated in studies, has emerged. This probiotic, screened from many **strains** of lactobacilli and named after its co-discoverers, Sherwood Gorbach and Barry Goldin, is known as Lactobacillus GG (LGG). LGG was demonstrated effective against psuedomembranous **colitis**, an infection of the colon by *Clostridium difficile* as a result of antibiotic overkill of beneficial bacteria, and against atopic **eczema** in children due to gut permeability. LGG was demonstrated to have positive results against Candida in mice, as well. Three patents have been awarded on LGG from June 1989 to May 1995. In 1987, a Finnish dairy cooperative, Valio, Ltd., was granted a license to conduct research. About 1992, Valio released a fermented milk product with LGG called Gefilus. In 1996, a division of an American corporation was formed, called CAG Functional Foods, which markets LGG as the product Culturelle. One source reported significant benefit from the use of

Culturelle when cultured in milk. Culturelle is currently available only in capsules, but a yogurt product is anticipated to be marketed soon.

Much of the research and marketing of proven probiotics is conducted outside the United States. One such research proven probiotic strain is Lactobacillus plantarum 299v. It has been particularly valuable in **irritable bowel syndrome** (IBS) and recovery from surgery. Its colonization ability was proven using biopsy.

Two proven beneficial strains marketed in the United States are *Lactobacillus reuteri,* a Swedish product proven effective against diarrhea in children due to a rotavirus (a virus transmitted from feces), available in the Stoncyfield brand of yogurt, and *Saccharomyces boulardii*, a yeast product available in capsules effective against antibiotic associated diarrhea.

Benefits

Probiotic foods and dietary supplements have been recommended as treatments for a variety of diseases and disorders, ranging from problems confined to the digestive tract to general health issues.

Intestinal complaints

To summarize, probiotic organisms, in particular the LGG strain, have been shown to be helpful in managing the following intestinal disorders:

- Pseudomembranous colitis, a potentially life-threatening inflammation of the colon caused by an overgrowth of the bacterium *Clostridium difficile* as a result of the patient's having taken antibiotics that causes profuse watery diarrhea, cramps, and low-grade fever.
- so-called "traveler's diarrhea"
- acute nonbacterial diarrhea
- rotaviral diarrhea
- irritable bowel syndrome (IBS)
- bacterial overgrowth in the small bowel by organisms such as Helicobacter pylori, implicated in gastric ulcers (studies have demonstrated benefit but not cure)

Lifestyle-related disorders

Some supporters of probiotics go beyond applications limited to treatment of intestinal disorders. In keeping with the theory of autointoxication, they maintain that probiotics are effective in treating a wide range of chronic and acute illnesses thought to result from a condition called intestinal dysbiosis, or poor intestinal health quality due to toxic buildup, putrefaction, and leaky gut syndrome. Intestinal dysbiosis is defined as an imbalance among the various microorganisms in the digestive tract. This imbalance is attributed to a combination of Western high-protein **diets**, **stress**, environmental pollution, and allopathic medications. Putrefaction is believed to result from a low fiber diet, chronic constipation or sluggish colon, and poor food combining leading to increased gut fermentation. Leaky gut syndrome is the term used to suggest that the effect of these toxins on the intestinal cell walls is damaging to intestinal integrity, and as a result, large molecules of relatively undigested food and toxins cross the intestinal membrane into the blood stream.

Some alternative practitioners maintain that the following diseases and disorders are directly related to intestinal dysbiosis or may also be beneficially treated with probiotics:

- mental health problems
- chronic fatigue syndrome
- muscular soreness and stiffness
- autoimmune disorders, including lupus, rheumatoid arthritis, ankylosing spondylitis, enteric arthritis, and Reiter's syndrome (by immune stimulation and repair of the leaking gut)
- lactose intolerance (by increasing the presence of lactase)
- infectious diseases
- high blood pressure (research has demonstrated a systolic blood pressure decrease of 10–20 mm Hg with the use of a fermented milk product
- high cholesterol (clinical studies have not been conclusive; as one source said, "evidence is not overwhelming")
- cancer (by decreasing exposure from gene altering substances)
- menopausal problems in women (by improving the liver's ability to detoxify and eliminate hormonal metabolites)
- vaginosis (once thought to be relatively benign, now implicated in easier transmission of sexual diseases, pelvic inflammatory disease, and pregnancy-related complications, improved by reducing vaginal pH which inhibits growth of unfavorable bacteria)
- allergies and asthma (a double-blind placebo-controlled study demonstrated a 50% drop in children followed up to two years of age)
- kidney stones, by inhibiting the absorption of oxalate from the intestines

More specifically, probiotic foods and dietary supplements are claimed to counteract intestinal dysbiosis in the following ways:

- production of vitamins. Friendly bacteria are said to manufacture vitamin B_3, vitamin B_6, and folic acid.
- anti-tumor and anti-cancer activity
- suppression of pathogenic microorganisms in favor of the non-pathogenic
- relief of anxiety symptoms through indirect detoxification
- protection against radiation and other environmental toxins
- support of the immune system, by reducing immune load
- recirculation of female hormones in the bloodstream by a cleaner liver and cleaner blood, thus maintaining higher levels of estrogen in menopausal women
- maintenance of smooth bowel functioning

Description

Products

Probiotics is a nutrition-based therapy and relies primarily on the addition of foods or supplements containing friendly bacteria to the diet. Some recommended foods are ordinary grocery store items that involve fermentation in their production; these include miso, pickles, sauerkraut and fermented dairy products such as yogurt and kefir. As mentioned, other food or food products called prebiotics, such as Jerusalem artichokes and FOS, are thought to support the growth of the beneficial bacteria in the intestines. Most users and recommenders of probiotics, however, encourage the use of loose powdered, refrigerated dietary supplements of friendly bacteria or LGG capsules. Some of these products are milk-based, while others are milk-free. Probiotic dietary supplements are over-the-counter (OTC) preparations that can be easily purchased at grocery or health food stores, or from European manufacturers over the Internet. The types of bacteria most often recommended are *Lactobacillus GG*, *Lactobacillus acidophilus*, *Lactobacillus bulgaricus*, and, especially for children *Bifidobacterium bifidum*. Breast milk is reported to contain nutrients that support bifidobacterium growth.

Dosage and administration

Some practitioners distinguish between a therapeutic dose of probiotic products, which is given for 10 days, and a maintenance dose, which is used afterward. One source gives 2–5 level tsp (5–10 g) of powdered supplement as the daily therapeutic dose if the patient is taking *L. acidophilus* or *B. bifidum*, 1–3 tsp

(3–6 g) if the patient is using *L. bulgaricus*. The maintenance dose of *L. acidophilus* is given as 0.5 tsp (1 g) daily; of *B. bifidum*, 2 tsp (4 g) daily; of *L. bulgaricus*, 0.5 tsp (1 g) with each meal. The recommended dose of LGG capsules is once daily. A dose two or three times daily may also be used initially to overcome acute symptoms.

Patients are advised to take these supplements with spring water, but not with juice or broth. These fluids are thought to stimulate the secretion of stomach acids that will destroy the friendly bacteria.

Preparation

The fact that probiotic products include some ordinary dairy and grocery items means that most people who use them do not think of them as medications and see no need to consult a health professional. Persons who are taking prescription medications and persons with compromised immune status, however, are advised to consult their doctors before using probiotic dietary supplements. These products often influence the bulk and frequency of bowel movements, thus increasing the elimination rate of some medications and necessitating a dose adjustment.

Some practitioners of nutritional therapies recommend cleansing the lower digestive tract with an enema or colonic treatment before beginning a course of probiotic supplements. Conversely, use of probiotics may be particularly recommended following colonic therapy as it is following antibiotic therapy.

Precautions

Although the bacteria in probiotic supplements are human-friendly, some persons may have food **allergies** or a digestive tract that is sensitive to miso, other fermented foods, or the milk powder that may be in some products. Vegetarians or persons who cannot digest milk-based products may prefer probiotic supplements with a rice base.

Product reliability is a concern because probiotic dietary supplements are not regulated by the Food and Drug Administration (FDA) and because study after study demonstrates the difficulty of maintaining a live probiotic culture, in or out of the body. One study of the microorganisms in 25 dairy products and 30 powdered products found that more than one third of these products contained no living microorganisms, and only 13% of the products contained all of the bacteria types listed on the label. One practitioner suggests the following guidelines for evaluating the effectiveness of probiotic products:

- Number of viable organisms. A number lower than 1 billion organisms per gram is considered inadequate for a therapeutic dosage.
- Type of organism. Single-strain products are considered more useful than multi-strain products on the grounds that the different bacteria in multi-strain products may compete with each other.
- Processing method. Products that have been put through a centrifuge or ultra-filtration system are thought to have fewer viable bacteria.
- Additives. Products that do not have hormones or other chemicals added to stimulate the growth of the bacteria are considered more effective.
- Form. Powdered supplements are considered preferable to liquids. Encapsulated powders are second-best, except in the case of LGG capsules.
- Storage. Probiotic products that are not refrigerated are thought to lose much of their effectiveness.

Side effects

The side effects of treatment with probiotics may include a condition called excessive drainage syndrome, which includes **headache**, diarrhea, bloating, or constipation. Another commonly reported side effect is intestinal **gas**. These side effects are attributed to the cleansing of toxins from the body and may last for some days. Practitioners recommend lowering the supplement dosage to reduce the side effects, or pretreating with colonic therapy, or stool softeners and fiber as tolerated or advised by a healthcare professional.

Research and general acceptance

More studies of probiotics have been done in Europe than in the United States, which is reflected in the fact that the leading manufacturers of probiotic supplements are presently based in Europe. Some mainstream researchers in Europe as well as in the United States are skeptical of some of the claims made for probiotics. Their reasons include the following considerations:

- The studies done in support of probiotics are mostly anecdotal or heavily reliant on test-tube experimentation rather than on clinical trials in human subjects. As of 2000, relatively few strains of probiotic bacteria have been shown to have clinical value. These strains are helpful in treating milk allergy and irritable bowel syndrome in humans, and in improving resistance to a yeast called *Candida* in immunocompromised mice.
- The basic concept of probiotics is based on a misunderstanding of the role of microflora in the human digestive tract.

KEY TERMS

Autointoxication—Self-poisoning by toxic products formed within the body during intestinal digestion. This term was coined around 1885 as part of a theory that regarded intestinal function as a central aspect of health.

Colon—The part of the large intestine that lies between the cecum and the rectum, and is divided by name into three parts, the ascending, transverse and descending colon. In a healthy person, the ascending colon rises upward intra-abdominally from above the right leg toward the right hip, the transverse colon crosses over to the left hip, and the descending colon segment joins the rectum intra-abdominally, near the top of the left leg. An unhealthy colon may droop, drape, or twist, and be enlarged or otherwise irregularly shaped.

Intestinal dysbiosis—An imbalance among the various microorganisms that live in the digestive tract.

Intestinal microflora—The bacteria and other microorganisms that live in the human gastrointestinal tract.

Miso—A fermented paste made from soybeans, salt, and rice or barley, used to flavor soups and sauces in Oriental cooking.

Pseudomembranous colitis—A potentially life-threatening inflammation of the colon, caused by a toxin released by the Clostridium difficile bacterium that multiplies rapidly following antibiotic treatment.

Traveler's diarrhea—Diarrhea caused by ingesting local bacteria to which one's digestive system has not yet adapted.

- It is difficult to see how bacteria taken by mouth can survive the process of human digestion. At present, only two species of lactobacilli, *L. GG* and *L. plantarum 299v*, have been shown to be able to colonize the human gut.

- Supporters of probiotics emphasize two types of bacteria, the lactobacilli and the bifidobacteria, and virtually ignore the hundreds of other species that live in the intestines.

More clinical studies examining the effects of probiotics on specific conditions are being conducted. One such study in the making will examine the effect of probiotics on hepatic steatosis, or fatty degeneration of the liver. An inclusion criteria was biopsy diagnosis of non-alcoholic fatty liver disease. The study is expected to be completed in October 2004.

Training and certification

As of 2000, there are no training or certification programs specifically for probiotics. Most practitioners who recommend probiotics have been trained as nutritionists or naturopathic physicians.

Resources

BOOKS

Chaitow, Leon, ND, and Natasha Trenev. *Probiotics.* Northampton, UK: Thorsons, 1990.

ORGANIZATIONS

American Academy of Alternative Medicine (AAAM). 16126 E. Warren, Box 24224. Detroit, MI 48224-0224. (313) 882-0641. Fax: (313) 882-0972.

Ontario College of Naturopathic Medicine. 60 Berl Avenue. Toronto, Ontario M8Y3C7.

OTHER

Bryan, Mike. "Probiotics and Prebiotics." 1997-2004. [cited June 4, 2004]. http://www.medicinalfoodnews.com/vol02/issue7/biotic.htm.

Clarke, Jane. "Bacteria." [cited June 4, 2004]. http://www.bbc.co.uk/cgi-bin/education.

"Frequently Asked Questions: Probiotics, New Zealand." 2001 [cited June 4, 2004]. http://www.probiotics.co.nz/faqsAnswrNtrn.sap?id = 5.

"History of Probiotic Research." June 27, 2001 [cited June 4, 2004]. http://www.phototour.minneapolis.mn.us/candida/history.html.

"Lactobacillus GG (LGG)." July 16, 2001 [cited June 4, 2004]. http://www.phototour.minneapolis.mn.us/candida/lgg.html.

"Lactobacillus plantarum 299v (Lp299v)." March 14, 2004. [cited June 4, 2004]. http://www.phototour.minneapolis.mn.us/candida/lp299v.html.

Mercola, M.D., Joseph. "One Third of Probiotics, 'Good Bacteria' Products Like Acidophilus, Found to be Worthless." July 11, 2001 [cited June 4, 2004]. http://www.mercola.com/2001/jul/11/probiotics.htm.

Solga, M.D., Steve. "Probiotics Effect on Hepatic Steatosis." September 2003 [cited June 4, 2004]. http://www.clinicaltrials.gov/ct/show.

"Summary of Probiotic Strains." April 30, 2002 [cited June 4, 2004]. http://www.phototour.minneapolis.mn.us/candida/summary.htm

"What Are Probiotics?" USProbiotics.org. 2004 [cited June 4, 2004]. http://www.usprobiotics.org/101.

Rebecca Frey, Ph.D.
Katherine E. Nelson, N.D.

Prolotherapy

Definition

Prolotherapy is the treatment of soft-tissue damage through the use of injections. The injections lead to inflammation in the area, and the body reacts by increasing the blood supply and sending more nutrients to the area, resulting in tissue repair. The term prolotherapy is derived from the word *prolo*, short for proliferation, as the therapy is intended to proliferate tissue growth in the damaged area.

Origins

The idea behind this therapy dates back more than 2000 years to Hippocrates, who used it to treat soldiers with injured shoulders. Instead of injections Hippocrates used a hot poker, which he speared into the shoulder joint, causing inflammation and stimulating the body to repair itself. Prolotherapy using injections was derived from a treatment developed by H.I. Biegeleisen called sclerotherapy, used to treat **varicose veins**. In the 1950s, George Hackett, often called a pioneer of prolotherapy, was experimenting with and touting the benefits of the procedure.

Benefits

Prolotherapy has been used to treat chronic neck and back **pain**, joint pain from arthritis, headaches, **fibromyalgia**, sports injuries, **carpal tunnel syndrome**, and partially torn tendons, ligaments, and cartilage.

The benefit of prolotherapy is that it is a nonsurgical procedure that can be administered in a clinic, saving patients from undergoing anesthesia and surgery followed by a long recovery period. It's also cheaper than surgery. The average back or neck surgery costs about $40,000, while a single prolotherapy treatment runs anywhere from $90–$200, though patients may need several treatments. Furthermore, with prolotherapy there is no loss of mobility as there is with back surgery, when doctors fuse together the vertebrae in an effort to create stability in the spine.

Another benefit is that prolotherapy takes patients off drugs. Patients escape the cost of pain killers and their side effects.

Description

In prolotherapy, a doctor injects a sugar water or salt water-based solution into the damaged ligament or tendon at the point where it attaches to the bone. The injection produces an inflammation, which

increases blood flow, swelling, and pain. The body then launches a course of repair and healing. The inflammation tricks the body into thinking another injury has occurred, so it sends in macrophages, which are cells that ingest and destroy the irritant solution. These cells clean up the area. The body then sends in fibroblasts, which are cells that help build fibrous tissue. The fibroblasts excrete collagen, a protein that makes the ligaments denser and stronger. The stronger ligaments provide more support for the joints, often alleviating the pain.

The length of treatment sessions varies and depends on the area being treated. For example, treatment of an injured elbow involves injections only in one site, whereas treatment of larger areas, like the neck and back, involves more injections. Treating an elbow may take only a few injections, whereas the back may involve up to 50 injections for one treatment. The more injections, the longer the treatment.

The treatment generally involves several sessions, usually three to six, which are separated by two or three-week intervals. Some practitioners space treatments four or six weeks apart.

Though doctors have practiced prolotherapy for more than a half-century, it is still considered an alternative treatment; therefore most insurance policies don't cover it.

Preparations

Analgesics and sedatives may be given before treatment to reduce discomfort. Many patients, however, forgo sedation because they cannot drive home afterward. Many doctors use topical freeze sprays, ice packs, or anaesthetic cream to reduce skin sensation.

It is recommended that patients drink plenty of water in the hours before the procedure because it helps with cell hydration.

Precautions

As with all procedures, there are risks. Patients are asked to sign a consent and waiver. Since the treatment involves inserting a needle into the body, there is a chance of puncture to arteries, nerves, or even lung tissue, depending on the area to be treated. Some patients may have allergic reactions to the substance injected.

Side effects

The most common side effects include pain during the injections and soreness and stiffness afterward. Patients are reminded not to take any anti-inflammatory drugs, such as ibuprofen, because these will impede the healing process prolotherapy aims to set in place.

Research and general acceptance

According to the Alternative Medicine Network, studies show prolotherapy relieves 92% of those treated; however, the therapy is relatively untested.

Opponents wonder how prolotherapists decide where to make their injections since areas of ligament weakening won't show up on an x ray. Others fear nervous system damage should the substance be injected too close to the nerves. Prolotherapy received a bad name in the 1950s when the *Lancet* reported three cases of paralysis and two deaths after treatment. It did not resurface for a number of years. As of 2000, there were only 400–500 U.S. doctors administering the treatment.

In the April 1997 issue of *Headache,* Dr. Irwin Abraham of Rochester, New York, reported preliminary findings of a study on prolotherapy to cure chronic headaches with **neck pain**. Of 17 patients, 11 said their symptoms were improved or relieved after treatment. At a two-year follow-up, nine reported complete relief, one had partial relief, and one's symptoms had relapsed.

Training and certification

Abraham stated in *Headache* that prolotherapy is a "safe, simple, and long-lasting treatment that any primary care physician can perform in the office setting." Doctors can learn prolotherapy through observation and instruction by a skilled prolotherapist.

The American Association of Orthopedic Medicine offers courses and workshops to train physicians and works to increase the number of physicians using the therapy.

Resources

PERIODICALS

Abraham, Irwin. "Prolotherapy for Chronic Headache." *Headache* (April 1997): 256.

Jennings, Suzanne. "The Prolotherapy Option." *Forbes* 152, no. 13 (December 1993): 248.

ORGANIZATIONS

American Association of Orthopedic Medicine. (800) 992-2062. http://www.aaomed.org.

OTHER

"Prolotherapy: The Natural Solution for Pain." *Mark T. Wheaton's Orthopedic Practice Page.* http://www.wheatons.com/Prolotherapy_CommonQuestions.htm. (June 2000).

"Prolotherapy defined." Prolotherapy.com http://www.prolotherapy.com/prolodefine.htm. (June 2000).

"The Thinking Person's Guide to Perfect Health: Sclerotherapy (Prololotherapy)." *The Alternative Medicine Network.* http://www.sonic.net/-nexus/sclero.html. (June 2000).

Lisa Frick

Prostate cancer

Definition

In prostate **cancer** cells of the prostate become abnormal and start to grow uncontrollably, forming tumors. Tumors that can spread to other parts of the body are called malignant tumors or cancers. Tumors incapable of spreading are said to be benign.

Description

As of 2007, prostate cancer was the most commonly diagnosed malignancy among adult males in Western countries. Although prostate cancer is often very slow growing, it can be aggressive, especially in younger men. Given its slow growing nature, many men with the disease die of other causes rather than from the cancer itself. In 2007, there were more than 218,000 new cases of prostate cancer and more than 27,000 deaths from the disease in the United States. More than 2 million men in the United States who have been diagnosed with prostate cancer at some

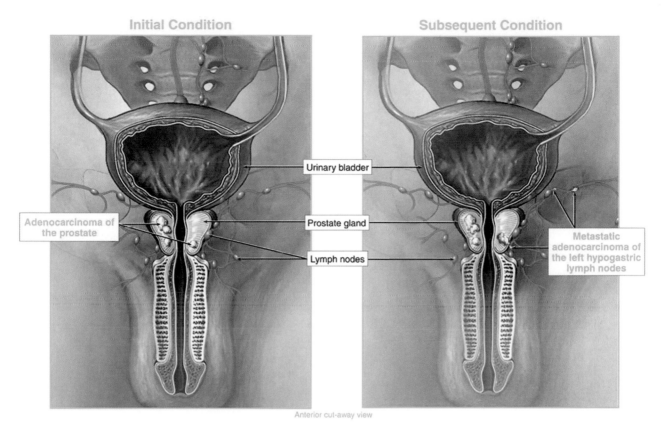

Initial Condition   Subsequent Condition

Adenocarcinoma of the prostate

Urinary bladder

Prostate gland

Lymph nodes

Metastatic adenocarcinoma of the left hypogastric lymph nodes

Anterior cut-away view

Progression of prostate cancer. *(© Nucleus Medical Art, Inc. / Alamy)*

point were still alive as of 2007, according to the American Cancer Society (ACS). The Canadian Cancer Society reported about 22,000 new cases of prostate cancer and 4,300 deaths in 2007. It is the number one cancer among Canadian men accounting for 27% of all cancers in males. Although prostate cancer may be very slow-growing, it is a heterogeneous disease and can be quite aggressive, especially in younger men. When the disease is slow-growing, it may often go undetected. Because it may take years for the cancer to develop, many men with the disease will probably die of other causes, rather than from the cancer itself.

Prostate cancer affects African American men twice as often as it does Caucasian men, and the mortality rate among African Americans is also two times higher. African Americans have the highest rate of prostate cancer in the world, whereas the rate in Asians is one of the lowest. However, although the rate of prostate cancer in native Japanese is low, the rate in Japanese Americans is closer to that of white American men. This pattern suggests that environmental factors and diet also play a role in prostate cancer.

The prostate, testicles, and seminal vesicles are the major male sex glands. These three glands together secrete the fluid that makes up semen. The prostate is about the size of a walnut and lies just behind the urinary bladder. A tumor in the prostate interferes with proper control of the bladder and normal sexual functions. Often, the first symptom of prostate cancer is difficulty in urinating. However, because the same symptom can be caused by a common, noncancerous condition of the prostate (benign prostatic hyperplasia), this symptom is insufficient in determining if prostate cancer is present.

As the prostate cancer grows, some of the cells break off and spread to other parts of the body through the lymph or the blood. The most common sites to which it spreads are the lymph nodes, the lungs, and various bones around the hips and the pelvic region.

Causes and symptoms

As of the late 2000s the cause of prostate cancer was not known; however, the disease is found mainly in men over the age of 55. The average age at diagnosis is 72. In fact, 80% of the prostate cancer cases occur in men over the age of 65. While only 1 in 100,000 men gets prostate cancer under the age of 40, the frequency rises to 1,326 cases per 100,000 for men between the ages of 70 and 74. Hence, age appears to be a risk factor for prostate cancer.

Some studies have shown that a family history of prostate cancer puts a man at higher risk for developing this disease. In addition, there is some evidence that a diet high in fat increases the risk of prostate cancer. Workers in the electroplating and welding industries who are exposed to the metal cadmium and rubber industry workers appear to have a higher than average risk of getting this disease. Research has indicated that men with high plasma testosterone levels also may be at an increased risk.

Frequently, prostate cancer has no symptoms, and the disease is diagnosed when the patient goes for a routine screening examination. However, occasionally, when the tumor becomes large or the cancer has spread to the nearby tissues, the following symptoms may be seen:

- weak or interrupted flow of the urine
- frequent urination (especially at night)
- difficulty starting urination
- inability to urinate
- pain or burning sensation when urinating
- blood in the urine
- persistent pain in lower back, hips, or thighs (bone pain)
- painful ejaculation

Diagnosis

Prostate cancer is curable when detected early. However, because the early stages of prostate cancer may not have any visible symptoms, it often goes undetected until the patient goes for a routine physical examination. Diagnosis of the disease is made using some or all of the following tests.

Digital rectal examination (DRE)

In order to perform this test, the doctor puts a gloved, lubricated finger into the rectum to feel for any lumps in the prostate. The rectum lies just behind the prostate gland, and a majority of prostate tumors begin in the posterior region of the prostate. If the doctor does detect an abnormality, then more tests are ordered to confirm the diagnosis.

BLOOD TESTS. Blood tests are used to measure the amounts of certain protein markers, such as the prostate-specific antigen (PSA), found circulating in the blood. The cells lining the prostate generally make this protein and a small amount can be detected in the bloodstream. However, prostate cancers produce a lot of this protein, and it can be easily detected in the blood. Hence, when PSA is found in the blood in higher than normal amounts for the patient's particular age group, cancer may be present.

TRANSRECTAL ULTRASOUND. A small probe is placed in the rectum, and sound waves are released from the probe. These sound waves bounce off the prostate tissue and an image is created. Since normal prostate tissue and prostate tumors reflect the sound waves differently, the test can be used quite efficiently to detect tumors. Though the insertion of the probe into the rectum may be slightly uncomfortable, the procedure is generally painless and takes only 20 minutes.

PROSTATE BIOPSY. If cancer is suspected from the results of any of the above tests, the doctor removes a small piece of prostate tissue with a hollow needle. This sample is then checked under the microscope for the presence of cancerous cells. Prostate biopsy is the most definitive diagnostic tool for prostate cancer.

If cancer is detected during the microscopic examination of the prostate tissue, the pathologist grades the tumor using the Gleason system, which means the pathologist scores the tumor on a scale of 1 to 10 to indicate how aggressive the tumor is. Tumors with a lower score are less likely to grow and spread than are tumors with higher scores. The Gleason system is different from staging the cancer. When doctors stage a cancer, they give it a number that indicates whether it has spread, as well as the extent of its spread. In Stage I, the cancer is localized, whereas in the last stage, Stage IV, the cancer cells have spread to other parts of the body.

X RAYS AND IMAGING TECHNIQUES. A chest x ray may be ordered to determine whether the cancer has spread to the lungs. Imaging techniques (such as computed tomography scans and magnetic resonance imaging), in which a computer is used to generate a detailed picture of the prostate and areas nearby, may be used to get a clearer view of the internal organs. A bone scan also may be used to check whether the cancer has spread to the bone.

Treatment

The doctor and the patient decide on the treatment mode after considering many factors. Such factors include the patient's age, the stage of the tumor, his general health, and the presence of any other illnesses. In addition, the patient's personal preferences and the risks and benefits of each treatment protocol are taken into account before any decision is made.

Various natural remedies used to treat noncancerous prostate problems can be implemented with the approval of a medical doctor along with the recommended medical care. **Prostate enlargement** is a precursor to prostate cancer, and many alternative treatments are available to alleviate benign prostate enlargement. Among these is the herb **saw palmetto**, which has shown to be highly effective in the treatment of prostate enlargement. In addition, treatments that focus on strengthening the immune system of the cancer patient can be helpful, using physiological and psychological therapies.

Lycopene, the antioxidant found in tomatoes and tomato products, has long been thought to help prevent prostate cancer. In the first clinical intervention trial of prostate cancer patients in 2001, lycopene supplementation slowed the progression of prostate cancer.

Visualization of a healthy, cancer-free body, and of cancer cells as weak and confused is believed to constitute healing imagery. Numerous studies affirm the power of a positive mental attitude in assisting conventional medical treatment to be more effective, while at the same time, minimizing undesirable side effects of chemotherapy or radiation.

Compounds contained in **maitake** mushrooms are believed to enhance the immune response and slow the growth of tumors. One study by a homeopathic physician, Abram Ber of Phoenix, Arizona, found that patients with prostate cancer treated with maitake mushroom tablets reported a decrease in the urge to urinate, along with improvement in the flow of urine.

Watchful waiting

Watchful waiting means no immediate treatment is recommended, but doctors keep the patient under careful observation. This option is generally used in older patients when the tumor is not very aggressive and the patients have other, more life-threatening illnesses. Prostate cancer in older men tends to be slow-growing. Therefore, the risk of the patient dying from prostate cancer, rather than from other causes, is relatively small.

Allopathic treatment

Surgery

For early stage prostate cancer, surgery is the best option and the most common one. Radical prostatectomy involves complete removal of the prostate.

During the surgery, a sample of the lymph nodes near the prostate is removed to determine whether the cancer has spread beyond the prostate gland. Because the seminal vesicles (the glands where sperm is made) are removed along with the prostate, **infertility** is a side effect of this surgery. In order to minimize the risk of **impotence** (inability to have an erection) and incontinence (inability to control urine flow), a procedure known as nerve-sparing prostatectomy is used.

In a different surgical method, known as the transurethral resection procedure (TURP), only the cancerous portion of the prostate is removed, by using a small wire loop that is introduced into the prostate through the urethra. This technique is most often used in men who cannot have a radical prostatectomy due to age or other illness, and it is rarely recommended.

RADIATION THERAPY. Radiation therapy involves the use of high-energy x rays to kill cancer cells or to shrink tumors. It can be used instead of surgery for early stages of cancer. The radiation can either be administered from a machine outside the body (external beam radiation), or small radioactive pellets can be implanted in the prostate gland in the area surrounding the tumor.

HORMONE THERAPY. Hormone therapy is commonly used when the cancer is in an advanced stage and has spread to other parts of the body. Prostate cells need the male hormone testosterone to grow. Decreasing the levels of this hormone, or inhibiting its activity, causes the cancer to shrink. Hormone levels can be decreased in several ways. Orchiectomy is a surgical procedure that involves complete removal of the testicles, leading to a decrease in the levels of testosterone. Alternatively, drugs (such as LHRH agonists or anti-androgens) that bind to the male hormone testosterone and block its activity can be given. Another method tricks the body by administering the female hormone estrogen. When this is given, the body senses the presence of a sex hormone and stops producing testosterone. However, there are some unpleasant side effects to hormone therapy. Depending on the doses of estrogen, men may have **hot flashes** (such as those symptomatic of **menopause**), enlargement and tenderness of the breasts, erectile dysfunction (ED) or loss of sexual desire, as well as a risk of **blood clots**, heart attacks, and strokes.

CHEMOTHERAPY. Chemotherapy is the use of drugs to treat a disease. The drugs can either be taken as a pill or injected into the body through a needle that is inserted into a blood vessel. This type of treatment is called systemic treatment because the drug enters the blood stream, travels through the whole body, and kills the cancer cells that are outside the prostate. Chemotherapy is sometimes used to treat prostate cancer that has recurred after other treatment. As of 2008, research was ongoing to find more drugs that are effective for the treatment of prostate cancer.

CRYOTHERAPY. Cryotherapy was still in the experimental stages in the United States as of early 2008. Cryosurgery destroys the cancer by freezing it and is under study as an alternative to surgery and radiation therapy. To avoid damaging healthy tissue, the doctor places a cryoprobe in direct contact with the tumor to freeze it. It is likely to be at least several years before cryotherapy is ready for general use in the United States. However, cryotherapy is in use in India as a primary treatment for localized or locally advanced prostate cancer.

Expected results

According to the American Cancer Society, the survival rate for all stages of prostate cancer combined increased from 50 to 87% between 1975 and 2005. Due to early detection and better screening methods, nearly 60% of the tumors are diagnosed while they are still confined to the prostate gland. The five-year survival rate for early stage cancers is almost 99%. Sixty three percent of the patients survive 10 years, and 51% survive 15 years after initial diagnosis.

Prevention

Because the cause of the cancer is not known, there is no definite way to prevent prostate cancer. However, the American Cancer Society recommends that all men over age 40 have an annual rectal exam and that men have an annual PSA test beginning at age 50. Those who have a higher than average risk, including African American men and men with a family history of prostate cancer, should begin annual PSA testing even earlier, starting at age 45.

Some evidence suggests that a diet high in fat increases the risk of prostate cancer. A diet high in fruits and vegetables may decrease the risk. Studies also suggest that nutrients such as soy isoflavones, **vitamin E**, **selenium**, **vitamin D**, and **carotenoids** (including lycopene, the red color agent in tomatoes and beets) may decrease prostate cancer risk. Further studies to find out whether men can reduce their risk of prostate cancer by taking certain dietary supplements were underway as of early 2008, according to the National Cancer Institute.

KEY TERMS

Anti-androgen drugs—Drugs that block the activity of the male hormone.

Benign—Not spreading, cancerous, or life-threatening.

Benign prostatic hyperplasia (BPH)—A noncancerous condition of the prostate that causes growth of the prostate tissue, thus enlarging the prostate and obstructing urination.

Biopsy—Surgical removal and microscopic examination of living tissue for diagnostic purposes.

Chemotherapy—Chemical (drug) treatment of disease; in cancer treatment, the use of synthetic drugs to destroy a tumor either by inhibiting the growth of the cancerous cells or by killing the cancer cells.

Estrogen—A female sex hormone.

Hormone therapy—In prostate cancer, treatment that involves reducing the levels of the male hormone testosterone, so that the growth of the prostate cancer cells is inhibited.

Lymph nodes—Small bean-shaped structures that are scattered along the lymphatic vessels. These nodes serve as filters and retain any bacteria or cancer cells that are traveling through the system.

Malignant—Capable of spreading, cancerous, and potentially life-threatening.

Prostatectomy—Surgical removal of the prostate gland.

Radiation therapy—Treatment using high energy radiation from x-ray machines, cobalt, radium, or other sources.

Rectum—The last 5 to 6 in (13-16 cm) of the intestine that leads to the anus.

Semen—A whitish, opaque fluid containing sperm released at ejaculation.

Seminal vesicles—The pouches above the prostate that store semen.

Testicles—Two egg-shaped glands that produce sperm and sex hormones.

Testosterone—A male sex hormone produced mainly by the testicles.

Trans-rectal ultrasound—A procedure in which a probe is placed in the rectum. High-frequency sound waves that cannot be heard by humans are sent out from the probe and reflected by the prostate. These sound waves produce a pattern of echoes which are then used by the computer to create sonograms, or pictures of areas inside the body.

Various research initiatives were underway as of early 2008 to discover new ways to treat and possibly prevent prostate cancer. Researchers were studying changes in genes that may increase the risk for developing prostate cancer. Some studies were looking at the genes of men who were diagnosed with prostate cancer at a relatively young age, such as less than 55 years old, and the genes of families who have several members with the disease. Other studies were trying to identify which genes, or combination of genes, are most likely to lead to prostate cancer. Much more work was needed, however, before scientists could say exactly how genetic changes relate to prostate cancer.

Scientists were also looking at ways to stop prostate cancer from returning in men who have already been treated for the disease. These approaches use drugs such as finasteride, flutamide, nilutamide, and LH-RH agonists that manipulate hormone levels. One study found that the combination of nilutamide and an experimental cancer vaccine was effective in reducing recurrence of prostate cancer. The experimental vaccine was designed to strengthen the body's natural defenses against prostate cancer. The experimental prostate cancer vaccine, called Provenge, was denied approval by the U.S. Food and Drug Administration (FDA) in 2007 because it failed to shrink prostate tumors during a trial in 127 men. The safety and effectiveness of a drug or vaccine are key measurements the FDA uses in approving or disapproving it. However, the study reported men who received the Provenge vaccine lived 4.5 months longer than men on conventional treatments. In 2007, an FDA advisory panel recommended approval of Provenge, finding that it was both safe and effective. In a rare move, the FDA rejected the advisory panel's approval recommendation, saying it wanted another study done. This study was expected to be completed in late 2008.

Resources

BOOKS

Ellsworth, Pamela, and Alan J. Wein. *100 Questions & Answers About Prostate Cancer*. Sudbury, MA: Jones & Bartlett Publishers, 2008.

Skarin, Arthur T., et al. *Prostate Cancer: Dana-Farber Cancer Institute Handbook*. Burlington, MA: Mosby, 2007.

Torrey, E. Fuller. *Surviving Prostate Cancer: What You Need to Know to Make Informed Decisions*. New Haven, CT: Yale University Press, 2008.

PERIODICALS

Albaugh, Jeffrey, and Eileen Danaher Hacker. "Measurement of Quality of Life in Men with Prostate Cancer." *Clinical Journal of Oncology Nursing* (February 2008): 81(6).

Babbington, Gabrielle. "Prostate Cancer Study Divides Experts." *Australian Doctor* (October 19, 2007): 6.

Bivins, Vincent Michael. "After the Prostate Cancer Diagnosis: Thanks to Advanced Technology, Treatment Options Can Lead to a Better Quality of Life." *Ebony* (February 2008): 50.

Doyle-Lindrud, Susan. "Prostate Cancer: A Chronic Illness." *Clinical Journal of Oncology Nursing* (December 2007): 857(5).

Faloon, William. "Lignans Protect Against Prostate Cancer." *Life Extension* (January 2008): N/A.

Katz, Aaron. "Life-Saving Advances in Prostate Cancer Testing." *Life Extension* (January 2008): N/A.

Ranjan, Pratyush, et al. "High Intensity Focused Ultrasound vs. Cryotherapy as Primary Treatment for Prostate Cancer." *Indian Journal of Urology* (January/March 2008): 16.

ORGANIZATIONS

American Cancer Society, 1599 Clifton Rd. NE, Atlanta, Georgia, 30329, (800) 227-2345, http://www.cancer.org.

American Prostate Society, PO Box 870, Hanover, MD, 21076, (410) 859-7335, http://www.americanprostatesociety.com.

American Urologic Association, 1000 Corporate Blvd., Suite 410, Linthicum, MD, 21090, (866) 746-4282, http://www.auanet.org.

Canadian Cancer Society, 10 Alcorn Ave., Suite 200, Toronto, ON, M4V 3B1, Canada, (888) 939-3333, http://www.cancer.ca.

National Cancer Institute, 9000 Rockville Pike, Bethesda, MD, 20892, (800) 422-6237, http://www.cancer.gov/.

Kathleen Wright
Ken R. Wells

Prostate enlargement

Definition

A non-cancerous condition that affects many men past 50 years of age, enlarged prostate makes eliminating urine more difficult by narrowing the urethra, a tube running from the bladder through the prostate gland. It can effectively be treated by surgery and, in the 2000s, by certain drugs.

Description

The common term for enlarged prostate is BPH, which stands for benign (non-cancerous) prostatic hyperplasia or hypertrophy. Hyperplasia means that the prostate cells are dividing too rapidly, increasing the total number of cells and therefore the size of the organ itself. Hypertrophy simply means enlargement. BPH is often part of the **aging** process. The actual changes in the prostate may start as early as the 30s but

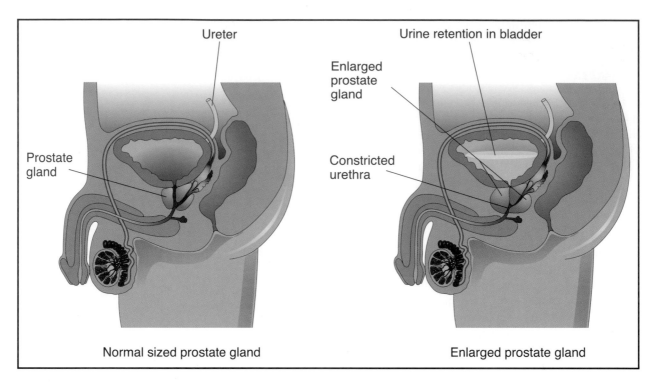

Ureter

Urine retention in bladder

Enlarged
prostate
gland

Prostate
gland

Constricted
urethra

Normal sized prostate gland

Enlarged prostate gland

An enlarged prostate is a non-cancerous condition in which the narrowing of the urethra makes the elimination of urine more difficult. It most often occurs in men over age 50. *(Iustration by Electronic Illustrators Group. Cengage Learning, Gale)*

take place very gradually, so that significant enlargement and symptoms usually do not appear until after age 50. Past this age the chances of the prostate enlarging and causing urinary symptoms become progressively greater. More than 40% of men in their 70s have an enlarged prostate. Symptoms generally appear between the ages of 55 and 75. About 10% of all men eventually require treatment for BPH.

BPH has been viewed as a rare condition in blacks, but this finding may partly be due to the fact that black patients may have less access to medical care. The condition also seems to be uncommon among the Chinese and other Asian peoples, for reasons that in the 2000s are not clear.

Causes and symptoms

The cause of BPH is a mystery, but age-related changes in the levels of hormones circulating in the blood may be a factor. Whatever the cause, an enlarging prostate gradually narrows the urethra and obstructs the flow of urine. Even though the muscle in the bladder wall becomes stronger in an attempt to push urine through the smaller urethra, in time, the bladder fails to empty completely at each urination. The urine that collects in the bladder can become infected and lead to stone formation. The kidneys themselves may be damaged by infection or by urine constantly backing up.

When the enlarging prostate gland narrows the urethra, a man will have increasing trouble starting the urine stream. Because some urine remains behind in the bladder, he will have to urinate more often, perhaps two or three times at night (nocturia). The need to urinate can become very urgent and, in time, urine may seep out. Other symptoms of BPH are a weak and sometimes a split stream and general aching or **pain** in the perineum (the area between the scrotum and anus). Some men may have considerable enlargement of the prostate before even mild symptoms develop.

If a man must strain to urinate, small veins in the bladder wall and urethra may rupture, causing blood to appear in the urine. If the urinary stream becomes totally blocked, the urine collecting in the bladder may cause severe discomfort, a condition called acute urinary retention. Urine that stagnates in the bladder can easily become infected. A burning feeling during urination and **fever** are clues that infection may have developed. Finally, if urine backs up long enough it may increase pressure in the kidneys, though this rarely causes permanent kidney damage.

Diagnosis

When a man's symptoms point to BPH, the physician first performs a digital rectal examination, inserting a finger into the anus to feel whether—and how much—the prostate is enlarged. A smooth prostate surface suggests BPH, whereas a distinct lump in the gland might mean **prostate cancer**. The next procedure is a blood test for a substance called prostate-specific antigen (PSA). Between 30–50% of men with BPH have an elevated PSA level. In fact, some studies indicate that the PSA level can be used as a predictor of a man's long-term risk of developing BPH. A high BPH level does not indicate **cancer** by any means, but other measures are needed to make sure that the prostate enlargement is benign.

An ultrasound examination of the prostate, which is entirely safe and delivers no radiation, can show whether the prostate is enlarged and may indicate if cancer is present.

If digital or ultrasound examination of the prostate raises the suspicion of cancer, most urologists recommend that a prostatic tissue biopsy be performed. This procedure is usually performed with a lance-like instrument that is inserted into the rectum. It pierces the rectal wall and, guided by the physician's finger, obtains six to eight pieces of prostatic tissue that are sent to the laboratory for microscopic examination.

A catheter placed through the urethra and into the bladder can show how much urine remains in the bladder after the patient urinates—a measure of how severe the obstruction is. Another and very simple test for obstruction is to have the man urinate into a uroflowmeter that measures the rate of urine flow. A very certain—though invasive—way of confirming obstruction from an enlarged prostate is to pass a special viewing instrument called a cystoscope into the bladder, but this is not often necessary.

It is routine to check a urine sample for an increased number of white blood cells, which may mean there is infection of the bladder or kidneys. The same sample may be cultured to show what type of bacterium is causing the infection and which antibiotics will work best. The state of the kidneys may be checked in two ways: imaging by either ultrasound or injecting a dye (the intravenous urogram, or pyelogram); or a blood test for creatinine, which collects in the blood when the kidneys cannot.

Treatment

An extract of the **saw palmetto** (*Serenoa repens* or *S. serrulata*) has been shown to stop or decrease the hyperplasia of the prostate. The herb is believed to inhibit the enzyme that converts one type of testosterone to another (significant in both prostate enlargement and prostate cancer), offering the same positive effects as the prescription drug Proscar or Propecia

(finasteride) without the negative side effects. Symptoms of BPH will improve after taking the herb for one to two months but continued use is recommended.

In 2006, researchers in San Francisco reported that a year-long study of saw palmetto to treat BPH showed it was no more effective than a placebo in controlling symptoms. The study of 225 men taking 160 mg of saw palmetto twice a day concluded that there clearly was no benefit of using saw palmetto to treat BPH. The researchers said that previous studies that showed saw palmetto effective in treating BPH involved a small number of participants and had a short duration. However, researchers said their study was not conclusive and urged further research. They also noted that other health practitioners believe a higher dose of saw palmetto is needed for it to be effective.

Zinc is also effective in shrinking an enlarged prostate. A 15–30 mg zinc supplement, or inclusion of pumpkin or sunflower seeds in the daily diet, can produce the desired effect. Prevention of prostate inflammation and swelling is thought to be aided by an increase in **essential fatty acids**. One source of these fatty acids is **flaxseed** oil, available in capsule or liquid form at most health food stores.

The increase in circulation to the groin achieved by certain **yoga** poses and exercises can ease prostate problems. The knee squeeze and the seated sun poses should become a part of the daily routine. The stomach lock **exercise**, performed in a supine position, involves taking a deep breath and then breathing out slowly as the buttocks, groin, and stomach muscles are pulled in. Experts believe this exercise can both prevent prostate problems and treat flare ups; however, this exercise is not recommended for those with **hypertension**, **heart disease**, **hiatal hernia**, or ulcers.

Imagery that involves picturing the prostate shrinking to normal size and sensing an even flow of urine, practiced twice a day, can be helpful. A **reflexology** session to relax the entire body, with special attention to the prostate and endocrine reflexes in the hands and feet, may help the body heal itself.

Allopathic treatment

A class of drugs called alpha blockers relaxes the muscle tissue surrounding the bladder outlet and lining the wall of the urethra to permit urine to flow more freely. These drugs improve obstructive symptoms but do not keep the prostate from enlarging. Examples of alpha-blockers include terazosin (Hytrin), doxazosin (Cardura), prazosin (Minipress), tamsulosin (Flomax), and alfuzosin (Uroxatral). Another class of drugs, called 5 alpha-reductase inhibitors, does shrink the prostate and may delay the need for surgery. Symptoms may not, however, improve until the drug has been used for three months or longer. One 5 alpha-reductase inhibitor, finasteride (Proscar and Propecia), has been shown to reduce the risk of developing prostate cancer by as much as 25%. Side effects occur in less than 10% of men using these drugs and include sexual problems such as a decrease in ejaculate volume, loss of sex drive, and erectile dysfunction. Another 5 alpha-reductase inhibitor is dutasteride (Avodart). Antibiotic drugs are given promptly whenever infection is diagnosed. Some medications, including antihistamines and some decongestants, can make the symptoms of BPH suddenly worse and even cause acute urinary retention and, therefore, should be avoided.

When drugs have failed to control symptoms of BPH but the physician does not believe that conventional surgery is yet needed, a procedure called transurethral needle ablation (TUNA) may be tried. The patient is given local anesthesia, and a needle is inserted into the prostate and radio frequency energy is applied to destroy the tissue that is obstructing urine flow. Another approach is microwave **hyperthermia**, using a device called the Prostatron to deliver microwave energy to the prostate through a catheter. This procedure is done at an outpatient surgery center.

For many years the standard operation for BPH has been transurethral resection (TUR) of the prostate. Under general or spinal anesthesia, a cystoscope is passed through the urethra and prostate tissue surrounding the urethra is removed using either a cutting instrument or a heated wire loop. The small pieces of prostate tissue are washed out through the scope. No incision is needed for TUR. There normally is some blood in the urine for a few days following the procedure. In a few men—less than 5% of all those having TUR—urine will continue to escape unintentionally. Other uncommon complications include a temporary rise in blood pressure with mental confusion, which is treated with salt solution. Erectile dysfunction—the inability to achieve lasting penile erections—does occur, but probably in fewer than 10% of patients. A narrowing or stricture rarely develops in the urethra, but this can be treated fairly easily.

Studies of men who undergo transurethral resection after acute urinary retention indicate that the general public remains not well informed about BPH. A majority of the men who were diagnosed with acute urinary retention said that they had had their symptoms for over a year. When asked why they did not seek treatment earlier, 35% said they were afraid of surgery, but 41% thought their symptoms were only a normal part of aging.

As of late 2007, a number of new treatments for BPH were being investigated, ranging from newly developed drugs to existing drugs used to treat other conditions. One of these new drugs, NX-1207, was undergoing clinical trials in the United States. Initial results showed the drug was extremely effective in treating BPH with minimal side effects and no sexual side effects, according to researchers at the Johns Hopkins University School of Medicine. Further studies were underway as of late 2007, and there was no estimated date when the drug might be ready to submit to the U.S. Food and Drug Administration for approval. Existing drugs that were being looked at as treatments for BPH include the anti-wrinkle drug botulinum toxin A (Botox), the over-the-counter pain relievers aspirin and ibuprofen, and the erectile dysfunction medications sildenafil (Viagra), vardenafil (Levitra), and tadalafil (Cialis).

Expected results

In several studies, 160 mg dose of saw palmetto given twice daily for 45 days achieved positive results in approximately 80% of the patients studied. That percentage increased when results were obtained after 90 days. People taking saw palmetto should use only standardized extracts that contain 85–95% fatty acids and sterols. Dosages vary depending on the type of saw palmetto used. A typical dose is 320 mg per day of standardized extract or 1–2 g per day of ground, dried, whole berries. It may take up to four weeks of use before beneficial effects are seen.

When BPH is treated by conventional TUR, there is a risk of complications but, in the great majority of men, urinary symptoms are relieved and the quality of life is much enhanced. It was anticipated that less invasive forms of surgical treatment would be increasingly used to achieve results as good as those of the standard operation.

Prevention

Whether BPH is caused by hormonal changes in aging men, there is no known way of preventing the condition as of early 2008. Once it does develop and symptoms are present that interfere seriously with the patient's life, timely medical or surgical treatment reliably prevents symptoms from getting worse. Also, if the condition is treated before the prostate has become grossly enlarged, the risk of complications is minimal. A potentially serious complication of BPH is urinary infection (and possible infection of the kidneys), which

KEY TERMS

Catheter—A rubber or plastic tube placed through the urethra into the bladder to remove excess urine when the flow of urine is cut off or to prevent urinary infection.

Creatinine—One of the waste substances normally excreted by the kidneys into the urine. When urine flow is slowed, creatinine may collect in the blood and cause toxic effects.

Hyperplasia—A condition in which cells, such as those making up the prostate gland, divide abnormally rapidly and cause the organ to become enlarged.

Hypertrophy—A term for enlargement, as in BPH (benign prostatic hypertrophy).

Urethra—The tube that conducts urine from the bladder outside the body; in male, the urethra extends from the bladder to the tip of the penis. When the urethra is narrowed by an enlarging prostate, symptoms of BPH develop.

Urinary retention—The result of progressive obstruction of the urethra by an enlarging prostate, causing urine to remain in the bladder even after urination.

can be prevented by using a catheter to drain excess urine out of the bladder so that it does not collect, stagnate, and become infected. There is no scientific evidence that diet or **nutrition** plays a direct role in the development of an enlarged prostate. However, a 2006 study reported that obese men were up to 3.5 times more likely to have an enlarged prostate than men with a normal weight.

Resources

BOOKS

Balch, Phyllis A. *Prescription for Nutritional Healing, fourth edition.* New York: Avery, 2007.

Katz, Aaron E. *Dr. Katz's Guide to Prostate Health: From Conventional to Holistic Therapies.* Topanga, CA: Freedom Press, 2005.

Moyad, Mark A., and Ian M. Thompson. *Complementary Medicine for Prostate Health.* Totowa, NJ: Humana Press, 2008.

PERIODICALS

Altshul, Sara. "Soothe His Prostate Problems." *Prevention* (January 2006): 80.

Bent, S., et al. "Saw Palmetto for Benign Prostatic Hyperplasia." *New England Journal of Medicine* (February 9, 2006): 557–566.

Cooperman, Ted. "Saw Palmetto for Benign Prostatic Hyperplasia." *Townsend Letter: The Examiner of Alternative Medicine* (June 2006): 94.

Giordano, Jill. "Prompt Diagnosis of BPH Can Prevent Complications." *American Family Physician* (May 1, 2006): 1632.

MacDougall, David S. "Obesity, Diabetes Increase BPH Risk; Enlarged Prostate More than Three Times as Likely in Obese Men than in Men with a Normal BMI." *Renal & Urology News* (July 2006): 29.

ORGANIZATIONS

American Institute of Homeopathy, 801 N. Fairfax St., Suite 306, Alexandria, VA, 22314, (888) 445-9988, http://www.homeopathyusa.org.

American Prostate Society, PO. Box 870, Hanover, MD, 21076, (410) 850-0818, http://www.americanprostatesociety.com.

American Urological Association, 1000 Corporate Blvd., Suite 410, Linthicum, MD, 21090, (866) 746-4282, http://www.auanet.org.

Canadian Urological Association, 1155 University, Suite 1155, MontrealQC, H3B 3A7, Canada, (514) 395-0376, http://www.cua.org.

Kathleen D. Wright
Ken R. Wells

Psoralea seeds

Description

Psoralea seed comes from the plant *Psoralea corylifolia*. *Psoralea corylifolia* grows in warm climates from the Middle East to China. This herb requires direct sunlight and moist, well-drained soil. In some parts of its habitat, it is considered a weed that competes with food crops. In other areas, especially in India, it is cultivated as a medicinal crop.

Psoralea corylifolia is an erect annual herb that grows to a height of about 20 to 40 inches (.6–1.2 m). It has broad, elliptical, slightly serrated leaves. The plant flowers from August to December and produces an elongated seed pod containing a single large, smooth, black seed. *Psoralea corylifolia* is a member of the bean family. Unlike some members of this family, the seeds have a bitter, unpleasant taste and are not used for food. They are, however, used extensively in healing. Occasionally the roots, leaves, and fruit (seed pod and seed) of the herb are also used medicinally.

Psoralea corylifolia is widely used in India, China, and Tibet and has more than a dozen different names. In **traditional Chinese medicine** (TCM) it is called bu gu zhi. In India some of its more common names are bakuchi, babachi, bawchi, bukchi, bemchi, barachi, bavachi, hakuch, latakasturi, and bodi. In English, it is sometimes called Malay tea or scruf pea.

General use

Psoralea seed is commonly used both internally and externally in Ayurvedic and traditional Chinese medicine. In both systems of healing, psoralea seed is used to treat similar conditions. An essential oil, when extracted from the seed, can be taken internally or applied to the skin. Seeds also can be ground into a powder and taken internally or mixed into a paste and used externally.

Psoralea seeds are most often used in the treatment of skin diseases, especially leucoderma and vitiligo. These are conditions in which the skin loses pigmentation. White patches begin as small spots, then merge into larger patches. Although rare in the United States, the condition is thought to affect between 1% and 2% of people in India. Leucoderma is treated both with the essential oil taken internally and a paste applied to the skin. It is thought to stimulate the production of new skin pigment. Other skin diseases such as **psoriasis**, alopecia (**hair loss**), **eczema**, and a variety of inflammatory skin diseases are also treated with psoralea seed. The herb is also used to treat leprosy, scorpion sting, and snake bite.

There is some scientific basis for the use of psoralea seed in treating skin disease. The seeds contain the compound psoralen. In traditional Western medicine, a compound containing psoralen is applied to the skin, and then the skin is exposed to ultraviolet (UV) light as a treatment for psoriasis and eczema. Research has also shown that psoralea seed extract has antibiotic and antifungal properties and is effective against some types of internal parasites.

In addition to treating skin diseases, psoralea seed oil or powder is used in TCM and **Ayurvedic medicine** to treat disorders of the urinary and male reproductive system, including **bedwetting**, frequent urination, premature ejaculation, low sex drive, and **impotence**. In TCM, psoralea is considered a general yang tonic.

Occasionally other parts of the plant are used besides the seed. Chewing the root is said to help control dental caries (cavities). The leaves are used to treat **diarrhea**, and the seed pod is used as a diuretic. Other claims for this herb are that it helps prevent **osteoporosis**, has anticancer properties, and can treat **tuberculosis**. There is little scientific evidence to support these uses, although much research was being done on this herb as of 2008 in China and India.

KEY TERMS

Ayurvedic medicine—A 5,000-year old system of holistic medicine developed in India. Ayurvedic medicine is based on the idea that illness results from a personal imbalance or lack of physical, spiritual, social, or mental harmony.

Diuretic—A substance that removes water from the body by increasing urine production.

Eczema—A disease in which the skin becomes dry, red, itchy, and thickened.

Osteoporosis—A condition found in older individuals in which bones decrease in density, become fragile, and are likely to break. It can be caused by lack of vitamin D and/or calcium in the diet.

Psoriasis—A disease in which the skin develops itchy, dry, scaly red patches.

Traditional Chinese medicine (TCM)—An ancient system of medicine based on maintaining a balance in vital energy or qi that controls emotions, spiritual, and physical wellbeing. Diseases and disorders result from imbalances in qi (the life force), and treatments such as massage, exercise, acupuncture, and nutritional and herbal therapy are designed to restore balance and harmony to the body.

Yang aspects—Qualities such as warmth, activity, and light.

Preparations

The traditional method of extracting the essential oil from psoralea seed was quite complicated and involved burying the seeds in a pottery crock and then building a fire over the crock to extract the oil. As of 2008, factories in India produce a standardized essential oil from the seeds by modern extraction methods. A powder for internal use is also available in capsule form. A paste for external use can be made in the proportions of 1 part alcoholic extract of psoralea seed, 2 parts chaulmugra oil, and 2 parts lanoline.

Precautions

No studies have been done on the safety of psoralea seed, so pregnant and breastfeeding women should avoid using this herb.

Side effects

The psoralen found in psoralea seed sensitizes the skin to sunlight. In about 5% of people, psoralea seed

---

oil or paste applied externally causes skin irritation and blistering. Internal use of psoralea seed may cause mild stomach upset.

Interactions

No studies have been done as of 2008 on interactions between psoralea seed and other herbs or traditional pharmaceuticals. Individuals who regularly take dietary supplements, herbs, or pharmaceutical drugs should discuss the use of psoralea seed with their healthcare provider before beginning treatment.

Resources

BOOKS

Pole, Sebastian. *Ayurvedic Medicine: The Principles of Traditional Practice.* Oxford: UK Churchill Livingston, 2006.

Premla, M. S. *Ayurvedic Herbs: A Clinical Guide to the Healing Plants of Traditional Indian Medicine.* New York: Routledge, 2006.

ORGANIZATIONS

Alternative Medicine Foundation, PO Box 60016, Potomac, MD, 20859, (301) 340-1960, http://www.amfoundation.org.

American Association of Oriental Medicine, PO Box 162340, Sacramento, CA, 95816, (866) 455-7999, (914) 443-4770, http://www.aaaomonline.org.

American Holistic Medical Association, PO Box 2016, Edmonds, WA, 98020, (425) 967-0737, http://www.holisticmedicine.org.

Centre for International Ethnomedicinal Education and Research (CIEER), http://www.cieer.org.

National Institute of Ayurvedic Medicine, 375 Fifth Ave., Fifth Floor, New York, NY, 10016, (212) 685-8600, http://niam.com/corp-web/index.htm.

Tish Davidson, A. M.

Psoriasis

Definition

Psoriasis is a chronic, non-contagious disease characterized by inflamed hyperproliferative lesions covered with silvery-white scabs of dead skin.

Description

Psoriasis, which affects at least four million Americans, is slightly more common in women than in men. Although the disease can develop at any time, 10–15% of all cases are diagnosed in children under 10, and the average age at onset of symptoms is 28 years of age.

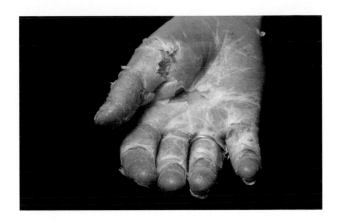

Hand with severe Psoriasis. (© *Medical-on-Line / Alamy*)

Psoriasis is most common in fair-skinned people and relatively rare in dark-skinned individuals, although the rate among African Americans appeared as of 2008 to be slowly rising.

Normal skin cells mature and replace dead skin every 28–30 days. Psoriasis causes skin cells to mature in less than a week. Because the body cannot shed the old skin as rapidly as new cells are rising to the surface, raised patches of dead skin develop on the arms, back, chest, elbows, legs, nails, folds between the buttocks, and scalp.

Psoriasis is considered mild if it affects less than 5% of the surface of the body, moderate if 5–30% of the skin is involved, and severe if the disease affects more than 30% of the body surface.

Types of psoriasis

Dermatologists distinguish different forms of psoriasis according to what part of the body is affected, how severe symptoms are, how long they last, and the pattern formed by the scales.

PLAQUE PSORIASIS. Plaque psoriasis (psoriasis vulgaris), the most common form of the disease, is characterized by small, red bumps that enlarge, become inflamed, and form scales. The top scales flake off easily and often, but those beneath the surface of the skin clump together. Removing these scales exposes tender skin, which bleeds and causes the plaques (inflamed patches) to grow.

Plaque psoriasis can develop on any part of the body, but most often occurs on the elbows, knees, scalp, and trunk.

SCALP PSORIASIS. At least 50 of every 100 people who have any form of psoriasis have scalp psoriasis. This form of the disease is characterized by scale-capped plaques on the surface of the skull.

NAIL PSORIASIS. The first sign of nail psoriasis is usually pitting of the fingernails or toenails. Size, shape, and depth of the marks vary, and affected nails may thicken, yellow, or crumble. The skin around an affected nail is sometimes inflamed, and the nail may peel away from the nail bed.

GUTTATE PSORIASIS. Named for the Latin word *gutta,* which means "a drop," guttate psoriasis is characterized by small, red, drop-like dots that enlarge rapidly and may be somewhat scaly. Often found on the arms, legs, and trunk and sometimes in the scalp, guttate psoriasis can clear up without treatment or disappear and resurface in the form of plaque psoriasis.

PUSTULAR PSORIASIS. Pustular psoriasis usually occurs in adults. It is characterized by blister-like lesions filled with non-infectious pus and surrounded by reddened skin. Pustular psoriasis, which can be limited to one part of the body (localized) or can be widespread, may be the first symptom of psoriasis or develop in a patient with chronic plaque psoriasis.

Generalized pustular psoriasis is also known as Von Zumbusch pustular psoriasis. Widespread, acutely painful patches of inflamed skin develop suddenly. Pustules appear within a few hours, then dry and peel within two days.

Generalized pustular psoriasis can make life-threatening demands on the heart and kidneys.

Palomar-plantar pustulosis (PPP) generally appears between the ages of 20 and 60. PPP causes large pustules to form at the base of the thumb or on the sides of the heel. In time, the pustules turn brown and peel. The disease usually becomes much less active for a while after peeling.

Acrodermatitis continua of Hallopeau is a form of PPP characterized by painful, often disabling, lesions on the fingertips or the tips of the toes. The nails may become deformed, and the disease can damage bone in the affected area.

INVERSE PSORIASIS. Inverse psoriasis occurs in the armpits and groin, under the breasts, and in other areas where skin flexes or folds. This disease is characterized by smooth, inflamed lesions and can be debilitating.

ERYTHRODERMIC PSORIASIS. Characterized by severe scaling, **itching**, and **pain** that affects most of the body, erythrodermic psoriasis disrupts the body's chemical balance and can cause severe illness. This particularly inflammatory form of psoriasis can be the first sign of the disease, but often it develops in patients with a history of plaque psoriasis.

PSORIATIC ARTHRITIS. About 10% of patients with psoriasis develop a complication called psoriatic arthritis. This type of arthritis can be slow to develop and mild, or it can develop rapidly. Symptoms of psoriatic arthritis include:

- joint discomfort, swelling, stiffness, or throbbing
- swelling in the toes and ankles
- pain in the digits, lower back, wrists, knees, and ankles
- eye inflammation

Causes and symptoms

The cause of psoriasis is unknown, but research related to the Human Genome Project was mapping the genetic component of the disease in the 2000s. In 2003, researchers at Washington University in St. Louis announced that three genes on chromosome 17 appear to be implicated in the development of psoriasis. Markers (indicators) for psoriasis have also been found on 10 other chromosomes, although specific genes for the diseases have not yet been discovered. Researchers believe that psoriasis is a multifactorial disorder, which means that it is the end result of a number of different factors. It appears to be caused by the combined action of multiple disease genes in a single individual that are triggered by irritants in the environment. Factors that increase the risk of developing psoriasis include:

- blood relatives with psoriasis
- stress
- exposure to cold temperatures
- injury, illness, or infection
- steroids and other medications
- mechanical stress (leaning on knees or skin exposure to chemicals, for example)

Trauma and certain bacteria may trigger psoriatic arthritis in patients with psoriasis.

Diagnosis

A medical history and physical examination is the basis for a diagnosis of psoriasis. In some cases, a microscopic examination of skin cells is also performed.

Blood tests can distinguish psoriatic arthritis from other types of arthritis.

Treatment

Psoriasis treatments include:

- Soaking in warm water and German chamomile (*Matricaria recutita*) or bathing in warm salt water

- Drinking as many as three cups a day of hot tea made with one or a combination of the following herbs: burdock root (*Arctium lappa*), dandelion (*Taraxacum mongolicum*) root, Oregon grape root (*Mahonia aquifolium*), sarsaparilla (*Smilax officinalis*), and balsam pear (*Momardica charantia*)
- Taking two 500–mg capsules of evening primrose oil (*Oenothera biennis*) a day. Pregnant women should not use evening primrose oil, and patients with liver disease or high cholesterol should use it only under a doctor's supervision.
- Eating a diet that includes plenty of fish, turkey, celery (for cleansing the kidneys), parsley, lettuce, lemons (for cleansing the liver), limes, fiber, and fruit and vegetable juices
- Eating a diet that eliminates animal products high in saturated and unsaturated fats, such as fried foods, dairy products, and fatty meats, that promote inflammation
- Drinking plenty of water (at least eight glasses) each day
- Regularly imagining clear, healthy skin

Other helpful alternative approaches include identifying and eliminating food allergens from the diet; enhancing liver function; augmenting the supply of hydrochloric acid in the stomach; and completing a **detoxification** program. Constitutional homeopathic treatment, if properly prescribed, can sometimes help resolve psoriasis.

Allopathic treatment

Age, general health, lifestyle, and the severity and location of symptoms influence the type of treatment used to reduce inflammation and decrease the rate at which new skin cells are produced. Because the course of this disease varies with each individual, doctors must experiment with or combine different treatments to find the most effective therapy for a particular patient.

Mild-moderate psoriasis

Steroid creams and ointments are commonly used to treat mild or moderate psoriasis, and steroids are sometimes injected into the skin of patients with a limited number of lesions. Two drugs, calcipotriene (Dovonex) and tazarotene (Tazorac) have been approved by the U.S. Food and Drug Administration (FDA) for the treatment of mile-to-moderate psoriasis.

Brief daily doses of natural sunlight can significantly relieve symptoms. **Sunburn**, however, has the opposite effect.

Certain moisturizers and bath oils can loosen scales, soften skin, and may eliminate the itch. (Often petroleum-based, coal tar-based, or other greasy ointments are used.) Adding a cup of oatmeal to a tub of bath water or using Aveeno in the bath can soothe the itch. Dilute, topical salicylic acid (an ingredient in aspirin) can be used to remove dead skin or increase the effectiveness of other therapies.

Moderate psoriasis

Administered under medical supervision, ultraviolet light B (UVB) is used to control psoriasis that covers many areas of the body or that has not responded to other treatment. Doctors combine UVB treatments with topical medications to treat some patients and sometimes prescribe home phototherapy, in which the patient administers his own UVB treatments.

Photochemotherapy (PUVA) is a medically supervised procedure that combines medication with exposure to ultraviolet light (UVA) to treat localized or widespread psoriasis. An individual with wide-spread psoriasis that has not responded to treatment may enroll in one of the day treatment programs conducted at special facilities throughout the United States. Psoriasis patients who participate in these intensive sessions are exposed to UVB and given other treatments for six to eight hours a day for two to four weeks.

Another form of treatment that has several advantages over standard phototherapy is therapy with an excimer laser system. Laser treatment for psoriasis uses a carefully focused beam of ultraviolet light that not only relieves symptoms quickly but also minimizes exposure of healthy skin to the ultraviolet rays.

Severe psoriasis

Methotrexate (MTX) can be given as a pill or as an injection to alleviate symptoms of severe psoriasis or psoriatic arthritis. Patients who take MTX must be carefully monitored by a doctor who checks blood liver enzymes to prevent liver damage. In the early years of its use, methotrexate was responsible for the death of a number of patients whose liver function had not been properly monitored.

Psoriatic arthritis can also be treated with nonsteroidal anti-inflammatory drugs (NSAIDs), such as acetaminophen (Tylenol) or aspirin. Hot compresses and warm water soaks may also provide some relief for painful joints.

Another medication used to treat severe psoriasis is etrentinate (Tegison), whose chemical properties are similar to those of **vitamin A**. Most effective in treating pustular or erythrodermic psoriasis, etrentinate also relieves some symptoms of plaque psoriasis. Etrentinate can enhance the effectiveness of UVB or

PUVA treatments and reduce the amount of exposure necessary.

Some doctors also use other systemic drugs that have not been approved specifically for the treatment of psoriasis. Among these so-called off-label drugs are isotretinoin (Accutane), hydroxyurea (Hydrea), mycophenolate mofetil, sulfasalazine, and 6-thioguanine. Accutane is a less effective psoriasis treatment than Tegison, but it can cause many of the same side effects, including **nosebleeds**, inflammation of the eyes and lips, **bone spurs**, **hair loss**, and birth defects. Tegison is stored in the body for an unknown length of time and should not be taken by a woman who is pregnant or planning to become pregnant. A woman should use reliable birth control while taking Accutane and for at least one month before and after her course of treatment.

Cyclosporin emulsion (Neoral) is used to treat stubborn cases of severe psoriasis. Cyclosporin is also used to prevent rejection of transplanted organs, and Neoral should be particularly beneficial to psoriasis patients who are young children or African Americans, or those who have diabetes. The drawback to cyclosporin, however, is that it has been implicated in an increased risk of **skin cancer** for psoriasis patients.

As of 2008, the latest drug approved by the FDA for use with psoriasis was a recombinant DNA (genetically engineered) product called alefacept (Amevive). Alefacept targets the T-cells that cause psoriasis without suppressing the patient's immune system. Not only does the new drug relieve the symptoms of psoriasis more rapidly than current treatments, but patients also remain symptom-free longer.

Other conventional treatments for psoriasis include:

- Capsaicin (*Capsicum frutecens*), an ointment that can stop production of the chemical that causes the skin to become inflamed and halts the runaway production of new skin cells. Capsaicin is available without a prescription but should be used under a doctor's supervision to prevent burns and skin damage.
- Hydrocortisone creams, topical ointments containing a form of vitamin D called calcitriol, and coal-tar shampoos and ointments can relieve symptoms but may cause such side effects as folliculitis (inflammation of hair follicles) and heightened risk of skin cancer.

Expected results

Most cases of psoriasis can be managed. However, some people who have psoriasis are so self-conscious and embarrassed about their appearance that they become depressed and withdrawn. The

---

KEY TERMS

Arthritis—An inflammation of the joints.

Cyclosporin—A drug that suppresses the immune system and has been used to treat severe psoriasis. Some research indicates that cyclosporin may increase the risk of skin cancer for psoriasis patients.

Plaque—An area or patch of inflamed skin. The most common form of psoriasis is plaque psoriasis.

Social Security Administration grants disability benefits to about 400 psoriasis patients each year.

Prevention

A doctor should be notified if any of the following occurs:

- Psoriasis symptoms appear or reappear after treatment.
- Pustules erupt on the skin and the patient experiences fatigue, muscle aches, and fever.
- Unfamiliar, unexplained symptoms appear.

Resources

BOOKS

Camisa, Charles. *Handbook of Psoriasis*. New York: Wiley-Blackwell, 2005.

Earls, Deirdre. *Your Healing Diet: A Quick Guide to Reversing Psoriasis and Chronic Diseases with Healing Foods*. Charleston, SC: BookSurge, 2006.

Langley, Richard G. B. *Psoriasis: Everything You Need to Know*. Westport, CT: Firefly Books, 2005.

Weinberg, Jeffrey M., ed. *Treatment of Psoriasis*. Basel: Berkhäuser, 2008.

PERIODICALS

Lowenthal, K. E., P. J. Horn, and R. E. Kalb. "Concurrent Use of Methotrexate and Acitretin Revisited." *Journal of Dermatological Treatment* (January 2008): 22–26.

Ormerod, A. D. "Adalimumab: A New Alternative Biologic Agent for Chronic Plaque Psoriasis." *British Journal of Dermatology* (March 2008): 435–436.

Su, Y. H., and J. Y. Fang. "Drug Delivery and Formulations for the Topical Treatment of Psoriasis." *Expert Opinion on Drug Delivery* (February 2008): 235–249.

Thass, J. J. "Siddha Medicine: Background and Principles and the Application for Skin Diseases." *Clinical Dermatology* (January/February 2008): 62–78.

ORGANIZATIONS

American Academy of Dermatology, PO Box 4014, Schaumburg, IL, 60618-4014, (866) 503-7546, http://www.aad.org.

American Skin Association, 346 Park Ave. South, 4th floor, New York, NY, 10010, (800) 499-SKIN, http://www.americanskin.org/frameset.htm.

National Psoriasis Foundation, 6600 SW Ninety-second Ave., Suite 300, Portland, OR, 97223-7195, (800) 723-9166, http://www.psoriasis.org.

Maureen Haggerty
Rebecca J. Frey, PhD
David Edward Newton, Ed.D.

Psychic healing *see* **Cayce systems**

Psychoneuroimmunology

Definition

Psychoneuroimmunology (PNI), is a relatively recent branch of science that enforces beliefs that physicians have held for many centuries, perhaps well before the times of the ancient Greeks. The premise is that a patient's mental state influences diseases and healing. Specifically, PNI studies the connection between the brain and the immune system.

Origins

The term psychoneuroimmunology was coined by Robert Ader, a researcher in the Department of Psychiatry at the University of Rochester Medical Center in Rochester, New York. In the 1970s, studies by Ader and other researchers opened up new understandings of how experiences such as **stress** and **anxiety** can affect a person's immune system.

In the 1970s, Ader performed experiments on lab rats, which showed that environmental factors could impact the immune system. Ader's work went against accepted scientific knowledge, which held that the immune system was not related to other bodily systems, and had no way to physically interact with the nervous system. However, other studies confirmed Ader's findings. The field of PNI blossomed, and hundreds of studies explored various interactions between the immune system and other mental and physical processes.

Many PNI studies have focused on how stress, hostility, and **depression** impact the immune system. Many conditions such as **heart disease**, **osteoporosis**, arthritis, delayed wound healing, and premature **aging**, are related to stress and negative emotions. Fewer studies have been aimed at showing the benefits

of happiness, or positive emotions, on health (perhaps because this is more difficult to test).

Many doctors have noted that a patient's desire to get well is related to the outcome of a disease. Clinical anecdotes recount cases of miraculous healing for no demonstrable reason, or cases where a terminally ill patient held on for months longer than expected to make it to a daughter's wedding or other important occasion. Faith in the physician (or shaman or other healer) has also long been thought to influence healing. The ancient Greek physician Galen wrote, "He cures most successfully in whom the people have the most confidence."

The **placebo effect** is also a curious aspect of healing. A placebo is a sugar pill or other non-active prescription, which might be given so that the patient thinks he or she is being treated medically. The actual incidence of the placebo effect is difficult to measure, but some researchers believe that as many as one-third of all patients will improve on a placebo.

Benefits

More than a particular therapy, PNI is a field of research. However, PNI has explored the benefits of many nontraditional or holistic approaches to healing. These include **psychotherapy** and counseling for people with **cancer**, and **biofeedback** and **relaxation** therapies to reduce stress. It is possible that PNI studies will lead to the discovery of new ways to enhance the immune system, just as it has already shown new ways the immune system can be suppressed. PNI gives credibility to many long-held folk beliefs about the effect of the mind on disease and healing. By demonstrating the physical means by which the mind influences the body, and vice versa, PNI provides a measure of validity to holistic approaches to healing.

Description

Psychoneuroimmunology provides a scientific framework for researchers to investigate the aspects of healing that go beyond standard clinical therapy. PNI researchers look for the physical links that allow the immune system to respond to psychological factors, such as the will to live to a certain date. They look at the ways that mental states, such as hopelessness, can signal the immune system to lower the body's defenses.

Research and general acceptance

Though many scientists were at first skeptical of the findings of PNI, by the start of the twenty-first century the field gained wider credibility. A great deal of new research is being carried out, and there are several academic journals devoted to PNI. Researchers emphasize that they are not simply providing scientific backing for beliefs that happy people live longer, or that people who hold in their anger give themselves cancer. Instead, they are discovering how the immune system communicates with the neurological and endocrine systems.

Some studies focus on the function of cytokines, which are substances secreted by cells of the immune system. The two main classes of cytokines are pro-inflammatory (producing inflammation) and anti-inflammatory (fighting inflammation). Studies of cytokines show that psychological factors such as stress depress the immune system, but that deviations in the immune system can also trigger psychological and behavioral changes. The communication goes both ways. A person, who is fighting infection, perhaps from a cold, undergoes behavioral changes like **fatigue**, irritability, and loss of appetite. PNI maps complex interactions among the body's systems. Factors studied include mood, illness, immune response, susceptibility to disease, and maintenance of health.

In the early years of the twenty-first century, the United States Public Health Service funded hundreds of research grants in the field of PNI. PNI has been particularly enlightening for researchers and caregivers who deal with people who have cancer, as well as depression.

Resources

PERIODICALS

"Cancer and the Mind." *Harvard Mental Health Letter* (July 2003): 1.

DeVito, Paul L. "The Immune System vs. Stress." *USA Today Magazine* (July 1994): 27.

Kiecolt-Glaser, Janice, K., et al. "Emotions, Morbidity, and Mortality." *Annual Review of Psychology*(2002): 83.

Sherwin, Nuland B. "The Uncertain Art." *American Scholar* (Summer 2001): 123.

Viljoen, M., et al. "Psychoneuroimmunology: From Philosophy, Intuition, and Folklore to a Recognized Science." *South African Journal of Science* (July/August 2003): 332–6.

ORGANIZATIONS

Association of Oncology Social Work. 1211 Locust Street, Philadelphia, PA 19107. (215) 599-6093. http://www.aosw.org.

OTHER

Azar, Beth. "Father of PNI Reflects on the Field's Growth." *APA Monitor Online*. June 1999 [cited May 11, 2004]. http://www.apa.org/monitor/jun99/pni.html

A. Woodward

Psychophysical integration *see* **Trager psychophysical integration**

Psychophysiology

Definition

Psychophysiology is the branch of physiology that is concerned with the relationship between mental (psyche) and physical (physiological) processes; it is the scientific study of the interaction between mind and body. The field of psychophysiology draws upon the work of physicians, psychologists, biochemists, neurologists, engineers, and other scientists.

A psychophysiological disorder is characterized by physical symptoms that are partly induced by emotional factors. Some of the more common emotional states responsible in forming illness include **anxiety**, **stress**, and fear. Common psychosomatic ailments include migraine headaches, attention deficit hyperactivity disorder (ADHD), arthritis, ulcerative **colitis**, and **heart disease**.

Origins

Historically, there has been a large chasm between the allopathic (mainstream) and alternative medical worlds with regard to views on psychophysiology. While the allopathic medical field continues to follow the Cartesian model of health, in which mind and body are seen as separate, the alternative medical field stands firmly on the notion that the mind and body are intricately connected. In general, treatment in the mainstream medical system is oriented toward fixing or curing isolated symptoms in the body. Alternative health providers strive to look at the symptoms, as well as the underlying pathology, or cause. While the first focuses on isolated parts of a whole system, the latter group strives to address the whole being, mind and body, emotions, and physical symptoms.

They believe that mental processes intricately affect bodily ones, and vice versa.

With a more holistic mentality, the population is experiencing an ever-progressing paradigm shift in which the body and mind are no longer viewed as separate, but rather as intricately interrelated. Medically, as well as culturally, Western society has reached the point at which the focus is increasingly on integrative mind/body healthcare. More patients and physicians are choosing to utilize therapies built upon the holistic models in which psyche (mind) and soma (physical body) are seen as one, or intimately related. They are utilizing such modalities as **meditation**, **yoga**, bodywork, and visualization techniques in efforts to relieve overall stress and to heal various psychosomatic illnesses.

Benefits

The field of psychophysiology is leading the way to an ongoing investigation into the intricacies of the mind/body relationship. Applied psychophysiology focuses on the effects of emotional states on the central nervous system, by observing and recording data on such physiological processes as sleep rhythms, heart rate, gastrointestinal functioning, immune response, and brain function. Techniques used to measure such factors include electroencephalograms (EEGs), magnetic resonance imaging (MRI), and computerized axial tomography (CAT) scans. In an effort to quantify the effectiveness of different treatment techniques, the science of psychophysiology is being applied to many areas of alternative medicine, from **psychotherapy** and hypnosis to bodywork and meditation. Studies of the effects of emotional states on various physiological processes abound. For instance, it has been shown that there is a relation between loneliness and heart disease, as well as a connection between post traumatic stress disorder, **irritable bowel syndrome**, and **fibromyalgia**. By documenting the effects of emotions on health, this field hopes to improve the healing capacities of treatments. Many of the studies done by psychophysiologists occur in research institutions and universities.

There are several interpretations of what a healthy psychophysiology may look like. However, there are common characteristics that speak of mind/body health. Ultimately, such a holistic state exists when internal and mental awareness becomes strong enough to create a sense of embodiment, balance, and presence in an individual's body. Disease may be present in such a state, yet with this underlying, holistic understanding there exists more fighting power by which to heal. Science is proving this fact. Therapies that

---

KEY TERMS

Paradigm shift—A philosophical or spiritual change in the pattern or model by which one lives and views the world.

Rolfing—Form of therapeutic bodywork that seeks to heal the mind by improving the physical structure of the body.

Ulcerative colitis—Autoimmune disease of the colon, classified as a psychosomatic disorder.

Visualization techniques—A form of meditation, contemplation, and imagination that seeks to alter physical processes and directions of behavior or outcomes by focused mental awareness on specific images.

---

integrate mind/body processes have been shown to aid the healing processes for numerous diseases.

When stresses, traumas, or debilitating emotional states are present, individuals may experience physiological unrest. For example, if an individual with a known allergy to bee **stings** receives such a sting, the natural reaction could be panic. As a result of this psychological response, blood pressure and heart rate increase, digestive functions decrease, and the person becomes dizzy. If emotional stresses or traumas of this kind remain in the body/mind for extended periods of time, an imbalance in the healthy system may eventually manifest, as when individuals under chronic stress succumb to illness or disease. The field of psychophysiology is showing that the most effective treatments are those that address the emotional states of disease as well as the physical aspects.

Treatments

Treatments for psychosomatic illnesses are being synthesized from both the allopathic and alternative medical worlds. Methods vary from drug therapy and **biofeedback** to the use of meditation, yoga, and **massage therapy**. Many treatments have been shown to be effective; individuals have the freedom and responsiblity to discover for themselves the treatments that have the most personal benefit. What is effective for one person may not work for another. Consumers of mind/body treatments are encouraged to evaluate options, practitioners, and their individual needs. The field of psychophysiology conducts research to improve the information available to consumers.

In general, treatments are selected if they complement and strengthen an individual's awareness of the body/mind relationship. Such practices are most effective in achieving overall states of health when addressing the mind to affect the body, and vice versa. For example, two disciplines that have proven effective in establishing this awareness are meditation, a mind-centered activity, and **Rolfing**, a form of therapeutic bodywork. Treatments that simultaneously work with both the physiology and the psychology are highly beneficial. This thorough approach may be achieved by pairing modalities that complement one another. Examples include combining psychotherapy with bodywork, and certain drug therapies with meditation, visualization, and yoga.

Mind/Body

Meditation is an age-old process that has great potential in quieting the mind, calming the emotions, and balancing the physiology. For centuries, Eastern peoples and their traditions have focused on the art of meditation. Meditative techniques vary from bringing one's attention to the breath, to chanting a mantra (a specifically pre-established word or phrase), or to focusing one's gaze on a specific, unchanging image (a visualization technique). Focusing awareness inward to bodily sensations may interrupt unhealthy thought patterns, thereby reducing or preventing the effects of stress on the physiology. Studies as well as experiential phenomena have shown that meditation decreases blood pressure, muscle **pain**, and **cholesterol**, while improving digestion, relieving anxiety and **depression**, improving immunity, and boosting energy levels. Ultimately, meditation may lead to knowing one's self, both psychologically and physiologically. It is out of this state of embodied presence and attention that healing occurs.

Body/Mind

Certain forms of bodywork have been successful in affecting the mind by working through the body. Emotions, thoughts, and feelings may reside in the body, just as much as they do in the mind. For example, a depressed person's body may reflect the emotional state by hunched shoulders, sad facial expressions, and slow movements. Psychology has shown that by adopting positive physical expressions such as a smile or improved posture, a person will experience corresponding and measurable effects in the mind. These relationships, through the science of psychophysiology, are being experimentally validated.

By manipulating the structure of the body during bodywork, a healer may directly or indirectly affect both physiological and psychological health. Benefits from this type of therapy come from both the new changes in the physiology, as well as the changes in the consciousness and awareness of physically existing patterns. By becoming aware of such body/mind relations, healer and client break up old patterns in the physical tissue, the mind, and the emotions. An overall body/mind freedom is enhanced, bringing with it a greater chance for a holistic state of health.

Research and general acceptance

Interest in the mind/body relationship is as ancient as it is vast, and the field of psychophysiology is researching and validating this connection. The allopathic medical world has achieved great breakthroughs in human health, particularly with regard to the treatment of traumatic and life-threatening injuries and diseases. Medically, socially, and environmentally, a more holistic and preventive approach to healthcare is being sought, one that integrates and balances the mind/body relationship. Much work is being done to develop new knowledge; the field of psychophysiology is a major contributor to the exploration.

Training and certification

A variety of health professionals, such as physicians and psychologists, incorporate the principles of psychophysiology into their work. One of the objectives of the Association for Applied Psychophysiology and Biofeedback (AAPB) is to promote professional standards of practice, ethics, and education for its members. Certifications exist for professionals such as massage therapists and others who perform specialized techniques that incorporate psychophysiology principles.

Resources

BOOKS

Andreassi, John L. *Psychophysiology: Human Behavior and Physiological Response*. Mahwah, NJ: Lawrence Erlbaum, 2000.

Borysenko, Joan, Ph.D. *The Power of the Mind to Heal*. Carlsbad, CA: Hay House, 1995.

Cacioppo, John T., ed. *Handbook of Psychophysiology*. Cambridge, UK: Cambridge University Press, 2000.

Chopra, Deepak, M.D. *Magical Health, Magical Body: Mastering the Mind/Body Connection for Perfect Health and Total Well-Being*. Chicago, IL: Nightengale-Conant, 2003.

ORGANIZATIONS

Association for Applied Psychophysiology and Biofeedback (AAPB). 10200 W. 44th Avenue, Suite 304. Wheat Ridge, CO 80033. (303) 422-8436. http://www.aapb.org.

Douglas Dupler

Psychosomatic medicine

Definition

Psychosomatic medicine is the study, diagnosis, and treatment of physical health conditions that stem from emotional problems. It emphasizes the unity of the mind and body in health and medicine. Many physicians believe understanding the psychological causes of illnesses is a key in understanding and treating the physical symptoms of the illnesses themselves.

Origins

Throughout recorded history, people are said to have been cured of diseases by various mystical practices, such as incantation, **prayer**, the laying on of hands, and other rituals. It is unclear exactly when medical practitioners made a connection between the mind and certain diseases, although records show that it dates back to at least the 1700s.

In 1774, German physician Franz Anton Mesmer (1734–1815) applied a scientific basis for mysticism when he waved magnets over some patients to cure them. He later discovered the magnets were not needed and he could get the same results by passing his hands over some patients. He called his technique "animal magnetism," and said it was based on the principle that illnesses occur when the body's flow of natural electromagnetic energy becomes blocked. He opened a practice in Vienna, Austria, and later went to Paris, where he lived and worked for six years, using magnetism and hypnosis to treat illnesses. He was eventually driven out of both cities and labeled a "quack" since his techniques did not always work.

Mesmer's work was studied by American scientist and statesman Benjamin Franklin (1706–1790) and French chemist Antoine Lavoisier (1743–1794), who became famous for isolating oxygen. Both spent years duplicating Mesmer's work, but with no successful results. However, the research led Franklin to conclude that the mind does have an influence over physical ailments; that in some patients, the belief that they will be cured actually cures them.

Further research into psychosomatic medicine was conducted by Austrian psychologist Sigmund Freud (1856–1939) in the late 1800s. Research continued, and by the 1960s the field had gained respect by the general medical community. Today, **biofeedback**, hypnosis, prayer, and humor are considered legitimate facets of psychosomatic medicine.

KEY TERMS

Biofeedback—The use of monitoring devices that display information about body functions, such as heart rate or blood pressure, to help patients learn to consciously control the functions.

Cholesterol—A compound found in animal tissue and blood of which high levels in the blood are linked to clogged arteries, heart disease, and gallstones.

Electromagnetic energy—Energy created by electromagnetism, the forces of electricity and magnetism.

Hypnosis—A sleeplike condition that can be artificially induced in people, in which they are susceptible to suggestions from the hypnotist.

Lipids—A group of organic compounds consisting of fats, oils, and related substances that, along with proteins and carbohydrates, are the structural components of living cells.

Meditation—Emptying the mind of thoughts, or concentrating on just one thing to help in relaxation.

Prostate—A gland in males that secretes a fluid into the semen that improves the movement and viability of sperm.

Psychoanalysis—A psychological theory and therapeutic method based on the idea that the mind works on conscious and unconscious levels and that childhood events have a psychological influence on people throughout their lives.

Psychosocial—Relating to both the psychological and the social aspects of a person.

Transendental Meditation—A focusing of the mind based in part on Hindu meditation techniques in which each person is given a word or phrase to meditate upon.

Benefits

The primary benefit of psychosomatic medicine is that it does not involve drugs, surgery, or other invasive treatments. It is also greatly beneficial in conditions created by the mind rather than a physical condition. In addition, in psychosomatic medicine, the patient has the greatest ability to control the healing process through various positive thinking techniques.

Description

In tne April 2002 issue of *Managed Healthcare Executive*, Dr. David Sobel, director of Patient Education and Health Promotions for Kaiser Permanente's

Northern California region, explained that one of the first things he noticed when he started practicing medicine is that a large number of his patients had problems that could not be explained by conventional medical and diagnostic techniques. He said that, "Up to 20% possess diagnosable psychiatric disorders but even more impressive is that upwards of 80% of the patients will be suffering significant levels of psychosocial distress." He went on to say "distress often expresses itself through physical or bodily symptoms...if not causing the symptoms, then certainly exacerbating them." He calls the condition a deficiency of mind-body regulation.

To address this, Kaiser Permanente developed a mind-body core program that includes teaching patients how to relax, manage **stress**, communicate more effectively, and think more positively.

Preparation

There is no preparation needed to undergo psychosomatic treatment, other than a willingness to believe it may be effective.

Precautions

Patients should be wary of psychosomatic practitioners who do not have degrees in medicine or psychology, or specialized training in either field. Some patients may also need conventional medical care or a combination of conventional and psychosomatic therapies.

Side effects

There are no known serious side effects of psychosomatic treatment in patients deemed suitable for the treatment by a qualified medical practitioner.

Research and general acceptance

A study published in 2002 by researchers at the Carnegie Mellon University Department of Psychology found that people with positive emotions were less likely to catch the **common cold**. A study by the University of California at San Francisco, published in 2002, reported that people with **AIDS** who had a positive attitude had a lower death rate from AIDS-related complications.

A Canadian study published in 2002 showed that people with breast or **prostate cancer**, who meditated and practiced **yoga** regularly, had an enhanced quality of life and reduced stress regarding their illness. A study published in 2000 by the Center for Health and **Aging** Studies at Maharishi University of Management

in Fairfield, Iowa, showed that people who practiced Transcendental **Meditation** significantly reduced their **cholesterol** levels. Meditation also improved brain and immune system functions of patients in a study by several universities, which was published in 2003.

Training and certification

Many colleges and universities have psychosomatic medicine departments or training programs for certification. Practitioners usually are certified physicians or psychiatrists, but can also be other medical professionals, such as psychologists and nurses. However, practitioners can also include those with no medical training, such as hypnotists, counselors, ministers, and yoga and meditation instructors.

Resources

BOOKS

Dreher, Henry. *Mind-Body Unity: A New Vision for Mind&-Body Science and Medicine*. Baltimore, MD: John Hopkins University Press, 2004.

Ramos, Denise. *The Psyche of the Body: A Jungian Paradigm in the Understanding of the Psyche-Body Phenomenon*. London, England: Brunner-Routledge, 2004.

Scarf, Maggie. *Secrets, Lies, Betrayals: The Body/Mind Connection*. New York, NY: Random House, 2004.

Taylor, Graeme J. *Psychosomatic Medicine and Contemporary Psychoanalysis (Stress and Health Series, Monograph 3)*. Guilford, CT: International Universities Press, 1987.

Ullman, Dana. *The One Minute (or So) Healer: 500 Simple Ways to Heal Yourself Naturally*. Berkeley, CA: North Atlantic Books, 2004.

PERIODICALS

Carlson, Linda E., et al. "Mindfulness-Based Stress Reduction in Relation to Quality of Life, Mood, Symptoms of Stress, and Immune Parameters in Breast and Prostate Cancer Outpatients." *Psychosomatic Medicine* (July-August 2003): 571–81.

Cohen, Sheldon, et al. "Emotional Style and Susceptibility to the Common Cold." *Psychosomatic Medicine* (July-August 2003): 652–7.

Davidson, Richard J., et al. "Alterations in Brain and Immune Function Produced by Mindfulness Meditation." *Psychosomatic Medicine* (July-August 2003): 564–70.

Jesitus, John. "Mind+Body Medicine: Putting Mind Over Health Matters." *Managed Healthcare Executive* (April 2002): 33–6.

Kroenke, Kurt. "Psychological Medicine: Integrating Psychological Care into General Medicine Practice." *British Medical Journal* (June 29, 2002): 1536–8.

Moskowitz, Judith Tedlie. "Positive Affect Predicts Lower Risk of AIDS Mortality" *Psychosomatic Medicine* (July-August 2003): 620–6.

Schneifer, R.H., et al. "Lower Lipid Peroxide Levels in Practitioners of the Transcendental Meditation Program." *Psychosomatic Medicine* (January-February 1998): 38–41.

ORGANIZATIONS

Academy of Psychosomatic Medicine. 5824 N. Magnolia, Chicago, IL 60660. (773) 784-2025. http://www.amp.org.

American Psychosomatic Society. 6728 Old McLean Village Drive, McLean, VA 22101. (703) 556-9222. http://www.psychosomatic.org.

Association for Psychosomatic Medicine. 4560 Delafield Ave., Bronx, NY 10471-3905. http://www.theamp.org.

OTHER

"Psychosomatic Medicine: The Puzzling Leap." National Library of Medicine. History of Medicine Division. *Emotions and Disease* [cited May 29, 2004] http://www.nlm.nih.gov/hmd/emotions/psychosomatic.html.

Ken R. Wells

Psychotherapy

Definition

Psychotherapy can be defined as a means of treating psychological or emotional problems such as neurosis or personality disorder through verbal and nonverbal communication. It is the treatment of psychological distress through talking with a specially trained therapist and learning new ways to cope rather than merely using medication to alleviate the distress. It is done with the immediate goal of aiding the person in increasing self-knowledge and awareness of relationships with others. Psychotherapy is carried out to assist people in becoming more conscious of their unconscious thoughts, feelings, and motives.

Psychotherapy's longer-term goal is making it possible for people to exchange destructive patterns of behavior for healthier, more successful ones.

Different approaches to psychotherapy

The psychodynamic approach was derived from principles and methods of psychoanalysis, and it encompasses psychoanalysis, Jungian analysis, Gestalt therapy, client-centered therapy, and somatic or body therapies, among other forms of psychotherapy. Psychoanalysis is therapy based upon the work of Austrian physician Sigmund Freud (1856–1939), and those who followed, Carl Jung, Alfred Adler, Erich Fromm, Karen Horney, and Erik Erikson. The basis of psychoanalytic therapy is the belief that behavior and personality develop in relation to unconscious wishes and conflicts from childhood. Gestalt therapy, developed by Frederick (Fritz) Perls, emphasizes the principles of self-centered awareness and accepting responsibility of one's own behavior. Client-centered therapy was formulated by Carl Rogers, and it introduced the idea that individuals have the resources within themselves for self-understanding and for change. Part of this concept is that the therapist exposes his or her own true feelings and does not adopt a professional posture, keeping personal feelings unclear. Somatic or body therapies include: dance therapy, holotropic breathwork, and Reichian therapy.

The behavioral approach encompasses various behavior modification techniques and theories, including assertiveness training/social skills training, operant conditioning, hypnosis/hypnotherapy, sex therapy, systematic desensitization, and others. Systematic desensitization was pioneered by Joseph Wolpe, after he became frustrated with psychoanalysis. This therapy is a combination of deep muscular **relaxation** and emotive imagery exercises, in which the client relaxes and the therapist verbally sets scenes for the client to imagine. These scenes include elements of the client's fears, building from the smallest fear toward the largest fear, and the therapist monitors the client and introduces the scenes, working to maintain the client's relaxed state.

The cognitive approach stresses the role that thoughts play in influencing behavior. Rational-emotive therapy and reality therapy are both examples of the cognitive approach. Rational-emotive therapy was pioneered by Albert Ellis in the mid-1950s. This therapy is based on the belief that events in and of themselves don't upset people, but people get upset about events because of their attitudes towards the events. Ellis's therapy set out to change people's attitudes about events through objective, firm direction from the therapist and talk therapy. Reality therapy, developed by William Glasser, is based upon the idea that humans seek to satisfy their complex needs, and the behaviors they adopt are to accomplish that satisfaction. In Glasser's theory, some people usually fulfill themselves and are generally happy, while others are unable to fulfill themselves and get angry or depressed.

The family systems approach includes family therapy in several forms and is the attempt to modify relationships within the family. Family therapy views behaviors and problems as the result of family interactions, rather than as belonging to a family member. One theory, developed by Murray Bowen, has become its own integrated system with eight basic concepts,

Types of psychotherapy

Type	Description	Disciplines	Proponents
Psychodynamic	Based on psychoanalysis, the psychodynamic approach believes behavior and personality stem from the unconscious wishes and conflicts from childhood.	Psychoanalysis, Jungian analysis, Gestalt therapy, Client-centered therapy, and somatic or body therapies.	Sigmund Freud, Carl Jung, Alfred Adler, Erich Fromm, Karen Horney, Erik Erikson, and Frederick (Fritz) Perls
Behavioral	Encompasses various behavior modification techniques and theories, but often includes the use of positive reinforcement in order to change attitudes and increase self-efficacy.	Assertiveness training/social skills training, operant conditioning, hypnosis/hypnotherapy, sex therapy, systematic desensitization, biofeedback, and stress management.	Joseph Wolpe
Cognitive	Focuses on the influence thoughts have on behavior.	Rational-emotive therapy and reality therapy	Albert Ellis, William Glasser
Family systems	Believes behavior is influenced by family dynamics and attempts to modify relationships within the family.	Family therapy	Murray Bowen

(Illustration by Corey Light. Cengage Learning, Gale)

including differentiation of self and sibling position. This system attempts to help an individual become differentiated from the family, while remaining in touch with the family system.

In the practical application of these approaches, psychotherapy can take many forms. Some of the most commonly practiced forms include:

- Counseling, the provision of both advice and psychological support, is the most elemental form of psychotherapy. Counseling can be short-term therapy done to assist a person in dealing with an immediate problem such as marital problems or family planning, substance abuse, bereavement, or terminal illness. Or it can be longer-term, more extensive treatment that addresses feelings and attitudes that impair success.

- Group psychotherapy requires less therapist time, and is thus less expensive. In fact, the interactions that occur between members of the group are expected to provide the change and healing each member receives. The therapist functions as a facilitator, or one who encourages and controls the group interchanges. Group therapy provides each member with the additional benefit of sharing and feedback from others experiencing similar emotional problems. This sharing and feedback has been found to be therapeutic, and the group can actually function as a trial social setting, allowing people to try out newly-learned behaviors.

- Family therapy began in the 1930s, when Freudian analyst Alfred Adler used it in working with his patients' entire families. Since the 1950s, it has been a widely used and highly respected means of therapy based upon the belief that the relationships and interactions within a family have a profound impact upon the patient's mental difficulties. Family therapy generally does not deal with internal conflicts, but rather encourages positive interactions between the various family members.

KEY TERMS

Behavioral therapy—A collection of techniques for treating mental disorders based upon changing abnormal behavior rather than attempting to analyze its fundamental basis. It is particularly used in phobic or obsessional disorders, and seeks to eliminate symptoms rather than treating the underlying psychological cause.

Magnetism—(Animal magnetism) A discredited theory put forth by Viennese physician Franz Anton Mesmer stating that all persons possess magnetic forces that can be used to influence magnetic fluid in other people and therefore effect healing. Mesmer opened a clinic in Paris in 1878, and appeared to cure people apparently suffering from hysterical conditions, such as emotionally caused paralysis.

Neurosis—A term commonly used to describe a range of relatively mild psychiatric disorders in which the sufferer remains in touch with reality. Neurotic disorders include mild depression, anxiety disorders (including phobias and obsessive compulsive disorders), somatization disorders, dissociative disorders, and psychosexual disorders.

Personality disorder—A group of conditions characterized by a general failure to learn from experience or adapt appropriately to changes, resulting in personal distress and impairment of social functioning.

All forms of psychotherapy require an atmosphere of absolute mutual trust and confidentiality. Without this total safety, no form of therapy will be successful.

Origins

Psychotherapy had its beginnings in the ministrations of some of the earliest psychologists, priests, magicians, and shamans of the ancient world. They attempted to determine the causes of the person's emotional distress by talking, counseling, and educating, and interpreting both behavior and dreams. Many of these practices became suspect as the work of charlatans, and fell into disrepute over the centuries. There was little change or progress in the treatment of mental illness over the centuries that followed.

Austrian physician Franz Anton Mesmer (1734–1815) began using what he termed *magnetism* and both the power of suggestion and hypnosis in 1772. Mesmer's treatments, too, fell into disrepute after his theories were rejected by a medical board of inquiry in 1784.

Then, nearly a century later, Mesmer's ideas were rediscovered by French neurologist Jean-Martin Charcot (1825–1893). Dr. Charcot used suggestion and hypnosis for treating psychological difficulties at Salpêtrière Hospital in Paris in the late nineteenth century. Mesmer is now known as the Father of Hypnosis.

In the late nineteenth and early twentieth century, Austrian physician Sigmund Freud studied Charcot's work, and came to believe that hypnosis was less a treatment for mental illness than a means of determining its underlying cause. Freud used hypnosis as one means of uncovering the often traumatic, not consciously recalled memories of his neurotic patients just as he used their dreams to evaluate their mental conflicts. He later abandoned hypnosis because he did not induce successful trances in his neurology patients. His *The Interpretation of Dreams*, published in 1899, made the point that a person's dreams were actually a window into the inner, unknown mind—the royal road to the unconscious. He used the information he obtained not only to help his patients, but also to collect data that eventually helped verify some of his psychodynamic assumptions.

Sigmund Freud theorized that the human personality is composed of three basic parts, the *id*, the *ego*, and the *superego*. The id is defined as the most elemental part, the one that unconsciously motivates people toward fulfilling instinctive urges. The ego is more related to intellect and judgment. It arbitrates between the internal, usually unrecognized desires all human beings have and the reality of the external world. The superego, unconscious controls dictated by moral or social standards outside of ourselves, is probably most easily described as another name for the conscience.

Freud believed that mental illness was the result of people being unable to resolve conflict, or inadequate settlement of disharmony among the ego, superego, and id. To deal with these internal psychic conflicts, people develop defense mechanisms, which is normally a healthy response. The defense mechanisms become harmful to mental health when overused, or used inappropriately. Freud further postulated that childhood psychic development is primarily based upon sexuality; he divided the first eighteen months of life into three sex-based phases: oral, anal, and genital.

Freud's earliest students, including Carl Jung and Alfred Adler, came to believe that Freud had overestimated the influence sexuality had on psychic development, and found other influences that helped to shape the personality. In the late 1800s and into the twentieth century, 1904 Nobel Prize winner Ivan

Petrovich Pavlov pioneered the research that would later result in behavioral therapies, such as the work of American behaviorist Burrhus Frederic Skinner. And in the 1930s, American psychologist Carl Ransom Rogers began his school of psychology that emphasized the importance of the relationship between the patient (or client, according to Rogers) and the therapist in bringing about positive psychic change.

Primal therapy, developed by Arthur Janov in the 1960s, is based upon the assumption that people must relive early life experiences with all the acuity of feeling that was somehow suppressed at the time in order to free themselves of compulsive or neurotic behavior. Primal therapy was a cathartic approach that many therapists now believe can impede progress because a person can become addicted to the release (even "high") associated with the catharsis and seek to keep repeating it for the momentary satisfaction. Transactional analysis, based on Eric Berne's work, came into favor in the 1970s, and supposes that all people function as either parent or child at various times, and teaches the person to identify which role he or she is filling at any given time and to evaluate whether this role is appropriate.

Benefits

The generally accepted aims of psychotherapy are:

- Increased insight or improved understanding of one's own mental state. This can range from simply knowing one's strengths and weaknesses to understanding that symptoms are signs of a mental illness and to deep awareness and acceptance of inner feelings.
- The resolution of disabling conflicts, or working to create a peaceful and positive settlement of emotional struggles that stop a person from living a reasonably happy and productive life.
- Increasing acceptance of self by developing a more realistic and positive appraisal of the person's strengths and abilities.
- Development of improved and more efficient and successful means of dealing with problems so that the patient can find solutions or means of coping with them.
- An overall strengthening of ego structure, or sense of self, so that normal, healthy means of coping with life situations can be called upon and used as needed.

Though there are no definitive studies proving that all five of these goals are consistently realized, psychotherapy in one form or other is a component of nearly all of both in-patient and community based psychiatric treatment programs.

Description

Classic Freudian psychotherapy is usually carried out in 50-minute sessions three to five times per week. The patient lies on a couch while he or she talks with the therapist. Freudian therapy characteristically requires ongoing treatment for several years, though in Freud's era it did not. Most other forms of individual psychotherapy, including Jungian, counseling, humanistic, Gestalt, or behavioral therapies, are carried out on a weekly basis (or more frequently, if necessary), in which the person meets with his or her therapist in the therapist's office, and may or may not continue for longer than a year.

Group therapy is held in a variety of settings. A trained group therapist chooses the people that presumably would benefit and learn from interactions with each other. The size of a group is usually five to 10 people, plus a specially trained therapist who guides the group discussion and provides examination of issues and concerns raised.

Child psychotherapy is done for the same reasons as adult psychotherapy—to treat emotional problems through communication. The obvious difference is that child psychotherapy must acknowledge the child's stage of development. This means that the therapist may use different techniques, including play, rather than only talking to the patient.

A newer direction in the treatment of mental disorders is the use of brief psychotherapy sessions, often combined with medication, to treat neurotic conditions. Another short-term psychotherapy is often termed crisis intervention, and is used to aid people in dealing with specific crises in their lives, such as the death of a loved one.

Research and general acceptance

Psychotherapy, in its many forms, has been accepted and used throughout the world for over one hundred years. It is normally covered as a valid treatment of mental disorder by both public and private health insurers. Because the various types of psychotherapy have different aims, and mental illnesses usually do not have absolute measurable signs of recovery, evaluating psychotherapy's effectiveness is difficult. As a general rule, the majority of people who undergo treatment with psychotherapy can expect to make appreciable gains. Studies have revealed, however, that not everyone who goes into therapy will be helped, or helped as much as others, and some will even be harmed.

Training and certification

Though the actual clinical practice of psychotherapy is very much the same among disciplines, therapists come from a variety of different fields, including medicine, psychology, social work, and nursing.

Psychiatrists are required to complete four years of medical school and one year of internship, followed by a three-year residency in psychiatry. In order to be a psychoanalyst, a minimum of three years further training at a psychoanalytic institute is necessary, along with personal ongoing analysis.

Psychologists earn a Ph.D. in clinical psychology followed by a year of supervised practice, and additionally may take specialized training at a specific psychotherapeutic school, including therapy for themselves.

Social workers who specialize in mental health must earn a master's degree or doctorate before being allowed to practice.

Psychiatric nurses generally earn a master's degree and practice in hospitals or community mental health centers.

Most states in the United States require a license to practice as a psychotherapist, and by law in the majority of the states, they are accountable only to the other members of their profession.

Resources

BOOKS

Clayman, Charles B., M.D. *American Medical Association Home Medical Encyclopedia*. New York: Random House, 1989.

Coleman, James C. *Abnormal Psychology and Modern Life*. Glenview, Illinois: Scott, Foresman and Company, 1972.

Engler, Jack, and Daniel Goleman. *The Consumer's Guide to Psychotherapy*. New York: Simon & Schuster, 1992.

Taber, Clarence Wilbur. *Taber's Cyclopedic Medical Dictionary*. F. A. Davis Co., 1997.

OTHER

American Group Psychotherapy Association. "About Group Psychotherapy." http//www.agpa.org (1999).

CNN. "A Century Later, Science Still Grapples with Freud." www.cnn.com.

Electric Library. "Group Psychotherapy." www.encyclopedia.com (1999).

Lucidcafe. "Sigmund Freud, Austrian Originator of Psycho-Analysis." www.lucidcafe.com.

Joan Schonbeck

Psyllium

Description

Psyllium is a seed used for medicinal purposes taken from the common fleawort, *Plantago psyllium* and related species. There are about 250 species of the genus *Plantago* found worldwide. The most common species producing seed for medicinal use, in addition to *P. psyllium,* are *P. afra*, *P. isphagula*, *P. ovata*, and *P. indica*.

Psyllium is extensively cultivated in many parts of the world. Shrubby perennial plants with narrow green leaves put up spikes of small flowers that mature into seedpods. The seeds and husks are harvested and used in healing. The seeds are small (1.5–2 cm) and brown or reddish-brown.

Psyllium has been used in **Ayurvedic medicine** in India and in **traditional Chinese medicine** for thousands of years. It has also been used in Europe for

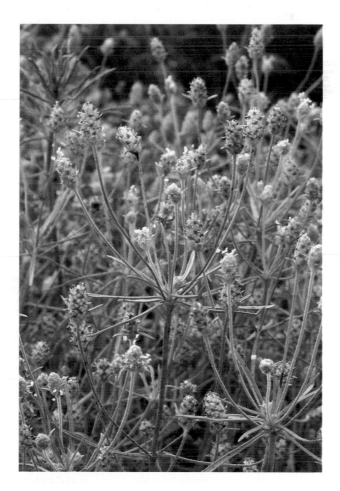

Psyllium plants. *(©PlantaPhile, Germany. Reproduced by permission.)*

many years, but it became common in North American healing in the second half of the twentieth century. However, by 21st century, psyllium was widely accepted by both alternative and traditional healthcare professionals.

General use

Psyllium has three major uses that have been well documented by modern scientific research. These include the treatment of **diarrhea**, the relief of **constipation**, and the lowering of serum **cholesterol** levels. Psyllium has other traditional uses that not been rigorously scientifically documented.

Psyllium seed is high in dietary fiber, making it a good bulk laxative for treating chronic constipation. It is also used to soften stools and ease bowel movements after operations involving the anus and rectum, when **hemorrhoids** or anal fissures are present, or during **pregnancy** to lessen the strain of bowel movements.

Psyllium seeds are coated with a substance called mucilage that swells or "bulks up" when exposed to water. This extra volume stimulates the movement of material through the bowel. In addition, the moist, gummy mucilage lubricates the lining of the intestine. Both United States health authorities and the German Federal Health Agency's Commission E, established in 1978 to independently review and evaluate scientific literature and case studies pertaining to herb and plant medications, approve the use of psyllium to treat constipation. Psyllium is the main ingredient in over-the-counter bulk laxatives such as Metamucil, Regulan, and Serutan.

Although it may at first seem contradictory, psyllium is also used to treat diarrhea and bouts of **irritable bowel syndrome**, a condition in which periods of diarrhea alternate with periods of constipation. As psyllium passes through the intestines, it absorbs water. This reduces the amount of fluid in the bowel and helps to control diarrhea. Both United States health authorities and the German Commission E have approved the use of psyllium to treat diarrhea.

German health authorities approved the use of psyllium to reduce serum cholesterol levels in the early 1990s, while the U. S. Food and Drug Administration (FDA) did not permit health claims to be made for psyllium content in foods until 1997. In that year, the FDA reviewed several scientific studies indicating that a daily intake of 10.2 grams of psyllium seed husk, combined with a diet low in saturated fats, consistently lowered blood cholesterol levels. Additional studies have confirmed the FDA's daily intake recommendation. Moreover, an improvement in the ratio of high-density lipoproteins (HDL, or "good"

cholesterol) to low-density lipoproteins (LDL, or "bad" cholesterol) occurs when psyllium is used on a daily basis. The beneficial effects of psyllium on blood cholesterol levels, however, are somewhat affected by sex and age. Other surveys have found that wellness programs in which psyllium intake is one component of personalized behavioral change recommendations are more effective in lowering blood cholesterol than simply taking psyllium by itself. The FDA allows psyllium to be added to foods such as cereals (e.g., Bran Buds, Heartwise). The FDA permits foods containing psyllium to make the health claim that as part of a diet low in saturated fat and cholesterol, psyllium may help to prevent coronary **heart disease**).

In addition to these approved therapeutic uses, psyllium is used in traditional Chinese medicine to treat stomach and intestinal ulcers, **heartburn**, and to help manage non-insulin dependent (type 2) diabetes. Studies done by traditional medical parishioners have shown that psyllium taken before meals may reduced the rise in blood glucose (blood sugar) that occurred after eating, suggesting a valid role for psyllium in diabetes management. Additional studies are being undertaken.

Psyllium is also used to help control appetite in individuals who are dieting. The idea behind this is that psyllium slows stomach emptying and makes the individual feel fuller sooner and longer.

Some early studies suggested that psyllium might protect against **colorectal cancer**. Larger, better-designed studies have found only a minimal association between dietary fiber intake (including psyllium) and decreased rates of colorectal **cancer**. As of 2008, the role of psyllium in cancer prevention was still being investigated.

In Ayurvedic medicine, psyllium is used to cleanse the body by absorbing toxins in the large intestine so that they can be eliminated from the body. Some herbalists believe this action helps reduce the risk of colon cancer. Psyllium is also used by Ayurvedic practitioners to treat urethritis.

Preparations

Psyllium is available in a large number of over-the-counter (OTC) formulations. In the United States, it is sold in mainstream pharmacies and supermarkets under a variety of brand names including Metamucil, Fiberall, and Naturacil. Many other common laxatives include psyllium as an ingredient. Psyllium is also added to some breakfast cereals to increase their fiber content. In health food stores, psyllium can be obtained as powdered husks or seeds. A common dosage for constipation is 2 tsp of psyllium (7 g) taken with at least one glass (8 oz) of water up to three times a day. The dose for diarrhea can be even higher—up to 40 grams per day.

Precautions

Psyllium is one of the safest laxatives available for long-term use. It is widely considered by the traditional medical community as very safe and effective when used in recommended doses for constipation and diarrhea.

People who are suspected of having an intestinal blockage or who suffer from narrowing of the esophagus or any other part of the intestinal tract should not use psyllium. People with diabetes, and children under age six should use psyllium only after talking to their doctor. Psyllium is generally accepted as safe to use throughout pregnancy and while breastfeeding. In rare cases psyllium can cause a severe allergic reaction. Allergic reaction is most common in people who have long-term workplace exposure to psyllium.

Although such accidents are unusual, cases have been reported of patients suffocating when a mass of psyllium blocked the upper airway. Although these incidents are most common in elderly patients or those with neurological disorders, anyone taking a psyllium preparation on a regular basis should drink a large glass of water or other liquid immediately following each dose.

Side effects

The use of psyllium may cause increased abdominal **gas**, stomach rumbling, and a feeling of bloating. A few patients may experience **nausea** and **vomiting**, but these side effects are rare.

Interactions

Psyllium slows the absorption from the intestine of some nutrients and may change the rate of absorption of some medications. Some nutrients that may be absorbed more slowly include **zinc**, **calcium**, **iron**, and vitamin B12. Carbohydrates are absorbed more slowly, which may make it necessary for insulin-dependent diabetics to adjust their insulin dose. Psyllium may also slow down or decrease the absorption of certain medications, including antibiotics, digoxin, lithium, tricyclic antidepressants, carbemazepine, and anti-diabetic medicines such as glyburide and metformin. Individuals taking any of these drugs should talk to their healthcare provider before beginning psyllium. Absorption problems can usually be avoided by taking psyllium an hour after taking other medications. Apart from affecting speed of absorption, as of 2008, psyllium is not known to interact with any standard pharmaceuticals.

Resources

BOOKS

Blumenthal, Mark, ed. *The Complete German Commission E Monographs: Therapeutic Guide to Herbal Medicines.* Boston: Integrative Medicine Communications, 1998.

Chevallier, Andrew. *Herbal Remedies.* New York: DK Publishing, 2007.

Foster, Steven and Rebecca Johnson. *National Geographic Desk Reference to Nature's Medicine.* Washington, DC: National Geographic Society, 2006.

PDR for Herbal Medicines, 4th ed. Montvale, NJ: Thompson Healthcare, 2007.

PERIODICALS

Jenkins, D. J., C. W. Kendall, V. Vuksan, et al. "Soluble Fiber Intake at a Dose Approved by the US Food and Drug Administration for a Claim of Health Benefits: Serum Lipid Risk Factors for Cardiovascular Disease Assessed in a Randomized Controlled Crossover Trial." *American Journal of Clinical Nutrition* 75 (May 2002): 834-839.

ORGANIZATIONS

Alternative Medicine Foundation. P. O. Box 60016, Potomac, MD 20859. (301) 340-1960. http://www.amfoundation.org.

Centre for International Ethnomedicinal Education and Research (CIEER). http://www.cieer.org.

OTHER

"Psyllium (Planto ovata, Planto isphagula)." *MedlinePlus.* October 1, 2006 [cited February 20, 2008]. http://www.nlm.nih.gov/medlineplus/druginfo/natural/patient-psyllium.html.

"Psyllium." *University of Maryland Medical Center.* April 1, 2002 [cited February 20, 2008]. http://www.umm.edu/altmed/articles/psyllium-000321.htm.

Tish Davidson, A. M.

Pukeweed *see* **Lobelia**

Pulmonary heart disease *see* **Heart disease**

Pulsatilla

Description

Pulsatilla nigricans, commonly known as pulsatilla, is a remedy derived from the plant commonly known as wind flower, pasque flower, or meadow anemone. The perennial plant is a member of the Ranunculaceae family and is native to central and northern Europe and southern England. This wild plant grows in sunny meadows, pastures, and fields.

A crown of leaves forms on the ground, from which a single flower grows in May and August. The stem reaches a height of about 6 in (15 cm) and has downy hairs that grow on it. The flower is colored dark violet-brown.

The plant was used medicinally during ancient times for eye ailments. During the 19th century, the eclectic physicians and contemporaries of Samuel Hahnemann, the father of **homeopathy**, noted pulsatilla's use in the treatment of melancholy, swelling of the knees, and nervous system disorders. In ancient times it was used as an external remedy for ulcers and eye inflammation.

The plant contains lactones, saponins, anemone camphor, tannins, and a volatile oil. It is antispasmodic and antibacterial and acts on the nervous system. When chewed, a caustic substance contained in the plant **burns** the tongue and throat. When applied topically, it may cause **blisters** on the skin. Though not used as widely as it was in the 19th century, pulsatilla may be used to treat painful periods, **insomnia**, headaches, **boils**, ovarian **pain**, and **asthma**.

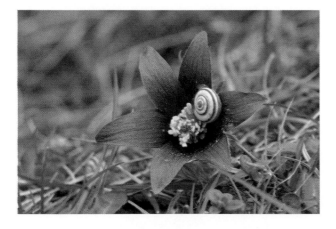

The pulsatilla plant contains lactones, saponins, anemone camphor, tannins, and a volatile oil. It is antispasmodic and antibacterial and acts on the nervous system. *(Chris Gomersall / Alamy)*

General use

Traditional Chinese medicine

Chinese anemone root (*Pulsatilla chinensis*) is a related herb used in **traditional Chinese medicine**. Bai tou weng, as it is referred to in Mandarin, is prescribed by Chinese medicine practitioners to clear heat and detoxify fire poison. It is used in damp heat conditions of the stomach and large intestine in dysentery. Dysentery is a disease marked by frequent watery stools and often accompanied by stomach pain, **fever** or dehydration. The herb has a bitter taste and is antimicrobial. The plant has also been used to treat **diarrhea**, **wounds**, and trauma.

Homeopathy

Homeopaths prescribe pulsatilla for acute ailments that are caused by grief, anger, fright, shock, consumption of rich foods, loss of vital fluids, exposure to the sun, suppression of **menstruation**, and mental strain. This herb is often called the queen of homeopathic remedies, as it is indicated in so many conditions. These conditions include arthritis, **bronchitis**, **chickenpox** with **cough** and low fever, colds, coughs, digestive troubles, eye and ear **infections**, fevers, headaches, **measles** with a cough and cold, **mumps** with swollen and painful glands, and menstrual difficulties.

Physical symptoms include thirstlessness, one-sided complaints, weakness, slow digestion, chilliness, and thick, yellow bodily discharges. The pains are cutting, stitching, or burning, and they wander from body part to body part. The lymph glands are often swollen, and the sweat and breath smell repugnant. The lips and mouth are dry, and a white or yellow-coated tongue is often present. The patient may crave butter, but dislikes bread, hot food and drinks, fats, rich food, and meat. These foods cause **indigestion** and **nausea**. The patient is chilly, often with cold hands and feet, but dislikes heat.

Pulsatilla is generally chosen because it acts so well on ailments that are of an emotional nature. The remedy is typically suited for mild, gentle, and timid women and children with blonde hair and blue eyes. Pulsatilla patients are generally emaciated persons who are sympathetic, sad, weepy, sensitive, easily offended, jealous, depressed, shy, introspective, and anxious. The patient desires affection and the company of others, and is often fearful of being alone, of the dark, or in a crowd. She may be filled with remorse or despair and may be suicidal. She cries easily and is not afraid to show her emotions.

A typical indication of the pulsatilla patient lies in her erratic emotional and physical behavior. Her moods are always changing: one minute she may be happy, the next may find her crying. Ailments are one-sided or change location. For instance, arthritic pain may stop in one joint and appear in another. Pulsatilla is a useful remedy for teething babies who are weepy, whiny, and want to be carried.

Symptoms are worse in the morning, in the evening before midnight, in cold air, when the feet are wet, and while standing or lying down. They are also aggravated by warmth, while lying on the painless side, during and after eating, eating warm foods, after sleep, by rapid motion, and before, during, and after menstruation. Conditions that improve the symptoms include fresh air, lying on the painful side, pressure, gentle motion, cold, and cold applications.

SPECIFIC INDICATIONS. Arthritic inflammations have little swelling or redness. The pains are pulling, sore, and bruised, and shift from joint to joint. They are relieved by the cold, fresh air, and slow movement. Symptoms are worse from heat, wet weather, upon beginning to move, or after the **common cold**. The patient often has a **dry mouth**, fever, and lacks thirst.

Back pains occur in the lower back or small of the back. The back feels tired and weak, like it was sprained, and the pains are aching and pressing. The pains are worse when bending down or rising after long periods of sitting, but are relieved from gentle motion and walking slowly. The backache often occurs before and during the menstrual period.

Bronchitis accompanied by a dry cough that is worse in the evening or when lying down is indicative of this remedy. The cough is loose in the morning and the mucous expelled is bitter or salty. The cough is better when sitting up or in cool air and worse after eating.

Pulsatilla is a useful remedy for breastfeeding mothers with an overabundant supply of milk. It is often indicated in postnatal **depression** accompanied by crying.

The cold indicative of pulsatilla is accompanied by **sneezing**, **chills**, fever, and sometimes **nosebleeds**. The patient catches cold easily. The nose is stuffed in a warm room and in the evening, and is watery in fresh air. The discharge is thick and yellow or green. The sense of smell and taste is lost. Symptoms are relieved by fresh air.

Conjunctivitis with redness and swelling of the eyelids is accompanied by a thick, yellow discharge that oozes from the eyes. In the morning the eyes are often stuck shut. The eyes are typically itchy and burning. The symptoms are better from cold applications or cold air.

Constipation with ineffective urging and a backache occurs with this remedy. When the patient does defecate, the stools are large and hard.

The cough typical of this remedy is an exhausting cough that occurs in fits. The cough is dry at night and loose in the morning. There is a loud rattling in the chest that often wakes the patient. A sticky, yellow or green mucus is present, but may be difficult to expel. The throat may become raw, sore, and painful from the cough. The cough is better from fresh air and sitting up, and worse from exertion, lying down, heat, or a stuffy room.

The diarrhea is a greenish-yellow color and is slimy and watery. There is a rumbling in the abdomen before it is expelled. The pains in the abdomen are cutting. The diarrhea is worse at night, after eating, after eating starchy or rich food, when overheated, or in a stuffy room.

Digestive disturbances are caused by eating rich or fatty foods, pork, ice cream, fruit, or cold foods. The patient lacks appetite or thirst and often suffers from nausea and **vomiting**. He may have a dry mouth and may feel as if a lump was behind the sternum. Indigestion is accompanied by bitter-tasting belches, stomach pains, and **heartburn**. Diarrhea may also be present. Symptoms are worse after eating or drinking and at night.

Pulsatilla types do not fare well in hot weather and often suffer from exhaustion. They are worse from the sun, a stuffy room, or mental exertion.

Pulsatilla is indicated in fevers in which the patient is not thirsty and has a dry mouth. The fever is hot and burning and is typically one-sided, i.e. the body may be hotter on one side than the other. The sweat produced may occur on one side of the body or be localized to one area. The patient may weep and moan while feverish. The fever is worse in heat, at night, under warm covers, in a stuffy room, or after washing. Intermittent fevers are worse between 2:00 p.m. and 3:00 p.m. These fevers are worse from heat and covering.

The **headache** pains occur in the front of the head or at the temples. The pains are throbbing, pressing, one-sided pains that are worse from movement, excessive sun, eating rich foods, hot drinks, bending over, standing, running, or blowing the nose.

Insomnia is caused by anxious dreams, a restless sleep, too much thinking, and a repetition of thoughts. When the feet become hot, the patient sticks them out of the bed. Then the patient is awakened because his feet are cold.

Menstrual difficulties are also indicative of this remedy and often occur as a result of suppressed menstruation. Menstruation is accompanied by vomiting, nausea, skin affections, sadness, weeping, and pain in the abdomen, liver, and back. The period is generally late. The flow may start and stop or be present only during the day. The pains are aching, dull, and wandering. They are better when the patient is doubled over. Symptoms are aggravated by wetting the feet.

Varicose veins are sore and stinging. They are worse while standing and better from walking and cold applications. They are also worse during **pregnancy** and when circulation in the limbs is poor.

Preparations

Pulsatilla nigricans is available in dried bulk form, and as a tincture. Pharmacies, health food stores, and Chinese herbal stores carry the various preparations. They are also available as prescribed by a herbalist, homeopathic doctor, and Chinese medicine practitioner.

The homeopathic preparation of pulsatilla is created in the following manner. The plant is collected when the flowers are in full bloom and pounded to a pulp. This pulp is soaked in alcohol, then strained and diluted. The final homeopathic remedy is created after the diluted mixture is succussed repeatedly. The remedy is available at health food and drug stores in various potencies in the form of tinctures, tablets, and pellets.

The dried plant combines well with **cramp bark** as a treatment for painful periods. For skin conditions it is combined with **echinacea**.

An infusion is made by pouring one cup of boiling water over 1/2 tsp of the dried plant. The mixture steeps for 10-15 minutes then should be strained. Pulsatilla can be drunk up to three times daily.

For use in traditional Chinese medicine, the herb should be soaked for one hour in warm water, then simmered for 30-120 minutes. It is usually used in combination with other herbs.

The tincture dosage is 1-2 ml three times daily.

Precautions

If symptoms do not improve after the recommended time period, a homeopath or health care practitioner should be consulted.

The recommended dose should not be exceeded.

Those seeking this remedy should not use the fresh plant.

Side effects

There are no known side effects.

Interactions

When taking any homeopathic remedy, use of **peppermint** products, coffee, or alcohol is discouraged. These products will cause the remedy to be ineffective.

Pulsatilla chinensis is contraindicated in chronic dysentery with a deficiency of Spleen and Stomach. It is only used for acute dysentery.

Resources

BOOKS

Cummings, M.D., Stephen, and Dana Ullman, M.P.H. *Everybody's Guide to Homeopathic Medicines*. New York, NY: Jeremy P. Tarcher/Putnam, 1997.

Kent, James Tyler. *Lectures on Materia Medica*. Delhi, India: B. Jain Publishers, 1996.

Jennifer Wurges

Pulse diagnosis

Definition

Pulse diagnosis is a diagnostic technique used in several healing systems to determine the health conditions and course of treatment for patients.

Acupuncture—Healing technique in traditional Chinese medicine utilizing the insertion of thin needles and other methods.

Ayurvedic medicine—Traditional healing system developed in ancient India and practiced around the world.

Diagnosis—Means of determining health problems and general condition in a patient.

Traditional Chinese medicine—Healing system developed in ancient China utilizing acupuncture, acupressure massage, herbal remedies, and other healing techniques.

Origins

As used in **Ayurvedic medicine** and **traditional Chinese medicine** (TCM), the techniques of pulse diagnosis have been developed over thousands of years, as these two systems of medicine are the world's oldest. **Acupuncture**, a branch of TCM, has long relied on pulse diagnosis as a main tool to determine the course of treatment. In Western medicine, every time a doctor checks the pulse of a patient and listens to the heartbeat with a stethoscope, the doctor is practicing a form of pulse diagnosis.

Benefits

Pulse diagnosis is a quick, inexpensive, and non-invasive diagnostic tool. When performed by trained professionals, it can be an effective means for determining the health conditions of patients.

Description

In conventional Western medicine, doctors check the pulse of patients by placing their hands on the wrist and by listening to the pulse at various points on the body with a stethoscope. Doctors check for abnormalities in rhythm and rate that may indicate heart problems, internal bleeding, and **fever**. Measuring blood pressure is essentially another pulse diagnosis, which indicates **hypertension**, circulatory conditions, and other problems.

In older healing systems, such as Ayurveda and TCM, doctors check the pulse just as Western doctors do, but they use a very intricate system of pulse measurements, and they rely on careful observations instead of diagnostic tools. Pulse diagnosis is considered as much an art as a science, and it takes physicians

many years of training to become experts. Doctors skilled in pulse diagnosis can often find health problems with a quick touch. Some published observations have documented the effectiveness of pulse diagnosis by trained experts, comparing their diagnoses with the diagnoses with modern technology.

In Ayurvedic medicine, pulse diagnosis is called *nadi parkiksha*. The principle measurement of pulse is taken at the radial artery, a blood vessel that is located on the inside of the wrist. Ayurvedic doctors use three fingers to feel the pulse, and particular conditions are indicated depending on the pulse characteristics that each finger feels. Doctors note heart rate, counting how many beats occur per minute and per breathing cycle of the patient. Doctors also take deep and shallow readings of the pulse, pressing hard or gently on the artery. Ayurvedic doctors believe that the pulse can indicate how *prana*, or life energy, is flowing through a patient's system, and can indicate the condition of internal organs. Doctors check the pulse on both wrists, because each side of the body gives different indications.

Ayurvedic doctors may take pulse readings at other points on the body as well. These points include the brachial artery on the inside of the arm above the elbow, the carotid artery at the base of the neck, the femoral artery that travels down the inside of the leg, and pulse points at the temples, at the ankles, and on the top of the feet. Ayurvedic physicians use other diagnostic tools in conjunction with pulse analysis, including interviewing the patient and closely observing the physical characteristics of the tongue, voice, skin, eyes, appearance, urine, and stool, in addition to utilizing conventional diagnostic methods.

Pulse diagnosis in traditional Chinese medicine (including acupuncture) shares some similarities with Ayurvedic medicine. In TCM, pulse diagnosis is used to check the condition of the blood and of *qi* (chi), which is the invisible life energy that travels in channels (meridians) throughout the body. Using pulse diagnosis, physicians determine the condition of the internal organs, and describe conditions according to yin and yang (cold or hot, empty or full, weak or strong, etc.). Pulse diagnosis tells acupuncturists where there are problems with the flow of energy in the body.

In TCM, there are several pulse diagnosis techniques, but the one most commonly used is checking the radial arteries on each wrist. Each wrist has six positions that are checked, and the 12 positions on both wrists correspond to the 12 internal organs. At each position, there are three depths that are checked.

LI SHIZ-HEN (1518-1593)

Li Shiz-hen was born in 1518 in the town of Kin Zhou (var. Qizhou) along the Yangtze River in the Hubei province of China. His family was renowned for its medical expertise. At age 14, Shiz-hen elected to study the family arts of medicine and pharmacology. As a medical student he distinguished himself with his scholarly writings.

Shiz-hen served as a pharmacist for the Ming Dynasty. His reputation was such that he was assigned to an official position at the Imperial Academy of Medicine in Peking. There he earned the respect of the prince of China. Between 1552 and 1578, with the express permission of the Imperial family, Shiz-hen engaged himself in studying the priceless ancient Chinese writings on medicinals, after which he undertook the massive task of reorganizing and classifying all of the information that was at his disposal. Shiz-hen incorporated information that he learned from his own family along with the knowledge from the treasured ancient writings collected by the Chinese monarchs for centuries. The result of his decades long project was a massive encyclopedic text, called the *Bencao gangmu.* Shiz-hen's work comprised 52 volumes, including all existing knowledge of botanicals and medicine that was available at the time. The books contained thousands of medical prescriptions and information on over 1,000 herbs. He presented the manuscript to the scholar Wang Shiz-hen, who wrote an introduction for the book.

Shiz-hen's voluminous work, also known as the *Great Herbal,* was the greatest written contribution from the Far East during the sixteenth century. In 1596, three years after Shiz-hen's death, the Emperor Shen Tsun declared the book to be the official medical reference of China.

In all, the pulse can have 36 different qualities. Some of the observations noted during pulse diagnosis include the position of the artery, whether it is deep or shallow, the hardness or softness of the artery, the diameter of the blood vessel, the rate and strength of the pulse, and the rhythm of the heartbeat. TCM practitioners may take the pulse at other points on the body, frequently including the carotid artery at the base of the neck.

In TCM and acupuncture, pulse diagnosis is used in conjunction with other diagnostic techniques. TCM doctors closely interview patients, and pay attention to seeing, hearing, and smelling the patient. TCM practitioners also observe the tongue, and palpate (touch) parts of the body to check for swelling, **pain**, temperature, moisture, and other characteristics. TCM practitioners may also use conventional diagnostic techniques such as blood tests, scans, and others.

Preparation

Pulse diagnosis should be performed on patients under normal conditions to insure accuracy. The pulse should not be diagnosed after **exercise**, physical exertion, bathing, massage, sex, eating or drinking, while the patient is very hungry, or in a room where the temperature is very hot or cold.

Precautions

Pulse diagnosis can be a quick and inexpensive means of diagnosis, but it should be performed by a trained specialist to be most effective. Pulse diagnosis is best used in conjunction with other diagnostic techniques, including conventional ones. For patients with severe, chronic, or undetermined conditions, getting more than one diagnosis or opinion is recommended.

Training and certification

Pulse diagnosis is a technique that requires careful training by specialists. Pulse diagnosis is taught at schools that teach Ayurvedic medicine, traditional Chinese medicine, and acupuncture.

Resources

BOOKS

Lad, Dr. Vasant. *Ayurveda: The Science of Self-Healing.* Wisconsin: Lotus Press, 1984.

Williams, Tom, Ph.D. *The Complete Illustrated Guide to Chinese Medicine.* Rockport, MA: Element, 1996.

ORGANIZATIONS

American Association of Acupuncture and Oriental Medicine. 433 Front St., Catasaugua, PA 18032. (610) 266-1433.

Ayurvedic Institute of Albuquerque. P.O. Box 23445, Albuquerque, NM 87192. (505) 291-9698.

Douglas Dupler

Purification therapy *see* **Panchakarma**

Purple coneflower *see* **Echinacea**

Pygeum *see* **Saw palmetto**

Pyridoxine

Description

Pyridoxine, or vitamin B_6, is a member of the water-soluble family of B vitamins. It is necessary in the metabolism of proteins, fats, and carbohydrates; to make hormones and neurotransmitters; and to support the immune system. It also plays a role in the production of normal, healthy red blood cells and some of the neurotransmitters needed for proper nervous system function. In conjunction with **folic acid** and cobalamin, it acts to reduce homocysteine levels, thus lowering the risk of developing **heart disease**.

General use

Mild deficiencies of pyridoxine are common, despite the low daily requirements. The Recommended Daily Allowance (RDA) for babies under six months of age is 0.1 milligram (mg), and for babies six months to one year old, it is 0.3 mg. The daily requirement is 0.5 mg for children one to three years old, 0.6 mg for those four to eight years old, and 1 mg for nine- to 13-year-olds. Males aged 14–18 years need 1 mg, and those 19 years and older need 1.3 mg. The RDA for females aged 14–18 years is 1.2 mg for females, and for females over the age of 19, 1.3 mg. Requirements are somewhat increased during **pregnancy** (1.9 mg) and lactation (2 mg).

Pyridoxine has numerous therapeutic uses apart from treating deficiency. It has a calming effect on the nervous system and may alleviate **insomnia** by increasing serotonin levels in the brain. Because of the calming effects of pyridoxine, it has been tried as a possible adjunctive treatment for **schizophrenia**. As of 2008, however, the findings were inconclusive although additional studies on the use of pyridoxine for dealing with mental illness were under way.

Evidence suggests that pyridoxine reduces **nausea** for about a third of pregnant women who experience **morning sickness**. In addition, pyridoxine does not have any harmful effects on the fetus. It is also used to decrease the risk of heart disease by lowering homocysteine levels. Taken in conjunction with **magnesium** supplements, pyridoxine has been found to have beneficial effects on some people with **autism**. The vitamin B_6 and magnesium combination can also help to prevent the recurrence of **calcium** oxalate **kidney stones** in susceptible people. Those who are affected by **depression** or gestational diabetes may benefit from a moderate addition of it, as well. One type of hereditary **anemia** and several metabolic diseases are effectively treated with high doses of pyridoxine. A few chemotherapeutic agents, including vincristine, can be taken with fewer side effects when pyridoxine is added to the patient's regimen. The data are equivocal on whether **asthma** is improved by vitamin B_6 supplementation, but high doses—50 mg, taken twice daily—were used in the studies performed, creating a risk of nerve injury. There is some question as to the benefit to taking it for PMS, **carpal tunnel syndrome**, or diabetic neuropathy, although there is no harm in a trial of additional B_6 at a modest level. Taking B_6 has some benefit for those suffering from **osteoporosis** and **epilepsy**. Nevertheless, the advice of a healthcare professional should be sought before undertaking this, and any, supplemental treatment.

Preparations

Natural sources

Meats are the best food source of pyridoxine, followed by dairy and eggs. Although some grains contain B vitamins, they are generally lost in processing. Bananas, potatoes, mangoes, and avocados have the highest vitamin B_6 value among vegetarian foods. Fresh foods should be used because freezing destroys much of this vitamin. Minimizing the amount of water used in cooking prevents pyridoxine and other water soluble vitamins from leaching into it.

Supplemental sources

Pyridoxine supplements are available in both oral and injectable forms. Pyridoxine is also added to many processed grain products. Individuals may consider taking a balanced B complex supplement rather than high doses of an individual vitamin unless given instructions by a medical doctor to do so. Supplements ought to be stored in a cool, dry place, away from light, and out of the reach of children.

Deficiency

Symptoms of pyridoxine deficiency are nonspecific but may include nervousness, irritability, muscle twitches, insomnia, confusion, weakness, loss of coordination, and anemia. Frequent **infections** are likely as well due to the importance of vitamin B_6 to the immune system.

Risk factors for deficiency

Since meats are the best source of pyridoxine, followed by dairy and eggs, vegans are one of the groups at risk for deficiency. A balanced B vitamin supplement is adequate to prevent deficiency. People with malabsorption syndromes, chronic illnesses, or hyperthyroidism may require somewhat larger amounts of vitamin B$_6$. Those who take birth control pills are more likely to have abnormally low levels and may benefit from a supplement of 25–50 mg per day. Elderly people are more likely to have a poor diet, and deficient pyridoxine will both increase their susceptibility to illness and prolong recovery. Alcoholics, smokers, and people who take certain medications, including estrogen, theophylline (for asthma), hydralazine (for **hypertension**), penicillamine (for **rheumatoid arthritis**), and isoniazid (for **tuberculosis**) are more likely to need extra pyridoxine. For asthmatics on theophylline, the side effects of this medication can also be reduced by the additional vitamin B$_6$. A healthcare professional ought to be consulted before individuals begin a program of supplementation.

Precautions

Allergic reactions to oral or injected pyridoxine are known to occur but are rare. It is possible to have toxic effects from large doses. At 2,000 mg daily, nerve damage may occur, causing numbness or tingling of the extremities and loss of coordination. These symptoms are usually, but not always, reversible. At 500 mg for daily dosages, there is possible toxicity if chronically taken many months or years. Finally, at 150 mg taken daily, there is rare, but possible, toxicity with long-term use. Thus, it is best to take no more than 50 mg a day unless under medical supervision to avoid the potential for toxicity. Chronic large doses may also cause photosensitivity. Pregnant women who take megadoses may create dependence in the newborn, who would be at risk for seizures. Nursing infants can also suffer adverse effects from large doses ingested in breast milk.

Side effects

High doses of pyridoxine may cause a rash in addition to the more serious complications listed under precautions.

Interactions

Optimal levels of **riboflavin**, **vitamin C**, magnesium, and **selenium** improve pyridoxine absorption. The effectiveness of levodopa is reduced by pyridoxine. Anyone taking levodopa, most commonly used to treat **Parkinson's disease**, should not take supplemental vitamin B$_6$. Other combination forms of medication for Parkinson's disease may not be affected. Phenytoin and phenobarbital, two medications sometimes used to

---

KEY TERMS

Chemotherapeutic agent—A medication used to treat disease, usually cancer.

Homocysteine—An amino acid produced from the metabolism of other amino acids. High levels are an independent risk factor for heart disease.

Neurotransmitter—One of a group of chemicals used by the nervous system to transmit messages between two neurons (nerve cells).

Serotonin—A neurotransmitter in the brain that helps to regulate moods, emotions, sleep, and appetite.

Vegan—A person who does not eat any animal products, including dairy and eggs.

---

control epilepsy, may also become less effective in the presence of extra vitamin B$_6$. Pyridoxine requirements are increased by the medications hydralazine, penicillamine, isoniazid, and some immunosuppressive agents. Both theophylline and estrogen containing medications, including birth control pills, block the metabolism of pyridoxine.

Resources

PERIODICALS

Cherniack, E. Paul. "The Use of Alternative Medicine for the Treatment of Insomnia in the Elderly." *Psychogeriatrics* (March 2006): 21–30.

"Folic Acid, Pyridoxine [vitamin B6] and Cyanocobalamin [vitamin B12] Improve Symptoms in Patients with Schizophrenia" *Inpharma* (September 2, 2006): 16.

Ozyurek, H., et al. "Pyridoxine and Pyridostigmine Treatment in Vincristine-induced Neuropathy." *Pediatric Hematology and Oncology* (September 2007): 447–452.

Sun, Y., et al. "Efficacy of Multivitamin Supplementation Containing Vitamins B6 and B12 and Folic Acid as Adjunctive Treatment with a Cholinesterase Inhibitor in Alzheimer's Disease: A 26-week, Randomized, Double-blind, Placebo-controlled Study in Taiwanese Patients." *Clinical Therapy* (October 2007): 2204–2214.

Yazdanpanah, N., et al. "Effect of Dietary B Vitamins on BMD and Risk of Fracture in Elderly Men and Women: The Rotterdam Study." *Bone* (December 2007): 987–994.

Judith Turner
Rebecca J. Frey, PhD
David Edward Newton, Ed.D.

Q

Qigong

Definition

Qigong (pronounced "chee-gung," also spelled *chi kung*) is translated from the Chinese to mean "energy cultivation" or "working with the life energy." Qigong is an ancient Chinese system of postures, exercises, breathing techniques, and meditations. Its techniques are designed to improve and enhance the body's *qi*. According to traditional Chinese philosophy, qi is the fundamental life energy responsible for health and vitality.

Origins

Qigong originated before recorded history. Scholars estimate qigong to be as old as 5,000–7,000 years. Tracing the exact historical development of qigong is difficult, because it was passed down in secrecy among monks and teachers for many generations. Qigong survived through many years before paper was invented, and it also survived the Cultural Revolutions in China of the 1960s and 1970s, which banned many traditional practices.

Qigong has influenced and been influenced by many of the major strands of Chinese philosophy. The Taoist philosophy states that the universe operates within laws of balance and harmony, and that people must live within the rhythms of nature—ideas that pervade qigong. When Buddhism was brought from India to China around the seventh century A.D., **yoga** techniques and concepts of mental and spiritual awareness were introduced to qigong masters. The Confucian school was concerned with how people should live their daily lives, a concern of qigong as well. The **martial arts** were highly influenced by qigong, and many of them, such as **t'ai chi** and kung fu, developed directly from it. **Traditional Chinese medicine** also shares many of the central concepts of qigong, such as the patterns of energy flow in the body. **Acupuncture** and **acupressure** use the same points on the body that qigong seeks to stimulate. In China, qigong masters have been renowned physicians and healers. Qigong is often prescribed by Chinese physicians as part of the treatment.

Due to the political isolation of China, many Chinese concepts have been shrouded from the Western world. Acupuncture was only "discovered" by American doctors in the 1970s, although it had been in use for thousands of years. With an increased exchange of information, more Americans have gained access to the once-secret teachings of qigong. In 1988, the First World Conference for Academic Exchange of Medical Qigong was held in Beijing, China, where many studies were presented to attendees from around the world. In 1990, Berkeley, California hosted the First International Congress of Qigong. In the past decade, more Americans have begun to discover the beneficial effects of qigong, which motivate an estimated 60 million Chinese to practice it every day.

Benefits

Qigong may be used as a daily routine to increase overall health and well-being, as well as for disease prevention and longevity. It can be used to increase energy and reduce **stress**. In China, qigong is used in conjunction with other medical therapies for many chronic conditions, including **asthma**, **allergies**, **AIDS**, **cancer**, headaches, **hypertension**, **depression**, mental illness, strokes, **heart disease**, and **obesity**.

Qigong is presently being used in Hong Kong to relieve depression and improve the overall psychological and social well-being of elderly people with chronic physical illnesses.

Description

Basic concepts

In Chinese thought, qi, or chi, is the fundamental life energy of the universe. It is invisible but present in

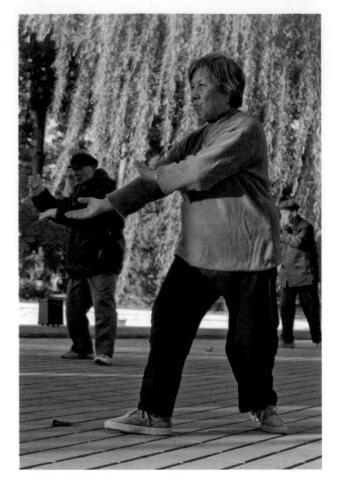

Beijing, woman in Ritan park using Qigong breathing exercise. *(© diyiming / Alamy)*

the meridians, and to increase the overall quantity and volume of qi. In qigong philosophy, mind and body are not separated as they often are in Western medicine. In qigong, the mind is present in all parts of the body, and the mind can be used to move qi throughout the body.

Yin and yang are also important concepts in qigong. The universe and the body can be described by these two separate but complementary principles, which are always interacting, opposing, and influencing each other. One goal of qigong is to balance yin and yang within the body. Strong movements or techniques are balanced by soft ones, leftward movements by rightward, internal techniques by external ones, and so on.

Practicing qigong

There are thousands of qigong exercises. The specific ones used may vary depending on the teacher, school, and objective of the practitioner. Qigong is used for physical fitness, as a martial art, and most frequently for health and healing. Internal qigong is performed by those wishing to increase their own energy and health. Some qigong masters are renowned for being able to perform external qigong, by which the energy from one person is passed on to another for healing. This transfer may sound suspect to Western logic, but in the world of qigong there are some amazing accounts of healing and extraordinary capabilities demonstrated by qigong masters. Qigong masters generally have deep knowledge of the concepts of Chinese medicine and healing. In China, there are hospitals that use medical qigong to heal patients, along with herbs, acupuncture, and other techniques. In these hospitals, qigong healers use external qigong and also design specific internal qigong exercises for patients' problems.

the air, water, food, and sunlight. In the body, qi is the unseen vital force that sustains life. We are all born with inherited amounts of qi, and we also get acquired qi from the food we eat and the air we breathe. In qigong, the breath is believed to account for the largest quantity of acquired qi, because the body uses air more than any other substance. The balance of our physical, mental, and emotional levels also affect qi levels in the body.

Qi travels through the body along channels called meridians. There are 12 main meridians, corresponding to the 12 principal organs as defined by the traditional Chinese system: the lung, large intestines, stomach, spleen, heart, small intestine, urinary bladder, kidney, liver, gallbladder, pericardium, and the "triple warmer," which represents the entire torso region. Each organ has qi associated with it, and each organ interacts with particular emotions on the mental level. Qigong techniques are designed to improve the balance and flow of energy throughout

There are basic components of internal qigong sessions. All sessions require warm-up and concluding exercises. Qigong consists of postures, movements, breathing techniques, and mental exercises. Postures may involve standing, sitting, or lying down. Movements include stretches, slow motions, quick thrusts, jumping, and bending. Postures and movements are designed to strengthen, stretch, and tone the body to improve the flow of energy. One sequence of postures and movements is known as the "Eight Figures for Every Day." This sequence is designed to quickly and effectively work the entire body, and is commonly performed daily by millions in China.

Breathing techniques include deep abdominal breathing, chest breathing, relaxed breathing, and holding breaths. One breathing technique is called the "Six Healing Sounds." This technique uses particular breathing sounds for each of six major organs. These sounds are believed to stimulate and heal the organs.

Meditations and mind exercises are used to enhance the mind and move qi throughout the body. These exercises are often visualizations that focus on different body parts, words, ideas, objects, or energy flowing along the meridians. One mental **exercise** is called the "Inner Smile," during which the practitioner visualizes joyful, healing energy being sent sequentially to each organ in the body. Another mental exercise is called the "Microscopic Orbit Meditation," in which the practitioner intently meditates on increasing and connecting the flow of qi throughout major channels.

Discipline is an important dimension of qigong. Exercises are meant to be performed every morning and evening. Sessions can take from 15 minutes to hours. Beginners are recommended to practice between 15–30 minutes twice a day. Beginners may take classes once or twice per week, with practice outside of class. Classes generally cost between $10–$20 per session.

Preparations

Qigong should be practiced in a clean, pleasant environment, preferably outdoors in fresh air. Loose and comfortable clothing is recommended. Jewelry should be removed. Practitioners can prepare for success at qigong by practicing at regular hours each day to promote discipline. Qigong teachers also recommend that students prepare by adopting lifestyles that promote balance, moderation, proper rest, and healthy **diets**, all of which are facets of qigong practice.

Precautions

Beginners should learn from an experienced teacher, as performing qigong exercises in the wrong manner may cause harm. Practitioners should not perform qigong on either full or completely empty stomachs. Qigong should not be performed during extreme weather, which may have negative effects on the body's energy systems. Menstruating and pregnant women should perform only certain exercises.

Side effects

Side effects may occur during or after qigong exercises for beginners, or for those performing exercises incorrectly. Side effects may include **dizziness**, **dry mouth**, **fatigue**, headaches, **insomnia**, rapid heartbeat, shortness of breath, heaviness or numbness in areas of the body, emotional instability, **anxiety**, or decreased concentration. Side effects generally clear up with rest and instruction from a knowledgeable teacher.

Research and general acceptance

Western medicine generally does not endorse any of the traditional Chinese healing systems that utilize the concept of energy flow in the body, largely because this energy has yet to be isolated and measured scientifically. New research is being conducted using sophisticated equipment that may verify the existence of energy channels as defined by the Chinese system. Despite the lack of scientific validation, the results of energy techniques including qigong and acupuncture have gained widespread interest and respect. One California group of qigong practitioners now conducts twice-yearly retreats to improve their skills and energy level. Furthermore, qigong masters have demonstrated to Western observers astounding control over many physical functions, and some have even shown the ability to increase electrical voltage measured on their skin's surface. Most of the research and documentation of qigong's effectiveness for medical conditions has been conducted in China, and is slowly becoming more available to English readers. Papers from the World Conferences for Academic Exchange of Medical Qigong are available in English, and address many medical studies and uses of qigong. A video is now available that presents the basic concepts of medical qigong as well as specific exercise prescriptions for the treatment of **breast cancer**. The exercise prescriptions consist of movements, postures, visualizations, and positive affirmations.

In terms of mainstream research in the United States, the first ongoing long-term study of qigong began in 1999 at the Center for Alternative and Complementary Medicine Research in Heart Disease at the University of Michigan; it focuses on the speed of healing of graft **wounds** in patients undergoing coronary bypass surgery. The National Center for Complementary and Alternative Medicine (NCCAM) has been funding studies of qigong since 2000. The first such study was conducted by a researcher in Arizona with patients using heart devices (pacemakers, etc.).

The breathing techniques of qigong are being studied intensively by Western physicians as of 2003 as a form of therapy for anxiety-related problems and for disorders involving the vocal cords. Qigong is also being used in the rehabilitation of patients with severe asthma or chronic obstructive pulmonary disease (COPD).

Training and certification

In China, qigong has been subject to much government regulation, from banning to increased requirements for teachers. In the United States at this time, qigong has not been regulated. Different schools may provide teacher training, but there are no generally accepted training standards. Qigong teachings may vary, depending on the founder of the school, who is often an acknowledged Chinese master. The organizations listed below can provide further information to consumers.

Resources

BOOKS

Lui, Dr. Hong, and Paul Perry. *Mastering Miracles: The Healing Art of Qi Gong as Taught by a Master.* New York: Warner Books, 1997.

MacRichie, Mames. *Chi Kung: Cultivating Personal Energy.* Boston: Element, 1993.

Pelletier, Kenneth R., MD. *The Best Alternative Medicine*, Part I: Sound Mind, Sound Body: Qi Gong. New York: Simon & Schuster, 2002.

Reid, Daniel. *A Complete Guide to Chi Gung.* Boston: Shambhala, 1998.

PERIODICALS

Baker, S. E.,C. M. Sapienza, and S. Collins. "Inspiratory Pressure Threshold Training in a Case of Congenital Bilateral Abductor Vocal Fold Paralysis." *International Journal of Pediatric Otorhinolaryngology* 67 (April 2003): 413–416.

Biggs, Q. M., K. S. Kelly, and J. D. Toney. "The Effects of Deep Diaphragmatic Breathing and Focused Attention on Dental Anxiety in a Private Practice Setting." *Dental Hygiene* 77 (Spring 2003): 105–113.

Emerich, K. A. "Nontraditional Tools Helpful in the Treatment of Certain Types of Voice Disturbances." *Current Opinion in Otolaryngology and Head and Neck Surgery* 11 (June 2003): 149–153.

Golden, Jane. "Qigong and Tai Chi as Energy Medicine." *Share Guide* (November-December 2001): 37.

Johnson, Jerry Alan. "Medical Qigong for Breast Disease." *Share Guide* (November-December 2001): 109.

Ram, F. S., E. A. Holloway, and P. W. Jones. "Breathing Retraining for Asthma." *Respiratory Medicine* 97 (May 2003): 501–507.

Tsang, H. W., C. K. Mok, Y. T. Au Yeung, and S. Y. Chan. "The Effect of Qigong on General and Psychosocial Health of Elderly with Chronic Physical Illnesses: A Randomized Clinical Trial." *International Journal of Geriatric Psychiatry* 18 (May 2003): 441–449.

ORGANIZATIONS

International Chi Kung/Qi Gong Directory. 2730 29th Street. Boulder, CO 80301. (303) 442-3131.

National Center for Complementary and Alternative Medicine (NCCAM) Clearinghouse. P.O. Box 7923, Gaithersburg, MD 20898-7923. (888) 644-6226. http://nccam.nih.gov.

Qi: The Journal of Traditional Eastern Health and Fitness. PO Box 221343. Chantilly, VA 22022. (202) 378 3859.

Qigong Human Life Research Foundation. PO Box 5327. Cleveland, OH 44101. (216) 475-4712.

Qigong Magazine. PO Box 31578. San Francisco, CA 94131. (800) 824-2433.

Douglas Dupler
Rebecca J. Frey, PhD

Quan yin

Definition

Quan yin is the English transliteration of the Chinese name for a Buddhist divine figure whose Sanskrit name is Avalokitesvara. The meaning of this name is usually given as "the lord who hears and sees all," or "the lord who is seen within [the believer's soul]." The Chinese name Quan yin is sometimes translated as "the one who hears prayers." Quan yin is also known in China as Guanshiyin; in Japan as Kannon, Kanzeon, or Kwannon; in southeastern Asia as Quon Am; in Bali as Kanin; and in Tibet as Chen-resigs or Spyan-ras-gzigs. Although some English-language sources refer to Quan yin as a "goddess" or "saint," these terms are somewhat misleading because of their association with Western religions. Peter Matthiessen's phrase, "mythical embodiment of Buddhahood," or bodhisattva, is a more accurate description. A bodhisattva is a spirit or person who has earned the right, through renunciation of passions and cravings, to escape from the cycle of reincarnation and enter nirvana, but chooses to postpone their own bliss until they have helped others to achieve enlightenment.

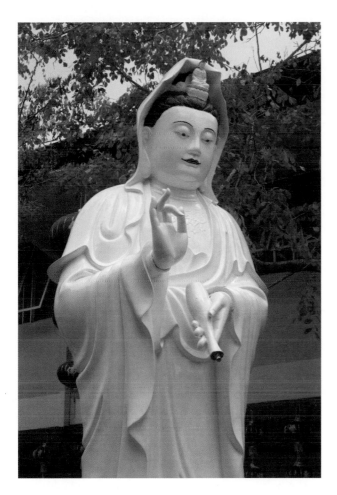

Devotion to Quan yin as the bodhisattva of infinite mercy and compassion is widespread in the Buddhist world, and can be dated as far back as the first centuries of the Christian era.
(Beaconstox / Alamy)

Origins

Devotion to Quan yin as the bodhisattva of infinite mercy and compassion is widespread in the Buddhist world, and can be dated as far back as the first centuries of the Christian era. It is important to note, however, that the notion of deity in Buddhism is quite different from Jewish and Christian concepts of God as creator and ruler of the universe. In classical Buddhist teachings, there are three forms or bodies of Buddhahood: the body of essence (Buddha as disembodied and impersonal absolute truth or reality; nirvana); the body of bliss (Buddha as a formless spirit with the power to save humans); and the body of emanation or transformation (Buddha assuming a human form to guide people to enlightenment). Avalokitesvara (Quan yin) is regarded as the embodiment of Buddha who guards the world between the appearance of Sakyamuni, the historical Siddhartha

Gautama (born in India about 500 B.C.), and Maitreya, the Buddha of the future.

Avalokitesvara was originally portrayed as a male among Indian Buddhists, because a female bodhisattva is impossible according to the oldest Buddhist texts. Devotion to Avalokitesvara in the form of Quan yin was introduced into China as early as the first century A.D., and into Japan in the sixth or seventh century. Prior to the twelfth century A.D., Quan yin was always portrayed as a male in Chinese and Japanese art. The reason for later artistic representations of her as a female is not completely understood. Some scholars attribute the change to the popularity of a passage in the Lotus Sutra that speaks of Avalokitesvara as having the power to grant children to childless women, and to assume a human body of either sex in order to guide others to nirvana. By the eighth century, the Lotus Sutra was honored in China and Japan above all other Buddhist sacred texts because it was understood to mean that women could also attain enlightenment.

Other scholars think that a Chinese legend about Quan yin may have also played a part in popular devotion to this bodhisattva as a woman. According to the legend, Quan yin was born into this world as the daughter of a king of the Chou Dynasty (1050–256 B.C.), who was sentenced to death by her father for refusing to marry. When the executioner tried to behead her, his sword shattered before he could touch her. The legend helps to explain why Quan yin has been regarded in some parts of Asia as a protector of women who offers life as a Buddhist nun as an alternative to marriage. In Japan, the princess Chujo-Hime (753–781 A.D.), who was persecuted by her stepmother and became a Buddhist nun at the age of seventeen, was thought to be a living incarnation of Kannon. A memorial service is held each year in Japan on May 14 for Chujo-Hime at the Tokushoji Temple.

In Japan, the Pure Land sect of Buddhism honored Kannon or Kanzeon as one of the principal attendants of Amida, the Buddha of the Western Paradise. Japanese religious art often portrays the so-called Amida Raigo triad, which depicts Amida himself; Kannon, who represents the Buddha's mercy; and the Seishi Bosatsu, a bodhisattva who represents the Buddha's strength and power. The three are often shown as descending on a cloud at the moment of a Buddhist's death to lead him or her to the Western Paradise.

Popular modern Buddhist art portrays Quan yin as a barefoot woman dressed in a long flowing white

KEY TERMS

Avalokitesvara—The Sanskrit name of Quan yin.

Bodhisattva—A Buddhist holy person who has attained enlightenment, but postpones nirvana in order to help others become enlightened.

Lotus sutra—One of the most sacred texts of Buddhism, regarded as a summary of the supreme Buddhist teaching that leads one directly to enlightenment.

Nirvana—In Buddhism, release from the cycle of reincarnation through conquering one's hatreds, passions, and delusions.

robe, often pouring a stream of water from a small vase. The water represents peace and healing. She may also be shown holding a lotus, which represents purity; pearls, which symbolize illumination; or a bowl of rice seed, which represents fertility. Some statues also show her with several pairs of arms, each holding a different cosmic symbol, which symbolize the universal embrace of Buddha's compassion. She is also depicted standing on a fish, which represents her role as the special protector of fishermen and travelers.

Benefits

The benefits of devotion to Quan yin, like those of Western religious practice, include inner peace, a feeling of love leading to acts of compassion for others, and a stronger sense that one's existence has meaning. According to the National Center for Complementary and Alternative Medicine (NCCAM), religious and spiritual practices that emphasize positive beliefs and attitudes help the human immune system, lower the impact of emotional **stress** on the body, and lower the risk of developing **anxiety** disorders and **depression**.

According to a Buddhist nun who claims to have been taught the Quan Yin Method for attaining enlightenment by a Himalayan master, those who practice this method will "gain a happy and more relaxed life, liberate [themselves from the cycle of reincarnation], and save five generations of [their] family."

Description

Devotion to Quan yin or Kannon is fairly informal in most parts of eastern Asia. Devotees may meditate on the bodhisattva's qualities of mercy and compassion, and strive to put these qualities into

action through service or acts of kindness toward others. In China, women sometimes offer small pieces of jade carved with images on Quan yin in her temples, or place them in domestic shrines. Other Buddhists may wear amulets with images of Quan yin or prayers of devotion. Peter Matthiessen tells of wearing an amulet made from a plum pit that was given to him by his Japanese spiritual teacher. The plum pit was inscribed with a ten-phrase **prayer** to Kanzeon in tiny Japanese characters. Some phrases from the prayer include: "Kanzeon! Devotion to Buddha! We are one with Buddha .... Our true Bodhisattva nature is eternal, joyful, selfless, pure. So let us chant each morning Kanzeon, with mindfulness! Every evening Kanzeon, with mindfulness!"

Some devotees go on pilgrimages to holy places associated with Quan yin. These include the mountainous island of Pu Tuo Shan off the coast of Shanghai, China, where Quan yin is said to have lived for nine years. At one time there were over a hundred shrines to Quan yin on the island, as well as a community of a thousand Buddhist monks. Japanese Buddhists may make the Bando Pilgrimage, which makes a circuit of 33 sites in eastern Japan sacred to Kannon. Visiting the shrines in the proper order is said to preserve the believer from hell and open the gate to the Western Paradise.

The Quan Yin Method for attaining nirvana requires 2-1/2 hours of **meditation** per day in addition to the following five precepts:

- Refraining from taking the life of any sentient beings. This precept requires strict adherence to a vegan or lactovegetarian diet.
- Refraining from speaking what is not true.
- Refraining from taking what is not offered.
- Refraining from sexual misconduct.
- Refraining from the use of intoxicants, which include gambling, pornography, and violent films or literature as well as alcohol, tobacco, and recreational drugs.

Preparations and precautions

There are no specific preparations necessary for devotion to Quan yin. Western readers, however, should obtain information about this bodhisattva from reliable histories of Buddhism or Asian religion rather than from popular New Age sources.

Research and general acceptance

No studies have been done as of 2004 comparing devotion to Quan yin to other forms of religious or spiritual practice. In the West, devotion to Quan yin is more common among women who have left mainstream Jewish or Christian groups than it is among men. Some of these women identify Quan yin with such mother goddesses as Isis or with such Christian saints as the Virgin Mary. Scholars of religion, however, regard these comparisons as misleading and historically inaccurate.

Training and certification

Although there are Buddhist monasteries and study centers in the United States, they do not offer certification for teachers comparable to ordination for Christian or Jewish clergy. Readers who are interested in learning more about Quan yin or Buddhism in general may contact the monastery listed under Resources below.

Resources

BOOKS

Matthiessen, Peter. *The Snow Leopard*. New York: Penguin Books, 1987.

Pelletier, Kenneth, M.D. *The Best Alternative Medicine*, Chapter 11, "Spirituality and Healing." New York: Simon & Schuster, 2002.

Stanley-Baker, Joan. *Japanese Art*. New York: Thames and Hudson, 1992.

Svoboda, Robert, and Arnie Lane. *Tao and Dharma*. Twin Lakes, WI: Lotus Press, 1995.

PERIODICALS

Hinohara, S. "Medicine and Religion: Spiritual Dimension of Health Care." *Humane Health Care* 1 (July-December 2001): E2.

ORGANIZATIONS

Buddhist Association of the United States (BAUS). 1384 Broadway, 19th Floor, New York, NY 10018. (212) 398-8886. http://www.baus.org.

Chuang Yen Monastery. 2020, Route 301, Carmel, NY 10512. (845) 225-1819 or (845) 228-4288.

National Center for Complementary and Alternative Medicine (NCCAM). National Institutes of Health (NIH), Bethesda, MD 20892. http://nccam.nih.gov.

Supreme Master Ching Hai International Association. P. O. Box 730247, San Jose, CA 95173-0247. http://www. godsdirectcontact.org.

OTHER

Glassman, Hank. "Chujo-Hime, Convents, and Women's Salvation." Lecture delivered at the International Symposium on Buddhist Convents, Columbia University, New York City, NY, 22 November 1998.

Rebecca Frey

Quercetin

Description

Quercetin is a widespread plant chemical, or phytochemical. Many food items contain quercetin. These include **garlic** and onions; broccoli, cauliflower, brussels sprouts, cabbage, and other brassica vegetables; leafy, green vegetables; apples, berries, and many other fruits; green and black tea; and red wine. This plant chemical is also found in commonly used medicinal herbal supplements such as St. John's wort (*Hypericum perforatum*) and *Ginkgo biloba*.

Quercetin is a particular type of phytochemical known as a flavonoid or bioflavonoid; more specifically, it is a member of a certain class of flavonoids called flavonols. Quercetin appears to have significant anti-inflammatory and antioxidant properties. **Antioxidants** act on free radicals, which are highly reactive molecules that initiate damaging chain reactions in the body. The body produces its own antioxidants that counter free radicals, but free radicals can still build up as a result of **stress**, age, pollution, cigarette smoke, or other causes. It is believed that the antioxidants found in fresh fruits and vegetables, sometimes by way of quercetin, may provide a protective effect. Practitioners of traditional medicine have long espoused the use of quercetin-containing plants to treat numerous medical conditions, including arthritis, **allergies**, **heart disease**, **cataracts**, cold sores, and **gout**, among others. Some practitioners also recommend quercetin supplements to treat **cancer**.

General use

For centuries, practitioners of traditional medicine in many different cultures have prescribed the intake of quercetin-containing plants to treat various illnesses. It was not until the 1930s, however, that Hungarian physiologist Albert Szent-Györgyi (1893–1986) first isolated flavonoids. His work introduced the scientific community to these phytochemicals.

At one point, scientists were concerned about quercetin because research had shown that it caused mutations in the DNA within bacteria and suggested that it might have a role in causing cancer in humans. Those concerns were allayed by subsequent studies in humans, as well as some in animals, that indicated quercetin instead may actually have a protective effect against cancer.

Cell-culture studies have indicated that quercetin both slows the growth of and encourages the programmed cell death (called apoptosis) of cancer cells.

The latter is especially important because cancer cells often do not undergo the programmed cell death that occurs in normal cells. In the late 2000s, the American Cancer Society, however, remained cautious with regard to quercetin because many of the studies of it had been performed on cell cultures or animals.

In addition to the cell-culture research, animal studies have also shown that quercetin may be effective in protecting against various cancers. In 2007, for instance, a research team published results from a small clinical trial that looked at quercetin's effects against colon cancer. Their results indicated that a combined treatment of quercetin and **curcumin**, a compound in curry, also worked against colon cancer in humans. In the study, published in *Clinical Gastroenterology & Hepatology*, the researchers provided the quercetin-containing supplement to five individuals who had a rare genetic condition, called familial adenomatous polyposis, which causes precancerous polyps to grow in their intestines and eventually leads to colon cancer. Over the course of the experiment, the researchers measured a 60% reduction in the number of polyps and a 50% decrease in the polyps' size. Another much larger study published in a 2006 issue of the *American Journal of Epidemiology*, however, showed no correlation between higher intakes of quercetin and other flavonols and a lower risk for colon cancer. This study reviewed self-reported dietary information as well as cancer incidence among 107,401 individuals. The researchers concluded that their results provided "little support for the hypothesis of an association between flavonoid intake and **colorectal cancer** risk, at least within the ranges of intakes consumed in the populations studied."

Another large cancer-related study published in a 2007 issue of the *American Journal of Epidemiology* indicated that quercetin seemed to have a preventive effect on pancreatic cancer, especially among smokers. This study's researchers estimated the intake of quercetin along with two other flavonols from self-reported dietary information collected from 183,518 individuals and then followed the participants for eight years to determine the incidence of pancreatic cancer. The researchers found that all three flavonols—the other two were kaempferol and myricetin—were associated with a significantly reduced risk of pancreatic cancer among current smokers, who have a comparatively high propensity for the disease.

Like the prostate-cancer study, many other studies have focused on fruit- and vegetable-rich **diets**, but not exclusively on quercetin. While such diets may be high in quercetin, the fact that they also contain many additional compounds makes it difficult for scientists to pinpoint the specific effects of quercetin.

The effects of quercetin on the cardiovascular system have also been studied. Animal studies have shown that quercetin prevents **hypertension** and cardiac hypertrophy (thickening of the heart muscle) in rats. In addition, numerous epidemiological studies point to a connection between quercetin and the prevention of **stroke** and cardiovascular disease, and a study in the November 2007 issue of the *Journal of Nutrition* reported that quercetin was able to reduce blood pressure in people who had hypertension.

Practitioners of traditional medicine may prescribe quercetin for various ailments, including **hay fever** and other allergies. It is thought that quercetin may reduce the amount of histamines that the body produces and releases in response to allergens, and this in turn may lessen the severity of allergy-related symptoms such as runny nose, watery eyes, and **hives**. This suspicion has also led to its use in treating insect **bites**. Quercetin is sometimes prescribed to treat arthritis, which is an inflammation of the joints, and to prevent **atherosclerosis** (sometimes called hardening of the arteries). It is also used treat or prevent cataracts and **macular degeneration**, which are thought to perhaps be related to the action of free radicals. Quercetin is also believed to lessen the burning **pain** associated with chronic prostatitis, which is an inflammation of the prostate, and to treat ulcers. Some users of quercetin assert that it helps **wounds** heal more quickly. In addition, practitioners may prescribe quercetin to help lower **cholesterol** levels, although research supporting this effect was lacking as of 2008.

Quercetin has potential implications in treatments for pain. According to a study in a 2003 issue of *Drug Development Research*, quercetin may alleviate some of the adverse effects that often occur with the use of morphine and other opioid drugs to treat moderate to severe pain. These adverse effects include drug tolerance, in which the effectiveness of the dose lessens over time, and drug dependence. The study, done on mice, showed that quercetin reversed the development of both morphine tolerance and dependence.

Various studies have shown that quercetin has antiviral properties. A study in a 2003 issue of the *Journal of Antimicrobial Chemotherapy*, for instance, reported that quercetin is a potential treatment for infection with the herpesvirus known as HSV-1. Indeed, some people use quercetin to treat cold sores, which are caused by HSV-1. The study also showed that quercetin counteracted a type of adenovirus. Adenoviruses infect numerous membranes in the body and are common causes of respiratory **infections**.

KEY TERMS

Bromelain—One or more enzymes found in pineapples and sometimes added to supplements to boost their effectiveness.

Flavonoids—Naturally occurring chemicals found in many fruits and vegetables that have potential beneficial effects on human health.

Phytochemicals—Plant chemicals.

Preparations

To help prevent cancer, the American Cancer Society recommends a daily diet that contains five or more servings of fruits and vegetables, but it does not have specific recommendations for any specific compound, including quercetin, that is contained within those fruits and vegetables.

Besides ingesting quercetin in foods, quercetin supplements are available in many health food stores as a powder and in capsule form. Quercetin supplements are sometimes combined with **bromelain**, which is an enzyme found in pineapple. This enzyme is thought to have anti-inflammatory properties, to fight allergies, and to heighten the activity of quercetin. Recommended dosages of quercetin can vary from 200–750 mg per day, often taken in several doses. Practitioners may also recommend that an individual increase his or her intake of the compound by taking various quercetin-containing extracts, such as *Ginkgo biloba*, or by consuming **green tea**, which is also high in quercetin.

Precautions

Major problems were unknown as of 2008, although some individuals may experience **nausea** from high doses of quercetin supplements.

Interactions

Persons taking quercetin supplements, particularly those containing bromelain, should consult their physician if they are taking other medications because possible drug interactions can occur. In addition, individuals who are undergoing chemotherapy should discuss this supplement with their doctors before taking it.

Resources

BOOKS

Mars, Brigitte. *The Desktop Guide to Herbal Medicine: The Ultimate Multidisciplinary Reference to the Amazing Realm of Healing Plants, in a Quick-study, One-stop Guide*. Laguna Beach, CA: Basic Health, 2007.

PERIODICALS

Cruz-Correa M., Daniel A. Shoskes, Patricia Sanchez, Rhongua Zhao, Linda Hylind, Steven Wexner, et al. "Combination Treatment with Curcumin and Quercetin of Adenomas in Familial Adenomatous Polyposis." *Clinical Gastroenterology & Hepatology* 4 (August 2006): 1035–1038.

Edwards, Randi L., Tiffany Lyon, Sheldon E. Litwin, Alexander Rabovsky, J. David Symons, and Thunder Jalili. "Quercetin Reduces Blood Pressure in Hypertensive Subjects." *Journal of Nutrition* 137 (November 2007): 2405–2411.

Lin, Jennifer, and Shumin M. Zhang. "Flavonoid Intake and Colorectal Cancer Risk in Men and Women." *American Journal of Epidemiology* 164, no. 7 (October 1, 2006): 644–651.

Nöthlings, Ute, Suzanne P. Murphy, Lynne R. Wilkens, Brian E. Henderson, Laurence N. Kolonel. "Flavonols and Pancreatic Cancer Risk: The Multiethnic Cohort Study." *American Journal of Epidemiology* 166, no. 8. (October 15, 2007): 924–931.

Leslie Mertz, Ph.D.

R

Rabies

Definition

Rabies is a viral illness that can affect any mammal but is most common in carnivores (flesh-eaters). It is sometimes referred to as a zoonosis, or disease of animals that can be communicated to humans. Rabies is usually transmitted in the saliva through a bite wound. The virus attacks the central nervous system, and is fatal once symptoms begin, with very rare exceptions.

Description

Rabies, also known as hydrophobia, belongs to the rhabdovirus family. Fewer than 10% of animal cases reported in the United States in 1998 were in domestic animals. Raccoons accounted for the largest number of cases in wild animals. Cases of rabies in humans are very infrequent in the United States, averaging one or two a year (down from over 100 cases annually in 1900), but the worldwide incidence is estimated to be between 30,000 and 50,000 cases each year. These figures are based on data collected by the World Health Organization (WHO) in 1997 and updated in 2002. Rabies is most common in developing countries in Africa, Latin America, and Asia, particularly India. Dog **bites** are the major origin of infection for humans in developing countries, but other important host animals may include the wolf, mongoose, and bat. Most deaths from rabies in the United States result from bat bites; the most recent victim was a man in Iowa who died in September 2002.

People whose work frequently brings them in contact with animals are considered to be at higher risk than the general population. This would include those in the fields of veterinary medicine, animal control, wildlife work, and laboratory work involving live rabies virus. People in these occupations and residents of or travelers to areas where rabies is a widespread problem should consider being immunized.

In late 2002, rabies re-emerged as an important public health issue. Dr. Charles E. Rupprecht, director of the World Health Organization (WHO) Collaborating Center for Rabies Reference and Research, has listed several factors responsible for the increase in the number of rabies cases worldwide:

- Rapid evolution of the rabies virus. Bats in the United States have developed a particularly infectious form of the virus.
- Increased diversity of animal hosts for the disease.
- Changes in the environment that are bringing people and domestic pets into closer contact with infected wildlife.
- Increased movement of people and animals across international borders. In one recent case, a man who had contracted rabies in the Philippines was not diagnosed until he began to feel ill in the United Kingdom.
- Lack of advocacy about rabies.

Causes and symptoms

The most common way to contract rabies is from the bite of an infected animal. Although bats are the most frequent source of human infection in the United States, dogs are the primary vector of rabies in most parts of the world. The disease may also be transmitted by tissues and body fluids other than saliva. Rare cases have occurred as a result of infection through corneal transplantation.

Rabies travels from the site of the bite along the peripheral nerves to the brain. The average incubation period in humans is 30–50 days, although it varies from 10 days to over a year. The initial symptoms are flu-like and nonspecific. They may include **fever, headache,** muscle **pain, sore throat, fatigue, nausea,** and **vomiting.** Altered sensation and muscle twitching in the area of the bite are signs that are more suspicious of rabies. When the virus reaches the brain, signs related to encephalitis (local or general inflammation of brain tissue)

KEY TERMS

Biopsy—The removal of a small sample of tissue for diagnostic purposes.

Direct fluorescent antibody test (dFA test)—A test in which a fluorescent dye is linked to an antibody for diagnostic purposes.

Encephalitis—Inflammation of the brain.

Rhabdovirus—A type of virus named for its rod- or bullet-like shape.

Vector—An animal or insect that carries a disease-producing organism.

Zoonosis (plural, zoonoses)—Any disease of animals that can be transmitted to humans. Rabies is an example of a zoonosis.

appear. This typically involves agitation, progressing to confusion, combativeness, seizures, and localized areas of paralysis. There may also be hypersensitivity to light, sound, and touch. The patient may be coherent at times, but less so as the disease progresses. Many viruses causing encephalitis may produce similar signs. The next stage is dysfunction of the brainstem. The well-known phenomenon of foaming at the mouth is caused by excessive saliva production combined with difficulty swallowing. Many patients will refuse liquids at this point due to the painful muscle contractions caused by swallowing. This is how rabies came to be known as hydrophobia, which means "fear of water." Coma ensues soon after brainstem involvement, and death occurs when the respiratory center is affected. The course of the disease is four to 20 days after symptoms appear, unless life support is used.

Diagnosis

Early in its course, and without a known history of an animal bite, rabies can be difficult to diagnose. Symptoms of the early encephalitic (brain tissue inflammation) phase are similar to those of most viral types of encephalitis. When signs of brainstem dysfunction appear shortly after this time, rabies becomes a more likely possibility. Several tests are available for rabies diagnosis, but none are extremely reliable in the living patient. Part of the challenge is that rabies is so limited to nerve tissue until the late phases of the disease. The examination of brain tissue reveals a characteristic known as a Negri body, which is diagnostic. Direct fluorescent antibody (dFA) staining of saliva, skin biopsy, and corneal impressions may also yield a diagnosis.

Treatment

Local wound cleansing is important. Anyone who has experienced an animal bite should wash it thoroughly with soap and water. Rabies is a fatal illness, so a bite that breaks the skin warrants a call to a health care provider for evaluation of whether post-exposure prophylaxis (PEP) is necessary. Alternative treatments are recommended as a complementary therapy to conventional treatment in the case of rabies. Observation of the animal for signs of rabies is recommended whenever possible.

Allopathic treatment

If a person is bitten by a domestic animal and the owner is known, vaccination status should be checked. People bitten by healthy, immunized animals are unlikely to need post-exposure prophylaxis (PEP). The animal can be confined for 10 days. If it is healthy at the end of that time, it is presumed not to have been capable of transmitting rabies at the time of the bite, so PEP for the person bitten is not necessary.

Wild animals that have bitten can be captured, destroyed, and tested for rabies. Postexposure vaccine and specific immune globulin can be given if deemed necessary. In the United States, if the person who was bitten has not had prophylactic immunization and has a high-risk bite, generally five rabies vaccinations and one injection of human rabies immune globulin are given. There have been no cases in this country of people contracting rabies after receiving correctly administered PEP.

Bites from mice, rats, or squirrels rarely require rabies prevention because these rodents are typically killed by any encounter with a larger, rabid animal, and would therefore be less likely to be carriers. Bites from raccoons, bats, or unvaccinated dogs or cats are more suspect. Anyone bitten by a bat in the United States should receive PEP unless the bat is captured and proven not to be rabid.

If a pet is bitten by an animal suspected to have rabies, its owner should contact a veterinarian immediately and notify the local animal control authorities. Domestic pets with current vaccinations should be revaccinated immediately; unvaccinated dogs, cats, or ferrets are usually euthanized (put to sleep). Further information about domestic pets and rabies is available on the American Veterinary Medical Association (AVMA) web site.

Expected results

Survival of rabies after the appearance of symptoms is exceedingly rare.

Prevention

The following precautions should be observed in environments where humans and animals may likely come into contact. Domesticated animals, including household pets, should be vaccinated against rabies. Booster shots, given according to the manufacturer's recommendations, are required to maintain immunity. Wild animals should not be touched or petted, no matter how friendly an animal may appear. It is also important not to touch an animal that appears ill or passive, or whose behavior seems odd, such as failing to show the normal fear of humans. These are all possible signs of rabies. Many animals, such as raccoons and skunks, are nocturnal and their activity during the day should be regarded as suspicious. People should not interfere with fights between animals. Because rabies is transmitted through saliva, a person should wear rubber gloves when handling a pet that has had an encounter with a wild animal. Windows and doors should be screened. Some victims of rabies have been attacked by infected animals, particularly bats, that entered through unprotected openings. Finally, garbage or pet food should not be left outside because it may attract wild or stray animals.

Members of the high-risk occupations mentioned above should consider prophylactic immunization. Those who receive this pre-exposure vaccine still require PEP in the event of a potentially infective episode, but they have several advantages. One is that they require fewer post-exposure vaccines. A second advantage is that the timing of the PEP may be less critical for people who are in remote areas, or don't have ready access to vaccine for other reasons. Last, some people may be exposed without being aware of it, and the prophylactic vaccine might protect them.

Resources

BOOKS

"Central Nervous System Viral Diseases: Rabies (Hydrophobia)." Section 13, Chapter 162 in *The Merck Manual of Diagnosis and Therapy*, edited by Mark H. Beers, MD, and Robert Berkow, MD. Whitehouse Station, NJ: Merck Research Laboratories, 1999.

Corey, Lawrence. "Rabies Virus and Other Rhabdoviruses." *Harrison's Principles of Internal Medicine*, edited by Anthony S. Fauci et al., 14th ed.; New York: McGraw-Hill, 1998.

PERIODICALS

Fooks, A. R., N. Johnson, S. M. Brookes, et al. "Risk Factors Associated with Travel to Rabies Endemic Countries." *Journal of Applied Microbiology* 94 (2003) (Supplement): 31S–36S.

"Human Rabies—Iowa, 2002." *Morbidity and Mortality Weekly Report* 52 (January 24, 2003): 47–48.

Messenger, S. L., J. S. Smith, L. A. Orciari, et al. "Emerging Pattern of Rabies Deaths and Increased Viral Infectivity." *Emerging Infectious Diseases* 9 (February 2003): 151–154.

Smith, J., L. McElhinney, G. Parsons, et al. "Case Report: Rapid Ante-Mortem Diagnosis of a Human Case of Rabies Imported Into the UK from the Philippines." *Journal of Medical Virology* 69 (January 2003): 150–155.

Stringer, C. "Post-Exposure Rabies Vaccination." *Nursing Standard* 17 (February 5-11, 2003): 41–42.

Weiss, R. A. "Cross-Species Infections." *Current Topics in Microbiology and Immunology* 278 (2003): 47–71.

ORGANIZATIONS

American Veterinary Medical Association (AVMA). 1931 North Meacham Road, Suite 100, Schaumburg, IL 60173-4360. http://www.avma.org.

Centers for Disease Control and Prevention. 1600 Clifton Rd., NE, Atlanta, GA 30333. (800) 311-3435, (404) 639-3311. http://www.cdc.gov

Institut Pasteur. 25-28, rue du Dr. Roux, 75015 Paris, France. +33 (0) 1 45 68 80 00. http://www.pasteur.fr/haut_ext.html.

OTHER

CDC. "Epidemiology of Rabies." http://www.cdc.gov/ncidod/dvrd/rabies/Epidemiology/Epidemiology.htm.

National Association of State Public Health Veterinarians, Inc. "Compendium of Animal Rabies Prevention and Control, 2003." *Morbidity and Mortality Weekly Report Recommendations and Reports* 52 (March 21, 2003) (RR-5): 1–6.

Judith Turner
Rebecca J. Frey, PhD

Radiation injuries

Definition

Radiation injuries are caused by ionizing radiation emitted by such sources as the sun, x-ray and other diagnostic machines, tanning beds, and radioactive elements released in nuclear power plant accidents and detonation of nuclear weapons during war and as terrorist acts.

Description

Ionizing radiation is made up of unstable atoms that contain an excess amount of energy. In an attempt to stabilize, the atoms emit the excess energy into the atmosphere, creating radiation. Radiation can either be electromagnetic or particulate.

Radiation sources

Natural sources

Radon gas	55%
Inside the body	11%
Rocks, soil, and groundwater	8%
Cosmic rays	8%

Artificial sources

Medical x-rays	11%
Nuclear medicine	4%
Consumer products (such as tobacco, televisions, and smoke detectors)	3%
Miscellaneous (including occupational exposure, nuclear fallout, and the production of nuclear materials for energy and weaponry)	<1%

(Illustration by Corey Light. Cengage Learning, Gale)

The energy of electromagnetic radiation is a direct function of its frequency. The high energy, high frequency waves that can penetrate solids to various depths cause damage by separating molecules into electrically charged pieces, a process known as ionization. X rays are a type of electromagnetic radiation. Atomic particles come from radioactive isotopes as they decay to stable elements. Electrons are called beta particles when they radiate. Alpha particles are the nuclei of helium atoms—two protons and two neutrons—without the surrounding electrons. Alpha particles are too large to penetrate a piece of paper unless they are greatly accelerated in electric and magnetic fields. Both beta and alpha particles are types of particulate radiation. When over-exposure to ionizing radiation occurs, there is chromosomal damage in deoxyribonucleic acid (DNA). DNA is very good at repairing itself; both strands of the double helix must be broken to produce genetic damage.

Because radiation is energy, it can be measured. There are a number of units used to quantify radiation energy. Some refer to effects on air, others to effects on living tissue. The roentgen, named after Wilhelm Conrad Roentgen, who discovered x rays in 1895, measures ionizing energy in air. A rad expresses the energy transferred to tissue. The rem measures tissue response. A

KEY TERMS

Bone marrow suppression—Decrease in production of blood components, including red blood cells, white blood cells, and platelets. This can result in anemia, increased susceptibility to infections, and excessive bleeding.

Cosmic radiation—Radiation of high penetrating power originating in outer space. It consists partly of high-energy atomic nuclei.

Dirty bomb—A bomb made with conventional explosives that also contains radioactive isotopes. When the bomb explodes, the radioactive material spreads contamination over a wide area.

DNA—Deoxyribonucleic acid. The chemical of chromosomes and hence the vehicle of heredity.

Esophagitis—Inflammation of the esophagus.

Isotope—An unstable form of an element that gives off radiation to become stable. Elements are characterized by the number of electrons around each atom. One electron's negative charge balances the positive charge of each proton in the nucleus. To keep all those positive charges in the nucleus from repelling each other (like the same poles of magnets), neutrons are added. Only certain numbers of neutrons work. Other numbers cannot hold the nucleus together, so it splits apart, giving off ionizing radiation. Sometimes one of the split products is not stable either, so another split takes place. The process is called radioactivity.

Melanoma—A highly malignant form of skin cancer associated with overexposure to ultraviolet radiation from sunlight.

Pneumonitis—Inflammation of the lungs.

roentgen generates about a rad of effect and produces about a rem of response. The gray and the sievert are international units equivalent to 100 rads and rems, respectively. A curie, named after French physicists who experimented with radiation, is a measure of actual radioactivity given off by a radioactive element, not a measure of its effect. The average annual human exposure to natural background radiation is roughly 3 milli-Sieverts (mSv).

Any amount of ionizing radiation will produce some damage; however, there is radiation everywhere, from the sun (cosmic rays) and from traces of radioactive elements in the air (radon) and the ground (uranium, radium, carbon-14, potassium-40 and many others). Earth's atmosphere protects us from most of the sun's radiation. Living at 5,000 feet altitude in Denver, Colorado, doubles exposure to radiation, and flight in a commercial airliner increases it 150-fold by lifting us above 80% of that atmosphere. Because no amount of radiation is perfectly safe and because radiation is ever present, arbitrary limits have been established to provide some measure of safety for those exposed to unusual amounts. Less than 1% of them reach the current annual permissible maximum of 20 mSv.

A 2001 ruling by the Federal Court of Australia indicated that two soldiers died from **cancer** caused by minimal exposure to radiation while occupying Hiroshima in 1945. The soldiers were exposed to less than 5 mSv of radiation. The international recommendation for workers is safety level of up to 20 mSv. The ruling and its support by many international agencies suggests that even extremely low doses of radiation can be potentially harmful.

Ultraviolet (UV) radiation exposure from the sun and tanning beds

UV radiation from the sun and tanning beds and lamps can cause skin damage, premature **aging**, and skin cancers. Malignant melanoma is the most dangerous of skin cancers and there is a definite link between type UVA exposure used in tanning beds and its occurrence. UVB type UV radiation is associated with **sunburn**, and while not as penetrating as UVA, it still damages the skin with over exposure. Skin damage accumulates over time, and effects do not often manifest until individuals reach middle age. Light-skinned people who most often burn rather than tan are at a greater risk of skin damage than darker-skinned individuals that almost never burn. The U.S. Food and Drug Administration (FDA) and the Centers for Disease Control (CDC) discourage the use of tanning beds and sun lamps and encourage the use of sunscreen with at least an SPF of 15 or greater. In addition, the rising incidence of melanoma in the United States has led the Environmental Protection Agency (EPA) to develop a sun safety education program for school-age children in order to begin changing public attitudes toward tanning.

Overexposure during medical procedures

Ionizing radiation has many uses in medicine, both in diagnosis and in treatment. X rays, CT scanners, and fluoroscopes use it to form images of the body's insides. Nuclear medicine uses radioactive isotopes to diagnose and to treat medical conditions. In the body, radioactive elements localize to specific tissues and give off tiny amounts of radiation. Detecting that radiation provides information on both anatomy and function. During the past 10 years, skin injuries caused by too much exposure during a medical procedure have been documented. In 1995, the FDA issued a recommendation to physicians and medical institutions to record and monitor the dosage of radiation used during medical procedures on patients in order to minimize the amount of skin injuries. The FDA suggested doses of radiation not exceed 1 Grey (Gy). (A Grey is roughly equivalent to a sievert.) As of 2001, the FDA was preparing further guidelines for fluoroscopy, the procedure most often associated with medical-related radiation skin injuries such as **rashes** and more serious **burns** and tissue death. Injuries occurred most often during angioplasty procedures using fluoroscopy.

CT scans of children have also been problematic. Oftentimes the dosage of radiation used for an adult isn't decreased for a child, leading to radiation overexposure. Children are more sensitive to radiation; a February 2001 study indicates 1,500 out of 1.6 million children under 15 years of age receiving CT scans annually will develop cancer. Studies show that decreasing the radiation by half for CT scans of children will effectively decrease the possibility of overexposure while still providing an effective diagnostic image. The benefits to receiving the medical treatment utilizing radiation is still greater than the risks involved; however, more stringent control over the amount of radiation used during the procedures will go far to minimize the risk of radiation injury to the patient.

Recent evidence suggests that some ethnic groups may be more vulnerable than others to radiation damage. A study done at New York University found that Jews are more likely to develop **ovarian cancer** as a delayed side effect of diagnostic x-rays of the abdomen than non-Jews. These findings require confirmation by further research, but they do indicate that ethnicity and other genetic factors are involved in susceptibility to radiation damage.

Side effects from radiation therapy to treat cancer

As many as half of all cancer patients receive some form of radiation therapy as a component of treatment. The therapy can be delivered from either an external or an internal source, although the former is more common. The machines used for external radiation have become more specialized to deliver the appropriate dose to either a superficial or a deep location on the body. Depending on the type and site of cancer being treated, internal sources of radiation can be injected, swallowed, or placed within the body in sealed containers. These are implanted into or near the tumor, either temporarily or permanently.

Some types of tumors may be eliminated by radiation therapy, if the patient is able to withstand the necessary dose. In other cases, radiation is used in conjunction with other methods of treatment. It may be given before surgery, to shrink a tumor to an operable size, or after surgery, to try to destroy any cancerous cells that may remain. Radiation can be used to make patients with incurable disease more comfortable by decreasing the bulk of tumors to reduce **pain** or pressure. Treatment that is given as a comfort measure only is known as palliation, or palliative therapy.

Occupational radiation exposure

Specialists in industrial and occupational health are increasingly aware of the rising number of injuries related to on-the-job radiation exposure. One study of Swedish workers exposed to high levels of low-frequency magnetic fields found an increased incidence of kidney, liver, and pituitary gland tumors among the men, and a higher rate of **leukemia** and brain tumors among the women.

Sadly, the delayed effects of occupational radiation exposure have also delayed the adoption of necessary protection for workers at risk. A study of the high rate of **lung cancer** among Navajo Indians who worked in uranium mines during World War II did not bring about even partial protection for the miners until 1962. It was not until 1990 that Congress passed the Radiation Exposure Compensation Act to provide care for the injured miners.

The effects of cosmic radiation on human beings are also being investigated because of concern for the safety of air crew. Although findings are still inconclusive as of 2002, recent reports of an increased incidence of cancer among airline pilots and cabin crew members have led epidemiologists to study the long-term effects of cosmic radiation at the altitudes of modern aircraft flight.

Radiation exposure from nuclear accidents, weaponry, and terrorist acts

Between 1945 and 1987, there were 285 nuclear reactor accidents, injuring over 1,550 people and killing 64. The most striking example was the meltdown of the graphite core nuclear reactor at Chernobyl in 1986, which spread a cloud of radioactive particles across the entire continent of Europe. Information about radiation effects is still being gathered from that disaster, however 31 people were killed in the immediate accident and 1,800 children have thus far been diagnosed with thyroid cancer. In a study published in May 2001

by the British Royal Society, children born to individuals involved in the cleanup of Chernobyl and born after the accident are 600% more likely to have genetic mutations than children born before the accident. These findings indicate that exposure to low doses of radiation can cause inheritable effects.

Since the terrorist attack on the World Trade Center and the Pentagon on September 11, 2001, the possibility of terrorist-caused nuclear accidents has been a growing concern. All 103 active nuclear power plants in the United States are on full alert, but they are still vulnerable to sabotage such as bombing or attack from the air. A no-fly zone of 12 miles below 18,000 feet has been established around nuclear power plants by the Federal Aviation Administration (FAA). There is also growing concern over the security of spent nuclear fuel—more than 40,000 tons of spent fuel is housed in buildings at closed plants around the country. Unlike the active nuclear reactors that are enclosed in concrete-reinforced buildings, the spent fuel is stored in non-reinforced buildings. Housed in cooling pools, the spent fuel could emit dangerous levels of radioactive material if exploded or used in makeshift weaponry. Radioactive medical and industrial waste could also be used to make "dirty bombs." Since 1993, the Nuclear Regulatory Commission (NRC) has reported 376 cases of stolen radioactive materials.

One response on the part of health care workers has been stepped-up training in radiation disaster management. Emergency department personnel are being trained as of 2002 to use radiologic monitoring and other specialized equipment for treating victims of a terrorist attack involving radiation.

Causes and symptoms

Radiation can damage every tissue in the body. The particular manifestation will depend upon the amount of radiation, the time over which it is absorbed, and the susceptibility of the tissue. The fastest growing tissues are the most vulnerable, because radiation as much as triples its effects during the growth phase. Bone marrow cells that make blood are the fastest growing cells in the body. A fetus in the womb is equally sensitive. The germinal cells in the testes and ovaries are only slightly less sensitive. Both can be rendered useless with very small doses of radiation. More resistant are the lining cells of the body—skin and intestines. Most resistant are the brain cells, because they grow the slowest.

The length of exposure makes a big difference in what happens. Over time the accumulating damage, if not enough to kill cells outright, distorts their growth and causes scarring and/or cancers. In addition to leukemias, cancers of the thyroid, brain, bone, breast, skin, stomach, and lung all arise after radiation. Damage depends, too, on the ability of the tissue to repair itself. Some tissues and some types of damage produce much greater consequences than others.

There are three types of radiation injuries.

- External irradiation: as with x-ray exposure, all or part of the body is exposed to radiation that either is absorbed or passes through the body.
- Contamination: as with a nuclear accident, the environment and its inhabitants are exposed to radiation. People are affected internally, externally, or with both internal and external exposure.
- Incorporation: dependent on contamination, the bodies of individuals affected incorporate the radiation chemicals within cells, organs, and tissues and the radiation is dispersed throughout the body.

Immediately after sudden irradiation, the fate of those affected depends mostly on the total dose absorbed. This information comes mostly from survivors of the atomic bomb blasts over Japan in 1945.

- Massive doses incinerate immediately and are not distinguishable from the heat of the source.
- A sudden whole-body dose over 50 Sv produces such profound neurological, heart, and circulatory damage that patients die within the first two days.
- Doses in the 10–20 Sv range affect the intestines, stripping their lining and leading to death within three months from vomiting, diarrhea, starvation, and infection.
- Victims receiving 6–10 Sv all at once usually escape an intestinal death, facing instead bone marrow failure and death within two months from loss of blood coagulation factors and the protection against infection provided by white blood cells.
- Between 2–6 Sv gives the person a fighting chance for survival if he or she is supported with blood transfusions and antibiotics.
- One or two Sv produces a brief nonlethal sickness with vomiting, loss of appetite, and generalized discomfort.

Side effects of radiation therapy

Damage caused to normal cells can show up either in the time frame shortly following radiation treatment, or as long as years after radiation has been completed. Symptoms that frequently occur soon after treatment include loss of appetite, **fatigue**, and skin changes. Less commonly, patients have **headache**, **nausea**, **vomiting**, **hair loss**, and weakness. In more severe cases, dehydration, seizures, and shock-type reactions can occur. The severity and type of effects will depend on the region of the body receiving treatment, the type of radiation used during the course of treatment, and the dose. There is also individual variation in the response. Skin rashes are common. They may take the form of redness, burn, dryness, **itching**, or soreness. Organs that were in the path of the beam may show changes, including scarring, functional changes (such as decrease in elasticity), and loss of cells. Tissues that have a rapid turnover of cells may be most severely affected, including the skin and lining of the gastrointestinal tract. More severe injuries may include long-term bone marrow suppression, and occasionally even other cancers, particularly sarcomas.

People who receive radiation in the region of the head and neck are likely to experience a dry and sore mouth to some degree. The skin may become dry, and the area under the chin may droop. Sense of taste can be altered or lost. Some may experience hair loss, earaches, or difficulty swallowing due to inflammation of the esophagus.

Radiation treatments given for or around the breast, chest, or lung can also cause esophagitis and accompanying trouble swallowing. Changes in the lung tissue may lead to pneumonitis or pulmonary fibrosis. The patient may develop a **cough**. Breast treatments may cause pain and swelling. Blood counts can decrease.

Side effects from treatment of the stomach and abdominal area can induce nausea and **diarrhea**. In the pelvic region, radiation may result in difficulties with urination, and **infertility** in both males and females. Women may also have symptoms of dryness, itching, or burning of the vagina.

Diagnosis

The various effects of radiation on the body are well recognized. Patients who are scheduled to undergo radioactive treatments should be informed of the potential side effects they will encounter based on the area being treated and the dose of radiation being used. Advice for coping with minor injuries should be given, as well as descriptions of what symptoms should prompt a call or a visit to the treating physician.

Treatment

It is clearly important to have some idea of the dose received as early as possible, so that attention can be directed to those victims in the 2-10 Sv range that might survive with treatment. Blood transfusions, protection from infection in damaged organs, and possibly the use of newer stimulants to blood formation can save many victims in this category.

Local radiation exposures usually damage the skin and require careful wound care, removal of dead tissue, and skin grafting if the area is large. Again infection control is imperative.

One of the best known, and perhaps even mainstream, treatments of radiation injury is the use of *Aloe vera* preparations on damaged areas of skin. It has demonstrated remarkable healing properties even for chronic ulcerations resulting from radiation treatment. Another topical herb that may be effective against skin inflammation following radiation therapy is **chamomile** cream. Studies support the benefits of chamomile for skin inflammation and wound healing. Additional topical herbs that may be helpful are **calendula** and **St. John's wort**. These therapies can prove very helpful since skin reaction is one of the most common side effects of radiation therapy.

Guided imagery is a method that may be used following radiation treatment, especially to help ease pain. Several nutritional supplements help with healing **wounds**. These include **essential fatty acids** (Omega 3 and 6), **vitamin A**, vitamin B, and magnesium/zinc.

If the tumor being treated is determined to be sensitive to radiation, there are a few herbs that are said to reduce the adverse effects of radiation exposure. Ginseng is one that research suggests may have this benefit. Other nutrients thought to have some protective effects are coenzyme Q10, **kelp**, **pantothenic acid**, and **glutathione** with L-cysteine and L-methionine. **Garlic** and **vitamin C** support immune function. **Grape seed extract** is a powerful antioxidant that protects against cell damage by free radicals. Any nutritional measures to support optimum health before treatment are beneficial.

Allopathic treatment

The type of treatment used depends on the area and severity of the injury. Something as serious as bone marrow suppression would require more intensive therapy, whereas more minor conditions are treated symptomatically. Radiation-induced esophagitis may necessitate intravenous or gastrostomy feeding for a time until the injury is healed. If a perforation or a stricture develops, surgery may be necessary. Products are available to keep the eyes (drops with vitamin A) and oral mucosa moist, as the cells producing mucus and tears are often damaged.

Expected results

Tissue damage resulting from radiation exposure tends to be chronic in nature, and may even be progressive. For the lesser and more common types of problems, long-term treatment of symptoms should be anticipated.

Prevention

Part of preventing radiation injury involves doing research on the condition being treated. It is a good idea to be certain that radiation is the best available treatment for a particular cancer type before embarking on a course of therapy.

Information on preventing or minimizing damage from radiation produced by terrorist devices or other nuclear emergencies is available in a series of fact sheets that can be downloaded from the Centers for Disease Control (CDC) web site. The fact sheets cover such topics as basic radiation facts, acute radiation sickness (ARS), dirty bombs, effects of radiation on health, possible effects of radiation on unborn children, and protective measures in the case of a nuclear event.

Resources

BOOKS

Altman, Robert, and Michael Sarg. *The Cancer Dictionary*, revised edition. New York: Checkmark Books, 2000.
Balch, James, and Phyllis Balch. *Prescription for Nutritional Healing*. New York: Avery Publishing Group, 1997.
Johns Hopkins University. *Johns Hopkins Family Health Book*. New York: HarperCollins Publishers, 1999.

PERIODICALS

Brugge, D., and R. Goble. "The History of Uranium Mining and the Navajo People." *American Journal of Public Health* 92 (September 2002): 1410-1419.
"'Dirty Bomb' Threat Puts Spotlight on Unprepared EDs: Do You Have a Plan?" *ED Management* 14 (September 2002): 97-100.
Fears, T. R., C. C. Bird, D. Guerry 4th, et al. "Average Midrange Ultraviolet Radiation Flux and Time Outdoors Predict Melanoma Risk." *Cancer Research* 62 (July 15, 2002): 3992-3996.
Grunwald, Michael and Peter Behr. "Are Nuclear Plants Secure? Industry Called Unprepared for Sept. 11-Style Attack." *Washington Post*, November 3, 2001, p. A01.
Hakansson, N., B. Floderus, P. Gustavsson, et al. "Cancer Incidence and Magnetic Field Exposure in Industries Using Resistance Welding in Sweden." *Occupational and Environmental Medicine* 59 (July 2002): 481-486.
Harlap, S., S. H. Olson, R. R. Barakat, et al. "Diagnostic X-Rays and Risk of Epithelial Ovarian Carcinoma in Jews." *Annals of Epidemiology* 12 (August 2002): 426-434.

Lim, M. K. "Cosmic Rays: Are Air Crew at Risk?" *Occupational and Environmental Medicine* 59 (July 2002): 428- 432.

Vergano, Dan. "'Dirty' Bombs Latest Fear." *USA Today*, November 3, 2001.

ORGANIZATIONS

American College of Occupational and Environmental Medicine (ACOEM). 1114 North Arlington Heights Road, Arlington Heights, IL 60004. (847) 818-1800. www.acoem.org.

Centers for Disease Control and Prevention (CDC). 1600 Clifton Road, Atlanta, GA 30333. (404) 639-3311. www.cdc.gov.

Judith Turner
Rebecca J. Frey, PhD

Radiesthesia

Definition

Radiesthesia is also commonly known as dowsing. It is regarded principally as a mystic art that has many facets and applications. Basically, it is the process of locating the presence of an object, or assessing the energy given off by a subject, with an implement known as a dowsing rod, which is a Y-shaped hazel, beech, or alder branch or a **copper** rod. Dowsers may also use a pendulum, which is often weighted with a crystal or some other heavy weight. It is said that the important factor is the length of the line to which the weight is attached.

Origins

The concept of radiesthesia was known to the ancient Egyptians and Chinese; their artwork bears witness to this fact. Some estimate that dowsing may date as far back as 7,000 years.

The British Society of Dowsers was formed in the 1930s. The art was given the name radiesthesia by French priest Alex Bouly, derived from the Latin words radiation and perception. However, to many people it is still called dowsing. Modern practitioners of radiesthesia claim that their art uses a "sense" that was once commonly acknowledged, but that has been lost with time. **Radionics** is the process of dowsing using specially designed electrical equipment.

Benefits

While some may call its usefulness to question, the least that can be said is that radiesthesia does no harm.

KEY TERMS

Divining—The act of locating an object using a special sense or instinct.

Geopathic stress—Any variation in normal energy patterns which some believe can cause illness.

Rates—The subtle emanations of energy which may be detected with radionic equipment.

It does not employ radiation, it does not involve the administration of chemicals, and it is noninvasive. Some radiesthesia practitioners claim that they can not only diagnose illness and potential illness, but that they can also cure the patient by altering their energy patterns.

Description

Many different types of objects have traditionally been found with the aid of radiesthesia. Perhaps water wells most readily spring to mind. However, the list is long and includes minerals, lost objects, and people, including bodies, animals, and plants.

Practitioners specializing in this field list several uses of radiesthesia for health purposes. They claim that, in addition to locating areas and causes of disease, dowsing can indicate energy levels before and after healing sessions.

Radiesthesia is used by some who follow a holistic way of life to detect how fresh fruit and vegetables are before they buy them, claiming that the freshest produce gives off more energy than that which is not so fresh. It can also be used to assess the quality of soil and indicate steps to improve soil quality, they say.

The basic concept of radiesthesia is that there is some kind of interaction between the mind of the dowser and the object or information being sought. Practitioners refer to this interaction as the use of a kind of sixth sense, or extra sensory perception. It has also been described as a particular kind of instinct. Some who practice radiesthesia say that as many as 80% of people have the ability to dowse but many are unaware of it.

Some practice radiesthesia without even a prosthesis (a divining rod or pendulum), they just instinctively sense things. When used, a diving rod or pendulum is described as an implement that will help the dowser to focus on the object at hand.

To measure a human energy field, it should first be ascertained that the subject is not wearing any jewelry or crystals. Then the therapist should stand three paces away, facing the patient. L-rods (divining rods) should be held parallel to the ground and pointing towards the patient. The dowser's mind should be focused and a conscious decision must be taken to measure the energy field of the patient's body.

Radiesthesia is also used to pick a location to build a house for example, so as to avoid certain situations such as groundwater, geopathic **stress**, or any other factor that is believed to be detrimental to health. In times gone by, important buildings such as churches, hospitals, palaces, castles and homes, were commonly built after consultation with a dowser regarding the best location.

Usually, when consulting with a radiesthesia practitioner, the patient will first be asked to provide a full case history prior to radiesthesia analysis. If radionic equipment is used, a detector pad will measure energy emanations, which are known as rates, and will be used in the analysis. These rates are said to correspond to organs, diseases, psychological condition, the elements, and even to indicate which alternative therapy would be best to treat the patient.

Preparations

The special equipment necessary for radiesthesia is the dowser's chosen divining implement, which may include specially designed electronic equipment. However, patients will be advised to remove jewelry and any crystals, and possibly anything metal attached to their clothes.

Precautions

Those who are seeking treatment for serious disease are advised to consult an alternative practitioner with regard to a radiesthesia consultation and to mention this to their allopathic physician.

Side effects

There are no known side effects associated with radiesthesia.

Research and general acceptance

Although there are many unexplained accounts of the successful use of radiesthesia, or dowsing, the practice is still the target of much ridicule and even contempt from some areas of the allopathic medical profession.

Training and certification

Since radiesthesia is considered an art, it is an acquired art more than a discipline that can be learned. However, the Radionics Institute, which was founded in 1988, offers various courses in addition to their world-wide training forum.

Resources

ORGANIZATIONS

The American Society of Dowsers. http://www.newhamp shire.com/dowsers.org/.

The British Society of Dowsers. Sycamore Cottage, Tamley Lane, Hastingleigh, Ashford, Kent TN26 5HW, United Kingdom.

The Radionics Association. Baerlein House, Goose Green, Deddington, Oxon. OX15 0SZ, United Kingdom. (01869) 338852. http://www.interlog.com/~radionic/ #institute.

Radionics Institute. 411 (W) 75 Eastdale, Toronto, Canada, M4C 5N3. http://www.mystical-www.co.uk/dowsing .html.

OTHER

"Introduction to dowsing." http://home.interstat.net/~slawcio/ dowsing.html.

Patricia Skinner

Radionics

Definition

Radionics is a highly controversial field that claims to detect and modulate life force using electronic devices. Patients can be diagnosed and treated without even meeting the practitioner, who uses a radionic "black box" to tune into "vibrational frequencies" from a sample of hair or blood. The device is then used to "broadcast" healing frequencies back to the patient, who may be hundreds of miles away.

Origins

The seeds of radionics can be found in **radiesthesia**, a diagnostic technique employing pendulums or dowsing rods developed by three French priests during the early 1900s. The founding father of radionics was Albert Abrams, an American neurologist (1864–1924) who believed that his machines could, from a sample of blood, hair, or even handwriting, determine a patient's sex, race, financial status, religion, and underlying causes of illness. His therapeutic machines were hermetically sealed and were not sold, only leased on the condition that they never be opened. Investigators who examined the devices around the time of Abrams' death found nothing inside to which they could attribute potential medical benefit. The principles of distance healing were developed by a U.S. chiropractor, Ruth Drown, during the 1930s. Drown also maintained that her devices could produce x-ray-like images of a patient's condition, based solely on a blood sample. A scientific committee that examined these images in 1950 detected no recognizable anatomic structures in them, and concluded they were simply "fog patterns."

Benefits

For legal reasons, most radionics practitioners and manufacturers of radionics equipment are cautious of making public pronouncements about specific health benefits. However, a journal published by radionics founder Albert Abrams claimed the technology was effective against diseases as serious as **cancer**, **tuberculosis**, and **syphilis**. Court testimony has indicated that similar claims are made by present-day practitioners.

Description

Radionics advocates believe that underlying causes of diseases emit radio-like frequencies that can be detected by their equipment. A bundle of hair or a card containing a few dried drops of blood is placed into a receptacle in the machine. This "witness" is then analyzed using either a moving pendulum or a detector pad on which changes in surface tension are noted. In this way, areas of "resonance" are detected. Treatment may employ both appropriate frequencies generated by the machine, as well as the extra-sensory abilities of the healer. During the 1990s, computerized "adaptive biofeedback-type" devices were developed, allegedly capable of monitoring and responding "every 200 millionths of a second" to changes in the patient's body. Radionic treatment may be supplemented by homeopathic remedies, **color therapy**, and herbal extracts.

Precautions

Patients need to understand that the claims of radionics are highly controversial and, in some cases, grandiose. One radionics organization based in Canada not only offers certification in 18 healing-related fields, but also advertises its willingness to advise on such diverse subjects as gambling, animal breeding, management consulting, gardening, financial investments, engineering, prospecting, and archeology. This institute claims that radionics has been proven "in hundreds of controlled studies over the past 80 years," but refuses to divulge the names of its graduates "given the controversial nature of radionics." Furthermore, this group will not correspond with any potential client until an initial fee of at least $300

has been paid in U.S. currency. Another manufacturer of radionics-type equipment claims the ability "to enter the mind of any person on this planet" and to "compel them to do your will." It is particularly important to carefully read the literature offered by radionics practitioners, which often contains revealing disclaimers. A medical opinion should be sought in all cases of serious illness.

Side effects

Radionic therapy is non-invasive and has no known side effects.

Research and general acceptance

Most physicians dismiss radionics as quackery, arguing that any observed benefits are caused only by **placebo effect**. In the United States, medical devices must be approved by the federal Food and Drug Administration (FDA), and a 1998 district court decision in Minnesota determined that the sale of an unapproved radionics "black box" device violated state laws against deceptive trade practices and consumer fraud. The sale of such equipment to terminally ill patients constituted "health quackery at its worst," said Hubert Humphrey III, the state's attorney general. "This deplorable conduct aimed at vulnerable, desperate consumers is health fraud in its darkest form and will not be tolerated in Minnesota," Humphrey said. Radionics advocates, on the other hand, say they suffer from systematic government oppression.

Training and certification

Home-study courses and/or certification in radionics are offered by institutions in the United States, Canada, and the United Kingdom. In some cases these institutes also market radionics equipment.

Resources

ORGANIZATIONS

The Radionic Association. Berlin House, Goose Green, Deddington, Oxford England OX5 4SZ.

David Helwig

Rashes

Definition

Rash is a popular term for a group of spots or an area of red, inflamed skin. A rash is usually a symptom of an underlying condition or disorder. Often only temporary, a rash is rarely a sign of a serious problem.

Description

A rash may occur on only one area of the skin, or it can cover almost all of the body. A rash may or may not itch. Depending on how it looks, a rash may be described as:

- blistering (raised oval or round collections of fluid within or beneath the outer layer of skin)
- macular (flat spots)
- nodular (small, firm, knotty rounded masses)
- papular (small, solid, slightly raised areas)
- pustular (pus-containing skin blisters)

Causes and symptoms

There are many theories as to why skin rashes occur. Sometimes the cause can be determined, and sometimes it cannot. Generally, a skin rash is an intermittent symptom, fading and reappearing. Rashes may accompany a range of disorders and conditions.

- Infectious illnesses. A rash is a symptom of many different infectious illnesses or conditions caused by bacteria, viruses, fungi, and other organisms. These include chickenpox, scarlet fever, Rocky Mountain spotted fever, ringworm, herpes, shingles, measles, scabies, and Lyme disease.
- Shared cosmetics and similar personal care items. It is not unusual for people to develop rashes from sharing face powder, mascara, and similar items with other family members or friends.
- Allergic reactions. One of the most common symptoms of an allergic reaction is an itchy rash. Contact dermatitis is a rash that appears after the skin is exposed to an allergen, such as metal, rubber, some cosmetics or lotions, or some types of plants (such as poison ivy, oak, or sumac). Drug reactions are another common allergic cause of rash. In this case, a rash is only one of a variety of possible symptoms, including fever, seizures, nausea and vomiting, diarrhea, heartbeat irregularities, and breathing problems. This rash usually appears soon after the first dose of the medicine is taken, although allergic reactions may be delayed for several days. Common culprits include such drugs as nevirapine, a medication used to treat

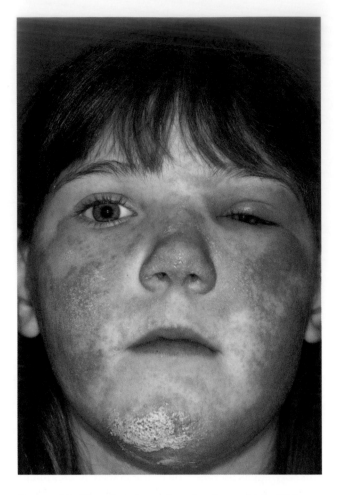

Young girl with poison ivy rash on her face, which she is treating with calamine lotion. (© *Scott Camazine / Alamy*)

HIV infection, and minocycline, a drug used to treat acne.

- Autoimmune disorders. Conditions in which the immune system attacks the body (like with systemic lupus erythematosus or purpura) often have a characteristic rash.
- Nutritional disorders. Scurvy, for example, is a disease caused by a deficiency of vitamin C and produces a rash as one of its symptoms.
- Cancer. A few types of cancer, such as chronic lymphocytic leukemia, can be the underlying cause of a rash.

Rashes in infants

Rashes are extremely common in infancy, are not usually serious, and can be treated at home most of the time.

Diaper rash is caused by prolonged skin contact with bacteria and the baby's waste products in a damp diaper. This rash has red, spotty sores and there may

KEY TERMS

Atopic dermatitis—An intensely itchy inflammation often found on the face of people prone to allergies. In infants and early childhood, it's called infantile eczema.

Dermatitis (dermatoses)—A general term for inflammation of the skin.

Eczema—A superficial type of inflammation of the skin that may be very itchy and weeping in the early stages; later, the affected skin becomes crusted, scaly, and thick. There is no known cause.

Psoriasis—A common chronic skin disorder that causes red patches anywhere on the body.

Purpura—A group of disorders characterized by purple, red, or brown areas of discoloration visible through the skin.

Scabies—A contagious parasitic skin disease characterized by intense itching.

Systemic lupus erythematosus—A chronic immune disorder that attacks multiple parts of the body, including skin, blood vessels, kidneys, and connective tissue. Patients sometimes have a butterfly rash.

be an ammonia smell. In most cases, the rash will respond to drying efforts within three days. A diaper rash that does not improve in this time may be a **yeast infection** requiring prescription medication. A doctor should be consulted if the rash is solid, bright red, and is associated with a **fever**, or if the skin develops **blisters**, **boils**, or pus.

Infants can also get a rash on their cheeks and chin caused by contact with food, saliva, and stomach contents. This rash will come and go, but usually responds to a good cleaning after meals. About one-third of all infants develop **acne**, usually after the third week of life, in response to their mothers' hormones before birth. This rash will disappear in a few weeks to a few months. Heat rash is a mass of tiny pink bumps on the back of the neck and upper back caused by blocked sweat glands. The rash usually appears during hot, humid weather, although a baby with a fever can also develop the rash.

A baby should been seen by a doctor immediately if a rash:

- appears suddenly and is purple or blood colored

- looks like a burn

- appears while the infant seems to be sick

Diagnosis

A family doctor, naturopathic doctor, or dermatologist (skin disease specialist) can diagnose and treat rashes. Diagnosis can be made based on the patient's medical history, the appearance of the rash, the location of the rash, and any other accompanying symptoms. In some cases, the doctor may take a biopsy (skin sample) of the rash to assist in the diagnosis.

Treatment

Alternative treatments for rashes focus on relieving symptoms, clearing the rash, and rejuvenating the skin. There are many forms of alternative medicine that have remedies for rashes.

Herbals

Herbal remedies are very common in the treatment of different types of rashes. **Shingles** may be relieved by taking 30–50 drops of **St. John's wort** tincture in water three to six times a day. A variety of different herbals can be applied to different kinds of rashes.

- agrimony (*Agrimonia eupatoria*) tea spray: hives and moist rashes

- aloe (*Aloe vera*) gel: weeping rash, shingles, burns, sunburn

- amaranth (*Amaranthus hypochondriacus*) tea wash: hives

- beech (*Fagus grandifolia*) tea wash: diaper rash and poison ivy or oak rash

- black walnut (*Juglans nigra*) leaf tea: rashes, rashes caused by parasites, scabies

- burdock (*Articum lappa*) decoction: hives, eczema

- calendula (*Calendula officinalis*) infusion: hives, burns, sunburn; calendula lotion: plant-contact dermatitis

- cattail (*Typha latifolia*) paste: poison ivy rash

- chamomile tea wash: poison ivy, oak, or sumac rash

- chickweed (*Stellaria media*) salve: severe rashes, hives

- comfrey (*Symphytum officinale*) ointment, cream, or lotion: inflamed rash; cold tea compress from comfrey root: plant-contact dermatitis

- heartsease (*Viola tricolor*) infusion: hives

- goldenseal (*Hydrastis canadensis*) wash: poison ivy rash, rash caused by infection, diaper rash

- jewelweed (*Impatiens pallida*) rub: poison ivy or oak rash and skin irritation caused by briars, brambles, or nettles

- nettle (*Urtica dioca*) infusion: hives

- oak bark (*Querus alba*) tea: rashes
- oatmeal bath: plant-contact dermatitis
- pennyroyal (*Hedeoma pulegiodes*) tea wash: hives, shingles, measles, scabies, mumps, chickenpox, diaper rash, and poison ivy or oak rash
- pine (*Pinus* species) ashes: measles, chickenpox, and mumps rash
- plantain (*Plantago major*) poultice: poison ivy rash
- poplar (*Populus candicans*) tea wash: rashes
- sage (*Salvia officinalis*) tea wash: poison ivy or oak rash, and moist, weepy rashes
- sassafras (*Sassafras albidum*) root tea: rashes, shingles
- slippery elm (*Ulmus fulva*) bark paste: rashes
- solomon's seal (*Polygonatum multiflorum*) mashed root: poison ivy or oak rash
- St. John's wort (*Hypericum perforatum*) oil: shingles, and dry, itchy rashes
- sumac (*Rhus glabra*) tea wash: poison ivy rash
- thyme (*Thymus vulgaris*) salve: rashes
- witch hazel (*Hamamelis virginiana*) tincture: poison ivy or oak rash, diaper rash, and weeping rash
- yellow dock (*Rumex crispus*) decoction: hives

It is a good idea, however, to be careful in using herbal remedies. Cases have been reported of patients developing body rashes from **allergies** to such herbs as **feverfew**.

Homeopathy

Homeopathic remedies are individually prescribed for each patient. Some possible homeopathic remedies include:

- calcium sulfide (*Hepar sulphuris*) for rash with pus
- graphite (*Graphites*) for dry, red, cracked, itchy rash in the skin folds
- honeybee (*Apis*) for swelling and hives from bee stings
- nosode (*Medorrhinum*) for sharply defined red, possibly shiny, rash suggesting yeast infection
- poison ivy (*Rhus toxicodendron*) for plant contact dermatitis, itching hives, and restlessness
- stinging nettle (*Urtica urens*) for stinging hives with little inflammation
- sulfur for dry, red, cracked, itchy rash anywhere, including around the anus.

Other treatments

Other rash remedies include:

- Aromatherapy. The essential oils thyme, lavender, jasmine, and German chamomile may relieve allergy-induced eczema.

- Ayurveda. Rashes and hives are treated by drinking fresh cilantro juice and applying the pulp onto the rash. Fresh coconut water, melon rind, or a paste of turmeric (one part) and sandalwood (two parts) in goat's milk can be applied to the affected area. Hot milk (1 cup) containing coriander (1 teaspoon), cumin (1/2 teaspoon), and raw sugar (1 teaspoon) can be ingested once or twice daily to heal rashes and hives and restore skin health.
- Chinese medicine. Hives are treated with herbal preparations, acupuncture, ear acupuncture, and cupping. Preparations applied to the skin to relieve the itching associated with hives include Jie Du Cha Ji (Resolve Toxin Smearing Liquid), Zhi Yang Po Fen (Relieve Itching Powder), and Zhi Yang Xi Ji (Relieve Itching Washing Preparation). Contact dermatitis and drug dermatitis are treated with herbal formulas comprised of herbs chosen specifically for the patient's symptoms.
- Diet. An increased intake of mackerel, salmon, and herring provides essential fatty acids that may decrease itching and inflammation.
- Hydrotherapy. Hives can be relieved by rubbing the affected area with an ice cube, taking a cool bath, or using a cold compress.
- Hypnosis. Emotional stress can trigger many different dermatoses including certain rashes. Hypnosis has been helpful in treating atopic dermatitis, herpes, itching, psoriasis, hives, and other dermatoses.
- Juice therapy. Red rashes are treated with fresh apple, dark grape, papaya, or pineapple juices drunk at room temperature between meals.
- Supplements. Rashes may be treated with skin-repairing vitamins A, C, B complex, and zinc. Vitamin E can reduce skin dryness (decreasing the itch).

Allopathic treatment

Treatment of rashes focuses on providing relief of the **itching** that often accompanies them. Soothing lotions, topical corticosteroids (such as hydrocortisone), or oral antihistamines (Benadryl) can provide some relief. Topical antibiotics may be administered if the patient, particularly a child, has caused an infection by scratching.

For diaper rash, the infant's skin should be exposed to the air as much as possible. Ointments are not needed unless the skin is dry and cracked. Experts also recommend switching to cloth diapers and cleaning affected skin with plain water.

Expected results

Most rashes that have an acute cause (such as an infection or an allergic reaction) will disappear as soon as the infection or irritant is removed from the system. Rashes that are caused by chronic conditions (such as autoimmune disorders) may remain indefinitely or may fade and then return periodically.

Prevention

Some rashes can be prevented, depending on the cause. A person known to be allergic to certain drugs or substances should avoid those things in order to prevent a rash. It is also a good idea to avoid sharing cosmetics and personal care items (including lip balms) with other family members or friends. Diaper rash can be prevented by using cloth diapers, keeping the diaper area very clean, breast-feeding, and changing diapers often. A person should launder clothing and rinse his or her skin first with rubbing alcohol and then with water after contact with a plant that can cause **contact dermatitis**.

Resources

BOOKS

"Rashes and Skin Problems." In *The Alternate Advisor: The Complete Guide to Natural Therapies and Alternative Treatments*. Richmond, VA: Time-Life Books, 1997.

Reichenberg-Ullman, Judyth, and Robert Ullman. *Homeopathic Self-Care: The Quick and Easy Guide for the Whole Family*. Rockland, CA: Prima Publishing, 1997.

Ying, Zhou Zhong, and Jin Hui De. *Clinical Manual of Chinese Herbal Medicine and Acupuncture*. New York: Churchill Livingston, 1997.

PERIODICALS

Bennett, Paul J., and Mukta Panda. "RHE1: It is Not Nice to Fool with Mother Nature: The Case of the Herbal-Induced Rash." *Southern Medical Journal* 94 (December 2001): S29-S30.

Disdier, Patrick, Brigitte Granel, et al. "A Teenager with Rash and Fever." *Lancet* 358 (December 15, 2001): 2046.

"Mommy, Did You Borrow My Blush?" *Consumer Reports* 66 (October 2001): 9.

Shenefelt, Philip D. "Hypnosis in Dermatology." *Archives of Dermatology* 136 (March 2000): 393–399.

ORGANIZATIONS

American Academy of Dermatology. 930 N. Meacham Rd., P.O. Box 4014, Schaumburg, IL 60168. (708) 330-0230. http://www.aad.org.

Belinda Rowland
Rebecca J. Frey, PhD

Raspberry

Description

Raspberry (*Rubus ideaeus*) is a deciduous bush from the Rosaceae family that grows up to 6 ft (2 m) high, with erect and thorny stems, a thin spine and perennial roots. The bush is well-known for its fruit, a red spherical berry that grows continuously on the branches. Cymes (clusters) of white flowers bloom in late spring to early summer. Raspberries can be grown in many temperate countries, in either dry or moist wooded areas.

General use

Raspberry leaves are used as an astringent and stimulant. High concentrations of tannin found in the plant are the source of its astringent effects. It also contains flavonoids, pectin, citric and malic acids, and a crystallizable fruit sugar and water. Raspberries are high in minerals, especially **iron**, **magnesium**, and **calcium**. Raspberry is well regarded as a women's herb. The leaves are brewed into a tea that is used during **pregnancy** as well as to increase breast milk after the baby is born. Some women use tea made from raspberry leaves to regulate their menstrual cycles and to decrease heavy menstrual flow. It is also used for gastrointestinal disorders, respiratory illness, the cardiovascular system and for sores in the mouth and throat. The fruit has been found be anticarcinogenic.

Pregnancy

Raspberry leaves have been used for centuries by women during pregnancy. But it wasn't until a 1941

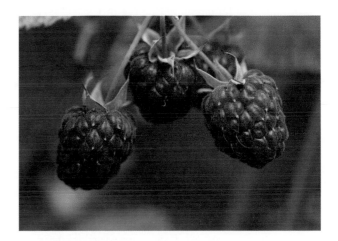

Raspberry. (© *blickwinkel / Alamy*)

study in the British medical journal *Lancet* that raspberry leaves were scientifically confirmed to contain a complex biochemical that is a uterine relaxant. Raspberry leaves are commonly used throughout pregnancy for many reasons, including helping **morning sickness**, preventing miscarriage, strengthening the uterus, regulating contractions, and relaxing the uterus during labor. Some pet breeders give a tincture of red raspberry leaves to pregnant cats who are likely to have difficulty in kittening.

Gastrointestinal disorders

Because it is an astringent, raspberry is a gentle antidiarrheal. It is also used to reduce **nausea** and **vomiting**, usually for morning sickness.

Mouth and throat sores

Raspberry tea is helpful for healing mouth and throat sores when used as a mouthwash or gargle. It can also be used for bleeding gums and other oral inflammations. Some herbalists recommend it for colds, **measles**, and coughs.

Cancer treatment

The fruit of the raspberry may help prevent **cancer**, according to a January 1999 report in *Cancer Weekly Plus*. "Ellagic acid in raspberries has been shown in previous studies to be effective in inhibiting cancers in rats and mice," the study detailed. "The compound is ... at especially high levels in blackberries and raspberries." Researchers at the Hollings Cancer Center at the Medical University of South Carolina in Charleston gave one cup of raspberries a day to each participant for one year. The study concluded that " ... eating red raspberries may possibly prevent cancer by inhibiting the abnormal division of cells and promoting the normal death of healthy cells."

A 2001 study has found that black raspberries appear to be as helpful as red raspberries in preveting or slowing the growth of cancer. Black raspberries, according to an article in the journal Cancer Research, help to protect against esophageal cancer, which is the sixth-leading cause of deaths from cancer worldwide. Esophageal cancer is one of the deadliest forms of the disease— five-year survival rates range from 8% to 12%. Researchers think that ellagic acid is not the only beneficial compound in raspberries, however, and are presently studying other substances found in the fruit.

Diabetes

Some studies have shown that raspberries may help reduce glucose levels and therefore may be helpful to people with diabetes.

Preparations

Raspberry leaf tea can be made by adding 1 tsp of the leaf to one cup of boiling water. The leaf should be infused for 10 min and then strained. The infusion can be taken once or twice a day. During pregnancy, use 0.5 oz of leaf to one pt of boiling water and drink once a day. For infant **diarrhea**, dilute this infusion by 50%. A tincture made of raspbery leaf can be taken three times a day, in 2–4 ml doses.

Precautions

Wilted raspberry leaves develop a mild poison that may make people ill. When picking the leaves for the tea, the user should make sure that the plant is flowering. Leaves used for steeping to make tea must be fully dried. Another important precaution is to be sure that the raspberries are not contaminated by a gastrointestinal parasite called *Cyclospora*. The parasite causes a disease called *cyclosporiasis,* which caused several serious outbreaks in the mid-1990s in the United States and Canada. The *Cyclospora* parasite was found in raspberries imported from Guatemala.

Side effects

Although raspberry is used as an antidiarrheal herb, overuse may actually cause diarrhea. In addition, some people may be allergic to raspberries and other berries. Lastly, the tea may sometimes be too tonifying in the early stages of pregnancy; it should be discontinued if contractions increase.

Interactions

No known adverse interactions with other medications have been reported.

Resources

BOOKS

Weiner, Michael. *Weiner's Herbal.* New York: Quantum Books, 1990.

PERIODICALS

Ackers, Marta-Louise, and Barbara L. Hervaldt. "An outbreak in 1997 of cyclosporiasis associated with imported raspberries." *New England Journal of Medicine* (May 29, 1997): 1545-9.

"Black Raspberries Show Multiple Defenses in Thwarting Cancer." *Cancer Weekly* (November 13, 2001): 24.

Henderson, Charles W. "Red Raspberries May Help Fight Cancer." *Cancer Weekly Plus* (January 18, 1999).

Katherine Y. Kim
Rebecca J. Frey, PhD

Raynaud's syndrome

Definition

Raynaud's syndrome is a disorder in which the fingers or toes (digits) suddenly experience decreased blood circulation. It is also called Raynaud's disease.

Description

Raynaud's syndrome can be classified as one of two types: primary, or idiopathic (of unknown cause) disease; and secondary, which is also called Raynaud's phenomenon.

Primary Raynaud's disease is milder and causes fewer complications. About half of all cases of Raynaud's disease are of this type. Women are four times more likely than men to develop primary Raynaud's disease, and the average age of diagnosis is between 20 and 40 years. About 30% of all cases of primary Raynaud's disease progress after diagnosis, while 15% of cases actually improve.

Secondary Raynaud's disease is more complicated, severe, and more likely to get worse over time. A number of medical conditions or other triggers predispose a person to secondary Raynaud's disease, but do not directly cause the disorder. These include:

• Scleroderma. Scleroderma is a serious disease of the connective tissue, in which tissues of the skin, heart, esophagus, kidney, and lung become thickened, hard, and constricted. About 30% of patients

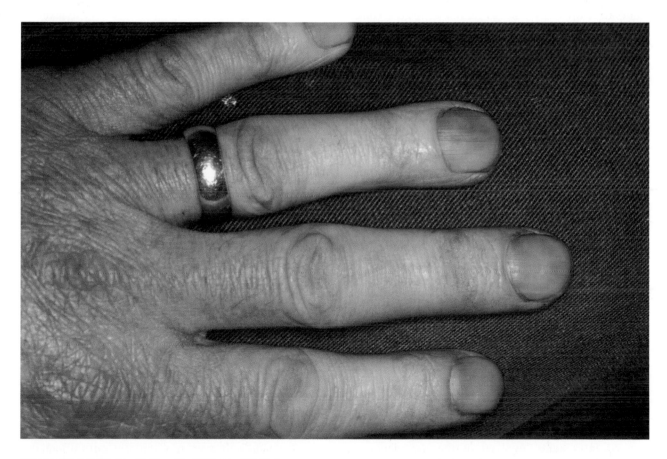

Raynaud's syndrome. *(© Hercules Robinson / Alamy)*

diagnosed with scleroderma will then develop Raynaud's disease.

- Other diseases of connective tissue. These include systemic lupus erythematosus, rheumatoid arthritis, dermatomyositis, and polymyositis.
- Diseases that cause arterial blockage. These include atherosclerosis or hardening of the arteries.
- A severe form of high blood pressure which is caused by diseased arteries in the lung, called pulmonary hypertension.
- Disorders of the nervous system. These include herniated discs in the spine, strokes, tumors within the spinal cord, polio, and carpal tunnel syndrome.
- Other blood disorders.
- Trauma. Injuries that lead to Raynaud's are typically caused by exposure to constant vibration (workers who use chainsaws, jackhammers, or other vibrating equipment); repetitive movements (keyboard instrumentalists, assembly line workers, typists); electric shock; repeated use of the lower side of the palm as a hammer; or extreme cold (frostbite).
- Environmental toxins. Workers in the plastics industry who are exposed to high levels of vinyl chloride may develop a scleroderma-like illness that includes Raynaud's syndrome.
- Prescription medications. Drugs that increase the risk of developing Raynaud's include those used for migraine headaches or high blood pressure, and some cancer chemotherapy agents. Cases have also been reported of Raynaud's disease developing in reaction to quinine.

Causes and symptoms

Causes

Both primary and secondary types of Raynaud's symptoms are believed to be due to overreactive arterioles, or small arteries. While cold normally causes the muscle which makes up the walls of arteries to contract (squeeze down to become smaller), in Raynaud's disease the degree is extreme. Blood flow to the area is severely restricted. Some attacks may also be brought on or worsened by **anxiety** or emotional distress.

Although the cause of primary Raynaud's is not known as of 2002, researchers are focusing on prostaglandin metabolism and the function of endothelial cells in the body. Prostaglandins are a group of unsaturated fatty acids involved in the contraction of smooth muscle and the control of inflammation and

body temperature. Endothelial cells form the layer of smooth tissue that lines the inside of the heart, blood vessels, and other body cavities.

Recent advances in gene mapping and sequencing indicate that Raynaud's may be linked to abnormal forms of a gene known as the Fibrillin-1 gene. This gene affects the composition of the protein molecules in human connective tissue.

Symptoms

Classically, there are three distinct phases to an episode of Raynaud's symptoms. When first exposed to cold, the arteries respond by contracting intensely. The digits in question, or in rare instances, the tip of the nose or tongue, become pale and white as they are deprived of blood flow and the oxygen carried by the blood. In response, the veins and capillaries dilate, or expand. Because these vessels carry deoxygenated blood, the digit becomes cyanotic, which means that it turns blue. The digit often feels cold, numb, and tingly. After the digit begins to warm up again, the arteries dilate. Blood flow increases significantly, and the digits turn a bright red. During this phase, the patient often describes the digits as feeling warm, and throbbing painfully.

Raynaud's disease may initially only affect the tips of the fingers or toes. When the disease progresses, it may eventually affect the entire finger or toe. Ultimately, all the fingers or toes may be affected. About 10% of the time, a complication called sclerodactyly may occur. In sclerodactyly, the skin over the affected digits becomes tight, white, thick, smooth, and shiny.

When the most serious complications of Raynaud's disease or phenomenon occur, the affected digits develop deep sores, or ulcers, in the skin. The tissue may even die, thus becoming gangrenous, and requiring amputation. This complication occurs only about 1% of the time in primary Raynaud's disease.

Diagnosis

While the patient's symptoms will be the first clue pointing to Raynaud's disease, a number of tests may also be performed to confirm the diagnosis. Special blood tests called the antinuclear antibody test (ABA) and the erythrocyte sedimentation rate (ESR) are often abnormal when an individual has a connective tissue disease.

When a person has connective tissue disease, his or her capillaries are usually abnormal. A test called a nailfold capillary study can demonstrate such abnormalities. In this test, a drop of oil is placed on the skin at the base of the fingernail. This allows the capillaries in that area to be viewed more easily with a microscope.

A cold stimulation test may also be performed. In this test, specialized thermometers are taped to each of the digits that have experienced episodes of Raynaud's disease. The at-rest temperature of these digits is recorded. The hand or foot is then placed completely into a container of ice water for 20 seconds. After removing the hand or foot from this water, the temperature of the digits is recorded immediately. The temperature of the digits is recorded every five minutes until they reach the same temperature they were before being put into the ice water. A normal result occurs when this pretest temperature is reached in 15 minutes or less. If it takes more than 20 minutes, the test is considered suspicious for Raynaud's disease or phenomenon.

Treatment

The first type of treatment for Raynaud's symptoms is simple prevention. Patients need to stay warm, and keep hands and feet well covered in cold weather. Patients who smoke cigarettes should stop, because nicotine worsens the problem. Most people—especially those with primary Raynaud's—are able to deal with the disease by taking these basic measures.

Because episodes of Raynaud's disease have also been associated with **stress** and emotional upset, the disease may be improved by helping a patient learn to manage stress. Regular **exercise** is known to decrease stress and lower anxiety. Hypnosis, **relaxation** techniques, and visualization are also useful methods to help a patient gain control of his or her emotional responses. **Biofeedback** training is a technique during which a patient is given continuous information on the temperature of his or her digits, and then taught to voluntarily control this temperature. **Acupuncture** is also used for treating these circulatory and heat distribution problems.

Some alternative practitioners believe that certain dietary supplements and herbs may be helpful in decreasing the vessel spasm of Raynaud's disease. Suggested supplements include **vitamin E** (found in fruits, vegetables, seeds, and nuts), **magnesium** (found in seeds, nuts, fish, beans, and dark green vegetables), and fish oils. Several types of herbs have been suggested, including peony (*Paeonia lactiflora*) and **dong quai** (*Angelica sinensis*). The circulatory herbs **cayenne** (*Capsicum frutescens*), **ginger** (*Zingiber officinale*), and prickly ash (*Zanthoxylum americanum*) can help enhance circulation to the extremities. Additionally, a tincture of one-half teaspoon of a combination of equal parts of *ginkgo biloba*, prickly ash, and ginger may be consumed three times daily.

Practitioners of **traditional Chinese medicine** (TCM) recommend certain formulas called *si ni*, which means cold extremities. TCM regards Raynaud's as an indication that the person is hypersensitive to cold outside the body because he or she is already cold inside. The Chinese practitioner will typically recommend various combinations of herbs regarded as warming to correct this condition. The *si ni* formulas contain different combinations of ginger, **aconite**, bupleurum, bitter orange, and honey-baked **licorice**.

Allopathic treatment

People with more severe cases of Raynaud's disease may need to be treated with medications to attempt to keep the arterioles relaxed and dilated. Some medications that are more commonly used to treat high blood pressure, such as calcium-channel blockers, or reserpine, are often effective for treatment of Raynaud's symptoms. Nitroglycerin paste can be used on the affected digits, and seems to be helpful in healing skin ulcers.

When a patient has secondary Raynaud's phenomenon, treatment of the coexisting condition may help control the Raynaud's as well. In the case of connective tissue disorders, this often involves treatment with corticosteroid medications.

Expected results

The prognosis for most people with Raynaud's disease is very good. In general, primary Raynaud's disease has the best prognosis, with a relatively small chance for serious complications (1%). In fact, about 50% of all patients do well by taking simple precautions, and never even require medications. The prognosis for people with secondary Raynaud's disease or phenomenon is less predictable. This prognosis depends greatly on the severity of the patient's other associated condition, such as scleroderma or lupus.

Prevention

As of 2002, there is no known way to prevent the development of Raynaud's disease. Once a person realizes that he or she suffers from this disorder, however, steps can be taken to reduce the frequency and severity of episodes.

Resources

BOOKS

Creager, Mark A., and Victor J. Dzau. "Vascular Disease of the Extremities." In *Harrison's Principles of Internal Medicine*, edited by Anthony S. Fauci, et al. 14th ed. New York: McGraw–Hill, 1998.

Pelletier, Kenneth R., MD. *The Best Alternative Medicine*. New York: Simon & Schuster, 2002.

"Raynaud's Disease and Phenomenon," Section 16, Chapter 212 in *The Merck Manual of Diagnosis and Therapy*, 17th edition, edited by Mark H. Beers, MD, and Robert Berkow, MD. Whitehouse Station, NJ: Merck Research Laboratories, 2003.

PERIODICALS

Agarwal, N., and B. Cherascu. "Concomitant Acral Necrosis and Haemolytic Uraemic Syndrome Following Ingestion of Quinine." *Journal of Postgraduate Medicine* 48 (July-September 2002): 197-198.

Dharmananda, Subhuti. "Raynaud's Disease: Chinese Medical Perspective." *Internet Journal of the Institute for Traditional Medicine and Preventive Health Care* 1 (July 2002): 1-7.

Heitmann, C., M. Pelzer, M. Trankle, et al. "The Hypothenar Hammer Syndrome." [in German] *Der Unfallchirurg* 105 (September 2002): 833-836.

Kodera, T., F. K. Tan, T. Sasaki, et al. "Association of 5 Untranslated Region of the Fibrillin-1 Gene with Japanese Scleroderma." *Gene* 297 (September 4, 2002): 61-67.

ORGANIZATIONS

American College of Rheumatology. 1800 Century Place, Suite 250, Atlanta, GA 30345. (404) 633-3777. www.rheumatology.org.

Institute of Traditional Medicine. 2017 SE Hawthorne Blvd., Portland, OR 97214. (503) 233-4907. www.itmonline.org.

National Institute of Arthritis and Musculoskeletal and Skin Diseases Information Clearinghouse. National Institutes of Health, 1 AMS Circle, Bethesda, MD 20892. (301) 495-4484 or (toll-free)(877) 22-NIAMS. www.niams.nih.gov.

OTHER

National Institutes of Health. *Questions and Answers About Raynaud's Phenomenon*. Bethesda, MD: National Institutes of Health, 2001. NIH Publication No. 01-4911.

"Raynaud's Disease." http://www.alternaticemedicine.com/digest/issue04/04354R00.sh.

Kathleen D. Wright
Rebecca J. Frey, PhD

Reconstructive therapy *see* **Prolotherapy**

Red cedar

Description

Red cedar, also called western red cedar or western redcedar, is the species *Thuja plicata*. It should not be confused with the eastern red cedar, *Juniperus virginiana*, or the Lebanon cedar, *Cedrus libani*, which are unrelated species. Eastern red cedar is toxic if taken internally.

Western red cedar is a tree that grows to a height of 125 ft (60 m) in moist soils in mixed coniferous forests. It has red-brown or gray-brown bark with thick longitudinal fissures that is easily peeled. Its foliage develops in sprays about 6 in (15 cm) long with small, highly aromatic leaves. The leaves, twigs, bark, and roots are all used medicinally.

Western red cedar is found in northwestern North America, in the United States and western Canada from Alaska through northern California and in the Rocky Mountains from British Columbia through Montana. Other names for *Thuja plicata* include giant red cedar, giant arborvitae, shinglewood, and canoe cedar. It is one of the most commercially important logging trees in the western United States.

A relative of the western red cedar, *Thuja orientalis* grows in the eastern part of the United States and

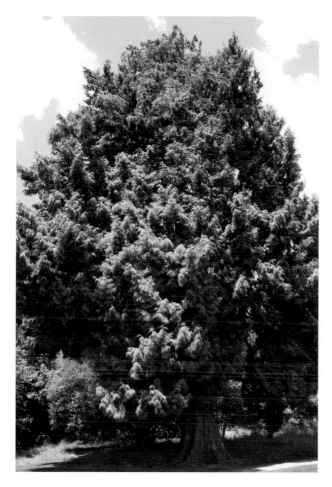

Red Cedar. (© *blickwinkel / Alamy*)

Canada as well as in China where it is called *ce bai ye or ya bai shu*. The naming of this species is confusing. It is called yellow cedar and sometimes also arbor vitae while *Thuja plicata* is sometimes called giant arbor vitae. More confusing, another relative, Chinese arbor vitae, is referred to in literature interchangeably as *Biota orientalis* and *Thuja orientalis*. It is used in **traditional Chinese medicine** in many of the same ways as *Thuja plicata*.

General use

Red cedar is of major cultural importance to Native American tribes living in the Pacific Northwest. The wood, bark, limbs, and roots were used to provide many of the needs of the tribe, ranging from shelter to cooking implements to medicine. Red cedar also has spiritual significance to some of these tribes and is used in ritual ways. Red cedar was a major medicinal herb for these Pacific Northwest cultures, although by the late 2000s it was not much used medicinally.

Native American tribes used the twigs, leaves, roots, bark, and leaf buds of red cedar to treat many different symptoms. Internal uses include:

- boiling limbs to make a tuberculosis treatment
- chewing leaf buds for sore lungs
- boiling leaves to make a cough remedy
- making a decoction of leaves to treat colds
- chewing leaf buds to relieve toothache pain
- making an infusion to treat stomach pain and diarrhea
- chewing the inner bark of a small tree to bring about delayed menstruation
- making a bark infusion to treat kidney complaints
- making an infusion of the seeds to treat fever
- using a weak infusion internally to treat rheumatism and arthritis

External uses include:

- making a decoction of leaves to treat rheumatism
- washing with an infusion of twigs to treat venereal disease, including the human papilloma virus and other sexually transmitted diseases
- making a poultice of boughs or oil to treat rheumatism
- making a poultice of boughs or oil to threat bronchitis
- making a poultice or oil from inner bark to treat skin diseases, including topical fungal infections and warts
- using shredded bark to cauterize and bind wounds

Scientific research supports some of these traditional uses of red cedar. Extracts of red cedar have been shown to have antibacterial properties against common bacteria. Compounds with antifungal properties have also been isolated. The aromatic and decay-resistant properties of western red cedar are attributed to organic compounds called tropolones.

Preparations

Most preparations of red cedar call for boiling the medicinal parts to make a decoction or for making a tea or infusion. As of 2008, little information existed on dosages.

An essential oil to be used topically can be prepared from red cedar. It is toxic if taken internally and has the ability to produce convulsions or even death if taken in even small quantities. A 1999 study done in Switzerland noted an increase in poisoning deaths from plant products, including *Thuja*, due possibly to an increase in people practicing herbal healing and **aromatherapy**.

Precautions

As noted above, the oil of all species of *Tthuja* can cause convulsions. Decoctions of the bark of red cedar can also cause miscarriage. Therefore, pregnant women should not use red cedar.

Side effects

Many people develop **asthma** and bronchial spasms from exposure to red cedar or red cedar dust. This response is an allergic reaction to plicatic acid present in the wood. Red cedar-induced asthma is a serious occupational hazard to loggers in western North America. Estimates of the number of loggers who develop occupational asthma due to red cedar exposure range from 4–13.5%. There are also reports of **contact dermatitis** (rash) caused by exposure to western red cedar heartwood.

Interactions

There were no studies and little observational evidence as of 2008 to indicate whether red cedar interacts with other herbs or with Western pharmaceuticals.

Resources

OTHER

"Thuja plicata." *Gymnosperm Database,* May 30, 2007. http://www.conifers.org/cu/th/plicata.htm. (February 16, 2008).

ORGANIZATIONS

Alternative Medicine Foundation, PO Box 60016, Potomac, MD, 20859, (301) 340-1960, http://www.amfoundation.org.

Tish Davidson, A. M.

Red clover

Description

Red clover (*Trifolium pratense*) is a familiar meadow herb, one of 250 species in the Leguminosae, or pea family. The Irish shamrock is another species in

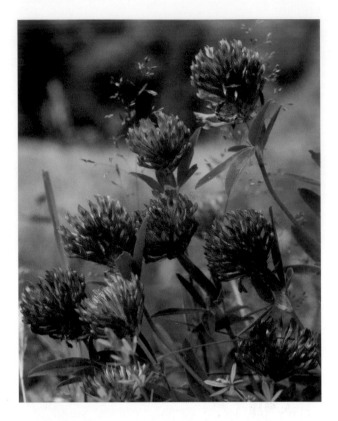

Red Clover. (© *Arco Images / Alamy*)

this family of plants. Red clover is a European native naturalized throughout North America and Canada. This familiar short-lived perennial grows wild along roadsides, in meadows, and in fields, and is extensively cultivated as a forage crop for cattle. It grows best in soils that are rich in **calcium**, **potassium**, and **phosphorus**. The common names for this sweet herb include wild clover, meadow trefoil, bee bread, trefoil, cow grass, purple clover, and three-leafed grass.

Red clover grows to about 2 ft (61 cm) high from a short, woody rootstock. The leaves are palmate and arranged alternately along the round, grooved, and hairy stem. They are divided into three oblong or oval leaflets, a characteristic that has given the genus its name. The dark green leaves often have a splash of a pale green or white on each leaflet. The leaf margins are toothed. The red-purple or magenta-hued blossoms comprise numerous florets that form a globe-shaped flower on the end of the stalk. Red clover blooms throughout the summer. The edible blossoms are sweet-tasting with a honey-like fragrance. Bees are attracted to clover blossoms, but seem to prefer the white blossoms of another common variety of clover, often growing nearby.

General use

In folk tradition, red clover was associated with the Christian doctrine of the Trinity because of its threefold leaflets. In England it was worn as a magic charm to protect against evil. The herb's value as a medicinal remedy was not well known until the herb made its way to North America. Native American herbalists soon found numerous medicinal uses for this common wayside beauty. Red clover was used as a **cancer** treatment; the blossoms, combined with other herbs, became commercially popular in the United States in the 1930s. Numerous so-called "Trifolium Compounds" were marketed as blood purifiers, or alteratives, to help clear the body of metabolic toxins. The herb was listed in the *National Formulary* of the United States until 1946.

Red clover has most often been used to treat such skin inflammations as **psoriasis** and **eczema**. It also acts as an expectorant and demulcent, and is helpful in the treatment of **bronchitis** and spasmodic coughs, particularly **whooping cough**. Red clover may stimulate the liver and gall bladder and has been used for **constipation** and sluggish appetite. The blossoms were smoked as a remedy for **asthma**. An infusion of red clover blossoms used as a skin wash, or a poultice prepared from fresh blossoms, may relieve the irritation of **athlete's foot** or insect **bites**. The infusion is also useful as an external skin wash in the treatment of persistent sores and ulcers, and may help speed healing. As an eyewash, red clover tincture diluted with fresh water may relieve **conjunctivitis**. An ointment prepared from red clover is helpful for lymphatic swellings, and a compress made with it may relieve the **pain** of arthritis and **gout**. More recently, red clover has been studied as an alternative remedy for **hot flashes** in menopausal women as well as hot flashes in men following surgery for **prostate cancer**.

Many of the chemical constituents present in red clover have been identified, including volatile oil, isoflavonoids, coumarin derivatives, and cyanogenic glycosides. Few scientific studies, however, have confirmed the folk use of red clover remedies. The genistein found in red clover has been found to contribute to the shrinking of cancerous tumors in vitro by preventing growth of the new blood vessels that feed the tumors. One of the first studies using purified extract of red clover, published in 1999, concluded that use of red clover in standardized extracts that include specific quantities of the four isoflavones genistein, daidzein, biochanin and formononetin, resulted in improved heart health in postmenopausal women. Red clover is considered by some herbalists to be a phytoestrogenic herb, useful in restoring estrogen balance in women. The chemical formononetin, found in red clover, acts on the body in a similar way as estrogen.

KEY TERMS

Alterative—A herb that changes one's physical condition, especially a blood cleanser.

Demulcent—A substance or agent used to soothe irritated mucous membranes.

Expectorant—A substance or medication that causes or eases the bringing up of sputum or phlegm from the respiratory tract.

Infusion—An herbal preparation made by adding herbs to boiling water and then steeping the mixture to allow the medicinal herb to infuse into the water.

Isoflavone—A type of phytoestrogen, or compound derived from plants that has weak estrogen-like activity. Red clover contains measurable quantities of four different isoflavones.

Palmate—A type of leaf that has lobes or leaflets radiating from a central point.

Tincture—A liquid extract of an herb prepared by steeping the herb in an alcohol and water mixture.

Preparations

Red clover blossoms are the medicinally active part of this herb. Fully open blossoms can be harvested throughout the flowering season. Pick the flower heads on a sunny day after the morning dew has evaporated. Spread the blossoms on a paper-lined tray to dry in a bright and airy room away from direct sun. The temperature in the drying room should be at least 70°F (21°C). When the blossoms are completely dry, store dried flowers in a dark glass container with an air-tight lid. The dried herb will maintain medicinal potency for 12–18 months. Clearly label the container with the name of the herb and the date and place harvested.

Tincture: Combine 4 oz of fresh or dried red clover blossoms with 1 pint of brandy, gin, or vodka in a glass container. The alcohol should be enough to cover the flowers. The ratio should be close to 50/50 alcohol to water. Stir and cover. Place the mixture in a dark cupboard for three to five weeks. Shake the mixture several times each day. Strain and store in a tightly capped, clearly labeled dark glass bottle. A standard dose is 1–3 mL of the tincture three times a day. Tinctures properly prepared and stored will retain medicinal potency for two years or longer.

Infusion: Place 2 oz fresh clover blossoms, less if dried, in a warmed glass container. Bring 2.5 cups of fresh nonchlorinated water to the boiling point and add it to the herbs. Cover the tea and steep for about 30 minutes, then strain. Drink cold, a few mouthfuls at a time throughout the day, up to one cup per day. The prepared tea may be kept for about two days in the refrigerator.

Ointment: Add fresh clover blossom to a glass pan of nonchlorinated water. Simmer on low heat or in a crock pot for two days. Strain. Allow most of the water to evaporate and combine the plant extract with an equal amount of melted beeswax. Pour while warm into small airtight containers.

Precautions

Red clover is a safe and mild remedy. No adverse effects have been reported in humans when taking therapeutic doses of the herb. Allergic reactions to red clover are rare but possible. Numerous reports of toxicity, even death, however, have been reported in cattle who overgraze in fields of clover.

Side effects

No side effects in humans have been reported for nonfermented red clover. Fermented extracts of red clover, however, may cause bleeding.

Interactions

No interactions have been reported between red clover and other herbs. It has, however, been reported to have adverse interactions with certain allopathic medications, particularly heparin, ticlopidine, and warfarin. Red clover also reduces the body's absorption of combined estrogens.

Resources

BOOKS

Coon, Nelson. *An American Herbal: Using Plants For Healing*. Emmaus, PA: Rodale Press, 1979.

Duke, James A., Ph.D. *The Green Pharmacy*. Emmaus, PA: Rodale Press, 1997.

Foster, Steven, and James A. Duke. *Peterson Field Guides, Eastern/Central Medicinal Plants*. Boston and New York: Houghton Mifflin Company, 1990.

Hoffmann, David. *The New Holistic Herbal,* 2nd ed. Boston: Element, 1986.

Hutchens, Alma R. *A Handbook of Native American Herbs*. Boston: Shambhala Publications, Inc., 1992.

PDR for Herbal Medicines. Montvale, NJ: Medical Economics Company, 1998.

Tyler, Varro E., Ph.D. *The Honest Herbal*. New York: Pharmaceutical Products Press, 1993.

Weiss, Gaea, and Shandor Weiss. *Growing & Using the Healing Herbs*. New York: Wings Books, 1992.

PERIODICALS

Howes, J., M. Waring, L. Huang, and L. G. Howes. "Long-Term Pharmacokinetics of an Extract of Isoflavones from Red Clover (*Trifolium pratense*)." *Journal of Alternative and Complementary Medicine* 8 (April 2002): 135-142.

Moyad, M. A. "Complementary/Alternative Therapies for Reducing Hot Flashes in Prostate Cancer Patients: Reevaluating the Existing Indirect Data from Studies of Breast Cancer and Postmenopausal Women." *Urology* 59 (April 2002) (4 Supplement 1): 20-33.

ORGANIZATIONS

American Botanical Council. 6200 Manor Road, Austin, TX 78714-4345. (512) 926-4900. www.herbalgram.org.

OTHER

Grieve, Mrs. M. *A Modern Herbal*. http://www.botanical.com.

Clare Hanrahan
Rebecca J. Frey, PhD

Red yeast rice extract

Description

Native to China, red yeast rice extract is the by-product of *Monascus purpureus* Went (red yeast) fermenting on rice. Part of the Monascaceae family, *Monascus purpureus* is identified by its ascospores. The color of the mycelium is initially white, but soon changes to pink and then yellow-orange due to an increase in acidity and the development of hyphae. They explain that as the culture ages, it is characterized by a dark crimson color at the substratum.

General use

Documented as early as 800 **A.D.**, Chinese red yeast rice was used in the preserving, flavoring, and coloring of food and wine. However, in addition to red yeast rice's culinary properties, it was soon discovered that red yeast rice possessed medicinal properties as well. The ancient Chinese pharmacopoeia, *Ben Cao Gang Mu-Dan Shi Bu Yi*, published during the Ming Dynasty (1368–1644), recorded a detailed description of red yeast rice and its manufacture. According to the pharmacopoeia, red yeast rice promotes blood circulation and stimulates the digestive system and spleen.

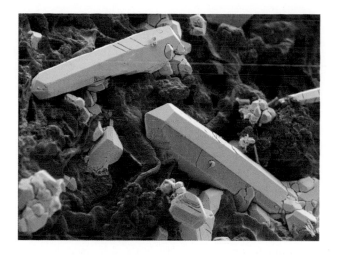

Red yeast rice results from fermenting regular rice with a fungus Monascus purpureus. *(Scimat / Photo Researchers, Inc.)*

Recent studies of red yeast rice indicate that it contains substances similar to those found in cholesterol-reducing (statin) prescription medications. In addition, research indicates red yeast rice may contain other cholesterol-reducing and be itself an agent useful in lowering **cholesterol**.

Traditional red yeast rice can be purchased in typical Chinese groceries. However, in this form, the extract possesses negligible to very low levels of statin compounds. Instead, manufacturers grow and process the *M. purpureus* Went under controlled conditions to increase the levels of statin. The powdered extract is then sold in capsule form.

In 2001, the Food and Drug Administration (FDA) determined that standardized red yeast rice extract (in this case, Cholestin®; developed by Pharmanex) possessed strong chemical similarities to the drug lovastatin, another cholesterol-reducing drug. Unfortunately, a pharmaceutical company, Merck & Co., trademarked lovastatin as Mevacor®. Because of the similarity, the FDA classified standardized red yeast rice extract as a drug. Under the Dietary Supplement Health Education Act of 1994, it could no longer be sold as a dietary supplement under penalty of law. As such, standardized red yeast rice extract has virtually disappeared from the United States marketplace.

Recent studies have indicated that taking the standardized dose (600 mg) of red yeast rice extract orally, two to four times per day, may assist in a significant reduction of total cholesterol (TC), low-density lipoprotein (LDL) cholesterol ("bad" cholesterol), and triglycerides (TG). It can also slightly increase levels of high-density lipoprotein (HDL) cholesterol ("good" cholesterol). Red yeast rice appears to achieve these benefits by reducing the

KEY TERMS

Ascomycete—Any class of higher fungi with septate hyphae and spores formed in the asci.

Ascospores—Any spores contained in the ascus, which is the oval or tubular spore case of an ascomycete.

Cholesterol—A waxy, fat-like substance, or lipid, required for important body functions. Excess cholesterol, however, can cause hardening of the arteries, which can lead to such serious health problems as heart disease. LDL cholesterol is considered "bad" because it can promote cholesterol build-up and hardened arteries. HDL cholesterol is considered "good" cholesterol because it helps break up cholesterol build-up.

HMG-CoA reductase—Hepetic hydroxy-methyl-glutaryl coenzyme A is an enzyme created in the liver that promotes the production of cholesterol.

Monacolin—An HMG-CoA reductase inhibitor, which assists in the lowering of cholesterol levels.

Rhabdomyolysis—The necrosis or disintegration of skeletal muscle.

Statin—An HMG-CoA reductase inhibitor, which assists in the lowering of cholesterol levels.

Triglycerides—A blood fat lipid that increase the risk of heart disease.

production of cholesterol in the liver. This cholesterol synthesis reduction stems from one ingredient in particular, monacolin, which acts as an inhibitor of the enzyme responsible for cholesterol production. (The enzyme is known as hepatic hydroxy-methyl-glutaryl coenzyme A (HMG-CoA) reductase.) By lowering high cholesterol levels and promoting blood circulation, red yeast rice may help reduce the risks of heart, coronary, and cerebral vascular diseases. As such, people suffering from high cholesterol (240 mg/dl or above) could benefit from using red yeast rice extract. According to the Natural Dietary Supplements Pocket Reference, a 20% decrease in total cholesterol has been documented for treatments longer than one month. Additionally, red yeast rice extract possesses antioxidant qualities.

Preparations

Although there have been several studies on red yeast rice extract, there remains little information regarding its safety for long-term usage. There are also certain medical risks associated with this extract. As such, it is strongly suggested that anyone considering

Red yeast rice extract

using red yeast rice extract for the prevention and treatment of high cholesterol consult with their physician before doing so. This is particularly important for people suffering from high cholesterol and/or **heart disease**. A baseline liver enzyme check is recommended beforehand, in addition to subsequent checks thereafter. In general, however, the recommended dose for adults is 600 mg (oral dose), two to four times per day.

Additionally, due to the 2001 FDA decision, only a doctor may legally prescribe standardized red yeast rice extract. As such, health-food stores now selling this product are doing so illegally. There are, however, several dietary supplements available to the public, which can be as effective as red yeast rice extract. Pharmanex, for example, has removed red yeast rice extract from their supplement, Cholestin®, and replaced it with other cholesterol-reducing, natural substances. It is advisable to consult with a physician regarding the available options.

Precautions

Due to the lack of medical evidence regarding red yeast rice extract's safety for use by youths and children, it is recommended that it not be given to people younger than age 20. Those at risk of or suffering from liver disease shouldn't take red yeast rice extract, as it may affect liver function. Due to the product's statin content, usage is also contraindicated for people with serious **infections** or physical disorders, who are pregnant or breastfeeding, or have had an organ transplant.

Side effects

Although the risks are low, usage can result in liver damage, kidney toxicity, and rhabdomyolysis (disintegration of skeletal muscle). Side effects are mild, including **headache**, **dizziness**, flatulence, **heartburn**, and stomachache. When the extract is no longer being taken, any side effects fade quickly.

Interactions

Because of its statin content, red yeast rice extract should not be taken with other HMG-CoA reductase inhibitors, such as atorvastatin and lovastatin. This interaction would increase the effects of these medications, thus increasing the risk of liver damage. However, **niacin** supplements can be safely used to enhance the cholesterol-lowering effects.

Due to the increased risk of rhabdomyolysis, red yeast rice extract should not be taken with high-dose nicotinic acid (more than 1,000 mg/per day). A physician should be contacted immediately if any muscle **pain**, tenderness, or weakness is experienced.

Alcohol consumption while using red yeast rice extract should not exceed two drinks a day. Also, grapefruit, grapefruit juice, and grapefruit products (like marmalade) should be strictly avoided. Grapefruit enhances the blood concentration of HMG-CoA reductase inhibitors by as much as 15 times, thus greatly increasing the risk of side effects and liver damage.

Resources

BOOKS

Burnham, T. H., S. L. Sjweain, and R. M. Short (eds.). *The Review of Natural Products*. Facts and Comparisons, 1997.

Kuhn, Winston. *Herbal Therapy and Supplements: A Scientific and Traditional Approach*. Lippincott, 2001.

McKenna, Dennis J., Kerry Hughes, and Kenneth Jones (eds.). *Natural Dietary Supplements Pocket Reference*. Institute for Natural Products Research, 2000.

PERIODICALS

Changling, Li, Zhu Yan, Wang Yinye, Jia-Shi Zhu, Joseph Chang, and David Kritchevsky. "Monascus Purpureus-fermented rice (red yeast rice): A natural food product that lowers blood cholesterol in animal models of hypercholesterolmia." *Nutrition Research* (February, 1998): 71–81.

Havel, Richard. "Dietary supplement or drug? The case of Cholestin." *American Journal of Clinical Nutrition* (February, 1999): 175–176.

Heber, David, A. Lembertas, Q. Y. Lu, S. Bowerman, and V. L. Go. "An analysis of nine proprietary Chinese red yeast rice dietary supplements: Implication of variability in chemical profile and contents." *The Journal of Alternative and Complementary Medicine* (April, 2001): 133–139.

Heber, David, Ian Yip, Judith Ashley, David Elashoff, Robert Elashoff, and Vay Go. "Cholesterol-lowering effects of a proprietary Chinese red-yeast-rice dietary supplement." *American Journal of Clinical Nutrition* (February, 1999): 231–236.

Juzlova, P., L. Martinkova, and V. Kren. "Secondary metabolites of the fungus Monascus: a review." *Journal of Industrial Microbiology* (March 1996): 163–170.

Wang, Junxian, Zongliang Lu, Jiamin Chi, et al. "Multicenter clinical trial of the serum lipid-lowering effects of a Monascus Purpureus (red yeast) rice preparation from traditional Chinese medicine." *Current Therapeutic Research* (December 1997): 964–978.

OTHER

"Red Yeast Rice." Health and Age. [cited June 5, 2004]. http://www.healthandage.com/html/res/com/ConsSupplements/RedYeastRicecs.html.

"Red Yeast Rice." Whole Health MD. [cited June 5, 2004]. http://www.wholehealthmd.com/refshelf/substances_view/1,1525,10054,00.html.

"Red Yeast Rice Analysis." Herbal Alternatives. [cited June 5, 2004]. http://www.dotcomtech.co.uk/content/herbal_remedies/cholesterol/redyeastanalysis.html.

Sharpe, Ed. "Red yeast rice: Cholesterol-busting superfood or just another pharmaceutical?" [cited June 5, 2004]. http://www.dclano.com/referencearticles/red-yeast-rice-sharpe.html.

Lee Ann Paradise

Reflexology

Definition

Reflexology is a therapeutic method of relieving **pain** by stimulating predefined pressure points on the feet and hands. This controlled pressure is designed to alleviate the source of the discomfort. In the absence of any particular malady or abnormality, reflexology may be as effective for promoting good health and for preventing illness as it may be for relieving symptoms of **stress**, injury, and illness.

Reflexologists work from maps of predefined pressure points that are located on the hands and feet. These pressure points are reputed to connect directly through the nervous system and to affect the bodily organs and glands. The reflexologist manipulates the pressure points according to specific techniques of reflexology therapy. By means of this touching therapy and the application of pressure at the respective foot or hand location, the reflexologist attempts to strengthen any part of the body that is the source of pain, illness, or potential debility.

Origins

Reflexology is a healing art of ancient origin. Although its origins are not well documented, it

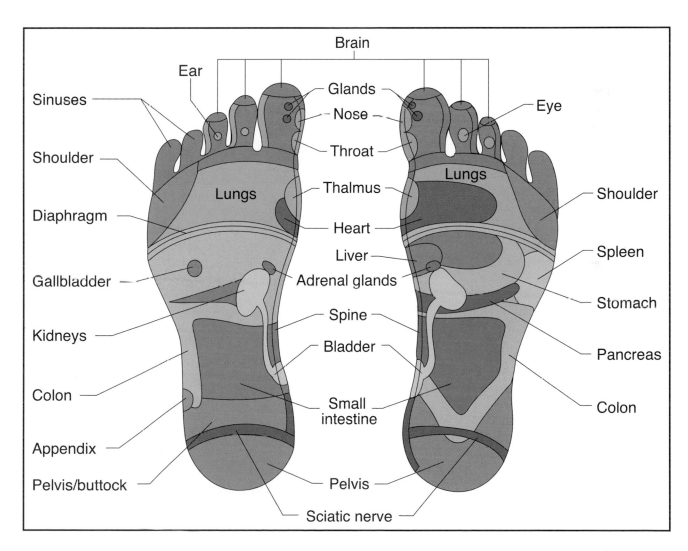

Reflexology employs the principle that the reflex points on the feet, when hand pressure is applied, will reflexively stimulate energy to a related muscle or organ in the body and promote healing. *(Illustration by GGS Information Services. Cengage Learning, Gale)*

dates to 4,000-plus years ago. Evidence of this exists in reliefs found on the walls of a Sixth Dynasty Egyptian tomb (c. 2450 B.C.) that depict two seated men receiving massage on their hands and feet. From Egypt, the practice may have entered the Western world during the conquests of the Roman Empire. The concepts of reflexology have also been traced to pre-dynastic China (possibly as early as 3000 B.C.) and to ancient Indian medicine. In addition, the Inca civilization may have subscribed to the theories of reflexology and passed on the practice of this treatment to the Native Americans in the territories that eventually became parts of the United States.

In modern times, Sir Henry Head first investigated the concepts underlying reflexology in England in the 1890s. Therapists in Germany and Russia were researching similar notions at approximately the same time, although with a different focus. Less than two decades later, the physician William H. Fitzgerald presented a similar concept that he called zone analgesia or zone therapy. Fitzgerald's zone analgesia was a method of relieving pain through the application of pressure to specific locations throughout the entire body. Fitzgerald divided the body into 10 vertical zones, five on each side, that extended from the head to the fingertips and toes, and from front to back. Every aspect of the human body appears in one of these 10 zones, and each zone has a reflex area on the hands and feet. Fitzgerald and his colleague, Edwin Bowers, demonstrated that by applying pressure on one area of the body, they could anesthetize or reduce pain in a corresponding part. In 1917, Fitzgerald and Bowers published *Relieving Pain at Home*, an explanation of zone therapy.

In the 1930s, the physical therapist Eunice D. Ingham explored the direction of the therapy and made the startling discovery that pressure points on the human foot were situated in a mirror image of the corresponding organs of the body with which the respective pressure points were associated. Ingham documented her findings, which formed the basis of reflexology, in *Stories the Feet Can Tell*, published in 1938. Although Ingham's work in reflexology was inaccurately described as zone therapy by some, there are differences between the two therapies of pressure analgesia. Among the more marked differences, reflexology defines a precise correlation between pressure points and afflicted areas of the body. Furthermore, Ingham divided each foot and hand into 12 respective pressure zones, in contrast to the 10 vertical divisions that encompass the entire body in Fitzgerald's zone therapy.

In 1968 two siblings, Dwight Byers and Eusebia Messenger, established the National Institute of

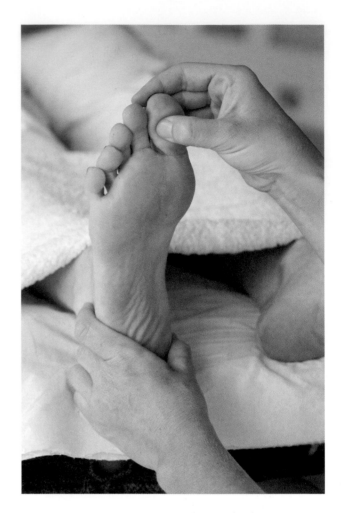

Reflexology foot massage. *(© Niall McDiarmid / Alamy)*

Reflexology. By the early 1970s the institute had grown and was renamed the International Institute of Reflexology.

Benefits

Reflexology promotes healing by stimulating the nerves in the body and encouraging the flow of blood. In the process, reflexology not only quells the sensation of pain but relieves the source of the pain as well.

Anecdotally, reflexologists claim success in the treatment of a variety of conditions and injuries. One condition is **fibromyalgia**. People with this disease are encouraged to undergo reflexology therapy to alleviate any of a number of chronic bowel syndromes associated with the condition. Frequent brief sessions of reflexology therapy are also recommended as an alternative to drug therapy for controlling the muscle pain related to fibromyalgia and for relieving difficult breathing caused by tightness in the muscles of the patient's neck and throat.

EUNICE D. INGHAM (1889–1974)

Eunice D. Ingham was born on February 24, 1889. A physical therapist by occupation, she was a colleague of Dr. Shelby Riley, who along with Dr. W. H. Fitzgerald actively developed zone therapy, a similar but distinct therapy from reflexology. Unlike reflexology, zone therapy does not connect the zones with the body as a whole. In the 1930s, Ingham discovered an unmistakable pattern of reflexes on the human foot; she subsequently devoted the rest of her life to publicizing the message of reflexology until shortly before her death on December 10, 1974.

Ingham traveled and lectured widely about reflexology, initially to audiences of extremely desperate or aging patients who had lost hope in finding relief. Because of their sometimes astonishing improvement, reflexology became better known and respected among the medical community and gained credibility for its therapeutic value. Ingham described her theories of reflexology in her 1938 book, entitled *Stories the Feet Can Tell*, which included a map of the reflex points on the feet and the organs that they parallel. The book was translated into seven languages, although it was erroneously published as *Zone Therapy* in some countries, an error which led to misunderstanding about the true nature of reflexology and inaccurately linked it to zone therapy.

Practitioners claim that when applied properly, reflexology can alleviate allergy symptoms, as well as stress, back pain, and chronic **fatigue**. The techniques of reflexology can be performed conveniently on the hand in situations in which a session on the feet is not practical, although practitioners consider the effectiveness of limited hand therapy to be less pronounced than with the foot pressure therapy.

Description

In a typical reflexology treatment, the therapist and patient engage in a preliminary discussion prior to therapy to enable the therapist to focus more accurately on the patient's specific complaints and to determine the appropriate pressure points for treatment.

A reflexology session involves pressure treatment that is most commonly administered in foot therapy sessions of approximately 40 to 45 minutes in duration. The foot therapy may be followed by a brief 15-minute hand therapy session. No artificial devices or special equipment are associated with this therapy. The human hand is the primary tool used in reflexology. The therapist applies controlled pressure with the thumb and forefinger, generally working toward the heel of the foot or the outer palm of the hand. Most reflexologists apply pressure with their thumbs bent; however, some also use simple implements, such as the eraser end of a pencil. Reflexology therapy is not massage, and it is not a substitute for medical treatment.

Reflexology is a complex system that identifies and addresses the mass of 7,000 nerve endings that are contained in the foot. Additional reflexology addresses the nerves that are located in the hand. This completely natural therapy is used to afford relief without the use of drugs.

Preparations

In order to realize maximum benefit from a reflexology session, the therapist as well as the patient should be situated so as to afford optimal comfort for both. Patients in general receive treatment in a reclining position, with the therapist positioned as necessary—to work on bare feet or on bare hands.

A reflexology patient removes both shoes and socks in order to receive treatment. No other preparation is involved. No prescription drugs, creams, oils, or lotions are used on the skin.

Precautions

Reflexology is completely safe. It may even be self-administered in a limited form whenever desired. The qualified reflexologist offers a clear and open disclaimer that reflexology does not constitute medical treatment in any form, nor is reflexology given as a substitute for medical advice or treatment. The ultimate purpose of the therapy is to promote wellness; fundamentally it is a form of preventive therapy.

People with serious and long-term medical problems are urged to seek the advice of a physician. Diabetes patients in particular are urged to approach this therapy cautiously. Likewise pregnant women are cautioned emphatically to avoid reflexology during the early phases of **pregnancy** altogether, as accidentally induced labor and subsequent premature delivery can result from reflexology treatment.

A consultation with a reflexologist is recommended in order to determine the safety and appropriateness of reflexology therapy for a specific health problem or condition.

Side effects

Because reflexology is intended to normalize the body functions, the therapy does not cause a condition to worsen. Most patients find that pain diminishes over the course of the therapy. It has been noted, however, that some patients experience greater discomfort in the second session than in the first session because a significant easing of pain and tension is generally associated with the initial therapy session. As a result, when pressure is reapplied to the tender points of the foot during the second session, the sensitivity has been heightened. This increase in sensitivity may cause minor additional discomfort for the patient.

Research and general acceptance

Reflexology is practiced worldwide at different levels of medical care. The Association of Reflexologists lists nearly six dozen professional organizations worldwide from the United States to the Japan, and from Ireland to India. These associations include:

- Academy of Reflexology Austria
- Reflexology Association of British Columbia
- China Reflexology Association
- Danish Reflexologists Association
- Holistic Association of Reflexologists Japan
- Polish Instytut of Reflexology (Polish language)
- Association of Reflexology Portugal
- South African Reflexology Society
- British Reflexology Association
- Reflexology Association of America

Several studies and/or reports have indicated the reflexology is effective in treating pain associated with child birth, **cancer**, and **multiple sclerosis**; in treating so-called "mousearm" arising from extended use of a computer mouse; and in treating back pain. Additional research, however, is necessary.

Regulatory status

Ongoing legislative debate ensued during the 1990s regarding the legal status of the reflexology trade. The reflexology community, along with legislators and other bodywork practitioners, engaged in reassessment of the reflexology business and its relationship to **massage therapy** and massage parlors. Organizations and individuals brought judicial appeals of certain court cases that threatened the legitimate licensing of reflexologists as practitioners of alternative medicine. Such professional reflexology interests as the RAA documented in detail the disparities between reflexology and massage, citing the purpose of reflexology, which is to stimulate internal body functions (glands and organs) as opposed to the topical muscular and joint relief associated with massage. In a status update in 1998 the association reported that 19 states had laws requiring the licensing of massage/reflexology therapists. Licensing laws established educational requirements and required candidates to pass written, oral, and/or practical examinations.

Also at issue was a trend among municipalities to license massage parlors (and reflexologists) under the business codes affecting adult entertainment business. B. Kunz and K. Kunz reported that judicial decisions in two states—Tennessee and New Mexico—had excluded the practice of reflexology practice from the laws pertaining to massage parlors. Those courts held that reflexology is a business separate and distinct from massage parlors and deserving of its own respective licensing standards. In Sacramento, California, reflexologists petitioned successfully to become licensed as practitioners of somatic therapy rather than as providers of adult entertainment. Likewise, in the Canadian province of Ontario, a nonprofit organization to register reflexology practitioners was established in order to define a distinct classification for therapists separate from erotic body rubbers, which was the original classification given to reflexologists. Work to legitimize reflexology was continuing as of 2008.

Training and certification

Reflexology is taught in seminars, classes, and training films. In the United States, certification is earned after students meet national standards for skill and knowledge by taking and passing an examination that has written, practical, and documentation components. The documentation component of the certification exam is the performance of reflexology sessions on clients. The exam is prepared by the independently organized American Reflexology Certification Board (ARCB), which certifies the competency of reflexology practitioners on an individual basis. To prepare for the exam, students frequently enroll in reflexology programs, but it lieu of that, the ARCB recommends the following:

- 40 hours of reflexology history, theory
- 55 hours of anatomy and physiology

KEY TERMS

Pressure points—Specific locations on the feet and hands that correspond to nerve endings. Pressure on these locations are used to connect to and affect the organs and glands of the human body via the spinal cord.

Zone therapy—Also called zone analgesia, a method of relieving pain by applying pressure to specific points on the body. It was developed in the early 20th century by William Fitzgerald.

- five hours of business ethics and standards

- 10 hours of supervised practicum

In addition, the ARCB makes a study guide available to students who apply for and are accepted for testing with the exam.

Individuals can only legally practice reflexology in the United States by abiding by any and all state, city, and county laws and regulations. According to the ARCB, only North Dakota and Tennessee had reflexology state-level laws regulating reflexology as of early 2008. The ARCB noted that other states had statewide massage laws that may refer to reflexology.

Once individuals are certified, they must pay an annual fee to the ARCB and obtain continuing education in the amount of 12 hours every two years to maintain the certification. If certification lapses in annual fee or continuing education for a certain period of time, they must retake the written and practical exams.

Resources

BOOKS

Kolster, Bernard C., and Astrid Waskowiak Inge. *The Reflexology Atlas*. Rochester, VT: Healing Arts Press, 2006.

Kunz, Barbara, and Kevin Kunz. *Complete Reflexology for Life*. London: DK Adult, 2007.

Muller, Marie-France. *Facial Reflexology: A Self-care Manual*. Rochester, VT: Healing Arts Press, 2005.

OTHER

American Reflexology Certification Board. "The Differences Between Reflexology and Massage." Reflexology Association of America. http://www.reflexology-usa.org/articles/differences.html (March 28, 2008).

ORGANIZATIONS

Association of Reflexologists, 5 Fore Street, Taunton Somerset, England, TA1 1HX, http://www.aor.org.uk.

International Institute of Reflexology, 5650 First Avenue North, PO Box 12642, St. Petersburg, FL, 33733-2642, (727) 343-4811, http://www.reflexology-usa.net/.

Reflexology Association of America, 4012 Rainbow St. KPMB#585, Las Vegas, NV, 89103-2059, (401) 578-6661, http://www.reflexology-usa.org/.

Gloria Cooksey
Leslie Mertz, Ph.D.

Reiki

Definition

Reiki is a form of therapy that uses simple hands-on, no-touch, and visualization techniques, with the goal of improving the flow of life energy in a person. Reiki (pronounced *ray-key*) means "universal life energy" in Japanese, and Reiki practitioners are trained to detect and alleviate problems of energy flow on the physical, emotional, and spiritual level. Reiki touch therapy is used in much the same way to achieve similar effects that traditional **massage therapy** is used—to relieve **stress** and pain, and to improve the symptoms of various health conditions.

Origins

Reiki was developed in the mid–1800s by Dr. Mikao Usui, a Japanese scholar of religion. According to the story that has been passed down among reiki teachers, Usui was a Christian who was intrigued by the idea that Christ could heal sick people by touching them with his hands. Searching for clues that would explain the secrets of healing with hands, Usui made a long pilgrimage around the world, visiting many ancient religious sects and studying ancient books. Some reiki teachers claim that Usui found clues leading back nearly 10,000 years to healing arts that originated in ancient Tibet. During his intense studies, Usui claimed he had a spiritual experience, which enabled him to heal with his own hands by becoming aware of and tapping into the universal life force. After that, he dedicated his life to helping the sick and poor. His reputation grew as he healed sick people for many years in Kyoto, Japan. Before his death, Usui passed on his healing insights using universal life energy to Dr. Chujiru Hayashi, a close acquaintance. Hayashi, in turn, passed on the healing techniques in 1938 to Hawayo Takata, a Japanese woman from Hawaii, whom he had cured of life-threatening illness using reiki methods. Takata became a firm believer and proponent of reiki, and during the 1970s formed an initiation program for training reiki masters to preserve Usui's teachings. Before she died, she prepared her granddaughter, Phyllis Lei Furumoto, to continue the lineage. Takata had personally trained 21 practitioners before she died at the age of 80 in 1980. Along with other reiki masters authorized by Takata, Furumoto formed the reiki Alliance. A faction led by Barbara Ray formed the American Reiki Association, which was known as Radiance Technique Association International. Today, there are over 1,000 reiki masters practicing around the world, whose methods can all be traced back directly to Dr. Usui.

Benefits

Reiki claims to provide many of the same benefits as traditional massage therapy, such as reducing stress, stimulating the immune system, increasing energy, and relieving the **pain** and symptoms of health conditions. Practitioners have reported success in helping patients with acute and chronic illnesses, from **asthma** and arthritis to trauma and recovery from surgery. Reiki is a gentle and safe technique, and has been used successfully in some hospitals. It has been found to be very calming and reassuring for those suffering from severe or fatal conditions. Reiki can been used by doctors, nurses, psychologists and other health professionals to bring touch and deeper caring into their healing practices.

Description

The basic philosophy of reiki

The basic concept underlying reiki is that the body has an energy field that is central to its health and proper functioning, and this energy travels in certain pathways that can become blocked or weakened. This idea of energy flow in the body is also a central concept in Ayurvedic medicine and **traditional Chinese medicine**, including acupuncture.

Reiki practitioners believe that everyone has the potential to access the universal life energy, but that over time most people's systems become blocked and the energy becomes weakened in them. A reiki practitioner is trained to be able to detect these blockages, and practitioners will use their hands, thoughts, and own energy fields to improve the energy flow in a patient. Reiki is one of the more esoteric alternative medical practices, because no one is sure exactly how it works on the physiological level. Practitioners claim that it works on very subtle energy levels, or possibly works on the *chakra* system. The chakras are the system of seven energy centers along the middle of

the body believed to be connected with the nervous and endocrine systems, as defined by **yoga** and Ayurvedic medicine. Reiki masters claim that healing energy can even be sent to a person from far away, noting that reiki works on the same principles that enables praying to work for some patients, although a practitioner needs advanced training to be able to send energy from afar.

According to the original principles of Usui, patients must also have a proper attitude for reiki to work most effectively. Patients must take responsibility for their own health, and must want to be healed. Furthermore, when energy is received from a reiki healer, patients must be willing to give back energy to others, and to compensate the healer in some way, as well. Finally, Usui claimed that a healing attitude was free from worry and fear, was filled with gratitude for life and for others, and placed emphasis on each person finding honest and meaningful work in their lives—all this, in order to complete the picture of overall health.

A reiki session

Reiki sessions can take various forms, but most commonly resemble typical bodywork appointments, where the receiver lies clothed on his or her back on a flat surface or massage table. A session generally lasts from an hour to an hour and a half. Reiki is a simple procedure, consisting of calm and concentrated touching, with the practitioner focusing on healing and giving energy to specific areas on the receiver's body. Practitioners place their hands over positions on the body where the organs and endocrine glands reside, and the areas that correspond to the chakra centers. Practitioners also use mental visualization to send healing energy to areas of the receiver's body that need it. In special cases or with injuries, a no-touch technique is used, in which the practitioner's hands are sometimes held just above the body without touching it. Advanced practitioners rely on intuition and experience to determine which areas of a body need the most energy healing.

The practitioner's hands are held flat against the receiver's body, with the fingertips touching. There can be over 20 positions on both sides of the body where the hands are placed. The positions begin at the crown of the head and move towards the feet. The receiver usually turns over once during the session. The practitioner's hands are held in each position for a usually five minutes, to allow the transfer of energy and the healing process to take place. In each position, the hands are kept stationary, unlike typical massage where the hands move, and both the giver and receiver attempt to maintain an attitude of awareness, openness, and caring.

Reiki practitioners recommend that those receiving reiki for the first time go through a series of three to four initial treatments over the course of about a week, to allow for cleansing and the initial readjustment of energy. Reiki sessions can cost from $30–100 per session. Insurance coverage is rare, and consumers should consult their individual policies as to whether or not such therapies are included.

Self-treatment with reiki

Although reiki practitioners believe that formal training is necessary to learn the proper methods of energy channeling and healing, individuals can still use some of the basic positions of reiki to relieve stress and to stimulate healing on themselves or another. The positions can be performed anywhere and for however long they are needed. Positions generally move from the top of the body down, but positions can be used wherever there is pain or stress. Mental attitude is important during reiki; the mind should be cleared of all stressful thoughts and concentrated on compassion, love, and peace as forms of energy that are surrounding, entering, and healing the body.

The following positions are illustrated in *Reiki: Energy Medicine:*

- Position one: Hands are placed on the top of the head, with the wrists near the ears and the fingertips touching on the crown of the head. Eyes should be closed. Hold for five minutes or more, until the mind feels clear and calm.

- Position two: Cup the hands slightly and place the palms over the closed eyes, with the fingers resting on the forehead.

- Position three: Place the hands on the sides of the head, with the thumbs behind the ear and the palms over the lower jaws, with the fingers covering the temples.

- Position four: Place one hand on the back of the neck, at the base of the skull, and put the other hand on the head just above it, parallel to it.

- Position five: Wrap the hands around the front of the throat, and rest them there gently with the heels of the hands touching in front.

- Position six: Place each hand on top of a shoulder, close to the side of neck, on top of the trapezius muscle.

- Position seven: Form a T-shape with the hands over the chest, with the left hand covering the heart and the right hand above it, covering the upper part of the chest.

- Position eight: The hands are placed flat against the front of the body with fingertips touching. Hold for five minutes or so, and repeat four or five times, moving down a hand-width each time until the pelvic region is reached, which is covered with a v-shape of the hands. Then, for the final position, repeat this technique on the back, beginning as close to the shoulders as the hands can reach, and ending by forming a T-shape with the hands at the base of the spine.

Side effects

Reiki generally has no side effects, as it is a very low-impact and gentle procedure. Some receivers report feeling tingling or sensations of heat or cold during treatment. Others have reported sadness or anxiety during treatment, which practitioners claim are buried or repressed emotions being released by the new energy flow.

Research and general acceptance

Reiki has been used in major clinics and hospitals as part of alternative healing practice, and doctors, dentists, nurses, and other health professionals have been trained to use its gentle touch techniques as part of their practice. It appears to offer particular benefits to special-care patients and their caregivers. Reiki has also become increasingly popular among veterinarians in small-animal practices for treating behavioral disorders as well as physical illnesses in dogs and cats. To date, the little scientific research that has been conducted with reiki implies that its techniques bring about the *relaxation response*, in which stress levels decrease, and immune response increases. Reiki practitioners claim that the most important measurement of their technique is whether the individual feels better after treatment. They also claim that science cannot measure the subtle energy changes that they are attempting to make.

MIKAO USUI (1865–1926)

Mikao Usui, born in the Gifu Prefecture (Japan), was an ethereal child who sought to unravel the mysteries of the universe. As an adult he developed an interest in the metaphysical healing talent of Buddha. Usui became determined to regenerate the healing secrets of Buddha in order to improve the lot of humanity. He traveled to many temples and spoke with holy people, but all said that the secret of Buddha's powers were lost to the world due to lack of use.

Eventually the abbot of a Zen monastery encouraged Usui to study the ancient writings containing the secrets on healing. Usui learned two new languages, Chinese and Sanskrit, in order to understand the writings better, and from his reading he obtained the formula for healing. The Sutras in particular provided the enlightenment that he sought.

Usui next set out to obtain the power to heal. It is widely believed that he developed that ability after spending 21 days in retreat and in fasting on the holy Mountain of Kori-yama, where he had a vision of light and received the knowledge of the symbols of reiki and their use in healing. He officially formulated Usui Reiki therapy in 1922 and touted as many as one million followers during his lifetime.

Prior to the transition (death) of Usui, he imparted the secrets of healing to 16 teachers in order that the secrets would not be lost again.

Training and certification

Reiki practitioners undergo a series of *attunements*, which are sessions with reiki masters that teach the basic methods of energy healing. Several organizations provide resources for reiki training. Reiki practitioners believe these attunements are necessary for correct technique. The masters teach each person how to activate the universal life energy in themselves before they can pass it on to others. These initiations often are held during weekend workshops. Trainees can achieve up to four levels of attunements, until they reach the level of master themselves. The certification process is not a formal one; masters approve students when they feel satisfied with their progress.

Resources

BOOKS

Baginski, B.J. and S. Sharamon. *Reiki: Universal Life Energy*. Mendocino, CA: LifeRhythm, 1988.

Barnett, Libby and Maggie Chambers. *Reiki: Energy Medicine*. Rochester, VT: Healing Arts Press, 1996.

Brown, Fran. *Living Reiki: Takata's Teachings*. Mendocino, CA: LifeRhythm, 1992.

PERIODICALS

Feary, A. M. "Touching the Fragile Baby: Looking at Touch in the Special Care Nursery (SCN)." *Australian Journal of Holistic Nursing* 9 (April 2002): 44-48.

Rexilius, S. J., et al. "Therapeutic Effects of Massage Therapy and Handling Touch on Caregivers of Patients Undergoing Autologous Hematopoietic Stem Cell Transplant." *Oncology Nursing Forum* 29 (April 2002): E35-E44.

ORGANIZATIONS

The International Association of Reiki Professionals. P.O. Box 481, Winchester, MA 01890. www.iarp.org.

OTHER

The American Reiki Masters Association (ARMA). P.O. Box 130, Lake City, FL 32056–0130. (904) 755–9638.

The Center for Reiki Training. 29209 Northwestern Highway, #592, Southfield, MI 48034. (800) 332–8112.

Global Reiki Healing Network. www.reiki.org.

Reiki Alliance. P.O. Box 41, Cataldo, ID 83810–1041. (208)682–3535.

Douglas Dupler
Rebecca J. Frey, PhD

Reishi mushroom

Description

Reishi mushrooms are some of the most widely used medicinal mushrooms in the world. Their scientific name is *Ganoderma lucidum*. In Chinese medicine, reishi mushrooms are known as *ling zhi*, which means spiritual plant as the Chinese believe the herb is healing for the spirit. Some Asians make good luck charms from the mushrooms in addition to using them as medicine.

The Latin name *Ganoderma* means shiny skin, which describes the reddish brown caps of the mushrooms. Reishi mushrooms are kidney-shaped and grow to 8 in (20 cm) or more in diameter. They grow in moist and temperate forest areas of Asia, Europe, South America, and the United States. Reishi mushrooms typically attach themselves to trees, particularly **oak** and plum trees.

Reishi mushrooms have a long history. They have been used in China and Japan for nearly 4,000 years as a

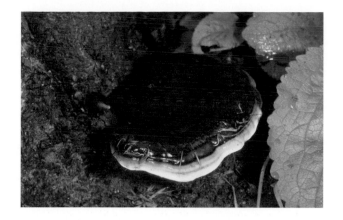

Reishi mushroom. *(© blickwinkel / Alamy)*

health tonic and as folk medicine for liver problems, heart conditions, **asthma**, **cancer**, high blood pressure, and arthritis. In **Traditional Chinese medicine**, reishi mushrooms are classified in a group of herbs known as *Fu Zheng*, which Chinese herbalists believe are the most powerful herbs for all-around strength, health, and longevity. Other Fu Zheng herbs include **Korean ginseng** and **astragalus**. Reishi mushrooms have been rare and expensive for most of their history because they are difficult to cultivate and find in the wild. In the 1980s, a Japanese man named Shigeaki Mori developed an intricate and effective method of cultivating them, which has made them widely available and affordable.

Reishi mushrooms have been well researched and tested, mostly in China and Japan. Scientists have isolated several chemicals in them that have pharmacological (medicinal) effects on the body. Reishi mushrooms contain compounds called polysaccharides, which have been shown to help the body fight cancerous tumors and also stimulate the immune system to combat **infections** and viruses. In studies on mice, reishi mushrooms have shown very strong results against cancerous tumors. One Japanese study suggests that reishi mushrooms may serve as a chemopreventive against colon cancer.

Other substances called triterpenes have been found in reishi mushrooms and shown to lower blood pressure and improve circulation. Reishi mushrooms also contain sterols, which may influence the hormonal system; and natural antihistamines, which reduce allergic reactions and inflammation in the body. More recently, reishi mushrooms have been identified as a source of **antioxidants**, which are enzymes or other organic compounds that counteract the damaging effects of oxidation on human tissue.

In Asia, numerous clinical studies with humans have documented reishi mushrooms' healing properties. They have shown significant results in treating **hepatitis**, chronic **bronchitis**, asthma, and **heart disease**. Reishi mushrooms have also been shown to lower blood pressure, lower **cholesterol**, increase white blood cell count, reduce allergic reactions, and have a calming effect on the central nervous system when given to humans in observed studies.

General use

Reishi mushrooms are recommended as a general tonic for health, energy, and longevity. They are prescribed for diseases including coronary heart disease, cancer, and **AIDS**; and for such chronic infections as bronchitis, hepatitis, and **mononucleosis**. Reishi mushrooms are also used to treat high blood pressure, asthma, nervous disorders, **chronic fatigue syndrome**, and arthritis. In China, they are used by mountain climbers to combat altitude sickness and are given as an antidote to patients who have eaten poisonous mushrooms.

Preparations

Reishi mushrooms are available dried and as powder, tinctures, tablets, capsules, and syrup. Reishi products can be found in health food stores, herb stores, and Chinese markets. The recommended daily dosage varies with conditions. For severe conditions such as cancer, heart disease, and chronic infections, 9–15 g daily in three equally divided dosages is recommended. For a general health tonic and for less severe conditions of asthma, high blood pressure, infections, and nervous disorders, 2–6 g can be taken daily, in three equal portions.

Tea can be made from dried mushrooms or powder, and the recommended ratio is 2–5 g of dried mushroom per liter of water. The mixture should be simmered on low heat for more than two hours, to extract all the active ingredients. The tea can be drunk twice daily. For severe health conditions or for an antidote to mushroom poisoning, some herbalists recommend a strong reishi tea mixture, with up to 20 g of dried mushrooms per liter of water.

Precautions

People with **allergies** to molds or fungi should use care with reishi mushrooms, although allergic reactions to them are generally rare. Consumers should search for reishi products that are made by reputable manufacturers. Some dried mushrooms have been sold as Reishi mushrooms when they were actually similar mushrooms by the scientific names of *Ganoderma oregonense* and *Ganoderma tsugae*. These resemble reishi mushrooms in appearance and taste and are in the same genus, but according to herbalists have different and less-effective healing properties.

Side effects

In clinical studies, reishi mushrooms have been shown to be nontoxic in high doses, and severe side effects have not been observed. Mild side effects may include stomach upset, **dry mouth**, **diarrhea**, and skin rash, and generally disappear after several days. Side effects can be alleviated by stopping use, or in the case of stomach upset and diarrhea, taking the supplement with meals.

Interactions

For treating severe conditions, large doses of **vitamin C**, from 1–10 g per day, may be prescribed in conjunction with reishi mushrooms. Prescribing vitamin C has been observed to reduce the side effect of diarrhea that may occur with patients who are given large doses of reishi mushrooms.

Reishi mushrooms have been reported to intensify the effects of blood-thinning (anticoagulant) drugs, including aspirin, dalteparin **sodium**, enoxaparin sodium, and warfarin. Patients taking these medications should not use tonics or other preparations containing reishi mushrooms without consulting their physicians.

Resources

BOOKS

Hobbs, Christopher. *Medicinal Mushrooms.* Loveland, CO: Botanica, 1986.

Lu, Henry C. *Chinese Herbal Cures.* New York: Sterling, 1994.

Willard, Terry, Ph.D. *Reishi Mushroom: Herb of Spiritual Potency and Medical Wonder.* Issaquah, Washington: Sylvan, 1990.

PERIODICALS

Bao, X. F., X. S. Wang, Q. Dong, et al. "Structural Features of Immunologically Active Polysaccharides from *Ganoderma lucidum*." *Phytochemistry* 59 (January 2002): 175-181.

Lu, H., E. Kyo, T. Uesaka, et al. "Prevention of Development of N,N'-Dimethylhydrazine-Induced Colon Tumors by a Water-Soluble Extract from Cultured Medium of *Ganoderma lucidum* (Rei-shi) Mycelia in Male ICR Mice." *International Journal of Molecular Medicine* 9 (February 2002): 113-117.

Shi, Y. L., A. E. James, I. F. Benzie, and J. A. Buswell. "Mushroom-Derived Preparations in the Prevention of H2O2-Induced Oxidative Damage to Cellular DNA." *Teratogenesis, Carcinogenesis, and Mutagenesis* 22 (2002): 103-111.

Wang, Y. Y., K. H. Khoo, S. T. Chen, et al. "Studies on the Immuno-Modulating and Antitumor Activities of *Ganoderma lucidum* (Reishi) Polysaccharides: Functional and Proteomic Analyses of a Fucose-Containing Glycoprotein Fraction Responsible for the Activities." *Bioorganic and Medicinal Chemistry* 10 (April 2002): 1057-1062.

ORGANIZATIONS

Herb Research Foundation. 1007 Pearl Street, Boulder, CO 80302. (303)449–2265.

Douglas Dupler
Rebecca J. Frey, PhD

Relaxation

Definition

Relaxation therapy is a broad term used to describe a number of techniques that promote **stress** reduction, the elimination of tension throughout the body, and a calm and peaceful state of mind.

Origins

Relaxation therapy as a general tern includes various forms: transcendental **meditation** (TM), **yoga**, t'ai chi, **qigong**, and vipassana (a Buddhist form of meditation meaning insight and also known as mindfulness meditation). Progressive relaxation, a treatment that is designed to rid the body of **anxiety** and related tension through progressive relaxation of the muscle groups, was first described by Edmund Jacobson in his book *Progressive Relaxation*, published in 1929. In 1975, Herbert Benson published his groundbreaking work *The Relaxation Response*, which described in detail the stress-reduction mechanism in the body that short-circuits the "fight-or-flight" response and lowers blood pressure, relieves muscle tension, and controls heart rate. This work gave further credence and legitimacy to the link between mind and body medicine. A number of relaxation techniques used commonly in the early 2000s, such as cue-controlled relaxation, are a direct result of Benson's work in this area.

Benefits

Stress and tension have been linked to numerous ailments, including **heart disease**, high blood pressure, **atherosclerosis**, **irritable bowel syndrome**, ulcers, anxiety disorders, **insomnia**, and **substance abuse**. Stress can also trigger a number of distinct physical symptoms, including **nausea**, **headache**, **hair loss**, **fatigue**, and muscle **pain**. Relaxation therapies have been shown to reduce the incidence and severity of stress-related diseases and disorders in many patients.

Description

A number of different relaxation methods are available. Some of the most widely taught and most frequently practiced by healthcare providers are progressive relaxation, cue-controlled relaxation, breathing exercises, **guided imagery**, and **biofeedback**.

Progressive relaxation

Progressive relaxation is performed by first tensing, and then relaxing, the muscles of the body, one group at a time. Muscle groups can be divided a number of different ways, but a common method is to use the following groupings: 1) Hands and arms; 2) head, neck, and shoulders; 3) torso, including chest, stomach and back; and 4) buttocks, thighs, lower legs, and feet. The patient lies or sits in a comfortable position and then starts with the first muscle group, focusing on the feeling of the muscles and the absence or presence of tension. The patient then tenses the first muscle in the group, holds the tension for approximately five seconds, and releases and relaxes for up to 30 seconds. The contrast allows the individual to notice difference between feelings of tension and those of relaxation. The procedure is repeated with the next muscle in the group and so on, until the first group is completed. The patient then starts on the next muscle group.

Progressive relaxation can be guided with verbal cues and scripts, either memorized by the patient or provided on instructional audiotapes. The procedure remains the same, but the individual is prompted on which muscles to flex and relax and given other cues about noticing the difference between the tense and relaxed state. Some individuals may prefer progressive relaxation that is prompted with a tape because it allows them to completely clear their minds and to just follow instructions.

Deep breathing exercises

Individuals under stress often experience fast, shallow breathing. This type of breathing, known as chest breathing, can lead to shortness of breath, increased muscle tension, and inadequate oxygenation of blood. Breathing exercises can both improve respiratory function and relieve stress and tension.

Before starting to learn breathing exercises, individuals should first become aware of their breathing patterns. This can be accomplished by placing one hand on the chest and one hand on the abdomen and observing which hand moves further during breathing. If it is the hand placed on the chest, then chest breathing is occurring, and breathing exercises may be beneficial.

Deep breathing exercises are best performed while lying flat on the back, usually on the floor with a mat. The knees are bent, and the body (particularly the mouth, nose, and face) is relaxed. One hand is placed on the chest and one on the abdomen to monitor breathing technique. The individual takes a series of long, deep breaths through the nose, attempting to raise the abdomen instead of the chest. Air is exhaled through the relaxed mouth. Deep breathing can be continued for up to 20 minutes. After the **exercise** is complete, the individual checks again for body tension and relaxation. Once deep breathing techniques have been mastered, an individual can use deep breathing at any time or place as a quick method of relieving tension.

Release-only relaxation

Like progressive relaxation, release-only relaxation focuses on relieving feelings of tension in the muscles. However, it eliminates the initial use of muscle tensing as practiced in progressive relaxation, focusing instead solely on muscle relaxation. Release-only relaxation is usually recommended as the next step in relaxation therapy after progressive relaxation has been mastered.

In release-only relaxation, breathing is used as a relaxation tool. The individual sits in a comfortable chair and begins to focus on breathing, envisioning tension leaving the body with each exhale. Once deep abdominal breathing is established, the individual begins to focus on releasing tension in each muscle group, until the entire body is completely relaxed.

Cue-controlled relaxation

Cue-controlled relaxation is an abbreviated tension-relief technique that combines elements of release-only relaxation and deep breathing exercises. It uses a cue, such as a word or mental image, to trigger immediate feelings of muscle relaxation. The cue must first be associated with relaxation in the individual's mind. Individuals choose the cue and then use it in breathing and release-only relaxation exercises repeatedly until the cue starts to automatically trigger feelings of relaxation outside the treatment sessions. Cues can be as simple as a given word such as "one" and are frequently used on relaxation audiotapes. They can also be a visual cue, such as a mental image of a white sand beach, a flower-filled meadow, or clear blue sky. Guided imagery also uses visualization exercises to produce feelings of relaxation.

Guided imagery

Guided imagery is a two-part process. The first component involves reaching a state of deep relaxation through breathing and muscle relaxation techniques. During the relaxation phase, individuals close their eyes and focuses on the slow in and out of their breath. Instead, individuals might focus on releasing the feelings of tension from their muscles, starting with the toes and working up to the top of the head. Relaxation tapes often feature soft music or tranquil, natural sounds such as rolling waves and chirping birds in order to promote feelings of relaxation.

Once complete relaxation is achieved, the second component of the exercise is the imagery, or visualization, itself. Relaxation imagery involves conjuring up pleasant images that rest the mind and body. These may be past experiences or idealized new situations.

The individual may also use mental rehearsal. Mental rehearsal involves imagining a situation or scenario and its ideal outcome. It can be used to reduce anxiety about an upcoming situation, such as **childbirth**, surgery, or even a critical event such as an important competition or a job interview. Individuals imagine themselves going through each step of the event, visualizing harmony and good will in the whole process and positive outcome.

Biofeedback

Biofeedback, or applied psychophysiological feedback, is a patient-guided treatment that teaches individuals to manipulate muscle tension through relaxation, visualization, and other cognitive techniques. The name biofeedback refers to the biological signals that are fed back, or returned, to the individual in order for him or her to develop the relaxation techniques.

During biofeedback, one or more special sensors are placed on the body. These sensors measure muscle tension, brain waves, heart rate, and body temperature, and translate the information into a visual and/or audible readout, such as a paper tracing, a light display, or a series of beeps. While viewing the instantaneous feedback from the biofeedback monitors, the individual begins to recognize what thoughts, fears, and mental images influence physical reactions. By monitoring this relationship between mind and body, the individual can then use thoughts and mental images deliberately to manipulate heart beat, brain wave patterns, body temperature, and other bodily functions, and to reduce feelings of stress. This is achieved through relaxation exercises, mental imagery, and other cognitive therapy techniques.

As the biofeedback response takes place, the individual can actually see or hear the results of the relaxation efforts instantly through the sensor readout on the biofeedback equipment. Once these techniques are learned and the individual is able to recognize the state of relaxation or visualization necessary to alleviate symptoms, the biofeedback equipment itself is no longer needed. The person then has a powerful, self-administered treatment technique for dealing with problem symptoms.

Dozens of other effective therapies promote relaxation, including hypnosis, meditation, yoga, **aromatherapy**, **hydrotherapy**, t'ai chi, massage, **art therapy**, and others. Individuals should choose a type of relaxation therapy based on their own interests and lifestyle requirements.

Preparations

When considering relaxation therapy to alleviate physical symptoms such as nausea, headache, high blood pressure, fatigue, or gastrointestinal problems, individuals should consult a doctor first to make sure that an underlying disorder or disease is not causing the symptoms. A complete physical examination and comprehensive medical history will be performed, and even if an organic cause for the symptoms is found, relaxation exercises may still be recommended as an adjunct, or complementary, treatment to relieve discomfort.

Relaxation therapy should always take place in a quiet, relaxing atmosphere in which the person has a comfortable place to sit or recline. Some people find that quiet background music improves their relaxation sessions. If an instructional audiotape or videotape is to be used, the appropriate equipment should be available.

The relaxation session, which can last anywhere from a few minutes to an hour, should be uninterrupted. Taking the phone off the hook, turning off cell phones, dimming the lights, and asking family members for privacy and silence can ensure a more successful and relaxing session.

Precautions

Most commonly practiced relaxation techniques are completely safe and free of side effects.

Relaxation techniques that involve special exercises or body manipulation such as massage, t'ai chi, and yoga should be taught or performed by a qualified healthcare professional or instructor. These treatments may not be suitable for individuals with certain health conditions such as arthritis or **fibromyalgia**. These individuals should consult with their healthcare professional before engaging in such therapies.

Biofeedback may not be recommended in some individuals who use a pacemaker or other implantable electrical devices. These individuals should inform their biofeedback therapist before starting treatments, as certain types of biofeedback sensors have the potential to interfere with implantable devices.

Relaxation therapy may not be suitable for some patients. Patients must be willing to take an active role in the treatment process and to practice techniques learned in treatment at home.

Some relaxation therapies may also be inappropriate for cognitively impaired individuals (e.g., patients with organic brain disease or a traumatic brain injury) depending on their level of functioning. Given the wide range of relaxation therapies available, if one type of relaxation treatment is deemed inappropriate for these patients, a suitable alternative can usually be recommended by a qualified healthcare professional.

Side effects

Relaxation therapy can induce sleepiness, and some individuals may fall asleep during a session. Relaxation therapy should not be performed while operating a motor vehicle or in other situations in which full and alert attention is necessary. Other than this, there are no known adverse side effects to relaxation therapy.

Research and general acceptance

Relaxation therapies are generally well-accepted by the medical community for relief of stress and anxiety.

Some research has also indicated that relaxation therapy may be useful for certain physiological conditions. One study, for example, reported results

indicating that relaxation therapy reduced the incidence of preterm labor in women at risk for delivering prematurely. It also found that women who discontinued relaxation exercises for whatever reasons delivered earlier and had lower birth-weight babies than those who continued the treatment. Positive benefits of relaxation therapy have also been reported for persons who have high blood pressure. Another study of 90 individuals who had previously experienced a **heart attack** reported a more favorable long-term outcome among the patients when they underwent both relaxation therapy and exercise training than exercise training alone. In 2006, researchers conducted a study of the therapy's impact on patients with chronic heart failure. For the study, 121 patients were split into control and experimental groups, with the experimental group receiving training in progressive muscle relaxation. The experimental group reported greater reduction in psychological distress compared to the control group. The researchers concluded that the training might be useful as part of a disease-management program for these patients, although further research would be necessary to discover if any other benefits could be attributed to the relaxation therapy.

Not all research supports relaxation therapy as a treatment option. A report published in 2001 reviewed numerous studies of the effectiveness of relaxation therapies on bronchial **asthma**. The report concluded that "little evidence in its favor has been presented." It noted, however, that healthcare professionals "continue to include relaxation training as a component in the nonpharmacological treatment of asthma."

Training and certification

Relaxation therapy techniques are used by many licensed therapists, counselors, psychologists, psychiatrists, and other healthcare professionals. Many self-help books, audiotapes, and videos are available that give instruction in relaxation techniques.

HERBERT BENSON (1935–)

Dr. Herbert Benson, the guru of mind/body medicine, was born in 1935. He graduated from Wesleyan University and the Harvard School of Medicine. He nurtured his interest in mind/body relationships and developed an expertise in behavioral medicine and spiritual healing. In his research, Benson straddled the thin line between medicine and religion. He conceived of what he called a three-legged approach to health care: self-care, pharmaceuticals, and medical treatment or surgery. His most significant work was his discovery of the relaxation response, which is the connection between lowered blood pressure and transcendental meditation. He was quoted by Daphne Howland of BeWell.com saying that "[B]elief is one of the most powerful healing tools we have in our therapeutic arsenal."

Benson served as the Mind/Body Institute Associate Professor of Medicine at Harvard School of Medical and worked as the Chief of the Division of Behavioral Medicine at the Beth Israel Deaconess Medical Center in Boston, Massachusetts. In 1988 he founded the Mind/Body Medical Institute in Boston, where he served as founding president. He lectured extensively about his work. On November 5, 1997 Benson addressed the Committee on Appropriations of the U.S. House of Representatives and spoke on the topic of "Healing and the Mind." Benson authored scores of scientific papers along with six books pertaining to his years of study, including *The Mind/Body Effect* in 1979, *Relaxation Response* in 1990, and *Timeless Healing: The Power and Biology of Belief* in 1996. Altogether his books sold over four million copies. Among his many honors and awards Benson received the John Templeton Spirituality and Medicine Curricular Award in 1999.

Resources

BOOKS

Davis, Martha et al. *The Relaxation & Stress Reduction Workbook*. 5th edition. Oakland, CA: New Harbinger Publications, Inc., 2000.

PERIODICALS

Yu, Doris. "Abstract 2506: Relaxation Therapy in Patients with Chronic Heart Failure: A Randomized Controlled Trial." *Circulation* 114, no. 2 (2007): 517.

ORGANIZATIONS

The American Psychological Association, 750 First St. NE, Washington, DC, 20002-4242, (800) 374-2721, http://www.apa.org.

Paula Ford-Martin
Leslie Mertz, Ph.D.

Rescue Remedy

Description

Rescue Remedy is the trademarked name of a combination of five **Bach flower essences** intended for use in emotional or psychological emergencies. It contains the essences of star of Bethlehem, rock rose, impatiens, cherry plum, and clematis. It is by far the most popular of the Bach preparations, and is available as a cream as well as in liquid form for internal use.

In terms of their history, the Bach flower essences are a variation of homeopathic remedies. Dr. Edward Bach (1886–1936), the English practitioner who first prepared them, was trained in both mainstream medicine and **homeopathy**. He worked as a bacteriologist and pathologist in the University College Hospital as well as the London Homoeopathic Hospital during the 1920s. Although Bach developed a series of homeopathic oral vaccines still known as the seven Bach nosodes, he was not satisfied with these preparations and decided that using plant material for homeopathic healing would be more effective than using disease organisms. He began experimenting around 1928 with flower extracts in order to treat personality problems and emotional conditions, which he thought had more important effects on a person's overall state of health than infectious diseases. He moved from London to a country setting in Oxfordshire in 1930 in order to devote himself fully to investigating the healing properties of local plants. By the time Bach died in 1936, he had discovered all of the 38 single flower essences presently in use. As of 2004, tinctures of the Bach **flower remedies** are still prepared at the Bach Centre in Mount Vernon, England.

Rescue Remedy is prepared in the same fashion as the Bach single flower essences, by either the sun method or by boiling. In the sun method, flower heads are floated in a clear glass bowl filled with natural spring water and allowed to soak in bright sunlight for three hours. The flowers are then removed and the water is mixed with brandy in a 50/50 ratio. In the boiling method, flowering twigs are boiled for half an hour in a large pan of spring water. After the water has cooled, the plant parts are removed and the remaining water is mixed with an equal part of brandy.

Flower essences included in rescue remedy

Clematis

Cherry plum

Impatiens

Rock rose

Star of Bethlehem

(Illustration by Corey Light. Cengage Learning, Gale)

General use

According to the Bach Centre, Dr. Bach intended Rescue Remedy "as an emotional first-aid kit and not as a quick replacement for the 38 individual remedies." The single remedies are selected according to the personality of the user and are said to take several weeks or months to bring about deeper changes in the person's feelings or behavior. For example, someone who is afraid of something specific and identifiable would be advised to take Mimulus, whereas someone who suffers from nameless **anxiety** would take Aspen. Bach is said to have chosen the five essences included in Rescue Remedy because he thought that they would act rapidly and cover most types of emotional crisis. His indications for the five flower essences in Rescue Remedy are as follows:

- Star of Bethlehem. For shock and emotional numbness resulting from trauma or bereavement.
- Rock rose. For terror, panic attacks, and hysteria; also recommended for recurrent nightmares.
- Impatiens. For those who tend to think and act impulsively, or become tense and irritable when upset.
- Cherry plum. For fear of losing physical or emotional control.
- Clematis. To prevent "spaciness" or passing out in crisis situations.

None of the Bach flower remedies are intended for use in treating infectious diseases or internal injuries.

Rescue Remedy cream is recommended for soothing such external skin problems as **sunburn**, windburn, scabs, minor **burns**, dryness, or **eczema**. It can also be applied after sports or **exercise** for discomfort caused by **bruises** or sore muscles.

Many people who use Rescue Remedy recommend it for pets and plants, as well as for humans. One alternative veterinarian suggests adding the remedy to a cat or dog's drinking water for such situations as a history of abuse or abandonment; recovery following veterinary surgery; fear of veterinarians; grief from losing a human caregiver or fellow pet; hyperactivity or aggressiveness; anxiety following a move or changes in the household; litter box problems; excessive self-grooming; and jealousy. The dose recommended for domestic pets is ten drops per gallon of water.

Preparations

The liquid form of Rescue Remedy is available in the United States for about $12 for a 20-mL bottle. Unlike the individual flower essences, which are taken two drops at a time, Rescue Remedy is taken in four-drop doses. It can be dropped directly on the tongue—care being taken not to touch the dropper —or added to a glass of water and sipped slowly. People who are concerned about the alcohol content of the tincture may add the Rescue Remedy to a cup of hot tea or other warm beverage, which will cause the alcohol to evaporate. Rescue Remedy is safe to use several times a day to treat emotional **stress**, as the flower essences in it are too dilute to cause any overdose effects.

Rescue Remedy cream contains crab apple in addition to the five flower essences in the liquid preparation. Crab apple was included in the mixture for its cleansing qualities. A 1-oz tube sells for about $11. The cream can be applied as often as needed.

Precautions

Rescue Remedy and the other Bach flower essences do not require any special precautions for use in most circumstances. The Bach Centre in England, however, does recommend that persons taking disulfiram (Antabuse) as part of treatment for alcohol abuse should consult their physician before using any of the Bach flower essences. Disulfiram works by changing the body's metabolism of alcohol in such a way that anyone taking the medication will experience **nausea**, **dizziness**, chest pains, and other unpleasant symptoms if they ingest even a small amount of alcohol. Although the amount of alcohol in four drops of Rescue Remedy is very small, it could conceivably trigger a reaction to disulfiram.

Unlike other homeopathic remedies, Bach flower essences are not affected by such substances as coffee, camphor, **eucalyptus**, or toothpaste and drinks containing **peppermint**. Practitioners of homeopathy refer to these substances and flavorings as antidotes, and advise their patients not to use them while taking prescribed remedies. Flower essences, however, can be taken with coffee, carbonated beverages, peppermint herbal tea, **cough** drops, or any other food flavored with peppermint or eucalyptus.

Side effects

No side effects from using the liquid form of Rescue Remedy have been reported as of 2004. Some practitioners of alternative medicine consider Rescue Remedy to be preferable to **kava kava** and other herbs used to treat anxiety, precisely because it is not dangerous in repeated doses, is not addictive, and does not affect the digestive tract or central nervous system.

Interactions

Apart from possible interactions with disulfiram due to its alcohol content, Rescue Remedy is not known to interact with prescription medications, herbal preparations, or other homeopathic remedies.

Resources

BOOKS

Stein, Diane. "Flower Remedies and Gem Elixirs." In *All Women Are Healers: A Comprehensive Guide to Natural Healing*. Freedom, CA: The Crossing Press, 1990.

PERIODICALS

Downey, R. P. "Healing with Flower Essences." *Beginnings* 22 (July-August 2002): 11–12.

Foster, Steven. "Herbal 911: Be Prepared for Any Emergency with an All-Natural Medicine Chest." *Better Nutrition* (January 2002): 24–25.

Gaeddert, Andrew. "Herbal Medicine Help People with Anxiety, Panic, and PTSD?—Ask the Herbalist—Post-Traumatic Stress Disorder." *Townsend Letter for Doctors and Patients* (August-September 2002): 4–5.

Reichenberg-Ullman, Judyth. "Homeopathy for Sports Injuries—Healing with Homeopathy." *Townsend Letter for Doctors and Patients* (July 2003): 2–3.

ORGANIZATIONS

Dr. Edward Bach Centre. Mount Vernon, Bakers Lane, Sotwell, Oxon United Kingdom OX10 0PZ. +44 (0) 1491-834-678. Fax: +44 (0) 1491-825-022. http://www.bachcentre.com.

Nelson Bach USA, Ltd. 100 Research Drive, Wilmington, MA 01887. (800) 319-9151 or (978) 988-3833. Fax: (978) 988-0233. http://www.nelsonbach.com/usa.html.

OTHER

Dr. Edward Bach Centre. *Frequently-Asked Questions.* [cited June 14, 2004]. http://www.bachcentre.com/centre/faq.htm.

Rebecca Frey

Restless leg syndrome

Definition

The condition known as restless leg syndrome (RLS) is a movement disorder caused by an irresistible urge to move the legs due to unpleasant sensations. It occurs primarily during times of **relaxation**, such as when a person is trying to go to sleep.

Description

RLS occurs most commonly in people over the age 40. Almost half of patients over age 60 who complain of **insomnia** are diagnosed with RLS. Those who have a family history of RLS may first experience the disorder as young adults, or even as children. It is not usually described as painful, although some people may complain of a disagreeable creeping, tugging, or aching sensation. A related condition, experienced by as many as 80% of RLS sufferers, is known as periodic limb movements of sleep (PLMS), or nocturnal myoclonus. In PLMS, jerky leg movements occur about every 20–40 seconds during sleep, and the arms may be affected as well.

Causes and symptoms

Although RLS appears to be familial in some cases, other causes should be ruled out and treated before starting medication. Certain diseases and conditions are more highly associated with RLS. People experiencing symptoms should be examined and tested for **anemia**, uremia, and electrolyte and vitamin imbalance. Renal failure is a major predisposing factor. RLS can also be associated with **pregnancy**. As many as one in seven pregnant women may experience RLS to some degree. The disorder usually disappears after delivery, but it can recur with subsequent pregnancies or later in life.

Many medications can induce or worsen the symptoms of RLS. A prescribed medication should not be discontinued without consulting a healthcare provider. Medications that may cause problems for some patients include some antidepressants, antihistamines, most anti-nausea medications, phenothiazine tranquilizers, sinemet, some **calcium** channel blockers used for **hypertension**, and a few antipsychotic drugs. Patients with RLS or PLMS should have a healthcare provider ask whether alternative medications are available if one is prescribed that may worsen RLS symptoms.

Most individuals with RLS experience mild symptoms. They may lie down to rest at the end of the day and, just before sleep, experience discomfort in their legs that prompts them to stand up, massage the leg, or walk briefly. Eighty-five percent of RLS patients either have difficulty falling asleep or wake several times during the night; almost half experience daytime **fatigue** or sleepiness. It is common for symptoms to be intermittent. They may disappear for several months and then return for no apparent reason. Two-thirds of patients report that their symptoms become worse with time. Some older patients claim to have had symptoms since they were in their early 20s but were not diagnosed until their 50s. Suspected underdiagnosis of RLS may be attributed to the difficulty experienced by patients in describing their symptoms. An estimated 2–15% of the population has some degree of RLS symptoms.

Diagnosis

A carefully taken history generally enables a physician to distinguish RLS from similar types of disorders that cause nighttime discomfort in the limbs, such as **muscle cramps**, circulatory diseases, and damage to nerves that detect sensations or cause movement (**peripheral neuropathy**).

The most important tool the doctor has in diagnosing RLS is the history obtained from the patient. Several common medical conditions are known either to cause or to be closely associated with RLS. A healthcare provider may link a patient's symptoms to one of these conditions, which include anemia, diabetes, disease of the spinal nerve roots (lumbosacral radiculopathy), **Parkinson's disease**, late-stage pregnancy, kidney failure (uremia), and complications of stomach surgery. In order to identify or eliminate such causes,

blood tests may be performed to determine the presence of serum ferritin, folate, **vitamin B$_{12}$**, creatinine, and thyroid-stimulating hormones. The physician may also ask if symptoms are present in any close family member, since it is common for RLS to run in families, and this type is sometimes more difficult to treat.

Treatment

The best alternative therapy combines both conventional and alternative approaches. Levodopa may be combined with a therapy that relieves **pain**, relaxes muscles, or focuses in general on the nervous system and the brain. Any such combined therapy that allows a reduction in dosage of levodopa is advantageous, since this approach will reduce the likelihood of unacceptable levels of drug side effects. Of course, the physician who prescribes the medication should monitor any combined therapy.

Acupuncture

Patients who also suffer from **rheumatoid arthritis** may benefit especially from **acupuncture** to relieve RLS symptoms. Acupuncture is believed to be effective in arthritis treatment and may stimulate those parts of the brain that are involved in RLS. Some practitioners also believe that acupuncture benefits RLS patients who do not have rheumatoid arthritis.

Homeopathy

Homeopaths believe that disorders of the nervous system are especially important because the brain controls so many other bodily functions. They tailor a remedy to the individual patient and base it on individual symptoms as well as on the general symptoms of RLS.

Reflexology

Reflexologists claim that the brain, head, and spine all respond to indirect massage of specific parts of the feet.

Nutritional supplements

Supplementation of the diet with **vitamin E**, calcium, **magnesium**, and **folic acid** may be helpful for people with RLS.

Allopathic treatment

If causes related to diet, metabolic abnormalities, and medication have been excluded or treated, therapeutic medications may be helpful. Some medications, including those mentioned above, may cause symptoms of RLS. Patients should check with a healthcare provider about these possible side effects, especially if symptoms first occur after starting a new medication.

In some people whose symptoms cannot be linked to a treatable associated condition, drug therapy may be necessary to provide relief and restore a normal sleep pattern. Prescription drugs that are normally used for RLS may include dopaminergic agents (such as levodopa and/or carbidopa, used to treat Parkinson's syndrome), dopamine agonists, opioids, benzodiazepines, anticonvulsants, **iron** (for anemic patients), and clonidine. Patient response is variable, so it is best to consult a healthcare provider to determine the best medication or combination regimen for the individual circumstances. Careful monitoring of side effects and good communication between patient and doctor can result in a flexible program of therapy that minimizes side effects and maximizes effectiveness.

Expected results

RLS usually does not indicate the onset of other neurological disease. It may remain static, although two-thirds of patients get worse with time. The symptoms usually progress gradually. Treatment with dopamine agonists is effective in moderate to severe cases that may include significant PLMS. These drugs, however, produce significant side effects, including sleepiness and **nausea**. An individually tailored treatment plan is optimal. The prognosis is usually best if RLS symptoms are recent and can be traced to another treatable condition that is associated with RLS.

Prevention

Diet is one factor that can prevent symptoms of RLS. A helpful diet includes an adequate intake of iron and the B vitamins, especially B_{12} and folic acid. Strict vegetarians should take vitamin supplements to obtain sufficient vitamin B_{12}. Ferrous gluconate may be easier to digest than ferrous sulfate, if iron supplements are prescribed. **Caffeine**, alcohol, and nicotine use should be minimized or eliminated. Even a hot bath before bed has been shown to prevent symptoms for some sufferers.

Resources

BOOKS

Buchfuhrer, Mark J., Wayne A. Hening, and Clete A. Kushida. *Restless Legs Syndrome: Coping with Your Sleepless Nights.* New York: Demos Medical, 2006.

Gunzel, Jill. *Restless Legs Syndrome: The RLS Rebel's Survival Guide.* Tucson, AZ: Wheatmark, 2006.

Hening, Wayne A., Mark J. Buchfuhrer, and Hochang B. Lee. *Clinical Management of Restless Legs Syndrome.* Caddo, OK: Professional Communications, 2007.

Ondo, William G, ed. *Restless Legs Syndrome: Diagnosis and Treatment.* London: Informa Healthcare, 2006.

PERIODICALS

Kushida, Clete, et al. "Burden of Restless Legs Syndrome on Health-related Quality of Life." *Quality of Life Research* (May 2007): 617–624.

Nineb, A., et al. "Restless Legs Syndrome Is Frequently Overlooked in Patients Being Evaluated for Polyneuropathies." *European Journal of Neurology* (July 2007): 788–792.

Pearson, V. E., et al. "Medication Use in Patients with Restless Legs Syndrome Compared with a Control Population." *European Journal of Neurology* (January 2008): 16–21.

Surani, Salim, and Alamgir Khan. "Sleep Related Disorders in the Elderly: An Overview." *Current Respiratory Medicine Reviews* (November 2007): 286–291.

ORGANIZATIONS

Restless Legs Syndrome Foundation, 1610 Fourteenth St NW, Suite 300, Rochester, MN, 55901, (877) INFO-RLS, http://www.rls.org.

Judith Turner
David Edward Newton, Ed.D.

Resveratrol

Description

Resveratrol (*trans*-3,5,4_-trihydroxy-*trans*-stilbene) is a phytochemical, or plant chemical, that is found in the skin of red grapes, in peanuts, blueberries, and in a variety of other fruits, seeds, and plants, as well as in wine and grape juice. Specifically, resveratrol is a phytoalexin, which is a compound made by the plants to fight microbes, in particular a pathogen called *Botrytis cinerea*, and in response to environmental stresses. Many phytoalexins, including resveratrol, have implications for treating various human health problems.

Resveratrol was first identified in 1940, when it was isolated from the roots of a plant called white hellebore (*Veratrum grandiflorum*), also known as Mao Ye Li Lu in China. White hellebore is native to China, where it is found in the Hubei, Hunan, Jiangxi, Sichuan, Yunnan, and Zhejiang provinces. In 1963, it was also discovered to be a component of Japanese knotweed (*Polygonum cuspidatum*), a plant that is native to Eurasia and was introduced to the New World. Since then, resveratrol has been found in more than 70 other plant species. The scientific world became especially interested in resveratrol in 1992 when research was published that suggested the phytochemical might be a reason why French people, who consume considerable amounts of wine as well as fatty foods, have a lower incidence of coronary **heart disease** than do persons in other Western populations. After that, numerous studies were conducted into resveratrol's potential health benefits.

General use

Foods and drinks containing resveratrol have been a historical part of the human diet, and wine has traditionally been associated with health. It was only after the 1992 study linking the phytochemical to a possible reduction in heart disease, however, that scientists and health experts began to explore the potential health benefits of resveratrol and resveratrol-containing foods and beverages for conditions ranging from the **common cold** to **cancer**. The results of many studies were available in the early 2000s.

Numerous studies in animals and in human cell cultures have shown that resveratrol has anti-cancer properties that affect the initiation and growth of tumors; curb the formation of blood vessels, called angiogenesis, that is involved in cancer progression; and suppress metastasis, or the spread of cancer. Research has indicated that resveratrol can act on various pathways involved in the progression of cancer, including the uncontrolled cell growth characteristic of cancers. Resveratrol is a strong antioxidant, and it is believed that this antioxidant activity is likely responsible for much of its anti-cancer effects.

One such research study into resveratrol in 1997 examined the effects of purified resveratrol from grapes and other foods on **skin cancer** in mice. The researchers found that resveratrol inhibited early cancerous lesions and reduced the number of tumors. Several additional studies on mice have also shown that the topical application of resveratrol seems to protect against the development of skin cancer.

Studies of resveratrol on various other cancers have also been conducted. For example, scientists gave mice resveratrol in their drinking water for seven weeks and reported in a 2000 study that they found a 70 percent reduction in the formation of small intestinal tumors, as well as the prevention of colon tumor development. It is believed that resveratrol, in part, works by turning off the genes that help tumor cells proliferate and turning on the genes that assist the body's immune system in battling cancer. Another colon cancer study, this time on rats, showed in 2006 that resveratrol reduced the occurrence of tumors and lesions and decreased the size of those tumors that did appear. Research in 2001 on the effects of resveratrol on **lung cancer** showed that the phytochemical was successful in reducing the size of tumors under certain conditions and in dampening their ability to spread. Other studies on additional cancers, including **prostate cancer** and **leukemia**, also showed that resveratrol appears to inhibit the proliferation of the cancers in lab experiments conducted on cancer cells. Additional research was under way as of 2008 that was expected to shed light on the phytochemical's potential impact on human cancers.

The benefits of resveratrol may extend beyond cancer. In 2002, for instance, a study conducted in Spain followed 4,300 people for one year, taking note of their susceptibility to colds and their consumption of beer, wine, and distilled spirits. While they found that beer and spirits provided no apparent protection against colds, wine consumption did. The research results showed that both men and women who drank an average of two or more glasses of wine a day had 40 percent fewer colds than those who did not drink any alcoholic beverages and revealed an even greater reduction if they drank red wine in particular. The researchers suggested that resveratrol could be one of the components of wine that may have a role in that reduction.

Resveratrol may also be useful against the flu. According to a study published in 2005, it blocked the **influenza** virus from multiplying.

Resveratrol has become increasingly well-known for its connection to longevity. Studies have shown increases in longevity for the yeast *Saccharomyces cerevisiae*, the nematode or roundworm known as *Caenorhabditis elegans*, the fruit fly (*Drosophila melanogaster*), and a vertebrate. The vertebrate was a type of fish, *Nothobranchius furzeri*, which has a short lifespan (no more than 13 weeks in captivity). The researchers supplemented the diet of the fish with different amounts of resveratrol. At 120 micrograms of resveratrol per gram of food, the median lifespan increased by 33 percent and the maximum lifespan by 27 percent. When the researchers increased the concentration of resveratrol to 600 micrograms, median and maximum lifespans increased by 56 and 59 percent respectively. The researchers noted that both males and females experienced the rise in longevity, that both remained fertile, and that the eggs from the fish developed and grew into normal adults. Beyond the hike in longevity, the researchers also reported results that indicated resveratrol had a positive influence on the decline in locomotor activity and on the cognitive deficit that typically occurs during **aging** in vertebrates. Although the researchers were unsure how resveratrol achieved its results, they reported, "(T)he observation that its supplementation with food extends vertebrate lifespan and delays motor and cognitive age-related decline could be of high relevance for the prevention of aging-related diseases in the human population." (Valenzano 4)

Another study in 2006 also noted an improvement in physical prowess in mice that were fed resveratrol. After receiving a diet containing resveratrol for 15 weeks, mice were able to run longer on a treadmill. No human studies of resveratrol on longevity or athletic prowess have been conducted to indicate how the phytochemical might work in people.

In addition to these potential health benefits, alternative-medicine practitioners sometimes recommend resveratrol to prevent heart attacks because the phytochemical has been shown to inhibit the aggregation of blood-clotting cells known as platelets.

Preparations

Resveratrol is available in a range of foods, as well as in beverages such as grape juice and wine. It is also available as a supplement in capsule form.

Precautions

Although several studies have indicated that resveratrol may fight **breast cancer**, some researchers believe that it may actually promote the disease. Some medical and alternative-medicine practitioners recommend certain people should avoid resveratrol. These include children under the age of 18 and women who are taking oral contraceptives, who are pregnant, or who are trying to become pregnant. In addition, individuals who have West Nile virus should consult their healthcare practitioner before taking resveratrol.

Side effects

No known side effects exist, although no research has been conducted on high doses in humans.

Interactions

Individuals who are being treated for West Nile virus and women who are taking oral contraceptives should consult their physician before taking resveratrol.

KEY TERMS

Phytoalexin—A compound made by some plants to fight various microbes, such as bacteria, viruses, and fungi, or as a response to environmental stress.

Phytochemical—A plant chemical.

Resources

BOOKS

Aggarwal, Bharat, and Shishir Shishodia, eds. *Resveratrol in Health and Disease (Oxidative Stress and Disease)*. Boca Raton, Fl: CRC, 2005.

Corder, Roger. *The Red Wine Diet*. Garden City Park, NY: Avery, 2007.

PERIODICALS

Athar, Mohammad, Jung Ho Back, Xiuwei Tang, Kwang Ho Kim, Levy Kopelovich, David R. Bickers, et al. "Resveratrol: A review of Preclinical Studies for Human Cancer Prevention." *Toxicology and Applied Pharmacology* 224, no. 3 (November 1, 2007): 274–283.

Palamara, Anna T., Lucia Nencioni, Katia Aquilano, Giovanna De Chiara, Leyanis Hernandez, Federico Cozzolino, et al. "Inhibition of Influenza: A Virus Replication by Resveratrol." *Journal of Infectious Diseases* 191, no. 10 (May 15, 2005): 1719–1729.

Stipp, David. "Can Red Wine Help You Live Forever?" *Fortune* January 19, 2007. http://money.cnn.com/2007/01/18/magazines/fortune/Live_forever.fortune/index.htm (April 13, 2008).

Valenzano, Dario R., Eva Terzibasi, Tyrone Genade, Antonino Cattaneo, Luciano Domenici, and Alessandro Cellerino. "Resveratrol Prolongs Lifespan and Retards the Onset of Age-Related Markers in a Short-Lived Vertebrate." *Current Biology* 16, no. 3 (February 7, 2006): 296–300.

Yang, M. R., S. R. Lee, W. Oh, E. W. Lee, J. Y. Yeh, J. J. Nah, et al. "West Nile Virus Capsid Protein Induces p53-Mediated Apoptosis Via the Sequestration of HDM2 to the Nucleolus." *Cellular Microbiology* 10, no. 1 (January 2008): 165–176.

OTHER

"Red Wine and Resveratrol: Good for Your Heart?" *MayoClinic.com* March 9, 2007. http://www.mayoclinic.com/health/red-wine/HB00089. (April 13, 2008).

"Resveratrol." *Micronutrient Nutrition Center, Linus Pauling Institute* March 4, 2005. http://lpi.oregonstate.edu/infocenter/phytochemicals/resveratrol/. (April 13, 2008).

Leslie Mertz, Ph.D.

Retinal detachment

Definition

Retinal detachment is a serious eye disorder in which the retina, a thin tissue of cells located in the back of the eye, separates from the underlying tissue layers.

Description

There are three layers of the eyeball. The outer, tough, white layer is called the sclera. Lining the sclera is the choroid, a thin membrane that supplies nutrients to part of the retina. The retina is located at the back of the eye and consists of three cellular layers.

The retina contains the light-sensitive receptors for sight and processes visual images. A retinal detachment occurs between the two outermost layers of the retina, the photoreceptor layer that receives light and the outermost pigmented epithelium. When a tear in the retina occurs, the fluids in the eye may leak and pull the retina out of place, or detach it from the layers. Because the choroid supplies the photoreceptors within the retina with nutrients, a detachment can basically starve the photoreceptors. If a detachment is not repaired within 24–72 hours, permanent damage may occur.

Causes and symptoms

Several conditions may cause retinal detachment:

- Scarring or shrinkage of the vitreous (substance comprising the insides of the eye) can pull the retina inward.
- Small tears in the retina allow liquid to seep behind the retina and push it forward.
- Injury to the eye can loosen the retina. Trauma is the most common cause of retinal detachment in children, although it is comparatively unusual in the adult population.

- Bleeding behind the retina, most often due to diabetic retinopathy or injury, can push it forward.
- Retinal detachment may be spontaneous. This occurs more often in the elderly or in very nearsighted (myopic) eyes.
- Cataract surgery causes retinal detachment 2% of the time.
- Myopia.
- Diabetes.
- Congenital factors (those that people are born with).
- Family history of retinal problems.
- High blood pressure.
- Stress.
- Tumors.

Retinal detachment will cause a sudden defect in vision. It may look as if a curtain or shadow has just descended before the eye. If most of the retina is detached, there may be only a small hole of vision remaining. If only a portion of the retina is involved, there will be a blind spot that may not even be noticed. Retinal detachment is often associated with *floaters*, which are little dark spots that float across the eye and can be mistaken for flies in the room. There may also be flashes of light. Anyone experiencing sudden flashes of light or floaters should contact their eye doctor immediately since these may be symptoms of detachment.

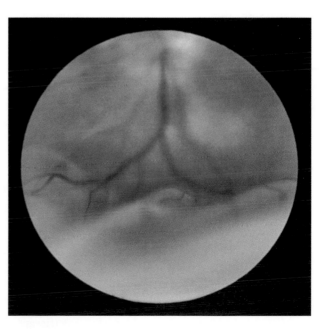

Opthalmoscope view of the inner eye, showing a detached retina. *(Paul Parker / Photo Researchers, Inc.)*

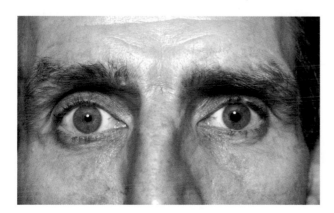

Retinal detachment. *(© Medical-on-Line / Alamy)*

KEY TERMS

Cauterize—To damage with heat or cold so that tissues shrink; used as a method to stop bleeding.

Diabetic retinopathy—A disorder of the eye associated with diabetes that damages the blood vessels in the back of the eye.

Ophthalmologist—A medical doctor who specializes in eye diseases and eye health; can prescribe drugs and perform surgery.

Optometrist—A professional who evaluates and tests sight for correction like glasses or contact lens.

Retina—The thin layer of tissue at the back of the eye that contains light-sensitive receptor cells and processes visual images.

Diagnosis

Diagnosis of retinal detachment should be done by an ophthalmologist. A person who has flashes, floaters, or has a curtain-like blockage of their visual field should see an ophthalmologist immediately because early treatment is required to prevent loss of sight. An optometrist may also diagnose retinal detachment during a routine eye examination.

Treatment

No alternative treatment is recommended for acute retinal detachment. Vision may be lost if the problem is not diagnosed and attended to promptly. However, some alternative therapies such as **behavioral optometry** prescribe eye **relaxation** exercises and use techniques that attempt to prevent and naturally heal **myopia** (near-sightedness). Nearsighted (myopic) people are at greatest risk for retinal detachment. Some alternative therapies that reduce **stress** to the eyes may promote general eye health. Also, alternative treatments to control high blood pressure such as diet, Chinese herbs, massage for stress relief, relaxation exercises, and **yoga**, may also indirectly prevent retinal damage by reducing high blood pressure and relieving stress. **Antioxidants** such as **bilberry** may also be used to decrease inflammation.

Allopathic treatment

Traditional treatment of retinal detachment involves immediate surgery to repair the retina. Small holes or tears may be sealed with a laser or with cryotherapy (freezing) under local anesthesia in a doctor's office. More extensive repairs are done in the hospital under general anesthesia.

These may involve injection of silicone oil to help the retina reattach.

Expected results

Retinal detachment is a serious condition that can result in blindness. If retinal detachment is diagnosed in its early stages and repair is made quickly, the patient's sight usually returns to normal. If the retina is fully detached, and extensive surgery is needed, the patient's sight may be partially or fully restored. The amount of restoration depends on the severity of the damage and how soon it is treated.

Prevention

To prevent retinal detachment, people should be keenly aware of eye function and diseases that may affect it. Regular eye examinations can detect changes that the patient may not notice. In such diseases as diabetes, with a high incidence of retinal disordes, routine eye examinations can detect early changes. Good control of diabetes can help prevent diabetic eye disease. High blood pressure and stress should be controlled daily. Blood pressure control can prevent **hypertension** from damaging the retinal blood vessels, and stress management techniques can also reduce blood pressure. Wearing eye protection can also prevent direct injury to the eyes.

Early treatment can prevent both progressing to detachment, and blindness from other events like hemorrhage. Other diseases can cause the tiny holes and tears in the retina through which fluid can leak. Preventive treatment uses a laser to cauterize the blood vessels so that they do not bleed and seals the holes so they do not leak.

Resources

PERIODICALS

Butler, T. K. H., A. W. Kiel, and G. M. Orr. "Anatomical and Visual Outcome of Retinal Detachment Surgery in Children." *British Journal of Ophthalmology* 85 (December 2001): 1437-1439.

"Eye Disorders: Retinal Detachment." *Harvard Health Letter* (December 1, 1998).

Jonas, Jost B., et al. "Retinal Redetachment After Removal of Intraocular Silicon Oil Tamponade." *British Journal of Ophthalmology* 85 (October 2001): 1203.

ORGANIZATIONS

American Academy of Ophthalmology. P.O. Box 7424, San Francisco, CA 94120-7424. (415) 561-8500.

American Optometric Association. 243 North Lindbergh Blvd., St. Louis, MO 63141. (314) 991-4100.

Angela Woodward
Rebecca J. Frey, PhD

Retinol *see* **Vitamin A**

Retinopathy

Definition

Retinopathy is a noninflammatory disease of the retina. There are many causes and types of retinopathy.

Description

The retina is the thin membrane that lines the back of the eye and contains light-sensitive cells (photoreceptors). Light enters the eye and is focused onto the retina. The photoreceptors send a message to the brain via the optic nerve. The brain then interprets the electrical message sent to it, resulting in vision. The macula is a specific area of the retina responsible for central vision. The fovea is about 1.5 mm in size and is located in the macula. The fovea is responsible for sharp vision. When looking at something, the fovea should be directed at the object.

Retinopathy, or damage to the retina, has various causes. A hardening or thickening of the retinal arteries is called arteriosclerotic retinopathy. High blood pressure in the arteries of the body can damage the retinal arteries and is called hypertensive retinopathy. Diabetes damages the retinal vessels resulting in a condition called diabetic retinopathy. **Sickle cell anemia** also affects the blood vessels in the retina. Exposure to the sun (or looking at the sun during an eclipse) can cause damage (solar retinopathy), as well as certain drugs (for example, chloroquine, thioridazine, and large doses of tamoxifen). The arteries and veins can become blocked, resulting in a retinal artery or vein occlusion. These are just some of the causes of the various retinopathies.

Retinopathies are divided into two broad categories: simple or nonproliferative retinopathies and proliferative retinopathies. The simple retinopathies include the defects identified by bulging of the vessel walls, bleeding into the eye, small clumps of dead retinal cells called cotton wool exudates, and closed vessels. This form of retinopathy is considered mild. The proliferative, or severe, forms of retinopathies include the defects identified by newly grown blood vessels, scar tissue formed within the eye, closed-off blood vessels that are badly damaged, and by the retina breaking away from its mesh of nourishing blood vessels (**retinal detachment**). These severe forms can cause blindness.

While each disease has its own specific effect on the retina, there is a general scenario for many of the retinopathies. However, not all retinopathies necessarily affect the blood vessels. Blood flow to the retina is disrupted, either by blockage or breakdown of the various vessels. This can lead to bleeding (hemorrhage)

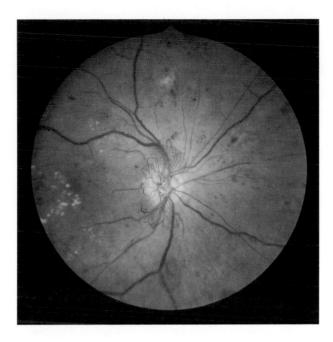

Opthalmoscope image of diabetic retinopathy, damage to the retina caused by diabetes. *(Paul Parker / Photo Researchers, Inc.)*

and fluids, cells, and proteins leak into the area (exudates). There can be a lack of oxygen to surrounding tissues (hypoxia) or decreased blood flow (**ischemia**). Chemicals produced by the body then can cause new blood vessels to grow (neovascularization); however, these new vessels generally leak and cause more problems. Neovascularization can even grow on the colored part of the eye (iris). The retina can swell and vision will be affected.

Diabetic retinopathy is the leading cause of blindness in people ages 20-74. Diabetic retinopathy will occur in 90% of people with type 1 diabetes (insulin dependent) and 65% of persons with type 2 diabetes (non-insulin dependent) by about 10 years after the onset of diabetes. In the United States, new cases of blindness are most often caused by diabetic retinopathy. Among these new cases of blindness, 12% are people between the ages of 20-44 years, and 19% are people between the ages of 45-64 years.

Causes and symptoms

There are many causes of retinopathy. Some of the more common ones are listed below.

Diabetic retinopathy

Diabetes is a complex disorder characterized by an inability of the body to properly regulate the levels of sugar and insulin (a hormone made by the pancreas) in the blood. As diabetes progresses, the blood vessels that feed the retina become damaged in different ways. The damaged vessels can have bulges in their walls (aneurysms) that can leak blood into the surrounding jelly-like material (vitreous) that fills the inside of the eyeball. They can become completely closed, or new vessels can begin to grow where there would not normally be blood vessels. Although these new blood vessels are growing in the eye, they can't nourish the retina and they bleed easily, releasing blood into the inner region of the eyeball, which can cause dark spots and cloudy vision. Diabetic retinopathy begins before any outward signs of disease are noticed. Once symptoms are noticed, they include poorer than normal vision, fluctuating or distorted vision, cloudy vision, dark spots, episodes of temporary blindness, or permanent blindness.

Hypertensive retinopathy

High blood pressure can affect the vessels in the eyes. Some blood vessels can narrow. The blood vessels can thicken and harden (arteriosclerosis). There will be flame-shaped hemorrhages and macular swelling (**edema**). This edema may cause distorted or decreased vision.

Sickle cell retinopathy

Sickle cell **anemia** occurs mostly in blacks and is a hereditary disease that affects the red blood cells. The sickle-shaped blood cell reduces blood flow. People will not have visual symptoms early in the disease; symptoms are more systemic. However, patients need to be followed closely in case new blood vessel growth occurs.

Retinal vein and artery occlusion

Retinal vein occlusion generally occurs in the elderly. There is usually a history of other systemic disease, such as diabetes or high blood pressure. The central retinal vein (CRV), or the retinal veins branching off of the CRV, can become compressed and stop the drainage of blood from the retina. This may occur if the central retinal artery hardens. Symptoms of retinal vein occlusion include a sudden, painless loss of vision or field of vision in one eye. There may be a sudden onset of floating spots (floaters) or flashing lights. Vision may be unchanged or decrease dramatically. Retinal artery occlusion is generally the result of an embolism that dislodges from somewhere else in the body and travels to the eye. Transient loss of vision may precede an occlusion. Symptoms of a central retinal artery or branch occlusion include a sudden, painless loss of vision or decrease in visual field. Ten percent of the cases of a retinal artery occlusion occur because of giant cell arteritis (a chronic vascular disease).

Solar retinopathy

Looking directly at the sun or watching an eclipse can cause damage. There may be a loss of the central visual field or decreased vision. The symptoms can occur hours to days after the incident.

Drug-related retinopathies

Certain medications can affect different areas of the retina. Doses of 20-40 mg a day of tamoxifen usually does not cause a problem, but much higher doses may cause irreversible damage. Patients taking chloroquine for lupus, **rheumatoid arthritis**, or other disorders may notice a decrease in vision. If so, discontinuing medication will stop, but not reverse, any damage. However, patients should never discontinue medication without the advice of their doctor. Patients taking thioridazine may notice a decrease in vision or color vision. These drug-related retinopathies generally only affect patients taking large doses. However, patients need to be aware if any medication they are taking will affect the eyes. Patients need to inform their doctors of any visual effects.

Diagnosis

The damaged retinal blood vessels and other retinal changes are visible to an eye doctor when an examination of the retina (fundus exam) is done. This can be done using a hand-held instrument called an ophthalmoscope. This allows the doctor to see the back of the eye. Certain retinopathies have classic signs (for example, peculiar fan shapes in sickle cell, dot and blot hemorrhages in diabetes, flame-shaped hemorrhages in high blood pressure). Patients may then be referred for other tests to confirm the underlying cause of the retinopathy. These tests include blood tests and measurement of blood pressure. Fluorescein angiography, where a dye is injected into the patient and the back of the eyes are viewed and photographed, helps to locate leaky vessels. Sometimes patients may become nauseated from the dye. Alternative practitioners often take thorough physical and psychological profiles of patients, considering lifestyle, **stress**, work habits, diet, emotional issues, and others to determine overall health factors that may be affecting the eyes and related organs.

Treatment

There are many alternative treatments available for retinopathy. When retina problems indicate other disorders such as diabetes, high blood pressure, or sickle cell anemia, those disorders are treated as well. **Holistic medicine** often treats eye disorders not only by promoting healing in the eyes but by strengthening the overall system on the physical, mental, and emotional levels.

Dietary and nutritional therapy

A diet to promote retinal healing includes plenty of fresh and raw vegetables, fruits, beans, peas, and whole grains. **Diets** should be low in fat, particularly fat from animal and dairy sources. Processed, artificial, and refined foods should be avoided, including sugar and white flour. Alcohol and **caffeine** intake should be reduced as well.

Certain foods may help heal retinopathies and injured blood vessels in the eye, especially food rich in **antioxidants** like **carotenoids** (found in some vegetables) and flavenoids (found in some fruits). Foods rich in carotenoids, such as carrots, tomatoes, melons, and green leafy vegetables, should be eaten often. **Lutein** and zeaxanthin are carotenoids found in spinach and collard greens, and support eye function and retinal healing. Lycopenes are similar compounds found in tomatoes, guava, watermelon, and pink grapefruit. The **bioflavonoids** rutin and **quercetin** promote healthy circulation in the blood vessels of the retina, and are found in red onions, grapes, citrus fruits, cherries, and blue-green algae. **Garlic** may also help retinal problems by reducing blood clotting. Blueberries and huckleberries are related to bilberries, the herb most used for retinal problems. **Green tea** also contains antioxidants that may help repair blood vessels in the retina. **Grape seed extract** and **pine bark extract** contain powerful bioflavenoid antioxidants called oligomeric proanthocyanidins (OPCs), which help repair blood vessels and increase circulation.

Nutritional supplements for retina support include the **amino acids** cysteine, taurine, alpha-lipoic acid, and **glutathione**. An essential fatty acid (EFA) supplement such as **flaxseed** oil or **evening primrose oil** is recommended. EFAs improve circulation and nerve function in the retina. Vitamins A, C, and E support retinal and blood vessel healing, as do the B-complex vitamins and the minerals **zinc** and **selenium**.

Herbal support

Bilberry is a strongly recommended herb, containing compounds called anthocyanocides, eye-tropic bioflavonoids, that have been shown to strengthen blood vessels and reduce bleeding in the retina. Ginkgo is also used regularly for retina problems, as it has antioxidant and circulation improving qualities. The herb marigold is a natural source of lutein. Other herbs used frequently

for retinopathy include agrimony, **milk thistle, dandelion, goldenseal**, and **eyebright**.

Traditional medicines

Traditional Chinese medicine utilizes **acupuncture, acupressure**, diet, and herbal remedies for eye problems. Chinese medicine views eye problems as related to liver dysfunction, and uses herbs such as ju hua, wood betony, burdock, **licorice**, dandelion, ginkgo, and **gotu kola** to strengthen both the eyes and liver. **Ayurvedic medicine** uses dietary and herbal therapies for retina problems. Low-fat vegetarian diets are recommended, which provide plenty of foods with sour, salty, and pungent flavors, and the herbs milk thistle, gingko, and others are used as well. **Fasting** is also practiced to cleanse the liver, improve circulation, and promote healing. **Homeopathy** prescribes the remedies **euphrasia** and **calendula** for eye disorders, and other remedies for systemic healing.

Allopathic treatment

Retinal specialists are ophthalmologists who specialize in retinal disorders. Retinopathy is a disorder of the retina that can result from different underlying systemic causes, so general doctors should be consulted as well. For drug-related retinopathies, the treatment is generally discontinuation of the drug (only under the care of a medical doctor). Surgery with lasers can help to prevent blindness or lessen any losses in vision. The high-energy light from a laser is aimed at the weakened blood vessels in the eye, destroying them. Scars will remain where the laser treatment was performed. For that reason, laser treatment cannot be performed everywhere. For example, laser photocoagulation at the fovea would destroy the area for sharp vision.

Panretinal photocoagulation may be performed. This is a larger area of treatment in the periphery of the retina, and the method is used to decrease neovascularization. Prompt treatment of proliferative retinopathy may reduce the risk of severe vision loss by 50%. Patients with retinal artery occlusion should be referred to a cardiologist. Patients with retinal vein occlusion need to be referred to a doctor because they may have an underlying disorder like high blood pressure.

In 2001, scientists reported that gene therapy may one day help halt or perhaps prevent blood vessel overgrowth that leads to diabetic retinopathy. Early studies indicate that the therapy will help prevent abnormal blood vessels from coming back after surgery.

Expected results

Nonproliferative retinopathy has a better prognosis than proliferative retinopathy. Prognosis depends upon the extent of the retinopathy, the cause, and promptness of treatment.

Prevention

Complete eye examinations done regularly can help detect early signs of retinopathy. Patients on certain medications should have more frequent eye exams. They also should have a baseline eye exam when starting the drug. People with diabetes must take extra care to be sure to have thorough, periodic eye exams, especially if early signs of visual impairment are noticed. Anyone experiencing a sudden loss of vision, decrease in vision or visual field, flashes of light, or floating spots should contact their eye doctor right away. Proper medical treatment for any of the systemic diseases known to cause retinal damage will help prevent retinopathy. For diabetics, maintaining proper blood sugar and blood pressure levels is important as well; however, over time some form of retinopathy will usually occur in diabetics. Eating properly, particularly for diabetics, and stopping **smoking** will also help delay retinopathy. Frequent, thorough eye exams and control of systemic disorders are the best prevention.

Having sound overall physical and mental health habits, including lifestyle, diet, **exercise**, and stress management, is good prevention for eye disorders. Overexposing the eyes to sunlight should be avoided by those with retina problems, and sunglasses are a necessity. Sound work habits such as reading in adequate lighting, and taking frequent breaks from televisions, computers, and intricate tasks, are recommended practices for those with eye disorders. Eye exercises, originally developed by Dr. William Bates, are also a good preventative and supportive measure for the eyes. Many books are available that illustrate these and other vision exercises.

Resources

BOOKS

Grossman, Marc, and Glen Swartwout. *Natural Eye Care: An Encyclopedia.* Los Angeles: Keats, 1999.

Horton, Jonathan, C. *Disorders of the Eye.* New York: McGraw-Hill, 1998.

PERIODICALS

"Gene Therapy May Be a Tool for Prevention." *Diabetes Week* (October 8, 2001).

ORGANIZATIONS

Cambridge Institute for Better Vision. 65 Wenham Rd., Topsfield, MA 01983.

The Foundation Fighting Blindness. Executive Plaza I, Suite 800, 11350 McCormick Rd., Hunt Valley, MD 21031-1014. (888) 394-3937. http://www.blindness.org.

Optometric Extension Program. 2912 South Daimler St., Santa Ana, CA 92705.

Prevent Blindness America. 500 East Remington Rd., Schaumburg, IL 60173. (800) 331-2020. http://www.prevent-blindness.org.

Prevent Blindness America (Diabetes and Eyesight). 500 East Remington Rd., Schaumburg, IL 60173. (800) 331-2020. http://www.diabetes-sight.org.

Douglas Dupler
Teresa Norris

Rheumatic fever

Definition

Rheumatic **fever** (RF) is an illness that occurs as a complication of untreated or inadequately treated **strep throat** infection. Rheumatic fever causes inflammation of tissues and organs and can result in serious damage to the heart valves, joints, central nervous system and skin.

Rheumatic fever is rare in the United States, though there were outbreaks in both New York City and in Utah in the 1990s. The disease is more prevalent in the developing world, where rheumatic fever is the leading cause of **heart disease**. In some countries, as many as one to two percent of children are afflicted with the disease.

Description

Though the exact cause of rheumatic fever is unknown, the disease usually follows the contraction of a throat infection caused by a member of the Group A streptococcus (strep) bacteria (called strep throat). The streptococcus A bacteria has also been linked to many serious diseases, including "flesh-eating" disease and **toxic shock syndrome**. About 9,700 cases of invasive diseases linked to strep A were reported in the United States in 1997. Rheumatic fever may occur in people of any age, but is most common in children between the ages of five and 15. Poverty, overcrowded living conditions, and inadequate access to medical care increase the likelihood of contracting the disease.

The initial strep throat is easily treated with a 10-day course of antibiotics taken orally. However, when a throat infection occurs without symptoms, or when a patient neglects to take the prescribed medication for the full 10-day course of treatment, there is up to an estimated 3% chance that he or she will develop rheumatic fever. Other types of strep **infections** (such as of the skin) do not put the patient at risk for RF

Causes and symptoms

Two different theories exist as to how a bacterial throat infection can result in rheumatic fever. One theory, less supported by research evidence, suggests that the bacteria produce some kind of poisonous chemical (toxin). This toxin is sent into circulation throughout the bloodstream, thus affecting other systems of the body. Research more strongly supports the theory that the disease is caused by an interaction between antibodies produced to fight the group A streptococcus bacteria and the heart tissue. The body produces immune cells (antibodies), that are specifically designed to recognize and destroy invading agents. The antibodies are able to recognize the bacteria because the bacteria contain special markers called antigens on their surface. Due to a resemblance between Group A streptococcus bacteria's antigens and antigens present on the body's own cells, the antibodies mistakenly attack the body itself, specifically heart muscle.

In 2002, a report announced that scientists had mapped the genome (genetic material) of an A streptococcus bacterium responsible for acute rheumatic fever. The discovery will help researchers map the factors in the strain of bacterium that help it overcome the body's defenses.

It is interesting to note that members of certain families seem to have a greater tendency to develop rheumatic fever than do others. This could be related to the above theory, in that these families may have cell antigens that more closely resemble streptococcal antigens than do members of other families.

Symptoms of rheumatic fever usually begin one to six weeks after a **sore throat**. Symptoms may include **fatigue** and fever, stomach **pain** and **vomiting**. In about 75% of all cases of RF one of the first symptoms is arthritis. The joints (especially those of the ankles, knees, elbows, and wrists) become red, hot, swollen, shiny, and extremely painful. Unlike many other forms of arthritis, symptoms may not occur symmetrically (affecting a particular joint on both the right and left sides, simultaneously). Rather, pain may move from joint to joint. The arthritis of RF rarely strikes the fingers, toes, or spine. The joints become so tender that even the touch of bedsheets or clothing is terribly painful.

A peculiar type of involuntary movement, coupled with emotional instability, occurs in about 10% of all RF patients (the figure used to be about 50%). The patient begins experiencing a change in coordination, often first noted by changes in handwriting. The arms or legs may flail or jerk uncontrollably. The patient seems to develop a low threshold for anger and sadness. This feature of RF is called Sydenham's chorea or St. Vitus' dance.

A number of skin changes are common in rheumatic fever patients. A rash called erythema marginatum develops (especially in those patients who will develop heart problems from their illness), which takes the form of pink splotches that may eventually spread into each other. The rash does not itch. Bumps the size of peas or larger may occur under the skin. These are called subcutaneous nodules; they are hard to the touch, but not painful. These nodules most commonly occur over the knee and elbow joint, as well as over the spine.

The most serious result of RF is called pancarditis (pan means total; carditis refers to inflammation of the heart). Pancarditis is an inflammation that affects all aspects of the heart, including the lining of the heart (endocardium), the sac containing the heart (pericardium), and the heart muscle itself (myocardium). Heart damage caused by RF has the most serious long-term effects. The valves within the heart (structures that allow the blood to flow only in the correct direction, and only at the correct time in the heart's pumping cycle) are frequently damaged, which may result in blood leaking back in the wrong direction, or being unable to pass a stiff, poorly moving valve. Damage to a valve can result in the heart having to work very hard in order to circulate the blood. The heart may not be able to "work around" the damaged valve, which may result in a consistently inadequate amount of blood entering the circulation. About 40-80% of all RF patients develop a form of carditis. Heart damage, however, may not be apparent until months or years after a bout with rheumatic fever. The effect of the disease on the heart also depends on the avoidance of recurrences. The severity of heart damage is often related to the number of attacks of RF a patient experiences.

Diagnosis

The initial description of diagnostic criteria for RF were created by William Cheadle in 1889, during a virulent outbreak of the disease in London. In the 1950s, T. Duckett Jones created a list of both major and minor diagnostics for RF. According to the "Jones Criteria," a patient can be diagnosed with RF if he or she exhibits either two major criteria (conditions), or one major and two minor criteria. In either case, it must also be proven that the individual has had a previous infection with streptococcus.

The major criteria include:

• carditis

• arthritis

• chorea

• subcutaneous nodules

• erythema marginatum

The minor criteria include:

• fever

• joint pain (without actual arthritis)

• evidence of electrical changes in the heart (determined by measuring electrical characteristics of the heart's functioning during a test called an electrocardiogram, or EKG)

• evidence (through a blood test) of the presence in the blood of certain proteins, which are produced early in an inflammatory/infectious disease

Tests are also performed to provide evidence of recent infection with group A streptococcal bacteria. The doctor may swab the throat and grow a culture to see if the bacteria will grow and multiply. The culture will be processed and examined to identify streptococcal bacteria. Blood tests can be performed to see if the patient is producing antibodies only made in response to a recent strep infection. A doctor may also do an electrocardiogram in order to check for abnormalities in the heartbeat. An echocardiogram, or ultrasound test, may be ordered to check the heart vales, cardiac function and the heart's structure.

Treatment

Though there are no proven effective alternative remedies for rheumatic fever itself, alternative methods may help patients with the results and symptoms of the disease, such as pain relief and improved cardiac function. **Rheumatoid arthritis** can be treated with a number of alternative therapies:

• Massage: A massage therapist uses gentle strokes to stimulate circulation in and around the joints.

• Aromatherapy: Often combined with massage, the essential oils of rosemary, benzoin, German chamomile, camphor, juniper, or lavender are used to help relieve pain. Oils of cypress, fennel, lemon, and wintergreen may be used to detoxify or reduce inflammation.

• Acupuncture: Uses small needles to stimulate appropriate acupoints for pain relief.

• Osteopathy: Recommends stretching and trigger point therapy to improve mobility, as well as craniofacial massage.

Allopathic treatment

Penicillin is still the most effective treatment for rheumatic fever. A 10-day course of penicillin by mouth, or a single injection of penicillin G is the first line of treatment for RF. Patients will need to remain on some regular dose of penicillin to prevent recurrence of RF. This can mean a small daily dose of penicillin by mouth, or an injection every three weeks. Some practitioners keep patients on this regimen for five years, or until they reach 18 years of age (whichever comes first). Other practitioners prefer to continue treating those patients who will be regularly exposed to streptococcal bacteria (teachers, medical workers), as well as those patients with known RF heart disease.

Of major concern to medical professionals is compliance in taking oral penicillin. A full course of penicillin must be taken to prevent rheumatic fever. However, it is not always easy for patients to follow such a strict regimen. Researchers have found that the time-honored practice of thrice-daily dosing may be unnecessary. Research has shown that twice-daily dosing is just as effective as more frequent doses, and compliance may be improved, since both doses can be administered at home.

Arthritis typically improves quickly when the patient is given a preparation containing aspirin, or some other anti-inflammatory agent (ibuprofen). Mild carditis will also improve with such anti-inflammatory agents; although more severe cases of carditis will require steroid medications. A number of medications are available to treat the involuntary movements of chorea, including diazepam for mild cases, and haloperidol for more severe cases.

Expected results

The long-term prognosis of an RF patient depends primarily on whether he or she develops carditis. This is the only manifestation of RF that can have permanent effects. Those patients with mild or no carditis have an excellent prognosis. Those with more severe carditis have a risk of heart failure, as well as a risk of future heart problems, which may lead to the need for valve replacement surgery.

Prevention

Initial prevention of rheumatic fever depends upon prompt medical attention. Patients should see a physician if they have sore throat that lasts for more than 24 hours and is accompanied by fever. Treatment of a streptococcal throat infection with an appropriate antibiotic will usually prevent the development of rheumatic fever. Prevention of RF recurrence requires continued antibiotic treatment, perhaps for life. Prevention of complications of already-existing RF heart disease require that the patient always take a special course of antibiotics when he or she undergoes any kind of procedure (even dental cleanings) that might allow bacteria to gain access to the bloodstream.

Because of the prevalence of the Strep A bacteria, it is difficult to completely eradicate rheumatic fever. However, progress in identifying a genetic marker for predisposition to the disease and in mapping the virulence (ability to overcome the body's defenses) or the bacteria that lead to rheumatic fever may help lead to a vaccine. Researchers are also seeking to develop a rapid test for strep which would mean earlier detection and more prompt treatment of strep. In addition, in 1999, testing began on a vaccine against group A streptococcus. The development of such a vaccine was halted in the 1970s after children who received the experimental vaccine developed rheumatic fever. In 1979, the Food and Drug Administration (FDA) prohibited group A strep vaccines from ever being licensed for use, the only vaccine to carry such a prohibition. Clinical trials have been approved by the FDA, however, it will be several years before a vaccine is approved. Doctors at the National Institute of Allergy and Infectious Diseases remain hopeful that a vaccine will someday be available.

Resources

BOOKS

Kaplan, Edward L. "Rheumatic Fever." In *Harrison's Principles of Internal Medicine*. edited by Anthony S. Fauci, et al. New York: McGraw-Hill, 1998.

Ryan, Kenneth. "Streptococci." In *Sherris Medical Microbiology: An Introduction to Infectious Diseases*. Norwalk, CT: Appleton and Lange, 1994.

Stoffman, Phyllis. *The Family Guide to Preventing and Treating 100 Infectious Diseases*. New York: John Wiley and Sons, Inc., 1995.

Todd, James. "Rheumatic Fever." In *Nelson Textbook of Pediatrics*. edited by Richard Behrman. Philadelphia: W.B. Saunders Co., 1996.

Woodham, Anne and Dr. David Peters. *Dorling Kindersley Encyclopedia of Healing Therapies*. New York: Dorling Kindersley, 1997.

PERIODICALS

Albert, Daniel A., et al. "The Treatment of Rheumatic Carditis: A Review and Meta-Analysis." *Medicine* 74, no. 1 (January 1995): 1+.

Bass, James W., Donald A. Person, and Debora S. Chan. "Twice Daily Oral Penicillin for Treatment of Streptococcal Pharyngitis: Less is Best." *Pediatrics 2000* 105 (February, 2000): 423-424.

Capizzi, Stephen A., et al. "Rheumatic Fever Revisited: Keep This Diagnosis on Your List of Suspects." *Postgraduate Medicine* 102, no. 6 (December 1997): 65+.

Eichbaum, Q.G., et al. "Rheumatic Fever: Autoantibodies Against a Variety of Cardiac, Nuclear, and Streptococcal Antigens." *Annals of the Rheumatic Diseases* 54, no. 9 (September 1995): 740+.

Harder, B. "Deciphering Virulence: Heart-Harming Bacteria Flaunt Unique Viral Genes." *Science News* 161, no. 13 (March 30, 2002): 197.

Markowitz, Milton. "Rheumatic Fever: A Half-Century Perspective." *Pediatrics* (July, 1998): 272-275.

Pollack, Andrew. "In the Works: Tests on Strep Vaccine Restart, Gingerly." *The New York Times* (July 20, 1999): Section F, Page 7, Column 1.

"Rheumatic Fever." In *Clinical Reference Systems* (July 1, 1999): 1264.

Stollerman, Gene H. "Rheumatic Carditis." *Lancet* 346, no. 8972 (August 12, 1995): 390+.

Stollerman, Gene H. "Rheumatic Fever." *Lancet* (March 29, 1997): 935-943.

ORGANIZATIONS

Centers for Disease Control and Prevention. (404) 332-4559. http://www.cdc.gov.

Amy Cooper
Teresa G. Odle

Rheumatoid arthritis

Definition

Rheumatoid arthritis (RA) is a chronic disease causing inflammation and deformity of the joints. Other systemic problems throughout the body may also develop, including inflammation of blood vessels (vasculitis), the development of bumps (rheumatoid nodules) in various parts of the body, lung disease, blood disorders, and weakening of the bones (**osteoporosis**).

Description

The skeletal system of the body is made up of different types of strong, fibrous tissue called connective tissue. Bone, cartilage, ligaments, and tendons are all forms of connective tissue that have different compositions and characteristics.

The joints are structures that hold two or more bones together. Synovial joints allow for movement between the bones being joined, the articulating bones. The simplest synovial joint involves two bones, separated by a slight gap called the joint cavity. The ends of each articular bone are covered by a layer of cartilage. Both articular bones and the joint cavity are surrounded by a tough tissue called the articular capsule. The articular capsule has two components: the fibrous membrane on the outside and the synovial membrane, or synovium, on the inside. The fibrous membrane may include tough bands of tissue called ligaments, which are responsible for providing support to the joints. The synovial membrane has special cells and many tiny blood vessels called capillaries. This

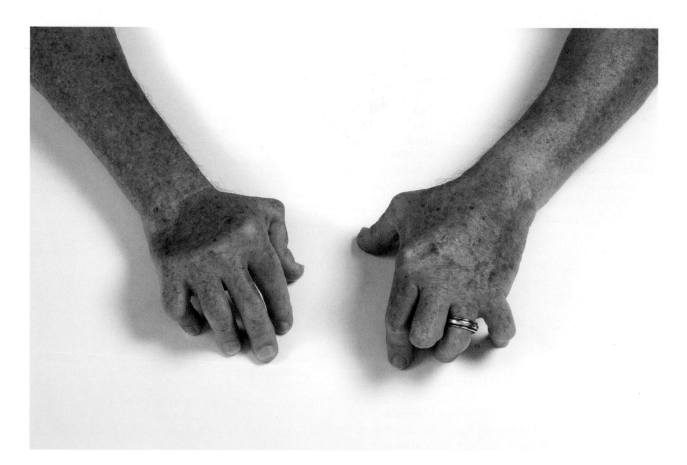

The hands of a 65 year old man with severe Rheumatoid arthritis. *(© jbcn / Alamy)*

Rheumatoid Arthritis

Risk Factors
  Family history

Physical Effects
  Affects joints
  Autoimmune disease
  Bony spurs
  Enlarged or malformed joints

Treatment Options
  Glucocorticoids
  Non-steroidal anti-inflammatory drugs
  MethotreXate
  Disease-modifying antirheumatic drugs

Pain Management
  Support groups
  Exercise
  Joint splitting
  Physical therapy
  Passive exercise
  Joint replacement
  Heat and cold
  Message therapy
  Acupuncture
  Psychological approaches
    (relaxation, visualization)
  Tai Chi
  Low stress yoga

(Illustration by Corey Light. Cengage Learning, Gale)

KEY TERMS

Articular bones—Two or more bones connected to each other via a joint.

Joint—Structures holding two or more bones together.

Synovial joint—A type of joint that allows articular bones to move.

Synovial membrane—The membrane that lines the inside of the articular capsule of a joint and produces a lubricating fluid called synovial fluid.

---

two million people suffer from the disease. Women are three times more likely than men to have RA. About 80% of people with RA are diagnosed between the ages of 35 and 50. RA appears to run in families, although certain factors in the environment may also influence the development of the disease.

Causes and symptoms

The underlying event that promotes RA in a person is unknown. Given the known genetic factors involved in RA, some researchers have suggested that an outside event occurs and triggers the disease cycle in a person with a particular genetic makeup. In late 2001, researchers announced discovery of the genetic markers that predict increased risk of RA. The discovery should soon aid research into diagnosis and treatment of the disease. Recent research has also shown that several autoimmune diseases, including RA, share a common genetic link. In other words, patients with RA might share common genes with family members who have other autoimmune diseases like systemic lupus, **multiple sclerosis**, and others.

Many researchers are examining the possibility that exposure to an organism (a bacteria or virus) may be the first event in the development of RA. The body's normal response is to produce cells that can attack and kill the organism, protecting the body from the foreign invader. In an autoimmune disease like RA, this immune cycle spins out of control. The body produces misdirected immune antibodies, which accidentally identify parts of the person's body as foreign. These immune cells then produce a variety of chemicals that injure and destroy parts of the body.

Reports in late 2001 suggest that certain **stress** hormones released during **pregnancy** may affect development of RA and other autoimmune diseases in women. Researchers have observed that women with autoimmune disorders will often show lessened symptoms during the third trimester of pregnancy. The

membrane produces a supply of synovial fluid that fills the joint cavity, lubricates it, and helps the articular bones move smoothly about the joint.

In rheumatoid arthritis, the synovial membrane becomes severely inflamed. Usually thin and delicate, the synovium becomes thick and stiff, with numerous infoldings on its surface. The membrane is invaded by white blood cells, which produce a variety of destructive chemicals. The cartilage along the articular surfaces of the bones may be attacked and destroyed, and the bone, articular capsule, and ligaments may begin to erode. These processes severely interfere with movement in the joint.

RA exists all over the world and affects men and women of all races. In the United States alone, about

symptoms then worsen in the year after pregnancy. Further, women appear to be at higher risk of developing new autoimmune disorders following pregnancy.

RA can begin very gradually or it can strike without warning. The first symptoms are **pain**, swelling, and stiffness in the joints. The most commonly involved joints include hands, feet, wrists, elbows, and ankles. The joints are typically affected in a symmetrical fashion. This means that if the right wrist is involved, the left wrist is also involved. Patients frequently experience painful joint stiffness when they first get up in the morning, lasting perhaps an hour. Over time, the joints become deformed. The joints may be difficult to straighten, and affected fingers and toes may be permanently bent. The hands and feet may also curve outward in an abnormal way.

Many patients also notice increased **fatigue**, loss of appetite, weight loss, and sometimes **fever**. Rheumatoid nodules are bumps that appear under the skin around the joints and on the top of the arms and legs. These nodules can also occur in the tissue covering the outside of the lungs and lining the chest cavity (pleura), and in the tissue covering the brain and spinal cord (meninges). Lung involvement may cause shortness of breath and is seen more in men. Vasculitis, an inflammation of the blood vessels, may interfere with blood circulation. This can result in irritated pits (ulcers) in the skin, **gangrene**, and interference with nerve functioning that causes numbness and tingling.

Diagnosis

There are no tests available that can absolutely diagnose RA. Instead, a number of tests exist that can suggest the diagnosis of RA. Blood tests include a special test of red blood cells, the erythrocyte sedimentation rate, which is positive in nearly 100% of patients with RA. However, this test is also positive in a variety of other diseases. Tests for **anemia** are usually positive in patients with RA, but can also be positive in many other unrelated diseases. Rheumatoid factor is an autoantibody found in about 66% of patients with RA. However, it is also found in about 5% of all healthy people and in 10–20% of healthy people over the age of 65. Rheumatoid factor is also positive in a large number of other autoimmune diseases and other infectious diseases.

A long, thin needle can be inserted into a synovial joint to withdraw a sample of the synovial fluid for examination. In RA, this fluid has certain characteristics that indicate active inflammation. The fluid will be cloudy, relatively thinner than usual, with increased protein and decreased or normal glucose. It will also contain a higher than normal number of white blood cells. While these findings suggest inflammatory arthritis, they are not specific to RA.

Treatment

There is no cure available for RA. However, treatment is available to combat the inflammation in order to prevent destruction of the joints and other complications of the disease. Efforts are also made to provide relief from the symptoms and to maintain maximum flexibility and mobility of the joints.

A variety of alternative therapies have been recommended for patients with RA. **Meditation**, hypnosis, **guided imagery**, **relaxation**, and **reflexology** techniques have been used effectively to control pain. **Acupressure** and **acupuncture** have also been used for pain; work on the pressure points should be done daily in combination with other therapies. Bodywork can be soothing and is thought to improve and restore chemical balance within the body. A massage with **rosemary** and **chamomile**, or soaking in a warm bath with these **essential oils**, can provide extra relief. Stiff joints may also be loosened up with a warm **sesame oil** massage, followed by a hot shower to further heat the oil and allow entry into the pores. Movement therapies like **yoga**, **t'ai chi**, and **qigong** also help to loosen up the joints.

A multitude of nutritional supplements can be useful for RA. Fish oils, the enzymes **bromelain** and pancreatin, and the **antioxidants** (vitamins A, C, and E, **selenium**, and **zinc**) are the primary supplements to consider.

Many herbs also are useful in the treatment of RA. Anti-inflammatory herbs may be helpful, including **turmeric** (*Curcuma longa*), **ginger** (*Zingiber officinale*), **feverfew** (*Chrysanthemum parthenium*), **devil's claw** (*Harpagophytum procumbens*), **Chinese thoroughwax** (*Bupleuri falcatum*), and **licorice** (*Glycyrrhiza glabra*). **Lobelia** (*Lobelia inflata*) and **cramp bark** (*Vibernum opulus*) can be applied topically to the affected joints.

Homeopathic practitioners recommend *Rhus toxicondendron* and **bryonia** (*Bryonia alba*) for acute prescriptions, but constitutional treatment, generally used for chronic problems like RA, is more often recommended. Yoga has been used for RA patients to promote relaxation, relieve stress, and improve flexibility. Nutritionists suggest that a vegetarian diet low in animal products and sugar may help to decrease both inflammation and pain from RA. Beneficial foods for patients with RA include cold water fish (mackerel, herring, salmon, and sardines) and flavonoid-rich berries (cherries, blueberries, **hawthorn** berries, blackberries, etc.). The enzyme bromelain, found in pineapple juice has also been found to have significant anti-inflammatory effects.

RA, considered an autoimmune disorder, is often connected with food **allergies** or intolerances. An elimination/challenge diet can help to decrease symptoms of RA as well as identify the foods that should be eliminated to prevent flare-ups and recurrences.

Hydrotherapy can help to greatly reduce pain and inflammation. Moist heat is more effective than dry heat, and cold packs are useful during acute flare-ups. Various yoga exercises done once a day can also assist in maintaining joint flexibility.

Allopathic treatment

Nonsteroidal anti-inflammatory agents and aspirin are used to decrease inflammation and to treat pain. While these medications can be helpful, they do not interrupt the progress of the disease. Low-dose steroid medications can be helpful at both managing symptoms and slowing the progress of RA, as well as other drugs called disease-modifying anti-rheumatic drugs. These include gold compounds, D-penicillamine, antimalarial drugs, and sulfasalazine. Methotrexate, azathioprine, and cyclophosphamide are all drugs that suppress the immune system and can decrease inflammation. All of the drugs listed have significant toxic side effects, which require healthcare professionals to carefully compare the risks associated with these medications to the benefits.

Total bed rest is sometimes prescribed during the very active, painful phases of RA. Splints may be used to support and rest painful joints. Later, after inflammation has somewhat subsided, physical therapists may provide a careful **exercise** regimen in an attempt to maintain the maximum degree of flexibility and mobility. Joint replacement surgery, particularly for the knee and the hip joints, is sometimes recommended when these joints have been severely damaged. Another surgery used to stop pain in a stiff joint, such as the ankle, is the fusion of the affected bones together (arthrodesis, or artificial anklylosis).

Prognosis

About 15% of all RA patients will have symptoms for a short period of time and will ultimately get better, leaving them with no long-term problems. A number of factors are considered to suggest the likelihood of a worse prognosis. These include:

- race and gender (female and Caucasian)
- more than 20 joints involved
- extremely high erythrocyte sedimentation rate
- extremely high levels of rheumatoid factor
- consistent, lasting inflammation

- evidence of erosion of bone, joint, or cartilage on x rays
- poverty
- older age at diagnosis
- rheumatoid nodules
- other coexisting diseases
- certain genetic characteristics, diagnosable through testing

Patients with RA have a shorter life span, averaging a decrease of three to seven years of life. Patients sometimes die when very severe disease, infection, and gastrointestinal bleeding occur. Complications due to the side effects of some of the more potent drugs used to treat RA are also factors in these deaths.

Prevention

There is no known way to prevent the development of RA. The most that can be hoped for is to prevent or slow its progress.

Resources

BOOKS

Aaseng, Nathan. *Autoimmune Diseases*. New York: F. Watts, 1995.

Lipsky, Peter E. "Rheumatoid Arthritis." *Harrison's Principles of Internal Medicine*. 14th ed. edited by Anthony S. Fauci, et al. New York: McGraw-Hill, 1998.

Schlotzhauer, M. *Living with Rheumatoid Arthritis*. Baltimore: Johns Hopkins University Press, 1993.

PERIODICALS

Akil, M., and R. S. Amos. "Rheumatoid Arthritis: Clinical Features and Diagnosis." *British Medical Journal*. 310 (March 4, 1995): 587+.

Gremillion, Richard B. and Ronald F. Van Vollenhoven. "Rheumatoid Arthritis: Designing and Implementing a Treatment Plan." *Postgraduate Medicine*. 103 (February 1998): 103+.

Moran, M. "Autoimmune Diseases Could Share Common Genetic Etiology." *American Medical News*. 44; no. 38: (October 8, 2001):38.

Ross, Clare. "A Comparison of Osteoarthritis and Rheumatoid Arthritis: Diagnosis and Treatment." *The Nurse Practitioner*. 22 (September 1997): 20+.

"Suspect Gene Mapped, May Lead to New Diagnostic Markers and Drug Targets." *Immunotherapy Weekly*. (December 26, 2001):24.

Vastag, Brian. "Autoimmune Disorders and Hormones." *JAMA, Journal of the American Medical Association*. 286, no. 19 (November 21, 2001):1.

ORGANIZATIONS

American College of Rheumatology. 60 Executive Park South, Suite 150, Atlanta, GA 30329. (404)633–1870. http://www.rheumatology.org. acr@rheumatology.org.

Arthritis Foundation. 1330 West Peachtree St., Atlanta, GA 30309. (404)872–7100. http://www.arthritis.org. help@arthritis.org.

Kathleen Wright
Teresa Norris

Rheumatoid spondylitis *see* **Ankylosing spondylitis**

Rhinitis

Definition

Rhinitis is inflammation of the mucous lining of the nose.

Description

Rhinitis is a nonspecific term that covers nasal congestion due to **infections**, **allergies**, and other disorders. In rhinitis, the mucous membranes of the nose become infected or irritated, producing a discharge, congestion, and swelling of the tissues.

The most widespread form of infectious rhinitis is the **common cold**. The common cold is the most frequent viral infection in the general population. Colds are self-limited, lasting about three to 10 days, although they are sometimes followed by a bacterial infection.

Causes and symptoms

Colds can be caused by as many as 200 different viruses which are transmitted by **sneezing** and coughing, by contact with soiled tissues or handkerchiefs, or by close contact with an infected person.

The onset of a cold is usually sudden. The virus causes the lining of the nose to become inflamed and produce large quantities of thin, watery mucus. The inflammation spreads from the nasal passages to the throat and upper airway, producing a dry **cough**, **headache**, and watery eyes. After several days, the nasal tissues becomes less inflamed and the watery discharge is replaced by a thick, sticky mucus. This change in the appearance of the nasal discharge helps to distinguish rhinitis caused by a viral infection from allergic rhinitis.

Allergies are another frequent cause of rhinitis which is called allergic rhinitis. Allergies occur when a person's immune system overreacts to a substance called an allergen. Airborne allergens can be just about anything but are commonly mold, pollen, dust mites,

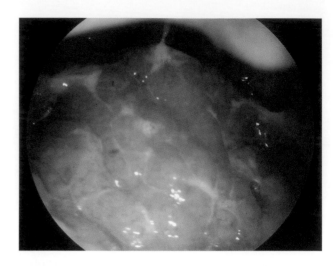

Posterior rhinoscopy showing acute rhinopharyngitis. *(Ism/ Phototake, Reproduced by permission.)*

and pet dander. Symptoms of allergy include watery eyes, nasal discharge, sneezing, and headache.

Diagnosis

Viral rhinitis is diagnosed based on symptoms. Symptoms that last longer than a week may require further testing to rule out a secondary bacterial infection, or an allergy. Allergies can be evaluated by blood tests, skin testing for specific substances, or nasal smears.

Treatment

The many alternative treatments for colds and allergies will not be addressed here. Treatments specifically for rhinitis, regardless of the cause, are described.

Herbal remedies

Flavonoids have anti-inflammatory activities and can be found in many plants including **licorice**, **parsley**, legumes (beans), onions, **garlic**, berries, and citrus fruits. Herbals which may help lessen the symptoms of rhinitis include:

- astragalus (*Astragalus membranaceous*) root
- baical skullcap (*Scutellaria baicalensis*) decoction
- echinacea (*Echinacea* spp.)
- elderflower (*Sambucus nigra*) tea
- garlic, which contains anti-inflammatory compounds
- goldenseal (*Hydrastis canadensis*)
- horehound (*Marrubium vulgare*) tea relieves congestion
- licorice (*Glycyrrhiza glabra*) has anti-inflammatory activity

KEY TERMS

Allergen—A substance that causes an allergic reaction because of a hypersensitive immune system.

Inflammation—A protective response caused by tissue damage that serves to destroy the offending agent. Inflammation is characterized by redness, swelling, pain, and fluid discharge.

- mullein (*Verbascum thapsus*) is a decongestant and soothes mucous membranes
- nettle (*Urtica dioica*) tea stops nasal discharge
- onion, which contains anti-inflammatory compounds
- thyme (*Thymus vulgaris*) tea, which is anti-inflammatory and soothes sore nasal tissues
- walnut (*Juglans nigra* or *regia*) leaf tea, which stops nasal discharge

Other remedies

Other natural remedies for rhinitis include those from **traditional Chinese medicine**. Chronic rhinitis is treated with **acupuncture**, ear acupuncture, and herbals taken internally or used externally. The most common rhinitis remedy is Bi Yan Pian (Bi is for nose.) There are many others, depending on the specific pattern of the patient. **Magnolia** flower and xanthium are commonly used herbs for rhinitis.

Less common Chinese remedies include Huo Dan Wan (**Agastache** and Pig's Gall Bladder Pill) taken three times daily. A decoction of Yu Xing Cao (*Herba houttuyniae*) may be taken internally. The patient can apply 30% Huang Lian Shui (**Coptis** Fluid), Huang Bai Shui (Phellodendron Fluid), Yu Xing Cao (*Herba houttuyniae*) juice, E Bu Shi Cao (*Herba centipedae*) decoction, or 1% ephedrine solution directly to the nose.

Colored **light therapy** is based upon the theory that an unhealthy body is lacking a specific color frequency. Green colored light therapy may relieve chronic rhinitis.

Homeopathic physicians prescribe any of 10 different remedies, depending on the appearance of the nasal discharge, the patient's emotional state, and the stage of infection.

Vitamin C is a natural antihistamine. **Vitamin A** and **zinc** may also be helpful.

Allopathic treatment

There is no cure for the common cold; treatment is given for symptom relief. Medications include aspirin or nonsteroidal anti-inflammatory drugs (NSAIDs) for headache and muscle **pain**, and decongestants to relieve stuffiness or runny nose. Antibiotics are ineffective against viral infections. Allergies are treated with antihistamines (Benadryl).

Expected results

Most colds resolve completely in about a week. Complications are unusual but may include sinusitis (inflammation of the nasal sinuses), bacterial infections, or infections of the middle ear. Allergies may resolve or may be lifelong.

Prevention

There is no vaccine effective against colds, and infection does not prevent one from getting colds. Prevention depends on washing hands often, minimizing contact with persons already infected, and not sharing hand towels, eating utensils, or water glasses. In 2002, researchers discovered a new antiseptic skin cleanser that may prevent hand-to-hand transmission of the rhinovirus that causes colds. The cleaner's active ingredient is salicylic or pyroglutamic acid, and each showed promising results for killing the virus on subject's hands.

Allergies may be prevented by avoiding the cause of the allergy, although this is not always possible or practical. Patients may become desensitized to the offending allergen by receiving a series of injections. In 2002, Australian researchers discovered a new potential vaccine that might boost immune response to allergens without the risk of side effects that come with some desensitizing vaccines available today.

Resources

BOOKS

Berman, Stephen, and Ken Chan. "Ear, Nose, & Throat." *Current Pediatric Diagnosis & Treatment*. Edited by William W. Hay, Jr., et al. Stamford, CT: Appleton & Lange, 1997.

Jackler, Robert K., and Michael J. Kaplan. "Ear, Nose, & Throat." In *Current Medical Diagnosis & Treatment 1998*, edited by Lawrence M. Tierney Jr., et al. Stamford, CT: Appleton & Lange, 1997.

King, Hueston C., and Richard L. Mabry. "Rhinitis." In *Current Diagnosis 9*, edited by Rex B. Conn, et al. Philadelphia: W. B. Saunders Company, 1997.

Ying, Zhou Zhong, and Jin Hui De. "Common Diseases of the Nose." *Clinical Manual of Chinese Herbal Medicine and Acupuncture*. New York: Churchill Livingston, 1997.

PERIODICALS

"Antispetic Skin Cleansers May Prevent Rhinovirus Transmission." *Clinical Infectious Diseases* (February 1, 2002): ii.

Cocilovo, Anna. "Colored Light Therapy: Overview of its History, Theory, Recent Developments and Clinical Applications Combined with Acupuncture." *American Journal of Acupuncture* 27 (1999): 71–83.

"Potential Vaccine Boosts Hope for Pollen Relief." *Immunotherapy Weekly* (March 6, 2002): 3.

Rebecca Frey
Belinda Rowland
Teresa G. Odle

Rhodiola rosea

Description

Siberian golden root *Rhodiola rosea* is native to the Altai Mountains of Siberia where it is known as *zolotov koren*. It is naturalized and widely distributed throughout higher elevations in Eastern Europe, Asia, and Scandinavia and in Ukraine's Carpathian Mountains where it was used to strengthen and protect against the harshness and **stress** of the arctic climate. It has been a folk remedy in these cold mountainous regions for centuries. An Alaskan variety has long been in common use as a staple food in the Eskimo diet, and various species of Rhodiola, some endangered, are found throughout the mountainous areas of North America. Wild *Rhodiola* is becoming a rare genetic resource.

The Greek physician Dioscorides mentioned the herb, then known as *rodia riza*, in the book *De Materia Medica*. The roots of this hardy plant exude a slight rose scent when freshly cut, a quality that inspired the Swiss botanist Linnaeus to assign it the scientific name *Rhodiola rosea*. Other common names are rose root, king's crown, and Sedum rhodiola. In Germany it is called *Rosenwurz*, in Japan *iwa-benkeior*, and in China, where it is a mainstay of traditional medicine, it is known as *Hong Jing Tian*. Researchers with the Swedish Herbal Institute, after decades of study, standardized a unique extract (SHR-5) of *Rhodiola rosea* marketed as Arctic Root.

Rhodiola rosea is a prized member of the *Crassulaceae*, or Stonecrop family, a worldwide family of succulents with about 25 genera and as many as 1,400 species. The genus *Rhodiola* has 200 or more related species. This perennial herb thrives on sunny mountain slopes, on sea cliffs, and in rock crevices and ledges at altitudes of 11,000 to 18,000 feet above sea level. In arctic areas the herb may grow among mats of moss. This drought-tolerant species can survive in sandy to clay soil; however, in soil rich with bird manure or near human habitat, the plant may grow lush and profuse.

The thick, fleshy and scaly aerial stems release a rose-like scent when cut and bear numerous simple leaves that last for a single season or less. Leaves are distributed alternately, sometimes whorl-like, along the stems. The succulent leaf blades, widening gradually from the base, are somewhat spoon shaped, without stalks. The veins are inconspicuous. There is a tap root and the ground-level or under-ground stems are horizontal or vertical and often branched. The plant is not self-fertile and requires bees and flies to pollinate. It is dioecious, bearing either male or female individual flowers. Both male and female plants are needed to propagate seed. The yellow flowers bloom from May to August and the seeds begin to ripen in July.

General use

The Vikings prized this Alpine herb and used it to bolster strength and stamina. In Norway, the herb was once planted on peat-moss roofs as a fire-protecting cover. In Mongolia it was used to treat **tuberculosis** and **cancer**. Russian cosmonauts used it to increase endurance on long space journeys, and Olympian athletes took the herb to increase strength and hasten recovery from physical exertion.

This beneficial mountain herb was mentioned in scientific writings in Iceland, Sweden, Norway, France, and Germany as early as the sixteenth century. It was listed in the first Swedish Pharmacopeia in 1775 and in the early 2000s is mentioned in the national pharmacopoeias of France, Sweden, Denmark, and the former USSR.

In Siberia, Rhodiola tea is said to promote long life. Those who drink it regularly are said to live beyond 100 years. The promise of such longevity motivated Chinese emperors to finance expeditions into Siberia to collect and bring back the plant, which became one the most popular medicinal herbs of middle Asia. *Rhodiola rosea* is commercially grown in Russia and China and in other suitable climates where its attributes have long been valued.

This beneficial tonic herb is classed as a superior herb in **traditional Chinese medicine**. It has been demonstrated as effective in the treatment of **Post-traumatic stress disorder** (PTSD), helping to alleviate typical symptoms such as **depression**, mood-swings, hyper vigilance, **insomnia**, nightmares, flashbacks, and panic attacks. During wartime, this potent herb was traditionally included in packages that families sent to soldiers on the front lines.

Clinical studies

Researchers in the former Soviet Union studied the beneficial effects of Siberian *Rhodiola rosea*, from as early as the 1930s, though much of this research was kept as a state secret, particularly during the cold war era. The Russian botanist and nutritionist, L. Utkin, discovered Rhodiola's effectiveness in enhancing physical strength in 1931. In 1947, the Russian scientist and professor Lazarev found that *Rhodiola rosea* could boost physical resistance to environmental stressors. Russian physician and scientist Dr. Israel Brekhman, coined the term *Adaptogen* to describe the biologically active properties of this prized traditional medicine.

Not all species have the adaptogenic properties of *R. rosea*, which contains a full spectrum of rosavin, rosarin, and rosin. These substances are derived from the plant rhizomes. Other phytochemical components include the phenylethanol derivatives salidroside and tyrosol, various flavonoids, monoterpernes, triterpenes, and phenolic and gallic acids. The biologically active compounds contained in the roots have large variation and potency varies among the species.

Since the mid-twentieth century there have been hundreds of research studies in Scandinavian countries. Much of the extensive research reported in Russian language journals was only made available in the late twentieth century for study by Western researchers, who replicated and confirmed some claims of the medicinal properties of *Rhodiola rosea*.

Benefits

- Promotes metabolic homeostasis by promoting cellular energy metabolism.
- Enhances physical endurance and recovery from exertion.
- Increases resistance to chemical, biological, and physical stressors.
- Improves memory, concentration, and hearing.
- Relieves anxiety and panic attacks.
- Restores sexual potency in males (through normalization of prostrate).
- Detoxifies the liver and eliminates toxins in muscle tissue.
- Regulates the heart beat, counteracting heart arrhythmias.

- Maintains optimal levels of serotonin and other neurotransmitters in the brain.
- Reduces the cortisol stress hormone, preventing many age-related diseases.
- Alleviates depression, improves sleep, and eliminates fatigue.
- Decreases risk of heart disease by reducing harmful blood lipids.
- Inhibits the spread of bacteria and viral agents.
- Inhibits the growth of tumors (anti-tumor effects demonstrated in animal studies), particularly in glandular tissue such as lungs and breasts.
- Reduces fat, improving the ratio of lean body mass to fat.
- Regulates blood sugar levels for diabetics.

Preparations

Rhodiola tincture is traditionally prepared by means of root decoction. The fresh rhizomes are soaked for a week in 40% alcohol to make a tincture known in the former Soviet Union as *nastojka*.

Native Eskimo people buried the roots for use when short of food and ate fermented stems, leaves, and young flower buds with walrus blubber or other oil. They consumed the young leaves and flowering stems as fresh salad, cooked them as a potherb, or prepared them as a kind of sauerkraut. As a remedy for intestinal discomfort, they steeped the flowers into ingest as a tea or ate them raw for a tuberculosis cure.

Commercially prepared tinctures, capsules, and teas are widely available. Clinical dosages are from standardized extracts containing effective amounts of active agents: Typically *Rhodiola rosea* is standardized to 3% Rosavins and 1% Salidroside, the ratio found in the natural root. An effective dose is from 200–600 mg/day.

Researchers also suggest varying dosage, depending upon the ratio of rosavin in the extract. For chronic use, the suggested daily dose is as follows:

- 360–600 mg daily of an extract standardized for 1% rosavin
- 180–300 mg daily of an extract standardized for 2% rosavin, or
- 100–170 mg of an extract standardized for 3.6% rosavin

A person may begin taking *Rhodiola rosea* several weeks before any expected increase in physiological, chemical, or biological stress and continue daily dosage throughout the duration of the stressful period.

KEY TERMS

Adaptogen—A plant with biologically active components that increase the adaptive ability of an organism stressed by internal and external factors; helps to counter and prevent damage from adverse physical, chemical, or biological stressors.

Antitumor—A property of plant chemistry that acts to prevent or inhibit the formation or growth of tumors.

Perennial—A plant with a lifecycle persisting more than two years, reoccurring year after year.

Rhizome—A fleshy plant stem that grows horizontally under or along the ground. Roots are sent out below this stem and leaves or shoots are sent out above it.

Succulent—Any type of drought-tolerant plant that stores water in its fleshy parts, such as stems and leaves.

Superior herb—The highest of three categories of herbal plants in traditional Chinese medicine. A superior herb is a non-toxic tonic that acts safely over time to assist the body in self-healing by eliminating toxins and nourishing, strengthening, and supporting cells, tissues, and organs and by supporting the immune system to maintain health and vitality.

Tonic—Herbal remedies with a slow, nourishing, gently stimulating and well-tolerated action in the body.

For circumstances of limited or short-term stress, a single dose, as high as three times the daily dose, may be beneficial in boosting the system to deal with the acute stress. *Rhodiola rosea* may be taken in appropriate dosages for only one day (acute administration) or with chronic conditions, daily up to four months.

Consumers should be aware that only the species *Rhodiola rosea* has been found to contain the full spectrum of the three pharmacologically active agents, rosavin, rosarin, and rosin. These agents, collectively known as rosavins, are believed to given the herb its beneficial effect.

Precautions

Rhodiola rosea is non-toxic. There are no known or suspected safety risks when it is taken in recommended doses. Though clinical trials have revealed no serious adverse effects, the safe use of *Rhodiola rosea*

by pregnant or nursing women, young children, or by people with severe liver or kidney disease has not been established. If individuals are prone to insomnia, it is advisable not to take the herb late at night, as it may disrupt sleep patterns. Consumers ought to consult a qualified herbalist or medical doctor before taking *Rhodiola* if they are also taking any prescription drug.

It would be prudent with chronic use of *Rhodiola rosea* to allow brief intervals without taking the herb, in keeping with established dosage patterns used with other plant adaptogens.

Resources

BOOKS

Winston, David, and Steven Maimes. *Adaptogens: Herbs for Strength, Stamina, and Stress Relief.* Rochester, VT: Healing Arts Press, 2007.

PERIODICALS

"Rhodiola." *Healthy for Men* (February/March 2006).
Tuttle, Dave. "Rhodiola: The Cellular Energy-Boosting Herb." *Life Extension* (February 2006).
Vastag, Brian. "Warming to a Cold War Herb." *Science News Online* 172, no. 12 (September 22, 2007).

OTHER

"Herbal Extract Found to Increase Lifespan." *ScienceDaily* (December 7, 2007). http://www.sciencedaily.com?/releases/2007/12/071205115232.htm (February 12, 2008).

ORGANIZATIONS

American Botanical Council, PO Box 144345, Austin, TX, 78714-4345, (512) 926-4900, http://abc.herbalgram.org.

Clare Hanrahan

Rhubarb root

Description

Rhubarb, also called sweet round-leaved dock or pieplant, is usually thought of as a fruit, but it is actually one of the few perennial vegetables in existence. Ordinary garden rhubarb carries the botanical name of *Rheum rhaponticum*, though there are other members of this botanical group that are also used for medicinal purposes. Chinese rhubarb, which is called *da huang* in traditional Chinese medicine, has the botanical name *Rheum palmatum*. Chinese rhubarb has a much stronger taste and properties than the common American variety. Rhubarb is a member of the same family as buckwheat, the Polygonaceae family. It originally came from Mongolia in northern Asia, but was

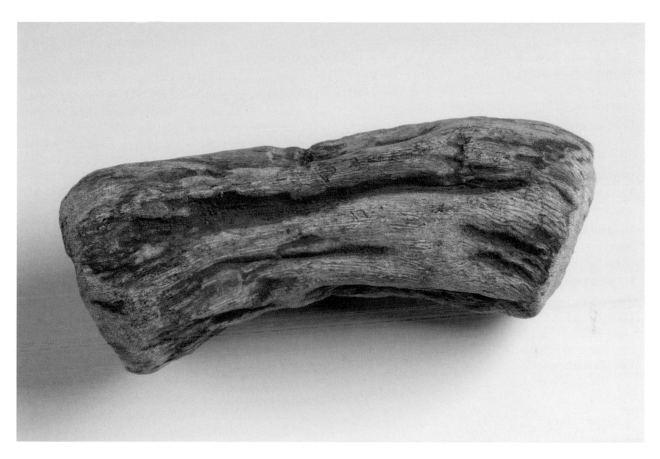

Rhubarb root. *(© Arco Images / Alamy)*

long ago introduced to both India and Turkey. It was formerly called India or Turkey rhubarb.

In the 1760s, in England, an Oxfordshire pharmacist named Hayward began developing and growing the type of rhubarb most commonly grown today. Records indicate that rhubarb was first grown as a market crop in England in 1810. But because it was unknown, few people purchased it. In the next one hundred years, its popularity grew tremendously.

The average life expectancy of rhubarb plants is five to eight years. Although rhubarb produces seeds, they can give birth to plants remarkably different from the parent plant. For this reason, rhubarb cultivation is usually done by cutting and replanting pieces of its large storage root.

Rhubarb is an early plant that is extremely hardy. It is relatively immune to attack by insects or disease. It puts out smaller feeder roots in early spring; even in colder regions, reddish bud-like projections appear in early April. These develop rapidly into long thick succulent stalks that can grow from 1–3 ft (approximately 30–90 cm) in length. Rhubarb stalks are generally ready for harvesting by late May. One very large spade-shaped leaf with curled edges grows at the tip of each stalk. There is considerable evidence that these leaves should be considered poisonous due to their high content of salts of oxalic acid. Oxalic acid is a powerful but toxic cleaning agent. Although M. Grieve reports that people have eaten both the leaves and the newly formed rhubarb buds without any problem, she also mentions several sources that listed several cases of death by rhubarb leaf poisoning around 1910. Rhubarb stalks have a tangy, sweet-sour taste much prized for the making of desserts, especially pies. Rhubarb stalks are a good source of ascorbic acid (**vitamin C**).

Chinese rhubarb produces a yellowish root with a distinctive network of white lines running along the outer surface. Chinese rhubarb root is much larger and more firmly textured than its Western relatives, and has much stronger laxative qualities, but it is also less astringent. The root of Western garden rhubarb is smaller, spongier, and is usually pinkish in color. It has sporadic star-shaped spots evident along its transverse sections.

KEY TERMS

Astringent—A substance that constricts or contracts the soft tissues or canals of the body. Rhubarb root has an astringent effect on the intestines.

Crohn's disease—A chronic inflammatory disease that can affect any part of the gastrointestinal tract from the mouth to the anus.

Diuretic—A group of drugs that help remove excess water from the body by increasing the amount lost in urine.

Electrolytes—Substances whose molecules split into electrically charged particles when dissolved or melted.

Hypokalemia—A condition in which the levels of potassium in the bloodstream are too low.

Oxalic acid—A poisonous white crystalline acid, used for bleaching, as a cleanser, and as a laboratory reagent. Rhubarb leaves contain small quantities of oxalic acid.

General use

Western herbalism

Rhubarb root has properties that make it a highly effective laxative. Its astringent qualities help to improve bowel tone after it has purged the intestines, making it an excellent agent for improving the tone and health of the digestive tract. Its laxative effects make it a valuable aid in the treatment of chronic **constipation**, hemorrhoids, and **gastroenteritis**. Skin eruptions caused by problems in elimination are also treated with rhubarb root. The Western rhubarb root, being milder, is used in treating infant digestive problems, constipation, or **diarrhea**.

Traditional Chinese medicine

Da huang, or Chinese rhubarb, is one of the most ancient and best known plants used in Chinese herbal medicine. Rhubarb and its wide range of uses were first documented in the *Divine Husbandman's Classic of Materia Medica*, which was written during the later Han Dynasty, around 200 A.D. The Chinese also used rhubarb root as a laxative and purgative for the treatment of both constipation and diarrhea, depending upon the dosage used. Larger doses cause purging that removes toxins from the intestinal tract, while smaller doses are believed to moisten the mucous membranes of the intestines and improve their tone. The tannins that are also found in the root may eventually cause binding of the bowel. Chinese rhubarb's laxative component normally works within eight hours.

Rhubarb root has been found useful in controlling gastrointestinal hemorrhage by promoting the formation of blood platelets. This increase in the number of platelets shortens blood clotting time and is helpful in treating **jaundice**. Recent studies in China and Japan demonstrated that rhubarb root can delay or stop the progression of chronic renal failure. One of the tannin components of rhubarb root, lindleyin, has been shown to act as an anti-inflammatory agent with fever-reducing properties similar to those of aspirin. Lindleyin is used in treating endometriosis and some menstrual problems. Emodin, another component of Chinese rhubarb root, has been found to inhibit the growth of cancer cells. Chinese herbalists have found rhubarb root helpful in external applications for **burns**, suppurative sores and ulcers, **conjunctivitis**, and traumatic injuries. There is some empirical evidence that *da huang* can reduce high blood pressure during **pregnancy**, although it should be used very cautiously in pregnancy. It has the ability to fight such anaerobic infectious agents as *Candida albicans*. Chinese herbalists also use rhubarb root for diseases and disorders in the upper body, including sinus and lung **infections**, nosebleeds, and eye infections. According to the principles of traditional Chinese medicine, rhubarb root makes the heat in the upper body discharge through the bowel.

More recently, Japanese researchers have suggested that rhubarb root is effective in treating the severe diarrhea associated with cholera. One of the tannins isolated from rhubarb root, galloyl-tannin, appears to counteract the toxin secreted by the bacterium that causes cholera.

Although some of the individual chemical compounds that can be isolated from rhubarb have been reported to cause **cancer**, there is no evidence as of 2002 that rhubarb by itself or herbal preparations containing it cause cancer in humans.

Preparations

Rhubarb root is usually taken from plants four or more years of age. It is dug up in the autumn, usually October, washed thoroughly, external fibers removed, and dried completely. The root is then pulverized and stored in a tightly closed container. Chinese rhubarb root usually comes from either China or Turkey. It can be purchased either in a powdered form or as a tincture. Putting 1.5–1 tsp (2.5–5 cc) of pulverized rhubarb root in 1 cup (240 cc) of water can make a decoction, or tea. This mixture is brought to a boil and then simmered at reduced heat for 10 minutes. Rhubarb tea can be taken twice a day. The tincture can be taken in a dose of 1–2 ml three times a day. Chinese herbal preparations of rhubarb root are individually compounded for each patient. Rhubarb root may be combined with other herbs.

Precautions

Chinese rhubarb should be prescribed only by a trained herbalist. It should not be taken by children under twelve years of age, or by pregnant or nursing women. It should also not be used by persons with acute and chronic inflammatory diseases of the intestine, including Crohn's disease, appendicitis, and intestinal obstruction. When rhubarb is used for its laxative-purgative qualities, the patient should be reminded that constipation is often caused by poor diet and lack of proper **exercise**. Correcting these patterns can improve bowel function without the use of any other therapy. People who use rhubarb root long-term for bowel problems may find that its effectiveness is decreased by extended use, and can also cause excessive loss of electrolytes from the intestinal tract. Loss of electrolytes, especially potassium, can lead to muscle weakness, and in extreme cases, cardiac arrhythmias. It should be noted that rhubarb root can color the urine either a deep yellow or even red. It is possible to become intoxicated from an overdose of rhubarb, though the plant is generally safe to take in the recommended doses and manner. Signs of overdosage include vertigo, nausea and **vomiting**, and severe abdominal cramps. Long-term use can lead to hypokalemia and cirrhosis of the liver.

Some specialists in internal medicine maintain that rhubarb should not be taken by people who are susceptible to **gallstones** or **kidney stones**.

Side effects

Severe abdominal cramping is a common side effect of rhubarb root. This problem can often be alleviated by reducing the dose.

Interactions

Due to the possible loss of **potassium**, rhubarb root should not be taken in combination with cardiac medications, diuretics, other laxatives or cathartics, or steroids. Loss of potassium from the system can be decreased by combining the rhubarb root with **licorice** root.

Resources

BOOKS

Grieve, M., and C. F. Leyel. *A Modern Herbal: The Medical, Culinary, Cosmetic and Economic Properties, Cultivation and Folklore of Herbs, Grasses, Fungi, Shrubs and Trees With All of Their Modern Scientific Uses.* New York: Barnes and Noble Publishing, 1992.

Hoffman, David, and Linda Quayle. *The Complete Illustrated Herbal: A Safe and Practical Guide to Making and Using Herbal Remedies.* New York: Barnes and Noble Publishing, 1999.

PERIODICALS

Mantani, N., N. Sekiya, S. Sakai, et al. "Rhubarb Use in Patients Treated with Kampo Medicines— A Risk For Gastric Cancer?" *Yakugaku Zasshi* 122 (June 2002): 403-405.

Oi, H., D. Matsuura, M. Miyake, et al. "Identification in Traditional Herbal Medications and Confirmation by Synthesis of Factors That Inhibit Cholera Toxin-Induced Fluid Accumulation." *Proceedings of the National Academy of Sciences of the United States* 99 (March 5, 2002): 3042-3046.

ORGANIZATIONS

American Association of Oriental Medicine. 5530 Wisconsin Avenue, Suite 1210, Chevy Chase, MD 20815. (301) 941-1064. www.aaom.org.

Rocky Mountain Herbal Institute. P. O. Box 579, Hot Springs, MT 59845. (406) 741-3811. www.rmhiherbal.org.

OTHER

Herbal Advisor. http://www2.AllHerb.com.

On Health. http://www.OnHealth.com.

Joan Schonbeck
Rebecca J. Frey, PhD

Rhus toxicodendron

Description

Rhus toxicodendron is the **homeopathy** remedy commonly known as poison ivy. This plant from the Anacardiaceae family grows in fields and wooded areas in North America. The plant is commonly identified by its pointy leaves that grow in threes.

There are two varieties of this plant. Poison ivy is a twining vine with a thick stem that branches out into slender stems. Poison **oak** is a shrub that reaches a height of 4 ft (1.2 m). The plant is also known as mercury vine or poison vine.

A main constituent of the plant is toxicodendric acid, a volatile substance that is most potent after dusk,

KEY TERMS

Polychrest—A homeopathic remedy that is used in the treatment of many ailments.

in damp or cloudy weather, or in June and July. This oil is poisonous when it comes in contact with the skin. Symptoms of poisoning include an itchy red rash that forms **blisters**, **fever**, loss of appetite, **nausea**, **headache**, delirium, swollen glands, and oral ulcers.

The medicinal use of poison ivy was discovered by accident. A French physician in the late eighteenth century discovered that a patient's chronic rash had been cured as a result of accidental poison ivy exposure. The doctor then went on to use the leaves and stalk of the plant in the treatment of skin disease, paralysis, and rheumatic complaints.

General use

Rhus toxicodendron (Rhus tox.) is a remedy frequently indicated for conditions that are accompanied by fever, swollen glands, inflammation of mucous membranes and/or muscles, skin conditions, and restlessness. Homeopaths prescribe Rhus tox. for a number of complaints including poison ivy, chicken pox, back **pain**, colds, herpes, **hives**, flu, **mumps**, **measles**, **sore throat**, nerve pain, muscle **strains** and **sprains**, **dermatitis**, arthritis, **bursitis**, carpal tunnel, rheumatism, and fevers. Ailments arise from overexertion, a change in weather, cold/damp weather, or from getting wet or chilled.

A portrait of the typical Rhus tox. patient is as follows. The patient has a red face, swollen glands, and dry lips. He may have **muscle cramps** or joint pains that are pressing, shooting, and sore. Because of his pains he is not comfortable unless he is moving. The patient may be hungry without having an appetite or have a **dry mouth** even though he is very thirsty. Drinking cold beverages may trigger nausea and **vomiting** and may cause pain in the stomach. Other symptoms include a gnawing pain in the stomach with a full and heavy feeling, a swollen liver that is painful when pressed, bladder weakness, inflammation of the glands of the abdomen and groin, and paralysis or numbing of limbs due to exposure to the cold.

The complaints are left-sided or move from the left side to right side. The patient's tongue is red-tipped, and he has a metallic taste in his mouth. He often has a violent thirst, but has difficulty swallowing solids. He dislikes the cold and is sensitive to dampness. He craves oysters, milk, and sweets and may have an aversion to meat. He is restless, anxious, confused, absent-minded, depressed, irritable, tearful, apprehensive, and often wants to be left alone.

The patient's ailments are generally worse in the morning and at night (particularly after midnight), while lying down, from physical exertion, from a change in weather, during wet weather, in open air, from touch, and from cold food or drinks. Symptoms are relieved by motion or a change in position, warmth, perspiration, or drinking hot beverages.

Specific indications

Rhus tox. is one of the major homeopathic remedies for mumps with hard swollen glands, fever, and a white or yellow coated tongue with a red tip. The left side will swell first or be worse on the left side. The glands are painful to the touch. Symptoms are better from heat and worse from cold.

Rhus tox. is one of the best remedies indicated in chronic or acute rheumatic or arthritic conditions. Sharp, aching pains are present in the bones. The joints are stiff and lame and the muscles, ligaments, and tendons feel sore and bruised. The pains are worse with movement, but are eased with gentle **exercise**. In acute arthritis, the joints are smooth and shiny with little redness. There is numbness or tingling in the affected part. In chronic arthritis conditions there is less swelling, but much stiffness of the joints. The pains may cause the patient to get up at night, causing sleeplessness. The symptoms are worse during damp weather, during fever, at night, or while chilled; continued movement and warmth makes them better.

Inflammations and conditions of the skin are common, and the patient may suffer from large blisters, hives, **eczema**, moist eruptions, or abscesses. Both men and women may have an eczematous rash in the genital area. Conditions of chicken pox, poison ivy, or poison oak are accompanied by red, itchy skin and inflamed blisters that are filled with an oozy pus or a clear fluid. Inflamed blisters are also common with herpes outbreaks. Cold sores appear on the lips. Hives may occur as a result of fever or getting wet. Hives are accompanied by a burning, **itching** rash that is worse from scratching or from cold conditions.

The headache typical of Rhus tox. is centered in the back of the head. The headache is of a pulsating nature with a buzzing in the ears. The head muscles are sore and the pains are sharp and stitching. The pain is improved by keeping the head warm. Walking around also improves the headache.

Inflammation of the eyes occurs as a result of exposure to cold conditions, damp weather, and through suppressing perspiration. The patient is sensitive to light and has sore, swollen, itchy, watery eyes. The lids are often glued together. Stitching pains in the eyes are made worse from moving the eyes. Restlessness and fever usually accompany these eye conditions.

Flu is accompanied by bone, joint, and leg pains. The patient has a fever, and suffers from **sneezing** and exhaustion.

A sore throat may be accompanied by a hoarse voice that is caused by talking or singing too much. The throat is dry and is worse from swallowing or cold drinks. It is made better from continued use.

The **cough** typical of Rhus tox. is an irritating, tickling cough that is better from hot drinks and worse from the cold. The cough is often brought on by swimming in cold water.

Rhus tox. is used to treat many kinds of fevers when all the symptoms match. The fever is of a dry and burning nature. A profuse sweat may occur at the slightest exertion. The patient may feel better from sweating but get chilled, which aggravates his symptoms. The fever is often on one side of the body. During typhoid fever, the abdomen is distended and painful.

A backache that is centered in the lower back or small of the back is made better from lying on a hard surface or from movement or heat. The back feels weak and tired. Caused by damp weather or injury, the ache is aggravated by wet weather or movement.

Nerve pain or **sciatica** may be present. It is ameliorated with movement or heat and made worse by lying on the painful side, bathing in cold water, or being exposed to the cold.

Preparations

The leaves and stalk of the plant are gathered when the poison is the most potent, generally at night. They are then pounded to a pulp and mixed with alcohol. The mixture is then strained and diluted.

Rhus tox. is available at health food and drug stores in various potencies in the form of tinctures, tablets, and pellets.

Precautions

If symptoms do not improve after the recommended time period, consult your homeopath or healthcare practitioner.

Do not exceed the recommended dose.

Side effects

The only side effects are individual aggravations that may occur with homeopathic remedies.

Interactions

When taking any homeopathic remedy, do not use **peppermint** products, coffee, or alcohol. These products may cause the remedy to be ineffective.

Resources

BOOKS

Cummings, M.D., Stephen, and Dana Ullman, M.P.H. *Everybody's Guide to Homeopathic Medicines.* New York, NY: Jeremy P. Tarcher/Putnam, 1997.

Kent, James Tyler. *Lectures on Materia Medica.* Delhi, India: B. Jain Publishers, 1996.

Jennifer Wurges

Riboflavin

Description

Riboflavin, also known as Vitamin B_2, is a water-soluble vitamin that the body needs to remain healthy. Humans cannot make riboflavin, so they must get it from foods in their diet. Riboflavin has many functions in common with the other members of the B complex family, including support of the immune and nervous systems and formation of healthy red blood cells. Riboflavin provides essential factors for the production of cellular enzymes that turn proteins, fats, and carbohydrates into energy. It also participates in cell reproduction, and keeps skin, hair, nails, eyes, and mucous membranes healthy. **Folic acid** (vitamin B_9) and **pyridoxine** (vitamin B_6) are activated by riboflavin.

Recent research has found that riboflavin is one of three vitamins involved in the regulation of circadian (daily) rhythms in humans and other mammals. Riboflavin helps to activate certain light-sensitive cells in the retina of the eye that synchronize the animal's daily biological rhythms with the solar light/darkness cycle.

General use

The United States Institute of Medicine (IOM) of the National Academy of Sciences has developed values called Dietary Reference Intakes (DRIs) for vitamins and minerals. The DRIs consist of three sets of numbers. The Recommended Dietary Allowance (RDA) defines the average daily amount of the

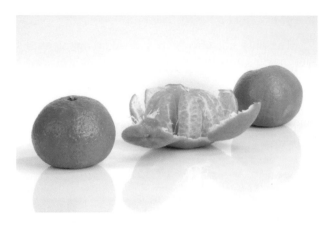

Clementines are a good source of Riboflavin. (© *imagebroker/Alamy*)

Recommended dietary allowance of riboflavin	
Age	**mg/day**
Children 0-6 mos.	0.3 (AI)
Children 7-12 mos.	0.4 (AI)
Children 1-3 yrs.	0.5
Children 4-8 yrs.	0.6
Children 9-13 yrs.	0.9
Boys 14-18 yrs.	1.3
Girls 14-18 yrs.	1.0
Men ≥ 19 yrs.	1.3
Women ≥19 yrs.	1.1
Pregnant women	1.4
Breastfeeding women	1.6
Foods that contain riboflavin	**mg**
Yogurt, low fat, 1 cup	0.52
Milk, 2%, 1 cup	0.40
Tempeh, cooked, 4 oz.	0.40
Beef tenderloin, broiled, 4 oz.	0.35
Milk, nonfat, 1 cup	0.34
Egg, boiled, 1 large	0.27
Almonds, roasted, 1 oz.	0.24
Spinach, cooked, 1/2 cup	0.21
Chicken, dark meat, roasted, 3 oz.	0.18
Salmon, broiled, 3 oz.	0.13
Asparagus, cooked, 1/2 cup	0.11
Chicken, light meat, roasted, 3 oz.	0.10
Broccoli, steamed, 1/2 cup	0.09
Bread, white, enriched, 1 slice	0.09
Bread, whole wheat, 1 slice	0.07

AI = Adequate Intake
mg = milligram

(Illustration by GGS Information Services. Cengage Learning, Gale)

nutrient needed to meet the health needs of 97–98% of the population. The Adequate Intake (AI) is an estimate set when there is not enough information to determine an RDA. The Tolerable Upper Intake Level (UL) is the average maximum amount that can be taken daily without risking negative side effects. The DRIs are calculated for children, adult men, adult women, pregnant women, and breastfeeding women.

The IOM has not set RDAs for riboflavin in children under one year old because of incomplete scientific information. Instead, it has set AI levels for this age group. No UL levels have been set for any age group because no negative (toxic) side effects have been found with large doses of riboflavin. RDAs for riboflavin measured in micrograms (mg).

The following are the RDAs and AIs for riboflavin for healthy individuals:

- children birth–6 months: AI 0.3 mg
- children 7–12 months: AI 0.4 mg
- children 1–3 years: RDA 0.5 mg
- children 4–8 years: RDA 0.6 mg
- children 9–13 years: RDA 0.9 mg
- boys 14–18 years: RDA 1.3 mg
- girls 14–18 years: RDA 1.0 mg
- women age 19 and older: RDA 1.1 mg
- men age 19 and older: RDA 1.3 mg
- pregnant women: RDA 1.4 mg
- breastfeeding women: RDA 1.6 mg

High doses of riboflavin, as much as 400 mg per day, have been shown to reduce the frequency of migraine headaches by half in susceptible people. The severity of the events was also reportedly decreased. This may be an effect of improved use of cellular energy in the brain. It is theorized that riboflavin may help decrease the odds of getting **cataracts**, but the evidence for this is not definitive. One large study had a group taking both **niacin** (vitamin B$_3$) and riboflavin, and while the group had a significantly lower total incidence of cataracts, they had a somewhat higher than average incidence of a specific cataract subtype. Memory may be improved by these supplements, according to some research done on older people. Riboflavin and **vitamin C** both help boost the body's level of **glutathione**, which is an antioxidant with many beneficial effects. There is not enough evidence to support the effectiveness of riboflavin for sickle-cell **anemia**, **canker sores**, or as an athletic performance aid.

Preparations

Natural sources

Beef liver is a very rich source of riboflavin, but dairy products also supply ample amounts. Higher fat sources contain less than those with low fat. In the United States starting in 1942, riboflavin, along with thiamin and niacin, has been added to flour. Some breakfast cereals are also fortified with riboflavin. Vegetable that are a good source of riboflavin include avocados, mushrooms, spinach, and other dark green, leafy vegetables. Nuts, legumes, nutritional yeast, and **brewer's yeast** contain riboflavin as well. Cooked foods provide as much of this vitamin as raw ones do, since the substance is heat stable. Light, however, does break down riboflavin. To preserve it dairy and grain products should be stored in something opaque or kept them away from light.

The following list gives the approximate riboflavin content for some common foods:

- spinach, cooked, 1/2 cup: 0.21 mg
- asparagus, cooked, 1/2 cup: 0.11 mg
- broccoli, steamed 1/2 cup: 0.09 mg
- milk, 2% 1 cup 0.40 mg
- milk, nonfat 1 cup: 0.34 mg
- yogurt, low fat: 1 cup: 0.52 mg
- egg, boiled, 1 large: 0.27 mg
- almonds, roasted, 1 ounce: 0.24 mg
- salmon, broiled, 3 ounces: 0.13 mg
- chicken, light meat, roasted, 3 ounces: 0.10 mg
- chicken, dark meat, roasted, 3 ounces: 0.18 mg
- beef tenderloin, broiled, 4 ounces: 0.35 mg
- tempeh, cooked, 4 ounces 0.4 mg
- bread, whole wheat, 1 slice: 0.07 mg
- bread, white, enriched, 1 slice 0.09 mg

Supplemental sources

Riboflavin is available as an oral single vitamin product. Individuals should consider taking a balanced B complex supplement rather than high doses of an individual vitamin unless there is a specific indication to do so. Supplements should be stored in a cool, dry place, away from light, and out of the reach of children.

Deficiency

Ariboflavinosis is the term for the condition of vitamin B_2 deficiency. Since small amounts can be stored in the liver and kidneys, a dietary inadequacy may not become apparent for several months. Insufficient levels of riboflavin have noticeable effects on several areas of the skin. Commonly the corners of the mouth are cracked. Facial skin and scalp tend to itch and scale, as does the scrotal skin. The eyes **fatigue** easily and are sensitive to light, and may also become watery, sore, or bloodshot. Trembling, neuropathy, **dizziness**, **insomnia**, poor digestion, slow growth, and

sore throat and tongue have also been reported. Anemia may develop if the deficiency is severe. People who are deficient in riboflavin are likely to be lacking in other B vitamins, and possibly additional nutrients, as well.

Recent studies done at the National **Cancer** Institute indicate that riboflavin deficiency increases a woman's risk of developing cervical cancer. Further studies of this connection are underway.

Risk factors for deficiency

Riboflavin deficiency is uncommon in developed countries, but some populations may need more than the RDA in order to maintain good health. War refugees are a population at high risk for riboflavin deficiency. Vegans and others who do not use dairy products may want to take a balanced B vitamin supplement; one study of Swedish vegans found that over 90% were not getting enough riboflavin in their diet. Those with increased need for riboflavin and other B vitamins may include people under high **stress**, including those experiencing surgery, chronic illnesses, liver disease, or poor nutritional status. Diabetics may have a tendency to be low on riboflavin as a result of increased urinary excretion. Athletes, and anyone else with a high-energy output may need additional vitamin B_2. This includes anyone who exercises with some regularity. The elderly are more likely to suffer from nutritional inadequacy as well as problems with absorption; the dietary preferences of many elderly people often exclude foods that are high in riboflavin. Smokers and alcoholics are at higher risk for deficiency as tobacco and alcohol suppress absorption. Birth control pills may possibly reduce riboflavin levels, as can phenothiazine tranquilizers, tricyclic antidepressants, and probenecid. Individuals should consult a health care professional to determine if supplementation is appropriate.

Recent advances in human genetics indicate that certain genotypes are at greater risk for riboflavin deficiency than others.

Precautions

Riboflavin should not be taken by anyone with a B vitamin allergy or chronic renal disease. Other populations are unlikely to experience any difficulty from taking supplemental B_2.

Side effects

Taking supplemental riboflavin causes a harmless intense orange or yellow discoloration of the urine.

KEY TERMS

Antioxidant—Any one of a group of substances that function to destroy cell-damaging free radicals in the body.

Genotype—The genetic makeup of an organism or group of organisms with respect to a biological trait or set of traits.

Migraine—A very severe headache, often accompanied by nausea and vomiting. It is usually experienced on one side of the head, and may be preceded by visual symptoms.

Neuropathy—Abnormality of the nerves which may be manifested as numbness, tingling, or weakness of the affected area.

Vegan—A vegetarian who omits all animal products from the diet.

Interactions

Probenecid (a drug treating **gout**) impairs riboflavin absorption, and propantheline bromide (a drug treating peptic ulcers) reportedly both delays and increases absorption. Phenothiazines (antipsychotic drugs) increase the excretion of riboflavin, thus lowering serum levels, and oral contraceptives may also decrease serum levels. Tricyclic antidepressants may lower the levels of riboflavin in the body. Long-term use of phenobarbitol seems to increase the rate of destruction of riboflavin by the liver. Supplementation should be discussed with a health care provider if these medications are being used. Absorption of riboflavin is improved when taken together with other B vitamins and vitamin C.

Riboflavin supplements may lower the effectiveness of chloroquine and other antimalarial medications. Riboflavin should not be taken at the same time as tetracycline antibiotics because it interferes with the absorption and effectiveness of these medications. It may also interfere with the effectiveness of sulfa-containing drugs used to treat bacterial **infections**.

Resources

BOOKS

Berkson, Burt and Arthur J. Berkson. *Basic Health Publications User&s Guide to the B-complex Vitamins.* Laguna Beach, CA: Basic Health Publications, 2006.

Bratman, Steven, and David Kroll. *Natural Health Bible.* Prima Publishing, 1999.

Feinstein, Alice. *Prevention's Healing with Vitamins.* Pennsylvania: Rodale Press, 1996.

Griffith, H. Winter. *Vitamins, Herbs, Minerals & Supplements: the complete guide.* Arizona: Fisher Books, 1998.

Jellin, Jeff, Forrest Batz, and Kathy Hitchens. *Pharmacist's letter/Prescriber's Letter Natural Medicines Comprehensive Database.* California: Therapeutic Research Faculty, 1999.

Lieberman, Shari and Nancy Bruning. *The Real Vitamin and Mineral Book: The Definitive Guide to Designing Your Personal Supplement Program,* 4th ed. New York: Avery, 2007.

PERIODICALS

Blanck, H. M., B. A. Bowman, M. K. Serdula, et al. "Angular Stomatitis and Riboflavin Status Among Adolescent Bhutanese Refugees Living in Southeastern Nepal." *American Journal of Clinical Nutrition* 76 (August 2002): 430-435.

Larsson, C. L., and G. K. Johansson. "Dietary Intake and Nutritional Status of Young Vegans and Omnivores in Sweden." *American Journal of Clinical Nutrition* 76 (July 2002): 100-106.

McNulty, H., M. C. McKinley, B. Wilson, et al. "Impaired Functioning of Thermolabile Methylenetetrahydrofolate Reductase Is Dependent on Riboflavin Status: Implications for Riboflavin Requirements." *American Journal of Clinical Nutrition* 76 (August 2002): 436-441.

Shahar, S., K. Chee, and W. C. Wan Chik. "Food Intakes and Preferences of Hospitalized Geriatric Patients." *BMC Geriatrics* 2 (August 6, 2002): 3.

Silberstein, S. D., and P. J. Goadsby. "Migraine: Preventive Treatment." *Cephalalgia* 22 (September 2002): 491-512.

Wolf, G. "Three Vitamins Are Involved in Regulation of the Circadian Rhythm." *Nutrition Reviews* 60 (August 2002): 257-260.

Ziegler, R. G., S. J. Weinstein, and T. R. Fears. "Nutritional and Genetic Inefficiencies in One-Carbon Metabolism and Cervical Cancer Risk." *Journal of Nutrition* 132 (August 2002): 2345S-2349S.

ORGANIZATIONS

American Dietetic Association, 216 West Jackson Blvd, Chicago, IL, 60606, (312) 899-0040, www.eatright.org.

Office of Dietary Supplements (ODS), National Institutes of Health, 6100 Executive Boulevard, Room 3B01, MSC 7517, Bethesda, MD, 20892, (301) 435-2920, www.ods.od.nih.gov.

Judith Turner
Rebecca J. Frey, PhD
Helen Davidson

Ringing ears *see* **Tinnitus**

Rolfing

Definition

Rolfing, also called Rolf therapy or structural integration, is a holistic system of bodywork that uses deep manipulation of the body's soft tissue to realign and

Following completion of a doctorate in biochemistry from Columbia University in 1920, Rolf studied atomic physics, mathematics, and homeopathic medicine in Europe. After 1928, when her father died and left her an inheritance that allowed her to pursue her own studies, she explored various forms of alternative treatment, including **osteopathy**, **chiropractic** medicine, tantric **yoga**, the **Alexander technique** of tension reduction through body movement, and Alfred Korzybski's philosophy of altered states of consciousness.

By 1940, Rolf had synthesized what she had learned from these various disciplines into her own technique of body movement that she called structural integration, which later became known as Rolfing. During the Second World War, Rolf continued to study with an osteopath in California named Amy Cochran. In the mid-1960s, Gestalt therapist Fritz Perls invited Rolf to Esalen, where she began to develop a following among people involved in the human potential movement. In 1977, she published *Rolfing: The Integration of Human Structures*, the definitive book on structural integration bodywork. She continued to refine the therapy until her death in 1979. Rolf's work is carried on through her Guild for Structural Integration, now known as the Rolf Institute of Structural Integration, which she founded in 1971 in Boulder, Colo.

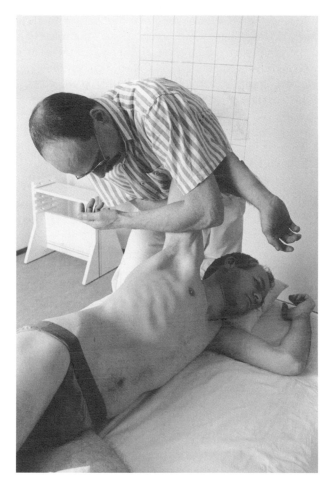

Therapist uses his elbows to give a deep massage to a patient as part of Rolfing therapy. *(Horacio Sormani / Photo Researchers, Inc.)*

balance the body's myofascial structure. Rolfing improves posture, relieves chronic **pain**, and reduces **stress**.

Origins

Ida Pauline Rolf (1896–1979) was a biochemist from New York who developed structural integration over the course of many years after an accident as a young woman. She was kicked by a horse's hoof on a trip out West and developed symptoms resembling those of acute **pneumonia**. She made her way to a hospital in Montana, where she was treated by a physician who called in an osteopath to assist in her treatment. After the osteopath treated her, she was able to breathe normally. After her return to New York, her mother took her to a blind osteopath for further treatment. He taught her about the body's structure and function, after which Rolf became dissatisfied with conventional medical treatment.

Benefits

Rolfing helps to improve posture and bring the body's natural structure into proper balance and alignment. This can bring relief from general aches and pains, improve breathing, increase energy, improve self-confidence, and relieve physical and mental stress. Rolfing has also been used to treat such specific physical problems as chronic back, neck, shoulder, and joint pain, and repetitive stress injuries, including **carpal tunnel syndrome**. Many amateur and professional athletes, including Olympic skaters and skiers, use Rolfing to keep in top condition, to prevent injuries, and to more quickly recover from injuries.

Description

Rolfing is more than just a massage of the body's surface. It is a system that reshapes the body's myofascial structure by applying pressure and energy, thereby freeing the body from the effects of physical and emotional traumas. Although Rolfing is used extensively to treat sports injuries and back pain, it is not designed as a therapy for any particular condition. Rather, it is a systematic approach to overall wellness. It works by counteracting the effects of gravity, which

KEY TERMS

Atrophy—A progressive wasting and loss of function of any part of the body.

Carpal tunnel syndrome—A condition caused by compression of the median nerve in the carpal tunnel of the hand, characterized by pain.

Fascia—The sheet of connective tissue that covers the body under the skin and envelops every muscle, bone, nerve, gland, organ, and blood vessel. Fascia helps the body to retain its basic shape.

Osteopathy—A system of medical practice that believes that the human body can make its own remedies to heal infection. It originally used manipulative techniques but also added surgical, hygienic, and medicinal methods when needed.

Parasympathetic nervous system—A part of the autonomic nervous system that is concerned with conserving and restoring energy. It is the part of the nervous system that predominates in a state of relaxation.

Structural integration—The term used to describe the method and philosophy of life associated with Rolfing. Its fundamental concept is the vertical line.

over time pulls the body out of alignment. This pull causes the body's connective tissue to become harder and stiffer, and the muscles to atrophy. Signs of this stiffening and contraction include slouching or an overly erect posture.

Rolfing identifies the vertical line as the ideal that the body should approximate. The mission statement of the Guild for Structural Integration describes Rolfing as "a method and a philosophy of personal growth and integrity . . . . The vertical line is our fundamental concept. The physical and psychological embodiment of the vertical line is a way of Being in the physical world [that] forms a basis for personal growth and integrity."

The basic ten

Basic Rolfing treatment consists of 10 sessions, each lasting 60–90 minutes and costing about $100 each. The sessions are spaced a week or longer apart. After a period of integration, specialized or advanced treatment sessions are available. A "tuneup" session is recommended every six months. In each session, the Rolfer uses his or her fingers, hands, knuckles, and elbows to rework the connective tissue over the entire body. The tissues are worked until they become pliable,

allowing the muscles to lengthen and return to their normal alignment. The deep tissue manipulation improves posture and agility, and increases the body's range of movement. Rolfers also believe that the blocked energy accumulated in the tissue from emotional tension is released through Rolfing treatment, causing the patient to feel more energetic and have a more positive frame of mind.

Clients are asked to wait for a period of six to 12 months before scheduling advanced work, known as the PostTen/Advanced Series. This period allows the body to integrate the work done in the "Basic Ten."

Rolfing movement integration

Rolfing movement integration, or RMI, is intended to help clients develop better awareness of their vertical alignment and customary movement patterns. They learn to release tension and discover better ways to use body movement effectively.

Rolfing rhythms

Rolfing rhythms are a series of exercises intended to remind participants of the basic principles of Rolfing: ease, length, balance, and harmony with gravity. In addition, Rolfing rhythms improve the client's flexibility as well as muscle tone and coordination.

Preparations

No pre-procedure preparations are needed to begin Rolfing treatment. The treatment is usually done on a massage table with the patient wearing only undergarments. Prior to the first session, however, the client is asked to complete a health questionnaire, and photographs are taken to assist with evaluation of his or her progress.

Precautions

Since Rolfing involves vigorous deep tissue manipulation, it is often described as uncomfortable and sometimes painful, especially during the first several sessions. In the past decade, however, Rolfers have developed newer techniques that cause less discomfort to participants. Since Rolfing is a bodywork treatment that requires the use of hands, it may be a problem for people who do not like or are afraid of being touched. It is not recommended as a treatment for any disease or a chronic inflammatory condition such as arthritis, and can worsen such a condition. Anyone with a serious medical condition, including **heart disease**, diabetes, or respiratory problems, should consult with a medical practitioner before undergoing Rolfing.

as it is called, frequently precedes the other manifestations on the skin. Telangiectasia may appear around the borders of the eyelid, the eyelids may be chronically inflamed, and small lumps called chalazious may develop. The cornea of the eye (the transparent covering over the lens) can also be affected, and in some cases vision will be affected. Most of these eye symptoms do not threaten sight, however.

Diagnosis

Diagnosis of rosacea is made by the presence of clinical symptoms. There is no specific test for the disease. Episodes of persistent flushing, redness (erythema) of the nose, cheeks, chin, and forehead, accompanied by pustules and papules are hallmarks of the disease. A dermatologist (skin disease specialist) will attempt to rule out a number of other diseases that have similar symptoms. Acne vulgaris is perhaps the disorder most commonly mistaken for rosacea, but acne patients do not have redness and spider-like veins. Blackheads and cysts are seen in acne patients, but not in those with rosacea.

Other diseases that produce some of the same symptoms as rosacea include perioral **dermatitis**, seborrheic dermatitis, and **systemic lupus erythematosus**.

Treatment

There is no cure for rosacea, but alternative and complementary treatments can be helpful in reducing the skin irritation and number of outbreaks associated with the disease. Green-tinted makeup can mask the redness associated with rosacea. Because rosacea may cause psychological distress, **psychotherapy** or support groups can be an important component of treatment.

Patients should avoid using skin care products that contain alcohol, **witch hazel**, **peppermint**, menthol, **eucalyptus** oil, or clove oil. Skin care products should be fragrance-free and have a smooth, non-grainy consistency. Men can shave with an electric razor to lessen skin irritation on the face.

Persons who are treated for rosacea with antibiotics over a long period are more prone to yeast **infections**. Long-term antibiotic use can decrease normal bacteria populations and increase the number of yeast. Eating a yeast-free diet (eliminating breads and other yeast products and sugars) can help to restore normal bacteria to the body.

Identifying food triggers

Certain foods are known to trigger an outbreak of rosacea. Although individual triggers vary, the following foods may aggravate rosacea: hot spices (pepper, paprika, and **cayenne**), marinated meat, soy sauce, vanilla, vinegar, red plums, peas, lima and navy beans, sharp cheeses, cider, Asian food dishes, canned fish products, processed beef and pork, chocolate, tomatoes, citrus fruit, alcohol, and hot beverages. Nitrates, sulfites, and certain drugs can also trigger outbreaks. Food **allergies** can also cause rosacea. The three foods that most often cause food allergies are wheat products, sugar, and dairy products.

Rosacea patients should keep a food diary to identify the specific foods that trigger rosacea outbreaks. Outbreaks can occur hours—or as long as a day—after the offending food has been eaten. The patient should stop eating a suspect food for a few months to observe the severity of the rosacea symptoms. If the rosacea improves, the patient can then eat a small amount of the offending food to confirm whether it triggers an outbreak. Once a rosacea trigger food is identified, it can be eliminated from the patient's diet.

Other treatments

Applying liquid-filled cold packs, a washcloth soaked in ice-cold water, or a compress of cold milk and ice-cold water to the neck and face can relieve flushing. Sucking on ice chips can also help relieve flushing. A cold compress of **chamomile** tea can soothe irritated skin. Applying ice to the face may feel good but it can cause **frostbite**, which would worsen the reddening.

Some practitioners advocate gentle circular massage for several minutes daily to the nose, cheeks, and forehead. However, controlled studies on the effectiveness of this technique are lacking.

A deficiency of hydrochloric acid (HCl) in the stomach may be a cause of rosacea, and supplementation with HCl capsules (taken after meals) may bring relief in some cases.

Hypnosis may reduce **stress**, promote healthful behavior, and control bad habits. **Hypnotherapy** is especially useful in treating skin disease that can be triggered by emotions, including rosacea. As a complementary therapy, hypnosis has been shown to improve rosacea, especially the flushing component.

Nutritionists recommend eating more dark green vegetables such as kale, broccoli, asparagus, and spinach. These foods, and others that contain high levels of vitamins A and C, **bioflavonoids**, and beta-carotene, can improve rosacea by increasing capillary strength and boosting the immune system. Apple juice and dark grape juice drunk at room temperature between meals can help persons with rosacea.

A deficiency of B-complex vitamins can lead to rosacea. Vitamin E's antioxidant properties can help prevent skin damage. **Zinc** can speed wound healing. Omega-3 and omega-6 fatty acid deficiencies can lead to dry, irritated skin, which can worsen rosacea. **Omega-3 fatty acids** can be found in **flaxseed** oil, cod liver oil, salmon, mackerel, and herring. Omega-6 fatty acid is found in **evening primrose oil**.

Allopathic treatment

The mainstay of treatment for rosacea is oral antibiotics. These appear to work by reducing inflammation in the small blood vessels and structure of the skin, not by destroying bacteria that are present. One of the more widely used oral antibiotics is tetracycline. In many patients, antibiotics are effective against the papules and pustules that can appear on the face. But antibiotics appear to be less effective against the background redness, and they have no effect on telangiectasia. Patients frequently take a relatively high dose of antibiotics until their symptoms are controlled, and then they slowly reduce their daily dose to a level that just keeps their symptoms in check. Other oral antibiotics used include erythromycin and minocycline.

Some patients are concerned about long-term use of oral antibiotics. For them, a topical agent applied directly to the face may be tried in addition to an oral antibiotic or in its place. Topical antibiotics are also useful for controlling the papules and pustules of rosacea, but do not control the redness, flushing, and telangiectasias. The newest of these topical agents is metronidazole gel, which can be applied twice daily.

Vitamin A derivatives called retinoids also appear useful in the treatment of rosacea. An oral retinoid called isotretinoin, which is used in severe cases of acne, reduces the pustules and papules in severe cases of rosacea that do not respond to antibiotics. Isotretinoin must be taken with care, particularly in women of childbearing age, because the drug is known to cause birth defects.

Topical vitamin A compounds may have a role in the treatment of rosacea. Accumulating evidence suggests that topical isotretinoin and topical azelaic acid can reduce the redness and pimples.

For later stages of the disorder, a surgical procedure may be needed to improve the appearance of the skin. To remove the telangiectasias, a dermatologist may use an electrocautery device to apply an electrical current to the blood vessel. This procedure **cuts** off the blood to the blood vessel, effectively destroying it and eliminating its appearance as a red line. Special lasers, called tunable dye lasers, can selectively destroy these tiny blood vessels. A variety of surgical techniques can be used to improve the shape and appearance of a bulbous nose. Surgeons may use a scalpel or laser to remove excess tissue from the nose and restore a more natural appearance.

Expected results

The prognosis is good for controlling symptoms of rosacea and improving the appearance of the face. Many people require lifelong treatment and achieve good results. There is no known cure for the disorder.

Prevention

Rosacea cannot be prevented, but once its is correctly diagnosed, outbreaks can be treated and repeated episodes can be limited. Patients can reduce outbreaks of rosacea by following this advice:

- Use mild soaps and cleansers. Avoiding anything that irritates the skin is a good preventive measure for persons with rosacea. Astringents and alcohol should be avoided.

- Learn what triggers flushing. Reducing factors in the diet and environment that cause flushing of the face is another good preventive strategy. The specific things that provoke flushing vary considerably from person to person and it usually takes some trial and error to figure these out.

- Cover the face. Limiting exposure of the face to excesses of heat and cold can also help. A sunscreen with a skin protection factor (SPF) of 15 or greater, used daily, can reduce rosacea outbreaks and limit the damage the sun causes to the skin and small blood vessels. Protective clothing (hats in the summer and scarves or ski masks in the winter) can reduce the skin's exposure to sun and cold temperatures.

Resources

BOOKS

Helm, Klaus F. and James G. Marks. *Atlas of Differential Diagnosis in Dermatology.* New York: Churchill Livingstone, 1998.

Macsai, Marian S., et al. "Acne Rosacea." In *Eye and Skin Disease.* Edited by Mark J. Mannis, et al. Philadelphia: Lippincott-Raven, 1996.

PERIODICALS

Jansen, Thomas and Gerd Plewig. "Rosacea: Classification and Treatment." *Journal of the Royal Society of Medicine* 90 (March 1997): 144–150.

Litt, Jerome Z. "Rosacea: How to Recognize and Treat an Age-Related Skin Disease." *Geriatrics* 52 (November 1997): 39 + .

Shenefelt, Philip D. "Hypnosis in Dermatology." *Archives of Dermatology* 136 (March 2000): 393–399.

Thiboutot, Diane M. "Acne Rosacea." *American Family Physician* 50 (December 1994): 1691–1697.

ORGANIZATIONS

American Academy of Dermatology. 930 N. Meacham Road, PO Box 4014, Schaumburg, IL 60168-4014. (847) 330-0230. http://www.aad.org.

National Rosacea Society. 800 S. Northwest Highway, Suite 200, Barrington, IL 60010. (888) 662-5874. http://www.rosacea.org.

OTHER

"Rosacea." MotherNature.com. http://www.mothernature.com/library/books/homeseniors/rosacea.asp.

Belinda Rowland

Rose hip

Description

Rose hips are the edible and nutritious fruit of the beautiful deciduous rose, a perennial member of the most extensive genus of classified plants. Botanists disagree on the number of species of rose, claiming 30–5,000, or more. There are more than 10,000 cultivated varieties of this fragrant native of Europe and the Middle East. Roses have been a garden favorite as far back as 2,600 B.C. during the time of the ancient Sumerians. This beneficial beauty was named the "Queen of Flowers" by the Greek poet Sappho writing in 600 B.C. Since that time legend and history have intertwined and volumes have been written about the cultivation and virtues of the much-loved rose. Garlands of roses decorated the statues of gods and goddesses in Greece and Rome. Early Christians considered rose hips to be sacred, and crafted the first rosary beads from rose hips. The rose is considered a symbol of love everywhere, despite, or perhaps because of, the thorny stems which can render a sharp prick to the unwary who are attracted to the fragrant and lovely blossoms.

Most species of rose grow as an upright shrub or a climbing vine. Wild roses often grow in thorny thickets or briers. The usually pinnate leaves are arranged alternately along the stems with two to four pairs of finely toothed, dark-green, oval leaflets and one terminal leaflet. The large blossoms of wild roses have five petals. They grow singly on the stem or in clusters of two or three. Cultivated varieties may have many more petals with colors as varied as white, yellow, pink, and many shades of red. A rose's true fruits are the numerous tiny achenes, each enclosing a single

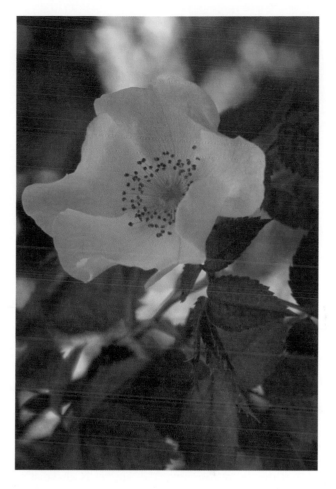

Rose hip blossom. *(©PlantaPhile, Germany. Reproduced by permission.)*

seed, contained within the hip. Rose hips develop from the stem tip that swells to enclose the hairy achenes. The smooth skin of the hip is first green, then turns shades of orange and, when fully ripe, a deep red.

Among the species of rose particularly valued for the hips are *Rosa rugosa*, known as Japanese rose; *R. canina*, known variously as wild briar, witches briar, dog rose, hip fruit, or hip tree; *R. acicularis*; and *R. cinnamomea*. The dog rose, so-named because of the belief that this wild briar could cure the bite of a rabid dog, thrives in stony ground, along embankments, in hedgerows, and on the edge of woods. The long and fibrous root and herbaceous trunk of this hardy species produces numerous shoots that divide into many thorny branches. The dagger-like thorns may also have inspired the common name, taken from the Old French word *dague* meaning dagger. The branches may reach 10 feet in length. They arch out and curve downward bearing an abundance of sweet-smelling, stalked flowers. The dog rose hips are said to contain the highest amounts of vitamin C of all the varieties, with 10 to 50 times that of an orange. In England, during the Second World War, the scarcity of citrus products led to a nationwide effort to harvest and process the nutritional hips of the dog rose. The dog rose hips, abundant in the countryside, provided the populace with adequate **vitamin C** to prevent the onset of the deficiency disease known as scurvy.

R. rugosa, also known as large-hip rose or wrinkled rose, is found growing wild in the northern United States and Canada, along coastal areas, and around seaside sand dunes. The dwarf shrub is valued for the size of the fleshy rose hips. This species is also distinguished by its very wrinkled leaves. This species is used in Chinese medicine. An infusion of the flowers, known as *mei gui hua*, is said to promote blood circulation, stimulate the flow of energy, and provide relief for stomach distress, liver stagnation, dysentery, mastitis, and leukorrhea.

General use

Rose petals and hips, and the seeds contained within the achenes, are medicinally valuable. The leaves are also sometimes used. Rose hips and seeds contain vitamins C, E, B, and K, tannin, pectin, carotene, malic and citric acid, flavonoids, fatty and volatile oils, and proteins. The vitamin content of the hips varies depending on the species, the growing conditions, the time and manner of harvest, and the care taken in drying and storage. The hips of roses grown in cooler climates have been found to have a higher content of vitamin C.

Rose hips are an abundant natural source of vitamin C, regarded as an important antioxidant. Used regularly as a tonic or food supplement, these compact, nutritious hips will help build the body's defense against colds and flu, catarrh, sore throats, and chest **infections**. Six to eight fresh raw rose hips, taken daily, will help prevent illness. Rose hip tea, taken following a course of antibiotic therapy, will help re-establish the beneficial bacteria in the digestive system. The natural balance of intestinal flora may have been disrupted or destroyed by the action of antibiotic drugs. Rose hip tea can also soothe the nervous system and relieve exhaustion. An infusion of the leaves and petals is said to help bring down fevers. A decoction of the seed is diuretic and is used for kidney ailments and problems with the lower urinary tract. The pectin and fruit acid content of the seeds have a laxative and mildly diuretic effect. Rose hip preparations can also ease the pelvic congestion and pain of **menstruation**.

The essential oil of rose, used in aromatherapy, has an uplifting effect, helpful in dispelling **depression**, **stress**, and nervous tension. The species generally used for oil distillation is a hybrid of *R.centifolia* and *R. gallica*. The oil is extracted from the fresh petals by water or steam distillation. Rose hip seed oil is vitamin rich and contains as much as 35% linoleic acid and 44% gamma-linolenic acid, or GLA. There are as many as 300 chemical constituents in rose oil, though only about one-third of these have been identified. This essential oil promotes tissue regeneration and is helpful in the treatment of **eczema**, **psoriasis**, and dry, sun-damaged, and aging skin. Newer methods of extracting the medicinal oil from rose hip seeds have yielded a purer product, without the need to evaporate the solvents used in older methods.

Preparations

Herbalists in centuries past, such as the Roman scholar Pliny the Elder, recorded numerous ways to prepare roses to extract their medicinal virtues. A variety of products using rose petals, hips, and seeds are commercially available, including perfumes and lotions, essential oil, rosewater, and tablets and tinctures.

The bright-red rose hips should be harvested in the fall after the first frost. The hips are cut lengthwise to facilitate drying and placed on a paper-lined tray in a warm and airy room out of direct sunlight. The irritant hairs on the dry hips can be winnowed by shaking the hips vigorously in a wire sieve. The hips should be stored in clearly labeled, dark glass containers in a cool location. The dried hips will retain medicinal potency for up to one year.

Decoction: Use about 2.5 tsp of thinly sliced, fresh or dried rose hips per 8 oz of cold water. Bring to a boil in a glass or ceramic pot. Reduce heat and simmer for about 10 minutes. Drink cold in small doses throughout the day.

Tincture: Combine 4 oz of finely cut fresh rose petals and hips, or 2 oz dry powdered herb with one pint of brandy, gin, or vodka, in a glass container. The alcohol should be enough to cover the plant parts. Cover and store the mixture away from light for about two weeks, shaking several times each day. Strain and store in a tightly capped, dark-glass bottle. A standard dose is 10–15 drops of the tincture in water, up to three times a day.

Rose hip syrup: Clean the freshly gathered hips by removing the seed-bearing achenes and any fine hairs. Prepare a strong decoction and mix with honey and/or sugar in a double boiler. Stir and simmer until the sugar is dissolved. Pour into small glass containers. Cool and seal with a tight-fitting lid. Refrigerate.

Precautions

It would be wise to use heavy gloves when harvesting the thorny rose. Pregnant women should not use essential oil of rose during the first four weeks of **pregnancy**.

Side effects

Some people may experience **diarrhea** or such allergic reactions as **hives** or throat swelling from large doses of rose hips. Patients who experience an allergic reaction should stop taking rose hips and contact their physician at once.

Interactions

No interactions with conventional prescription medications have been reported as of 2002.

Resources

BOOKS

Duke, James A. *The Green Pharmacy*. Emmaus, PA: Rodale Press, 1997.

McIntyre, Anne. *The Medicinal Garden*. New York: Henry Holt and Company, Inc., 1997.

Medical Economics Company. *PDR for Herbal Medicines*. Montvale, NJ: Medical Economics Company, 1998.

"Rose Hips." In: *Organic Gardening Collection, No. 4* Rodale, Inc., 1999.

PERIODICALS

Daels-Rakotoarison, D. A., B. Gressier, F. Trotin, et al. "Effects of *Rosa canina* Fruit Extract on Neutrophil Respiratory Burst." *Phytotherapy Research* 16 (March 2002): 157-161.

Szentmihalyi, K., P. Vinkler, B. Lakatos, et al. "Rose Hip (*Rosa canina L.*) Oil Obtained from Waste Hip Seeds by Different Extraction Methods." *Bioresource Technology* 82 (April 2002): 195-201.

ORGANIZATIONS

American Herbalists Guild. 1931 Gaddis Road, Canton, GA 30115. (770) 751-6021. www.americanherbalistsguild.com.

American Rose Society. P. O. Box 30000, Shreveport, LA 71130. (318) 938-5402. www.ars.org.

Clare Hanrahan
Rebecca J. Frey, PhD

Rosemary

Description

Rosemary, a herb whose botanical name is *Rosmarinus officinalis*, is a sun-loving shrub, native to the south of France and other Mediterranean regions. It is widely cultivated for its aromatic and medicinal properties. This pine-scented evergreen of the Lamiaceae, or mint, family, can grow to 5 ft (1.5 m) in height in favorable settings. Rosemary thrives in chalky or sandy soil in full sun. The herb grows wild on dry, rocky slopes near the sea. Its name is derived from the Latin *ros marinus*, meaning "sea dew." Other common names for the herb include polar plant, compass-weed, or compass plant. The specific name, *officinalis*, refers to the herb's inclusion in official Western listings of medicinal herbs. Rosemary was a favored herb in early apothecary gardens.

Legend abounds around this lovely perennial known as the "herb of remembrance." It is said that rosemary will grow particularly well in gardens tended by strong-willed women. Young brides traditionally carried a sprig of rosemary in their wreaths or wedding bouquets. The young couple may even have been brought together with the magic of a touch of rosemary, as in the refrain of an old ballad: "Young men and maids do ready stand/With sweet rosemary in their hands." Greek scholars wore a bit of the pungent herb in their hair when engaged in study as an aid to increase concentration. The fragrant herb was exchanged between friends as a symbol of loyalty, and tossed onto the graves of departed loved ones. Gypsy travelers sought rosemary for its use as a rinse for highlighting dark hair, or as a rejuvenating face wash. In the fourteenth century, Queen Isabella of Hungary used an alcohol extract of the flowering herb to treat **gout**. In ancient Egypt the herb was buried with the pharaohs. Rosemary was believed to

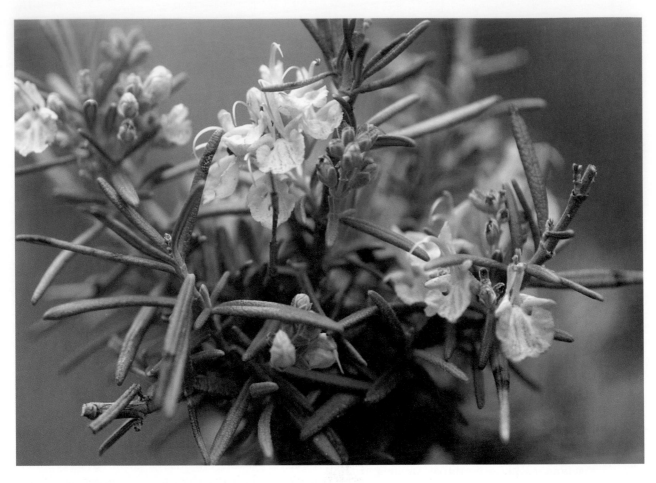

Rosemary blooming. *(© blickwinkel / Alamy)*

have magical powers to banish evil spirits. It was burned in sick rooms as a disinfectant, and was used to ward off the plague.

Rosemary's deep, woody taproot produces stout, branching, scaly, light brown stalks covered with simple, sessile narrow leaves about 1 in long and opposite, growing in whorls along the square stalks. Rosemary leaves are dark green on top and pale green on the underside with a distinctive mid vein. They curl inward along the margins. Tiny two-lipped, light blue or violet flowers grow in a cluster of five to seven blossoms each on a pair of short, opposite spikes. Each pair of flower spikes alternates along the sides of the stalk. This graceful aromatic herb blooms in late spring and early summer bearing two tiny seeds in each flower. Bees are attracted to rosemary flowers.

General use

Rosemary can be used to make an essential oil, a fixed oil, or teas and tinctures. These different products have different uses.

Volatile oil of rosemary

The volatile oil in rosemary leaves and blossoms, called a "sovereign balm" by the seventeenth-century herbalist Nicholas Culpeper, has a long history of medicinal uses in the West. Other chemical constituents of rosemary include **bitters**, borneol, linalol, camphene, camphor, cineole, pinene, resin, tannins, and rosmarinic acid, which acts as an antioxidant. Research has yielded promising results regarding the cancer-inhibiting effects of this antioxidant component of rosemary oil. In addition, rosemary is a circulatory stimulant. It has been shown to increase coronary blood flow, and is useful in treatment of blood pressure problems. A flavonoid known as diosmin in the volatile oil of rosemary can restore strength to fragile capillaries. Many of the traditional uses for this healing herb, discovered through trial and error and passed down through the generations, have not been clinically verified. Rosemary is still, however, officially listed as a medicinal herb in the *United States Pharmacopoeia*.

KEY TERMS

Carminative—A substance or medication that causes gas to be expelled from the stomach and intestines.

Carnosol—An antioxidant compound found in rosemary that appears to have anticancer properties.

Emmenagogue—A medication that helps to bring on menstruation or increase menstrual flow.

Flavonoids—Plant pigments that have a variety of effects on human physiology. The diosmin contained in rosemary is a flavonoid.

Sessile—Attached directly at the base without an intermediate stalk; issuing directly from the main stem of a plant.

Simple—A type of leaf that is not divided into parts.

Essential oil of rosemary

The essential oil of rosemary has potent antibacterial and antifungal effects. It was burnt as an incense in rituals, and used in sick rooms to provide protection from disease and infection. The herb has also been used as a digestive stimulant and liver tonic. It increases the flow of bile through its ability to relax the smooth muscle in the digestive tract and gallbladder. Rosemary's astringent properties, due to its tannin content, may help in the treatment of **diarrhea**, and reduce excessive menstrual flow. Rosemary can be used as a carminative (gas-relieving medication) to ease the discomfort of **colic** and dyspeptic disorders. The pungent herb has an energizing effect; it is used in **aromatherapy** to improve memory and focus, dispel **depression**, and relieve **migraine headache**. An external application of essential oil of rosemary, as a component in liniments, can ease **pain** in rheumatism. An infusion of rosemary, combined with **sage** (*Salvia officinale*), makes a good **sore throat** gargle. When used as a hair rinse, rosemary will stimulate hair follicles, and may help to reduce **dandruff**. A poultice of the herb may be applied to soothe **eczema**, or to speed the healing of **wounds**. Essential oil of rosemary is a component of many commercially available lotions, perfumes, liniments, soaps, and mouthwash preparations. Lastly, dried rosemary is used widely as a culinary herb.

More recently, carnosol, a naturally occurring antioxidant compound found in rosemary, has been studied for its anticancer properties. Carnosol appears to be effective against **cancer** by reducing inflammation and by inhibiting the expression of cancer genes. Carnosic acid, another compound found in rosemary, appears to reduce the risk of **skin cancer** by protecting skin cells against the effects of ultraviolet radiation.

Preparations

Dried: Rosemary leaves and blossoms may be harvested during the second year of growth. Carefully trim the branches in 4 in (10 cm) lengths, leaving at least two-thirds of the shrub intact. Strip the leaves from the stems and spread out on a tray, or hang the branches in bunches away from direct sunlight in a bright, airy room. Store the dried herb in tightly sealed dark containers.

Infusion: In a glass teapot, combine 1 oz (28.35 g) of fresh or dried flowering tops with 1 pt of non-chlorinated water that has been brought just to the boiling point. Steep the mixture in a covered container for 10–15 min. Strain. Drink the tea warm up to three cups per day.

Oil infusion: Pack a quart jar with fresh rosemary leaves and flowering tops. Pour enough olive oil in the jar to cover the herbs completely. Seal and place on a sunny windowsill for 2–3 weeks. Strain the oil through cheesecloth into a large glass container. Squeeze the remaining oil from the cloth. Pour this first oil infusion over additional fresh herbs in a jar to cover. Seal and place on a sunny window sill for an additional two weeks. Strain again through cheesecloth. Store this second oil infusion in tightly sealed, clearly labeled, dark glass containers.

Compress: Soak a cotton pad with the hot infusion of rosemary leaf and apply to **bruises** or **sprains**, or as an aid in the healing of wounds and skin irritations.

Precautions

Rosemary should not be used in medicinal preparations during **pregnancy** or breast-feeding, although it is safe to use in cooking in small quantities to season foods. Persons with high blood pressure, **epilepsy** or diverticulosis, chronic ulcers, or **colitis**, should not take rosemary internally for medicinal purposes. Rosemary acts as an emmenagogue, stimulating the flow of menstrual blood. The essential oil of rosemary was once used in folk practice in attempts to induce abortion. As with all **essential oils**, only small amounts of it should be used, either topically or internally. An overdose of essential oil of rosemary may lead to deep coma, **vomiting**, spasms, uterine bleeding, **gastroenteritis**, kidney irritation, and even death, according to the *PDR for Herbal Medicines*. No documented cases have been reported, however.

Side effects

No side effects are known when rosemary is used in designated therapeutic doses, properly harvested, prepared, and administered. Some persons, however, may be allergic to rosemary or its oils, and experience **nausea** and vomiting.

Interactions

Relatively few interactions between rosemary and Western pharmaceuticals have been reported. Rosemary appears to increase the effects of doxorubicin, a cancer medication. Although further studies are necessary, as of 2002 patients taking doxorubicin are advised to consult their physician before taking rosemary.

Resources

BOOKS

McIntyre, Anne. *The Medicinal Garden*. New York: Henry Holt and Company, 1997.

Ody, Penelope. *The Complete Medicinal Herbal*. New York: Dorling Kindersley, 1993.

PDR for Herbal Medicines. Montvale, NJ: Medical Economics Company, 1998.

Polunin, Miriam, and Christopher Robbins. *The Natural Pharmacy*. New York: Macmillan Publishing Company, 1992.

Prevention's 200 Herbal Remedies, 3rd ed. Emmaus, PA: Rodale Press, Inc., 1997.

Price, Shirley. *Practical Aromatherapy*. London: Thorsons/ HarperCollins, 1994.

Weiss, Gaea, and Shandor Weiss. *Growing & Using The Healing Herbs*. New York: Wings Books, 1992.

PERIODICALS

Lo, A. H., Y. C. Liang, S. Y. Lin-Shiau, et al. "Carnosol, an Antioxidant in Rosemary, Suppresses Inducible Nitric Oxide Synthase Through Down-Regulating Nuclear Factor-KappaB in Mouse Macrophages." *Carcinogenesis* 23 (June 2002): 983-991.

Offord, E. A., J. C. Gautier, O. Avanti, et al. "Photoprotective Potential of Lycopene, Beta-Carotene, Vitamin E, Vitamin C and Carnosic Acid in UVA-Irradiated Human Skin Fibroblasts." *Free Radicals in Biology and Medicine* 32 (June 15, 2002): 1293-1303.

ORGANIZATIONS

American Botanical Council. PO Box 144345. Austin, TX 78714-4345.

International Aromatherapy and Herb Association. 3541 West Acapulco Lane. Phoenix, AZ 85053-4625. (602) 938-4439. http://www.aztec.asu.edu./iaha/.

Clare Hanrahan
Rebecca J. Frey, PhD

Rosen method

Definition

Rosen method bodywork is a gentle hands-on approach to **relaxation** and awareness that was developed by Marion Rosen through her 30 years of experience as a physical therapist. Rosen method movement consists of playful, low impact exercises designed to move all of the joints in the body and facilitate breathing.

Origins

Rosen method is one of many somatic, or bodywork, therapies which later developed out of the partnership between physical therapists and psychoanalysts between the two World Wars. Born in Germany, Marion Rosen originally studied "breath therapy." After fleeing Nazi Germany, Rosen trained in physical therapy and emigrated to the United States. In 1944 she graduated from a physical therapy program at the Mayo Clinic. After working in Kaiser Permanente Hospital, she opened a private physical therapy practice in Oakland, California.

Over the years Rosen treated many individuals who continued to experience chronic **pain** from earlier injuries, although there was now no evidence of physical injury or trauma. She began to see that the people who talked about their injuries healed faster. Gradually she developed the theory that all trauma—physical, mental, and emotional—is held in the body as chronic muscle tension. She observed that as her patients relaxed, they often experienced thoughts and emotions that had been held unconsciously in their bodies over long periods of time.

Rosen developed a reputation in the medical community as someone who could successfully treat patients that failed to respond to conventional medical treatment. Patients with **asthma**, chronic pain and psychosomatic illnesses responded favorably. Besides treating patients with injuries or physical complaints, Rosen became interested in the restorative and transformational potential of her approach for people who were basically healthy.

In 1972, she began to teach her method to a few individuals, and in 1980 she expanded to teaching public classes. Rosen method now has 13 centers for training practitioners. There are approximately 600 practitioners from 15 countries in North America, Europe, and Australia.

Rosen method movement classes were created in response to patients' requests for exercises to decrease injuries. Marion developed an enjoyable way to move all of the joints in the body by setting to music the range of motion tests used by physical therapists.

Benefits

According to the *Clinician's Complete Reference to Complementary and Alternative Medicine*, Rosen method is considered "ideally suited" for arthritis, back pain, chronic **fatigue**, headaches and **stress**. It is "one of the better therapies" for asthma, **colic**, **hypertension**, **insomnia**, **constipation**, menstrual cramps, **osteoarthritis**, preconception, and **restless leg syndrome**. It is considered a "valuable adjunctive therapy" for **allergies**, **colitis** and **Crohn's disease**, **emphysema**, postpartum care, **pregnancy** and **childbirth**, and **premenstrual syndrome**. Rosen method is also experienced as a valuable complement to **psychotherapy**. Some people are drawn to this approach for emotional and spiritual growth.

Rosen method movement classes help to improve range of motion, increase breathing capacity and encourage ease in movement. The exercises are especially helpful for people who are recovering from injuries or seldom **exercise**.

Description

Rosen method bodywork sessions are conducted on a massage table. The patient is partially clothed and covered with a blanket. During a session the practitioner uses gentle, direct, non-manipulative touch to bring awareness to chronically tight muscles in the body. The practitioner responds to subtle changes in the breath and muscles with touch and words. This allows the client to recognize the memories and feelings which have unconsciously been "held down" by muscle tension. As the tight muscles relax, the breath moves with ease and the client may feel invigorated and have a greater sense of well-being.

Rosen method bodywork sessions last from fifty to sixty minutes and are usually received once every week or every other week. The number and frequency of the sessions depend upon the goals of the client. Strict confidentiality is always maintained. With the consent of the client, a Rosen practitioner may consult with other mental health or medical professionals.

Certified Rosen method practitioners charge 60-90 dollars for a session. Lower cost sessions are frequently available from Rosen interns. Rosen method is not specifically covered by medical insurance.

In Rosen method movement classes, the exercises are done to music with a partner or by oneself. Some exercises are done on the floor. Students wear comfortable clothes for moving. Movement classes last 50-60 minutes and cost from seven to 10 dollars per class.

Precautions

Rosen method practitioners do not work with people with a history of serious mental illness and psychosis or those who need strong defenses to get through the circumstances of life. Rosen method is not recommended during the early stages (less than one year) of recovery from alcohol or drug addiction. It is also not recommended during the acute phase of any physical or emotional trauma. People with medical conditions or in psychotherapy are advised to consult their physicians or therapists before receiving sessions.

Research and general acceptance

No scientific studies have been conducted concerning the benefits of Rosen method. Although Rosen was honored by the International **Somatics** Congress in 1999 for her contribution to the field of somatics, Rosen method is not well-known by the general public or health care professionals.

Training and certification

Certification in Rosen method requires two years of classroom instruction, followed by an internship of 350 patient hours and 55 hours of supervision and review. This internship period requires a minimum of nine months and may last up to 18 months. Classroom instruction is offered either through weekly classes or an intensive format. Many Rosen practitioners are certified or licensed massage therapists.

Certification as a Rosen method movement teacher requires 125 hours of instruction either through weekly classes or intensives and completion of an internship involving teaching, observation, and supervision.

Linda Chrisman

Royal jelly

Description

Royal jelly, which is sometimes called bee's milk, is a thick creamy liquid secreted by special glands in young worker bees who serve as "nurses" to the hive.

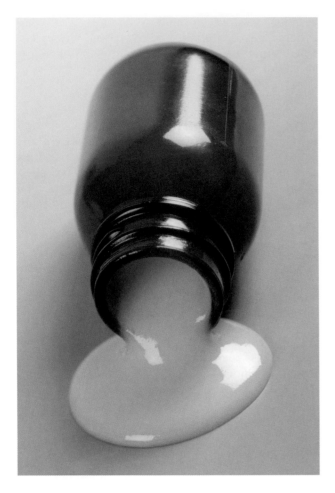

Royal jelly is a liquid secreted by special glands in young worker bees. *(Bon Appetit / Alamy)*

General use

Proponents of **apitherapy** (which also includes the use of other hive products, such as **bee pollen**, propolis, and bee venom) make many claims for the virtues of royal jelly. Among other things, it is said to increase appetite and general vigor; retard **aging**; boost longevity; accelerate healing; strengthen the immune system; and exhibit antibiotic and antiviral properties. Specific claims for royal jelly have been made in connection with **Parkinson's disease** and other nervous disorders; arthritis; and reproductive and sexual functioning.

Clinical studies over the last several decades have reported evidence supporting some of these claims, including shrinking tumors in mice, reducing **cholesterol** levels in humans, fighting microbial and viral **infections**, and reducing the trembling associated with Parkinson's disease. These accounts are case reports only, however, and not the results of controlled clinical trials.

Preparations

Royal jelly is available in various forms. In its pure state, it is a jelly that must be kept under refrigeration. It is also found in honey, which works to preserve it naturally. Royal jelly may be purchased in a freeze-dried form in capsules or tablets, sometimes combined with other bee products; it is also available as a liquid. In addition, royal jelly may appear as an ingredient in cosmetics, skin care products, and assorted ointments and salves.

Synthetic royal jelly has also been manufactured and marketed, but according to some sources, it does not produce the same effects, on either bees or human subjects, in clinical trials.

Precautions

Although apitherapy proponents maintain that royal jelly is not only entirely safe but almost miraculously beneficial, a number of deaths have been linked to its use. Australian researchers have reported cases of **asthma** said to have been induced by royal jelly (including at least

All bee larvae are fed a small amount of royal jelly mixed with honey for the first three days of their lives. Starting on day four, however, most of the bees are weaned from this diet and develop into worker bees. But one bee, hatched from an egg identical to the rest, is fed exclusively on royal jelly. That bee becomes the queen. She will grow, on average, 40% larger than her fellow bees, perhaps 50% heavier, and live up to 40 or 50 times as long. And all the while, she will be producing enormous numbers of eggs, equal to more than twice her own body weight, every single day.

This phenomenon has led numerous researchers and practitioners to explore both the chemical composition and the potential therapeutic uses of royal jelly, particularly over the last several decades. Among other things, the complex substance has been found to be rich in **amino acids** (including the eight essential to human life), **essential fatty acids**, vitamins, minerals, RNA, DNA, and many other elements of clinically proven usefulness. Other compounds in royal jelly have yet to be identified.

one death), and a Japanese report blames royal jelly for causing a case of **gastroenteritis**. More research is needed, however, to clearly determine the connection between royal jelly and potential allergic reactions.

Side effects

Some side effects have been reported for royal jelly, including occasional central nervous system symptoms, agitation, heart palpitations, **insomnia**, and **anxiety**.

Interactions

No instances of interactions with other medications have been reported.

Resources

BOOKS

Cassileth, Barrie R. *The Alternative Medicine Handbook*. New York: W. W. Norton & Company, 1998.

ORGANIZATIONS

American Apitherapy Society. 5390 Grande Road, Hillsboro, OH 45133. (937) 364-1108. http://www.apitherapy. org/.

Peter Gregutt

Rubella

Definition

Rubella is a highly contagious viral disease, spread through contact with discharges from the nose and throat of an infected person. A person infected with the rubella virus is contagious for about seven days before any symptoms appear and continues to spread the disease for about four days after the appearance of symptoms. Rubella has an incubation period of 12–23 days.

Description

Rubella is also called German **measles** or the three-day measles. This disease was once a common childhood illness, but its occurrence has been drastically reduced since vaccine against rubella became available in 1969. In the three decades following the introduction of the vaccine, reported rubella cases dropped 99.6%. Only 229 cases of rubella were reported in the United States in 1996. A recent study indicates, however, that the age group pattern of rubella is shifting. As of 2002, the number of cases reported in people aged 15 years or

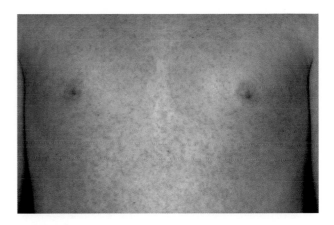

View of a chest rash in a child suffering from Rubella (German measles). *(Dr. P. Marazzi / Photo Researchers, Inc.)*

younger is dropping, while the number of cases in people between 25 and 45 is rising.

People of any age who have not been vaccinated or previously caught the disease can become infected. Having rubella once or being immunized against rubella normally gives lifetime immunity. This is why vaccination is so effective in reducing the number of rubella cases. The United States had a public health goal of eliminating all rubella within its borders by the year 2000; however, this goal was not attained because of new **strains** of the rubella virus entering the country from the Caribbean and Central America. The availability of molecular typing indicates that three separate strains of the virus caused localized outbreaks that were quickly contained. As of 2002, cases of rubella in the United States are more common among Hispanics than among Caucasians, Native Americans, or African Americans.

Women of childbearing age who do not have immunity against rubella should be the most concerned about infection. Rubella infection during the first three months of **pregnancy** can cause a woman to miscarry or cause the baby to be born with severe birth defects, including mental retardation and sensory impairments. In addition, recent studies indicate that infants exposed to rubella in utero (in the womb) are at increased risk of developing **schizophrenia** as adults.

Although it has been practically eradicated in the United States, rubella is still common in less developed countries because of poor immunization penetration, creating a risk to susceptible travelers. Some countries have chosen to target rubella vaccination to females only. As a result, outbreaks among foreign-born males have occurred on cruise ships and at summer camps in the United States. The United Kingdom is considering targeting immigrants of either sex from underdeveloped countries for rubella immunization following several cases of babies born with congenital rubella syndrome.

Causes and symptoms

Rubella is caused by the rubella virus (*Rubivirus*). Symptoms are generally mild, and complications are rare in anyone who is not pregnant.

The first visible sign of rubella is a fine red rash that begins on the face and rapidly moves downward to cover the whole body within 24 hours. The rash lasts about three days, which is why rubella is sometimes called the three-day measles. A low **fever** and swollen glands, especially in the head (around the ears) and neck, often accompany the rash. Joint **pain** and sometimes joint swelling can occur, more often in women. It is quite common to get rubella and not show any symptoms (subclinical infection).

Symptoms disappear within three to four days, except for joint pain, which may linger for a week or two. Most people recover fully with no complications. Although rubella causes only mild symptoms of low fever, swollen glands, joint pain, and a fine red rash in most children and adults, it can have severe complications for women in their first trimester of pregnancy. Babies may be miscarried or stillborn and a high percentage are born with birth defects. Birth defects are reported to occur in 50% of women who contract the disease during the first month of pregnancy, 20% of those who contract it in the second month, and 10% of those who contract it in the third month. The most common birth defects resulting from congenital rubella infection are eye defects, such as **cataracts**, **glaucoma**, and blindness, deafness, congenital heart defects, and mental retardation. Taken together, these conditions are called congenital rubella syndrome (CRS). The risk of birth defects drops after the first trimester, and by the fifth month, there are rarely any complications.

Diagnosis

The rash caused by the rubella virus and the accompanying symptoms are so similar to other viral infections that it is impossible for a physician to make a confirmed diagnosis on visual examination alone. The only sure way to confirm a case of rubella is by checking for antibodies with a blood test or in a laboratory culture.

When the body is infected with the rubella virus, it produces both immunoglobulin G (IgG) and immunoglobulin M (IgM) antibodies to fight the infection. Once IgG exists, it persists for a lifetime, but the special IgM antibody usually wanes over six months. A blood test can be used either to confirm a recent infection (IgG and IgM) or determine whether a person has immunity to rubella (IgG only). The lack of antibodies indicates that a person is susceptible to rubella.

All pregnant women should be tested for rubella early in pregnancy, whether or not they have a history of vaccination. If the woman lacks immunity, she is counseled to avoid anyone with the disease and to be vaccinated after giving birth.

Treatment

Rather than vaccinating a healthy child against rubella, some alternative practitioners recommend allowing the child to contract the disease naturally at the age of five or six years, since the immunity conferred by contracting the disease naturally lasts a lifetime. It is, however, difficult for a child to contract rubella naturally when everyone around him or her has been vaccinated.

Ayurvedic practitioners recommend making the patient comfortable and giving the patient **ginger** or clove tea to hasten the progress of the disease. **Traditional Chinese medicine** uses a similar approach. Believing that inducing the skin rash associated with rubella hastens the progress of the disease, traditional Chinese practitioners prescribe herbs such as **peppermint** (*Mentha piperita*) and chai hu (*Bupleurum chinense*). **Cicada** is often prescribed as well. Western herbal remedies may be used to alleviate rubella symptoms. Distilled **witch hazel** (*Hamamelis virginiana*) helps calm the **itching** associated with the skin rash and an eyewash made from a filtered diffusion of **eyebright** (*Euphrasia officinalis*) can relieve eye discomfort. Antiviral western herbal or Chinese remedies can be used to assist the immune system in establishing equilibrium during the healing process. Depending on the patient's symptoms, among the remedies a homeopath may prescribe are *Belladonna, Pulsatilla,* or *Phytolacca*. These can be used with or with out **bilberry**.

Allopathic treatment

There is no drug treatment for rubella. Bed rest, fluids, and acetaminophen or Motrin for pain and temperatures over 102°F (38.9°C) are usually all that is necessary.

Babies born with suspected CRS are isolated and cared for only by people who are sure they are immune to rubella. Congenital heart defects are treated with surgery.

Expected results

Complications from rubella infection are rare in children, pregnant women past the fifth month of pregnancy, and other adults.

Prevention

Vaccination is the best way to prevent rubella and is normally required by law for children entering school. Rubella vaccine is usually given in conjunction with measles and **mumps** vaccines in a shot referred to as MMR (mumps, measles, and rubella). Children receive one dose of MMR vaccine at 12–15 months and another dose at four to six years. The MMR vaccine has aroused some controversy since early 2000 because of media reports that it increases the risk of **wheezing** and lower respiratory tract disorders in young children. A recent study of vaccine safety has concluded, however, that there is no connection between the MMR vaccine and a reported rise in the incidence of wheezing in children.

Pregnant women should not be vaccinated; women who are not pregnant should avoid conceiving for at least three months following vaccination. To date, however, accidental rubella vaccinations during pregnancy have not clearly been associated with the same risk as the natural infection itself. Women may be vaccinated while they are breast-feeding. People whose immune systems are compromised, either by the use of such drugs as steroids or by disease, should discuss possible complications with their doctor before being vaccinated.

Resources

BOOKS

Cooper, Louis Z. "Rubella." In *Rudolph's Pediatrics*, 21st ed., edited by M. M. Rudolph, J. I. E. Hoffman, and C. D. Rudolph. Stamford, CT: McGraw-Hill, 2002.

Gershon, Anne. "Rubella (German Measles)." In *Harrison's Principles of Internal Medicine*, 15th ed., edited by Anthony S. Fauci. New York: McGraw-Hill, 2001.

PERIODICALS

Brown, A. S., and E. S. Susser. "In Utero Infection and Adult Schizophrenia." *Mental Retardation and Developmental Disabilities Research and Review* 8 (January 2002): 51–7.

Carvill, S., and G. Marston. "People with Intellectual Disability, Sensory Impairments and Behaviour Disorder: A Case Series." *Journal of Intellectual Disability Research* 46 (March 2002): 264–72.

Case Definitions for Infectious Conditions under Public Health Surveillance. *Morbidity and Mortality Weekly Report* 46 (1997): 30.

Dixon, B. "Triple Vaccine Fears Mask Media Efforts at Balance." *Current Biology* 12 (March 5, 2002): R151-R152.

Mullooly, J. P., J. Pearson, L. Drew, et al. "Wheezing Lower Respiratory Disease and Vaccination of Full-Term Infants." *Pharmacoepidemiology and Drug Safety* 11 (January-February 2002): 21–30.

Reef, S. E., T. K. Frey, K. Theall, et al. "The Changing Epidemiology of Rubella in the 1990s: On the Verge of Elimination and New Challenges for Control and Prevention." *Journal of the American Medical Association* 287 (January 23, 2002): 464–72.

Sheridan E., C. Aitken, D. Jeffries, et al. "Congenital Rubella Syndrome: A Risk in Immigrant Populations." *Lancet* 359 (February 23, 2002): 674–675.

ORGANIZATIONS

March of Dimes Resource Center. 1275 Mamaroneck Avenue, White Plains, NY 10605. (888) 663-4637. http://www.modimes.org.

National Organization of Rare Disorders. 55 Kenosia Avenue PO Box 1968 Danbury, CT 06813-1968. (800) 999-6673. orphan@rarediseases.org. http://www.rarediseases.org.

Kathleen Wright
Rebecca J. Frey, PhD

Rubenfeld synergy

Definition

The Rubenfeld synergy method is a hybrid of various bodywork and **psychotherapy** techniques, aimed at accessing stored emotions and memories. This psychophysical approach uses talk, touch, and movement to remove tensions, imbalances, and energy blocks.

Origins

Rubenfeld synergy is a trademarked system for mind-body integration. It was developed during the early 1960s by former orchestra and choral conductor Ilana Rubenfeld. A graduate of the Juilliard School of Music, where she studied with Pablo Casals, Rubenfeld played viola, oboe, and piano. Later, she became a conductor and served as assistant to well-known conductor Leopold Stokowski (1882–1977). When she experienced back and shoulder spasms from her work, Rubenfeld began seeking ways to promote her own healing and eventually developed a system to help others as well. Her method incorporates elements from the following:

- Body/mind teachings of Frederick M. Alexander and Moshe Feldenkrais
- Hypnotherapy methods of Milton Erickson
- Gestalt psychotherapy approach and techniques of Fritz and Laura Perls

Rubenfeld was an Alexander teacher and trainer who studied with the Perls, trained also with Moshe **Feldenkrais**, and became one of his first teachers in the United States. Her synthesis of the various elements became the Rubenfeld Synergy Method in the 1970s.

Benefits

Reported benefits of the Rubenfeld synergy method include recovery from physical and emotional trauma, release of tension, improved ease of movement, and **pain** management, as well as improved body image, self-esteem, and mind-body awareness.

Description

A typical Rubenfeld synergy session lasts between 45 and 50 minutes. A practitioner determines the number and frequency of patient visits to match the individual's needs. Patients may remain fully clothed during the sessions, which combine gentle touch and talk. Clients may sit or lie down or may move about during the session. A wide range of techniques may be used by the practitioner, including dream work, aura analysis, sound, imagination, breathing exercises, humor, **spirituality**, and verbal expression. Practitioners say that motions, memories, and suppressed or denied emotions can be stored in any part of the body as energy blocks, tensions, and imbalances that can affect physical and emotional well-being. For example, practitioners may suggest that sexually abused women store memories from their negative experiences in the pelvis.

A patient undergoing Rubenfeld synergy therapy is considered an equal partner in the healing process. The practitioner may place considerable emphasis on a lifestyle governed by choices instead of habits.

Precautions

Rubenfeld synergy may involve substantial physical contact. Patients should be aware that traditional psychotherapists often frown upon such touching because of the risk of inducing improper fantasies. As with all therapies involving touch, it is important to ensure that a practitioner is certified to reduce risk of improper behavior.

Side effects

There are few, if any, known side effects.

Research and general acceptance

Some aspects of Rubenfeld synergy method, including psychotherapy techniques and **stress** management, are known and generally respected by the medical establishment. Other aspects, such as aura analysis, are well outside the boundaries of traditional medicine.

Training and certification

Training and certification are offered through the Omega Institute in Rhinebeck, New York, or at a conference site near Philadelphia. Admission in the program carries no formal prerequisites; applicants need only submit two letters of recommendation, an application form, and a non-refundable application fee. Training takes place over four years and consists of three seven-day sessions and three weekend regional meetings each year. Besides the weeklong sessions and weekend meetings, the program requires that trainees must themselves experience the Rubenfeld method and participate in 20 private sessions a year with a Rubenfeld practitioner. Graduate practitioners are referred to as Rubenfeld synergy practitioners or synergists. Practitioners must be recertified every three years.

Resources

BOOKS

Rubenfeld, Ilana. *The Listening Hand: Self-Healing through the Rubenfeld Synergy Method of Talk and Touch*. New York: Bantam Doubleday Dell, 2001.

ORGANIZATIONS

International Association of Rubenfeld Synergists (INARS), 7 Kendall Rd., Kendall Park, NJ, 08824, (877) RSM-2468, http://www.rubenfeldsynergy.com.

OTHER

"Rubenfeld Synergy Method." American Cancer Society, May 23, 2007. http://www.cancer.org/docroot/ETO/content/ETO_5_3X_Rubenfeld_Synergy_Method.asp?(March 4, 2008).

David Helwig
Leslie Mertz, Ph.D.

Rubeola *see* **Measles**
Rudbeckia *see* **Echinacea**
Runny nose *see* **Rhinitis**

Russian massage

Definition

Russian massage is a system of therapeutic and **sports massage** developed in the former Soviet Union. It uses a variety of manipulations of the body's soft tissues to achieve benefits, including **stress** reduction and relief from muscle aches.

Origins

Many cultures around the world developed forms of **massage therapy**, including the ancient peoples of China, India, and Greece. One early advocate was Hippocrates, the Greek physician widely considered to be the father of medicine. Per Henrik Ling, a nineteenth-century Swedish physician who employed vigorous massage to stimulate circulation of the blood and lymph, is usually considered the founder of modern European massage. Massage was not studied or used scientifically in Russia until 1860. Treatment methods were developed further after World War II when pharmaceuticals were in short supply. The Soviet Union employed physiatrists—medical doctors with Ph.D. degrees in physical therapy—to research the benefits of using natural healing modalities. They developed a form of petrissage to reverse atrophy in muscles and help stimulate new growth. Russian physiologists found all movements of massage function on the basis of neurohormone and neuroendocrine reflexes. Unlike other massage therapies, Russian massage is based on the physiology of a dysfunction rather than on anatomy as the principal guideline for treatment.

Benefits

Practitioners say that Russian massage is useful for a wide range of musculoskeletal, cardiovascular, gastrointestinal, neurological, gynecological, internal disorders, and in post-surgical situations. In Russia, massage therapists are regarded as medical professionals. The massage therapy department is often the largest in Russian hospitals and clinics because it is crucial to rehabilitation. Patients describe it as "waking up" both body and mind. It has been used to increase circulation of blood and lymphatic flow, to stimulate production of endorphins, control physical and mental stress, and to increase range of movement. Ailments said to benefit from massage therapy include **asthma**, **insomnia**, arthritis, **bursitis**, **carpal tunnel syndrome**, hip **sprains and strains**, rotator cuff injuries, myofascial **pain**, temporomandibular joint (TMJ) problems, **headache**, spastic colon, **colic**, **constipation**, and immune

function disorders. Because of its gentle, non-invasive nature, Russian massage is considered especially suitable for seniors.

Description

Russian massage is considered less invasive and more relaxing than many other forms of massage therapy. It uses four principal techniques:

- petrissage, a stretching or kneading motion
- effleurage, a gliding, relaxing stroke
- friction, a rubbing action
- vibration, a continuous-motion stroke ranging from very fast to very slow

Treatments may be as short as 15 minutes or as long as almost one hour. They may be repeated daily or every other day, but may also be interrupted after a dozen or so treatments to ensure that patient does not become dependant on massage.

Precautions

Like other types of massage therapy, Russian massage involves intimate personal contact. To lessen the possibility of unprofessional conduct, it is important to ensure that practitioners belong to a known regulatory body.

Massage should not be used on **burns**, in cases of deep vein thrombosis (**blood clots**), infectious diseases, or in other situations in which it is clearly inappropriate. In **cancer** patients, there is no evidence that massage causes the disease to spread. However, it is nonetheless advisable to avoid direct pressure at tumor sites. There is controversy over the advisability of massage following a **heart attack**. Some studies have suggested that the heart is not unduly strained by gentle massage, but this issue should be discussed with a physician. Massage is also not recommended in cases of **phlebitis**.

Side effects

Adverse effects from massage therapy are quite rare, and are usually related to unusually vigorous methods or used when contraindicated.

Research and general acceptance

The usefulness of Russian and other forms of massage therapy is acknowledged by most medical professionals, some of whom have undertaken massage training themselves. One 1995 study found that 54% of family practitioners and primary-care doctors in the United States were prepared to recommend therapeutic massage to their patients, and 34% would refer patients to a massage therapist. Many health insurance plans now cover prescribed massage therapy.

Training and certification

In Russia, massage therapists are highly trained health professionals who start with a college degree in nursing or some related discipline such as physiotherapy, then undertake months of specialized training. In the United States, massage therapists are regulated in at least 29 states. There are numerous regulatory bodies, including the American Massage Therapy Association, which recommends a minimum 500 hours of classroom instruction. The U.S. National Certification Board for Therapeutic Massage and Bodywork administers a national certification examination. In the United Kingdom, there are also a number of regulatory organizations, of which some are members of the British Complementary Medicine Association, that conducts regular membership reviews. The International Therapy Examinations Council conducts examinations for would-be massage therapists.

Resources

ORGANIZATIONS

American Massage Therapy Association. 820 Davis St., Suite 100, Evanston, IL 60201-4444. 847-864-0123. http://www.amtamassage.org.

British Massage Therapy Council. 17 Rymers Lane, Oxford OX4 3JU. 01865-774123. http:\\www.bmtc.co.uk.

David Helwig

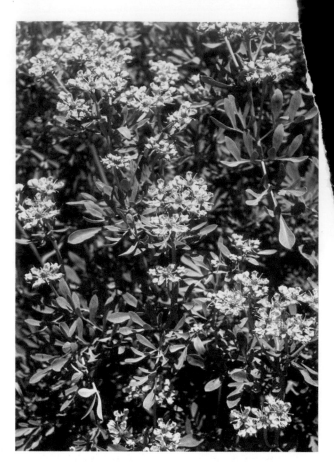

Ruta graveolens blooming. (© *blickwinkel / Alamy*)

Ruta

Description

Ruta is today primarily a homeopathic remedy made from the plant *Ruta graveolens*. This plant is also called rue, herb of grace, herb of repentance, bitter herb, or rue bitterwort. It grows to a height of about 3 ft (1 m) and has fleshy leaves and yellowish flowers. Ruta is native to southern Europe, but it is cultivated worldwide. The plant has a strong, unpleasant odor.

Chemical compounds found in ruta include rutin, a flavonoid; alkaloids, including graveoline and rutacridine; lignans in the root; and furocoumarins, which are compounds that are toxic to both animals and humans. Symptoms of ruta poisoning in humans include **nausea**, **vomiting**, stomach **pain**, exhaustion, and convulsions. Animals that eat ruta while grazing develop tremors, frequent urination, difficulty breathing, loss of coordination, and inability to stand up.

General use

Homeopathic medicine operates on the principle that "like heals like." This means that a disease can be cured by treating it with products that produce the same symptoms as the disease. These products follow another homeopathic law, the Law of Infinitesimals. In opposition to traditional medicine, the Law of Infinitesimals states that the *lower* a dose of curative, the more effective it is. To achieve a very low dose, the curative is diluted many, many times until only a tiny amount remains in a huge amount of the diluting liquid.

KEY TERMS

Abortifacient—A medication or other substance that causes a miscarriage or abortion.

Emmenagogue—A preparation given to bring on a woman's menstrual period.

Furocoumarins—Toxic compounds found in ruta that can cause nausea, vomiting, and convulsions in humans.

Periosteum—The specialized layer of connective tissue that covers all bones in the body.

Rectal prolapse—A condition where the lining of the rectum, the last part of the large intestine, protrudes through the anus.

Rutin—A bright greenish-yellow flavonoid (plant pigment) found in ruta that has been credited with antioxidant properties.

Sciatica—Pain extending from the buttocks to the foot caused by pressure on the sciatic nerve.

In homeopathic medicine, ruta is used as a first-aid remedy. It is used to treat **strains** and **sprains**, injuries of the cartilage and tendons around the joints, injuries to tissues lying over the bone, injuries of the periosteum, and **sciatica**. Ruta is often used for pain and stiffness in the hands, wrists, feet, and legs.

Ruta is also a remedy for eyestrain. It is primarily used when the eyes feel hot, red, or are burning after periods of close work such as reading or sewing. Ruta is also used to treat **headache** that results from eyestrain.

In homeopathic dentistry, ruta is used to relieve pain. It is also used to treat infection of the tooth socket after a tooth is pulled. Other homeopathic uses for ruta include treatment of plantar **warts** on the feet, blood and mucus in stools, pain in the rectum, rectal prolapse, and general weakness and **depression**.

In homeopathic medicine, the fact that certain symptoms get better or worse under different conditions is used as a diagnostic tool to indicate what remedy will be most effective. Symptoms that benefit from treatment with ruta get worse with heavy use of the eyes; in cold, damp weather; with rest or lying down; and by stooping or crouching. Symptoms improve with movement.

Homeopathy also ascribes certain personality types to certain remedies. People with the ruta personality are said to be depressed, chronically dissatisfied, quarrelsome, and apt to contradict others. They may be anxious and lack a sense of personal satisfaction.

They exhibit restlessness, but still feel unmotivated and despairing.

In addition to homeopathic use, ruta has been used by folk herbalists for centuries. The ancient Greeks used it for coughs. In the Middle Ages, this herb was used as a charm against witchcraft. It was also used as an abortifacient and an emmenagogue, or preparation to bring on a woman's menstrual period. Michelangelo (1475-1564) and artists of his time believed ruta improved eyesight. Because of its intense odor, ruta was used to ward off plague, repel flies, kill fleas, and prevent the spread of typhus. It has also been used to treat mushroom poisoning, snake **bites**, poisonous insect **stings**, **epilepsy**, and internal parasites.

Preparations

Ruta is prepared from the whole plant, picked before it flowers, and is then dried. For homeopathic remedies, the dried plant material is finely ground then prepared by extensive dilutions. There are two homeopathic dilution scales: the decimal (x) scale with a dilution of 1:10 and the centesimal (c) scale with a dilution of 1:100. Once the mixture is diluted, shaken, strained, then rediluted many times to reach the desired degree of potency, the final mixture is added to lactose (a type of sugar) tablets or pellets. These are then stored away from light. Ruta is available commercially in tablets in many different strengths. Dosage depends on the symptoms being treated.

Homeopathic and orthodox medical practitioners agree that by the time the initial remedy solution is diluted to strengths used in homeopathic healing, it is likely that very few molecules of the original remedy remain. Homeopaths, however, believe that these remedies continue to work through an effect called "potentization" that has not yet been explained by mainstream scientists.

Precautions

Pregnant women should not use ruta because it stimulates contraction of the uterus and can cause miscarriage. Many people get **contact dermatitis** (skin **rashes**) from handling fresh ruta. People should wear gloves when harvesting this plant to prevent this rash.

Side effects

When taken in the recommended dilute form, no side effects have been reported, except for individual aggravations that can occur with homeopathic remedies. Concentrated quantities of ruta can cause miscarriage.

Interactions

Ruta has been reported to cause negative interactions with **sodium** warfarin, a blood-thinning medication.

Resources

BOOKS

Chevallier, Andrew. *Encyclopedia of Medicinal Plants*. Boston: DK Publishers, 1996.

Hammond, Christopher. *The Complete Family Guide to Homeopathy*. London: Penguin Studio, 1995.

Jonas, Wayne B., and Jennifer Jacobs. *Healing with Homeopathy*. New York: Warner Books, 1996.

Lockie, Andrew, and Nicola Geddes. *The Complete Guide to Homeopathy*. London: Dorling Kindersley, 1995.

Ullman, Robert, and Judyth Reichenberg-Ullman. *Homeopathic Self-Care*. Rocklin, CA: Prima Publishing, 1997.

PERIODICALS

Bernardo, L. C., M. B. de Oliveira, C. R. da Silva, et al. "Biological Effects of Rutin on the Survival of *Escherichia coli* AB1157 and on the Electrophoretic Mobility of Plasmid PUC 9.1 DNA." *Cellular and Molecular Biology* 48 (July 2002): 517-520.

el Agraa, S. E., S. M. el Badwi, and S. E. Adam. "Preliminary Observations on Experimental *Ruta graveolens* Toxicosis in Nubian Goats." *Tropical Animal Health and Production* 34 (July 2002): 271-281.

ORGANIZATIONS

Foundation for Homeopathic Education and Research. 21 Kittredge St., Berkeley, CA 94704. (510) 649-8930.

International Foundation for Homeopathy. P. O. Box 7, Edmonds, WA 98020. (206) 776-4147.

National Center for Homeopathy. 801 N. Fairfax St., Suite 306, Alexandria, VA 22314. (703) 548-7790.

Tish Davidson
Rebecca J. Frey, PhD